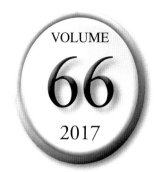

VOLUME

66

2017

INSTRUCTIONAL COURSE LECTURES

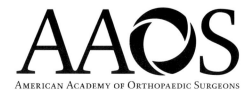

AMERICAN ACADEMY OF ORTHOPAEDIC SURGEONS

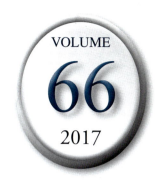

VOLUME
66
2017

INSTRUCTIONAL COURSE LECTURES

Edited by

Tad L. Gerlinger, MD
Assistant Professor
Midwest Orthopaedics at Rush
Rush University Medical Center
Chicago, Illinois
Associate Professor
Uniformed Services
University of the Health Sciences
Bethesda, Maryland

Javad Parvizi, MD, FRCS
Professor
Director and Vice Chairman of Research
Department of Orthopaedic Surgery
The Rothman Institute at Thomas Jefferson University
Philadelphia, Pennsylvania

Published 2017 by the
American Academy
of Orthopaedic Surgeons
9400 West Higgins Road
Rosemont, IL 60018

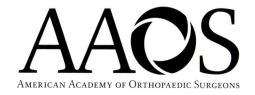

AMERICAN ACADEMY OF ORTHOPAEDIC SURGEONS

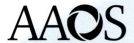

AAOS
AMERICAN ACADEMY OF
ORTHOPAEDIC SURGEONS

Instructional Course Lectures, Volume 66

The material presented in the *Instructional Course Lectures, Volume 66* has been made available by the American Academy of Orthopaedic Surgeons for educational purposes only. This material is not intended to present the only, or necessarily best, methods or procedures for the medical situations discussed, but rather is intended to represent an approach, view, statement, or opinion of the author(s) or producer(s), which may be helpful to others who face similar situations.

Some drugs or medical devices demonstrated in Academy courses or described in Academy print or electronic publications have not been cleared by the Food and Drug Administration (FDA) or have been cleared for specific uses only. The FDA has stated that it is the responsibility of the physician to determine the FDA clearance status of each drug or device he or she wishes to use in clinical practice.

Furthermore, any statements about commercial products are solely the opinion(s) of the author(s) and do not represent an Academy endorsement or evaluation of these products. These statements may not be used in advertising or for any commercial purpose.

Published 2017 by the
American Academy of Orthopaedic Surgeons
9400 West Higgins Road
Rosemont, IL 60018

Copyright 2017
by the American Academy of Orthopaedic Surgeons

ISBN: 978-1-62552-565-9

ISSN: 0065-6895

Printed in the USA

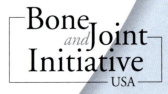

Acknowledgments

Editorial Board
Instructional Course Lectures, Volume 66
Tad L. Gerlinger, MD
Editor

Javad Parvizi, MD, FRCS
Assistant Editor

Section Editors
Susan V. Bukata, MD
Tumor and Metastatic Disease

J. Chris Coetzee, MD
Foot and Ankle

Paul J. Duwelius, MD
Adult Reconstruction: Hip

Thomas J. Errico, MD
Spine

Martin Joseph Herman, MD
Pediatrics

Kerwyn Jones, MD
Practice Management

Sanjeev Kakar, MD
Hand and Wrist

Mark D. Lazarus, MD
Shoulder and Elbow

Adolph V. Lombardi Jr, MD
Adult Reconstruction: Knee

Bradley J. Nelson, MD
Sports Medicine and Arthroscopy

Robert D. Zura, MD
Trauma

Editorial Board Members
Thomas R. Hunt III, MD
Richard W. Kruse, DO
Michael P. Mott, MD

Explore the full portfolio of AAOS educational programs and publications across the orthopaedic spectrum for every stage of an orthopaedic surgeon's career, at www.aaos.org/store. The AAOS, in partnership with Jones & Bartlett Learning, also offers a comprehensive collection of educational and training resources for emergency medical providers, from first responders to critical care transport paramedics. Learn more at www.aaos.org/ems.

Contributors

Joshua M. Abzug, MD
Associate Professor, Departments of Orthopedics and Pediatrics, University of Maryland School of Medicine, Director, University of Maryland Brachial Plexus Clinic, Director of Pediatric Orthopedics, University of Maryland Medical Center, Deputy Surgeon-in-Chief, University of Maryland Children's Hospital, Baltimore, Maryland

Mark R. Adams, MD
Assistant Professor, Department of Orthopaedics, Rutgers New Jersey Medical School, Newark, New Jersey

Nirav H. Amin, MD
Associate Professor, Department of Orthopedic Surgery, Loma Linda University, Loma Linda, California

Thomas An, AB
Medical Student, Vanderbilt University Medical School, Nashville, Tennessee

Robert B. Anderson, MD
Team Orthopaedist, Carolina Panthers, Founder, OrthoCarolina Foot and Ankle Institute, Charlotte, North Carolina

Afshin A. Anoushiravani, MD
Clinical Research Fellow, Department of Orthopaedic Surgery, NYU Langone Medical Center, Hospital for Joint Diseases, New York, New York

Mohammad Humza Ansari, BS
Mayo Clinic College of Medicine, Mayo Clinic, Rochester, Minnesota

Robert Arciero, MD
Professor of Orthopaedics, Department of Orthopaedics, University of Connecticut, Farmington, Connecticut

Elizabeth A. Arendt, MD
Professor and Vice Chair, Department of Orthopaedic Surgery, University of Minnesota, Minneapolis, Minnesota

Alexandre Arkader, MD
Division of Orthopaedic Surgery, Children's Hospital of Philadelphia, Associate Professor of Orthopaedic Surgery, Perelman School of Medicine at University of Pennsylvania, Philadelphia, Pennsylvania

Donald S. Bae, MD
Associate Professor of Orthopaedic Surgery, Department of Orthopaedic Surgery, Boston Children's Hospital and Harvard Medical School, Boston, Massachusetts

Andrea Sesko Bauer, MD
Assistant Professor, Department of Orthopaedic Surgery, Boston Children's Hospital/Harvard Medical School, Boston, Massachusetts

Michael S. Bednar, MD
Professor, Department of Orthopaedic Surgery and Rehabilitation, Loyola University–Chicago, Maywood, Illinois

Michael Benvenuti, BS
Medical Student, School of Medicine, Vanderbilt University, Nashville, Tennessee

Richard A. Bernstein, MD
The Orthopaedic Group, Connecticut Orthopaedic Specialists, Assistant Clinical Professor of Orthopaedic Surgery, Yale University School of Medicine, New Haven, Connecticut

Randy Bindra, MD, FRACS
Professor of Orthopaedic Surgery, Griffith University School of Medicine, Gold Coast University Hospital, Southport, Queensland, Australia

Laurel C. Blakemore, MD
Chief and Associate Professor, Pediatric Orthopaedics, University of Florida College of Medicine, Gainesville, Florida

Christopher M. Brusalis, BA
Benjamin Fox Orthopaedic Surgery Research Fellow, Department of Orthopaedic Surgery, Children's Hospital of Philadelphia, Philadelphia, Pennsylvania

Quinlan Buchlak, MPsych, MBIS
Neuroscience Research Scholar, Neuroscience Institute, Virginia Mason Medical Center, Seattle, Washington

Aaron J. Buckland, MBBS, FRACS
Assistant Professor, Department of Orthopaedic Surgery, NYU Langone Medical Center, New York, New York

Dwight W. Burney III, MD
Head, Section on Safety Education, Patient Safety Committee, American Academy of Orthopaedic Surgeons, Rosemont, Illinois

Patrick J. Cahill, MD
Associate Professor, Department of Orthopaedic Surgery, Perelman School of Medicine, University of Pennsylvania and Children's Hospital of Philadelphia, Philadelphia, Pennsylvania

John J. Callaghan, MD
The Lawrence & Marilyn Dorr Chair, Department of Orthopaedics and Rehabilitation, University of Iowa, Iowa City, Iowa

Monique C. Chambers, MD, MSL
Clinical and Translational Research Fellow, Department of Orthopaedic Surgery, Southern Illinois University, Springfield, Illinois

Timothy P. Charlton, MD
Associate Professor of Orthopaedic Surgery, Cedars-Sinai Medical Center, Los Angeles, California

Brian J. Chilelli, MD
Orthopaedic Surgeon, Department of Orthopaedics, Northwestern Medicine, Warrenville, Illinois

Steven Claes, MD, PhD
Doctor, Department of Orthopaedic Surgery, AZ St Elisabeth Herentals, Herentals, Belgium

Brian J. Cole, MD, MBA
Associate Chairman and Professor, Department of Orthopedics, Chairman, Department of Surgery, Rush OPH, Midwest Orthopedics at Rush, Rush University Medical Center, Chicago, Illinois

James H. Conway, MD
Professor of Pediatrics, Division of Pediatric Infectious Diseases, University of Wisconsin–Madison, School of Medicine and Public Health, Madison, Wisconsin

Lawson A. Copley, MD, MBA
Professor, Department of Orthopaedic Surgery, University of Texas Southwestern, Texas Scottish Rite Hospital, Dallas, Texas

Chris A. Cornett, MD, MPT
Assistant Professor of Orthopaedic Surgery, Department of Orthopaedic Surgery, University of Nebraska Medical Center, Omaha, Nebraska

Roger Cornwall, MD
Associate Professor, Division of Orthopaedic Surgery, Cincinnati Children's Hospital Medical Center, Cincinnati, Ohio

Dana L. Cruz, MD
Research Fellow, Spine Research Institute, NYU Hospital for Joint Diseases, New York, New York

Fred D. Cushner, MD
Chief, Department of Orthopedics, Southside Hospital, Bay Shore, New York

Diane L. Dahm, MD
Professor, Department of Orthopedic Surgery, Mayo Clinic, Rochester, Minnesota

Timothy A. Damron, MD
Professor, Department of Orthopedic Surgery, State University of New York Upstate Medical University, Syracuse, New York

David Dejour, MD
Orthopaedic Surgeon, Department of Knee Surgery, Lyon Ortho Clinic, Lyon, France

Clinton James Devin, MD
Assistant Professor of Orthopaedic Surgery, Department of Orthopaedic Surgery, Vanderbilt University Medical Center, Nashville, Tennessee

Giovanni Di Giacomo, MD
Medical Doctor, Department of Orthopaedics, Concordia Hospital, Rome, Italy

Karan Dua, MD
Resident Physician, Department of Orthopaedic Surgery and Rehabilitation Medicine, State University of New York Downstate Medical Center, Brooklyn, New York

Paul J. Duwelius, MD
Adjunct Associate Professor of Orthopedics, Oregon Health and Science University, Clinical Attending Orthopedics, Orthopedic and Fracture Specialists, St. Vincent Hospital and Medical Center, Portland, Oregon

Mouhanad M. El-Othmani, MD
Associate Clinical Researcher, Musculoskeletal Institute of Excellence, Orthopaedics and Sports Medicine, Detroit Medical Center, Detroit, Michigan

Sean M. Esmende, MD
Orthopedic Spine Surgery Fellow, Department of Orthopedic Surgery, University of Pittsburgh Medical Center, Pittsburgh, Pennsylvania

Jonathan Falakassa, MD
Clinical Instructor, Department of Orthopaedic Surgery, Spine Service, Stanford University, Palo Alto, California

Frances A. Farley, MD
Professor, Department of Orthopaedic Surgery, University of Michigan, Ann Arbor, Michigan

Jack Farr, MD
Professor of Orthopedic Surgery, Indiana University School of Medicine, Director, Cartilage Restoration Center, OrthoIndy Hospital, Indianapolis, Indiana

Richard D. Ferkel, MD
Director of Sports Medicine Fellowship, Southern California Orthopedic Institute, Assistant Clinical Professor of Orthopedic Surgery, University of California–Los Angeles, Center for the Health Sciences, Van Nuys, California

James R. Ficke, MD, FACS
Professor and Chair, Johns Hopkins Medicine, Baltimore, Maryland

Reza Firoozabadi, MD, MA
Director of Orthopaedic Trauma Research, Assistant Professor, Department of Orthopaedic Surgery, Harborview Medical Center, University of Washington, Seattle, Washington

Theodore J. Ganley, MD
Associate Professor, Department of Orthopaedic Surgery, Children's Hospital of Philadelphia, Philadelphia, Pennsylvania

Emmett Gannon, MD
Orthopaedic Surgery Resident, Department of Orthopaedic Surgery, University of Nebraska Medical Center, Omaha, Nebraska

Dia Eldean Giebaly, MBChB, MSc, MRCS
Trainee Trauma and Orthopaedic Surgeon, West of Scotland, Glasgow Royal Infirmary, Glasgow, Scotland

Eric Giza, MD
Associate Professor of Orthopaedic Surgery, Chief, Foot and Ankle Surgery, Department of Orthopaedics, University of California–Davis, Sacramento, California

Jenna Godfrey, MD, MSPH
Fellow, Department of Orthopaedic Surgery, Cincinnati Children's Hospital, Cincinnati, Ohio

Andreas H. Gomoll, MD
Associate Professor of Orthopedic Surgery, Department of Orthopedic Surgery, Brigham and Women's Hospital, Harvard Medical School, Boston, Massachusetts

Daniel W. Green, MD, MS
Professor of Orthopaedic Surgery, Hospital for Special Surgery, New York, New York

Fares S. Haddad, FRCS (Orth)
Professor, Department of Orthopaedics, University College London Hospitals, London, United Kingdom

George J. Haidukewych, MD
Chief of Orthopedic Trauma and Complex Adult Reconstruction, Level One Orthopedics, Orlando Health, Orlando, Florida

Ginger E. Holt, MD
Professor of Orthopaedic Surgery, Department of Orthopaedic Surgery, Vanderbilt University Medical Center, Nashville, Tennessee

Serena S. Hu, MD
Professor and Vice Chair, Department of Orthopedic Surgery, Stanford University, Stanford, California

Bradley P. Jaquith, MD
Orthopaedic Sports Medicine Fellow, Campbell Clinic, Memphis, Tennessee

Claudius D. Jarrett, MD
Hand and Upper Extremity Surgery, Orthopaedic Surgery, Wilmington Health Associates, Wilmington, North Carolina

William A. Jiranek, MD, FACS
Professor and Chief of Adult Reconstruction, Abbott and Allison Byrd Chair in Orthopaedic Surgery, Department of Orthopaedic Surgery, Virginia Commonwealth University Health System, Richmond, Virginia

Lynne C. Jones, PhD
Associate Professor, Department of Orthopaedic Surgery, Johns Hopkins University, Baltimore, Maryland

James D. Kang, MD
Thornhill Family Professor of Orthopaedic Surgery, Harvard Medical School, Chairman, Department of Orthopaedic Surgery, Brigham and Women's Hospital, Boston, Massachusetts

Lori A. Karol, MD
Professor, Department of Orthopaedics, University of Texas–Southwestern, Assistant Chief of Staff, Texas Scottish Rite Hospital for Children, Dallas, Texas

Harpal S. Khanuja, MD
Chief and Associate Professor, Johns Hopkins Bayview, Department of Orthopaedic Surgery, Johns Hopkins University, Baltimore, Maryland

Elliott Kim, MD
Orthopaedic Surgery Resident, Department of Orthopaedic Surgery, Vanderbilt Orthopaedics, Nashville, Tennessee

Eric O. Klineberg, MD
Associate Professor, Department of Orthopaedic Surgery, University of California–Davis Medical Center, Sacramento, California

Mininder S. Kocher, MD, MPH
Professor of Orthopaedic Surgery, Harvard Medical School, Associate Director, Division of Sports Medicine, Boston Children's Hospital, Boston, Massachusetts

Kenneth L. Koury, MD
Orthopaedic Trauma Fellow, Department of Orthopaedic Surgery, Rutgers University–New Jersey Medical School, Newark, New Jersey

Philip J. Kregor, MD
Director of Orthopedic Trauma, The Hughston Clinic at Skyline Medical Center, Nashville, Tennessee

Aaron J. Krych, MD
Associate Professor, Department of Orthopedic Surgery, Mayo Clinic, Rochester, Minnesota

Richard F. Kyle, MD
Professor of Orthopaedic Surgery, University of Minnesota, Department of Orthopaedic Surgery, Hennepin County Medical Center, Minneapolis, Minnesota

Laurent Lafosse, MD
Orthopaedic Surgeon, Department of Orthopaedics, Alps Surgery Institute–Clinique Generale, Annecy, France

Christian Latterman, MD
Professor, Vice-Chair for Clinical Research, Department of Orthopaedic Surgery and Sports Medicine, University of Kentucky, Lexington, Kentucky

Joon Yung Lee, MD
Associate Professor, Department of Orthopaedic Surgery, University of Pittsburgh Medical Center, Pittsburgh, Pennsylvania

Jean-Christophe Leveque, MD
Neurosurgeon, Department of Neurosurgery, Virginia Mason Medical Center, Seattle, Washington

Adam S. Levin, MD
Assistant Professor, Department of Orthopaedic Surgery, Johns Hopkins University, Baltimore, Maryland

Valerae O. Lewis, MD
Professor and Chair, Department of Orthopaedic Oncology, MD Anderson Cancer Center, Houston, Texas

Jay R. Lieberman, MD
Professor and Chairman, Department of Orthopaedic Surgery, Keck School of Medicine of University of Southern California, Los Angeles, California

Jess H. Lonner, MD
Associate Professor of Orthopaedic Surgery, Rothman Institute, Sidney Kimmel School of Medicine at Thomas Jefferson University, Philadelphia, Pennsylvania

Bilal Mahmood, MD
Orthopaedic Surgery Resident, Department of Orthopaedic Surgery, Cleveland Clinic Foundation, Cleveland, Ohio

Michael R. Marks, MD, MBA
President, Marks Healthcare Consulting, Westport, Connecticut

J. Bohannon Mason, MD
Orthopedic Surgeon, OrthoCarolina, Hip and Knee Center, Charlotte, North Carolina

Dustin H. Massel, BS
Research Coordinator, Department of Orthopaedic Surgery, Rush University Medical Center, Chicago, Illinois

Richard L. McGough, MD
Chief, Division of Musculoskeletal Oncology, Department of Orthopaedic Surgery, University of Pittsburgh, Pittsburgh, Pennsylvania

Rodrigo Góes Medéa de Mendonça, MD
Orthopaedic Spine Surgery, Department of Traumatology and Orthopedics, Pavillion Fernandinho Simonsen, Sao Paulo, Brazil

Alan J. Micev, MD
Fellow, The Philadelphia Hand Center, Thomas Jefferson University, Philadelphia, Pennsylvania

Megan Mignemi, MD
Assistant Professor of Orthopaedics and Rehabilitation, Department of Orthopaedics and Rehabilitation, Vanderbilt Medical Center, Nashville, Tennessee

William M. Mihalko, MD, PhD
Professor and J.R. Hyde Chair, Campbell Clinic Department of Orthopaedic Surgery and Biomedical Engineering, University of Tennessee and Campbell Clinic Orthopaedics, Memphis, Tennessee

Ryan Miyamoto, MD
Orthopaedic Surgeon, Fair Oaks Orthopaedics, Fairfax, Virginia

Berton R. Moed, MD
Professor and Chairman, Department of Orthopaedic Surgery, Saint Louis University School of Medicine, St. Louis, Missouri

Carol D. Morris, MD, MS
Division Chief, Department of Orthopaedic Oncology, Johns Hopkins, Baltimore, Maryland

Michael J. Morris, MD
Joint Implant Surgeons, New Albany, Ohio

Brian A. Mosier, MD
Department of Orthopaedic Surgery, Allegheny Health Network, Pittsburgh, Pennsylvania

Michael P. Mott, MD
Division Head of Musculoskeletal Oncology, Department of Orthopaedic Surgery, Henry Ford Health System, Detroit, Michigan

John W. Munz, MD
Assistant Professor, Department of Orthopaedic Surgery, The University of Texas McGovern Medical School at Houston, Houston, Texas

Zan A. Naseer, BS
Clinical Research Fellow, Department of Orthopaedic Surgery, Johns Hopkins University, Baltimore, Maryland

Venu M. Nemani, MD, PhD
Cervical and Reconstructive Spine Surgery, Raleigh Orthopaedic Clinic, Raleigh, North Carolina

Philippe Neyret, MD
Professor, Department of Orthopaedic Surgery, Hôpital Croix Rousse Lyon–Centre Albert Trillat, Lyon, France

Kenneth Noonan, MD
Orthopaedic Surgeon, Department of Orthopaedics, University of Wisconsin, Madison, Wisconsin

Martin J. O'Malley, MD
Attending Surgeon, Foot and Ankle Service, Hospital for Special Surgery, New York, New York

A. Lee Osterman, MD
Director, The Philadelphia Hand Center, Thomas Jefferson University, Philadelphia, Pennsylvania

William Pannell, MD
Resident Physician, Department of Orthopaedic Surgery, Keck School of Medicine of University of Southern California, Los Angeles, California

Loukia K. Papatheodorou, MD, PhD
Orthopaedic Surgeon, Department of Orthopaedic Surgery, University of Pittsburgh, Orthopaedic Specialists–University of Pittsburgh Medical Center, Pittsburgh, Pennsylvania

Wayne G. Paprosky, MD, FACS
Orthopaedic Surgeon, Midwest Orthopaedics at Rush University Medical Center, Chicago, Illinois, Cadence Health–Central DuPage Hospital, Winfield, Illinois

Shital N. Parikh, MD, FACS
Associate Professor of Orthopaedic Surgery, Division of Orthopaedic Surgery, Cincinnati Children's Hospital Medical Center, Cincinnati, Ohio

Rakesh D. Patel, MD
Assistant Professor, Department of Orthopaedic Surgery, University of Michigan, Ann Arbor, Michigan

David M. Prior, MD
Fellow, Department of Orthopaedic Surgery, University of California–Davis Medical Center, Sacramento, California

Themistocles Protopsaltis, MD
Assistant Professor, Department of Orthopaedic Surgery, NYU Langone Medical Center, New York, New York

Adam Rana, MD
Orthopedic Surgeon, Department of Orthopedics and Sports Medicine, Maine Medical Center, Portland, Maine

Afshin E. Razi, MD
Clinical Assistant Professor, Department of Orthopaedic Surgery, NYU Langone Hospital for Joint Diseases, New York, New York

Lauren H. Redler, MD
Assistant Professor of Orthopaedic Surgery, Adult and Pediatric Sports Medicine, Columbia University Medical Center, New York, New York

Christian Refakis, BA
Clinical Research Fellow, Department of Pediatric Orthopaedics, Children's Hospital of Philadelphia, Philadelphia, Pennsylvania

Mark C. Reilly, MD
Professor and Chief of Orthopaedic Trauma Service, Department of Orthopaedics, Rutgers–New Jersey Medical School, Newark, New Jersey

Andrew Barrister Richardson, MD
Adult Hip and Knee Reconstruction Fellow, Joint Implant Surgeons, New Albany, Ohio

Anthony A. Romeo, MD
Professor, Department of Orthopedic Surgery, Rush University Medical Center, Chicago, Illinois

Andrew J. Rosenbaum, MD
Assistant Professor, Division of Orthopaedic Surgery, Albany Medical College, New York, New York

Scott B. Rosenfeld, MD
Director, Hip Preservation Program, Pediatric Orthopedic Surgery, Texas Children's Hospital, Associate Professor of Orthopaedic Surgery, Baylor College of Medicine, Houston, Texas

Khaled J. Saleh, MD, MSc, FACSC, MHCM, CPE
Executive in Chief, Department of Orthopaedics, Detroit Medical Center, Detroit, Michigan

Michael Isiah Sandlin, MD
Orthopaedic Surgery Foot and Ankle Fellow, Department of Orthopaedic Surgery, Cedars-Sinai Medical Center, Los Angeles, California

Zain Sayeed, MSc, MHA
Researcher, Chicago Medical School, North Chicago, Illinois

Andrew H. Schmidt, MD
Chief, Department of Orthopaedic Surgery, Hennepin County Medical Center, Minneapolis, Minnesota

Jonathan Schoenecker, MD, PhD
Assistant Professor, Department of Orthopaedics, Vanderbilt University, Nashville, Tennessee

Gregory D. Schroeder, MD
Spine Research and Clinical Fellow, Rothman Institute, Thomas Jefferson University, Philadelphia, Pennsylvania

Travis Scudday, MD
Resident, Department of Orthopedic Surgery, Loma Linda University Medical Center, Loma Linda, California

Rajiv Sethi, MD
Clinical Associate Professor, Chair of the Neuroscience Institute, Departments of Neurosurgery and Orthopaedics, Virginia Mason Medical Center, Department of Health Services, University of Washington, Seattle, Washington

Kern Singh, MD
Associate Professor, Department of Orthopaedic Surgery, Rush University Medical Center, Chicago, Illinois

James Slover, MS, MD
Associate Professor, Department of Orthopaedic Surgery, NYU Langone Medical Center, New York, New York

Dean G. Sotereanos, MD
Clinical Professor of Orthopaedic Surgery, University of Pittsburgh School of Medicine, Orthopaedic Specialists–University of Pittsburgh Medical Center, Pittsburgh, Pennsylvania

Kurt P. Spindler, MD
Vice Chairman of Research, Director of Orthopaedic Clinical Outcomes, Academic Director, Cleveland Clinic Sports Health, Orthopaedic and Rheumatologic Institute, Cleveland Clinic, Cleveland, Ohio

Eileen Storey, BA
Clinical Research Coordinator, Department of Orthopaedics, The Children's Hospital of Philadelphia, Philadelphia, Pennsylvania

Michael D. Stover, MD
Professor, Department of Orthopaedic Surgery, Northwestern University, Feinberg School of Medicine, Chicago, Illinois

Adam B. Strohl, MD
Instructor, Philadelphia Hand Center, Thomas Jefferson University Hospital, Department of Orthopaedic Surgery, Department of Surgery–Division of Plastic Surgery, Philadelphia, Pennsylvania

Michael J. Stuart, MD
Professor and Chair, Division of Sports Medicine, Department of Orthopedic Surgery, Mayo Clinic, Rochester, Minnesota

Matthew P. Sullivan, MD
Assistant Professor, Department of Orthopaedic Surgery, State University of New York, Upstate Medical University, Syracuse, New York

Cyrus E. Taghavi, MD
Foot and Ankle Fellow, Department of Orthopaedic Surgery, Cedars-Sinai Medical Center, Los Angeles, California

David B. Thordarson, MD
Professor, Department of Orthopedics, Cedars-Sinai Medical Center, Los Angeles, California

Robert J. Thorsness, MD
Shoulder and Elbow, Sports Medicine, Hinsdale Orthopaedics, Joliet, Illinois

Beverlie Ting, MD
Orthopaedic Surgeon, Seattle Hand Surgery Group, Seattle, Washington

John M. Tokish, MD
Fellowship Director, Steadman Hawkins Clinic of the Carolinas, Professor, University of South Carolina School of Medicine, Department of Orthopaedics, Greenville Health System, Steadman Hawkins Clinic of the Carolinas, Greenville, South Carolina

Robert T. Trousdale, MD
Professor of Orthopedics, Department of Adult Reconstruction, Orthopedic Surgery, Mayo Clinic, Rochester, Minnesota

Alexander R. Vaccaro, MD, PhD, MBA
Richard H. Rothman Professor and Chairman, Department of Orthopaedic Surgery, Professor of Neurosurgery, Co-Director, Delaware Valley Spinal Cord Injury Center, Co-Chief of Spine Surgery, Sidney Kimmel Medical Center at Thomas Jefferson University, President, Rothman Institute, Philadelphia, Pennsylvania

Nikhil N. Verma, MD
Professor and Director, Division of Sports Medicine, Fellowship Director, Sports Medicine, Department of Orthopedics, Rush University Medical Center, Midwest Orthopedics at Rush, Team Physician, Chicago White Sox and Chicago Bulls, Chicago, Illinois

Shaleen Vira, MD
Orthopedic Surgery Resident, NYU Hospital for Joint Diseases, New York University, New York, New York

William C. Warner Jr, MD
Professor of Orthopaedics, Department of Orthopaedics, University of Tennessee and Campbell Clinic, Memphis, Tennessee

Daniel C. Wascher, MD
Professor, Department of Orthopaedic Surgery, University of New Mexico School of Medicine, Albuquerque, New Mexico

Kristy Weber, MD
Professor, Department of Orthopaedic Surgery, University of Pennsylvania, Philadelphia, Pennsylvania

Adam M. Wegner, MD, PhD
Resident, Department of Orthopaedic Surgery, University of California–Davis Medical Center, Sacramento, California

Scott D. Weiner, MD
Chair and Medical Director, Department of Orthopaedic Surgery, Summa Health, Akron, Ohio

Roger F. Widmann, MD
Chief of Pediatric Orthopaedic Surgery, Hospital for Special Surgery, Professor of Clinical Orthopaedic Surgery, Weill Cornell Medical College, New York, New York

Craig S. Williams, MD
Hand and Upper Extremity, Illinois Bone and Joint Institute, Des Plaines, Illinois

Brian R. Wolf, MD, MS
Congdon Professor and Vice-Chairman, Department of Orthopaedics and Rehabilitation, University of Iowa, Iowa City, Iowa

Rick W. Wright, MD
Professor and Executive Vice Chair, Department of Orthopaedic Surgery, Washington University, St. Louis, Missouri

Theresa O. Wyrick, MD
Associate Professor, Department of Orthopaedic Surgery, Arkansas Children's Hospital, Little Rock, Arkansas

Vijay Yanamadala, MD
Fellow, Spine Surgery, Virginia Mason Medical Center, Seattle, Washington

David S. Zelouf, MD
Assistant Clinical Professor, Thomas Jefferson University Hospital, Department of Orthopaedic Surgery, The Philadelphia Hand Center, Philadelphia, Pennsylvania

Preface

The Instructional Course Lectures (ICLs) presented at the 2016 American Academy of Orthopaedic Surgeons (AAOS) Annual Meeting in Orlando, FL, were a resounding success, as was the entire meeting under the leadership of David Teuscher, MD. This volume of ICLs includes 54 chapters on topics presented at the 2016 Annual Meeting.

Instructional Course Lectures, Volume 66 (ICL 66) was produced through the hard work and dedication of many different groups: the Central Instructional Courses Committee, the specialty Instructional Course committees, the contributing authors, and the AAOS editorial staff. The efforts of the Central Instructional Courses Committee resulted in the outstanding organization and excellent array of topics presented at the Annual Meeting and the ICLs presented in this publication. I would like to thank the previous chairs of the Central Instructional Courses Committee, beginning with my predecessors, Thomas (Quin) Throckmorton, 2015 chair; and Craig J. Della Valle, 2014 chair; as well as the upcoming chairs, Jay Parvizi, 2017 chair; and James Huddleston, 2018 chair. The specialty Instructional Course committee chairs and members assisted in the selection of the ICLs for the Annual Meeting and functioned as section editors and editorial board members for this volume. The authors of ICL 66 dedicated many hours of hard work to contribute chapters on important topics; without these individuals, this publication would not be possible. Last but not least, a debt of gratitude is owed to the outstanding AAOS staff, including April Holmes, Nicole Williams, and Domenic Picardo, who continue to be essential resources for the Central Instructional Courses Committee. My sincerest gratitude also goes to Michelle Wild, Lisa Claxton Moore, Kathleen Anderson, Genevieve Charet, and Katie Hovany, all of whom work with a large group of surgeon-volunteers to ensure that deadlines are met and to achieve an organized and well-written textbook and a useful video supplement. Finally, I would like to offer a special thank you to Paul Tornetta, MD, the outgoing Annual Meeting Committee Chair, for his amazing vision, tireless efforts, and endless dedication to improving the Annual Meeting and the education of AAOS members.

It is my sincerest hope that AAOS members use this volume and the many resources of the AAOS to continue to provide patients with the highest level of care and to pursue solutions to questions that remain unanswered.

Tad L. Gerlinger, MD
Chicago, Illinois

Table of Contents

Section 4: Adult Reconstruction: Hip and Knee

Section 5: Foot and Ankle

Section 10: The Practice of Orthopaedics

Video Abstracts

Chapter 1 Acetabular Fractures: A Problem-Oriented Approach

Video 1.1: Moed BR: *Performance of the EUA.* St. Louis, MO, 2016. (1 min)

This video demonstrates an examination of the hip joint of a patient under anesthesia. The patient is positioned supine on a radiolucent surgical table. With the hip in full extension and neutral rotation, the hip joint is slowly flexed past 90°, with progressive manual force applied through the hip along the longitudinal axis of the femur. Concurrently, the hip is visualized with use of C-arm image intensifier fluoroscopic imaging. If the hip joint remains congruent during this assessment, the examination is repeated with the addition of approximately 20° of adduction and approximately 20° of internal rotation. In general, the examination is performed twice, once with the use of the anteroposterior fluoroscope projection and once with the use of the obturator oblique fluoroscope projection.

Video 1.2: Moed BR, Stover MD: *Ballottable Fluid Wave.* St. Louis, MO, and Chicago, IL, 2016. (10 sec)

This video demonstrates the ballottable fluid wave that can be elicited in a patient with a Morel-Lavallée lesion. Note that the overlying skin of the patient is intact.

Video 1.3: Moed BR, Stover MD: *Percutaneous Débridement.* St. Louis, MO, and Chicago, IL, 2016. (23 sec)

The patient shown in this video was struck and run over by a truck. The fluid collection observed 8 hours postinjury is shown, and a percutaneous débridement technique is demonstrated.

Chapter 7 Cubital Tunnel Syndrome

Video 7.1: Sotereanos DG: *Cubital Tunnel Syndrome.* Pittsburgh, PA, 2016. (4 min)

This video demonstrates a partial medial epicondylectomy in a patient with cubital tunnel syndrome. The skin incision is made 5 cm proximal and 5 cm distal to the medial epicondyle. The ulnar nerve is identified under the medial intermuscular septum, which is released and excised. The ulnar nerve is then decompressed around the medial epicondyle. Care is taken to preserve the medial antebrachial cutaneous nerve via more distal dissection. The Osborne band is released, and the ulnar nerve is decompressed distally with care taken to preserve the flexor carpi ulnaris branch of the ulnar nerve. The blood supply of the nerve must be preserved. An ulnar nerve subluxation is observed in the patient shown in this video. The medial epicondyle is identified. A subperiosteal epicondylar exposure is performed. A partial medial epicondylectomy is performed with the use of an osteotome. The excised fragment is shown. Bone wax is applied at the osteotomy site. No ulnar nerve subluxation is observed in the patient shown in this video after partial medial epicondylectomy. A subperiosteal flap closure is performed, and the suture is buried. Again, no ulnar nerve subluxation is observed in the patient shown in this video after partial medial epicondylectomy.

Chapter 20 Achilles Tendon Rupture in Elite Athletes

Video 20.1: Charlton TP: *Achilles Tendon Rupture in Athletes.* Los Angeles, CA, 2016. (3 min)

This video demonstrates a minimally invasive technique for repair of a ruptured Achilles tendon. Postoperative rehabilitation is discussed.

Chapter 21 Lisfranc Injuries in the Elite Athlete

Video 21.1: Anderson RB: *Lisfranc Injuries in the Elite Athlete.* Charlotte, NC, 2016. (9 min)

This video discusses the importance of a Lisfranc injury to the midfoot in elite athletes. Incidence and the indirect mechanism of injury are discussed. Lisfranc injuries are primarily a twisting injury rather than a contact injury or the result of axial loading. An open surgical approach rather than a percutaneous approach is recommended for management of a Lisfranc injury. The use of solid screws rather than cannulated screws is recommended. The use of bridge plates is recommended. Postoperative rehabilitation is discussed.

Chapter 23 Management of Osteochondral Lesions of the Talus

Video 23.1: Giza E: *Ankle and Cartilage Treatment in the Athlete.* Sacramento, CA, 2016. (3 min)

This video discusses allograft cartilage extracellular matrix scaffold as an augment for microfracture. The technique for the application of allograft cartilage extracellular matrix scaffold is demonstrated, and case examples are discussed. Matrix-induced autologous chrondrocyte implantation is discussed.

Chapter 26 Surgical Management of Cervical Spondylotic Myelopathy

Video 26.1: Cornett CA: *Surgical Management of Cervical Spondylotic Myelopathy.* Omaha, NE, 2016. (3 min)

This video demonstrates surgical management of cervical spondylotic myelopathy via laminectomy with fusion. Standard positioning for posterior cervical procedures generally includes positioning in Mayfield tongs and a slight reverse Trendelenburg position to prevent venous bleeding. A midline approach is outlined and undertaken. The fascia is divided in the midline with care taken to avoid strain into the muscle to prevent bleeding and to facilitate closure of the fascia at the end of the procedure. Good visualization of the posterior bony elements is achieved after the muscle is reflected off the posterior spine. Dissection is carried out to the lateral aspect of the lateral masses in question. Care is taken to avoid disruption of the junctional ligaments above and below the area that is to be visualized. The instrumentation is then performed, placing lateral mass screws in a standard fashion, which are angled superiorly and laterally to avoid the vertebral artery and the nerve roots. After the lateral mass screws have been placed, lateral rods are connected, the set screws are placed, and the spine is stabilized across those areas. Decortication of the facet joints with the use of a burr is advised at this stage of the procedure. The spinous processes are then removed to facilitate use of the burr for laminectomy. A laminectomy is then performed, creating full-thickness troughs at the junction of the lamina and the lateral mass bilaterally so that the spinous process and the lamina can be removed en bloc after division of the ligamentum flavum with the use of a small Kerrison rongeur. After the spinous process and the lamina have been removed, the margins are cleaned up with the use of a small Kerrison rongeur. Hemostasis is ensured, after which bone grafting in the facet joints can be performed. Typically, a drain is placed, and a multilayer closure is performed.

Chapter 34 Pediatric Phalanx Fractures

Video 34.1: Abzug JM: *Pediatric Phalanx Fracture.* Timonium, MD, 2016. (19 sec)

This video demonstrates the assessment of a child in whom a pediatric phalanx fracture is suspected. The digital cascade must be assessed and compared with that of the uninjured hand to determine if any malrotation or substantial deviation is present. An assessment of the digital cascade during active and passive range of motion via tenodesis grasp and release will provide surgeons with the most useful information.

Chapter 42 The Four Most Common Types of Knee Cartilage Damage Encountered in Practice: How and Why Orthopaedic Surgeons Manage Them

Video 42.1: Farr J: *Autologous Chondrocyte Implantation.* Indianapolis, IN, 2016. (3 min)

This video demonstrates autologous chondrocyte implantation in a patient with a chondral defect of the knee. The medial femoral condyle is approached via a medial parapatellar arthrotomy. Care is taken to not harm the medial meniscus or the articular surfaces. Retractors are placed, and the knee is flexed to observe the defect. A No. 15 blade is used to create vertical walls, and a curette is used to clear the base. The defect is measured, the tourniquet is deflated, fibrin glue is applied, and digital pressure is maintained to achieve hemostasis. The measurements of the defect are transferred to a template. The template is cut to fit the exact dimensions of the defect and is marked for orientation. A type I/III collagen patch is hydrated; it has a rough surface and a smooth surface. The smooth surface is labeled "UP." The template is then transferred to the hydrated type I/III collagen patch, and the patch is cut to fit. Maintenance of adequate hydration of the type I/III collagen patch is necessary. Cells are resuspended, and in this video, the cells are seeded on the rough surface of the type I/III collagen patch. After 10 minutes, the cells will be adherent. During that time, the cells are protected.

After hemostasis has been achieved and reconfirmed, the seeded patch is placed into the defect with the rough seeded area facing bone. Any extraneous patch is removed, after which the patch is sutured into place with the use of 6-0 absorbable suture. Sutures are placed at 3- to 4-mm intervals and are then further sealed with fibrin glue. A second vial of cells is injected, after which the injection site is sutured and further sealed with fibrin glue. After approximately 10 minutes, the area is irrigated, and the incision is closed in layers.

Video 42.2: Farr J: *Anteromedialization.* Indianapolis, IN, 2016. (2 min)

This video demonstrates anteromedialization of the tibial tubercle, which typically is performed in combination with tibial tubercle osteotomy. In this video, a longer incision is used to allow for concomitant cartilage restoration. Proximally, a lateral lengthening is performed. The incision is carried along the lateral aspect of the tuberosity, and the anterior compartment musculature is elevated. An incision is made along the medial border of the patellar tendon and is continued obliquely as it courses distally. A cutting guide with a jig is applied. The slope arm selects the point at which the saw will exit along the lateral wall. The retractor helps protect neurovascular structures. The saw exits onto the retractor and is located above or anterior to the posterior wall of the tibia. The jig is removed. The saw is then inserted into the cut, and the cut is used as a capture guide to continue the proximal and distal extents of the osteotomy. Proximally, the osteotomy is completed with the use of an osteotome, changing directions as it is moved from posterior to anterior. The free tuberosity is then elevated and medialized, after which it is temporarily held in place with the use of a pin. After the tuberosity is in the desired position, it is fixed using a standard interfragmentary technique; typically, two 4.5-mm screws are used. The sharp proximal-medial aspect of the tuberosity is trimmed. The amount of anteriorization and medialization are directly measured. The lateral compartment musculature is lightly reapproximated to tamponade the cancellous bone posteriorly. Proximally, the lateral lengthening is reapproximated.

Video 42.3: Farr J: *Lateral Lengthening.* Indianapolis, IN, 2016. (2 min)

This video demonstrates lateral lengthening, which typically is performed in combination with tibial tubercle osteotomy, in a patient with recurrent lateral patellar dislocations. In addition to recurrent dislocations, a static component of lateral subluxation is present. The patient has normal medial displacement of the patella but excessive lateral displacement of the patella. Arthroscopy demonstrates patellar and trochlear chondrosis. Therefore, the goal is to improve the static position of the patella (ie, improve the contact area in an attempt to slow chondrosis progression). Because the position and rotation of the tuberosity are within normal limits, the static subluxation pattern will be managed via concomitant lateral lengthening and medial patellofemoral ligament reconstruction. The superficial oblique fibers of the lateral retinaculum as they course from the iliotibial band are identified and elevated from the deeper transverse fibers. The deeper transverse fibers are then cut approximately 1.5 cm posterior to the patella. The superficial fibers are reflected, after which, the deeper fibers of the patient shown in this video are grasped using the forceps. These two layers are then reapproximated, which will allow for approximately 1.5 cm of lengthening in most patients. To improve clarity, the reapproximation site is marked, after which the lateral aspect of the patella is marked. The distance between the reapproximation site and the lateral aspect of the patella in the patient shown in this video is approximately 18 mm. Postoperative radiographs demonstrate improved central positioning of the patella.

Video 42.4: Farr J: *Medial Patellofemoral Ligament Reconstruction.* Indianapolis, IN, 2016. (4 min)

This video demonstrates two-incision medial patellofemoral ligament reconstruction, which can be performed in combination with tibial tubercle osteotomy in select patients. An incision is made adjacent to the patella through the superficial and middle layers of the knee. The interval between the middle and deep layers of the knee is bluntly dissected, which allows for the insertion of a hemostat. Digital palpation is used to confirm that no adhesions are present. An incision is made along the medial border of the patella. A superficial trough is made, and the area is decorticated to encourage healing with cancellous bone. A first suture anchor is placed in the mid-waist of the patella, after which a shape memory device is inserted and expanded. The inserter is then removed, and the suture anchor should be secure. A second suture anchor is then placed proximally in the same bony trough. A posterior incision is made over the femoral attachment of the medial patellofemoral ligament. The superficial and medial layers of the knee are incised, and a hemostat should be able to course from the first incision so that it exits posteriorly though the second incision. The first approximation of the anatomic attachment site of the medial patellofemoral ligament is made using the anatomic references of the adductor tendon and the epicondyle. The second approximation of the anatomic attachment site of the medial patellofemoral ligament is made using a true lateral fluoroscopic image to identify the Amos point. A drill pin is then inserted in the Amos point. The third approximation of the anatomic attachment site of the medial patellofemoral ligament is made to measure the distance changes between the two attachment sites. Sutures are drawn from the patella to the drill pin, after which the sutures are secured with the use of a hemostat with the knee in 20° of flexion. Further flexion of the knee decreases the distance, and, thus, the sutures will be loose. With the knee in 20° of flexion, the sutures are out to length. After the anatomic attachment site of the medial patellofemoral ligament has been confirmed, a blind socket is created at the attachment site. A graft is then trimmed to fit precisely into the socket. A graft pusher is inserted at the doubled area of the graft, and the graft is placed into the base of the socket. A memory shape interference device is then inserted and impacted until it is level with the cortex. After expansion, the graft should be secure. The graft is then passed through the tunnel to the patella, after which the graft is secured with the use of the sutures with the graft out to length and with the knee in 20° of flexion. After this initial fixation is complete, the graft is doubled back upon itself, and each arm of the graft is secured. After both arms of the graft are secured, the superficial and middle layers of the knee are reapproximated adjacent to the patella. Patellar displacement is then assessed; the patient shown in this video has 1+ medial and lateral patellar displacement, as desired. Patellar tracking is then assessed from the front and the lateral aspect; the patient shown in this video has smooth and central patellar tracking, and no restriction to full flexion or extension is present.

Video 42.5: Farr J: *Patellofemoral Arthroplasty.* Indianapolis, IN, 2016. (9 min)

This video demonstrates patellofemoral arthroplasty in the right knee of a patient who underwent patellofemoral arthroplasty of the contralateral knee. The patient's right knee has marked lateral joint space narrowing, whereas the tibiofemoral joints in both knees are intact and asymptomatic. A midline skin incision allows for exposure of the lateral retinaculum. The lateral retinaculum is prepared via lateral lengthening, first incising the superficial oblique fibers and then the deep transverse fibers. By reapproximating these fibers, the lateral retinaculum is lengthened approximately 1.5 cm. Lateral lengthening is an alternative to recession or lateral release. A medial parapatellar arthrotomy is performed to expose the trochlea. In the patient shown in this video, exposed bone is present in the central lateral portion of the trochlea and also at the patella. Fat is removed to expose the patellar and quadriceps tendon attachments. In the patient shown in this video, osteophytes are present at the margins of the patella. The patella is measured, which will allow for reapproximation of the thickness of the original patella at the end of the procedure, and then cut from medial to lateral. The cut is gradually increased until the bone thickness is approximately 13 mm. An area of exposed bone and eburnated bone remains laterally. The lug holes are created, after which the lateralmost aspect of the exposed bone and fibrous tissue over some of the eburnated bone are removed. Multiple drill holes are made, and the area is irrigated. A trial button is attached. Soft tissue, including synovium and fat, is removed immediately proximal to the trochlea because the flange of the final implant will extend approximately 1 cm proximally. Osteophytes around the notch are removed. The nose of the implant must not be placed over osteophytes. The goal is to place the nose of the femoral implant approximately 2 cm above the roof of the notch. A step drill is used to create a socket, which will be used as a reference for the following jigs. The area is then sized, attempting to accommodate the morphology and size of the bone. After the size has been selected, the next jig is applied, and the stepped portion of the jig is inserted into the socket. The placement of the jig is confirmed with an osteotome. After rotation is deemed acceptable, the jig is attached with the use of temporary screws and rechecked. The proximal arm of the jig prevents the femur from being notched. The anterior bone is then removed. A second jig with a step is then applied; the step ensures that the final implant will be flush with the surrounding distal articular cartilage. A forceps is used to check the distance between the jig and the underlying articular cartilage, ensuring that it is equal. After the distance is confirmed to be equal on both sides, the jig is secured into position. A router is then used to remove bone to the depth of the final implant. The router must be maintained along the peripheral guides. After the routing is complete, the jig is removed.

The elevated soft tissues are then removed, and the trial trochlear implant is positioned and impacted. The goal is to position the trial trochlear implant so that it is either equal to or slightly recessed from the adjacent articular cartilage; this is checked with an osteotome. After the desired position of the trial trochlear implant is confirmed, a drill guide, which is used to create the lug holes, is attached. Each lug hole is then created with the use of a drill bit. After the three lug holes have been created, the jig is removed. The patellar button is reattached to the patella, and the knee is brought through a range of motion to ensure smooth tracking of the patella and that the patella remains central. After this is confirmed, the trials are removed, and the cut bone is copiously irrigated with pulsatile lavage. Standard drilling is performed at both the trochlea and patella. The surgeon should put on a new set of gloves. The components are inspected. Three lugs are noted on the back of the trochlear component, and three lugs are noted on the back of the all-polyethylene patellar component. High-viscosity cement is applied to the backside of the trochlear and patellar implants. Cement is then applied to the cut bone at the trochlea. The trochlear implant is inserted. Initial excess cement is removed, after which the implant is impacted, and final excess cement is removed around the margins of the implant. The patella is irrigated, suctioned, and dried. Cement is applied to the patella, after which the patellar all-polyethylene button is applied digitally and then with the use of a clamp. Excess cement is removed. After the cement has cured, the medial arthrotomy is reapproximated (in the patient shown in this video, barbed running suture is used for reapproximation), and the lateral lengthening is reapproximated. The knee is brought through a range of motion after reapproximation and after the skin is closed; in the patient shown in this video, patellar tracking is smooth and the patella remains central from both the lateral aspect and the front. Postoperative radiographs of the right knee of the patient shown in this video reveal a properly positioned patellofemoral arthroplasty.

Video 42.6: Farr J: *High Tibial Valgus Osteotomy.* Indianapolis, IN, 2016. (7 min)

This video demonstrates high tibial valgus osteotomy in a 55-year-old man with progressive medial knee pain, which has been present since he underwent a medial meniscectomy in 2004, and 8° of varus. The patient was seeking an alternative to arthroplasty. Standing AP and Rosenberg plain radiographs revealed some degree of moderate joint space remaining. Alignment radiographs revealed 8° of mechanical axis varus. An incision is made between the tibial tuberosity and the posterior border of the tibia, beginning at the joint line and extending approximately 6 cm distally. The incision is made to the level of the fascia. Subcutaneous dissection allows for mobilization of the incision window. The medial border of the patellar tendon and the pes group are identified. An incision is made along the medial border of the patellar tendon just proximal to its attachment to the tuberosity. The interval is developed, and a retractor is placed to protect it from harm. Next, a reverse L cut is made parallel to the tibial crest in line with the medial border of the patellar tendon and then anterior to posterior; this is then elevated subperiosteally. The sleeve is then elevated and retracted posteriorly, which allows a digit to be slipped from the medial border of the tibia to the fibular head. A Cobb elevator is used to perform subperiosteal dissection, after which it is replaced with a blunt Hohmann elevator. A temporary guide pin is placed just proximal to the patellar tendon attachment. Note that with gentle deflexion, the medial tibial plateau is collinear. The saw is adjusted so that the plane of the saw cut will be coplanar with the tibial plateau. Note that this medial to lateral cut is made under direct visualization, and that the patellar tendon is protected with the Army-Navy retractor. The posterior cut is then made with the use of a thin osteotome. The Hohmann elevator protects posterior neurovascular structures, and during each step, the knee is checked and rechecked. The posterior margin of the osteotome is palpated during the final advancement. The osteotomy is then slowly opened with the use of standard osteotomes. After the opening is approximately 4 mm, removal of the posterior osteotome and insertion of a small trial (in the patient shown in this video, a 6-mm trial is inserted) are possible. The trial is advanced slowly, and the osteotomy opening is observed via fluoroscopy. After an opening has been achieved with the use of the smaller trial, an anterior spacer is added, after which a final trial (in the patient shown in this video, a 13-mm final trial is used) is inserted very slowly. Fluoroscopy is used to confirm the trial position and that no fracture exists laterally or proximally. An alignment rod placed from the hip to the ankle is checked to ensure that it is in the lateral tibial spine at the knee, as desired. The surgeon should put on a new set of gloves. The trial is then exchanged for a permanent tricalcium phosphate wedge, which is a biplanar wedge that does not change the slope and also fits the contour of the posterior aspect of the tibia. A plate is used to compress and hold the tricalcium phosphate wedge in position. The lateral opening can be filled with tricalcium phosphate granules. The template is removed, and the final implant is inserted. Fine tuning is then performed with the use of an impactor. The tricalcium phosphate wedge should be flush with the medial cortex, which is verified fluoroscopically. A temporary pin is placed through the plate to hold it in position while the drill holes are made. The drill guides are attached to the plate. The drill is advanced to approximately 50 mm, which is verified with a depth gauge and then confirmed fluoroscopically. A reamer is used to prepare the hole for the final screw, which is a locking screw that is inserted with the use of a torque screwdriver. After both proximal screws have been fully seated, the temporary pin is removed. A compression loading drill guide is then placed onto the distal aspect of the plate. It should be labeled "DOWN." The drill hole is made, after which a screw is placed to compresses the plate against the wedge. After the screw has been seated, two locking screws are placed in the plate distally in the same manner as those that were placed proximally, after which the compression loading screw is removed. Tricalcium phosphate granules are used to fill the void on the lateral aspect of the osteotomy. The final construct is then assessed on both AP and lateral fluoroscopic images. In the patient shown in this video, fluoroscopic images demonstrate good positioning of the wedge, granules, plate, and screws. The elevated sleeve followed by the subcutaneous tissue are reapproximated. In the patient shown in this video, a zip line was used to reapproximate the skin incision.

Trauma

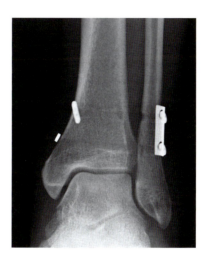

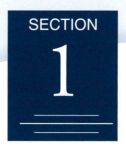

Acetabular Fractures: A Problem-Oriented Approach

Berton R. Moed, MD
Philip J. Kregor, MD
Mark C. Reilly, MD
Michael D. Stover, MD

Abstract

The main goals of acetabular fracture management are to restore the congruity and stability of the hip joint. These goals are the same for all patients who have an acetabular fracture, regardless of the morphology or etiology of the fracture. Nevertheless, certain acetabular fracture types and several patient factors pose management challenges for surgeons. Therefore, surgeons who manage acetabular fractures must understand the distinctive features of acetabular fractures as well as the soft-tissue and patient-related factors that play a critical role in patient outcomes. Particular challenges in the management of acetabular fractures include acetabular fracture types that involve the posterior wall, acetabular fractures with soft-tissue concerns, acetabular fractures in patients with multiple injuries, and acetabular fractures in the geriatric population. Although the well-known protocols that were established by Judet and Letournel continue to be important guidelines for the management of acetabular fractures, the injury characteristics of acetabular fractures, the demographics of the patients in whom acetabular fractures occur, and the treatment options for acetabular fractures have evolved. Therefore, surgeons must be aware of new and more recently published information on acetabular fractures.

Instr Course Lect 2017;66:3–24.

Most surgeons agree that displaced acetabular fractures that are left untreated result in poor outcomes, such as residual joint instability or incongruity between the femoral head and the weight-bearing area of the acetabulum.[1-4] Poor outcomes in patients with acetabular fractures that are left untreated were substantiated by the seminal studies of Judet and Letournel.[5,6] These studies proposed and refined the radiographic method used to analyze acetabular fractures as well as the classification of acetabular fractures, both of which continue to be used.[5,6] The analysis and classification of acetabular fractures (**Figure 1**; **Table 1**) is based on three radiographic views, which are supplemented by two-dimensional CT scans (**Figures 2, 3, 4** and **5**). Simulated radiographs and three-dimensional images that are generated from two-dimensional CT scans have recently become readily available.[7-10] Despite these advances in imaging, the diagnosis and classification of acetabular fractures continue to be primarily determined by an analysis of three radiographic views

Dr. Moed or an immediate family member has received royalties from Biomet and serves as a board member, owner, officer, or committee member of AO North America and the AO Foundation. Dr. Kregor or an immediate family member is a member of a speakers' bureau or has made paid presentations on behalf of Medtronic and serves as a paid consultant to or is an employee of Acumed. Dr. Reilly or an immediate family member is a member of a speakers' bureau or has made paid presentations on behalf of Stryker and serves as a paid consultant to or is an employee of Stryker. Dr. Stover or an immediate family member is a member of a speakers' bureau or has made paid presentations on behalf of the AO Foundation and Stryker and has stock or stock options held in Radlink.

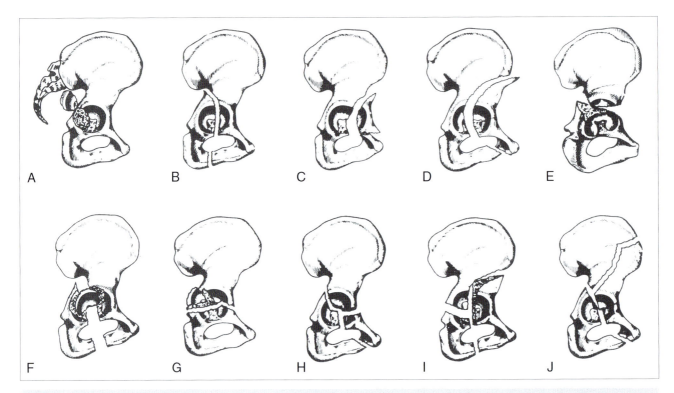

Figure 1 Schematic illustrations show the Letournel and Judet classification of acetabular fractures. **A,** Posterior wall fracture. **B,** Posterior column fracture. **C,** Anterior wall fracture. **D,** Anterior column fracture. **E,** Transverse fracture. **F,** Posterior wall and posterior column fracture. **G,** Transverse and posterior wall fracture. **H,** T-shaped fracture. **I,** Anterior column and posterior hemitransverse fracture. **J,** Both-column fracture. (Adapted from Matta JM, Merritt PO: Trauma: Pelvis and acetabulum, in Fitzgerald RH Jr, ed: *Orthopaedic Knowledge Update,* ed 2. Park Ridge, IL, American Academy of Orthopaedic Surgeons, 1987, pp 341-356.)

Table 1

Letournel and Judet Classification of Acetabular Fractures

Elementary Acetabular Fracture Types	Associated Acetabular Fracture Types
Posterior wall	Posterior column and posterior wall
Posterior column	Transverse and posterior wall
Anterior wall	T-shaped
Anterior column	Anterior column or wall with posterior hemitransverse
Transverse	Both-column

(actual radiographs or CT-generated radiographs) and two-dimensional CT scans.[9-11] The use of a standardized method for the analysis of imaging studies is helpful in the diagnosis and classification of acetabular fractures.[12,13]

Although the well-known protocols that were established by Letournel and Judet continue to be important guidelines for the management of acetabular fractures, alterations in the management of certain acetabular fracture types and several injury patterns have occurred. In addition, the demographics of the patients in whom acetabular fractures occur have changed. Furthermore, certain acetabular fracture types and several patient-related factors continue to pose management challenges for surgeons. Particular challenges in the management of acetabular fractures include fracture types that involve the posterior wall, fractures with associated damage of the surrounding soft-tissue envelope, acetabular fractures in patients with multiple injuries, and acetabular fractures in the geriatric population.

Acetabular Fracture Types That Involve the Posterior Wall

Acetabular fractures that involve the posterior wall are some of the most common types of acetabular fractures, accounting for approximately 50% of all acetabular fractures.[6,14] Isolated posterior wall acetabular fractures are

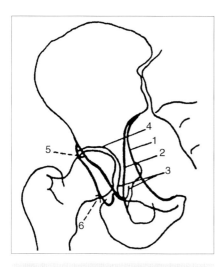

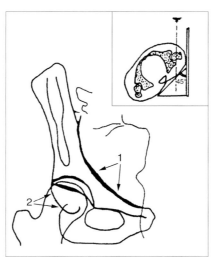

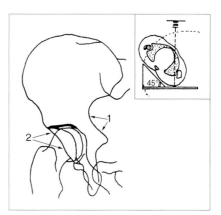

Figure 2 Schematic illustration of a hip shows the six basic acetabular landmarks observed on an AP radiograph: iliopectineal line (1), ilioischial line (2), radiographic U or teardrop (3), acetabular roof (4), anterior acetabular rim (5), and posterior acetabular rim (6). (Reproduced from Templeman DC, Olson S, Moed BR, Duwelius P, Matta JM: Surgical treatment of acetabular fractures. *Instr Course Lect* 1999;48:481-496.)

Figure 3 Schematic illustration of a hip shows the iliopectineal line (1) and the posterior acetabular rim (2) as observed on an obturator oblique radiograph. The obturator ring is observed en face. To obtain a properly oriented obturator oblique radiograph (inset), the patient should be rotated so that the tip of the coccyx lies just above the center of the ipsilateral femoral head. (Adapted from Templeman DC, Olson S, Moed BR, Duwelius P, Matta JM: Surgical treatment of acetabular fractures. *Instr Course Lect* 1999;48:481-496.)

Figure 4 Schematic illustration of a hip shows the posterior border of the innominate bone (1) and the anterior acetabular rim (2) as observed on an iliac oblique radiograph. The iliac wing is observed en face. The anterior acetabular rim can be best observed on an iliac oblique radiograph. To obtain an iliac oblique radiograph (inset), a patient should be rotated so that the tip of the coccyx lies just above the center of the contralateral femoral head. (Adapted from Templeman DC, Olson S, Moed BR, Duwelius P, Matta JM: Surgical treatment of acetabular fractures. *Instr Course Lect* 1999;48:481-496.)

the most common type of acetabular fracture, accounting for approximately one-fourth of all acetabular fractures.[6] Unfortunately, elementary posterior wall, associated posterior column and posterior wall, and associated transverse and posterior wall fractures have been reported to result in some of the worst clinical outcomes. Based on the modified Merle d'Aubigné and Postel clinical scoring system, which is used to evaluate pain, ambulation, and range of motion, more than 30% of elementary posterior wall acetabular fractures result in unsatisfactory clinical outcomes.[14-17] Only 5% of elementary transverse acetabular fractures result in unsatisfactory outcomes; however, 26% of transverse acetabular fractures result in unsatisfactory outcomes if they occur in association with a posterior wall

fracture. Similarly, only 9% of elementary posterior column fractures result in unsatisfactory outcomes; however, 53% of posterior column fractures result in unsatisfactory outcomes if the posterior wall is involved.[6] Therefore, acetabular fractures that involve the posterior wall, despite a relatively simple radiographic appearance, are a management challenge for surgeons.[6,18,19]

Mechanism of Injury and Fracture Patterns

Most acetabular fractures are sustained as a result of a motor vehicle accident or a similar high-energy mechanism of injury.[6,14,18,19] Acetabular fracture patterns depend on the location and the

direction of the applied force as well as the position of the hip at the time of impact.[6] Isolated posterior wall acetabular fractures result from a force that is applied to the flexed knee along the axis of the femoral shaft with the hip positioned in neutral to 25° of adduction.[6] Likewise, the posterior acetabular column becomes involved if the hip is positioned in 15° of abduction.[6] The associated transverse and posterior wall acetabular fracture results from a force that is applied to the greater trochanter along the axis of the femoral neck with the hip positioned in approximately 50° of internal rotation.[6] The degree of hip flexion at the time of impact determines the level of the posterior wall acetabular fracture.[6]

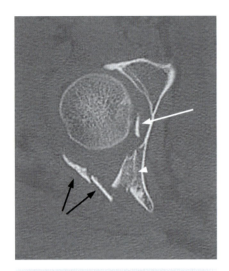

Figure 5 Axial CT scan of a section through an acetabulum demonstrates a posterior wall fracture (black arrows) with marginal impaction (white arrowhead). An intra-articular loose body (white arrow) is present between the femoral head and the acetabulum. (Copyright Berton R. Moed, MD, St. Louis, MO.)

Initial Management

Initial management of posterior wall acetabular fractures is extremely important. Therefore, identifying the injury and making the specific diagnosis early are critical.[18,20] Patients who have a fracture that involves the posterior wall of the acetabulum do not always report hip pain. Therefore, treating physicians must have a high level of suspicion for any lower extremity injury that may cause abnormal loading to the hip joint. Although the clinical findings may be obscure, the radiographic findings are straightforward. On an AP radiograph, the rim of the posterior wall approximates a straight line and is more vertical compared with the anterior wall. Any break or deficit in this line indicates fracture or displacement of the posterior rim of the posterior acetabulum (**Figure 6, A**). Signs of hip dislocation on an AP radiograph include a break

in the Shenton line, proximal migration of the lesser trochanter, a relatively smaller affected femoral head (caused by the femoral head being closer to the radiographic cassette), and a bony double-density observed above the femoral head. The bony double-density is the posterior acetabular wall fragment (**Figure 6, A**), which often is observed atop the dislocated femoral head and may appear similar to normal joint space, potentially resulting in a misdiagnosis. An obturator oblique radiograph is especially helpful in the diagnosis of a posterior wall acetabular fracture because it places the posterior wall almost perpendicular to the x-ray beam and minimizes the overlay of the anterior acetabular wall (**Figure 3**).

Dislocation of the femoral head occurs in more than 85% of patients who have a posterior wall fracture.[18] The failure to timely relocate the femoral head greatly increases the risk for osteonecrosis of the femoral head.[18] In 2002, Moed et al[18] reported that a delay in relocation of the femoral head of more than 12 hours was an independent risk factor for a poor clinical outcome. More recently, a meta-analysis that was conducted by Kellam and Ostrum[20] substantiated the findings reported by Moed et al[18] and indicated that they also apply to other acetabular fractures that involve a posterior dislocation of the femoral head. Therefore, urgent reduction of any associated hip dislocation is one of the most important interventions that a physician can perform in the treatment of patients who have an acetabular fracture that involves the posterior wall. Often, reduction of any associated hip dislocation can be performed in the emergency department with the use of adequate sedation and pain medication. Closed

reduction in the operating room with the use of general anesthesia is indicated if an initial attempt at closed reduction in the emergency department fails, if contraindications to the use of conscious sedation exist, or because of surgeon preference. Radiographs should be obtained immediately after reduction to confirm adequate reduction of the hip dislocation (**Figure 6, B**). Although a CT scan usually is not required to confirm a concentric hip reduction, it provides valuable additional information and, generally, is required to plan subsequent treatment. A dislocated hip that cannot be reduced via closed means requires urgent open reduction, which, usually, is followed by internal fixation of the acetabular fracture.

Video 1.1: Performance of the EUA. Berton R. Moed, MD (1 min)

Definitive Management

Acetabular fractures that have an incongruent or unstable relationship with the femoral head require open reduction and internal fixation (ORIF). Nonsurgical management can be considered for stable, concentrically reduced acetabular fractures. Acetabular roof arc angle measurements have been used to determine if the remaining intact acetabulum is sufficient to maintain a stable and congruent relationship with the femoral head (**Figure 7**). Vrahas et al[21] reported that acetabular fractures with a medial roof arc angle of more than 45°, an anterior roof arc angle of more than 25°, and a posterior roof arc angle of more than 70° have sufficient intact acetabulum for nonsurgical management. However, in a subsequent biomechanical study, Matityahu et al[22] suggested that, with the acetabulum

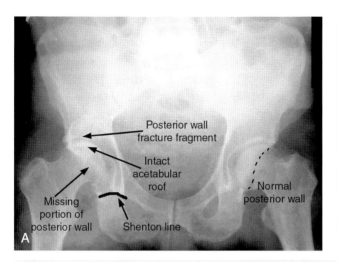
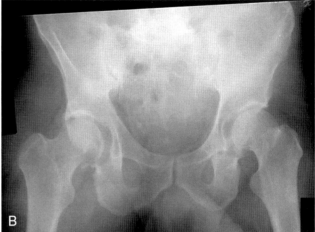

Figure 6 AP radiographs of a pelvis demonstrate initial management of an acetabular fracture with an associated hip dislocation. **A,** Radiograph demonstrates a dislocated right hip and a posterior wall acetabular fracture. **B,** Radiograph demonstrates adequate reduction of the hip dislocation. (Copyright Berton R. Moed, MD, St. Louis, MO.)

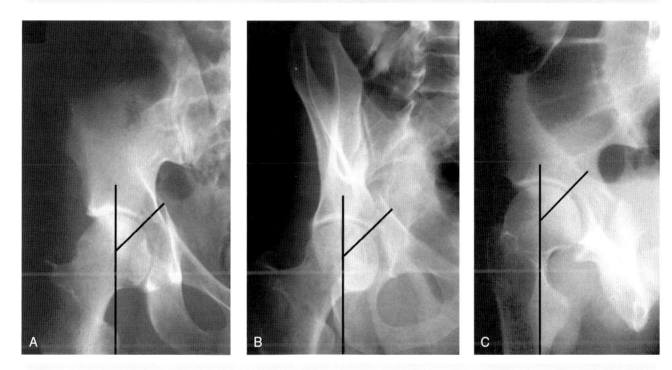

Figure 7 AP (**A**), obturator oblique (**B**), and iliac oblique (**C**) radiographs of a hip with a transverse acetabular fracture demonstrate an acetabular roof arc angle of approximately 50° (as indicated by the black lines) on each view. (Copyright Berton R. Moed, MD, St. Louis, MO.)

subjected to sit-to-stand loading rather than single-leg-stance loading, the critical angles are significantly higher, requiring a medial roof arc angle of 90.9°, an anterior roof arc angle of 67.3°, and a posterior roof arc angle of 101.4° to have sufficient intact acetabulum for nonsurgical management. Regardless, these roof arc angle measurements, which may be helpful to assess the stability of the fractured columns of the acetabulum, are unreliable if a posterior wall fracture is present.[21,23] In addition, although certain risk factors for hip instability, such as a history of associated hip dislocation at the time of initial injury and a fracture that extends within 5 mm of the acetabular dome,[24] have been reported in patients who have a posterior wall acetabular fracture, none have been reported to be independent

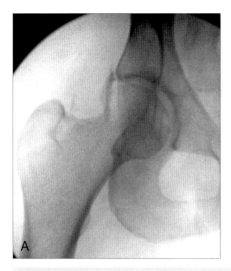
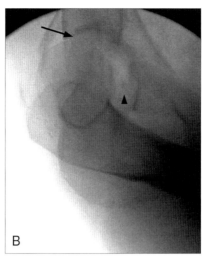

Figure 8 Fluoroscopic images of the hip of a patient taken during an examination that was performed with the use of general anesthesia show a small posterior wall acetabular fracture. **A,** Obturator oblique fluoroscopic image taken with the hip in neutral rotation and flexed to approximately 90° shows a located and congruent hip joint. **B,** Obturator oblique fluoroscopic image subsequently taken with the hip in neutral rotation and flexed to approximately 90° with an axial load applied shows gross subluxation with loss of hip joint parallelism and joint congruity (arrow) as well as gross enlargement of the medial clear space (arrowhead). (Reproduced with permission from Moed BR, Ajibade DA, Israel H: Computed tomography as a predictor of hip stability status in posterior wall fractures of the acetabulum. *J Orthop Trauma* 2009;23[1]:7-15.)

or reliable indicators (Jay Patel, MD, St. Louis, MO, and Berton R. Moed, MD, St. Louis, MO, unpublished data, 2016). Furthermore, a small-sized posterior wall fracture fragment does not reliably indicate a stable hip joint.[24,25] Reagan and Moed[25] reported that hip joint instability may be present even in patients who have posterior wall acetabular fractures that involve less than 20% of the joint surface; this finding was later confirmed by Firoozabadi et al.[24] Currently, a dynamic stress fluoroscopic examination that is performed with the use of general anesthesia (EUA) is the only reliable method to determine the stability of the hip joint in patients who have a posterior wall fracture.[24-26]

Surgeons who wish to measure the size of a posterior acetabular wall fragment should use the method described by Moed et al.[24,27] In general, posterior wall acetabular fractures that involve more than 50% of the articular surface are considered unstable and require ORIF. Fractures that involve less than 50% of the articular surface but have a congruent relationship between the femoral head and the acetabulum should be further evaluated via an EUA to determine the stability of the hip joint. This EUA can be quickly performed using the method that was described by Moed et al[27] and Grimshaw and Moed.[26] Posterior subluxation of the femoral head, which is observed as widening of the medial clear space or loss of joint parallelism, indicates dynamic hip instability and should be managed via ORIF (**Figure 8**). Nonsurgical treatment can be considered in patients with maintained joint

congruity.[26,28] Good to excellent mid-term outcomes (minimum follow-up of 2 years) have been reported in patients who undergo EUA-directed nonsurgical management of isolated posterior wall fractures.[26,28]

Numerous risk factors have been proposed for the poor outcomes reported in patients with a posterior wall or a posterior wall–associated acetabular fracture. These risk factors include extensive wall comminution, marginal impaction, injury to the femoral head articular surface, osteonecrosis of the femoral head, delay in time to reduction of an associated dislocation of the femoral head, and older age of the patient.[18,23] Total hip arthroplasty (THA) has been suggested as a better initial treatment option for high-risk patients compared with ORIF; a recently proposed nomogram (**Figure 9**), which prognosticates reconstructive hip surgery within 2 years after ORIF, attempted to better define this high-risk patient group.[29] Although the nomogram proposed by Tannast et al[29] may help predict the clinical outcome of patients with other types of acetabular fractures, it does not include sufficient information to predict the clinical outcome of patients with posterior wall fractures who undergo ORIF or to determine the appropriate surgical management for patients who have posterior wall fractures.[30] The quality of acetabular fracture reduction has consistently been reported to be an important factor with regard to clinical outcomes.[18,19,23] Therefore, the two most important interventions that the treating physician can perform to achieve the best possible clinical outcome are urgent reduction of any associated hip dislocation within 12 hours of injury and anatomic reduction of the acetabular fracture.

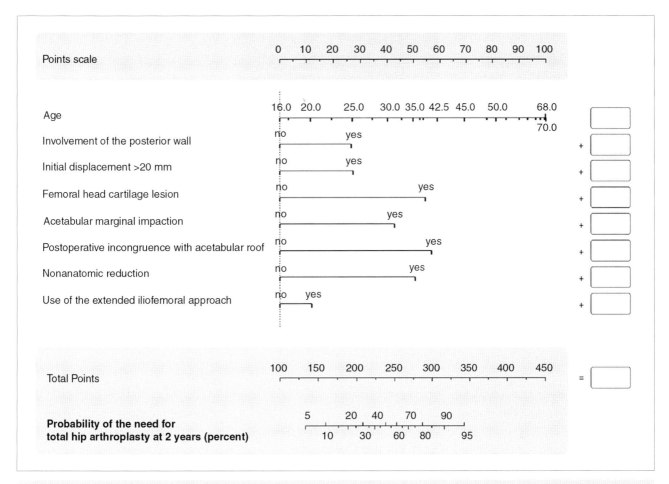

Figure 9   Nomogram proposed by Tannast et al,[29] which is used to predict the early need for total hip arthroplasty (or hip arthrodesis) within 2 years after open reduction and internal fixation (ORIF) of an acetabular fracture. To use the nomogram, the surgeon draws a straight line from the appropriate age of the patient on the age scale to the points scale; this determines how many points the patient receives based on his or her age. This process is repeated for each predictor variable. The surgeon then adds the points for the predictor variables and locates this sum total on the total points scale. The surgeon then draws a straight line from this location on the total points scale to the probability scale; this determines the predicted probability of the need for total hip arthroplasty within 2 years after ORIF of an acetabular fracture. (Adapted with permission from Tannast M, Najibi S, Matta JM: Two to twenty-year survivorship of the hip in 810 patients with operatively treated acetabular fractures. *J Bone Joint Surg Am* 2012;94[17]:1559-1567.)

In the presence of all the reported risk factors (especially fracture comminution and marginal impaction), however, achieving anatomic reduction is not easy. Often, initial critical errors are made preoperatively by not appreciating the complexity of the fracture or the need to carefully address each fracture component. Excellent acetabular fracture reduction can be achieved with careful attention to detail and the use of standard fixation techniques. After full exposure of the acetabular fracture is attained via an appropriate standard surgical approach (eg, the Kocher-Langenbeck approach, the modified Gibson approach, or a trochanteric flip osteotomy), the femoral head is distracted, the hip joint is cleared of debris, and the acetabular fracture is visually assessed (**Figure 10, A**). Intra-articular free fragments are removed from the joint and cleared of debris. If sufficient cancellous bone remains attached to the intra-articular free fragments and their articular surface is intact, these intra-articular free fragments should be retained for reinsertion in their anatomic position later in the procedure. All of the fracture margins are cleared of debris. After anatomic reduction and initial fixation (with the use of lag screws or plates, as required) of any associated acetabular column fractures, all of the marginally impacted areas are elevated into their anatomic position. The femoral head,

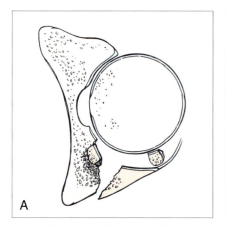 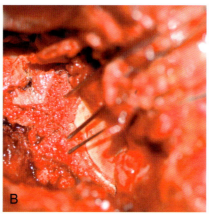 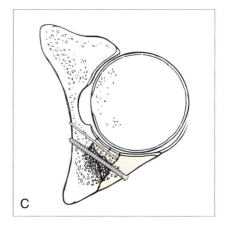

Figure 10 Images demonstrate anatomic reduction and fixation of a comminuted posterior wall acetabular fracture. **A,** Cross-sectional illustration of an acetabulum shows a posterior wall fracture with an area of marginal impaction and an osteochondral free fragment. **B,** Intraoperative photograph of a comminuted posterior wall fracture similar to that illustrated in panel **A** taken after elevation and temporary Kirschner wire fixation of the impacted intra-articular fragments shows that the residual underlying cancellous bone defect has been filled with freeze-dried cancellous allograft bone. **C,** Cross-sectional illustration of the comminuted posterior wall fracture illustrated in panel **A** shows the two-level construct method for fixation. (Copyright Berton R. Moed, MD, St. Louis, MO.)

which is no longer held in a distracted position, can be used as a template for this reduction. These reduced marginally impacted areas are temporarily fixed with the use of smooth Kirschner wires (typically, 1.6 mm), and the residual underlying cancellous bone defect is filled (typically with freeze-dried cancellous allograft bone; **Figure 10, B**). Any osteochondral free fragments are replaced sequentially and temporarily fixed in a similar fashion. For permanent fixation, the Kirschner wires are exchanged for subchondral 2.0-mm miniscrews or 1.5-mm bioabsorbable pegs. This method of fragment stabilization is more dependable compared with relying on fracture interdigitation alone.[31] The overlying posterior acetabular wall fragments are then reduced and fixed with the use of a standard lag screw technique (**Figure 10, C**). The entire acetabular fracture is buttressed and neutralized with the use of well-described fixation constructs (**Figure 11**). Good to excellent clinical results have been reported in more than 88% of patients who undergo this two-level method of posterior wall acetabular fracture fixation.[18,19,31]

Acetabular Fractures With Soft-Tissue Concerns

As previously discussed, the assessment of a patient with an acetabular fracture includes an examination of three radiographic views and a two-dimensional CT scan. A concurrent and complete evaluation of a patient's associated injuries and comorbidities also is extremely important. The importance of a careful evaluation of the surrounding soft tissues cannot be overestimated because the status of the soft tissues can alter the surgical approach and tactic, affect the rate of complications, and influence overall patient outcomes.[32] Therefore, injury to the surrounding soft-tissue envelope, injury to the soft tissues in the pelvic ring, and preexisting obesity should be considered in the discussion of treatment options and expected outcomes with patients who have acetabular fractures.

Obesity

In the United States, more than 35% of adults are obese, which is defined as a body mass index greater than 30 kg/m^2.[33] Adequate-quality radiographs may be difficult to obtain in patients with obesity. CT-generated simulated plain radiographs may aid surgeons in obtaining images that allow for adequate evaluation of an acetabular fracture in these patients.[10] CT-generated radiographs provide surgeons with the same information as high-quality plain radiographs with regard to the classification of acetabular fractures and eliminate the need for patient repositioning or repeat radiographs (**Figure 12**). Obesity has been reported to increase surgical times and associated estimated blood loss.[34,35] Furthermore, patients with an acetabular fracture who have a body mass index greater than 30 kg/m^2 have an increased risk for surgical site infection.[34,35] In addition, fracture reduction is more difficult to achieve in patients with obesity.[36] Moreover, despite the

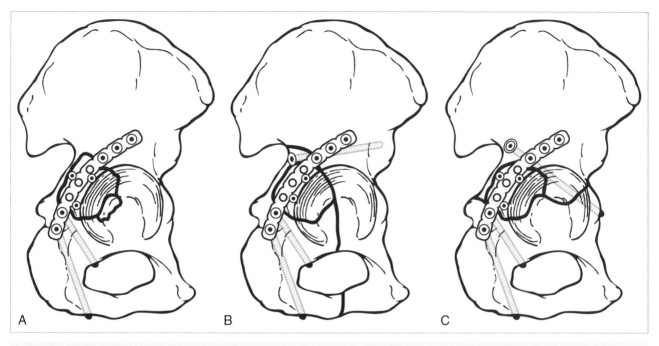

Figure 11   Illustrations of an innominate bone show the typical completed fixation constructs for an elementary posterior wall acetabular fracture (**A**), an associated posterior wall and posterior column acetabular fracture (**B**), and an associated transverse and posterior wall acetabular fracture (**C**). (Copyright Berton R. Moed, MD, St. Louis, MO.)

use of postoperative prophylactic measures, patients with obesity have a higher risk for extensive heterotopic bone formation.[37] Because of these increased surgical risks, some studies have advocated for less-invasive procedures to stabilize displaced acetabular fractures in patients with obesity;[38] however, measures can be taken to minimize some of these surgical risks in patients with obesity.

Improving antibiotic availability to the local soft tissues, which may help decrease the risk for wound complications, can be achieved via weight-based antibiotic dosing.[39] Currently, the local administration of antibiotics is being evaluated and has been reported to be effective in patients who undergo obesity surgery[40] as well as some orthopaedic procedures.[41,42] Maintenance of adequate postoperative patient oxygenation and nutrition (providing supplements as required) may be important,

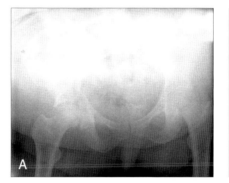
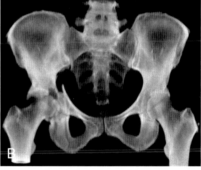

Figure 12   AP radiograph (**A**) and CT-generated AP radiograph (**B**) of the pelvis of a patient with a body mass index of 35 kg/m² demonstrate an acetabular fracture. (Reproduced with permission from Sinatra PM, Moed BR: CT-generated radiographs in obese patients with acetabular fractures: Can they be used in lieu of plain radiographs? *Clin Orthop Relat Res* 2014;472(11):3362-3369.)

especially in patients with obesity.[43] A mean perioperative blood glucose level greater than 220 mg/dL is associated with an increased risk for infection in patients with orthopaedic trauma and no known history of diabetes mellitus.[44] Therefore, careful attention to a

patient's blood glucose level may lessen the risk for infection in the postoperative period. In addition, postoperative incisional negative pressure therapy via a wound vacuum system may help decrease the risk for surgical site infection.[45]

Video 1.2: Ballottable Fluid Wave. Berton R. Moed, MD; Michael D. Stover, MD (10 sec)

Video 1.3: Percutaneous Débridement. Berton R. Moed, MD; Michael D. Stover, MD (23 sec)

Abrasions and Contusions

Ipsilateral abrasions and contusions to the lateral thigh or buttock region commonly occur in patients who have acetabular fractures. As soon as 6 hours postinjury, skin abrasions cannot be decontaminated with the use of routine surgical preparations.[46] Therefore, an abrasion or contusion in the area of the planned skin incision is an indication for a surgeon to consider an alteration in the surgical plan. Modification of the skin incision or alteration of the entire surgical approach may be prudent to decrease the risk for wound contamination.[47] The more severe, closed soft-tissue degloving injuries, which were first described in the mid-1800s by Morel-Lavallée,[48] also commonly occur in the lateral thigh and hip region in patients who have acetabular fractures. The area of degloving can occur over the trunk, buttock, or thighs.[49] Letournel and Judet[6] referred to these degloving injuries over the region of the greater trochanter as Morel-Lavallée lesions.

Morel-Lavallée lesions are caused by a combination of shear and compression forces, which result in traumatic separation of the skin and subcutaneous tissues from the underlying, unyielding fascia.[50] This separation disrupts the segmental vessels and lymphatics as they perforate the fascia and creates a potential space that subsequently fills with blood, serosanguineous fluid, and necrotic fat, which further jeopardizes the vascular supply to the overlying contused skin.[50] Morel-Lavallée lesions can evolve, and, initially, the overlying soft tissue may appear uninjured. Therefore, many Morel-Lavallée lesions are initially missed or disregarded.[51] The diagnosis of Morel-Lavallée lesions is more of a challenge in patients with a body mass index greater than 30 kg/m². Nickerson et al[52] did not report a statistically significant association between Morel-Lavallée lesions and increased body mass index; however, Carlson et al[53] reported that 18 of 22 patients who were admitted or referred to a trauma center for the management of Morel-Lavallée lesions were overweight or obese.

Regardless, the early diagnosis of Morel-Lavallée lesions is a key factor with regard to their management.[49,54] Despite otherwise minimal initial clinical findings, the diagnosis of Morel-Lavallée lesions often can be made via the observation of a fluid wave in the cavity that is formed by a collection of hematoma or serosanguineous fluid superficial to the fascia. Evaluation with the use of ultrasonography, CT, and MRI usually is diagnostic. Untreated Morel-Lavallée lesions or Morel-Lavallée lesions that result from an injury with a predominant crush component may involve the overlying skin. In a study of 87 Morel-Lavallée lesions, Nickerson et al[52] reported that eight of the lesions (9%) required débridement for skin involvement. Despite the presence of intact overlying skin, a bacterial colonization rate as high as 46% has been reported in patients who have Morel-Lavallée lesions, which is extremely problematic for both patients and surgeons.[49]

Multiple options have been proposed for the management of Morel-Lavallée lesions. In 1997, Hak et al[49] recommended open irrigation and débridement of the degloved areas, obtaining tissue cultures, open packing of the wound, and delayed primary or secondary wound closure. The authors delayed ORIF of acetabular fractures if a patient's overlying soft tissue was abraded or if evidence of skin necrosis was present. Otherwise, ORIF of acetabular fractures and Morel-Lavallée lesion débridement were performed concurrently. In their study of 24 patients with Morel-Lavallée lesions, Hak et al[49] reported positive cultures in 11 of the patients (46%) and a deep infection in three of the patients (13%). The authors recommended against the percutaneous management of Morel-Lavallée lesions; however, 23 of the 24 patients were not treated until 4 days postinjury, and most of the patients did not undergo débridement until 1 week or more postinjury.

In 2006, Tseng and Tornetta[54] described a percutaneous débridement and irrigation technique for the management of Morel-Lavallée lesions in 19 patients. For this technique, small incisions are made at the proximal and distal extent of a Morel-Lavallée lesion, and the fluid is evacuated. Through these small incisions, a coarse, plastic, disposable canal brush is used to débride the areas of necrotic fat. Next, the area is irrigated with the use of pulsed lavage. The incisions are closed over deep drains, which are maintained until drainage is less than 30 mL in 24 hours (**Figure 13**). Acetabular fracture fixation is delayed until at least 24 hours after drain removal. In three

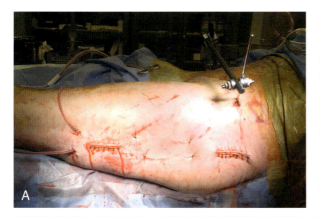 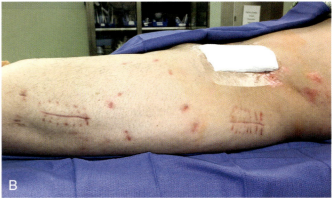

Figure 13 Photographs of the hip of a patient who underwent percutaneous débridement and irrigation for the management of Morel-Lavallée lesions. **A,** Intraoperative photograph taken immediately after surgery shows that the surgical wounds were closed over drains, and that four fascial-to-skin sutures were placed to eliminate dead space. **B,** Clinical photograph taken 6 weeks postoperatively shows that the wounds have healed and the external fixator has been removed. (Copyright Michael D. Stover, MD, Chicago, IL, and Berton R. Moed, MD, St. Louis, MO.)

of the six patients who underwent surgical acetabular fracture fixation, Tseng and Tornetta[54] performed ORIF via an incision through the degloving injury. One of these three patients had wound drainage complications that required a return to the operating room. The authors reported bacterial growth in 3 of the 16 Morel-Lavallée lesions (19%) in which cultures were obtained; however, no infections occurred. Of critical importance in this study, all of the patients were treated within 3 days postinjury, and none of the patients had full-thickness skin lesions.

In 2007, Carlson et al[53] described a technique in which any required definitive ORIF was performed immediately after open débridement and irrigation of a Morel-Lavallée lesion. The Morel-Lavallée lesion cavity is closed with the use of facial-to-dermal sutures or sutures that are placed from the fascia through the skin and tied over bolsters. In their series of 22 patients who had different types of injuries, Carlson et al[53] used this technique in three of five patients during the initial surgical approach to the acetabular fracture.

The authors reported no deep infections postoperatively.

Another technique for the management of Morel-Lavallée lesions has recently been described. This technique involves ORIF and closure of the fascia, after which negative pressure therapy (ie, vacuum sealing) is used on the cutaneous tissues until drainage has been documented as less than 20 mL per day.[55,56] Delayed primary wound closure or skin grafting is then performed. In these two small series,[55,56] no deep infections were reported. Recent studies have proposed algorithms that may aid in the management of Morel-Lavallée lesions (**Figure 14**);[52,57,58] however, a high index of suspicion and early intervention are the most important factors in the management of Morel-Lavallée lesions. Regardless, patients with these lesions may report body contour abnormalities or other symptoms many years postinjury.

Open Acetabular Fractures
Open acetabular fractures are very rare. In some case studies, open acetabular fractures were managed with

débridement, reduction, fixation, and wound closure;[59] however, the role of repeat débridement after internal fixation is uncertain. In general, and similar to the recommendations for the management of other intra-articular fractures, the management of open acetabular fractures should be based on the extent of soft-tissue injury, the amount of wound contamination, and the presence of any associated organ injuries.

Nerve Injury
Because of the proximity of the sciatic nerve to the posterior pelvic structures, peripheral nerve injuries frequently are associated with acetabular fractures. In a review of the German Pelvic Trauma Registry records of 2,073 patients with acetabular fractures, Lehmann et al[60] reported that 4% of the patients had a peripheral neurologic deficit at the time of hospital admission. The authors reported that peripheral neurologic deficits were more common in patients who had acetabular fractures that involved the posterior wall (ie, posterior wall, posterior column and posterior wall,

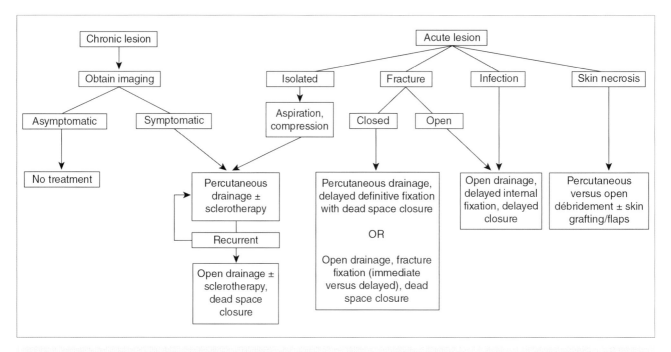

Figure 14 Example of an algorithm that shows the decision-making process for the management of Morel-Lavallée lesions. (Adapted with permission from Greenhill D, Haydel C, Rehman S: Management of the Morel-Lavallée lesion. *Orthop Clin North Am* 2016;47[1]:115-125.)

and transverse and posterior wall). The authors reported that iatrogenic neurologic deficits were more common in patients who underwent surgical treatment via the Kocher-Langenbeck approach. In addition, 7% of the patients had a neurologic deficit at the time of hospital discharge.

Bogdan et al[61] reviewed 137 patients from eight centers who had an acetabular fracture and a peripheral nerve injury. The most common acetabular fracture types were transverse and posterior wall, posterior wall, and both-column. The authors reported nerve injuries based on the nerve root levels that were involved rather than by the specific peripheral nerve. The L5 nerve root level was the most common nerve root level involved. Overall, deficits were identified preoperatively in 57% of the patients, as iatrogenic in 19% of the patients, and postoperatively with no preoperative examination in

24% of the patients. Overall, only 29% of the patients had a full recovery, 37% of the patients had a partial recovery, and 34% of the patients had no recovery (no return of function). No return of function was reported in 43% of the patients with S1 neurologic injuries and 29% of the patients with L5 neurologic injuries. No return of function was reported in 55% of the patients who had iatrogenic neurologic injuries.

Arterial Injury

Historically, injury to or embolization of the superior gluteal artery was believed to be a contraindication to the surgical management of acetabular fractures via an extended approach, such as the extended iliofemoral approach.[62] A further study showed that complete necrosis of the abductors does not occur in patients with superior gluteal artery disruption who undergo surgical treatment for acetabular fractures via the

extended iliofemoral approach;[63] however, an associated decrease in muscle mass and histologic evidence of muscle necrosis have been reported.[63] The extended iliofemoral approach has been reported to be safe and effective.[64,65] Therefore, this approach can be used for acetabular fracture reduction, if required, in patients with a superior gluteal artery injury.

Acetabular Fractures in Patients With Multiple Injuries

As previously discussed, acetabular fractures, particularly those that occur in younger patients, frequently result from high-energy trauma.[6,14,18,19] Therefore, these fractures are commonly encountered in the treatment of patients who have multiple injuries. The definitive management of an acetabular fracture rarely is a priority in the treatment of patients who have multiple injuries or patients with

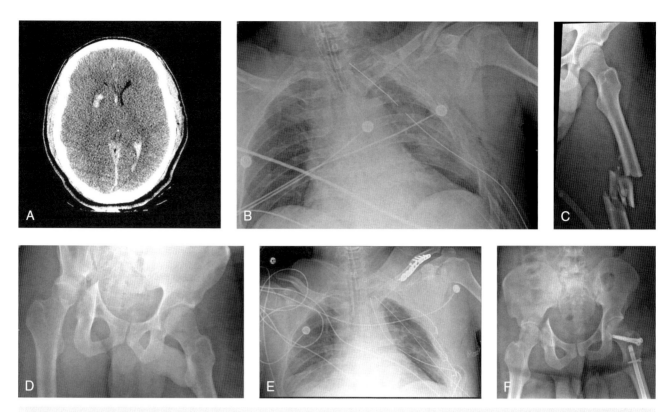

Figure 15   Images of a 28-year-old man who fell from scaffolding and sustained severe injuries. **A,** Axial CT scan of the patient's head demonstrates a severe closed head injury. **B,** AP radiograph of the patient's chest demonstrates a flail chest as well as ipsilateral scapular and clavicular fractures. **C,** AP radiograph of the patient's hip and proximal femur demonstrates a comminuted femoral shaft fracture. **D,** AP radiograph of the patient's pelvis demonstrates a pelvic ring disruption, an associated transverse and posterior wall acetabular fracture, and an ipsilateral hip dislocation. The patient emergently underwent a craniectomy and partial temporal lobectomy, external fixation of the femur, and closed reduction of the hip. **E,** AP radiograph of the patient's chest taken 2 days postinjury and after the flail chest was surgically stabilized because the patient's ventilatory status continued to worsen and impending acute respiratory distress syndrome was suspected. Clavicular fracture fixation also was performed because gross motion was noted during fixation of the ribs. Six days postinjury, the patient's pulmonary function improved sufficiently to allow for additional surgical intervention. **F,** AP radiograph of the patient's pelvis taken after intramedullary nailing of the femur and fixation of a nondisplaced basilar neck fracture that was discovered intraoperatively. The patient's pulmonary function deteriorated postoperatively. Note that the patient's right hip remains located.

hemodynamic instability. Dissimilar to pelvic ring injuries, acetabular fractures usually are not the cause of acute traumatic hemodynamic instability;[66,67] however, certain displaced acetabular fractures are more frequently associated with arterial lacerations that require prompt management. Acetabular fractures with substantial displacement of the superior portion of the greater sciatic notch may result in superior gluteal artery injury.[65] Similarly, acetabular fractures with displacement of the

obturator canal may result in obturator artery injury.[68]

Associated Displaced Fractures or Dislocations of the Pelvic Ring

Acetabular fractures may occur in combination with displaced fractures or dislocations of the pelvic ring. Patients in whom this combination of injuries occur have sustained high-energy trauma, have a greater likelihood of multisystem injury, have a higher Injury Severity

Score, have greater blood transfusion requirements, and present with a lower blood pressure.[66,69-71] In a recent review of 40 patients who had acetabular fractures in combination with pelvic ring disruptions, Osgood et al[70] reported that the most common type of pelvic ring disruptions were anteroposterior compression injuries (**Figure 15, A** through **H**) followed by those that were caused by a lateral compression force vector. The acetabular fracture component of this injury combination is commonly a

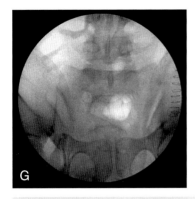
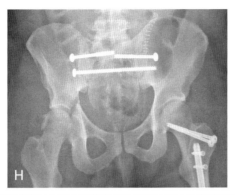
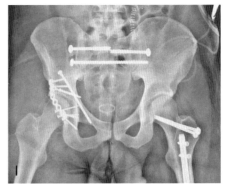

Figure 15 (*continued*)   **G,** AP fluoroscopic image of the patient's pelvis taken during an intraoperative examination performed 13 days postinjury, at which time the patient's respiratory function had improved sufficiently to allow for additional surgical intervention, shows bilateral sacroiliac joint injuries. **H,** AP radiograph of the patient's pelvis taken 13 days postinjury demonstrates successful open reduction of the right sacroiliac joint, closed reduction of the left sacroiliac joint, and fixation with the use of iliosacral and transsacral screws. Note the indirect reduction of the transverse acetabular fracture, which was achieved via reduction of the sacroiliac joint dislocations. **I,** AP radiograph of the patient's pelvis taken after definitive acetabular fixation, which was delayed until 24 days postinjury because of aspiration pneumonia with leukocytosis and a fever, demonstrates anatomic reduction of the fracture. Because of the chronicity of the acetabular fracture, sequential anterior and posterior surgical approaches were used. A supine intrapelvic (Stoppa) approach was used to allow for débridement of callus formation anteriorly, after which a prone Kocher-Langenbeck approach was used to allow for débridement of callus formation posteriorly and to accomplish reduction and fixation of the acetabular fracture.

transverse type.[70,71] Stabilization of the pelvic ring with the use of antishock sheets or a pelvic binder may aid in initial hemodynamic management;[69-71] however, these circumferential wraps may cause increased malreduction of the associated acetabular fracture.[69] In addition, external fixation of the pelvis in an area of a subsequent surgical approach to the acetabulum may increase a patient's risk for infection.[69] Skeletal traction is an important adjunctive treatment because it may improve bony pelvic and acetabular alignment. Often, angiography is used in patients with multiple injuries who are hemodynamically unstable. However, the use of angiography with embolization is not free of potential complications; it has been shown to be an independent risk factor for deep infection after acetabular fracture.[72,73] Regardless, diagnostic angiography and possible embolization are indicated in patients who have persistent hemodynamic instability without an identifiable source of hemorrhage. In the definitive surgical treatment of patients who have acetabular fractures in combination with pelvic ring disruptions, optimal reduction of an acetabular fracture requires the accurate reduction of the posterior pelvic ring injury (**Figure 15, G** and **H**).[6,70]

Associated Hip Dislocations

As previously discussed, a hip dislocation that occurs in combination with an acetabular fracture requires urgent management, even in patients who have multiple injuries.[18,20] In general, surgeons believe that the expeditious reduction of a femoral head protects articular cartilage from ongoing damage that is caused by wear against the bony surface of an acetabular fracture. Expeditious reduction also eliminates the risk for sciatic nerve palsy that may be caused by direct pressure of a dislocated femoral head. Usually, closed reduction of a hip that is performed with the use of conscious sedation or general anesthesia is successful[18,19] (**Figure 15, A** through **D** and **Figure 15, F**). Unsuccessful closed reduction is an indication for urgent open reduction of the hip;[74] however, the decision to proceed with open reduction depends on a patient's resuscitation status, a surgeon's familiarity with acetabular fracture surgery and surgical approaches to the acetabulum, and the anticipated risk associated with delayed reduction. Reduction of a hip dislocation is extremely unlikely with the use of skeletal traction alone, and skeletal traction alone should not be used in lieu of closed or open reduction; however, traction often is applied and is effective to maintain the position of the femoral head after successful closed reduction (**Figure 15, F**).

Associated Long-Bone Fractures

Long-bone fractures commonly occur in combination with acetabular fractures.[74] Typically, long-bone fractures take precedence in patients who have multisystem injuries (**Figure 15, A** through **F**), and the definitive management of an acetabular fracture is performed after the patient is metabolically stable. If possible, damage-control limb surgery should avoid interfering with future planned surgical approaches to the acetabulum. Diaphyseal femur fractures are well suited for external fixation or retrograde nailing, both of which avoid compromising definitive anterior or posterior approaches to the acetabulum. If doubt exists with regard to whether definitive fixation of an associated lower limb injury may interfere with future surgical approaches to the acetabulum, temporary external fixation should be considered. Temporary external fixation is especially appealing if definitive long-bone surgery can easily be accomplished at the time of definitive surgical acetabular fracture fixation.

Surgeons who will manage all of a patient's orthopaedic injuries should carefully consider the order in which the fractures are addressed. For example, a diaphyseal femur fracture in association with a widely displaced transverse fracture may be exceedingly difficult to manage with the use of an antegrade intramedullary nail because the appropriate starting point may be inaccessible as a result of medial subluxation of the femoral head. In patients who have a hip joint that is very unstable, retrograde nailing may cause additional damage to the articular cartilage of the femoral head if the hip repeatedly subluxates during the nailing process. In this circumstance, provisional stabilization of the femur with the use of an external fixator followed by reduction and fixation of the acetabulum may be

preferred before definitive fixation of the femoral shaft. Rarely, surgeons may find it advantageous to reduce and fix a transverse acetabular fracture first and then stabilize the femoral fracture with the use of an antegrade nail via the same posterior surgical approach.

Definitive Management of Acetabular Fractures in Patients With Multiple Injuries

The optimal timing for the definitive management of an acetabular fracture is controversial. Recent studies have reported improved acetabular fracture reduction quality and improved outcomes in patients definitively treated within 48 hours postinjury.[75,76] Unfortunately, this often is not feasible in patients who have multiple injuries. Head, chest, or abdominal injuries may preclude early definitive acetabular fracture management. Staged injury management is typical, and definitive acetabular fracture management often must be delayed until a patient is medically optimized (**Figure 15**). Trauma system modifications that allow patients who have multiple injuries to be taken directly to a level I trauma center as well as the standardization of the clearance protocols at trauma centers that govern the timing of acetabular fracture management have been reported to improve patient outcomes.[77,78]

Acetabular Fractures in the Geriatric Population

The United States has a growing but aging population.[79] As of 2013, 44.7 million individuals in the United States were at least age 65 years, which is an increase of 8.8 million individuals (24.7%) since 2003 and represents 14.1% of the total US population or approximately one in every seven Americans.[80]

Elderly individuals are expected to represent approximately 22% of the US population by 2040.[80] Given this expected increase in the number of elderly individuals, an increase in the number of fractures in elderly patients also is expected. Similar to other osteoporotic fractures in this age group, the number of acetabular fractures in elderly individuals also is increasing.[81-85] Ferguson et al[85] reported a 2.4-fold increase in the number of acetabular fractures that occurred in patients older than 60 years in a comparison of the first half and second half of the time period between 1980 and 2007.

Mechanism of Injury and Fracture Patterns

Ferguson et al[85] reported that 50% of the acetabular fractures that occurred between 1980 and 2007 in patients older than 60 years were caused by simple falls.[85] According to the Letournel and Judet classification of acetabular fractures (**Table 1**), the predominant fracture pattern that results from a low-energy mechanism type of injury such as this is an anterior column, an anterior column or wall with posterior hemitransverse, or a both-column acetabular fracture.[6,81,82,85,86] In a recent meta-analysis of 15 studies that included 414 patients older than 55 years with an acetabular fracture, Daurka et al[82] reported that 11.4% of the patients had an anterior column acetabular fracture, 19.4% of the patients had an anterior column or wall with a posterior hemitransverse acetabular fracture, and 23% of the patients had a both-column acetabular fracture. Acetabular fractures that result from a high-energy mechanism of injury, such as a motor vehicle accident, also occur in elderly patients.[85] Any fracture pattern is possible in elderly patients who sustain an acetabular fracture as a result of a high-energy mechanism of injury. Therefore, in the meta-analysis previously discussed, Daurka et al[82] unsurprisingly reported that 11.4% of the patients had a transverse acetabular fracture, 10.9% of the patients had a T-shaped acetabular fracture, 8% of the patients had an associated transverse and posterior wall acetabular fracture, and 8.2% of the patients had an elementary posterior wall acetabular fracture.

Treatment

The primary goals in the treatment of an elderly patient who has an acetabular fracture are preservation of life and early ambulation or mobilization without excessive dependence on pain medication.[81-83,87-91] These goals are no different from those of an elderly patient who has a hip fracture (ie, intertrochanteric or femoral neck).[92-97] Often, elderly patients are frail and have cardiac and pulmonary issues; therefore, considerable blood loss and fluid shifts are not well tolerated. Acetabular fractures in elderly patients are associated with additional challenges, including underlying osteoporosis, complex fracture patterns, fracture comminution, impaction fracture of the weight-bearing acetabular articular dome, fracture of the acetabular quadrilateral surface, and previous surgery (eg, vascular bypass or herniorrhaphy) in the area of the planned surgical appoach.[6,14,29,81-83,88-91,98,99] A secondary goal is maintenance of the native hip socket; however, in a small percentage of patients, early or delayed THA is the only viable option.

Letournel and Judet[6] highlighted that articular surface impaction may be present in patients who have

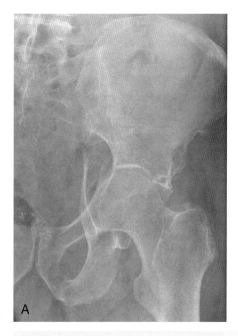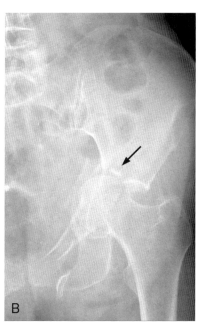

Figure 16   **A,** AP radiograph of the hip of a 73-year-old man who misstepped as he was descending stairs demonstrates a typical anterior column acetabular fracture. Note that the femoral head is medial and superior. The external rotation of the anterior column and the internal rotation of the quadrilateral surface allow the femoral head to move in this direction. **B,** AP radiograph of the hip of an 82-year-old man who sustained a left anterior column acetabular fracture after a fall demonstrates an example of a true gull sign, which is impaction of the superomedial aspect of the acetabular articular dome (arrow).

anterior-type acetabular fractures (ie, anterior column, anterior column or wall with posterior hemitransverse, and both-column acetabular fractures). The gull sign is a true separation and impaction of the superomedial aspect of the acetabular articular dome and is a predictor of poor maintenance of the native hip socket.[90] The gull sign should be differentiated from a simple translation of the articular surface with displacement of the anterior acetabular column (**Figure 16**). Other poor prognostic factors for maintenance of the native hip socket after acetabular fracture fixation include advancing age, femoral head impaction, poor fracture reduction, and loss of hip joint congruency.[6,14,29,82]

The treatment options for elderly patients who have an acetabular fracture can be simply grouped into nonsurgical treatment, internal fixation, and THA. Hip joint congruency should be a prerequisite for nonsurgical treatment. In addition, early mobilization, at least into a wheelchair, is important to avoid the well-known complications of bed immobilization that occur in elderly patients who have hip fractures. The radiographic appearance of an acetabular fracture may be less than ideal; however, elderly patients can improve rapidly. Often, the low functional demands of elderly patients preclude the need for future surgical treatment. If nonsurgical treatment is selected, early and frequent radiographs should be obtained because fracture displacement and rapid deterioration of the hip joint can occur (**Figure 17**).

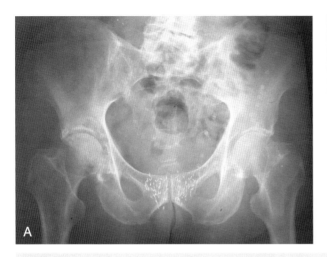
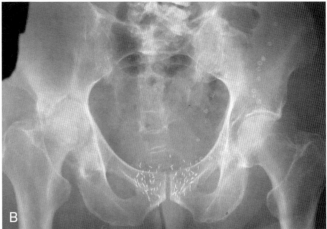

Figure 17 AP radiographs of the pelvis of an 88-year-old man who sustained a right acetabular fracture after a low-energy fall. **A,** Radiograph taken 2 weeks postinjury demonstrates an anterior column acetabular fracture with superior joint impaction. **B,** Radiograph taken 4 weeks later demonstrates extensive superior migration of the femoral head and complete loss of hip joint congruency.

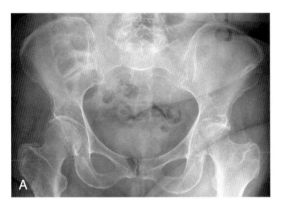
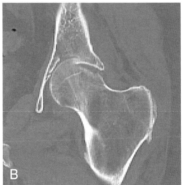
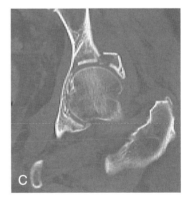

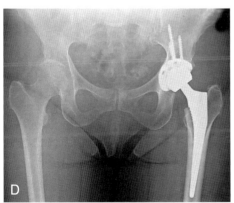

Figure 18 Images of a 56-year-old woman who sustained an acetabular fracture after a low-energy fall. **A,** AP radiograph of the patient's pelvis taken at the time of injury demonstrates a posterior wall acetabular fracture. **B,** Coronal CT reconstruction through the acetabular dome of the patient's hip taken at the time of injury shows femoral head impaction. **C,** Coronal CT reconstruction through the posterior wall of the patient's hip taken at the time of injury shows fracture and impaction of the posterior wall. **D,** AP radiograph of the patient's pelvis taken 4 months postinjury demonstrates that total hip arthroplasty was performed. The total hip arthroplasty was performed soon after the injury via an anterior surgical approach. Total hip arthroplasty was required because of articular surface impaction. The patient was allowed to bear weight immediately without hip flexion precautions.

Surgical management should be selected if the fracture or femoral head displacement precludes a viable hip socket and/or the pain from the fracture does not allow for mobilization of the patient. In deciding whether an elderly patient should undergo ORIF or THA, surgeons should not rely on limited weight bearing to protect the fixation. This strategy is not viable and is inconsistent with the physical and mental capacity of an elderly patient. Immediate THA may be very helpful in elderly patients who have severe articular impaction and a femoral head injury[100,101] (**Figure 18**); however, the impaction of a THA acetabular cup component into an unfixed acetabular fracture is technically challenging and may be associated with early acetabular cup loosening.[102-104] Closed reduction and percutaneous screw fixation of acetabular fractures in elderly patients also has been reported. In a study of 43 patients aged at least 60 years with an acetabular fracture, Gary et al[105] reported no difference in the functional outcomes of the patients who underwent closed reduction and percutaneous screw fixation compared with those of the patients who underwent ORIF. The authors reported that conversion to THA was performed in 31% of the patients.[105]

An anterior column fracture with quadrilateral surface involvement is a common acetabular fracture pattern in elderly patients. In patients with this fracture pattern, the anterior column externally rotates, the quadrilateral surface internally rotates, and the femoral head medializes (**Figure 19, A** and **B**). In elderly patients who undergo ORIF, successful correction of anterior acetabular column displacement is achieved via multiple steps: (1) the femoral head is brought distal and lateral with the use of a Schanz pin that is inserted in the proximal femur or with the use of a traction table; (2) the anterior column is derotated with the use of a Schanz pin that is inserted in (or a bone reduction clamp that is placed on) the anterior column fragment; (3) one tine of a bone reduction clamp is placed on the inner aspect of the anterior column fragment, and the other tine is placed on the outer aspect of the innominate bone; and (4) an undercontoured plate is placed along the pelvic brim to aid in pushing the anterior column distal and posterior, which is achieved with the use of a screw that is inserted through the plate just superior to the fracture

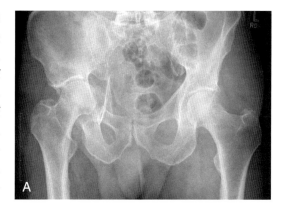
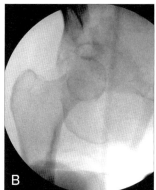
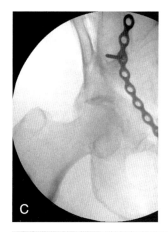
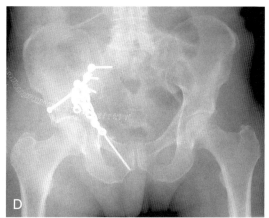

Figure 19   Images of a 71-year-old woman who sustained an acetabular fracture after a fall. **A,** AP radiograph of the patient's pelvis taken at the time of injury demonstrates an anterior column acetabular fracture. Note the medial and superior displacement of the femoral head and the considerable displacement of the quadrilateral surface. **B,** Intraoperative obturator oblique fluoroscopic image of the patient's hip shows considerable displacement of the anterior acetabular column. **C,** Intraoperative obturator oblique fluoroscopic image of the patient's hip shows the anterior column reduction, which was aided by the use of an undercontoured pelvic brim plate. A screw inserted just superior to the fracture line was directed toward the strong sciatic buttress bone to help reduce the acetabular fracture. **D,** Postoperative AP radiograph of the patient's pelvis taken after final anatomic reduction of the acetabular fracture demonstrates that two plates were placed on the inner pelvic surface, and an intrapelvic plate was used to support the quadrilateral surface.

line (**Figure 19, C** and **D**). Considerable anterior column displacement with articular impaction is common in elderly patients who have underlying osteoporosis. These patients should undergo anterior column fixation with the use of an undercontoured plate that is placed on the internal pelvic brim (**Figure 19, C**) in combination with THA that is performed via an anterior surgical approach. In these patients, the Levine anterior approach allows for sequential reduction and fixation of an acetabular fracture as well as anterior THA via the same incision.[106]

Complications

Complications in elderly patients who undergo treatment for an acetabular fracture can be substantial and frequent.

Similar to the treatment of an elderly patient who has a standard hip fracture (ie, proximal femur), a multidisciplinary approach with early intervention may help minimize these complications. In a meta-analysis of 15 studies overall that included a total of 414 patients older than 55 years with an acetabular fracture, Daurka et al[82] reported an overall mortality rate of 19.1% and a nonfatal complication rate of 39.8% at a mean follow-up of 64 months. In a retrospective study of 176 patients aged at least 60 years with an acetabular fracture, Bible et al[107] reported a 1-year mortality rate of 8.1%. In the meta-analysis previously discussed, Daurka et al[82] reported conversion to THA in 23.1% of the patients who underwent internal fixation of an acetabular fracture. Unfortunately, conversion to THA is not a panacea. Morison et al[108] reported that the risk for infection, hip dislocation, and heterotopic ossification is significantly higher in patients who undergo THA after failed acetabular fracture surgery compared with patients who undergo primary THA.

Summary

The goals of acetabular fracture management are restoration of hip joint congruity and stability. In general, displaced acetabular fractures require ORIF; however, many mitigating factors are involved. Particular challenges in the management of acetabular fractures include posterior wall acetabular fractures, fractures associated with damage to the surrounding soft-tissue envelope, acetabular fractures in patients with multiple injuries, and acetabular fractures in the geriatric population. Although these challenges are complex and demanding, knowledgeable and experienced surgeons can achieve excellent outcomes in patients who undergo treatment for acetabular fractures.

References

1. Knight RA, Smith H: Central fractures of the acetabulum. *J Bone Joint Surg Am* 1958;40(1):1-16, passim.

2. Rowe CR, Lowell JD: Prognosis of fractures of the acetabulum. *J Bone Joint Surg Am* 1961;43(1):30-92.

3. Stewart MJ: Discussion: Prognosis of fractures of the acetabulum. *J Bone Joint Surg Am* 1961;43(1):59.

4. Stewart MJ, Milford LW: Fracture-dislocation of the hip; an end-result study. *J Bone Joint Surg Am* 1954;36(2):315-342.

5. Judet R, Judet J, Letournel E: Fractures of the acetabulum: Classification and surgical approaches for open reduction. Preliminary report. *J Bone Joint Surg Am* 1964;46(8):1615-1675.

6. Letournel E, Judet R: *Fractures of the Acetabulum,* ed 2. New York, NY, Springer-Verlag, 1993.

7. Martinez CR, Di Pasquale TG, Helfet DL, Graham AW, Sanders RW, Ray LD: Evaluation of acetabular fractures with two- and three-dimensional CT. *Radiographics* 1992;12(2):227-242.

8. Kuszyk BS, Heath DG, Bliss DF, Fishman EK: Skeletal 3-D CT: Advantages of volume rendering over surface rendering. *Skeletal Radiol* 1996;25(3):207-214.

9. O'Toole RV, Cox G, Shanmuganathan K, et al: Evaluation of computed tomography for determining the diagnosis of acetabular fractures. *J Orthop Trauma* 2010;24(5):284-290.

10. Sinatra PM, Moed BR: CT-generated radiographs in obese patients with acetabular fractures: Can they be used in lieu of plain radiographs? *Clin Orthop Relat Res* 2014;472(11):3362-3369.

11. Beaulé PE, Dorey FJ, Matta JM: Letournel classification for acetabular fractures: Assessment of interobserver and intraobserver reliability. *J Bone Joint Surg Am* 2003;85(9):1704-1709.

12. Prevezas N, Antypas G, Louverdis D, Konstas A, Papasotiriou A, Sbonias G: Proposed guidelines for increasing the reliability and validity of Letournel classification system. *Injury* 2009;40(10):1098-1103.

13. Ly TV, Stover MD, Sims SH, Reilly MC: The use of an algorithm for classifying acetabular fractures: A role for resident education? *Clin Orthop Relat Res* 2011;469(8):2371-2376.

14. Matta JM: Fractures of the acetabulum: Accuracy of reduction and clinical results in patients managed operatively within three weeks after the injury. *J Bone Joint Surg Am* 1996;78(11):1632-1645.

15. Chin FY, Lo WH, Chen TH, Chen CM, Huang CK, Ma HL: Fractures of posterior wall of acetabulum. *Arch Orthop Trauma Surg* 1996;115(5):273-275.

16. Saterbak AM, Marsh JL, Nepola JV, Brandser EA, Turbett T: Clinical failure after posterior wall acetabular fractures: The influence of initial fracture patterns. *J Orthop Trauma* 2000;14(4):230-237.

17. Aho AJ, Isberg UK, Katevuo VK: Acetabular posterior wall fracture: 38 cases followed for 5 years. *Acta Orthop Scand* 1986;57(2):101-105.

18. Moed BR, WillsonCarr SE, Watson JT: Results of operative treatment of fractures of the posterior wall of the acetabulum. *J Bone Joint Surg Am* 2002;84(5):752-758.

19. Moed BR, Carr SE, Gruson KI, Watson JT, Craig JG: Computed tomographic assessment of fractures of the posterior wall of the acetabulum after operative treatment. *J Bone Joint Surg Am* 2003;85(3):512-522.

20. Kellam P, Ostrum RF: Systematic review and meta-analysis of avascular necrosis and posttraumatic arthritis after traumatic hip dislocation. *J Orthop Trauma* 2016;30(1):10-16.

21. Vrahas MS, Widding KK, Thomas KA: The effects of simulated transverse, anterior column, and posterior column fractures of the acetabulum on the stability of the hip joint. *J Bone Joint Surg Am* 1999;81(7):966-974.

22. Matityahu A, McDonald E, Buckley JM, Marmor M: Propensity for hip dislocation in gait loading versus sit-to-stand maneuvers: Implications for redefining the dome of the

acetabulum needed for stability of the hip during activities of daily living. *J Orthop Trauma* 2012;26(8):e97-e101.

23. Matta JM, Merritt PO: Displaced acetabular fractures. *Clin Orthop Relat Res* 1988;230:83-97.

24. Firoozabadi R, Spitler C, Schlepp C, et al: Determining stability in posterior wall acetabular fractures. *J Orthop Trauma* 2015;29(10):465-469.

25. Reagan JM, Moed BR: Can computed tomography predict hip stability in posterior wall acetabular fractures? *Clin Orthop Relat Res* 2011;469(7):2035-2041.

26. Grimshaw CS, Moed BR: Outcomes of posterior wall fractures of the acetabulum treated nonoperatively after diagnostic screening with dynamic stress examination under anesthesia. *J Bone Joint Surg Am* 2010;92(17):2792-2800.

27. Moed BR, Ajibade DA, Israel H: Computed tomography as a predictor of hip stability status in posterior wall fractures of the acetabulum. *J Orthop Trauma* 2009;23(1):7-15.

28. McNamara AR, Boudreau JA, Moed BR: Nonoperative treatment of posterior wall fractures of the acetabulum after dynamic stress examination under anesthesia: Revisited. *J Orthop Trauma* 2015;29(8):359-364.

29. Tannast M, Najibi S, Matta JM: Two to twenty-year survivorship of the hip in 810 patients with operatively treated acetabular fractures. *J Bone Joint Surg Am* 2012;94(17):1559-1567.

30. Moed BR, McMahon MJ, Armbrecht ES: The acetabular fracture prognostic nomogram: Does it work for fractures of the posterior wall? *J Orthop Trauma* 2016;30(4):208-212.

31. Giannoudis PV, Tzioupis C, Moed BR: Two-level reconstruction of comminuted posterior-wall fractures of the acetabulum. *J Bone Joint Surg Br* 2007;89(4):503-509.

32. Tornetta P III: Displaced acetabular fractures: Indications for operative and nonoperative management. *J Am Acad Orthop Surg* 2001;9(1):18-28.

33. Flegal KM, Carroll MD, Kit BK, Ogden CL: Prevalence of obesity and trends in the distribution of body mass index among US adults, 1999-2010. *JAMA* 2012;307(5):491-497.

34. Porter SE, Russell GV, Dews RC, Qin Z, Woodall J Jr, Graves ML: Complications of acetabular fracture surgery in morbidly obese patients. *J Orthop Trauma* 2008;22(9):589-594.

35. Karunakar MA, Shah SN, Jerabek S: Body mass index as a predictor of complications after operative treatment of acetabular fractures. *J Bone Joint Surg Am* 2005;87(7):1498-1502.

36. Porter SE, Graves ML, Maples RA, Woodall J Jr, Wallace JG, Russell GV: Acetabular fracture reductions in the obese patient. *J Orthop Trauma* 2011;25(6):371-377.

37. Mourad WF, Packianathan S, Shourbaji RA, et al: The impact of body mass index on heterotopic ossification. *Int J Radiat Oncol Biol Phys* 2012;82(5):e831-e836.

38. Bates P, Gary J, Singh G, Reinert C, Starr A: Percutaneous treatment of pelvic and acetabular fractures in obese patients. *Orthop Clin North Am* 2011;42(1):55-67, vi.

39. Polso AK, Lassiter JL, Nagel JL: Impact of hospital guideline for weight-based antimicrobial dosing in morbidly obese adults and comprehensive literature review. *J Clin Pharm Ther* 2014;39(6):584-608.

40. Alexander JW, Rahn R: Prevention of deep wound infection in morbidly obese patients by infusion of an antibiotic into the subcutaneous space at the time of wound closure. *Obes Surg* 2004;14(7):970-974.

41. Keating JF, Blachut PA, O'Brien PJ, Meek RN, Broekhuyse H: Reamed nailing of open tibial fractures: Does the antibiotic bead pouch reduce the deep infection rate? *J Orthop Trauma* 1996;10(5):298-303.

42. Kang DG, Holekamp TF, Wagner SC, Lehman RA Jr: Intrasite vancomycin powder for the prevention of surgical site infection in spine surgery: A systematic literature review. *Spine J* 2015;15(4):762-770.

43. Pierpont YN, Dinh TP, Salas RE, et al: Obesity and surgical wound healing: A current review. *ISRN Obes* 2014;638936.

44. Karunakar MA, Staples KS: Does stress-induced hyperglycemia increase the risk of perioperative infectious complications in orthopaedic trauma patients? *J Orthop Trauma* 2010;24(12):752-756.

45. Reddix RN Jr, Leng XI, Woodall J Jr, Jackson B, Dedmond B, Webb LX: The effect of incisional negative pressure therapy on wound complications after acetabular fracture surgery. *J Surg Orthop Adv* 2010;19(2):91-97.

46. Jeray KJ, Banks DM, Phieffer LS, et al: Evaluation of standard surgical preparation performed on superficial dermal abrasions. *J Orthop Trauma* 2000;14(3):206-211.

47. Moed BR: The modified gibson posterior surgical approach to the acetabulum. *J Orthop Trauma* 2010;24(5):315-322.

48. Morel-Lavallée M: Decollements traumatiques de la peau et des couches sousjacentes. *Arch Gen Med* 1863;1: 20-38, 172-200, 300-332.

49. Hak DJ, Olson SA, Matta JM: Diagnosis and management of closed internal degloving injuries associated with pelvic and acetabular fractures: The Morel-Lavallée lesion. *J Trauma* 1997;42(6):1046-1051.

50. Kottmeier SA, Wilson SC, Born CT, Hanks GA, Iannacone WM, DeLong WG: Surgical management of soft tissue lesions associated with pelvic ring injury. *Clin Orthop Relat Res* 1996;329:46-53.

51. Hudson DA, Knottenbelt JD, Krige JE: Closed degloving injuries: Results following conservative surgery. *Plast Reconstr Surg* 1992;89(5):853-855.

52. Nickerson TP, Zielinski MD, Jenkins DH, Schiller HJ: The Mayo Clinic experience with Morel-Lavallée lesions: Establishment of a practice management guideline. *J Trauma Acute Care Surg* 2014;76(2):493-497.

53. Carlson DA, Simmons J, Sando W, Weber T, Clements B: Morel-lavalée lesions treated with debridement and meticulous dead space closure: Surgical technique. *J Orthop Trauma* 2007;21(2):140-144.

54. Tseng S, Tornetta P III: Percutaneous management of Morel-Lavallee

lesions. *J Bone Joint Surg Am* 2006;88(1):92-96.

55. Wei D, Wang Y, Yuan J, et al: One-stage operation for pelvis and acetabular fractures combined with Morel-Lavallée injury by internal fixation associated with vacuum sealing drainage. *Zhongguo Xiu Fu Chong Jian Wai Ke Za Zhi* 2014;28(1):38-42.

56. Köhler D, Pohlemann T: Operative treatment of the peripelvic Morel-Lavallée lesion. *Oper Orthop Traumatol* 2011;23(1):15-20.

57. Shen C, Peng JP, Chen XD: Efficacy of treatment in peri-pelvic Morel-Lavallee lesion: A systematic review of the literature. *Arch Orthop Trauma Surg* 2013;133(5):635-640.

58. Greenhill D, Haydel C, Rehman S: Management of the Morel-Lavallée lesion. *Orthop Clin North Am* 2016;47(1):115-125.

59. Georgiadis GM: The displaced open acetabular fracture: Treatment with immediate open reduction and internal fixation. *J Trauma* 1999;47(2):389-392.

60. Lehmann W, Hoffmann M, Fensky F, et al: What is the frequency of nerve injuries associated with acetabular fractures? *Clin Orthop Relat Res* 2014;472(11):3395-3403.

61. Bogdan Y, Tornetta P III, Jones C, et al: Neurologic injury in operatively treated acetabular fractures. *J Orthop Trauma* 2015;29(10):475-478.

62. Bosse MJ, Poka A, Reinert CM, Brumback RJ, Bathon H, Burgess AR: Preoperative angiographic assessment of the superior gluteal artery in acetabular fractures requiring extensile surgical exposures. *J Orthop Trauma* 1988;2(4):303-307.

63. Tabor OB Jr, Bosse MJ, Greene KG, et al: Effects of surgical approaches for acetabular fractures with associated gluteal vascular injury. *J Orthop Trauma* 1998;12(2):78-84.

64. Griffin DB, Beaulé PE, Matta JM: Safety and efficacy of the extended iliofemoral approach in the treatment of complex fractures of the acetabulum. *J Bone Joint Surg Br* 2005;87(10):1391-1396.

65. Reilly MC, Olson SA, Tornetta P III, Matta JM: Superior gluteal artery in the extended iliofemoral approach. *J Orthop Trauma* 2000;14(4):259-263.

66. Magnussen RA, Tressler MA, Obremskey WT, Kregor PJ: Predicting blood loss in isolated pelvic and acetabular high-energy trauma. *J Orthop Trauma* 2007;21(9):603-607.

67. Džupa V, Grill R, Fridrich F, Krbec M, Skála-Rosenbaum J, Báča V: Pelvic injuries and acetabular fractures: Differences in their severity. *Acta Chir Orthop Traumatol Cech* 2013;80(1):60-63.

68. Ebraheim NA, Liu J, Lee AH, Patil V, Nazzal MM, Sanford CG Jr: Obturator artery disruption associated with acetabular fracture: A case study and anatomy review. *Injury Extra* 2008;39(2):44-46.

69. Halvorson JJ, Lamothe J, Martin CR, et al: Combined acetabulum and pelvic ring injuries. *J Am Acad Orthop Surg* 2014;22(5):304-314.

70. Osgood GM, Manson TT, O'Toole RV, Turen CH: Combined pelvic ring disruption and acetabular fracture: Associated injury patterns in 40 patients. *J Orthop Trauma* 2013;27(5):243-247.

71. Suzuki T, Smith WR, Hak DJ, et al: Combined injuries of the pelvis and acetabulum: Nature of a devastating dyad. *J Orthop Trauma* 2010;24(5):303-308.

72. Manson TT, Perdue PW, Pollak AN, O'Toole RV: Embolization of pelvic arterial injury is a risk factor for deep infection after acetabular fracture surgery. *J Orthop Trauma* 2013;27(1):11-15.

73. Sagi HC, Dziadosz D, Mir H, Virani N, Olson C: Obesity, leukocytosis, embolization, and injury severity increase the risk for deep postoperative wound infection after pelvic and acetabular surgery. *J Orthop Trauma* 2013;27(1):6-10.

74. Moed BR, Reilly MC: Acetabulum fractures, in Court-Brown CM, Heckman JD, McQueen MM, et al, eds: *Rockwood and Green's Fractures in Adults,* ed 8. Philadelphia, PA, Wolters Kluwer Health, 2015, pp 1891-1981.

75. Vallier HA, Wang X, Moore TA, Wilber JH, Como JJ: Timing of orthopaedic surgery in multiple trauma patients: Development of a protocol for early appropriate care. *J Orthop Trauma* 2013;27(10):543-551.

76. Vallier HA, Cureton BA, Ekstein C, Oldenburg FP, Wilber JH: Early definitive stabilization of unstable pelvis and acetabulum fractures reduces morbidity. *J Trauma* 2010;69(3):677-684.

77. Vallier HA, Moore TA, Como JJ, et al: Teamwork in trauma: System adjustment to a protocol for the management of multiply injured patients. *J Orthop Trauma* 2015;29(11):e446-e450.

78. Morshed S, Knops S, Jurkovich GJ, Wang J, MacKenzie E, Rivara FP: The impact of trauma-center care on mortality and function following pelvic ring and acetabular injuries. *J Bone Joint Surg Am* 2015;97(4):265-272.

79. Ortman JM, Velkoff VA, Hogan H: An aging nation: The older population in the United States. Current Population Reports. Washington, DC, United States Census Bureau, 2014, pp 25-1140. Available at: https://www.census.gov/prod/2014pubs/p25-1140.pdf. Accessed July 27, 2016.

80. US Department of Health and Human Services, Administration for Community Living: Administration on Aging (AoA): Aging statistics. Available at: http://www.aoa.gov/Aging_Statistics. Accessed April 9, 2016.

81. Buller LT, Lawrie CM, Vilella FE: A growing problem: Acetabular fractures in the elderly and the combined hip procedure. *Orthop Clin North Am* 2015;46(2):215-225.

82. Daurka JS, Pastides PS, Lewis A, Rickman M, Bircher MD: Acetabular fractures in patients aged > 55 years: A systematic review of the literature. *Bone Joint J* 2014;96(2):157-163.

83. Henry PD, Kreder HJ, Jenkinson RJ: The osteoporotic acetabular fracture. *Orthop Clin North Am* 2013;44(2):201-215.

84. Tosounidis TH, Giannoudis PV: What is new in acetabular fracture fixation? *Injury* 2015;46(11):2089-2092.

85. Ferguson TA, Patel R, Bhandari M, Matta JM: Fractures of the acetabulum in patients aged 60 years

and older: An epidemiological and radiological study. *J Bone Joint Surg Br* 2010;92(2):250-257.

86. Miller AN, Prasarn ML, Lorich DG, Helfet DL: The radiological evaluation of acetabular fractures in the elderly. *J Bone Joint Surg Br* 2010;92(4):560-564.

87. Gary JL, Paryavi E, Gibbons SD, et al: Effect of surgical treatment on mortality after acetabular fracture in the elderly: A multicenter study of 454 patients. *J Orthop Trauma* 2015;29(4):202-208.

88. Archdeacon MT, Kazemi N, Collinge C, Budde B, Schnell S: Treatment of protrusio fractures of the acetabulum in patients 70 years and older. *J Orthop Trauma* 2013;27(5):256-261.

89. Jeffcoat DM, Carroll EA, Huber FG, et al: Operative treatment of acetabular fractures in an older population through a limited ilioinguinal approach. *J Orthop Trauma* 2012;26(5):284-289.

90. Anglen JO, Burd TA, Hendricks KJ, Harrison P: The "Gull Sign": A harbinger of failure for internal fixation of geriatric acetabular fractures. *J Orthop Trauma* 2003;17(9):625-634.

91. Helfet DL, Borrelli J Jr, DiPasquale T, Sanders R: Stabilization of acetabular fractures in elderly patients. *J Bone Joint Surg Am* 1992;74(5):753-765.

92. Kates SL: Hip fracture programs: Are they effective? *Injury* 2016;47(suppl 1):S25-S27.

93. Kates SL, Behrend C, Mendelson DA, Cram P, Friedman SM: Hospital readmission after hip fracture. *Arch Orthop Trauma Surg* 2015;135(3):329-337.

94. Kates SL, Mendelson DA, Friedman SM: The value of an organized fracture program for the elderly:

Early results. *J Orthop Trauma* 2011;25(4):233-237.

95. Suhm N, Rikli D, Schaeren S, Studer P, Jakob M, Kates SL: Recent aspects on outcomes in geriatric fracture patients. *Osteoporos Int* 2010;21(suppl 4):S523-S528.

96. Schnell S, Friedman SM, Mendelson DA, Bingham KW, Kates SL: The 1-year mortality of patients treated in a hip fracture program for elders. *Geriatr Orthop Surg Rehabil* 2010;1(1):6-14.

97. Marsland D, Colvin PL, Mears SC, Kates SL: How to optimize patients for geriatric fracture surgery. *Osteoporos Int* 2010;21(suppl 4):S535-S546.

98. Collinge CA, Lebus GF: Techniques for reduction of the quadrilateral surface and dome impaction when using the anterior intrapelvic (modified Stoppa) approach. *J Orthop Trauma* 2015;29(suppl 2):S20-S24.

99. Carroll EA, Huber FG, Goldman AT, et al: Treatment of acetabular fractures in an older population. *J Orthop Trauma* 2010;24(10):637-644.

100. Mears DC, Velyvis JH: Acute total hip arthroplasty for selected displaced acetabular fractures: Two to twelve-year results. *J Bone Joint Surg Am* 2002;84(1):1-9.

101. Mears DC, Velyvis JH: Primary total hip arthroplasty after acetabular fracture. *Instr Course Lect* 2001;50:335-354.

102. von Roth P, Abdel MP, Harmsen WS, Berry DJ: Total hip arthroplasty after operatively treated acetabular fracture: A concise follow-up, at a mean of twenty years, of a previous report. *J Bone Joint Surg Am* 2015;97(4):288-291.

103. Makridis KG, Obakponovwe O, Bobak P, Giannoudis PV: Total hip

arthroplasty after acetabular fracture: Incidence of complications, reoperation rates and functional outcomes. Evidence today. *J Arthroplasty* 2014;29(10):1983-1990.

104. Ranawat A, Zelken J, Helfet D, Buly R: Total hip arthroplasty for posttraumatic arthritis after acetabular fracture. *J Arthroplasty* 2009;24(5):759-767.

105. Gary JL, VanHal M, Gibbons SD, Reinert CM, Starr AJ: Functional outcomes in elderly patients with acetabular fractures treated with minimally invasive reduction and percutaneous fixation. *J Orthop Trauma* 2012;26(5):278-283.

106. Beaulé PE, Griffin DB, Matta JM: The Levine anterior approach for total hip replacement as the treatment for an acute acetabular fracture. *J Orthop Trauma* 2004;18(9):623-629.

107. Bible JE, Wegner A, McClure DJ, et al: One-year mortality after acetabular fractures in elderly patients presenting to a level-1 trauma center. *J Orthop Trauma* 2014;28(3):154-159.

108. Morison Z, Moojen DJ, Nauth A, et al: Total hip arthroplasty after acetabular fracture is associated with lower survivorship and more complications. *Clin Orthop Relat Res* 2016;474(2):392-398.

Video References

1.1. Moed BR: Video. *Performance of the EUA*. St. Louis, MO, 2016.

1.2. Moed BR, Stover MD: Video. *Ballottable Fluid Wave*. St. Louis, MO, and Chicago, IL, 2016.

1.3. Moed BR, Stover MD: Video. *Percutaneous Débridement*. St. Louis, MO, and Chicago, IL, 2016.

Challenges and Controversies of Foot and Ankle Trauma

Cyrus E. Taghavi, MD
Michael Isiah Sandlin, MD
David B. Thordarson, MD

Abstract

Traumatic injury to the foot and ankle can result in long-term disability, which may have substantial negative implications on a patient's functional outcomes and quality of life. The diagnosis and appropriate management of these challenging injuries are not always agreed on or straightforward. In particular, the appropriate diagnosis and management of distal tibiofibular syndesmotic injuries as well as the surgical approach and role of primary subtalar arthrodesis for intra-articular calcaneal fractures are controversial.

Instr Course Lect 2017;66:25–37.

Traumatic injury to the foot and ankle can be devastating for patients, often resulting in long-term disability, which may have substantial negative implications on a patient's functional outcomes and quality of life. The diagnosis and appropriate management of traumatic foot and ankle injuries are not always agreed on or straightforward. Surgeons should understand the challenges and controversies associated with the orthopaedic care of distal tibiofibular syndesmotic injuries and intra-articular calcaneal fractures. Surgeons should be aware of, in particular, the debate with regard to syndesmotic fixation as well as the surgical approach and role of primary subtalar arthrodesis for intra-articular calcaneal fractures.

Syndesmotic Injuries

Five percent to 10% of all ankle sprains[1,2] and 23% of all ankle fractures[3] are associated with syndesmotic injury. In a study on data from the National Collegiate Athletic Association's Injury Surveillance System, Hunt et al[4] reported that 24.6% of all ankle sprains in National Collegiate Athletic Association football players involved injury to the syndesmosis. Syndesmotic injury can critically destabilize an ankle joint, which can lead to substantial disability as well as lost time from work and sporting activity. Both syndesmotic injury and malreduction can substantially affect ankle dynamics. Just 1 mm of lateral talar shift decreases the tibiotalar contact area by 42% and substantially increases contact pressure,[5] which, ultimately, can lead to early arthritic changes and decreased quality of life.

Although the prevalence of syndesmotic injuries is high and the long-term consequences can be quite debilitating, no consensus among orthopaedic surgeons exists with regard to appropriate management. Several variations in fixation techniques, including the size and number of screws used, the number of cortices engaged, and the indications for screw removal, have been developed. Recent attention has been directed toward the role of flexible fixation of the syndesmosis with the use of a suture-button construct.

Anatomy

The distal tibiofibular syndesmosis is stabilized by four distinct ligamentous

Dr. Thordarson or an immediate family member has received royalties from OrthoHelix; serves as a paid consultant to Bio2 Medical, Biomet, Paragon28, and Stryker; has stock or stock options held in Bio2 Medical and Paragon28; and serves as a board member, owner, officer, or committee member of the American Orthopaedic Foot and Ankle Society. Neither of the following authors nor any immediate family member has received anything of value from or has stock or stock options held in a commercial company or institution related directly or indirectly to the subject of this chapter: Dr. Taghavi and Dr. Sandlin.

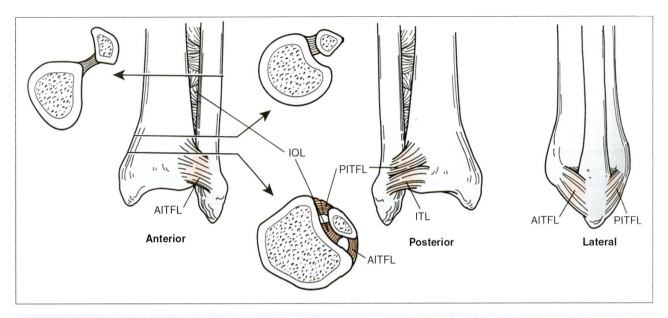

Figure 1 Illustrations show the anatomy of the distal tibiofibular syndesmosis, which includes the anteroinferior tibiofibular ligament (AITFL), the posteroinferior tibiofibular ligament (PITFL), the interosseous ligament (IOL), and the inferior transverse ligament (ITL). (Reproduced with permission from Van Heest TJ, Lafferty PM: Injuries to the ankle syndesmosis. *J Bone Joint Surg Am* 2014;96[7]:603-613.)

structures: the anteroinferior tibiofibular ligament (AITFL), the posteroinferior tibiofibular ligament (PITFL), the interosseous ligament, and the inferior transverse ligament (**Figure 1**). The AITFL originates from the anterolateral tubercle (Tillaux-Chaput) of the tibia and inserts at the anterior tubercle (Wagstaffe) of the fibula. Although the AITFL is the weakest of the ligaments, it has been reported to provide the greatest resistance against external rotation.[6] The accessory AITFL, which also is known as the Bassett ligament, runs at the inferior border and can be a substantial cause of anterior impingement. The PITFL originates from the posterior tubercle (Volkmann) of the tibia and inserts at the posterior aspect of the lateral malleolus. The PITFL is the strongest of the ligaments, and injury often involves avulsion of the posterior malleolus. The interosseous ligament, which is a thickened continuation of the interosseous membrane, acts as a spring that allows slight widening of the mortise with dorsiflexion. The inferior transverse ligament, which runs anterior to the PITFL, acts as a labrum analogue for the talus and often is considered the deep portion of the PITFL. At the medial aspect of the ankle, the deltoid ligament, which is composed of deep and superficial layers, acts as the primary stabilizer of the ankle.

Mechanism of Injury

Syndesmotic injuries can be purely ligamentous or can occur in conjunction with ankle fractures. Surgeons should have a high index of suspicion for syndesmotic involvement in patients with supination external rotation (Weber type B), pronation external rotation (Weber type C), or high fibular (Maisonneuve) fractures. Typically, the mechanism of injury for syndesmotic injury involves forced external rotation of the foot with simultaneous internal rotation of the leg. The mechanism of injury for syndesmotic injury also may involve hyperdorsiflexion or calcaneal eversion.[7-9] A notable rate of syndesmotic injuries occur in patients who participate in activities that involve rigid fixation of the feet, such as skiing and wakeboarding.

Diagnosis

History and Physical Examination

A thorough history and physical examination are essential to the diagnosis of syndesmotic injury. The critical elements of a patient's history include the mechanism of injury and any symptoms of instability. Patients will have an antalgic gait as well as pain with step-off and dorsiflexion and may exhibit a steppage gait with circumduction. Patients will have very localized pain over the syndesmosis and may have ecchymosis above the ankle. Substantial tenderness and ecchymosis over the medial ankle also will be present in patients who have an associated deltoid ligament injury.

Even with a complete physical examination, as many as 20% of syndesmotic injuries may go undetected.

Specific clinical tests may facilitate the diagnosis of syndesmotic injury. A positive squeeze test, which is performed by compressing the patient's fibula to the tibia proximal to the midpoint of the calf, results in pain at the syndesmosis.[10] The external rotation test is performed with the patient's knee bent at 90° and the leg stabilized. A positive external rotation test results in pain at the syndesmosis if an external rotation force is applied to the foot.[11] The crossed-leg test is a self-administered test in which the patient crosses his or her injured leg over his or her noninjured leg, which allows gravity to elicit pain at the syndesmosis. Gentle downward force also may be applied to the patient's knee to help trigger pain.[12] The syndesmosis compression test is performed by applying forced dorsiflexion to the patient's foot or by having the patient perform a single leg heel raise. The syndesmosis compression test is repeated after applying compression to the syndesmosis with the use of athletic tape. Decreased pain indicates a syndesmotic injury.[13] The syndesmosis compression test is useful only in patients who have questionable instability because it is too painful in patients who have a fracture.

Imaging

Radiographic evaluation consists of AP, mortise, and lateral views of the ankle as well as AP and lateral views of the tibia and fibula. Radiographs should be scrutinized for any fractures, and three specific measurements should be taken. The tibiofibular overlap, which is measured 1 cm proximal to the tibial plafond, should be greater than 6 mm on AP radiographs and greater than

1 mm on mortise radiographs. The tibiofibular clear space should be less than 6 mm. The medial clear space should be less than 4 mm or less than or equal to the clear space between the talar dome and the tibial plafond[14-17] (**Figure 2**). The tibiofibular clear space is the most reliable of these measurements because it does not substantially change from 5° of external rotation to 25° of internal rotation.[14]

Unfortunately, static radiographs are not reliable for the detection of subtle syndesmotic injury.[15,18,19] Stress radiographs, such as those obtained with the use of the external rotation stress test, may reveal an occult injury but are limited in a patient who is awake because substantial pain will be elicited. Gravity external rotation stress radiographs may cause limited discomfort but can aid in the detection of any associated deltoid ligament injury. Gill et al[20] reported that gravity stress radiographs were equivalent to manual stress examinations with regard to the detection of deltoid ligament injuries in patients who had isolated fibular fractures. Additional imaging modalities, such as CT and MRI, may be useful for the assessment of suspected syndesmotic disruption.

CT aids in the detection of minor syndesmotic diastasis. The ability to directly compare the injured extremity with the contralateral extremity is invaluable for the detection of minute variations in sagittal alignment and rotational deformity or malreduction.[18] MRI is highly sensitive for the detection of subtle ligamentous injuries, occult osteochondral defects, loose bodies, stress fractures, and other pathology.[21-23] In a study that compared imaging modalities with regard to the detection of syndesmotic injury, Takao et al[24] reported that MRI had a 96%

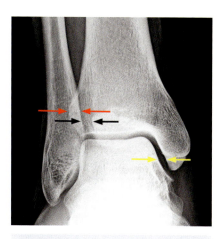

Figure 2 AP radiograph of an ankle demonstrates the measurements used to detect syndesmotic injury, including tibiofibular overlap (red arrows), tibiofibular clear space (black arrows), and medial clear space (yellow arrows).

accuracy for the detection of syndesmotic injury.

Intraoperatively, the syndesmosis can be stressed with the use of the external rotation or hook (Cotton) stress tests (**Figure 3**). Diastasis or medial joint space widening greater than 2 mm is considered a positive test. Mild and moderate injuries may be difficult to detect, even with the use of a stress test. In a study that compared the external rotation and Cotton stress tests, Matuszewski et al[25] reported that the external rotation test resulted in 37% greater medial clear space widening. Unfortunately, both tests have limited sensitivity.[26] If any doubt with regard to diagnosis exists, arthroscopy allows for direct visualization of any diastasis and has been reported to detect more than two times the number of syndesmotic injuries compared with those detected via intraoperative stress examinations.[27]

Syndesmotic Sprains

Syndesmotic sprains, which also are known as high ankle sprains, are

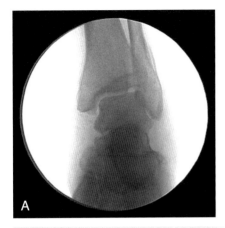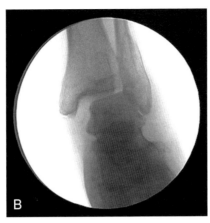

Figure 3   AP radiographs of an ankle taken before (**A**) and after (**B**) the application of external rotation stress.

syndesmotic ligamentous injuries in the absence of a fracture. Syndesmotic sprains occur in as many as 17.6% of patients who sustain an ankle sprain and result in a substantially longer recovery time.[28] In a study that compared the outcomes of National Hockey League players who sustained a syndesmotic sprain with those that sustained a lateral ankle sprain, Wright et al[29] reported that National Hockey League players who had a syndesmotic sprain took an average of 45 days to return to play, whereas National Hockey League players who had a lateral ankle sprain took an average of 1.4 days to return to play. Grade I syndesmotic sprains involve injury to the AITFL; grade II syndesmotic sprains involve injury to the AITFL and the interosseous ligament; grade III syndesmotic sprains involve injury to the AITFL, the interosseous ligament, and the PITFL; and grade IV syndesmotic sprains involve complete syndesmotic injury and a deltoid ligament tear.[30]

Patients who have grade I or grade II syndesmotic sprains may be treated nonsurgically with the use of a three-phase treatment plan. Phase I of the nonsurgical treatment plan involves ankle protection and pain management with rest, ice, compression, and elevation. After a few days, phase II of the nonsurgical treatment plan, which involves strengthening and proprioceptive exercises, may begin. Patients who are able to jog and hop without substantial pain are transitioned to phase III of the nonsurgical treatment plan, which involves rigorous strengthening and sport-specific movements.[13] Patients who have grade III or grade IV syndesmotic sprains require surgical treatment to achieve symptomatic relief and restore syndesmotic stability.

Treatment

Surgical Indications
To examine the stability of the lower extremity and the necessity of a syndesmosis screw to supplement fixation, Boden et al[31] sectioned the syndesmosis of cadaver models into 1.5-cm intervals. Testing was performed in cadaver models that had both intact and sectioned deltoid ligaments. The authors reported minimal widening in the cadaver models that had intact deltoids and did not observe tibiofibular widening greater than 2 mm until the degree of injury

was 4.5 cm proximal to the tibial plafond. The authors concluded that syndesmotic stabilization is not necessary in patients with rigid fixation of the medial malleolus and patients with a fixed fibular fracture that is within 4.5 cm of the ankle joint. Yamaguchi et al[32] applied the criteria described by Boden et al[31] to 18 patients (10 of whom were available for follow-up) in a clinical setting and reported no diastasis at a follow-up of 1 to 3 years.

The criteria described by Boden et al[31] are based on two assumptions: (1) fixation of the medial malleolus is equivalent to an intact deltoid, and (2) the level of an interosseous membrane tear is limited to the level of the fibular fracture. Tornetta[33] challenged these assumptions in a study that illustrated that concurrent deltoid injury can occur in patients who have a medial malleolus fracture and is commonly observed in patients who have an anterior colliculus fracture. In a study of 238 patients who had unstable supination external rotation (Weber type B) fractures, Stark et al[34] reported evidence of syndesmotic instability on the external rotation stress tests of 39% of the patients who underwent malleolar fixation, which illustrates that unstable syndesmotic injuries can occur distal to 4.5 cm from the tibial plafond.

Nielson et al[35] further refuted the criteria described by Boden et al[31] in an MRI study of the interosseous membrane of 73 patients who had fibular fractures. The authors reported that the interosseous membrane tears of 33% of the patients did not correspond with the level of fibular fracture, and, in fact, the interosseous membrane tears of 23% of the patients were more proximal to the level of fibular fracture. This study further illustrates that surgeons cannot consistently estimate the need for syndesmotic fixation based on the level of fibular fracture. Even for experienced surgeons, consistent detection of syndesmotic injury is limited. Preoperative radiographs and biomechanical criteria are unable to routinely predict the presence or absence of syndesmotic instability. Currently, intraoperative stress examinations and fluoroscopy are the best practical tools for the detection of unstable syndesmotic injury.

Syndesmotic Reduction

Anatomic reduction of the tibiofibular syndesmosis is a major predictor of clinical outcome, with syndesmotic malreduction being the most common indication for revision surgery.[35,36] Minimal degrees of syndesmotic malreduction can lead to substantial increased articular contact pressures and early posttraumatic degeneration. Unfortunately, malreduction is observed on the postoperative CT scans of as many as 52% of patients who undergo syndesmotic reduction.[37,38] One-half of syndesmotic malreductions are undetected on standard radiographs.[38]

In a cadaver model study, Miller et al[39] used postreduction CT to compare reduction clamp positioning at 0°, 15°, and 30° in relation to the intermalleolar axis. The authors reported that reduction clamping at 15° and 30° resulted in substantial external rotation of the fibula, whereas reduction clamping at the neutral anatomic axis (0°) resulted in the most accurate syndesmotic reduction; however, all reduction clamp positions resulted in slight overcompression. In an effort to reduce overcompression, some orthopaedic surgeons manually reduce the syndesmosis, which is held in place with the use of two divergent Kirschner wires.

Direct visualization of syndesmotic reduction via release of the extensor retinaculum from the anterior aspect of the fibula allows for improved accuracy and has been reported to decrease the rate of syndesmotic malreduction to 15%.[40]

Intraoperative assessment of syndesmotic reduction can be a challenge. External rotation of the fibula up to 30° and internal rotation of the fibula up to 10° cannot be reproducibly detected with the use of fluoroscopy.[41] Using mortise and lateral fluoroscopic images of the uninjured extremity, Summers et al[42] evaluated the accuracy of intraoperative assessment of syndesmotic reduction in 18 patients who had suspected syndesmotic injuries. Syndesmotic reductions were subsequently verified with the use of intraoperative CT. The authors reported that syndesmotic reduction was satisfactory (discrepancy of less than 2 mm) in 17 of the 18 patients.

An intraoperative O-arm has been reported to be a valuable tool for difficult syndesmotic reductions, allowing for real-time evaluation of fibular length, rotation, and displacement and for direct comparison with the contralateral extremity. If available, the use of an intraoperative O-arm is fast (approximately 2 minutes) and may prevent the need for a revision procedure.[43]

Syndesmotic Fixation

Debate with regard to the technique used for syndesmotic fixation (**Figure 4**), including the size and number of screws used; the number of cortices engaged; the position of the foot during fixation; fixation of the posterior malleolus; subsequent syndesmotic screw removal; and, more recently, the use of flexible fixation, currently exists.

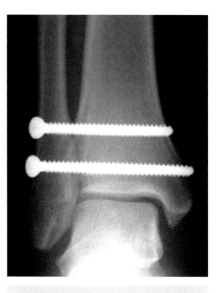

Figure 4 AP radiograph of an ankle demonstrates rigid syndesmotic fixation with the use of two 4.5-mm screws across four cortices.

Screw Size

Biomechanical and clinical studies have reported no differences in patients who undergo syndesmotic fixation with the use of either 3.5-mm or 4.5-mm screws.[44] The larger head of a 4.5-mm screw may facilitate screw removal in the physician's office at a later date but also may cause local irritation.

Number of Screws or Cortices

No substantial biomechanical or clinical differences have been reported with regard to screw failure, loss of reduction, or the need for hardware removal in patients who undergo syndesmotic fixation with the use of either one or two screws or three or four cortices.[45,46]

Foot Position

Because of the trapezoidal shape of the talus, the intermalleolar space widens 1.5 mm with the foot in dorsiflexion. Because of this, surgeons believed that a syndesmosis that was fixed with the ankle positioned in plantar flexion would

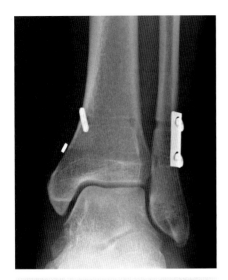

Figure 5 AP mortise radiograph of an ankle with syndesmotic instability that was managed with the use of two suture-button constructs that were passed through a two-hole fibular plate.

overcompress and limit range of motion; however, Tornetta et al[47] disproved this notion in a cadaver model study. Most surgeons now elect to fix the syndesmosis with the ankle positioned in neutral or plantar flexion.

Posterior Malleolus Fixation

In general, most surgeons fix posterior malleolus fractures if they involve more than 25% of the articular surface; however, in patients with syndesmotic instability, posterior malleolus fractures often are associated with an intact PITFL.[40] Fixation of the posterior malleolus fragment, regardless of its size, has been reported to restore the tibial incisura, which acts as a buttress for more symmetric syndesmotic reduction. Fixation of the posterior malleolus in patients who have an intact PITFL also has been reported to result in more stability compared with traditional syndesmotic fixation.[48]

Screw Removal

Syndesmotic fixation is required for 6 weeks or more to allow for adequate healing. Syndesmotic fixation for more than 6 weeks may limit normal fibular biomechanics, which can result in screw breakage after increased weight bearing and activity are initiated. In fact, better American Orthopaedic Foot and Ankle Society (AOFAS) scores have been reported in patients with retained broken screws compared with patients with intact screws.[49] Many surgeons elect to routinely remove syndesmotic screws 10 to 12 weeks after syndesmotic fixation; however, additional risks and costs are associated with hardware removal. Hardware removal is further confounded by studies that report no substantial clinical benefit of routine screw removal.[46] Based on these findings, an increased trend to remove only symptomatic hardware currently exists.

Flexible Syndesmotic Fixation

Flexible syndesmotic fixation with the use of a suture-button construct is a recent subject of debate (**Figure 5**). Flexible syndesmotic fixation with the use of a suture-button construct is gaining popularity and currently represents approximately 10% of all of the syndesmotic repairs performed in the United States.[50] The purported advantages of a suture-button construct include flexible syndesmotic fixation, which may be more advantageous for ligamentous healing; physiologic motion that allows for maintenance of reduction; less symptomatic hardware and, subsequently, a decreased need for hardware removal; earlier return to activity; and a decreased rate of malreduction.[51,52]

Early biomechanical studies have reported that syndesmotic fixation with the use of a screw is stronger but more dependent on bone quality compared with syndesmotic fixation with the use of a suture-button construct, which results in sufficient strength with failure that depends on the implant rather than bone quality.[53] Thornes et al[54] reported significantly higher mean AOFAS scores at 3 and 12 months postoperatively and earlier return to work in patients who underwent syndesmotic fixation with the use of a suture-button construct compared with those who underwent syndesmotic fixation with the use of a 3.5-mm screw. In a prospective controlled study, Laflamme et al[55] randomized 70 patients to either syndesmotic fixation with the use of a 3.5-mm screw that crossed four cortices (36 patients) or syndesmotic fixation with the use of a suture-button construct (34 patients). The authors reported that the patients in the suture-button fixation group had significantly better Olerud-Molander scores but similar AOFAS scores at 12 months postoperatively compared with the patients in the screw fixation group. The authors reported greater range of motion and no failures in the patients in the suture-button fixation group, whereas diastasis developed in four patients in the screw fixation group. These studies demonstrate that flexible syndesmotic fixation with the use of a suture-button construct is equivalent, if not superior, to rigid syndesmotic fixation.

Studies have hypothesized that flexible syndesmotic fixation with the use of a suture-button construct may decrease the high rate of syndesmotic malreduction and, subsequently, negative clinical outcomes. In a cohort study that compared the postoperative CT scans of 46 patients who underwent syndesmotic fixation with the use of either a screw or a suture-button construct, Naqvi et al[56] reported that, at a mean follow-up of 2.5 years, the patients in the screw fixation group had a 22% rate of late diastasis, whereas no patients in the suture-button fixation group had diastasis; however, no differences in AOFAS scores were reported between the patients in the two groups. In a cadaver model study, Westermann et al[52] simulated malreduction with the use of off-axis clamping. The authors then fixed the malreduced cadaver syndesmoses with the use of either a single 4.5-mm screw that was placed across four cortices or a suture-button construct. The malreduced cadaver syndesmoses in the suture-button fixation group had a significantly decreased degree of malreduction compared with the malreduced cadaver syndesmoses in the screw fixation group. The authors hypothesized that the inherent flexibility of the suture-button construct allowed the syndesmosis to reduce into its anatomic position.

Intra-Articular Calcaneal Fractures

Calcaneal fractures are the most common tarsal bone fractures, representing approximately 60% of all tarsal fractures. As many as 75% of calcaneal fractures involve intra-articular extension.[57] The long-term effects of intra-articular calcaneal fractures, which cause residual disability and pain in patients, can be quite devastating. The complex anatomy and challenges associated with the optimal management of intra-articular calcaneal fractures is a topic of extensive debate and investigation. Surgeons should understand recent advances in the management of intra-articular calcaneal fractures.

Diagnosis

History and Physical Examination

Most intra-articular calcaneal fractures are associated with a high-energy mechanism of injury and concurrent injuries, particularly spine, femoral neck, and other extremity fractures. Typically, the etiology of an intra-articular calcaneal fracture involves a fall from a height or a motor vehicle collision that results in a supraphysiologic axial load. Typically, the deformity associated with an intra-articular calcaneal fracture is a shortened, wide heel and varus malalignment. Important factors that may further compromise a patient's outcomes include a history of diabetes mellitus, peripheral vascular disease, tobacco use, or an ongoing workers' compensation claim.

Any associated injuries should be ruled out during the physical examination. Special attention must be paid to the soft-tissue envelope in particular to assess for any open wounds, the degree of swelling, and compromised tissues secondary to fracture morphology and displacement. Often, the wrinkle test is used to assess a patient's readiness for surgical treatment.

Imaging

The initial radiographic evaluation of intra-articular calcaneal fractures includes AP, lateral, and axial Harris views of the hindfoot, all of which allow for a general appreciation of the degree of displacement and intra-articular involvement. Lateral radiographs can help assess the degree of joint surface depression and allow for measurement of the Böhler angle. Although different patient populations have variable Böhler angles, any Böhler angle measurement below the accepted range of 20° to 40° has a sensitivity and specificity of 99%

for intra-articular calcaneal fracture.[58] The presence and extent of hindfoot varus malalignment can be evaluated on Harris axial radiographs.

The wide availability of CT allows for substantially improved visualization of fracture morphology, which aids in both the classification and creation of a management plan for intra-articular calcaneal fractures. The Sanders classification of intra-articular calcaneal fractures is based on the number of articular fragments observed from the posterior facet through the sustentaculum tali on a coronal CT scan[59] (**Figure 6**). The Sanders classification of intra-articular calcaneal fractures is prognostically important because patients with higher grades of intra-articular calcaneal fractures have poorer prognoses.[59] Many studies advocate primary subtalar arthrodesis for patients who have Sanders type IV and some Sanders type III intra-articular calcaneal fractures because a large number of these patients ultimately require salvage subtalar arthrodesis.[59-61]

Treatment

The optimal management for intra-articular calcaneal fractures is controversial. Several studies have compared the nonsurgical and surgical management of intra-articular calcaneal fractures and reported varying results.[62-66] In a prospective study of 30 patients with Sanders type II or type III intra-articular calcaneal fractures who were randomized to either nonsurgical treatment, which consisted of early mobilization and delayed weight bearing, or surgical treatment, which consisted of open reduction and fixation (ORIF) via an expansile L-shaped lateral approach, Thordarson et al[62] reported that the patients in the surgical group achieved

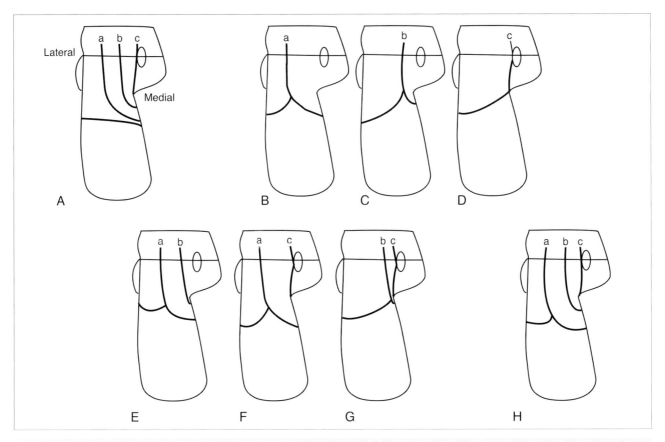

Figure 6 Illustration shows the Sanders classification of intra-articular calcaneal fractures. Lines a, b, and c indicate the presence of different nondisplaced fractures. **A,** Type I. **B,** Type IIA. **C,** Type IIB. **D,** Type IIC. **E,** Type IIIAB. **F,** Type IIIAC. **G,** Type IIIBC. **H,** Type IV. (Adapted with permission from Kim TS: Fractures of the calcaneus, in Chou LB, ed: *Orthopaedic Knowledge Update: Foot and Ankle*, ed 5. Rosemont, IL, American Academy of Orthopaedic Surgeons, 2014, pp 319-332.)

significantly better AOFAS hindfoot scores, which indicated greater function and decreased pain, compared with the patients in the nonsurgical group. In a prospective multicenter study of 424 patients with 471 displaced intra-articular calcaneal fractures who were randomized to either nonsurgical treatment or surgical treatment, Buckley et al[63] reported no significant differences in Medical Outcomes Study 36-Item Short Form or visual analog scale scores at a minimum follow-up of 2 years between the nonsurgical and surgical groups as a whole. Further stratification, however, revealed significantly higher satisfaction scores for the patients in the surgical group who were not receiving workers'

compensation. Women in the surgical group also had significantly higher Medical Outcomes Study 36-Item Short Form scores compared with women in the nonsurgical group.

Nonsurgical Management

Traditionally, the high complication rates associated with the surgical management of intra-articular calcaneal fractures led many surgeons to manage a large number of intra-articular calcaneal fractures nonsurgically. Nonsurgical management of intra-articular calcaneal fractures is appropriate for patients who have a nondisplaced intra-articular calcaneal fracture and may be considered in patients who have relative

contraindications to the surgical management of an intra-articular calcaneal fracture, including advanced physiologic age, heavy tobacco use, poorly controlled diabetes mellitus, massive comminuted fracture, or work-related injury. Nonsurgical management of intra-articular calcaneal fractures typically consists of rest, ice, elevation, and short-term immobilization in a well-padded splint. Gentle range of motion of the ankle and hindfoot should begin within 10 days postinjury to help decrease stiffness. Patients should adhere to a strict non–weight-bearing protocol for 6 to 10 weeks postinjury, after which patients may gradually progress to full weight bearing. Ultimately, patients may require custom orthotics or a delayed procedure, such as a lateral wall exostectomy for subfibular impingement or subtalar arthrodesis.[63,65,67]

Surgical Management

The most common approach in the past 25 years to achieve sufficient visualization of the fracture fragments and restore calcaneal anatomy involves an extensile L-shaped lateral incision; however, this approach may place the vascular supply to the hindfoot from the lateral calcaneal branch of the peroneal artery at risk. The greatest complications associated with an extensile L-shaped lateral approach are wound-healing problems and infection.[59,63,68-72] The risk for wound complications is further increased in patients who have comorbidities, such as poorly controlled diabetes mellitus, tobacco use, and peripheral vascular disease.

Recently, less invasive techniques for the surgical management of intra-articular calcaneal fractures, in particular the sinus tarsi approach, have gained favor.[73-75] In a study of 20 patients (22 intra-articular calcaneal fractures) who underwent surgical treatment via the sinus tarsi approach, Kikuchi et al[73] reported significant restoration of the Böhler angle and calcaneal width; however, superficial wound infection, which was managed with oral antibiotics and local wound care, developed in three of the intra-articular calcaneal fractures (13.7%). In a retrospective review that compared 79 intra-articular calcaneal fractures that were managed surgically via an extensile approach with 33 intra-articular calcaneal fractures that were managed surgically via the sinus tarsi approach, Kline et al[75] reported that the intra-articular calcaneal fractures in the extensile group had a wound complication rate of 29%, whereas the intra-articular calcaneal fractures in the sinus tarsi group had a wound complication rate of 6%. The authors reported no significant differences in foot function index or visual analog scale scores between the intra-articular calcaneal fractures in the two groups. A 100% fusion rate was achieved in the intra-articular calcaneal fractures in the two groups, and no significant differences in the final Böhler angle or Gissane angle were reported between the intra-articular calcaneal fractures in the two groups.

Less invasive techniques may allow for the earlier surgical management of intra-articular calcaneal fractures, decreased wound complications, decreased postoperative pain, and earlier rehabilitation. Less invasive techniques also may provide patients who have relative contraindications to the surgical management of an intra-articular calcaneal fracture with a safer treatment option.

Sinus Tarsi Approach

The patient is positioned in the lateral position, and a thigh tourniquet is applied. A 2- to 4-cm incision is made from the tip of the fibula to the base of the fourth metatarsal. The extensor digitorum brevis is elevated dorsally to expose the sinus tarsi (**Figure 7**). The posterior facet of the calcaneus should be able to be visualized. A Schanz pin is placed in the calcaneal tuberosity to aid with fracture manipulation and reduction. Traction and manipulation of the Schanz pin allows for restoration of both calcaneal length and alignment. The posterior facet is reduced by elevating the fragments with the use of a Cobb or Freer elevator. After reduction is attained, temporary fixation can be achieved with the use of Kirschner wires until appropriate plate or screw fixation is complete.

Primary Subtalar Arthrodesis

The role of primary subtalar arthrodesis in patients who have substantial articular and cartilaginous destruction is a topic of investigation. As many as 17% of patients with intra-articular calcaneal fractures who undergo ORIF require salvage subtalar arthrodesis for the management of symptomatic subtalar arthritis.[59,76,77] The rate of poor functional outcomes in patients who have intra-articular calcaneal fractures and the increased need for salvage subtalar arthrodesis corresponds with the degree of articular involvement.[59,63,78,79] Sanders et al[59] reported that 23% of patients who had Sanders type III intra-articular calcaneal fractures and 73% of patients who had Sanders type IV intra-articular calcaneal fractures ultimately required salvage subtalar arthrodesis. Patients with Sanders type IV intra-articular calcaneal fractures have been reported to be 5.5 times more likely to require salvage subtalar arthrodesis compared with patients with Sanders type II intra-articular calcaneal fractures.[78] Furthermore, outcomes after salvage subtalar arthrodesis are suboptimal. In a study on the outcomes of 40 patients who underwent salvage subtalar arthrodesis for the management of intra-articular calcaneal fractures in which primary management failed, Thermann et al[80] reported that 41% of the patients had fair or poor AOFAS scores, decreased ankle range of motion, and painful arthritis in adjacent joints at a mean follow-up of 5.2 years.

Subtalar arthrodesis alone does not address associated loss of calcaneal height and varus deformity. The

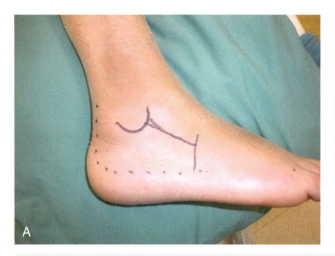
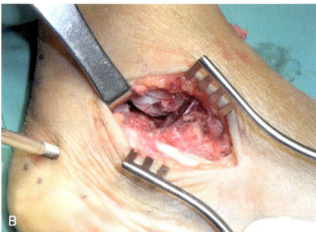

Figure 7 Intraoperative photographs of an ankle show the sinus tarsi approach for the surgical management of intra-articular calcaneal fractures. **A,** A skin incision is made from the tip of the fibula to the base of the fourth metatarsal. The dotted line indicates the location of the extensile lateral approach for the surgical management of intra-articular calcaneal fractures. **B,** Exposure attained via the sinus tarsi approach.

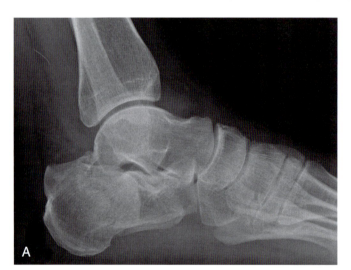
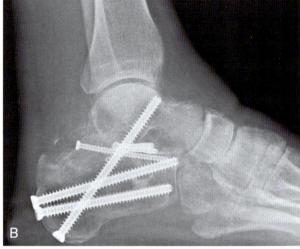

Figure 8 Lateral radiographs of an ankle with a comminuted intra-articular calcaneal fracture that was managed with the use of open reduction and internal fixation (**A**) and primary subtalar arthrodesis (**B**). (Courtesy of Clifford Jeng, MD, Baltimore, MD.)

surgeon must restore as much native anatomic alignment as possible with ORIF in combination with salvage subtalar arthrodesis.[81] The substantial necessity for salvage subtalar arthrodesis as well as the prolonged duration of disability, loss of productivity, financial and emotional burdens, and overall cost to society associated with salvage subtalar arthrodesis of intra-articular calcaneal fractures have led to an increased trend to perform ORIF in combination with primary subtalar fusion in patients who have highly comminuted intra-articular calcaneal fractures (**Figure 8**).

Summary

Many challenges are involved in the appropriate diagnosis and management of syndesmotic injuries. Regardless of the specific type of fixation used, anatomic reduction of the syndesmosis is the most important element to achieve a satisfactory outcome. The specific indications for flexible syndesmotic fixation have yet to be fully elucidated but will likely be revealed as more long-term outcomes of patients who underwent flexible syndesmotic fixation become available.

Intra-articular calcaneal fractures can be extremely debilitating and life-changing injuries. The optimal management of intra-articular calcaneal fractures can be quite challenging for orthopaedic surgeons. Improved understanding of the fracture morphology and outcomes associated with intra-articular calcaneal fractures as well as the advances in the surgical management of intra-articular calcaneal fractures have encouraged surgeons to perform less invasive procedures in appropriate patients. An increased focus on the reduction of salvage procedures, which is associated with morbidity, by decreasing wound complications and performing primary subtalar arthrodesis in patients who have highly comminuted intra-articular calcaneal fractures also exists. Additional large, prospective, long-term outcome studies are necessary to determine the optimal management for intra-articular calcaneal fractures.

References

1. Kellett JJ: The clinical features of ankle syndesmosis injuries: A general review. *Clin J Sport Med* 2011;21(6):524-529.

2. Dubin JC, Comeau D, McClelland RI, Dubin RA, Ferrel E: Lateral and syndesmotic ankle sprain injuries: A narrative literature review. *J Chiropr Med* 2011;10(3):204-219.

3. Purvis GD: Displaced, unstable ankle fractures: Classification, incidence, and management of a consecutive series. *Clin Orthop Relat Res* 1982;165:91-98.

4. Hunt KJ, George E, Harris AH, Dragoo JL: Epidemiology of syndesmosis injuries in intercollegiate football: Incidence and risk factors from National Collegiate Athletic Association injury surveillance system data from 2004-2005 to 2008-2009. *Clin J Sport Med* 2013;23(4):278-282.

5. Ramsey PL, Hamilton W: Changes in tibiotalar area of contact caused by lateral talar shift. *J Bone Joint Surg Am* 1976;58(3):356-357.

6. Ogilvie-Harris DJ, Reed SC: Disruption of the ankle syndesmosis: Diagnosis and treatment by arthroscopic surgery. *Arthroscopy* 1994;10(5):561-568.

7. Edwards GS Jr, DeLee JC: Ankle diastasis without fracture. *Foot Ankle* 1984;4(6):305-312.

8. Norkus SA, Floyd RT: The anatomy and mechanisms of syndesmotic ankle sprains. *J Athl Train* 2001;36(1):68-73.

9. Brosky T, Nyland J, Nitz A, Caborn DN: The ankle ligaments: Consideration of syndesmotic injury and implications for rehabilitation. *J Orthop Sports Phys Ther* 1995;21(4):197-205.

10. Hopkinson WJ, St Pierre P, Ryan JB, Wheeler JH: Syndesmosis sprains of the ankle. *Foot Ankle* 1990;10(6):325-330.

11. Boytim MJ, Fischer DA, Neumann L: Syndesmotic ankle sprains. *Am J Sports Med* 1991;19(3):294-298.

12. Kiter E, Bozkurt M: The crossed-leg test for examination of ankle syndesmosis injuries. *Foot Ankle Int* 2005;26(2):187-188.

13. Williams GN, Jones MH, Amendola A: Syndesmotic ankle sprains in athletes. *Am J Sports Med* 2007;35(7):1197-1207.

14. Pneumaticos SG, Noble PC, Chatziioannou SN, Trevino SG: The effects of rotation on radiographic evaluation of the tibiofibular syndesmosis. *Foot Ankle Int* 2002;23(2):107-111.

15. Beumer A, van Hemert WL, Niesing R, et al: Radiographic measurement of the distal tibiofibular syndesmosis has limited use. *Clin Orthop Relat Res* 2004;423:227-234.

16. Zalavras C, Thordarson D: Ankle syndesmotic injury. *J Am Acad Orthop Surg* 2007;15(6):330-339.

17. Harper MC, Keller TS: A radiographic evaluation of the tibiofibular syndesmosis. *Foot Ankle* 1989;10(3):156-160.

18. Ebraheim NA, Lu J, Yang H, Mekhail AO, Yeasting RA: Radiographic and CT evaluation of tibiofibular syndesmotic diastasis: A cadaver study. *Foot Ankle Int* 1997;18(11):693-698.

19. Nielson JH, Gardner MJ, Peterson MG, et al: Radiographic measurements do not predict syndesmotic injury in ankle fractures: An MRI study. *Clin Orthop Relat Res* 2005;436:216-221.

20. Gill JB, Risko T, Raducan V, Grimes JS, Schutt RC Jr: Comparison of manual and gravity stress radiographs for the evaluation of supination-external rotation fibular fractures. *J Bone Joint Surg Am* 2007;89(5):994-999.

21. Oae K, Takao M, Naito K, et al: Injury of the tibiofibular syndesmosis: Value of MR imaging for diagnosis. *Radiology* 2003;227(1):155-161.

22. Vogl TJ, Hochmuth K, Diebold T, et al: Magnetic resonance imaging in the diagnosis of acute injured distal tibiofibular syndesmosis. *Invest Radiol* 1997;32(7):401-409.

23. Roemer FW, Jomaah N, Niu J, et al: Ligamentous injuries and the risk of associated tissue damage in acute ankle sprains in athletes: A cross-sectional MRI study. *Am J Sports Med* 2014;42(7):1549-1557.

24. Takao M, Ochi M, Oae K, Naito K, Uchio Y: Diagnosis of a tear of the tibiofibular syndesmosis: The role of arthroscopy of the ankle. *J Bone Joint Surg Br* 2003;85(3):324-329.

25. Matuszewski PE, Dombroski D, Lawrence JT, Esterhai JL Jr, Mehta S: Prospective intraoperative syndesmotic evaluation during ankle fracture fixation: Stress external rotation versus lateral fibular stress. *J Orthop Trauma* 2015;29(4):e157-e160.

26. Pakarinen H, Flinkkilä T, Ohtonen P, et al: Intraoperative assessment of the stability of the distal tibiofibular joint in supination-external rotation injuries of the ankle: Sensitivity, specificity, and reliability of two clinical tests. *J Bone Joint Surg Am* 2011;93(22):2057-2061.

27. Lui TH, Ip K, Chow HT: Comparison of radiologic and arthroscopic diagnoses of distal tibiofibular syndesmosis disruption in acute ankle fracture. *Arthroscopy* 2005;21(11):1370.

28. Nussbaum ED, Hosea TM, Sieler SD, Incremona BR, Kessler DE: Prospective evaluation of syndesmotic ankle sprains without diastasis. *Am J Sports Med* 2001;29(1):31-35.

29. Wright RW, Barile RJ, Surprenant DA, Matava MJ: Ankle syndesmosis sprains in national hockey league players. *Am J Sports Med* 2004;32(8):1941-1945.

30. Sikka RS, Fetzer GB, Sugarman E, et al: Correlating MRI findings with disability in syndesmotic sprains of NFL players. *Foot Ankle Int* 2012;33(5):371-378.

31. Boden SD, Labropoulos PA, McCowin P, Lestini WF, Hurwitz SR: Mechanical considerations for the syndesmosis screw: A cadaver study. *J Bone Joint Surg Am* 1989;71(10):1548-1555.

32. Yamaguchi K, Martin CH, Boden SD, Labropoulos PA: Operative treatment of syndesmotic disruptions without use of a syndesmotic screw: A prospective clinical study. *Foot Ankle Int* 1994;15(8):407-414.

33. Tornetta P III: Competence of the deltoid ligament in bimalleolar ankle fractures after medial malleolar fixation. *J Bone Joint Surg Am* 2000;82(6):843-848.

34. Stark E, Tornetta P III, Creevy WR: Syndesmotic instability in Weber B ankle fractures: A clinical evaluation. *J Orthop Trauma* 2007;21(9):643-646.

35. Nielson JH, Sallis JG, Potter HG, Helfet DL, Lorich DG: Correlation of interosseous membrane tears to the level of the fibular fracture. *J Orthop Trauma* 2004;18(2):68-74.

36. Ovaska MT, Mäkinen TJ, Madanat R, Kiljunen V, Lindahl J: A comprehensive analysis of patients with malreduced ankle fractures undergoing re-operation. *Int Orthop* 2014;38(1):83-88.

37. Sagi HC, Shah AR, Sanders RW: The functional consequence of syndesmotic joint malreduction at a minimum 2-year follow-up. *J Orthop Trauma* 2012;26(7):439-443.

38. Gardner MJ, Demetrakopoulos D, Briggs SM, Helfet DL, Lorich DG: Malreduction of the tibiofibular syndesmosis in ankle fractures. *Foot Ankle Int* 2006;27(10):788-792.

39. Miller AN, Barei DP, Iaquinto JM, Ledoux WR, Beingessner DM: Iatrogenic syndesmosis malreduction via clamp and screw placement. *J Orthop Trauma* 2013;27(2):100-106.

40. Miller AN, Carroll EA, Parker RJ, Boraiah S, Helfet DL, Lorich DG: Direct visualization for syndesmotic stabilization of ankle fractures. *Foot Ankle Int* 2009;30(5):419-426.

41. Marmor M, Hansen E, Han HK, Buckley J, Matityahu A: Limitations of standard fluoroscopy in detecting rotational malreduction of the syndesmosis in an ankle fracture model. *Foot Ankle Int* 2011;32(6):616-622.

42. Summers HD, Sinclair MK, Stover MD: A reliable method for intraoperative evaluation of syndesmotic reduction. *J Orthop Trauma* 2013;27(4):196-200.

43. Hsu AR, Gross CE, Lee S: Intraoperative O-arm computed tomography evaluation of syndesmotic reduction: Case report. *Foot Ankle Int* 2013;34(5):753-759.

44. Thompson MC, Gesink DS: Biomechanical comparison of syndesmosis fixation with 3.5- and 4.5-millimeter stainless steel screws. *Foot Ankle Int* 2000;21(9):736-741.

45. Nousiainen MT, McConnell AJ, Zdero R, McKee MD, Bhandari M, Schemitsch EH: The influence of the number of cortices of screw purchase and ankle position in Weber C ankle fracture fixation. *J Orthop Trauma* 2008;22(7):473-478.

46. Moore JA Jr, Shank JR, Morgan SJ, Smith WR: Syndesmosis fixation: A comparison of three and four cortices of screw fixation without hardware removal. *Foot Ankle Int* 2006;27(8):567-572.

47. Tornetta P III, Spoo JE, Reynolds FA, Lee C: Overtightening of the ankle syndesmosis: Is it really possible? *J Bone Joint Surg Am* 2001;83(4):489-492.

48. Gardner MJ, Brodsky A, Briggs SM, Nielson JH, Lorich DG: Fixation of posterior malleolar fractures provides greater syndesmotic stability. *Clin Orthop Relat Res* 2006;447:165-171.

49. Hamid N, Loeffler BJ, Braddy W, Kellam JF, Cohen BE, Bosse MJ: Outcome after fixation of ankle fractures with an injury to the syndesmosis: The effect of the syndesmosis screw. *J Bone Joint Surg Br* 2009;91(8):1069-1073.

50. Bava E, Charlton T, Thordarson D: Ankle fracture syndesmosis fixation and management: The current practice of orthopedic surgeons. *Am J Orthop (Belle Mead NJ)* 2010;39(5):242-246.

51. Schepers T: Acute distal tibiofibular syndesmosis injury: A systematic review of suture-button versus syndesmotic screw repair. *Int Orthop* 2012;36(6):1199-1206.

52. Westermann RW, Rungprai C, Goetz JE, Femino J, Amendola A, Phisitkul P: The effect of suture-button fixation on simulated syndesmotic malreduction: A cadaveric study. *J Bone Joint Surg Am* 2014;96(20):1732-1738.

53. Seitz WH Jr, Bachner EJ, Abram LJ, et al: Repair of the tibiofibular syndesmosis with a flexible implant. *J Orthop Trauma* 1991;5(1):78-82.

54. Thornes B, Shannon F, Guiney AM, Hession P, Masterson E: Suture-button syndesmosis fixation: Accelerated rehabilitation and improved outcomes. *Clin Orthop Relat Res* 2005;431:207-212.

55. Laflamme M, Belzile EL, Bédard L, van den Bekerom MP, Glazebrook M, Pelet S: A prospective randomized multicenter trial comparing clinical outcomes of patients treated surgically with a static or dynamic implant for acute ankle syndesmosis rupture. *J Orthop Trauma* 2015;29(5):216-223.

56. Naqvi GA, Cunningham P, Lynch B, Galvin R, Awan N: Fixation of ankle syndesmotic injuries: Comparison of tightrope fixation and syndesmotic screw fixation for accuracy of syndesmotic reduction. *Am J Sports Med* 2012;40(12):2828-2835.

57. Hildebrand KA, Buckley RE, Mohtadi NG, Faris P: Functional outcome measures after displaced intra-articular calcaneal fractures. *J Bone Joint Surg Br* 1996;78(1):119-123.

58. Isaacs JD, Baba M, Huang P, et al: The diagnostic accuracy of Böhler's angle in fractures of the calcaneus. *J Emerg Med* 2013;45(6):879-884.

59. Sanders R, Fortin P, DiPasquale T, Walling A: Operative treatment in 120

displaced intraarticular calcaneal fractures: Results using a prognostic computed tomography scan classification. *Clin Orthop Relat Res* 1993;290:87-95.

60. Huefner T, Thermann H, Geerling J, Pape HC, Pohlemann T: Primary subtalar arthrodesis of calcaneal fractures. *Foot Ankle Int* 2001;22(1):9-14.

61. Buch BD, Myerson MS, Miller SD: Primary subtaler arthrodesis for the treatment of comminuted calcaneal fractures. *Foot Ankle Int* 1996;17(2):61-70.

62. Thordarson DB, Krieger LE: Operative vs. nonoperative treatment of intra-articular fractures of the calcaneus: A prospective randomized trial. *Foot Ankle Int* 1996;17(1):2-9.

63. Buckley R, Tough S, McCormack R, et al: Operative compared with nonoperative treatment of displaced intra-articular calcaneal fractures: A prospective, randomized, controlled multicenter trial. *J Bone Joint Surg Am* 2002;84(10):1733-1744.

64. Randle JA, Kreder HJ, Stephen D, Williams J, Jaglal S, Hu R: Should calcaneal fractures be treated surgically? A meta-analysis. *Clin Orthop Relat Res* 2000;377:217-227.

65. Agren PH, Wretenberg P, Sayed-Noor AS: Operative versus non-operative treatment of displaced intra-articular calcaneal fractures: A prospective, randomized, controlled multicenter trial. *J Bone Joint Surg Am* 2013;95(15):1351-1357.

66. Ibrahim T, Rowsell M, Rennie W, Brown AR, Taylor GJ, Gregg PJ: Displaced intra-articular calcaneal fractures: 15-year follow-up of a randomised controlled trial of

conservative versus operative treatment. *Injury* 2007;38(7):848-855.

67. Sharr PJ, Mangupli MM, Winson IG, Buckley RE: Current management options for displaced intra-articular calcaneal fractures: Non-operative, ORIF, minimally invasive reduction and fixation or primary ORIF and subtalar arthrodesis. A contemporary review. *Foot Ankle Surg* 2016;22(1):1-8.

68. Abidi NA, Dhawan S, Gruen GS, Vogt MT, Conti SF: Wound-healing risk factors after open reduction and internal fixation of calcaneal fractures. *Foot Ankle Int* 1998;19(12):856-861.

69. Griffin D, Parsons N, Shaw E, et al: Operative versus non-operative treatment for closed, displaced, intra-articular fractures of the calcaneus: Randomised controlled trial. *BMJ* 2014;349:g4483.

70. Veltman ES, Doornberg JN, Stufkens SA, Luitse JS, van den Bekerom MP: Long-term outcomes of 1,730 calcaneal fractures: Systematic review of the literature. *J Foot Ankle Surg* 2013;52(4):486-490.

71. Al-Mudhaffar M, Prasad CV, Mofidi A: Wound complications following operative fixation of calcaneal fractures. *Injury* 2000;31(6):461-464.

72. Benirschke SK, Kramer PA: Wound healing complications in closed and open calcaneal fractures. *J Orthop Trauma* 2004;18(1):1-6.

73. Kikuchi C, Charlton TP, Thordarson DB: Limited sinus tarsi approach for intra-articular calcaneus fractures. *Foot Ankle Int* 2013;34(12):1689-1694.

74. Abdelgawad AA, Kanlic E: Minimally invasive (sinus tarsi) approach for open reduction and internal fixation

of intra-articular calcaneus fractures in children: Surgical technique and case report of two patients. *J Foot Ankle Surg* 2015;54(1):135-139.

75. Kline AJ, Anderson RB, Davis WH, Jones CP, Cohen BE: Minimally invasive technique versus an extensile lateral approach for intra-articular calcaneal fractures. *Foot Ankle Int* 2013;34(6):773-780.

76. Zwipp H, Tscherne H, Thermann H, Weber T: Osteosynthesis of displaced intraarticular fractures of the calcaneus: Results in 123 cases. *Clin Orthop Relat Res* 1993;290:76-86.

77. Raymakers JT, Dekkers GH, Brink PR: Results after operative treatment of intra-articular calcaneal fractures with a minimum follow-up of 2 years. *Injury* 1998;29(8):593-599.

78. Csizy M, Buckley R, Tough S, et al: Displaced intra-articular calcaneal fractures: Variables predicting late subtalar fusion. *J Orthop Trauma* 2003;17(2):106-112.

79. Rammelt S, Zwipp H, Schneiders W, Dürr C: Severity of injury predicts subsequent function in surgically treated displaced intraarticular calcaneal fractures. *Clin Orthop Relat Res* 2013;471(9):2885-2898.

80. Thermann H, Hüfner T, Schratt E, Held C, von Glinski S, Tscherne H: Long-term results of subtalar fusions after operative versus nonoperative treatment of os calcis fractures. *Foot Ankle Int* 1999;20(7):408-416.

81. Clare MR, Sanders RW: Open reduction and internal fixation with primary subtalar arthrodesis for Sanders type IV calcaneus fractures. *Tech Foot Ankle Surg* 2004;3(4):250-257.

Current Management of Talar Fractures

Matthew P. Sullivan, MD

Reza Firoozabadi, MD, MA

Abstract

Talar fractures are some of the most challenging injuries that orthopaedic traumatologists manage. The current knowledge of functional alterations with regard to malreduction of talar fractures is well established. Decision making with regard to timing, approach, and implant selection as well as strategies to help achieve accurate restoration of talar anatomy substantially affect outcomes and must be carefully considered. Perfect anatomic talar reconstruction should always be attempted, and orthopaedic surgeons should have a strong working knowledge of the vascular, three-dimensional, and radiographic anatomy of the talus before performing talar surgery. Almost the entire talus is surgically accessible via several approaches, all of which surgeons should be clinically familiar with to optimize reduction and fixation and safely preserve the soft-tissue envelope. Furthermore, surgeons must appreciate the plantarmedial vascular area of the talus, which must be avoided during dissection. The complication rates in patients who have talar fractures are high, particularly in those who have talar neck and talar body fractures; therefore, patients should be counseled on their expected outcome, with a specific discussion on the risk of osteonecrosis and subtalar arthritis.

Instr Course Lect 2017;66:39–49.

Talar fractures are relatively uncommon, accounting for less than 1% of all adult fractures described in the orthopaedic literature.[1-3] The overall effect that talar fractures have on an individual's quality of life continues to be substantial, and the importance of surgical management cannot be overstated. The literature heavily supports perfect surgical restoration of talar anatomy because it affects foot mechanics and clinical outcomes.

Historical Importance

Before the advent of safe, aseptic surgical technique and plain radiography, limited knowledge of the anatomy and function of the talus existed. A historical review of the literature reveals the devastating effect that talar fractures had with regard to quality of life and mortality. The first report of a patient with an open talar dislocation dates back to 1608,[2] and the earliest accessible publications that describe talar injuries, in which the authors describe fracture-dislocations that were managed with talectomy and resulted in poor outcomes, date back to the 1840s.[4,5] In 1843, Smart[4] reported an open talus fracture-dislocation in a 50-year-old man who sustained a farm injury. The author managed the open talus fracture-dislocation with talectomy, and the patient died from sepsis within 6 days postinjury.

More than 100 years after Smart's[4] case report, the first modern, scientific work on traumatic talar injuries was published.[2] Coltart's[2] experience as a surgeon in the Royal Air Force during World War II provided readers with a unique perspective on

Dr. Firoozabadi or an immediate family member serves as a paid consultant to or is an employee of Smith & Nephew. Neither Dr. Sullivan nor any immediate family member has received anything of value from or has stock or stock options held in a commercial company or institution related directly or indirectly to the subject of this chapter.

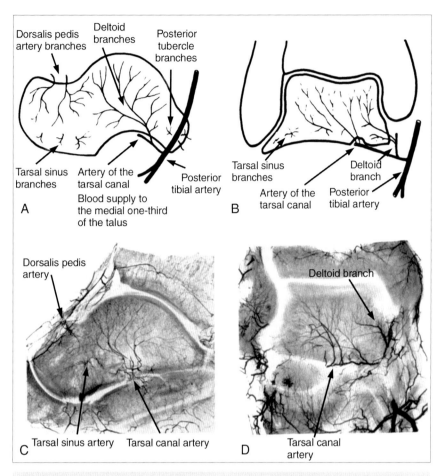

Figure 1   Images show talar blood flow. Sagittal (**A**) and coronal (**B**) view illustrations show blood flow to the talus. Sagittal (**C**) and coronal (**D**) histologic injection images show peri-talar vasculature. (Reproduced with permission from Mulfinger GL, Trueta J: The blood supply of the talus. *J Bone Joint Surg Br* 1970;52[1]:160-167.)

the mechanism of injury and the morphology of talar fracture-dislocations, and his case series of 228 talar injuries that were managed by surgeons in the Royal Air Force created the framework for the current understanding of talar injury patterns and pathoanatomy.

Anatomy

An understanding of talar anatomy is critical to the creation of a sound treatment plan. The talus is unique in that most of it is covered with articular cartilage, ligamentous structures, and joint capsule, and it has no muscular attachments. The talar body is

the most cephalad extent of the talus and broadly articulates with the tibial plafond, forming the ankle joint. The talar body is trapezoidal shaped and is wider anteroinferiorly than posteriorly, which makes ankle dorsiflexion inherently more stable than plantar flexion. The location of the lateral process, which is tucked between the fibula and the calcaneus, allows it to play an important role in lateral ankle stability because it not only articulates with the fibula and calcaneus but also serves as the attachment site for the lateral talocalcaneal ligament. The posterior process is composed of posteromedial and

posterolateral tubercles between which the flexor hallucis longus tendon glides. The talus intimately associates with the calcaneus via three articulations: the posterior facet joint, the middle facet joint, and the anterior facet joint. The talar neck is generally void of cartilage and bridges the talar body to the talar head. The talar head is the most anterior structure of the talus and plays an important role in midfoot-hindfoot motion as a result of its contribution to the talonavicular joint.

A discussion on the ligamentous anatomy of the talus, which is extremely complex, is beyond the scope of this chapter; however, surgeons should be familiar with the general ligamentous attachment sites to avoid unnecessary ligament damage during open reduction and internal fixation.

The vascular supply to the talus has been a topic of much investigation[6,7] (**Figure 1**). Although the vascular anatomy of the talus is quite variable from patient to patient, the talus can be divided into the talar head/neck and the talar body. The talar head/neck predominantly receives its blood supply from the medial and lateral talar branches of the dorsalis pedis artery, which enter the talus dorsomedially along the talar neck. The talar body predominantly receives its blood supply from the posterior tibial artery via the artery of the tarsal canal. The artery of the tarsal canal has medial and lateral plantar arteries as well as deltoid branches. The branches of the posterior tibial artery must be carefully protected during open talar surgery. The artery of the tarsal canal is located between the middle and posterior facets of the subtalar joint on the caudal aspect of the nonarticulating surface of the medial talar wall and must be avoided during the anteromedial approach to the talus. The artery of the sinus tarsi, which is a branch of the perforating peroneal vessel, supplies the lateral process and the inferior neck.

Biomechanics, Pathomechanics, and Mechanism of Injury

The tibiotalar and subtalar joints have highly complex geometry and biomechanics. At heel strike during normal ambulation, the hindfoot rests in a valgus position and the talonavicular and calcaneocuboid joints lie parallel to one another, which allows for substantial motion through the midtarsal joints. The opposite is true during toe-off. At toe-off during normal ambulation, the hindfoot takes on a varus position and the midtarsal and subtalar joints become rigid, which results in a long lever arm for forward propulsion. The importance of this phenomenon can be observed in patients who have talar neck varus malunion. In these patients, the hindfoot takes on a constitutively varus and supinated alignment, and the subtalar and midfoot joints remain rigid throughout the gait cycle, which likely leads to pain and posttraumatic arthrosis.[8,9] In addition to loss of motion, subtalar contact characteristics were reported to be substantially altered in simulated talar neck fractures with translational malreduction of as little as 2 mm.[10]

Pathologic forces associated with talar injuries are closely correlated with the anatomic structure that has been injured.[2,11] Talar neck fractures are the result of forced dorsiflexion, during which the anterior articular margin of the tibial plafond wedges into the nonarticular surface of the talar neck, causing a coronal plane fracture. Concomitant hindfoot inversion and forefoot adduction result in the classic pattern of dorsomedial neck comminution with or without medial malleolar fracture. Isolated lateral process fractures are uniquely observed in snowboarders (15 times more often than in the general population).[3,12] Funk et al[11] reported that lateral process injuries result from a forceful axial load with ankle dorsiflexion and hindfoot eversion, which is often observed in snowboarders as a result of a lateral fall toward the lead leg. The authors' findings refuted earlier expert opinions that the primary mechanism of injury for lateral process fractures was hindfoot inversion.[13-17]

Fracture Classification and Patterns

Talar neck fractures account for approximately one-half of all talar fractures, and talar body fractures account for approximately one-fourth to one-third of all talar fractures. Lateral process, posterior process, and talar head fractures account for the remaining talar fractures.[18]

Talar Neck and Talar Body Fractures

The Hawkins classification of talar fractures, which was modified by Canale and Kelly,[19] is the system most commonly used to classify talar neck injuries. Hawkins sought to correlate the severity of talar neck injury with a higher risk of osteonecrosis. The Hawkins classification describes vertical talar neck fractures that exit plantarly between the posterior and middle articular facets. Type I talar neck fractures are nondisplaced, without an associated dislocation. Type II talar neck fractures are displaced and have subluxation or dislocation of the posterior facet of the subtalar joint. Type III talar neck fractures are displaced and have both subtalar and tibiotalar dislocation. Frequently, the talar body shifts posteromedially between the Achilles tendon and the posterior aspect of the tibia adjacent to the tarsal tunnel neurovascular structures. Canale and Kelly[19] added a type IV injury in which a talar neck fracture is present with either a subtalar or ankle dislocation and a talonavicular joint disruption (**Figure 2**).

Talar body fractures are distinguished from talar neck fractures in that a talar body fracture extends into or posterior to the lateral process. In addition, talar body fractures are intra-articular injuries that involve both the tibiotalar and subtalar joints.

Lateral Process Fractures

As many as 40% of lateral process fractures are missed on initial presentation.[20] If a high index of suspicion for a lateral process fracture exists, advanced imaging with CT or MRI should be performed because failed diagnosis or insufficient management of a lateral process fracture can result in long-term disability, specifically subtalar arthrosis.[11,13,21] Multiple lateral process fracture classification systems exist;[11,13] however, their clinical utility appears to be limited.

Posterior Process Fractures

Posterior process fractures have received limited attention in the orthopaedic literature, and the available literature on posterior process fractures is almost entirely composed of case reports and case series.[22-25] Posterior process fractures are rare injuries that are often missed on plain radiographs. The posterior process is composed of medial and lateral tubercles; posterior process

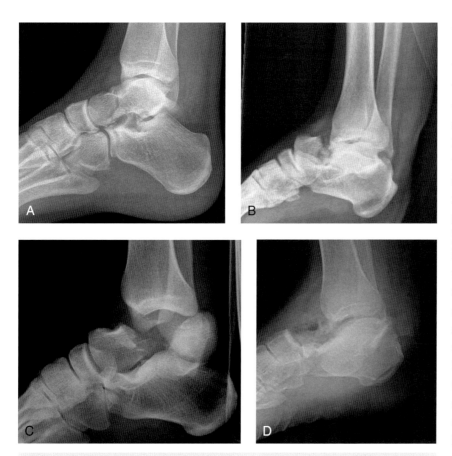

Figure 2 Lateral ankle radiographs demonstrate the Hawkins classification of talar neck fracture-dislocations. **A,** Type I nondisplaced talar neck fracture. **B,** Type II talar neck fracture with subtalar dislocation. **C,** Type III talar neck fracture with subtalar and tibiotalar dislocation. **D,** Type IV talar neck fracture with subtalar, tibiotalar, and talonavicular dislocation.

fractures most commonly involve one isolated tubercle. CT is essential in planning the surgical approach for and defining the anatomy of posterior process fractures. An os trigonum should not be mistaken for a posterior process fracture.

Extruded Talus Fractures

Extruded talus fractures, which are defined as any situation in which the talar body exits the soft-tissue envelope of the hindfoot, also have received limited attention in the literature.[26,27] Extruded talus fractures may or may not include an associated fracture of the talar neck or talar body. Likewise, the extruded component may or may not have any remaining soft-tissue attachments (ligamentous or vascular structures). Initial management of extruded talus fractures involves intravenous antibiotics and irrigation of the extruded component with successive antibacterial solutions, followed by urgent/emergent reimplantation.

Imaging

Standard imaging of the ankle, including mortise and lateral plain radiographic views, should be obtained. In addition, a Canale radiograph may better characterize the talar neck. A Canale radiograph is obtained by positioning the ankle in maximal plantar flexion and 15° of pronation and angling the x-ray 75° cephalad from the horizon (**Figure 3**). Because of the complex anatomy of the talus, a CT scan of the ankle after successful reduction is extremely helpful for surgical planning.[28-30] Advanced imaging should not be obtained in patients with an unreduced talus fracture-dislocation. A Broden radiograph is obtained to assess the subtalar joint; however, this radiographic view is less commonly obtained because of the widespread use of CT. A Broden radiograph is obtained by placing the foot on film cassette in 45° of internal rotation. The x-ray should be directed at the lateral malleolus, and images should be obtained with sequential angling of the x-ray from 10° to 40° of cephalic tilt until an accurate image of the middle facet, the posterior facet, or both facets is obtained (**Figure 4**).

Management
Nonsurgical Management
Nonsurgical and surgical indications for talar fractures can be deduced from both biomechanical and clinical studies on talar fractures. Nonsurgical management of talar neck and talar body fractures is rare because most talar fractures have some degree of malalignment or comminution. The talus poorly tolerates even the smallest amount of malalignment. In the 1980s, surgical management became the standard of care for talar fractures.[31] Pressure testing analyses of subtalar facets in cadaver models demonstrated substantial alterations in contact pressures with talar neck malalignment of as little as 2 mm,[10] and that for every 3° of varus malalignment, 1° of subtalar joint motion was lost in the coronal plane.[9] Multiple clinical studies have reported improved function in

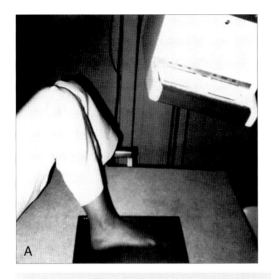
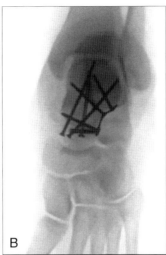

Figure 3   **A,** Photograph shows the method for obtaining a Canale radiograph of the talar neck. The ankle is pronated 15° and placed in equinus over the film cassette. The x-ray is oriented 75° cephalad. **B,** Intraoperative fluoroscopic Canale radiograph demonstrates an anatomically reduced and fixed talar neck fracture. (Reproduced with permission from Canale ST, Kelly FB Jr: Fractures of the neck of the talus: Long-term evaluation of seventy-one cases. *J Bone Joint Surg Am* 1978;60[2]:143-156.)

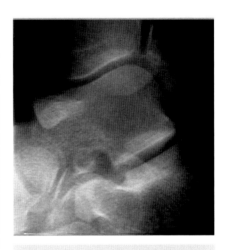

Figure 4   Intraoperative Broden radiograph of a subtalar joint.

patients who undergo open anatomic talar neck and talar body reduction compared with patients who undergo less precise reduction.[32,33] Furthermore, talar body fractures are true periarticular injuries, which warrant anatomic reduction and absolute stability fixation. Contralateral imaging can help surgeons determine the overall alignment of the talus if substantial medial and lateral comminution is present.

Surgical Management

The current literature has not determined whether an optimal time exists from injury to closed reduction or open reduction and internal fixation for talar neck fracture-dislocations with regard to preventing complications such as osteonecrosis and posttraumatic arthritis.[32-36] The general standard of care for talar neck fracture-dislocations includes an emergent attempt at closed reduction and, if closed reduction attempts are unsuccessful, urgent open reduction.[37]

Approaches

Many surgical approaches are available for open reduction of talar injuries. Because each talar fracture pattern is different, advanced imaging should be scrutinized preoperatively to identify the ideal surgical approach(s) based on the specific fracture morphology and surgeon comfort. Most talar neck, talar head, and anterior talar body fractures can be successfully accessed via a standard dual-incision technique that includes the anterolateral and anteromedial approaches.[38,39]

Anterolateral and Anteromedial Approaches

The anterolateral approach to the talus is an extension of the anterolateral approach to the ankle.[40] The skin incision is made in line with the fourth ray of the foot and is centered over the talar neck. The branches of the superficial peroneal nerve will often traverse the superficial dissection. After the deep interval made between the extensor digitorum

longus (medial) and the extensor digitorum brevis (lateral) is traversed, the joint capsule that overlies the talar neck will be immediately apparent. The joint capsule should be incised sharply and thoroughly débrided off the talar neck to allow for adequate visualization of the fracture. The surgeon can follow the lateral talar neck plantar into the sinus tarsi and posterolaterally around the lateral process.

The skin incision for the anteromedial approach to the talus is made between the tip of the medial malleolus and the base of the first metatarsal and is centered between the tibialis posterior tendon and the tibialis anterior tendon. After dissection through the superficial interval, the joint capsule that overlies the medial neck will be immediately apparent. The joint capsule should be traversed sharply and débrided proximally, distally, and dorsally to allow for adequate visualization of the fracture. The surgeon must avoid plantar dissection along the medial talar neck because it is the location of the talar body vascular supply.

The authors of this chapter advocate for reduction and fixation of talar

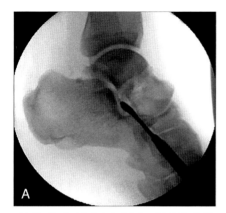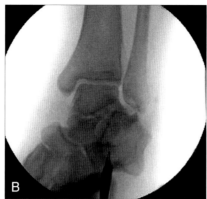

Figure 5 Lateral (**A**) and AP (**B**) fluoroscopic images of an ankle show the sinus tarsi approach for management of a talar injury. Note that the incision is centered over the lateral aspect of the subtalar joint in the immediate vicinity of the lateral process.

neck fractures via both the anterolateral and anteromedial approaches simultaneously. Surgeons should avoid performing reduction via only one of the two approaches because it can result in malalignment.

Posteromedial Approach

The posteromedial approach to the talus is extremely versatile and can be performed with the patient positioned supine with the surgical leg placed in a figure-of-4 or prone position. The surgeon must confirm that the ipsilateral hip has enough external rotation capacity to allow for supine positioning. The skin incision should be made just off the posteromedial border of the tibia and gently curve anterior at the tip of the medial malleolus. The value of the posteromedial approach lies in the use of multiple deep intervals, which allow the surgeon to see almost completely around to the lateral aspect of the ankle, depending on the fracture pattern. If the fracture pattern requires an interval posterior to the posterior tibial tendon, the tarsal tunnel should be opened, and the posterior tibial neurovascular bundle should be identified and protected.

The creation of a deep interval between the flexor hallucis longus and the neurovascular bundle allows for visualization of almost all of the posterior talar body. Alternatively, the patient can be positioned prone, and the incision can be made just off the medial border of the Achilles tendon with the creation of a deep interval between the Achilles tendon and the flexor hallucis longus. Both supine and prone positioning allow for excellent visualization of the posterior talar body and the posterior process.

Posterolateral Approach

The posterolateral approach to the talus requires prone positioning of the patient and is an extension of the posterolateral approach to the ankle. The skin incision is made between the Achilles tendon and the posterolateral border of the fibula. Deep dissection traverses the interval between the peroneal tendons and the flexor hallucis longus.

Sinus Tarsi Approach

The sinus tarsi approach to the talus can be used if the lateral process and subtalar joints need to be well visualized. The skin incision for the sinus tarsi

approach is made approximately 2 cm plantar and parallel to the skin incision for the anterolateral approach. The sinus tarsi approach should be visualized fluoroscopically before the incision is made. A deep interval is made just lateral to the flexor digitorum brevis (**Figure 5**). The sinus tarsi approach does not allow for adequate visualization of the anterolateral talar neck.

Medial Malleolar Osteotomy

The use of medial malleolar osteotomy is well described but infrequently used for the management of talar fractures. The anteromedial approach is carried proximal to the medial malleolus. The authors of this chapter find it most effective to predrill and then place and remove definitive fixation (3.5-mm cortical or cannulated screws) before performing the osteotomy. The osteotomy should be created perpendicular to the orientation of the fixation screws and enter the ankle at the anteromedial shoulder of the tibial plafond. In a fashion similar to that of an olecranon osteotomy, a microsagittal saw should be used for approximately 75% of the osteotomy, which is then completed with the use of an osteotome.

Fixation Strategies
Talar Neck Fractures

Talar neck fracture-dislocations are challenging injuries. In Hawkins type III and type IV fracture patterns, the talar body often dislocates posteromedially out of the ankle joint and into the space between the posteromedial border of the tibia and the Achilles tendon and is usually buttonholed between the flexor tendons. Hawkins type III and type IV fracture patterns are almost impossible to reduce in a closed manner without the use of general anesthesia with complete paralysis. Plantar flexion of the patient's foot will relax the flexor tendons and may reduce the talar body back into the ankle joint. If a closed reduction attempt in the operating room is unsuccessful, medial and lateral distractors with pins placed in the calcaneus and tibia should be applied, and a dual-incision approach will need to be performed.

An understanding of the common morphology and pitfalls of talar neck fractures will help surgeons prevent malreduction. Classic talar neck and very anterior talar body fracture patterns involve lateral tension failure and dorsomedial compression failure with comminution, which can result in a varus deformity.

Multiple intraoperative tools can be used to assess talar neck reduction. Because of the circumferential nature of talar neck fractures, surgeons should never be confident with regard to a talar neck reduction before both the anteromedial and anterolateral approaches are fully laid out. In general, a cortical read will be present at the location that the talar neck failed in tension, which can help establish length. After length is established, talar neck alignment may be assessed fluoroscopically. On both AP and lateral fluoroscopic views, the body-neck axis of the talus should be in line with the first metatarsal. In addition, all subtalar facets should be congruent (**Figure 6**). Provisional fixation is achieved with the use of modified pointed reduction clamps and Kirschner wires. Talar neck and anterior talar body fractures should be definitively fixed with 2.0- to 2.7-mm implants. A nonlocking 2.0-mm flexible plate, which provides excellent fixation transversely across the talar head and posteriorly into the

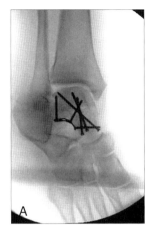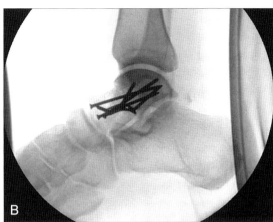

Figure 6   AP (**A**) and lateral (**B**) fluoroscopic images of an ankle show intraoperative assessment of talar neck reduction. On both AP and lateral views, the body-neck axis of the talus is in line with the first ray. The lateral view demonstrates concentrically reduced middle and posterior subtalar facets.

dense bone of the posterior process, can be aggressively contoured to 90° and applied from the lateral talar neck to the lateral process. Typically, the medial talar neck is transfixed with the use of anterior-to-posterior positional screws that are countersunk into the cartilage of the talar head; however, some talar fractures may have enough room on the medial talar neck for plate fixation. Surgeons should be extremely careful to not compress across comminution during medial talar neck fixation, which can result in a varus malreduction.

A mechanical analysis reported better load-to-failure for two posterior-to-anterior 4.0-mm partially threaded lag screws compared with traditional lateral 2.0-mm plating and a single medial anterior-to-posterior 2.7-mm screw.[41] The main disadvantage of the posterior-to-anterior screw technique is that anatomic reduction of the talar neck is impossible via a posterior approach and, in many patients, symmetric compression across the talar fracture will result in an unacceptable angular deformity. Therefore, the authors of this chapter recommend that talar neck

fractures be managed with the use of a dual anterior incision approach that allows for direct visualization of the fracture.

Talar Body Fractures
Simple sagittally oriented talar body fractures can be managed via a single anterior-based approach in which plantar flexion of the foot allows for visualization of much of the talar body.[35] Occasionally, a medial malleolar osteotomy may be required to place medial-to-lateral lag screws across the fracture. In general, posterior talar body and posterior process injuries require the use of a posterior approach. Flexion of the knee and dorsiflexion of the ankle as well as the use of a commercially available distractor or external fixator can help provide adequate visualization of a fracture fixed via a posterior approach (**Figure 7**).

In a study on the mechanical stability of talar fixation, Swanson et al[42] reported that posterior-to-anterior independent screw fixation was more mechanically sound compared with anterior-to-posterior screw

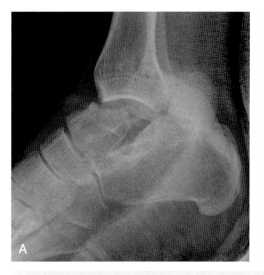 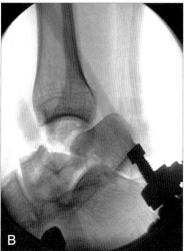 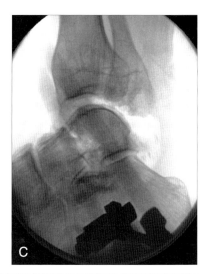

Figure 7 **A,** Lateral ankle radiograph demonstrates a type III Hawkins fracture-dislocation that failed initial closed reduction. Final reduction required general endotracheal anesthesia with complete muscle paralysis. **B** and **C,** Lateral fluoroscopic images of the ankle show that medial and lateral distraction was obtained via a transcalcaneal and anterior external fixator and a 5-mm threaded pin with the knee in flexion to reduce the posteromedially dislocated talus.

fixation; the authors of this chapter have found this to be most true for posterior talar body fractures. 2.0-mm flexible plates are a good option for fixation of posterior talar body fractures, if amenable, because they can be placed plantar to the articular surface of the posterior talar body with screws directed perpendicular to the fracture plane (**Figure 8**).

Occasionally, osteochondral body fragments may be free floating, and great measures should be taken to preserve these fragments. An attempt should be made to interdigitate any remaining subchondral bone into its parent location. The tibial plafond will serve as a template during the healing phase if fixation cannot be attained through the fragment. Bone loss in the talar neck and talar body should be addressed with the use of allograft. Tricortical, structural allograft can be fashioned into a wedge to address angular deformity in patients who have severe talar neck bone loss (**Figure 9**).

Lateral Process Fractures

Management of lateral process fractures is essential because the lateral process plays an important role in ankle stability. In addition, lateral process fractures may be associated with debris in the posterior facet of the subtalar joint. Lateral process fractures can be managed via the anterolateral approach as well as the sinus tarsi approach. Standard 2.0-mm lateral plating is frequently acceptable for fixation of lateral process fractures (**Figure 10**).

Postoperative Management

Talar injuries may be associated with considerable soft-tissue trauma; therefore, great care should be taken to avoid iatrogenic soft-tissue damage. The authors of this chapter close the talar neck capsule and then close the skin with 3-0 nylon suture that is sequentially tied using the Allgöwer-Donati suture technique. Patients are fitted with a splint and remain non–weight bearing for 10 to 12 weeks postoperatively, after

which they are gradually returned to full weight bearing.

Outcomes and Complications

Posttraumatic arthrosis is the most common sequela of talar fractures.[19,31,34,36,43] Reported rates of subtalar and tibiotalar arthrosis vary greatly in the literature and range from 40% to 90% in patients who have talar neck and/or talar body fractures.[19,33,35,43] Although the literature varies greatly with regard to which talar joint is most commonly affected by arthrosis, two recent systematic reviews, each of which included more than 900 patients who had talar neck fractures, suggested that arthrosis most commonly develops in the subtalar joint.[31,34] Arthrosis is uncommon in the talonavicular joint. The presence of an open talar injury appears to be associated with the development of posttraumatic arthrosis.[43]

Numerous published studies have described osteonecrosis rates in relation to the Hawkins classification of talar fractures.[19,34,35,44] Almost all of these studies include fewer than 100 patients (some include far fewer), which makes determining the actual risk for osteonecrosis difficult. Two recent systematic reviews, each of which included more than 900 patients who had talar neck fractures, reported osteonecrosis rates as follows: 5.7% to 8% in patients who had type I talar neck fractures, 18.4% to 21% in patients who had type II talar neck fractures, 45% in patients who had type III talar neck fractures, and 12.1% to 36% in patients who had type IV talar neck fractures.[31,34] Vallier et al[36] modified the Hawkins classification of talar fractures to distinguish between subluxated (type IIA) and dislocated (type IIB) subtalar joint fractures. Interestingly, the authors noted considerable protection from osteonecrosis in patients who had preservation (type I) and relative preservation (type IIA) of the subtalar joint. The authors reported no osteonecrosis in all patients who had type I and type IIA fracture patterns but reported a 25% osteonecrosis rate in patients who had type IIB fracture patterns (subtalar dislocation). One hypothesis for this finding is that the medial and lateral branches of the artery of the tarsal canal in patients who have type IIA and type IIB displaced talar neck fractures are likely disrupted; however, relative preservation of the subtalar joint (type IIA) allows the deltoid branch to remain viable, which protects the talar body from osteonecrosis.[45] Concomitant talar head and talar body fractures result in the highest rate of osteonecrosis (>50%).[43] The development of osteonecrosis substantially affects functional outcomes as well as increases the risk for a required secondary reconstructive procedure.[32]

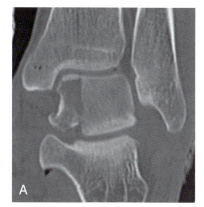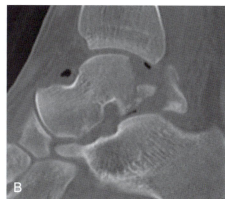
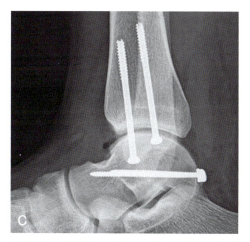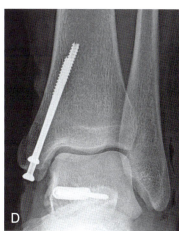

Figure 8   Coronal (**A**) and sagittal (**B**) CT scans of an ankle demonstrate a posteromedial talar body fracture. Lateral (**C**) and AP (**D**) ankle radiographs demonstrate posterior-to-anterior fixation plantar to the articular surface of the talar body. Both talar and medial malleolar fixation was applied through the same posteromedial incision.

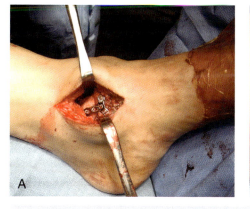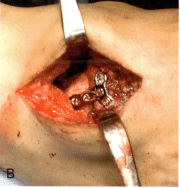

Figure 9   **A**, Intraoperative photograph of an ankle shows a tricortical iliac crest bone graft, which was used as a structural graft to gain length in an area of bone loss and comminution, via the anteromedial approach. **B**, Intraoperative photograph of the same ankle shown in panel **A** shows a close-up view of the allograft.

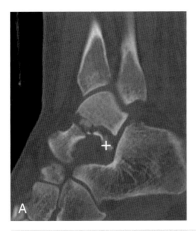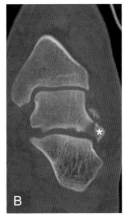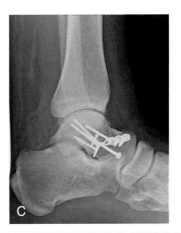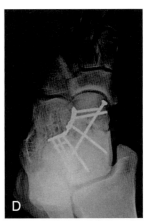

Figure 10 Images show a talar neck fracture with a concomitant lateral process fracture. Coronal (**A**) and sagittal (**B**) CT scans of an ankle demonstrate debris in the subtalar joint (+) and lateral process comminution (*). This fracture pattern demonstrates an excellent example of the utility of a dual-incision approach (the anteromedial approach and the sinus tarsi approach). Lateral (**C**) and AP (**D**) radiographs demonstrate lateral process stabilization via an aggressively contoured 2.4-mm T-plate.

The Hawkins sign has long been an area of radiographic interest. The Hawkins sign is an area of subchondral lucency that is appreciated on both AP and lateral plain radiographs of the talus that are taken between 6 and 8 weeks postoperatively. In general, the Hawkins sign is considered a favorable sign of talar vascularity; however, its absence does not reliably predict osteonecrosis, and its presence does not guarantee that osteonecrosis will not develop.[32,38]

Revascularization is an important process to consider in counseling patients on the prognosis of their talar injury. Coltart,[2] whose work dates back to the 1950s, reported that complete revascularization after posttraumatic osteonecrosis occurred between 16 and 34 weeks postinjury. Revascularization in patients without collapse occurs at a rate close to 40% to 50% and within 9 to 12 months postinjury.[35,36,43]

Anatomic reduction and alignment is likely the most important surgeon-controlled factor that influences the functional outcomes of patients who undergo treatment for talar neck factures. Varus malalignment substantially affects both joint-specific and general functional outcomes.[32,33] Surgeons must scrutinize intraoperative fluoroscopic images for malalignment before leaving the operating room.

Nonunion is an infrequent complication in patients who undergo treatment for talar fractures. Nonunion rates of approximately 5% to 10% have been reported in the literature, with risk factors for nonunion being open fracture and poor surgical reduction.[32,34]

Summary

Talar fractures have received considerable attention in the orthopaedic literature in the past two to three decades. Talar fractures are challenging injuries because the anatomy of the talus is complex, their management requires a high surgeon skill level, and complication rates, particularly for subtalar arthrosis and osteonecrosis, are extremely high. Many factors affect the outcomes of patients who have talar fractures. Although some of these factors cannot be controlled, surgeons have the ability to influence patients' functional return by accurately restoring anatomy, which, in turn, restores the normal biomechanics of the hindfoot.

References

1. Court-Brown CM, Caesar B: Epidemiology of adult fractures: A review. *Injury* 2006;37(8):691-697.

2. Coltart WD: Aviator's astragalus. *J Bone Joint Surg Br* 1952;34(4):545-566.

3. Vlahovich AT, Mehin R, O'Brien PJ: An unusual fracture of the talus in a snowboarder. *J Orthop Trauma* 2005;19(7):498-500.

4. Smart TW: Compound dislocation of the astragalus. *Prov Med J Retrosp Med Sci* 1843;6(153):470-471.

5. Spry EJ: Case of simple fracture and dislocation of the greater portion of the right astragalus, forwards and outwards. *Prov Med Surg J* 1847;11(17):456-458.

6. Mulfinger GL, Trueta J: The blood supply of the talus. *J Bone Joint Surg Br* 1970;52(1):160-167.

7. Gelberman RH, Mortensen WW: The arterial anatomy of the talus. *Foot Ankle* 1983;4(2):64-72.

8. Sproule JA, Glazebrook MA, Younger AS: Varus hindfoot deformity

after talar fracture. *Foot Ankle Clin* 2012;17(1):117-125.

9. Daniels TR, Smith JW, Ross TI: Varus malalignment of the talar neck: Its effect on the position of the foot and on subtalar motion. *J Bone Joint Surg Am* 1996;78(10):1559-1567.

10. Sangeorzan BJ, Wagner UA, Harrington RM, Tencer AF: Contact characteristics of the subtalar joint: The effect of talar neck misalignment. *J Orthop Res* 1992;10(4):544-551.

11. Funk JR, Srinivasan SC, Crandall JR: Snowboarder's talus fractures experimentally produced by eversion and dorsiflexion. *Am J Sports Med* 2003;31(6):921-928.

12. Kirkpatrick DP, Hunter RE, Janes PC, Mastrangelo J, Nicholas RA: The snowboarder's foot and ankle. *Am J Sports Med* 1998;26(2):271-277.

13. Hawkins LG: Fracture of the lateral process of the talus. *J Bone Joint Surg Am* 1965;47:1170-1175.

14. Cantrell MW, Tarquinio TA: Fracture of the lateral process of the talus. *Orthopedics* 2000;23(1):55-58.

15. Fjeldborg O: Fracture of the lateral process of the talus: Supination-dorsal flexion fracture. *Acta Orthop Scand* 1968;39(3):407-412.

16. McCrory P, Bladin C: Fractures of the lateral process of the talus: A clinical review. "Snowboarder's ankle". *Clin J Sport Med* 1996;6(2):124-128.

17. Heckman JD, McLean MR: Fractures of the lateral process of the talus. *Clin Orthop Relat Res* 1985;199:108-113.

18. Browner BD, Jupiter JB, Krettek C, Anderson PA: *Skeletal Trauma: Basic Science, Management, and Reconstruction,* ed 5. Philadelphia, PA, Saunders, 2014.

19. Canale ST, Kelly FB Jr: Fractures of the neck of the talus: Long-term evaluation of seventy-one cases. *J Bone Joint Surg Am* 1978;60(2):143-156.

20. Mills HJ, Horne G: Fractures of the lateral process of the talus. *Aust N Z J Surg* 1987;57(9):643-646.

21. Ebraheim NA, Skie MC, Podeszwa DA, Jackson WT: Evaluation of process fractures of the talus using computed tomography. *J Orthop Trauma* 1994;8(4):332-337.

22. Mehrpour SR, Aghamirsalim MR, Sheshvan MK, Sorbi R: Entire posterior process talus fracture: A report of two cases. *J Foot Ankle Surg* 2012;51(3):326-329.

23. Iyakutty PP, Singaravadivelu V: Fracture of the entire posterior process of the talus: A case report. *J Foot Ankle Surg* 2000;39(3):198-201.

24. Nasser S, Manoli A II: Fracture of the entire posterior process of the talus: A case report. *Foot Ankle* 1990;10(4):235-238.

25. Chen YJ, Hsu RW, Shih HN, Huang TJ: Fracture of the entire posterior process of talus associated with subtalar dislocation: A case report. *Foot Ankle Int* 1996;17(4):226-229.

26. Smith CS, Nork SE, Sangeorzan BJ: The extruded talus: Results of reimplantation. *J Bone Joint Surg Am* 2006;88(11):2418-2424.

27. Marsh JL, Saltzman CL, Iverson M, Shapiro DS: Major open injuries of the talus. *J Orthop Trauma* 1995;9(5):371-376.

28. He F, Huang H, Deng YM, et al: Application of spiral CT image 3D reconstruction in severe talar neck fracture. *Chin J Traumatol* 2007;10(1):18-22.

29. Haapamaki VV, Kiuru MJ, Koskinen SK: Ankle and foot injuries: Analysis of MDCT findings. *AJR Am J Roentgenol* 2004;183(3):615-622.

30. Shi Z, Zou J, Yi X: Posteromedial approach in treatment of talar posterior process fractures. *J Invest Surg* 2013;26(4):204-209.

31. Dodd A, Lefaivre KA: Outcomes of talar neck fractures: A systematic review and meta-analysis. *J Orthop Trauma* 2015;29(5):210-215.

32. Lindvall E, Haidukewych G, DiPasquale T, Herscovici D Jr, Sanders R: Open reduction and stable fixation of isolated, displaced talar neck and body fractures. *J Bone Joint Surg Am* 2004;86(10):2229-2234.

33. Sanders DW, Busam M, Hattwick E, Edwards JR, McAndrew MP, Johnson KD: Functional outcomes following displaced talar neck fractures. *J Orthop Trauma* 2004;18(5):265-270.

34. Halvorson JJ, Winter SB, Teasdall RD, Scott AT: Talar neck fractures:

A systematic review of the literature. *J Foot Ankle Surg* 2013;52(1):56-61.

35. Vallier HA, Nork SE, Barei DP, Benirschke SK, Sangeorzan BJ: Talar neck fractures: Results and outcomes. *J Bone Joint Surg Am* 2004;86(8):1616-1624.

36. Vallier HA, Reichard SG, Boyd AJ, Moore TA: A new look at the Hawkins classification for talar neck fractures: Which features of injury and treatment are predictive of osteonecrosis? *J Bone Joint Surg Am* 2014;96(3):192-197.

37. Patel R, Van Bergeyk A, Pinney S: Are displaced talar neck fractures surgical emergencies? A survey of orthopaedic trauma experts. *Foot Ankle Int* 2005;26(5):378-381.

38. Mayo KA: Fractures of the talus: Principles of management and techniques of treatment. *Tech Orthop* 1987;2(3):42-54.

39. Vallier HA, Nork SE, Benirschke SK, Sangeorzan BJ: Surgical treatment of talar body fractures. *J Bone Joint Surg Am* 2004; 86(pt 2, suppl 1):180-192.

40. Mehta S, Gardner MJ, Barei DP, Benirschke SK, Nork SE: Reduction strategies through the anterolateral exposure for fixation of type B and C pilon fractures. *J Orthop Trauma* 2011;25(2):116-122.

41. Charlson MD, Parks BG, Weber TG, Guyton GP: Comparison of plate and screw fixation and screw fixation alone in a comminuted talar neck fracture model. *Foot Ankle Int* 2006;27(5):340-343.

42. Swanson TV, Bray TJ, Holmes GB Jr: Fractures of the talar neck: A mechanical study of fixation. *J Bone Joint Surg Am* 1992;74(4):544-551.

43. Vallier HA, Nork SE, Benirschke SK, Sangeorzan BJ: Surgical treatment of talar body fractures. *J Bone Joint Surg Am* 2003;85(9):1716-1724.

44. Hawkins LG: Fractures of the neck of the talus. *J Bone Joint Surg Am* 1970;52(5):991-1002.

45. Alton T, Patton DJ, Gee AO: Classifications in brief: The Hawkins Classification for talus fractures. *Clin Orthop Relat Res* 2015;473(9):3046-3049.

4

Fractures of the Calcaneus

Mark R. Adams, MD
John W. Munz, MD
Kenneth L. Koury, MD

Abstract

Calcaneal fractures are potentially devastating injuries. To effectively manage calcaneal fractures, surgeons must understand the anatomy of the calcaneus as well as the surgical techniques necessary to restore normal biomechanics of the foot. Surgeons also must understand calcaneal fracture patterns and classifications; initial management techniques, surgical indications and rationale, temporizing management techniques, surgical approaches, definitive management techniques, and postoperative management for calcaneal fractures; as well as outcomes and common complications of calcaneal fractures.

Instr Course Lect 2017;66:51–61.

Calcaneal fractures are relatively rare injuries, with an estimated annual incidence of 11.5 per 100,000 injuries.[1] Calcaneal fractures represent approximately 1% to 2% of all fractures that occur each year. Regardless, an increased interest in calcaneal fracture management exists because calcaneal fractures are complex, life-altering injuries that are difficult to manage. In the past 20 to 30 years, orthopaedic surgeons have attempted to improve surgical techniques for the management of displaced calcaneal fractures to help minimize the devastating and economic effects of these severe injuries on patients and society, respectively.[2-7] Increased attention to the calcaneus has resulted in new calcaneal fracture classifications, new methods via which appropriate surgical candidates are selected, and modified surgical approaches.[8-11] Surgeons must understand the anatomy and biomechanics of the calcaneus; calcaneal fracture patterns and classifications; initial management techniques, surgical indications and rationale, temporizing management techniques, surgical approaches, definitive management techniques, and postoperative management for calcaneal fractures; as well as outcomes and common complications of calcaneal fractures.

Anatomy and Biomechanics

The calcaneus is the largest tarsal bone and has a unique and complex morphology, which can be observed by the posterior tuberosity, the medial sustentaculum tali, and the anterior and superior articulations. The calcaneus plays a critical role in weight bearing because it is included in the longitudinal arch and the lateral column of the foot, and because it is the site of the plantar fascia and the triceps surae attachments. The calcaneus has four articulations: calcaneocuboid, anterior facet, middle facet, and posterior facet (**Figure 1**). The calcaneus articulates with the cuboid at the anteriormost aspect of the anterior process, which forms a connection with the lateral column of the foot. The anterior, middle, and posterior facets on the anterosuperior portion of the calcaneus articulate with similarly named

Dr. Munz or an immediate family member is a member of a speakers' bureau or has made paid presentations on behalf of Synthes. Neither of the following authors nor any immediate family member has received anything of value from or has stock or stock options held in a commercial company or institution related directly or indirectly to the subject of this chapter: Dr. Adams and Dr. Koury.

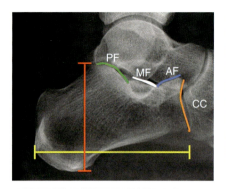

Figure 1 Lateral radiograph of a calcaneus demonstrates normal anatomy. Height (red line) is measured from the superiormost aspect of the posterior facet (PF; green line) to the plantarmost aspect of the tuberosity. Length (yellow line) is measured from the posteriormost aspect of the tuberosity to the anteriormost aspect of the anterior process at the calcaneocuboid (CC; orange line) joint. AF = anterior facet (blue line), MF = middle facet (white line).

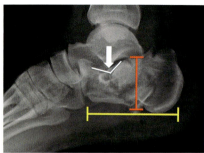

Figure 2 Lateral radiograph of a calcaneus demonstrates a joint depression fracture with loss of height (red line), loss of length (yellow line), and depression of the subtalar joint with talar impingement (arrow and white lines).

facets on the talus to form the subtalar joint. The anterior and middle facets of the calcaneus may coalesce to form one articulation or remain two distinct articulations at the superior aspect of the sustentaculum tali. The posterior facet is the largest of the three facets and functions as the primary weight-bearing articulation. The surface of the posterior facet is convex, which creates a dome on the calcaneal side of the joint.

The calcaneus is an important site of muscular and ligamentous attachments. The tuberosity is the site of the triceps surae and the plantar fascia attachments. The Achilles tendon inserts into the calcaneus posteriorly and inferiorly. The Achilles tendon attachment is continuous with the plantar fascia attachment. The height of the calcaneus, which is measured from superior to inferior on a lateral radiograph of the foot, is an important component

of lever arm function, which affects the function of the gastrocnemius-soleus complex. Ligamentous attachments that are located medial to the sustentaculum tali include the superomedial spring ligament, which is an important stabilizer of the longitudinal arch, and the tibiocalcaneal portion of the deltoid ligament. The calcaneofibular ligament attaches to the calcaneus laterally and contributes to ankle stability.[12,13]

Several relevant soft-tissue structures that course near the calcaneus are important to consider in the management of calcaneal fractures.[12,13] The peroneal tendons course along the lateral wall of the calcaneus and can become impinged in patients who sustain lateral wall blowout. The sural nerve and the arterial blood supply to the skin on the lateral heel, which also course along the lateral wall of the calcaneus, are important structures to consider during the extensile lateral approach to the calcaneus. Medially, the flexor hallucis longus courses inferior to the sustentaculum tali, which makes it susceptible to tethering on screws that are placed lateral to medial during fixation.

The shape of the calcaneus contributes to the biomechanics of the foot; therefore, disruption of calcaneal anatomy can alter the biomechanics of foot. The height of the calcaneus is measured on a lateral radiograph from the superior aspect of the posterior facet to the inferior border of the calcaneus (**Figure 1**). Loss of calcaneal height can lead to a diminished gastrocnemius-soleus complex lever arm and, subsequently, anterior tibiotalar impingement. Similarly, loss of calcaneal length, which is measured from anterior to posterior, can lead to shortening of the lateral column and, subsequently, forefoot abduction, pes planus, and talar impingement[14] (**Figure 2**). Conversely, calcaneal fractures can lead to calcaneal widening from medial to lateral (**Figures 3** and **4**) and, subsequently, peroneal irritation, calcaneofibular ligament abutment, sural nerve entrapment, and difficulties with normal shoe wear. Posterior facet displacement and step-off can lead to subtalar arthrosis.

Fracture Patterns and Classifications

Typically, calcaneal fractures result from axial loading of the calcaneus that is caused by either a fall from height or a high-speed motor vehicle accident.[15] The primary fracture line begins at the lateral aspect of the sinus tarsi, runs across the posterior facet, and exits the medial wall posterior to the sustentaculum tali. Thus, the calcaneus is separated into two fragments: anteromedial and posterolateral. The posterolateral fragment consists of the tuberosity, the lateral portion of the posterior facet, and the lateral wall. The anteromedial fragment consists of the medial portion of the posterior facet, the sustentaculum tali, and the middle and anterior facets. Typically, the sustentaculum tali retains its relationship with the talus; therefore, it is considered the constant fragment.

Essex-Lopresti[15] categorized calcaneal fractures into two subtypes based on the orientation of the secondary fracture line. Joint depression-type calcaneal fractures result from more posterior axial loading of the calcaneus, which causes a secondary fracture that separates the tuberosity from the posterior facet. Conversely, tongue-type calcaneal fractures result from a more anterior and inferior force, which causes a secondary fracture that separates the tuberosity without disrupting the posterior facet or the superior portion of the tuberosity.[15-17]

Secondary fractures in the anterior process that extend into the calcaneocuboid joint also may exist. Typically, the anterolateral fragment is displaced dorsally into the sinus tarsi as the foot pronates during impact. Shortening of calcaneal height and length as well as a corresponding increase in calcaneal width occur as a result of the secondary fracture that separates the posterior facet and the tuberosity. In addition, displacement of the tuberosity as an intact unit results in varus deformity of the calcaneus.

Tongue-type calcaneal fractures have a distinct split in the tuberosity fragment, which causes superior displacement of the superior portion of the tuberosity as a result of the pull of the Achilles tendon. Surgeons must recognize superior displacement of the tuberosity, which creates an area of focal pressure on the skin and may lead to erosion. Timely recognition and urgent management of tongue-type calcaneal fractures can help minimize soft-tissue complications.[18]

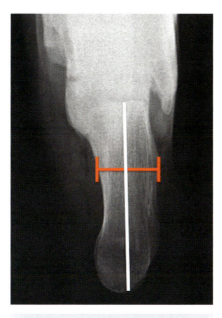

Figure 3 Axial heel radiograph of a calcaneus demonstrates normal anatomy. Calcaneal width (red line) is measured from medial to lateral. Varus and valgus (white line) are based on the angulation of the tuberosity relative to the subtalar joint.

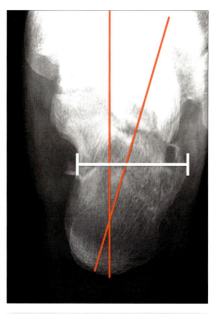

Figure 4 Axial heel radiograph of a calcaneus demonstrates a calcaneal fracture with calcaneal widening (white line) and varus deformity (red lines).

Measurements made on lateral radiographs of the calcaneus can be used to assess the amount of joint depression. The Böhler angle is the angle formed by a line drawn between the superiormost aspect of the anterior process and the posterior facet and a line drawn along the superior border of the tuberosity on a lateral radiograph. Typically, a normal Böhler angle ranges from 20° to 40°; a decreased Böhler angle indicates posterior facet displacement and a loss of overall calcaneal height.[19] The angle of Gissane is the angle drawn between the two cortical columns that are inferior to the lateral process of the talus on a lateral radiograph, which correlates with the sinus tarsi. Typically, a normal angle of Gissane ranges from 95° to 110°; an increased angle of Gissane correlates with posterior facet displacement.[20]

Studies have attempted to further classify calcaneal fractures based on the amount and location of posterior facet comminution observed on CT scans.[6,8,21] The benefit of this further classification of calcaneal fractures is a subject of debate.[2,22] However, axial, coronal, and sagittal CT scans allow surgeons to further assess the calcaneal fracture pattern, which aids in planning surgical treatment.[23]

Initial Management Techniques

The initial management of calcaneal fractures is critical to overall patient outcomes. The primary focus of the initial management of calcaneal fractures involves minimization of soft-tissue insult and optimization of the patient for definitive treatment. The secondary focus of the initial management of calcaneal fractures involves obtaining patient information and imaging studies necessary for definitive surgical treatment.

In patients with both joint depression-type and tongue-type calcaneal fractures, soft-tissue management is essential to achieve good outcomes. Patients with joint depression-type calcaneal fractures rarely have soft-tissue injury that requires early surgical management unless an open calcaneal fracture is present. Patients who have open calcaneal fractures, which typically occur medially, require emergent antibiotics, assessment for tetanus, urgent débridement, irrigation, and temporary fixation.[24,25] Patients with open calcaneal fractures have an increased risk for foot compartment syndrome, specifically in the calcaneal compartment, as a result of bleeding in the tight fascial envelope. Therefore, surgeons should have a heightened awareness for foot compartment syndrome in patients with open calcaneal fractures because these patients may require acute compartment release.[26,27]

In most patients who have calcaneal fractures, initial management consists of the application of a layered compression wrap, after which a splint is applied to help minimize the anticipated swelling associated with calcaneal fractures. Patience with regard to the soft tissues is essential, especially in patients who have lateral skin blistering.[28,29] Surgeons must wait for swelling to subside, which may take several weeks, before open reduction is considered. The use of a medially-based external fixator to help stabilize the calcaneus and skin in patients who have severe calcaneal fractures is discussed later.

Patients who have tongue-type calcaneal fractures may require urgent treatment to prevent catastrophic soft-tissue injury.[18] The superior displacement of the tuberosity from the pull of the Achilles tendon can lead to posterior heel skin erosion. Therefore, patients who have tongue-type calcaneal fractures must be evaluated and treated with urgent, percutaneous reduction to prevent soft-tissue compromise.[18] If urgent, percutaneous reduction is not performed, swelling control and careful attention to padding of the heel are prudent. Splinting of the foot in equinus is beneficial in patients who have tongue-type calcaneal fractures because forced dorsiflexion can increase the risk for posterior heel skin erosion.

In addition to an evaluation of the foot and ankle for potentially emergent and urgent injuries, surgeons also must evaluate patients who have calcaneal fractures for injuries that are commonly associated with axial loading, such as ipsilateral and contralateral talar, tibial plafond, tibial plateau, pelvis, and lumbar spine injuries. Surgeons may overlook associated injuries in patients who have calcaneal fractures because of the severity of injury and pain in the hindfoot.[1,30,31]

Radiographs and CT scans should be obtained in patients with joint depression-type and tongue-type calcaneal fractures. As previously discussed, lateral radiographs are necessary to determine the calcaneal fracture subtype as well as to evaluate the severity of calcaneal deformity and posterior facet displacement. Harris heel radiographs allow surgeons to assess displacement of the tuberosity, increased width of the heel, and varus deformity. Broden radiographs also allow surgeons to assess posterior facet displacement.[32] Multiple radiographic views aid in the initial evaluation of patients who have calcaneal fractures and, more importantly, can be compared against radiographs obtained postoperatively. CT scans of the calcaneus allow surgeons to assess the number of fracture fragments as well as displacement, which aids in planning surgical treatment.

Surgeons should evaluate if patients with calcaneal fractures are appropriate surgical candidates before open reduction is considered. Buckley et al[9] and Tufescu and Buckley[33] reported that advanced age, tobacco use, male sex, workers' compensation status, and manual labor were predictive of poorer outcomes in patients with calcaneal fractures who underwent surgical treatment. Although these factors do not preclude patients who have calcaneal fractures from surgery, they should be looked for during the initial evaluation and considered in the discussion of treatment options with a patient.

Surgical Indications and Rationale

Despite advances in imaging, implant designs, biologics, and intraoperative techniques, the surgical management of displaced calcaneal fractures is controversial.[7,34-38] The literature on the management of displaced calcaneal fractures provides surgeons with some guidance; however, variations exist with regard to the design and quality of these studies. These variations include comparisons of different types of calcaneal fractures, different treatment methods, different levels of surgeon experience, and different outcome measures. In addition, most studies on the management of displaced calcaneal fractures lack necessary long-term follow-up and are underpowered.[2,6,7,9,35-37,39-46] Furthermore, most studies on the management of displaced calcaneal fractures are retrospective. Most surgeons agree that the nonsurgical management of calcaneal fractures is poorly tolerated by patients, and that some type of surgical management is necessary; however, the execution of surgical management is the subject of debate.

The natural history of displaced calcaneal fractures includes deformity, antalgic gait, painful shoe wear, and altered hindfoot mechanics,[2,3,6,44,47,48] all of which are related to loss of calcaneal height, increased calcaneal width, loss of lateral column length, varus tuberosity positioning, and joint incongruity. The goals of the surgical management of displaced calcaneal fractures are restoration of calcaneal anatomy, maintenance of function across the tibiotalar and subtalar joints, and normal shoe wear. The decision-making process for the surgical management of displaced calcaneal fractures is complex, and multiple factors require careful consideration.[7,33,39] Patient-related factors, fracture-related factors, soft-tissue integrity, and surgeon experience must be closely assessed before surgical treatment is considered. A patient's social history should be carefully examined during the initial evaluation. Tobacco use, illicit drug abuse, and alcoholism must be documented and considered in the decision-making process. A patient's medical history also plays an important role in the decision-making process. Although psychiatric problems, diabetes mellitus, peripheral vascular disease, and neuropathy do not preclude patients who have displaced calcaneal fractures from surgical treatment, they should be considered in the decision-making process.

A patient who undergoes nonsurgical treatment of a calcaneal fracture and sustains a malunion is preferred to a patient who undergoes surgical treatment of a calcaneal fracture and sustains an infection that cannot be eradicated. However, the outcomes of certain patients who undergo surgical treatment of a calcaneal fracture are substantially better compared with those of patients who undergo nonsurgical treatment of a calcaneal fracture. Studies have reported that patients with displaced calcaneal fractures have poorer outcomes compared with patients who have non-displaced calcaneal fractures. In addition, patients with increased amounts of posterior facet displacement, increased fracture lines, and comminution tend to have poorer outcomes.[42] The integrity of the soft tissue is paramount in determining appropriate surgical management. Open calcaneal fractures, heel pad injuries, and plantar wounds, which tend to be associated with higher complication rates, may influence a surgeon's approach and fixation strategies.[18,24,31,49] All of these factors must be considered in the selection of appropriate surgical candidates. A patient's social/medical history, expectations, bony pathology, and soft-tissue integrity as well as a surgeon's experience must be considered in the selection of appropriate surgical candidates and to achieve a successful outcome.

Temporizing Management Techniques

Calcaneal fractures that result from high-energy trauma involve injury to not only the osseous anatomy of the hindfoot but also the soft-tissue envelope. Definitive management of osseous injury must be delayed until soft-tissue swelling has subsided and skin blisters or open wounds have re-epithelialized; however, the displacement of fracture fragments can hinder soft-tissue healing.[18] Temporary external fixation is advantageous because it grossly reduces displaced fracture fragments, which may minimize the time to definitive management (formal open reduction and internal fixation), and facilitates incisional wound closure. In patients who have joint depression-type calcaneal fractures with substantial depression, medial external fixation can be used to allow for soft-tissue healing and may aid in future reconstruction.[24]

Medial external fixation involves the use of a medially based external fixator to help stabilize the lateral soft tissues for lateral exposure after soft-tissue swelling subsides. The patient is placed in the supine position with the injured extremity elevated on a radiolucent ramp. A medial stab wound is made over the medial cuneiform with the use of fluoroscopic guidance. A 5- × 170-mm Schanz pin is placed across the medial, intermediate, and lateral cuneiforms. A second 5- × 170-mm Schanz pin is placed in the medial tibia via a percutaneously placed stab wound to provide a point of fixation on the tibia. Large external fixation clamps are then applied, and a bar is placed from the Schanz pin in the cuneiforms to the medial tibial Schanz pin. A third 5- × 170-mm Schanz pin is placed in the calcaneal tuberosity via a medial stab wound. Distraction is performed between the medial tibial Schanz pin and the calcaneal tuberosity Schanz pin to restore calcaneal height. Distraction is performed along the bar that connects the calcaneal tuberosity Schanz pin and the Schanz pin in the cuneiforms to restore appropriate calcaneal length. Both the calcaneal tuberosity Schanz pin and the Schanz pin in the cuneiforms are pulled in a medial direction to correct varus tuberosity positioning and pronation of the foot, respectively. The medial tibial Schanz pin is connected to the Schanz pin in the cuneiforms with a bar, which is used to maintain the foot in a plantigrade position. After gross correction of the deformity is achieved, standard radiographs (AP, axial heel, and lateral views) are obtained to evaluate alignment.

In patients who have tuberosity avulsion injuries, which are known as hatchet fractures, the posterosuperior skin can become impinged, which may result in an open injury. Tuberosity avulsion injuries are considered an orthopaedic emergency and should be handled expeditiously.[18] The patient is placed in the lateral or prone position, and a percutaneous clamp is applied across the fracture line with the use of stab wounds. One clamp tine is placed on the superiorly displaced tuberosity, and the other clamp tine is placed deep to the heel pad. An AO elevator is used to disimpact the tuberosity fragment near the posterior facet if the calcaneal fracture extends more distally. A 4- × 150-mm Schanz pin is placed from posterior to anterior to manipulate the tuberosity into position. Provisional Kirschner wire (K-wire) fixation is used to maintain the reduction, after which 3.5- or 4.5-mm interfragmentary lag screws are used to achieve fixation. In patients who have poor bone quality, a small plate, which acts as a washer to help secure the tuberosity, also can be used.

Definitive Management Techniques
Approaches
Surgical fixation of calcaneal fractures can be achieved via many methods. Percutaneous and limited open surgical techniques as well as internal and external fixation methods have been described in the literature. If an open surgical technique is indicated, medial, lateral, or combined approaches are advocated.

Medial Approach
The medial approach allows for direct visualization of the primary fracture line and the application of a buttress plate from the tuberosity to the sustentaculum tali fragment.[11,40,46] The primary fracture, which exits along the medial wall, tends to have sharp fracture exit points, which allow for precise cortical reduction confirmation. A 4- to 5-cm incision is made in the midportion of the heel between the medial malleolus and the plantar skin junction. The incision can be shifted either anteriorly or posteriorly, depending on the fracture exit point and displacement. Fluoroscopic guidance can aid in planning the incision. After the skin and fascia have been incised, the neurovascular bundle should be identified and carefully retracted. The abductor hallucis and quadratus plantae muscles are retracted, after which the medial wall should be able to be visualized.

The osteology of the medial calcaneus as well as the surrounding neurovascular structures and the flexor hallucis tendon make implant application difficult. Other limitations of the medial approach include the inability to visualize the entire subtalar joint or address lateral pathology. The medial approach is more appropriate for direct reduction of isolated sustentaculum tali fractures or calcaneal body fractures with minimal or no articular involvement.

Lateral Extensile Approach
The lateral extensile approach is considered the mainstay for the surgical fixation of calcaneal fractures because it allows access to the entire calcaneus.[2] The lateral extensile approach allows visualization of lateral wall blowout, the anterior process, fracture extension into the calcaneocuboid joint, and the entire subtalar joint. The lateral extensile approach requires indirect reduction of the tuberosity to the sustentaculum tali fragment at the medial wall. The lateral extensile approach allows easier implant application along the lateral calcaneal surface as well as multiple fixation options.

A J- or L-shaped incision, depending on laterality, is made, with the vertical limb of the incision made parallel to the Achilles tendon. The incision begins 1 cm anterior to the Achilles tendon. The sural nerve, which courses from approximately 2 cm posterior to the distal tip of the lateral malleolus to the base of the fifth metatarsal, is located anterior to the vertical limb of the incision and is contained in the osteocutaneous flap. The plantar limb of the incision is made in the transition zone between the lateral skin and the thicker glabrous plantar skin. The plantar limb of the incision is made across the calcaneocuboid joint. The apex of the incision is curved sharply, after which full-thickness dissection is carried down to the lateral calcaneus. The surgeon must avoid beveling the skin edge or incising the skin too superficially as the incision is curved. The sural nerve, peroneal tendons, and calcaneofibular ligament are raised as a full-thickness osteocutaneous flap. Dissection is carried anteriorly until the subtalar joint is visualized; extension of dissection superior to the tuberosity is rarely necessary. The superior limb of the incision should be made carefully so that the lateral calcaneal branch of the peroneal artery, which supplies most of the osteocutaneous flap, is not injured.[50] The lateral calcaneal branch of the peroneal artery is identified intraoperatively with the use of a Doppler probe and avoided. After the lateral aspect of the calcaneus has been exposed, retraction is performed with the use of retractors or K-wires that are inserted in the talus and fibula.

Sinus Tarsi Approach

The sinus tarsi approach has gained popularity because of concerns for wound healing in patients who undergo surgical fixation of calcaneal fractures via the lateral extensile approach and is used in patients who have more complex calcaneal fractures.[40] The sinus tarsi approach is commonly used for subtalar reconstructive procedures. A 4- to 5-cm incision is made distal to the tip of the lateral malleolus and parallel to the sinus tarsi. The posterior aspect of the incision should be made carefully so that the sural nerve is not injured. The peroneal tendons are mobilized, after which the posterior facet should be able to be directly visualized from a top-down vantage point. Dissection is carried anteriorly to the angle of Gissane and onto the anterolateral process. Lateral wall blowout is dissected free in the inferior aspect of the incision. Limitations of the sinus tarsi approach include the inability to directly débride the fracture site and reduce plantar fracture involvement. In addition, compared with the lateral extensile approach, fixation options are limited with the sinus tarsi approach.

Reduction

After lateral extensile exposure is achieved, the entire lateral aspect of the calcaneus should be able to be visualized. The lateral wall is either hinged plantarward or removed from the surgical site and placed on a back table, after which the posterior facet, which was covered by the displaced lateral wall, should be able to be visualized. Typically, the displaced tuberosity, which has lost height and length as a result of axial loading, crowds the space available for reduction of the anterior process and the posterior facet. Space for reduction of the displaced posterior facet will only become available after the tuberosity has been restored to a more appropriate height and length.

Realignment of the tuberosity can be performed via several methods. A 4.0-mm Schanz pin, with either a universal chuck with T-handle or a 4.5-mm drill guide placed over the shaft of the pin, is inserted from lateral to medial in the posterior aspect of the tuberosity to facilitate realignment of the tuberosity fragment. Alternatively, a lamina spreader, with one tine placed on the tuberosity and the other tine placed on the cancellous bone of the intact posterior facet, can be used. Spreading of the tines of the lamina spreader will drive the tuberosity toward the proper height and length but also will create a varus force on the tuberosity. The realigned tuberosity is maintained with the use of at least two 1.6-mm K-wires that are percutaneously placed from the tuberosity into the intact sustentaculum tali (**Figure 5, A**).

After the tuberosity has been realigned, the anterior process is reduced. Dedicated, deliberate dissection with the use of a No. 15 blade will result in exposure of the dorsal cortical bone

from the anterior process to the medial facet, which is necessary for accurate reduction and fixation of any secondary fractures that involve the anterior process. The anterior process, which is frequently displaced in an anterior position and separated from the intact sustentaculum tali by a fracture that runs through the angle of Gissane, requires manipulation to match the intact sustentaculum tali and the remaining intact posterior facet. Pressure on the dorsal surface of the anterior process in a plantar direction is achieved with the use of an elevator or a small bone hook. Multiple K-wires that are 1.25 mm or smaller in diameter are inserted at the dorsolateral corner of the anterior process toward the intact sustentaculum tali to maintain provisional fixation. Lateral and AP radiographs should be obtained to evaluate reduction of the anterior process. To obtain an AP radiograph of the anterior process of a patient who is placed in the lateral decubitus position, the radiology technician must direct the fluoroscope across the surgical table as the surgeon flexes the patient's hip and knee and plantarflexes the patient's foot. Imaging of the patient in this manner should result in an AP radiograph that distinctly shows the calcaneocuboid joint.

After accurate reduction of the anterior process has been confirmed, the posterior facet fragments are reduced to the intact posterior facet and the newly reestablished sinus tarsi. The displaced posterior facet fragment(s) are frequently débrided extracorporeally to completely remove any interposed tissue and hematoma. Preparation of the displaced posterior facet fragment(s) with the use of 1.0-mm K-wires, which are used as tools for manipulation as well as for provisional/definitive fixation,

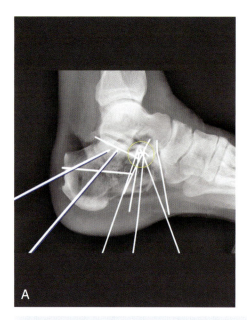 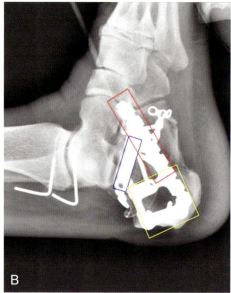 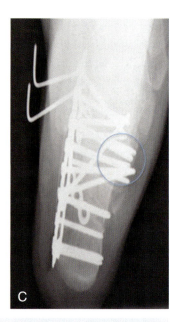

Figure 5 Intraoperative radiographs of a calcaneus demonstrate definitive surgical management of a calcaneal fracture. **A,** Lateral radiograph demonstrates the placement of Kirschner wires (K-wires) to maintain reduction. The K-wires highlighted with the blue lines were used to reduce the tuberosity to the posterior facet fragment. The K-wires in the yellow circle were used to reduce the anterior process to the sustentaculum tali. Similar K-wires may be used to support and reduce the posterior facet to the sustentaculum tali fragment; however, such fixation was not required in this patient. **B,** Lateral radiograph demonstrates final fixation. The plate has three main components. The screws in the red rectangle compress from lateral to medial and reduce the anterior process as well as the middle facet to the sustentaculum tali fragment. The screws in the blue rectangle support and reduce the posterior facet to the sustentaculum tali fragment. The screws in the yellow square pull the tuberosity out of varus. **C,** Axial heel radiograph demonstrates appropriate narrowing of the calcaneus, with the plate acting as a washer. The screw tips in the blue circle are aimed toward the sustentaculum tali fragment. K-wires were placed in the fibula to hold the subluxated peroneal tendons in place after reduction.

before reinsertion is helpful. Direct visualization is essential to achieving and maintaining accurate posterior facet fracture reduction. Several options exist for patients who have more than one displaced posterior facet fragment. If possible, reduction and fixation of the displaced posterior facet fragment(s) should be performed outside of the wound, which, in effect, results in one large posterior facet fragment that is maintained by K-wires. This large posterior facet fragment is then reduced to the intact medial posterior facet. If reduction is performed in the wound, the medial facet fragment is reduced to the intact posterior facet. K-wires that are used to maintain the reduction of the medial facet fragment must be directed

away from the reduction of the lateral posterior facet fragment, which is performed next. Alternatively, the medial facet fragment can be reduced to the intact posterior facet with the use of a small-diameter flat-head lag screw. The lag screw is concealed after the lateral posterior facet fragment is reduced. Provisional fixation of the posterior facet is achieved with the use of 1.0-mm K-wires, which also serve as an adjunct for definitive fixation. Lag screws are placed either independently or, preferably, through a plate and directed slightly toward the sustentaculum tali to maintain reduction of the posterior facet. Lateral, axial heel, and Broden radiographs should be obtained to evaluate posterior facet reduction and fixation.

After accurate reduction of the posterior facet and anterior process has been confirmed, the tuberosity reduction is reevaluated. The superior aspect of the tuberosity and the cortical bone that is posterior to the posterior facet are used to evaluate reduction of the tuberosity in patients without comminution. Because the posterior facet and the tuberosity are in continuity in patients who have tongue-type calcaneal fractures, reduction of the posterior facet will realign the tuberosity to its proper position. The lateral wall should be replaced after its normal flat contour has been restored. Interdigitation of the restored fragments at the periphery of the lateral wall confirms that the tuberosity has been restored to the proper height and length. Axial heel and lateral radiographs of the contralateral limb are obtained for comparison. Particular attention should be paid to the Böhler angle, the overall pitch of the calcaneus, and varus tuberosity positioning. Any final adjustments to provisional reduction and fixation should be made before plate application.

Fixation

Plate fixation of calcaneal fractures relies on screw purchase in several key areas. Body weight is unevenly distributed in the calcaneus, which makes the lateral side of the calcaneus far less important with regard to supporting body weight compared with the medial side of the calcaneus. The medial side of the calcaneus, therefore, consists of substantially denser bone, which is used to attain screw purchase. In particular, this dense bone is present in the sustentaculum tali, the trabecular bone that is plantar to the posterior facet, the cancellous bone that is near the insertion of the Achilles tendon, and the dorsal one-half of the anterior process.

A broad-based lateral plate is important for the maintenance of reduction because it links the disparate calcaneal fragments into a single construct. Appropriate narrowing of the calcaneus is achieved with the use of lateral to medial screws (the plate acts as a large washer), which attain excellent purchase in the dense medial cortex and poor purchase in the thin lateral cortex. After appropriate narrowing of the calcaneus has been achieved, lag screws are placed through the plate to support the posterior facet. At this point, the plate has a broad base of screw purchase in the sustentaculum tali and, therefore, is well positioned to reduce the tuberosity. Any residual varus tuberosity positioning

should be eliminated before the lateral tuberosity is reduced to the straight, stiff lateral plate (**Figure 5, B** and **C**). Screws that are placed into the anterior process through the plate should be aimed toward the dorsomedial corner because considerably dense bone exists in this area. The radiographic views that were obtained to evaluate the reduction also should be obtained to evaluate the fixation. An AP fluoroscopic image of the foot helps guide the lateral to medial screws that are aimed toward the sustentaculum tali and the lateral to medial screws that are placed in the anterior process, which should be posterior to the calcaneocuboid joint.

Postoperative Management and Outcomes

Typically, a suction drain that is set at 80 to 100 mm Hg is placed under the osteocutaneous flap to remove tension from the two-layer closure that is used for the lateral extensile approach. The foot is placed in a well-padded, molded plaster splint that includes medial and lateral support as well as a posterior slab with a toe plate. Early active motion of the tibiotalar and subtalar joints should begin after the wound is sealed, preferably before the stitches are removed. If possible, early active motion of the tibiotalar and subtalar joints should begin on postoperative day 5, at which time the plaster splint is exchanged for a removable, padded, aluminum splint. Passive manipulation of the toes is an essential early component of the physical therapy program. After 12 weeks postoperatively, the patient can be transitioned from non–weight bearing, to partial progressive–weight bearing, and, finally, to full–weight bearing. Typically, weight bearing begins in a boot, after which the patient is transitioned to a

shoe over the course of 4 to 6 weeks. In some patients, 15 mm Hg compression socks and insoles that support the longitudinal arch may provide additional gait support. Although many patients will not require an assistive device for walking after 4 to 6 months postoperatively, complete recovery may not be achieved until approximately 1 year postoperatively. Counseling of patients with regard to proper expectations is an essential component of postoperative management. Patients must be educated with regard to stiffness of the subtalar joint and its implications, possible long-term pain, and the potential for posttraumatic arthritis. Patients who perform manual laborer, particularly those who perform activities that require prolonged standing, walking, and/or climbing, may never return to their preoperative level of activity.

Complications

The surgical management of calcaneal fractures avoids the complications associated with the nonsurgical management of calcaneal fractures, especially malunion;[47] however, particular complications, namely infection and wound issues, are associated with the surgical management of calcaneal fractures.[50] The skin about the lateral calcaneus effectively contracts before calcaneal fractures are managed surgically because the tuberosity is not the appropriate length or height. Acute restoration of the tuberosity to the appropriate length and height places the wound under tension, which, in certain patients, likely contributes to delayed healing or skin flap necrosis as well as infection. The rate of delayed healing and skin flap necrosis in patients who undergo the surgical management of calcaneal fractures is approximately 8% to 9%. The infection rate in patients who undergo the surgical management of calcaneal fractures is approximately 2% to 3%.[2] For most patients in whom delayed healing, skin flap necrosis, or an infection occurs, supportive care typically is provided until fracture union is attained. Antibiotics are used in a suppressive manner in patients in whom an infection develops. Antibiotics are discontinued after fracture union is attained, at which point the hardware is removed and the bone is débrided. The risk for delayed healing, skin flap necrosis, and infection is higher in patients who have diabetes mellitus, open fractures, and a history of tobacco use; therefore, preoperative counseling of these patients with regard to their increased risk for these complications is essential.

Summary

The calcaneus has a complex shape, which affects the biomechanics of the foot in a variety of ways. Disruption of calcaneal anatomy can alter the biomechanics of the foot. Reduction and fixation of the calcaneus is the only option to restore calcaneal anatomy and, potentially, proper foot biomechanics. Several factors affect whether a patient with a calcaneal fracture is an appropriate candidate for surgical treatment. In patients with calcaneal fractures who are indicated for surgery, the proper timing of surgical management is essential to increase the likelihood of a successful outcome. Calcaneal fractures can be surgically managed via a variety of approaches; however, accurate reduction and stable fixation always is the goal. Complications, particularly problems related to the skin, are not infrequent in patients who undergo surgical treatment for calcaneal fractures.

References

1. Mitchell MJ, McKinley JC, Robinson CM: The epidemiology of calcaneal fractures. *Foot (Edinb)* 2009;19(4):197-200.

2. Barei DP, Bellabarba C, Sangeorzan BJ, Benirschke SK: Fractures of the calcaneus. *Orthop Clin North Am* 2002;33(1):263-285, x.

3. Sanders R: Displaced intra-articular fractures of the calcaneus. *J Bone Joint Surg Am* 2000;82(2):225-250.

4. Benirschke SK, Sangeorzan BJ: Extensive intraarticular fractures of the foot: Surgical management of calcaneal fractures. *Clin Orthop Relat Res* 1993;292:128-134.

5. Thordarson DB, Krieger LE: Operative vs. nonoperative treatment of intra-articular fractures of the calcaneus: A prospective randomized trial. *Foot Ankle Int* 1996;17(1):2-9.

6. Zwipp H, Tscherne H, Thermann H, Weber T: Osteosynthesis of displaced intraarticular fractures of the calcaneus: Results in 123 cases. *Clin Orthop Relat Res* 1993;290:76-86.

7. Brauer CA, Manns BJ, Ko M, Donaldson C, Buckley R: An economic evaluation of operative compared with nonoperative management of displaced intra-articular calcaneal fractures. *J Bone Joint Surg Am* 2005;87(12):2741-2749.

8. Sanders R, Fortin P, DiPasquale T, Walling A: Operative treatment in 120 displaced intraarticular calcaneal fractures: Results using a prognostic computed tomography scan classification. *Clin Orthop Relat Res* 1993;290:87-95.

9. Buckley R, Tough S, McCormack R, et al: Operative compared with nonoperative treatment of displaced intra-articular calcaneal fractures: A prospective, randomized, controlled multicenter trial. *J Bone Joint Surg Am* 2002;84(10):1733-1744.

10. Stephenson JR: Surgical treatment of displaced intraarticular fractures of the calcaneus: A combined lateral and medial approach. *Clin Orthop Relat Res* 1993;290:68-75.

11. Burdeaux BD: Calcaneus fractures: Rationale for the medial approach technique of reduction. *Orthopedics* 1987;10(1):177-187.

12. Riegger CL: Anatomy of the ankle and foot. *Phys Ther* 1988;68(12):1802-1814.

13. Schneck CD: Anatomy and kinesiology of the ankle and foot. *J Back Musculoskelet Rehabil* 1992;2(3):1-16.

14. Sangeorzan BJ, Mosca V, Hansen ST Jr: Effect of calcaneal lengthening on relationships among the hindfoot, midfoot, and forefoot. *Foot Ankle* 1993;14(3):136-141.

15. Essex-Lopresti P: The mechanism, reduction technique, and results in fractures of the os calcis. *Br J Surg* 1952;39(157):395-419.

16. Carr JB, Hamilton JJ, Bear LS: Experimental intra-articular calcaneal fractures: Anatomic basis for a new classification. *Foot Ankle* 1989;10(2):81-87.

17. Wülker N, Zwipp H, Tscherne H: Experimental study of the classification of intra-articular calcaneus fractures. *Unfallchirurg* 1991;94(4):198-203.

18. Gardner MJ, Nork SE, Barei DP, Kramer PA, Sangeorzan BJ, Benirschke SK: Secondary soft tissue compromise in tongue-type calcaneus fractures. *J Orthop Trauma* 2008;22(7):439-445.

19. Böhler L: Diagnosis, pathology, and treatment of fractures of the os calcis. *J Bone Joint Surg Am* 1931;13(1):75-89.

20. Gissane W: News notes: The British Orthopaedic Association. *J Bone and Joint Surg Am* 1947;29 (1):254-255.

21. Crosby LA, Fitzgibbons T: Computerized tomography scanning of acute intra-articular fractures of the calcaneus: A new classification system. *J Bone Joint Surg Am* 1990;72(6):852-859.

22. Swords MP, Alton TB, Holt S, Sangeorzan BJ, Shank JR, Benirschke SK: Prognostic value of computed tomography classification systems for intra-articular calcaneus fractures. *Foot Ankle Int* 2014;35(10):975-980.

23. Richardson ML, Van Vu M, Vincent LM, Sangeorzan BJ, Benirschke SK: CT measurement of the calcaneal varus angle in the normal and

fractured hindfoot. *J Comput Assist Tomogr* 1992;16(2):261-264.

24. Mehta S, Mirza AJ, Dunbar RP, Barei DP, Benirschke SK: A staged treatment plan for the management of Type II and Type IIIA open calcaneus fractures. *J Orthop Trauma* 2010;24(3):142-147.

25. Benirschke SK, Kramer PA: Wound healing complications in closed and open calcaneal fractures. *J Orthop Trauma* 2004;18(1):1-6.

26. Fakhouri AJ, Manoli A II: Acute foot compartment syndromes. *J Orthop Trauma* 1992;6(2):223-228.

27. Myerson M, Manoli A: Compartment syndromes of the foot after calcaneal fractures. *Clin Orthop Relat Res* 1993;290:142-150.

28. Varela CD, Vaughan TK, Carr JB, Slemmons BK: Fracture blisters: Clinical and pathological aspects. *J Orthop Trauma* 1993;7(5):417-427.

29. Giordano CP, Koval KJ: Treatment of fracture blisters: A prospective study of 53 cases. *J Orthop Trauma* 1995;9(2):171-176.

30. Walters JL, Gangopadhyay P, Malay DS: Association of calcaneal and spinal fractures. *J Foot Ankle Surg* 2014;53(3):279-281.

31. Worsham JR, Elliott MR, Harris AM: Open calcaneus fractures and associated injuries. *J Foot Ankle Surg* 2016;55(1):68-71.

32. Broden B: Roentgen examination of the subtaloid joint in fractures of the calcaneus. *Acta radiol* 1949;31(1):85-91.

33. Tufescu TV, Buckley R: Age, gender, work capability, and worker's compensation in patients with displaced intraarticular calcaneal fractures. *J Orthop Trauma* 2001;15(4):275-279.

34. Rammelt S, Zwipp H: Fractures of the calcaneus: Current treatment strategies. *Acta Chir Orthop Traumatol Cech* 2014;81(3):177-196.

35. Buckley R, Leighton R, Sanders D, et al: Open reduction and internal fixation compared with ORIF and primary subtalar arthrodesis for treatment of Sanders type IV calcaneal fractures: A randomized multicenter trial. *J Orthop Trauma* 2014;28(10):577-583.

36. Buckley RE: Evidence for the best treatment for displaced intra-articular calcaneal fractures. *Acta Chir Orthop Traumatol Cech* 2010;77(3):179-185.

37. Swanson SA, Clare MP, Sanders RW: Management of intra-articular fractures of the calcaneus. *Foot Ankle Clin* 2008;13(4):659-678.

38. Rammelt S, Zwipp H: Calcaneus fractures: Facts, controversies and recent developments. *Injury* 2004;35(5):443-461.

39. Buckley R: Operative care did not benefit closed, displaced, intra-articular calcaneal fractures. *J Bone Joint Surg Am* 2015;97(4):341.

40. Carr JB: Surgical treatment of intra-articular calcaneal fractures: A review of small incision approaches. *J Orthop Trauma* 2005;19(2):109-117.

41. Buckley RE, Tough S: Displaced intra-articular calcaneal fractures. *J Am Acad Orthop Surg* 2004;12(3):172-178.

42. Csizy M, Buckley R, Tough S, et al: Displaced intra-articular calcaneal fractures: Variables predicting late subtalar fusion. *J Orthop Trauma* 2003;17(2):106 112.

43. Sanders R, Gregory P: Operative treatment of intra-articular fractures of the calcaneus. *Orthop Clin North Am* 1995;26(2):203-214.

44. Macey LR, Benirschke SK, Sangeorzan BJ, Hansen ST: Acute calcaneal fractures: Treatment options and results. *J Am Acad Orthop Surg* 1994;2(1):36-43.

45. Sanders R: Intra-articular fractures of the calcaneus: Present state of the art. *J Orthop Trauma* 1992;6(2):252-265.

46. Stephenson JR: Treatment of displaced intra-articular fractures of the calcaneus using medial and lateral approaches, internal fixation, and early motion. *J Bone Joint Surg Am* 1987;69(1):115-130.

47. Howard JL, Buckley R, McCormack R, et al: Complications following management of displaced intra-articular calcaneal fractures: A prospective randomized trial comparing open reduction internal fixation with nonoperative management. *J Orthop Trauma* 2003;17(4):241-249.

48. Carr JB: Mechanism and pathoanatomy of the intraarticular calcaneal fracture. *Clin Orthop Relat Res* 1993;290:36-40.

49. Heier KA, Infante AF, Walling AK, Sanders RW: Open fractures of the calcaneus: Soft-tissue injury determines outcome. *J Bone Joint Surg Am* 2003;85(12):2276-2282.

50. Harvey EJ, Grujic L, Early JS, Benirschke SK, Sangeorzan BJ: Morbidity associated with ORIF of intra-articular calcaneus fractures using a lateral approach. *Foot Ankle Int* 2001;22(11):868-873.

Shoulder and Elbow

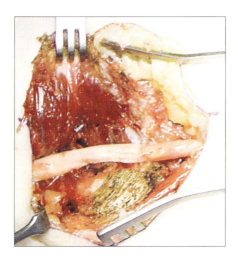

Diagnosis and Management of the Biceps-Labral Complex

Robert J. Thorsness, MD
Anthony A. Romeo, MD

Abstract

The long head of the biceps tendon (LHBT) is a common source of pathology. The biceps-labral complex (BLC) is the collective anatomic and clinical features shared by the biceps tendon and the superior labrum. LHBT pathology can be caused by inflammation, instability, or trauma. Numerous tests can be performed to determine the existence of biceps tendon and superior labrum anterior to posterior (SLAP) lesions; however, many of these tests do not have high sensitivity and specificity, which limit their clinical utility. Because it is difficult to diagnose both LHBT and SLAP pathology, management strategies are best guided by a strong clinical suspicion and imaging findings on either MRI or ultrasonography. Initial nonsurgical management of LHBT and SLAP pathology includes focused physical therapy, anti-inflammatory medications, and corticosteroid injections. If nonsurgical management fails, surgical techniques for the management of LHBT pathology include biceps anchor reattachment (SLAP repair), biceps tenotomy, and biceps tenodesis. Techniques for biceps tenodesis, which can be performed in either an arthroscopic or open manner, include soft-tissue tenodesis, suprapectoral tenodesis, and subpectoral tenodesis. If appropriately managed, patients with LHBT pathology often have excellent clinical outcomes.

Instr Course Lect 2017;66:65–77.

Anatomy

The anatomy of the long head of the biceps tendon (LHBT) involves a complex interplay between the LHBT and its stabilizing pulley, the superior labrum, and the glenoid. The authors of this chapter prefer to use the term "biceps-labral complex" (BLC) to comprehensively describe the clinically relevant anatomy. The BLC has three clinically relevant zones: the inside, the junction, and the bicipital tunnel.[1] The inside component includes both the superior labrum and the LHBT anchor at the supraglenoid tubercle. The junction includes the intra-articular LHBT and its stabilizing pulley. Both the inside and junction components of the BLC can be visualized during standard glenohumeral arthroscopy. The bicipital tunnel, which is an extra-articular component of the BLC, includes the LHBT beginning at the articular margin of the humeral head adjacent to the pulley and extending to the subpectoral region and incorporates the fibro-osseous bicipital tunnel that stabilizes the LHBT within the groove[1,2] (**Figure 1**).

Inside Component

The inside component of the BLC consists of the superior labrum and the LHBT anchor at the supraglenoid tubercle. The superior labrum and

Dr. Romeo or an immediate family member has received royalties from Arthrex; is a member of a speakers' bureau or has made paid presentations on behalf of Arthrex; serves as a paid consultant to or is an employee of Arthrex; has received research or institutional support from Arthrex, DJO Surgical, Smith & Nephew, and Ossur; has received nonincome support (such as equipment or services), commercially derived honoraria, or other non-research–related funding (such as paid travel) from Arthrex; and serves as a board member, owner, officer, or committee member of the American Orthopaedic Society for Sports Medicine and the American Shoulder and Elbow Surgeons. Neither Dr. Thorsness nor any immediate family member has received anything of value from or has stock or stock options held in a commercial company or institution related directly or indirectly to the subject of this chapter.

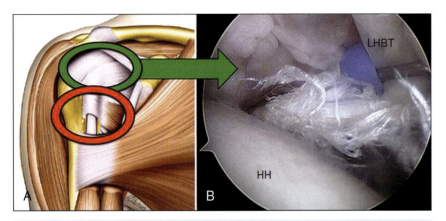

Figure 1   Images show the anatomy of the biceps-labral complex (BLC). **A,** Illustration of a shoulder shows that the BLC exists in continuum and consists of both an intra-articular component (green circle) and an extra-articular component (red circle). **B,** Arthroscopic image of a left shoulder shows examination of the long head of biceps tendon (LHBT). A probe is used to pull the LHBT intra-articularly, which allows the surgeon to assess for abnormalities, such as the partial tearing seen here. HH = humeral head. (Reproduced with permission from Taylor SA, Kahir MM, Gulota LV, et al: Diagnostic glenohumeral arthroscopy fails to fully evaluate the biceps-labral complex. *Arthroscopy* 2015;31[2]:215-224.)

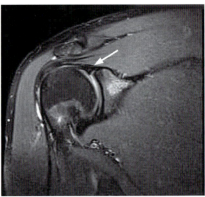

Figure 2   Coronal T2-weighted noncontrast MRI of a shoulder demonstrates a type II superior labrum anterior to posterior tear (arrow).

biceps anchor demonstrate heterogeneity with respect to their attachments. Compared with the inferior labrum, the superior labrum has a loose, more meniscal attachment to the glenoid.[3] The biceps anchor is most often posterior or posterior-dominant to its origin.[4-6] Surgeons must recognize that the superior labrum has an anatomic recess with respect to the glenoid, which represents normal synovial reflection and should not be mistaken for a tear.[7]

Superior labrum anterior to posterior (SLAP) lesions are the predominant pathologic entity that affect the inside component of the BLC. SLAP tears are believed to be caused by superior migration of the humeral head, biceps tension, or peelback as a result of internal impingement.[8] SLAP lesions were first described and classified by Snyder et al[9] and have been modified[10] to include seven distinct pathologic variants, with the most common variant being type II SLAP lesions (**Figure 2**).

Junction

The junction of the BLC includes the intra-articular component of the LHBT and its stabilizing pulley. A hypovascular watershed region of the intra-articular LHBT, which represents an area at high risk for rupture, exists near the articular margin of the humeral head.[11] The stabilizing pulley is composed of fibers of the superior glenohumeral ligament, coracohumeral ligament, subscapularis, and supraspinatus[12] (**Figure 3**). The pulley stabilizes the LHBT within the proximal portion of the bicipital groove as it enters the groove from its intra-articular position. Tears of the capsuloligamentous pulley complex destabilize the LHBT and can result in subluxation or dislocation of the tendon.[13]

Pathologic entities that affect the junction of the BLC include LHBT tears, LHBT incarceration,[14] biceps chondromalacia (humeral head chondral damage as a result of pathologic

motion of the LHBT),[15] hourglass biceps,[16] and pulley lesions.

Bicipital Tunnel

The bicipital tunnel is the fibro-osseous confinement of the extra-articular component of the LHBT. The bicipital tunnel extends from the articular margin of the humeral head to the subpectoral region. The bicipital tunnel often contains LHBT lesions that are hidden and unable to be appreciated via diagnostic glenohumeral arthroscopy, even if a probe is used to pull the LHBT into the joint[1] (**Figure 4**). The proximal aspect of the bicipital tunnel consists of a bony groove that extends from the articular margin of the humeral head to just distal to the subscapularis. The bony groove has variable anatomy and is a common location for osteophyte formation.[17,18] Traditionally, it was believed that a structure defined as the "transverse humeral ligament" ran over the bony groove to stabilize the LHBT; however, recent studies have suggested that the transverse humeral ligament is not a separate structure but is composed of the superficial fibers of the

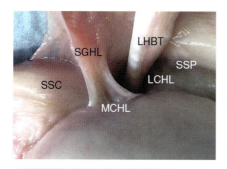

Figure 3 Clinical photograph shows a gross specimen of the stabilizing pulley of the long head of the biceps tendon (LHBT). LCHL = lateral coracohumeral ligament, MCHL = medial coracohumeral ligament, SGHL = superior glenohumeral ligament, SSC = subscapularis, SSP = supraspinatus. (Reproduced with permission from Martetschläger F, Tauber M, Habermeyer P: Injuries to the biceps pulley. *Clin Sports Med* 2016;35[1]:19-27.)

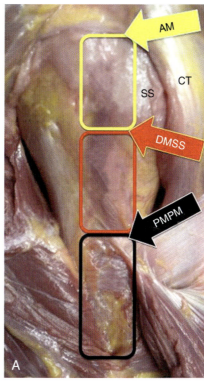

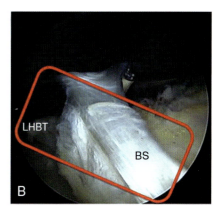

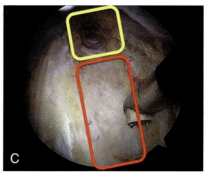

Figure 4 Images show the bicipital tunnel. A soft-tissue sheath consistently covers the long head of the biceps tendon (LHBT) to the level of the proximal margin of the pectoralis major tendon (PMPM) and contributes to the roof of the bicipital tunnel. The soft-tissue sheath is clearly visible during open procedures (**A**) and within the subdeltoid space during extra-articular arthroscopic procedures (**B** and **C**). **A,** Intraoperative photograph shows that the fibro-osseous bicipital tunnel consists of three distinct anatomic zones. Zone 1 (yellow box), which represents the traditional bony bicipital groove, begins at the articular margin (AM) and ends at the distal margin of the subscapularis tendon (DMSS). Zone 2 (red box), which represents a no-man's-land because it is not viewable via arthroscopy from above or via subpectoral exposure from below, extends from the DMSS to the PMPM. Zone 3, which represents the subpectoral region, is distal to the PMPM. **B** and **C,** Arthroscopic images show that the soft-tissue sheath that overlies zone 2 can be robust. BS = bicipital sheath, CT = conjoint tendon, D = deltoid, SS = subscapularis. (Reproduced with permission from Taylor SA, Fabricant PD, Bansal M, et al: The anatomy and histology of the bicipital tunnel of the shoulder. *J Shoulder Elbow Surg* 2015;24[4]:511-519.)

subscapularis that blend with the superficial fibers of the supraspinatus and the coracohumeral ligament.[19,20]

The bicipital tunnel may contain LHBT lesions that are unable to be appreciated via glenohumeral arthroscopy because it is too distal to allow for enough excursion of the LHBT within the glenohumeral joint. Numerous LHBT lesions, including LHBT tears, loose bodies, and tenosynovitis, have been reported in the bicipital tunnel.[1] The osseous floor of the bicipital tunnel is shallow and covered by blending fibers of the latissimus dorsi and periosteum. The roof of the bicipital tunnel is composed of a tendon sheath for the LHBT that is distinct from the overlying falciform ligament, which is an extension of the sternal head of the pectoralis major.[2]

During biceps tenodesis, the surgeon should stabilize the LHBT at a physiologic length-tension relationship to minimize the likelihood of weakness,

fatigue, cramping, and a Popeye deformity. Therefore, the surgeon must locate the musculotendinous junction of the biceps to be able to reliably re-create the length-tension relationship. Although the location of the musculotendinous junction of the biceps may vary, studies have shown it to be approximately 3.2 cm distal to the proximal margin of the pectoralis major tendon and

approximately 3.3 cm distal to the inferior margin of the pectoralis major tendon.[21]

Physical Examination

Physical examination of the shoulder may be difficult; however, distinguishing biceps pain from other causes of pain may be more of a challenge because pain generators may be referred to multiple anatomic locations in the shoulder.[22] Further, patients with biceps lesions and pain often have concomitant pathology, such as a rotator cuff tear, which can confound physical examination findings.[23,24] To further complicate the physical examination, patients with SLAP lesions may have symptoms similar to those of patients with biceps lesions. SLAP lesions have a multitude of physical examination findings and are notoriously difficult to diagnose with a clinical examination alone. Therefore, surgeons should have a thorough understanding of the various pathologies that cause shoulder pain and should consider a number of pathologic conditions in the differential diagnosis.

The physical examination should begin with a thorough assessment of range of motion (ROM) and a neurovascular examination that includes strength testing of all of the rotator cuff muscles. Special attention should be paid to the subscapularis because lesions on the upper part of the tendon are often correlated with biceps tendon lesions and LHBT instability. Subscapularis tests include the belly-press test, the lift-off test, and the bear hug test.

Biceps rupture will often present with a tearing sensation anteriorly if sustained acutely; however, some patients may have a sagging biceps muscle belly or a Popeye deformity, which are often associated with swelling and ecchymosis in the arm if biceps rupture was sustained acutely. The deformity can be exaggerated by having the patient flex his or her biceps, which can then be compared with the contralateral side. Surgeons should not rule out more serious causes of atraumatic swelling in the upper limb, such as soft-tissue tumor.[25]

Patients with biceps disorders will often have localized pain in the bicipital groove. The optimal position for palpation of the biceps within the bicipital groove is 10° of internal rotation with the arm in adduction and the elbow flexed.[26] The tendon can be more reliably palpated by externally rotating the arm from this optimal position while flexing and extending the elbow; however, simple palpation has poor sensitivity and specificity for the diagnosis of biceps lesions.[27] The Speed test is performed with the elbow extended, forearm supinated, and the shoulder in forward flexion. The patient is asked to resist a downward force on the arm in this position; anterior shoulder pain is elicited in a positive test. The Speed test has an overall sensitivity of 57% and specificity of 52% with regard to the diagnosis of both biceps tendon disorders and SLAP lesions.[27] For the Yergason test, which is performed with the elbow flexed 90° and pronated, the patient is asked to resist supination of the arm by an examiner; pain is referred to the anterior shoulder in a positive test. Multiple studies have suggested that the Yergason test is not a reliable predictor of biceps pathology or SLAP tears.[28-30]

Biceps tendon instability is often associated with rotator cuff tears, especially those of the upper border of the subscapularis.[27,31] Although static instability can be appreciated on advanced imaging studies, such as MRI, dynamic instability may be more readily appreciated with the use of ultrasonography.[32] Boileau et al[16] described biceps entrapment, in which the biceps tendon is hypertrophied and can become trapped during arm elevation, which limits motion and causes pain. Biceps entrapment cannot be reliably

diagnosed with a physical examination alone and can only be diagnosed accurately via diagnostic arthroscopy.

Although many tests for the diagnosis of SLAP lesions exist, diagnosis remains challenging with a physical examination alone. In addition, SLAP lesions are difficult to diagnose arthroscopically because although intraobserver reliability is generally good, interobserver reliability remains relatively poor.[33,34] The O'Brien active compression test and the dynamic labral shear test have demonstrated reasonable diagnostic utility for SLAP lesions; however, both tests are controversial.

The O'Brien active compression test[35] is performed with the patient's arm forward flexed to 90°, adducted 10°, and maximally internally rotated. The patient is asked to resist a downward directed force by the examiner; pain or clicking indicates a positive test. Next, the patient is asked to externally rotate the arm so that his or her palm faces upward, and the test is repeated. A SLAP tear is suggested if the pain lessens with the arm in this position. O'Brien et al[35] reported remarkably excellent results for the diagnostic utility of the O'Brien active compression test; however, subsequent studies were not as promising, with a meta-analysis suggesting that the O'Brien active compression test is not diagnostic of SLAP tears.[36]

The dynamic labral shear test, which was first described by Cheung and O'Driscoll,[37] is performed with the patient's arm in abduction and external rotation. The examiner, who stands behind the patient, applies an anterior directed force on the patient's shoulder as the patient's arm is moved from approximately 70° to 120° of elevation; pain in the posterosuperior shoulder indicates a positive test. Cheung and O'Driscoll[37] as well as a subsequent study by Kibler et al[38] reported excellent results for the diagnostic utility of the dynamic labral shear test; however, further studies were not as enthusiastic.[39] Although controversial, the dynamic labral shear test remains promising with regard to its diagnostic utility for SLAP tears; however, further studies are necessary.

Imaging

Biceps tendinitis and SLAP tears, in particular, may be difficult to diagnose with a physical examination alone. Advanced imaging studies can facilitate the diagnosis of biceps tendinitis and SLAP tears; however, studies on the accuracy of MRI with regard to the diagnosis of BLC lesions report conflicting results. Most MRI studies demonstrate reasonable sensitivity and specificity for the diagnosis of SLAP tears, biceps rupture, and other inside lesions; however, junctional lesions and bicipital tunnel lesions are poorly identified via MRI.[40-44] Therefore, surgeons must have a low threshold to address a chronically symptomatic LHBT at the time of surgery in patients with negative or equivocal MRI studies.

Nonsurgical Management

Nonsurgical management of LHBT disorders remains controversial because there are no current studies in the literature on the clinical response of LHBT disorders to nonsurgical management, including corticosteroid injections. Therefore, nonsurgical management remains driven by individual surgeon experience.

After a LHBT disorder is identified as either tendinitis, instability, or a tear, nonsurgical management

typically begins with NSAIDs, activity modifications, and corticosteroid injections.[45] Although corticosteroid injections will likely provide patients with short-term improvement in their symptoms, they pose a risk of biceps tendon rupture if they are injected into the tendon.[46] Ultrasonographic-guided injection may be preferred because it allows for a more accurate injection into the biceps sheath.[47] Other modalities that can be used for the nonsurgical management of LHBT disorders include iontophoresis, phonophoresis, ultrasonography, extracorporeal shock wave therapy, and laser therapy; however, these nonsurgical modalities have demonstrated conflicting results in the literature.[48,49] Clinical outcomes on the use of regenerative injection therapy, including the use of platelet-rich plasma, are promising but remain inconclusive.[50] Although physical therapy may help improve overall shoulder strength, ROM, and function, there are no studies in the literature on the outcomes of physical therapy for the management LHBT disorders.

Surgical Management

Surgical management of BLC injuries is reserved for patients in whom nonsurgical management fails or patients who have an acute injury such as an acute, symptomatic type II SLAP lesion.

SLAP Repair

Because SLAP lesions occur in multiple patient populations, including manual laborers and overhead athletes, and outcome studies are plagued with confounding variables and low-level evidence, appropriate surgical management for SLAP lesions remains controversial. The ideal candidate for a SLAP repair is a young, active patient who has

a history, a physical examination, and imaging studies that are consistent with a type II SLAP lesion. Surgeons should exercise caution in overhead athletes who undergo SLAP repair because clinical outcomes in these patients can be unpredictable, especially with regard to the ability of an athlete to return to his or her preinjury level of play.

Typically, the patient is placed in the beach-chair position; however, some surgeons place the patient in the lateral decubitus position because it allows for better access to the anterior, posterior, and inferior labrum in patients in whom the tear extends beyond the superior labrum. Standard diagnostic arthroscopy is performed from a standard posterior portal, with careful attention paid to the superior labrum to clearly identify fiber failure rather than labral recess, which is physiologic. The biceps tendon should be carefully probed and mobilized to identify concomitant pathology. An adjunctive biceps tenodesis may be indicated if the patient's history, physical examination, and arthroscopic findings indicate concomitant LHBT tendinitis, tear, or instability.

Portal placement allows the surgeon to gain access to the superior labrum for glenoid preparation, anchor placement, and suture passage. The authors of this chapter prefer to use a standard anterior portal through the rotator interval and an accessory anterosuperior portal through the musculotendinous junction of the supraspinatus (medial to the rotator cable) for anchor placement. Portals can be placed with the use of a small cannula or percutaneously to minimize iatrogenic trauma to the supraspinatus.

Through the anterior portal, the labral footprint is débrided, and a burr or bone-cutting shaver is used to prepare the bone to a bleeding base for

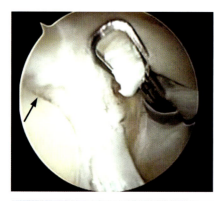

Figure 5 Arthroscopic image taken from the posterior portal in a right shoulder of a man (who worked as a manual laborer) placed in the beach-chair position shows biceps tenotomy, which was followed by tenodesis, of a symptomatic type II superior labrum anterior to posterior lesion (arrow).

healing. The authors of this chapter prefer to place anchors posterior to the biceps origin to prevent stiffness, which may occur with anchors that are placed anterior to the biceps origin. The suture anchor is placed through an accessory portal, and a suture shuttling device is used through the anterior portal for suture passage. Alternatively, a spinal needle can be used through the Neviaser portal for suture shuttling. Knots are tied off the glenoid face to prevent knot abrasion. Alternatively, knotless systems that prevent knot abrasion are available for SLAP repair.

Postoperatively, patients progress through a graduated rehabilitation program. An initial protective phase that lasts for 6 weeks includes full-time sling wear; shoulder, elbow, and hand ROM, as tolerated; and passive ROM exercises. Patients then graduate to phase 2, which includes active ROM, isotonic strengthening of the rotator cuff, and scapular stabilization exercises. Patients should avoid biceps strengthening during phase 2. At 12 weeks postoperatively,

patients typically progress to active strengthening and maintenance of full ROM, with throwing, if indicated, beginning at approximately 4 months postoperatively. The patient then progresses to a sport-specific rehabilitation protocol.

Biceps Tenotomy

Biceps tenotomy is a viable option and has long been the surgical management strategy of choice in Europe for the management of LHBT pathology. Surgeons must consider a patient's age, body habitus, and concerns for cosmesis in the decision of whether to perform tenotomy or tenodesis. Surgical time also is a factor for patients in whom other concomitant procedures are necessary.

A biceps tenotomy is a relatively quick and simple procedure. The patient is placed in the beach-chair or lateral decubitus position, a standard posterior portal is established, and an anterior portal is established through the rotator interval. An arthroscopic biter, scissors, or radiofrequency ablation device is introduced into the anterior portal, and the biceps tendon is released from its origin and allowed to retract into the bicipital groove. The surgeon can resect a small amount of superior labrum with the LHBT to create a stump, which may lead to autotenodesis of the LHBT at the articular margin and prevent it from sliding down into the bicipital groove (**Figure 5**).

Biceps Tenodesis

Biceps tenodesis, whether performed in either an arthroscopic or open manner, is an option for patients who have anterior shoulder pain in the bicipital groove, a provocative physical examination, and, possibly, corroborative

imaging findings. An ideal patient for biceps tenodesis has concern for the cosmetic appearance of a Popeye deformity, is a laborer or active individual who may report biceps muscle cramping, and is compliant and willing to undergo the prolonged rehabilitation and protective phase necessitated by biceps tenodesis.

Arthroscopic Biceps Tenodesis

Arthroscopic biceps tenodesis can be performed with the use of multiple techniques. The biceps can be tenodesed to the rotator interval or the anterior supraspinatus tendon (soft-tissue tenodesis), or it can be tenodesed to bone high in the bicipital groove or, alternately, above the pectoralis insertion (suprapectoral tenodesis). Some surgeons have adopted suprapectoral arthroscopic tenodesis because of persistent bicipital groove pain, which can occur with a more proximally located tenodesis.[51,52]

For arthroscopic tenodesis, the authors of this chapter prefer to use an interference screw technique in the suprapectoral location. Diagnostic arthroscopy is performed as previously discussed; however, the biceps tendon is tagged with a monofilament suture before tenotomy to control the tendon and maintain its length-tension relationship during tenodesis. Attention is then turned to the subacromial space, and a more anterior-based lateral working portal is established to access the anterolateral subdeltoid space. The patient's arm is positioned in forward flexion, the suprapectoral location is identified, and the tenodesis site is prepared with the use of a shaver and a radiofrequency ablation device. A separate anterior portal is made lower than the standard anterior portal and in line with the bicipital groove. The guide pin and reamer are introduced through this portal after the biceps tendon is mobilized away from the bicipital groove with the use of a monofilament suture for control. The tenodesis screw is inserted, and the biceps tendon is secured just proximal to the pectoralis insertion. The remaining proximal tendon is then removed (**Figure 6**). Additional suture fixation through the superior pectoralis can be used as necessary.

Open Subpectoral Biceps Tenodesis

Open subpectoral biceps tenodesis (OBT) is advantageous compared with arthroscopic tenodesis techniques, which leave all or a portion of the biceps within the bicipital groove, because it avoids the possibility of residual pain postoperatively. The biceps tendon contains a dense network of sensory nerve fibers, with more innervation at the proximal aspect of the tendon.[53] OBT allows for the removal of a larger amount of the LHBT and the tenodesis site that is distal to the bicipital groove, which helps reduce the risk of residual pain postoperatively.

OBT can be performed with the use of multiple surgical techniques and fixation constructs. The authors of this chapter use an interference screw technique because it has demonstrated superior biomechanical properties compared with the use of bone tunnels, suture anchors, and cortical buttons[54-60] and allows for intramedullary healing of the tendon inside the cortex of the humerus rather than to the cortical surface. The authors of this chapter place the patient in the beach-chair position and perform a standard tenotomy as previously discussed, which is followed by concomitant procedures as indicated. At the end of the arthroscopic portion

of the procedure, attention is turned to the anterior arm.

The arm and axilla are reprepared with chlorhexidine. A 2- to 3-cm incision is made within the axillary skin crease, overlying the pectoralis major tendon. Blunt dissection is carried to the level of the short head of the biceps and the adjacent pectoralis major. The interval between the short head of the biceps and the adjacent pectoralis major is explored, and the LHBT is reliably located within the interval. The surgeon's finger is used to free the LHBT, which is then pulled into the wound. The authors of this chapter use a narrow pointed Hohmann retractor laterally around the humerus, a Chandler retractor medially around the humerus, and an Army-Navy retractor superiorly in the wound to expose the tenodesis site. The LHBT is then whipstitched with No. 2 braided composite suture, and the tendon is cut approximately 2 cm from the musculotendinous junction to optimize the length-tension relationship. The tenodesis site is then prepared and drilled, and the LHBT is fixed in the tenodesis site with a single polyetheretherketone interference screw. The suture is then tied over the screw for additional fixation (**Figure 7**).

Nonsurgical and Surgical Management of LHBT Lesions in Overhead Athletes

Overhead athletes who have LHBT lesions deserve special attention because they have unique shoulder mechanics and clinical expectations. Baseball pitchers, in particular, have a high risk for SLAP tears. The baseball pitch is the fastest described human motion, often exceeding 7,000° per second; this places a large force, often more than 1,000 N, on the shoulder in professional baseball

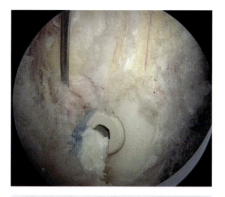

Figure 6 Arthroscopic image of a shoulder shows final arthroscopic biceps tenodesis with interference screw fixation that was supplemented with suture.

pitchers.[61] Several theories on the pathomechanism of SLAP tears in baseball pitchers, including tension during the deceleration phase or peelback during the late cocking phase of throwing, both of which are often exacerbated by anterior microinstability or posterior capsular contracture and glenohumeral internal rotation deficit, have been proposed.[62-64] The management of SLAP tears in overhead athletes is controversial, and some SLAP tears may be physiologic adaptations to throwing kinematics, most of which are asymptomatic in this patient population.[65]

Nonsurgical management of SLAP tears in overhead athletes includes the use of NSAIDs as well as an initial trial of physical therapy to improve glenohumeral internal rotation deficit, strengthen the rotator cuff and scapular stabilizers, and improve throwing mechanics. Surgery is indicated for patients in whom nonsurgical management fails. Surgical options for the management of SLAP tears in overhead athletes include labral débridement, SLAP repair, biceps tenotomy, and biceps tenodesis.[66]

Inability to return to play is the most common complication in overhead

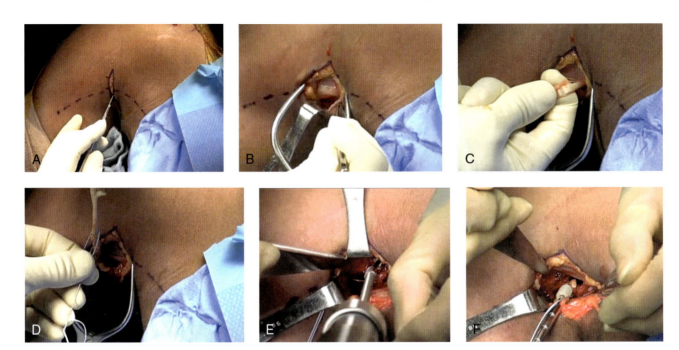

Figure 7 Intraoperative photographs of a shoulder show open subpectoral biceps tenodesis. **A,** A 2-cm incision is made longitudinally over the pectoralis insertion (dashed line) in the axillary crease. **B,** The pectoralis is identified. **C,** The subpectoral region is bluntly explored, and the long head of the biceps tendon (LHBT) is retrieved manually. **D,** The LHBT is whipstitched with No. 2 braided composite suture. The tenodesis site is then prepared (**E**), and the LHBT is fixed in the tenodesis site with a tenodesis screw (**F**).

athletes who undergo SLAP repair. Inability to return to play is likely caused by multiple factors, including continued pain, loss of ROM, and changes in proprioception and shoulder mechanics.[67] In a recent systematic review of patients who underwent SLAP repair, Gorantla et al[68] reported a 64% rate of return to preinjury level of play; however, Fedoriw et al[69] reported a rate of return to preinjury level of play as low as 7% in the specific evaluation of overhead athletes who underwent SLAP repair. Overhead athletes who undergo nonsurgical treatment for SLAP tears also have poor return to play outcomes but demonstrate improvements in pain, function, and quality of life.[70]

OBT has resulted in excellent clinical outcomes in patients with biceps pathology and good outcomes in patients in whom SLAP repair fails.[71-73] OBT has demonstrated equivocal clinical

outcomes and return to play compared with those of SLAP repair;[71,74,75] however, a recent motion analysis study reported that pitchers who underwent OBT had more normal pitching mechanics compared with those who underwent SLAP repair.[67] Although OBT may be appropriate for patients who have SLAP tears and concomitant biceps tendinitis,[76] further studies are necessary to determine the appropriate surgical management strategy for overhead athletes. Therefore, an initial trial of nonsurgical management that includes extensive physical therapy is imperative in overhead athletes, and caution should be maintained in overhead athletes in whom surgery is indicated.

Clinical Outcomes

In general, good outcomes have been reported in patients who undergo SLAP

repair; however, those outcomes are substantially worse in specific patient populations, including patients older than 35 years, workers' compensation patients, and overhead athletes, with reports of recalcitrant pain and stiffness.[68,77,78] Salvage options in patients with recalcitrant pain and stiffness are typically limited to tenodesis because revision repair has been associated with poor outcomes.[72,79-81]

In general, outcomes of arthroscopic biceps tenodesis are favorable with respect to improvements in clinical outcomes scores, pain, and function. Although studies comparing arthroscopic biceps tenodesis with OBT have reported no substantial difference with regard to postoperative clinical outcome scores,[71,82-87] Werner et al[86] suggested an increased risk of early postoperative stiffness in patients who undergo arthroscopic biceps tenodesis.

Clinical outcomes of OBT are good, with patients demonstrating substantial improvements in pain and functional outcomes scores.[73,85,86] Studies comparing tenotomy with tenodesis have not demonstrated a clear difference with regard to clinical outcomes;[88-95] this is likely confounded by multiple variables, one of which is that tenotomy and tenodesis are often performed concomitant with other procedures, including rotator cuff repair, which makes it difficult to isolate only the outcomes of tenotomy and tenodesis. Although recent meta-analyses have reported that, compared with tenotomy, tenodesis is associated with a substantially decreased risk of Popeye deformity and cramping biceps muscle pain, the meta-analyses reported no difference between the two procedures with respect to Constant assessment score, flexion strength, or supination strength.[96,97] Compared with tenotomy, tenodesis is more technically challenging and is associated with longer surgical time, longer rehabilitation time, and the need to protect the repair postoperatively.[96] Therefore, surgeons should counsel patients on expectations when choosing between the two procedures. The ideal candidate for tenotomy is older, has lower functional demands, and does not have cosmetic concern for the possibility of a Popeye deformity.

Complications

Studies have reported that patients who undergo OBT have an increased risk for iatrogenic injury to adjacent neurovascular structures as well as humeral fracture,[98,99] with an overall complication risk of approximately 2%.[100] Although these complications are uncommon, surgeons must be mindful of retractor placement, especially the medial retractor, during OBT. To minimize fracture risk, surgeons must position the tenodesis site in the center of the bicipital groove with the use of a concentrically placed tenodesis screw.[101] In addition, patients should adhere to postoperative activity restrictions to minimize stress on the tenodesis site.

The potential complications of arthroscopic biceps tenodesis mirror those described for OBT, including residual postoperative groove pain and injury to the surrounding neurovascular structures. Compared with patients who undergo OBT, patients who undergo arthroscopic biceps tenodesis have a lower risk for fracture and neurovascular injury because of the more proximal location of the tenodesis in the metaphyseal bone.[66,98,100] However, Werner et al[86] reported an increased risk of early postoperative stiffness in patients who underwent arthroscopic biceps tenodesis.

Summary

The LHBT is a common source of disease and shoulder pain. Etiologies of LHBT disease include inflammation, instability, and trauma. Although there are numerous diagnostic tests to evaluate for superior labral and LHBT pathology, most lack the reliability necessary for diagnosis, which requires surgeons to rely on MRI and other supplemental diagnostic strategies. Initial nonsurgical treatment of LHBT and SLAP pathology includes guided physical therapy, anti-inflammatory medications, and corticosteroid injections. If nonsurgical management fails, surgical techniques for the management of BLC pathology include SLAP repair, biceps tenotomy, and biceps tenodesis. Techniques for biceps tenodesis, which can be performed in either an arthroscopic or open manner, include soft-tissue tenodesis, suprapectoral tenodesis, and subpectoral tenodesis. If appropriately treated, patients with LHBT pathology often have excellent clinical outcomes. Surgeons must be aware of the risk for iatrogenic neurologic complications and fracture. These complications, although rare, may be devastating but, fortunately, can be avoided in most patients with the use of sound surgical technique.

References

1. Taylor SA, Khair MM, Gulotta LV, et al: Diagnostic glenohumeral arthroscopy fails to fully evaluate the biceps-labral complex. *Arthroscopy* 2015;31(2):215-224.

2. Taylor SA, Fabricant PD, Bansal M, et al: The anatomy and histology of the bicipital tunnel of the shoulder. *J Shoulder Elbow Surg* 2015;24(4):511-519.

3. Cooper DE, Arnoczky SP, O'Brien SJ, Warren RF, DiCarlo E, Allen AA: Anatomy, histology, and vascularity of the glenoid labrum: An anatomical study. *J Bone Joint Surg Am* 1992;74(1):46-52.

4. Tuoheti Y, Itoi E, Minagawa H, et al: Attachment types of the long head of the biceps tendon to the glenoid labrum and their relationships with the glenohumeral ligaments. *Arthroscopy* 2005;21(10):1242-1249.

5. Vangsness CT Jr, Jorgenson SS, Watson T, Johnson DL: The origin of the long head of the biceps from the scapula and glenoid labrum: An anatomical study of 100 shoulders. *J Bone Joint Surg Br* 1994;76(6):951-954.

6. Pal GP, Bhatt RH, Patel VS: Relationship between the tendon of the long head of biceps brachii and the glenoidal labrum in humans. *Anat Rec* 1991;229(2):278-280.

7. Connell DA, Potter HG, Wickiewicz TL, Altchek DW, Warren RF: Noncontrast magnetic resonance imaging of superior labral lesions: 102 cases confirmed at arthroscopic surgery. *Am J Sports Med* 1999;27(2):208-213.

8. Hwang E, Carpenter JE, Hughes RE, Palmer ML: Effects of biceps tension and superior humeral head translation on the glenoid labrum. *J Orthop Res* 2014;32(11):1424-1429.

9. Snyder SJ, Karzel RP, Del Pizzo W, Ferkel RD, Friedman MJ: SLAP lesions of the shoulder. *Arthroscopy* 1990;6(4):274-279.

10. Maffet MW, Gartsman GM, Moseley B: Superior labrum-biceps tendon complex lesions of the shoulder. *Am J Sports Med* 1995;23(1):93-98.

11. Cheng NM, Pan WR, Vally F, Le Roux CM, Richardson MD: The arterial supply of the long head of biceps tendon: Anatomical study with implications for tendon rupture. *Clin Anat* 2010;23(6):683-692.

12. Habermeyer P, Magosch P, Pritsch M, Scheibel MT, Lichtenberg S: Antero-superior impingement of the shoulder as a result of pulley lesions: A prospective arthroscopic study. *J Shoulder Elbow Surg* 2004;13(1):5-12.

13. Braun S, Horan MP, Elser F, Millett PJ: Lesions of the biceps pulley. *Am J Sports Med* 2011;39(4):790-795.

14. Verma NN, Drakos M, O'Brien SJ: The arthroscopic active compression test. *Arthroscopy* 2005;21(5):634.

15. Byram IR, Dunn WR, Kuhn JE: Humeral head abrasion: An association with failed superior labrum anterior posterior repairs. *J Shoulder Elbow Surg* 2011;20(1):92-97.

16. Boileau P, Ahrens PM, Hatzidakis AM: Entrapment of the long head of the biceps tendon: The hourglass biceps—a cause of pain and locking of the shoulder. *J Shoulder Elbow Surg* 2004;13(3):249-257.

17. Cone RO, Danzig L, Resnick D, Goldman AB: The bicipital groove: Radiographic, anatomic, and pathologic study. *AJR Am J Roentgenol* 1983;141(4):781-788.

18. Pfahler M, Branner S, Refior HJ: The role of the bicipital groove in tendopathy of the long biceps tendon. *J Shoulder Elbow Surg* 1999;8(5):419-424.

19. Gleason PD, Beall DP, Sanders TG, et al: The transverse humeral ligament: A separate anatomical structure or a continuation of the osseous attachment of the rotator cuff? *Am J Sports Med* 2006;34(1):72-77.

20. MacDonald K, Bridger J, Cash C, Parkin I: Transverse humeral ligament: Does it exist? *Clin Anat* 2007;20(6):663-667.

21. LaFrance R, Madsen W, Yaseen Z, Giordano B, Maloney M, Voloshin I: Relevant anatomic landmarks and measurements for biceps tenodesis. *Am J Sports Med* 2013;41(6):1395-1399.

22. Gerber C, Galantay RV, Hersche O: The pattern of pain produced by irritation of the acromioclavicular joint and the subacromial space. *J Shoulder Elbow Surg* 1998;7(4):352-355.

23. Murthi AM, Vosburgh CL, Neviaser TJ: The incidence of pathologic changes of the long head of the biceps tendon. *J Shoulder Elbow Surg* 2000;9(5):382-385.

24. Chen CH, Hsu KY, Chen WJ, Shih CH: Incidence and severity of biceps long head tendon lesion in patients with complete rotator cuff tears. *J Trauma* 2005;58(6):1189-1193.

25. Tantisricharoenkul G, Tan EW, Fayad LM, McCarthy EF, McFarland EG: Malignant soft tissue tumors of the biceps muscle mistaken for proximal biceps tendon rupture. *Orthopedics* 2012;35(10):e1548-e1552.

26. Matsen FA III, Kirby RM: Office evaluation and management of shoulder pain. *Orthop Clin North Am* 1982;13(3):453-475.

27. Gill HS, El Rassi G, Bahk MS, Castillo RC, McFarland EG: Physical examination for partial tears of the biceps tendon. *Am J Sports Med* 2007;35(8):1334-1340.

28. Holtby R, Razmjou H: Accuracy of the Speed's and Yergason's tests in detecting biceps pathology and SLAP lesions: Comparison with arthroscopic findings. *Arthroscopy* 2004;20(3):231-236.

29. Parentis MA, Glousman RE, Mohr KS, Yocum LA: An evaluation of the provocative tests for superior labral anterior posterior lesions. *Am J Sports Med* 2006;34(2):265-268.

30. Oh JH, Kim JY, Kim WS, Gong HS, Lee JH: The evaluation of various physical examinations for the diagnosis of type II superior labrum anterior and posterior lesion. *Am J Sports Med* 2008;36(2):353-359.

31. Walch G, Nové-Josserand L, Boileau P, Levigne C: Subluxations and dislocations of the tendon of the long head of the biceps. *J Shoulder Elbow Surg* 1998;7(2):100-108.

32. Gandolfo N, Bianchi S, Martinoli C, Derchi LE: Long biceps brachii instability: Role of ultrasonography. *Radiol Med* 1998;96(1-2):18-22.

33. Gobezie R, Zurakowski D, Lavery K, Millett PJ, Cole BJ, Warner JJ: Analysis of interobserver and intraobserver variability in the diagnosis and treatment of SLAP tears using the Snyder classification. *Am J Sports Med* 2008;36(7):1373-1379.

34. Jia X, Yokota A, McCarty EC, et al: Reproducibility and reliability of the Snyder classification of superior labral anterior posterior lesions among shoulder surgeons. *Am J Sports Med* 2011;39(5):986-991.

35. O'Brien SJ, Pagnani MJ, Fealy S, McGlynn SR, Wilson JB: The active compression test: A new and effective test for diagnosing labral tears and acromioclavicular joint abnormality. *Am J Sports Med* 1998;26(5):610-613.

36. Hegedus EJ, Goode AP, Cook CE, et al: Which physical examination tests provide clinicians with the most value when examining the shoulder? Update of a systematic review with meta-analysis of individual tests. *Br J Sports Med* 2012;46(14):964-978.

37. Cheung E, O'Driscoll S: The dynamic labral shear test for superior labral anterior posterior tears of the shoulder. Presented at the 76th Annual Meeting of the American Academy of Orthopaedic Surgeons, San Diego, CA, February 14-18, 2007.

38. Ben Kibler W, Sciascia AD, Hester P, Dome D, Jacobs C: Clinical utility of traditional and new tests in the diagnosis of biceps tendon injuries and superior labrum anterior and posterior lesions in the shoulder. *Am J Sports Med* 2009;37(9):1840-1847.

39. Cook C, Beaty S, Kissenberth MJ, Siffri P, Pill SG, Hawkins RJ: Diagnostic accuracy of five orthopedic clinical tests for diagnosis of superior labrum

anterior posterior (SLAP) lesions. *J Shoulder Elbow Surg* 2012;21(1):13-22.

40. Taylor SA, Newman AM, Nguyen J, et al: Magnetic resonance imaging currently fails to fully evaluate the biceps-labrum complex and bicipital tunnel. *Arthroscopy* 2016;32(2):238-244.

41. Mohtadi NG, Vellet AD, Clark ML, et al: A prospective, double-blind comparison of magnetic resonance imaging and arthroscopy in the evaluation of patients presenting with shoulder pain. *J Shoulder Elbow Surg* 2004;13(3):258-265.

42. Houtz CG, Schwartzberg RS, Barry JA, Reuss BL, Papa L: Shoulder MRI accuracy in the community setting. *J Shoulder Elbow Surg* 2011;20(4):537-542.

43. Reuss BL, Schwartzberg R, Zlatkin MB, Cooperman A, Dixon JR: Magnetic resonance imaging accuracy for the diagnosis of superior labrum anterior-posterior lesions in the community setting: Eighty-three arthroscopically confirmed cases. *J Shoulder Elbow Surg* 2006;15(5):580-585.

44. Dubrow SA, Streit JJ, Shishani Y, Robbin MR, Gobezie R: Diagnostic accuracy in detecting tears in the proximal biceps tendon using standard nonenhancing shoulder MRI. *Open Access J Sports Med* 2014;5:81-87.

45. Nho SJ, Strauss EJ, Lenart BA, et al: Long head of the biceps tendinopathy: Diagnosis and management. *J Am Acad Orthop Surg* 2010;18(11):645-656.

46. Nichols AW: Complications associated with the use of corticosteroids in the treatment of athletic injuries. *Clin J Sport Med* 2005;15(5):370-375.

47. Hashiuchi T, Sakurai G, Morimoto M, Komei T, Takakura Y, Tanaka Y: Accuracy of the biceps tendon sheath injection: Ultrasound-guided or unguided injection? A randomized controlled trial. *J Shoulder Elbow Surg* 2011;20(7):1069-1073.

48. Childress MA, Beutler A: Management of chronic tendon injuries. *Am Fam Physician* 2013;87(7):486-490.

49. Andres BM, Murrell GA: Treatment of tendinopathy: What works,

what does not, and what is on the horizon. *Clin Orthop Relat Res* 2008;466(7):1539-1554.

50. Moon YL, Ha SH, Lee YK, Park YK: Comparative studies of platelet-rich plasma (PRP) and prolotherapy for proximal biceps tendinitis. *Clin Shoulder Elbow* 2011;14(2):153-158.

51. Romeo AA, Mazzocca AD, Tauro JC: Arthroscopic biceps tenodesis. *Arthroscopy* 2004;20(2):206-213.

52. David TS, Schildhorn JC: Arthroscopic suprapectoral tenodesis of the long head biceps: Reproducing an anatomic length-tension relationship. *Arthrosc Tech* 2012;1(1):e127-e132.

53. Alpantaki K, McLaughlin D, Karagogeos D, Hadjipavlou A, Kontakis G: Sympathetic and sensory neural elements in the tendon of the long head of the biceps. *J Bone Joint Surg Am* 2005;87(7):1580-1583.

54. Patzer T, Santo G, Olender GD, Wellmann M, Hurschler C, Schofer MD: Suprapectoral or subpectoral position for biceps tenodesis: Biomechanical comparison of four different techniques in both positions. *J Shoulder Elbow Surg* 2012;21(1):116-125.

55. Tashjian RZ, Henninger HB: Biomechanical evaluation of subpectoral biceps tenodesis: Dual suture anchor versus interference screw fixation. *J Shoulder Elbow Surg* 2013;22(10):1408-1412.

56. Richards DP, Burkhart SS: A biomechanical analysis of two biceps tenodesis fixation techniques. *Arthroscopy* 2005;21(7):861-866.

57. Mazzocca AD, Bicos J, Santangelo S, Romeo AA, Arciero RA: The biomechanical evaluation of four fixation techniques for proximal biceps tenodesis. *Arthroscopy* 2005;21(11):1296-1306.

58. Arora AS, Singh A, Koonce RC: Biomechanical evaluation of a unicortical button versus interference screw for subpectoral biceps tenodesis. *Arthroscopy* 2013;29(4):638-644.

59. Sethi PM, Rajaram A, Beitzel K, Hackett TR, Chowaniec DM, Mazzocca AD: Biomechanical performance of subpectoral biceps tenodesis: A comparison of

interference screw fixation, cortical button fixation, and interference screw diameter. *J Shoulder Elbow Surg* 2013;22(4):451-457.

60. Werner BC, Lyons ML, Evans CL, et al: Arthroscopic suprapectoral and open subpectoral biceps tenodesis: A comparison of restoration of length-tension and mechanical strength between techniques. *Arthroscopy* 2015;31(4):620-627.

61. Fleisig GS, Andrews JR, Dillman CJ, Escamilla RF: Kinetics of baseball pitching with implications about injury mechanisms. *Am J Sports Med* 1995;23(2):233-239.

62. Andrews JR, Carson WG Jr, McLeod WD: Glenoid labrum tears related to the long head of the biceps. *Am J Sports Med* 1985;13(5):337-341.

63. Bey MJ, Elders GJ, Huston LJ, Kuhn JE, Blasier RB, Soslowsky LJ: The mechanism of creation of superior labrum, anterior, and posterior lesions in a dynamic biomechanical model of the shoulder: The role of inferior subluxation. *J Shoulder Elbow Surg* 1998;7(4):397-401.

64. Burkhart SS, Morgan CD, Kibler WB: Shoulder injuries in overhead athletes: The "dead arm" revisited. *Clin Sports Med* 2000;19(1):125-158.

65. Lesniak BP, Baraga MG, Jose J, Smith MK, Cunningham S, Kaplan LD: Glenohumeral findings on magnetic resonance imaging correlate with innings pitched in asymptomatic pitchers. *Am J Sports Med* 2013;41(9):2022-2027.

66. Provencher MT, LeClere LE, Romeo AA: Subpectoral biceps tenodesis. *Sports Med Arthrosc* 2008;16(3):170-176.

67. Chalmers PN, Trombley R, Cip J, et al: Postoperative restoration of upper extremity motion and neuromuscular control during the overhand pitch: Evaluation of tenodesis and repair for superior labral anterior-posterior tears. *Am J Sports Med* 2014;42(12):2825-2836.

68. Gorantla K, Gill C, Wright RW: The outcome of type II SLAP repair: A systematic review. *Arthroscopy* 2010;26(4):537-545.

69. Fedoriw WW, Ramkumar P, McCulloch PC, Lintner DM: Return to play after treatment of superior labral tears in professional baseball players. *Am J Sports Med* 2014;42(5):1155-1160.

70. Edwards SL, Lee JA, Bell JE, et al: Nonoperative treatment of superior labrum anterior posterior tears: Improvements in pain, function, and quality of life. *Am J Sports Med* 2010;38(7):1456-1461.

71. Boileau P, Parratte S, Chuinard C, Roussanne Y, Shia D, Bicknell R: Arthroscopic treatment of isolated type II SLAP lesions: Biceps tenodesis as an alternative to reinsertion. *Am J Sports Med* 2009;37(5):929-936.

72. Gupta AK, Bruce B, Klosterman EL, McCormick F, Harris J, Romeo AA: Subpectoral biceps tenodesis for failed type II SLAP repair. *Orthopedics* 2013;36(6):e723-e728.

73. Mazzocca AD, Cote MP, Arciero CL, Romeo AA, Arciero RA: Clinical outcomes after subpectoral biceps tenodesis with an interference screw. *Am J Sports Med* 2008;36(10):1922-1929.

74. Ek ET, Shi LL, Tompson JD, Freehill MT, Warner JJ: Surgical treatment of isolated type II superior labrum anterior-posterior (SLAP) lesions: Repair versus biceps tenodesis. *J Shoulder Elbow Surg* 2014;23(7):1059-1065.

75. Denard PJ, Lädermann A, Parsley BK, Burkhart SS: Arthroscopic biceps tenodesis compared with repair of isolated type II SLAP lesions in patients older than 35 years. *Orthopedics* 2014;37(3):e292-e297.

76. Gupta AK, Chalmers PN, Klosterman EL, et al: Subpectoral biceps tenodesis for bicipital tendonitis with SLAP tear. *Orthopedics* 2015;38(1):e48-e53.

77. Erickson J, Lavery K, Monica J, Gatt C, Dhawan A: Surgical treatment of symptomatic superior labrum anterior-posterior tears in patients older than 40 years: A systematic review. *Am J Sports Med* 2015;43(5):1274-1282.

78. Sayde WM, Cohen SB, Ciccotti MG, Dodson CC: Return to play after Type II superior labral anterior-posterior lesion repairs in athletes: A systematic review. *Clin Orthop Relat Res* 2012;470(6):1595-1600.

79. Park S, Glousman RE: Outcomes of revision arthroscopic type II superior labral anterior posterior repairs. *Am J Sports Med* 2011;39(6):1290-1294.

80. McCormick F, Nwachukwu BU, Solomon D, et al: The efficacy of biceps tenodesis in the treatment of failed superior labral anterior posterior repairs. *Am J Sports Med* 2014;42(4):820-825.

81. Werner BC, Pehlivan HC, Hart JM, et al: Biceps tenodesis is a viable option for salvage of failed SLAP repair. *J Shoulder Elbow Surg* 2014;23(8):e179-e184.

82. Boileau P, Krishnan SG, Coste JS, Walch G: Arthroscopic biceps tenodesis: A new technique using bioabsorbable interference screw fixation. *Arthroscopy* 2002;18(9):1002-1012.

83. Nord KD, Smith GB, Mauck BM: Arthroscopic biceps tenodesis using suture anchors through the subclavian portal. *Arthroscopy* 2005;21(2):248-252.

84. Lutton DM, Gruson KI, Harrison AK, Gladstone JN, Flatow EL: Where to tenodese the biceps: Proximal or distal? *Clin Orthop Relat Res* 2011;469(4):1050-1055.

85. Werner BC, Evans CL, Holzgrefe RE, et al: Arthroscopic suprapectoral and open subpectoral biceps tenodesis: A comparison of minimum 2-year clinical outcomes. *Am J Sports Med* 2014;42(11):2583-2590.

86. Werner BC, Pehlivan HC, Hart JM, et al: Increased incidence of postoperative stiffness after arthroscopic compared with open biceps tenodesis. *Arthroscopy* 2014;30(9):1075-1084.

87. Gombera MM, Kahlenberg CA, Nair R, Saltzman MD, Terry MA: All-arthroscopic suprapectoral versus open subpectoral tenodesis of the long head of the biceps brachii. *Am J Sports Med* 2015;43(5):1077-1083.

88. Delle Rose G, Borroni M, Silvestro A, et al: The long head of biceps as a source of pain in active population: Tenotomy or tenodesis? A comparison of 2 case series with isolated lesions. *Musculoskelet Surg* 2012;96(suppl 1):S47-S52.

89. De Carli A, Vadalà A, Zanzotto E, et al: Reparable rotator cuff tears with concomitant long-head biceps lesions: Tenotomy or tenotomy/tenodesis? *Knee Surg Sports Traumatol Arthrosc* 2012;20(12):2553-2558.

90. Wittstein JR, Queen R, Abbey A, Toth A, Moorman CT III: Isokinetic strength, endurance, and subjective outcomes after biceps tenotomy versus tenodesis: A postoperative study. *Am J Sports Med* 2011;39(4):857-865.

91. Shank JR, Singleton SB, Braun S, et al: A comparison of forearm supination and elbow flexion strength in patients with long head of the biceps tenotomy or tenodesis. *Arthroscopy* 2011;27(1):9-16.

92. Koh KH, Ahn JH, Kim SM, Yoo JC: Treatment of biceps tendon lesions in the setting of rotator cuff tears: Prospective cohort study of tenotomy versus tenodesis. *Am J Sports Med* 2010;38(8):1584-1590.

93. Boileau P, Baqué F, Valerio L, Ahrens P, Chuinard C, Trojani C: Isolated arthroscopic biceps tenotomy or tenodesis improves symptoms in patients with massive irreparable rotator cuff tears. *J Bone Joint Surg Am* 2007;89(4):747-757.

94. Zhang Q, Zhou J, Ge H, Cheng B: Tenotomy or tenodesis for long head biceps lesions in shoulders with reparable rotator cuff tears: A prospective randomised trial. *Knee Surg Sports Traumatol Arthrosc* 2015;23(2):464-469.

95. Cho NS, Cha SW, Rhee YG: Funnel tenotomy versus intracuff tenodesis for lesions of the long head of the biceps tendon associated with rotator cuff tears. *Am J Sports Med* 2014;42(5):1161-1168.

96. Frost A, Zafar MS, Maffulli N: Tenotomy versus tenodesis in the management of pathologic lesions of the tendon of the long head of the biceps brachii. *Am J Sports Med* 2009;37(4):828-833.

97. Gurnani N, van Deurzen DF, Janmaat VT, van den Bekerom MP: Tenotomy or tenodesis for pathology of the long head of the biceps brachii: A systematic review and meta-analysis. *Knee Surg Sports Traumatol Arthrosc* 2015.

98. Rhee PC, Spinner RJ, Bishop AT, Shin AY: Iatrogenic brachial plexus injuries associated with open subpectoral biceps tenodesis: A report of 4 cases. *Am J Sports Med* 2013;41(9):2048-2053.

99. Sears BW, Spencer EE, Getz CL: Humeral fracture following subpectoral biceps tenodesis in 2 active, healthy patients. *J Shoulder Elbow Surg* 2011;20(6):e7-e11.

100. Nho SJ, Reiff SN, Verma NN, Slabaugh MA, Mazzocca AD, Romeo AA: Complications associated with subpectoral biceps tenodesis: Low rates of incidence following surgery. *J Shoulder Elbow Surg* 2010;19(5):764-768.

101. Euler SA, Smith SD, Williams BT, Dornan GJ, Millett PJ, Wijdicks CA: Biomechanical analysis of subpectoral biceps tenodesis: Effect of screw malpositioning on proximal humeral strength. *Am J Sports Med* 2015;43(1):69-74.

Patients in Whom Arthroscopic Bankart Repair is Not Enough: Evaluation and Management of Complex Anterior Glenohumeral Instability

John M. Tokish, MD
Laurent Lafosse, MD
Giovanni Di Giacomo, MD
Robert Arciero, MD

Abstract

Arthroscopic Bankart repair has become the most common treatment option for patients who have anterior shoulder instability. Although arthroscopic Bankart repair is generally an effective treatment method, it may be insufficient for the treatment of many patients who have anterior shoulder instability. Risk factors for failure of arthroscopic Bankart repair include younger age, level and type of sport, and shoulder specific risks, such as ligamentous laxity and the presence of bone loss. Recently, researchers have defined the limits of arthroscopic Bankart repair and more clearly defined treatment options for patients who have a high risk for failure after arthroscopic Bankart repair. Surgeons must recognize patients with anterior shoulder instability in whom a more aggressive surgical approach should be considered as well as patients who have a high risk for failure after arthroscopic Bankart repair to optimize outcomes in this patient population.

Instr Course Lect 2017;66:79–89.

Dr. Tokish or an immediate family member is a member of a speakers' bureau or has made paid presentations on behalf of Arthrex; serves as a paid consultant to or is an employee of Arthrex, DePuy, and Mitek; and serves as a board member, owner, officer, or committee member of the Arthroscopy Association of North America. Dr. Lafosse or an immediate family member has received royalties from DePuy; is a member of a speakers' bureau or has made paid presentations on behalf of DePuy; serves as a paid consultant to or is an employee of DePuy; has stock or stock options held in OrthoSpace and Innovative Shoulder Technology; and has received nonincome support (such as equipment or services), commercially derived honoraria, or other non-research–related funding (such as paid travel) from DePuy. Dr. Di Giacomo or an immediate family member has received royalties from Arthrex; is a member of a speakers' bureau or has made paid presentations on behalf of Arthrex; serves as a paid consultant to or is an employee of Arthrex; and serves as a board member, owner, officer, or committee member of the International Society of Arthroscopy, Knee Surgery and Orthopaedic Sports Medicine. Dr. Arciero or an immediate family member is a member of a speakers' bureau or has made paid presentations on behalf of Arthrex and Mitek; serves as a paid consultant to or is an employee of Biomet, Mitek, and Soft Tissue Regeneration; has stock or stock options held in Soft Tissue Regeneration; has received research or institutional support from Arthrex; and serves as a board member, owner, officer, or committee member of the American Orthopaedic Society for Sports Medicine.

Although arthroscopic management of anterior shoulder instability continues to increase,[1] it is clear that isolated arthroscopic Bankart repair may be insufficient for the treatment of many patients who have anterior shoulder instability. Risk factors for failure of arthroscopic Bankart repair can be demographic (eg, younger age and chosen sport) as well as anatomic (eg, ligamentous laxity and the presence of bone loss). Recent advances in the workup and treatment of patients who have shoulder instability have helped define the limits of arthroscopic Bankart repair and the treatment options for patients who have a high risk for failure after arthroscopic Bankart repair.

The Limits of Arthroscopic Bankart Repair

Although early results have demonstrated that arthroscopic Bankart repair has a higher failure rate compared

Table 1
The Instability Severity Index Score[a]

Prognostic Factor	Points
Age at time of surgery (yr)	
≤20	2
>20	0
Degree of preoperative sport participation	
Competitive	2
Recreational or none	0
Type of preoperative sport participation	
Contact or forced overhead	1
Other	0
Shoulder hyperlaxity	
Anterior or inferior shoulder hyperlaxity	1
Normal laxity	0
Hill-Sachs lesion on AP radiograph	
Visible in external rotation	2
Not visible in external rotation	0
Glenoid loss of contour on AP radiograph	
Loss of contour	2
No lesion	0
Total points	**10**

[a]The Instability Severity Index Score is based on a preoperative questionnaire, clinical examination, and radiographs.

Adapted with permission from Balg F, Boileau P: The instability severity index score: A simple pre-operative score to select patients for arthroscopic or open shoulder stabilisation. *J Bone Joint Surg Br* 2007;89(11):1470-1477.

with open Bankart repair,[2,3] many have argued that, with improved techniques and materials, arthroscopic Bankart repair would eventually result in similar outcomes compared with those of open surgery. Several studies have reported similar outcomes for arthroscopic Bankart repair and open surgery; however, Burkhart and De Beer[4] reported that significant bone loss, which was defined as an inverted pear-shaped glenoid, increased the rate of failure after arthroscopic Bankart repair from 4% to 67% and that participation in contact sports and significant bone loss increased the rate of arthroscopic failure from 6.5% to 89%. As a result of the Burkhart and De Beer study,[4] an increased emphasis has been placed on determining the proper indications for arthroscopic Bankart repair. Independent risk factors for failure after arthroscopic Bankart repair include younger age, generalized laxity, type and level of sport, and the presence of bone loss.[5] Balg and Boileau[5] included these risk factors in a 10-point Instability Severity Index Score to help guide decision making for the surgical treatment of patients who have anterior glenohumeral instability[5] (**Table 1**). The authors reported that patients with an Instability Severity Index Score higher than 6 had a failure rate of 70% after arthroscopic Bankart repair.[5] More recently, an Instability Severity Index Score higher than 3 has been reported to result in a failure rate of 70% after arthroscopic Bankart repair.[6] Few of the risk factors for failure after arthroscopic Bankart repair are modifiable or correctable.

Younger age is recognized as the most important risk factor for recurrent shoulder dislocation after arthroscopic Bankart repair.[6-8] Unfortunately, the age of a patient who has anterior shoulder instability is not modifiable, except via benign neglect. Although benign neglect may be appropriate for a very young patient,[9] it has been associated with recurrent dislocations as well as worse functional and clinical outcomes in young athletes.[10,11] Further, although anterior shoulder instability occurs in patients of many ages, it is primarily a condition that affects young, active athletes whose primary goal is return to play.

Shoulder hyperlaxity also is a well-recognized risk factor for recurrent shoulder instability and failure after arthroscopic Bankart.[5,12] Cho et al[12] reported that shoulder hyperlaxity was a risk factor for failed arthroscopic Bankart repair that required revision to an open procedure. Balg and Boileau[5] reported that patients with shoulder hyperlaxity and patients without shoulder hyperlaxity had an 18.9% and 4.9% failure rate, respectively, after arthroscopic Bankart repair. The authors included shoulder hyperlaxity, which was measured with the use of the Gagey test, in the Instability Severity Index Score, giving it a score of 1 point.[5] Although shoulder hyperlaxity is not modifiable, many studies recommended that it can be addressed with a rotator interval closure,[13,14] which limits inferior translation in the adducted position; however, other studies have reported that an arthroscopic rotator interval closure adds little value to most shoulder instability procedures.[15] Thus, an open rotator interval closure, or at least its arthroscopic equivalent, should be considered in patients who have substantial shoulder hyperlaxity, especially in the setting of other risk factors.

The type and level of sport in which a patient who has anterior shoulder instability participates is a critical factor for determining an appropriate surgical approach. Several studies have reported that contact athletes have a substantially higher rate of failure after arthroscopic Bankart repair. Cho et al[16] reported that collision athletes and noncollision athletes had a recurrence risk of 28.6% and 6.7%, respectively, after arthroscopic Bankart repair. Rhee et al[17] reported that contact athletes with anterior shoulder instability who were treated with an arthroscopic Bankart repair had a failure rate of 25% compared with those with anterior shoulder instability who were treated with open Bankart repair (12.5% failure rate). In the Instability Severity Index Score, Balg and Boileau[5] assigned 2 points to competitive athletes and 1 point to athletes who participated in contact or overhead sports.

Of all the risk factors for failure after arthroscopic Bankart repair, the presence of bone loss is nonpareil.[4] Burkhart and De Beer[4] definitively established the presence of glenohumeral bone loss as a primary determinant of outcome after arthroscopic Bankart repair. The authors reported a 6.5% recurrence rate in contact athletes without significant bone loss, which rose to 89% in contact athletes who had significant bone loss. In a follow-up study of a similar patient population, Burkhart et al[18] reported a 4.9% recurrence rate and a mean Constant score of 94.4 in patients who underwent an open Latarjet procedure. Pagnani[19] also reported a low recurrence rate (2%) in patients who underwent an open capsular repair, many of whom had significant bone loss that did not affect their outcomes. As surgeons began to appreciate the effects of bone loss, it was reported more frequently. Shaha et al[20] reported that patients with anterior shoulder instability had a mean glenoid bone loss of 13.4%. The prevalence of glenoid erosion or glenoid rim fracture in patients with anterior shoulder instability has been reported to range from 8% to 95%.[21-23]

In a study of 161 patients who had anteroinferior shoulder dislocation, Rowe et al[24] reported that 73% of the patients had damage to the glenoid rim, and 44% of the patients had fractures of the glenoid rim, 51% of which involved more than one-quarter of the glenoid diameter. Methods used to measure glenoid bone loss have been described in the literature. Huijsmans et al[25] described the most popular method used to measure glenoid bone loss, which assumes that the inferior two-thirds of the glenoid is a circle. Bone loss is calculated by dividing the radius of bone loss by the diameter of the circle. In patients with recurrent anterior shoulder dislocation who underwent three-dimensional (3D; best-fit circle) reconstruction, Sugaya et al[26] reported that 40% of patients had erosion-type bone loss, 50% of patients had fragment-type bone loss, and 10% of patients had intact bone. Conversely, smaller glenoid rim avulsions may occur after low-energy trauma that is associated with less axial load and more translation and shearing of the humeral head over the glenoid rim. A similar mechanism of injury also may be responsible for the compression fractures without bony fragments that are associated with attritional or erosive bone loss, which is caused by repeated recurrent episodes of shoulder instability.[27,28]

Boileau et al[29] reported that an episode of shoulder instability leads to glenoid rim avulsion without substantial stretching of the joint capsule if the joint capsule is strong and of good quality. Conversely, a weak joint capsule will be subject to elongation and, thus, recurrent subluxations or dislocations that can lead to compression and erosion of the glenoid rim. Therefore, in the clinical context, traumatic anterior shoulder instability can lead to only two types of glenoid lesions: glenoid rim fractures or avulsions and compression fractures or erosive bone loss. A wide range of noninvasive imaging methods have been used to evaluate and quantify glenoid bone loss, but it is very hard to define the size of a glenoid rim avulsion or a compression fracture. The importance of accurate measurement of glenoid bone loss has become increasingly recognized. Further investigation has suggested that patients who have even smaller amounts of bone loss may be at risk for failure after isolated arthroscopic Bankart repair. Shaha et al[20] redefined bone loss in a group of 72 active-duty military patients. The authors reported that as little as a 13.5% glenoid defect resulted in poor outcomes, based on Western Ontario Shoulder Instability Index and Single Assessment Numeric Evaluation scores, after arthroscopic Bankart repair even though the patients did not report recurrence.

Surgeons must distinguish between the normal anatomic structures of the

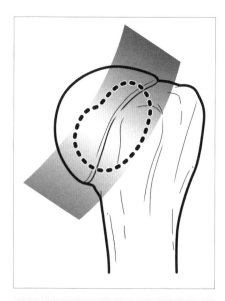

Figure 1 Illustration of a humeral head shows the glenoid track (shaded area). The dotted line represents the superimposed glenoid through range of motion.

posterior humeral head and the features characteristic of Hill-Sachs lesions. Richards et al[30] reported that the bare spot of the humeral head has no direct attachment to the rotator cuff tendons and is the anatomic groove of the humeral head that continues caudally to the humeral shaft.

Hill-Sachs Lesion Orientation

Burkhart and De Beer[4] reported that a nonengaging Hill-Sachs lesion has a long axis that is not parallel to the anterior glenoid with the shoulder in abduction and external rotation. In a shoulder with a nonengaging Hill-Sachs lesion, the articular surfaces are in continual contact and the lesion does not engage with the anterior glenoid. Conversely, an engaging Hill-Sachs lesion has a long axis that is parallel to the anterior glenoid with the shoulder in abduction and external rotation, such that the lesion engages with the corner of the anterior glenoid. A shoulder with an engaging

Hill-Sachs defect is at risk for recurrent dislocation and subluxation even after arthroscopic repair.

Hill-Sachs Lesion Position

Yamamoto et al[31] proposed the concept of the "glenoid track" in a 3D CT study on the contact areas between the humeral head and the glenoid. The authors reported that, with the shoulder in abduction and external rotation, the contact area between the humeral head and the glenoid shifted from the inferomedial to the superolateral side of the posterior articular surface, which the authors defined as the glenoid track (**Figure 1**). Bony stability increased if no substantial bone loss was present and the glenoid track was intact. The authors reported that the glenoid track was 18.4 mm or 84% of the glenoid width with the arm in 60° of abduction to the scapula or 90° of abduction to the trunk.[31] The integrity of the glenoid track and the location of the medial margin of a Hill-Sachs lesion are essential to correctly treat patients.[32,33]

Hill-Sachs Lesion Size

Both Boileau et al[29] and Rowe et al[24,34] identified large Hill-Sachs lesions as a risk factor for recurrent shoulder instability; however, neither of the studies quantified what constituted a large Hill-Sachs defect. Similarly, Cho et al[35] reported that engaging Hill-Sachs lesions were wider and deeper compared with nonengaging Hill-Sachs lesions and demonstrated a close correlation between the size of a Hill-Sachs lesion and its engagement. In a biomechanical study, Kaar et al[36] reported that glenohumeral stability was less prevalent in patients who had a Hill-Sachs defect that constituted five-eighths of the humeral head radius. In contrast, Sekiya

et al[37] reported that glenohumeral stability decreased in patients who had a Hill-Sachs defect that constituted 25% of the humeral head.

Bipolar Bone Loss

In separate laboratory studies, both Itoi et al[38] and Greis et al[39] reported that a 21% glenoid defect increased glenohumeral translation and adversely affected Bankart repair. Similarly, in separate studies, Sekiya et al[37] and Kaar et al[36] reported that a 25% humeral head defect increased glenohumeral translation. In many clinical situations, both glenoid and humeral head defects are present; therefore, consideration of whether much smaller lesions can compromise arthroscopic Bankart repair is warranted. The concept of the glenoid track[32] accounts for the size and location of both glenoid and humeral head defects. The amount of the humeral head that is congruent with the remaining intact glenoid can be estimated with the use of 3D CT and arthroscopy to determine whether bone defects are substantial enough to compromise traditional soft-tissue repair. A determination of whether a Hill-Sachs lesion is on track or off track can then guide decision making (**Figure 2**). Recently, Cook et al[40] reported that a determination of whether a Hill-Sachs lesion is on track or off track was highly accurate in predicting the success of arthroscopic Bankart repair. The authors reported that patients with on-track Hill-Sachs lesions that were fixed with arthroscopic Bankart repair alone had a failure rate of 8.2%, and patients with off-track Hill-Sachs lesions that were fixed with arthroscopic Bankart repair alone had a failure rate of 75%.

In a recent biomechanical study, Arciero et al[41] simultaneously evaluated

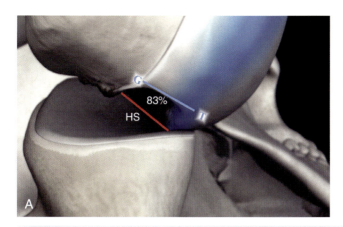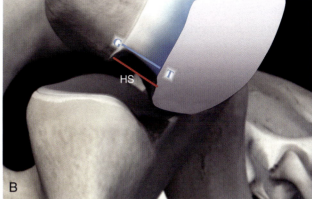

Figure 2   Three-dimensional illustrations of a shoulder show an on-track Hill-Sachs (HS) lesion (**A**) and an off-track HS lesion (**B**). Line G-T = glenoid track. (Reproduced with permission from Di Giacomo G, Itoi E, Burkhart SS: Evolving concept of bipolar bone loss and the Hill-Sachs lesion: From "engaging/non-engaging" lesion to "on-track/off-track" lesion. *Arthroscopy* 2014;30[1]:90-98.)

both glenoid and humeral head defects and their effect on glenohumeral translation with and without Bankart repair. Based on 3D CT scans of 142 patients who had recurrent shoulder instability, the authors used a 3D printer to model the defects. The authors reported that as little as a 2-mm glenoid defect (8% defect) in combination with a medium-sized humeral head lesion reduced the ability of the Bankart repair to resist translation by 26%. The authors concluded that the effect of lesions on both the glenoid and humeral head have an additive adverse effect on glenohumeral stability.

Revision Surgery After Failed Stabilization

Revision surgery after failed shoulder stabilization is underappreciated because the failure rate of revision surgery with the use of an arthroscopic soft-tissue approach has been unacceptable.[42-44] It should be emphasized that revision arthroscopic stabilization procedures have a high recurrence rate. **Table 2** lists several recent studies on the outcomes of revision arthroscopic

stabilization.[42-46] These studies were performed by surgeons who have known expertise in arthroscopic shoulder surgery. In one study, the recurrence rate was 36% even though revision arthroscopic stabilization was performed with the use of the remplissage procedure.[43] An arthroscopic revision surgery must have an ideal demographic, clinical, radiographic, arthroscopic, and technical scenario to result in good long-term outcomes. Specifically, the ideal scenario for arthroscopic revision surgery includes a patient with an acute substantial traumatic reason for recurrence and who is an older noncollision athlete with no midrange apprehension, little bone loss (<13% on the glenoid), and no engaging Hill-Sachs lesions (observed via imaging and arthroscopy). Further, at arthroscopy in the ideal scenario, the tissue must be in excellent condition, a minimum of three to four anchors (preferably double-loaded) must be used, and additional tensioning of the inferior glenohumeral ligament would be required. A remplissage procedure may contribute to the stability of the construct, especially in patients

who have smaller lesions and in patients who have little, if any, glenoid bone loss. Despite careful selection criteria that excluded patients who had bone loss, patients who were contact athletes, and patients who had multidirectional instability, Arce et al[44] reported a 22% failure rate after arthroscopic revision surgery.

Treatment Approaches for Complex Shoulder Instability

There are several alternative surgical approaches for the management of shoulder instability (**Figure 3**). An isolated arthroscopic Bankart repair should be considered in patients who have an on-track Hill-Sachs lesion and glenoid bone loss that is less than 20%. The authors of this chapter recommend an augmented procedure, such as an open Bankart repair/inferior capsular shift or a Latarjet procedure, in patients who have an on-track Hill-Sachs lesion and glenoid bone loss that exceeds 20%; however, bone grafting with either iliac crest, distal clavicle autograft, or distal tibia allograft is recommended in patients who have severe glenoid bone loss. An isolated arthroscopic Bankart

Table 2

Results of Revision Arthroscopic Stabilization[a]

Authors (Year)	No. of Patients/ Shoulders	Procedure or Approach	Mean Patient Age in Years (Range)	Mean Follow-up in Months (Range)	Results
Ryu and Ryu[46] (2011)	15 patients	Revision arthroscopic Bankart repair with double-loaded suture anchors	27.5 (17–44)	22 (18–70)	4 failures (27%): 2 with recurrent dislocation, 2 with atraumatic subluxations
Arce et al[44] (2012)	16 patients	Revision arthroscopic Bankart repair with single- or double-loaded suture anchors	26.8 (16–35)	31 (24–46)	3 with recurrent instability; 2 with ongoing pain
Blackman et al[42] (2014)	15 patients	Revision anterior shoulder stabilization	16.6 (14–18)	50 (22–102)	5 failures (33%), all recurrent dislocations
Friedman et al[45] (2014)	388 shoulders	Latarjet (49 shoulders), arthroscopic Bankart repair (191 shoulders), open Bankart repair (73 shoulders), and other open procedures (75 shoulders)	28.2 (NA)	44.2 (NA)	Latarjet: 7 failures (14.3%) Arthroscopic Bankart repair: 28 failures (14.7%) Open Bankart repair: 4 failures (5.5%) Other open procedures: 32 failures (42.7%)
McCabe et al[43] (2014)	11 patients	Revision arthroscopic repair with remplissage	23 (16.9–44.8)	41 (24–68)	4 failures (36%) had a mean postoperative Rowe score of 51

NA = not available.

[a]All studies are level IV evidence.

repair and a remplissage procedure are reasonable for patients who have an off-track Hill-Sachs lesion and glenoid bone loss that is less than 20%. The authors of this chapter recommend the Latarjet procedure or glenoid bone stock augmentation in patients who have severe glenoid bone loss.

Open Bankart Repair and Inferior Capsular Shift

In a classic study on Bankart repair for the treatment of 161 patients who had anterior shoulder instability, Rowe et al[24] ignored glenoid bone loss and reported a recurrence rate of 3.5%. In a more recent study, Pagnani[19] performed capsular repair without a bone block procedure for the management of anterior shoulder instability in 119 patients, 84% of whom had Hill-Sachs lesions

(27% of which were engaging) and 14% of whom had substantial glenoid bone loss. The authors reported an overall recurrence rate of 2% in the 103 patients who were available at a minimum follow-up of 2 years. Other studies have reported similar results.[12,24]

Latarjet Procedure

The Latarjet procedure transfers the coracoid process with its attached conjoined tendon to the anterior glenoid in the region of a glenoid osseous defect. A bone block is fixed over the inferior one-half of the subscapularis. The Latarjet procedure is advantageous for stabilization of an anteriorly unstable shoulder because fixation of the coracoid to the glenoid creates a bony extension of the articular arc, transfer of the coracoacromial ligament reinforces the

anterior capsular structures, and transfer of the conjointed tendon creates a sling effect on the lower subscapularis during abduction and external rotation. Despite the favorable results of the Latarjet procedure,[18,47-50] concern exists for the relatively high complication rate (25%).[51] Delaney et al[52] reported a 21% incidence of nerve deficit (mostly transient) after the Latarjet procedure.

Lafosse et al[53] recently described an arthroscopic approach for the Latarjet procedure (**Figure 4**), which has several potential advantages compared with the open Latarjet procedure. The arthroscopic Latarjet procedure allows for improved visualization of the bone graft; this helps avoid graft malposition, which has been correlated with recurrent shoulder instability if the graft is placed too medially and with

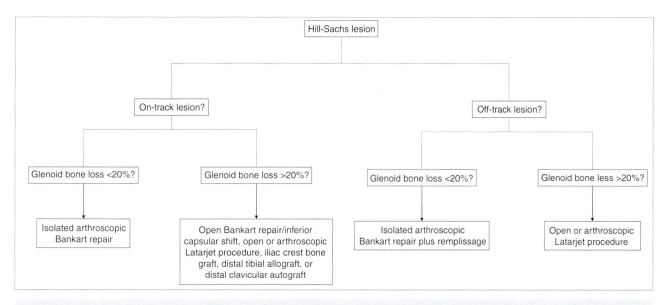

Figure 3 Algorithm shows the surgical treatment approaches for patients who have recurrent anterior/inferior shoulder instability.

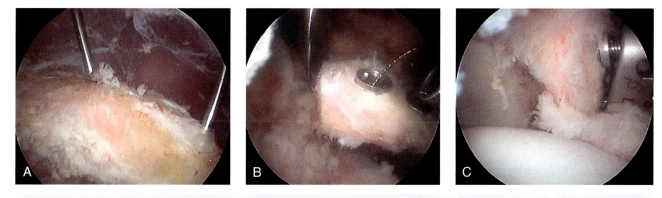

Figure 4 Arthroscopic images of a shoulder show the arthroscopic Latarjet procedure. **A,** The coracoid is exposed. **B,** A coracoid osteotomy is performed. **C,** The coracoid is seated against the glenoid.

osteoarthritis if the graft is placed too laterally. The arthroscopic Latarjet procedure allows the surgeon to address concomitant pathology that may go unrecognized with the open Latarjet procedure. Because the arthroscopic Latarjet procedure is a true muscle-sparing approach, it may result in less morbidity, fewer adhesions, and fewer patients who have early stiffness. The arthroscopic Latarjet procedure also may result in an improved cosmetic appearance. In a study of 87 patients who underwent the arthroscopic Latarjet

procedure (64 of whom were available for follow-up), Dumont et al[54] reported a 1.6% recurrence rate and a mean Western Ontario Shoulder Instability Index score of 90.6% at mean follow-up of 76.4 months. The authors reported complications, including hematoma (three patients), graft fracture (one patient), and transient musculocutaneous nerve palsy (one patient), in 15.6% of the patients, excellent outcomes in 91% of the patients, good outcomes in 9% of the patients, and a high return to sport.[55]

Iliac Crest Bone Grafting
Popularized by Warner et al,[56] a bulk iliac crest bone graft can be fashioned to re-create the contour of the glenoid, provide bone stock, and restore glenoid bone loss in patients who have recurrent shoulder instability. Iliac crest bone grafting, which is a modification of the Eden-Hybbinette procedure, is advantageous for the stabilization of an anteriorly unstable shoulder because the graft can be substantially large and may heal better than other graft sources because it is an autograft. In a study

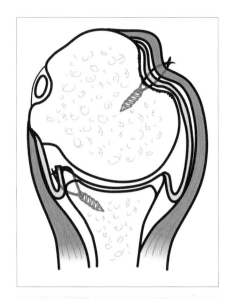

Figure 5 Illustration of a humeral head shows the remplissage procedure.

of 11 patients who underwent iliac crest bone grafting, Warner et al[56] reported no recurrence and no substantial arthropathy based on short-term radiographic imaging at a mean follow-up of 33 months. Disadvantages of iliac crest bone grafting include no cartilage on the graft and concern for arthritis as a result of contact between the graft and the humeral head.

Other Bone Grafting Procedures

Provencher et al[57] described the use of a fresh allograft source from the distal tibia, which is an excellent source of bone quality and has a radius of curvature that closely matches the native glenoid. A distal tibia allograft is advantageous for the stabilization of an anteriorly unstable shoulder because it provides the shoulder with a viable chondral graft source and restores anatomy. Concern exists for resorption of the allograft in the shoulder; however, distal tibia allografts are fresh rather than frozen or irradiated. Short-term results of the use of distal tibia allograft are promising. Tokish et al[58] described the use of distal clavicle autograft for the management of glenoid bone loss. Although only short-term results have been reported on the use of distal clavicle autograft for the stabilization of an anteriorly unstable shoulder, it is advantageous because it is an osteochondral graft that is readily available and cost effective.

Remplissage Procedure

The remplissage procedure, which was described by Purchase et al,[59] is an arthroscopic transfer of the infraspinatus and posterior capsule into a Hill-Sachs lesion. Originally described by Connolly[60] as an open procedure, the transferred infraspinatus prevents the glenoid from falling into the Hill-Sachs defect (**Figure 5**). Results of the remplissage procedure are promising. In a study of 47 patients who underwent arthroscopic Bankart repair and a remplissage procedure, Boileau et al[61] reported that, at a mean follow-up of 24 months, 98% of the patients had a stable shoulder, 90% of the patients returned to sport (68% at same level as preinjury), and all of the patients demonstrated healing of the tendon on postoperative imaging. Similarly, Zhu et al[62] reported an 8.2% failure rate in a study of 49 patients who underwent arthroscopic Bankart repair and a remplissage procedure, and Park et al[63] reported a 15% recurrence rate in a study of 20 patients who underwent arthroscopic Bankart repair and a remplissage procedure. In a study on the effect of adding the remplissage procedure to arthroscopic Bankart repair, Franceschi et al[64] compared the outcomes of 25 patients who underwent only an arthroscopic Bankart repair with those of 25 patients who underwent arthroscopic Bankart repair and the remplissage procedure. At minimum follow-up of 2 years, 20% of the patients who underwent only an arthroscopic Bankart repair experienced a recurrence, and none of the patients who underwent arthroscopic Bankart repair and the remplissage procedure experienced a recurrence. The authors reported no differences in range of motion between the patients in the two groups. Conversely, in a study that compared the outcomes of patients who underwent arthroscopic Bankart repair with or without the remplissage procedure, Nourissat et al[65] reported no difference in the rate of recurrence between the patients in the two groups, but noted that one-third of the patients who underwent arthroscopic Bankart repair and the remplissage procedure had posterosuperior pain.

Summary

The treatment options for anterior glenohumeral instability continue to be refined. Although technology aided in the creation of more anatomic and less invasive procedures, studies have shown that more invasive and adjunctive procedures are still the best treatment options in many clinical scenarios. Arthroscopic Bankart repair should be considered with caution in young athletic patients who have bone loss and shoulder hyperlaxity. Surgeons and patients should have a vested interest in correctly managing anterior glenohumeral instability with a primary procedure because revision surgery is problematic and results in poorer outcomes and higher recurrence rates compared with primary surgery. Meticulous attention to detail with regard to the clinical workup and the technical aspects of surgery is the best tool available for the management of anterior shoulder instability in young athletes.

References

1. Wasserstein D, Dwyer T, Veillette C, et al: Predictors of dislocation and revision after shoulder stabilization in Ontario, Canada, from 2003 to 2008. *Am J Sports Med* 2013;41(9):2034-2040.

2. Karlsson J, Magnusson L, Ejerhed L, Hultenheim I, Lundin O, Kartus J: Comparison of open and arthroscopic stabilization for recurrent shoulder dislocation in patients with a Bankart lesion. *Am J Sports Med* 2001;29(5):538-542.

3. Cole BJ, L'Insalata J, Irrgang J, Warner JJ: Comparison of arthroscopic and open anterior shoulder stabilization: A two to six-year follow-up study. *J Bone Joint Surg Am* 2000;82(8):1108-1114.

4. Burkhart SS, De Beer JF: Traumatic glenohumeral bone defects and their relationship to failure of arthroscopic Bankart repairs: Significance of the inverted-pear glenoid and the humeral engaging Hill-Sachs lesion. *Arthroscopy* 2000;16(7):677-694.

5. Balg F, Boileau P: The instability severity index score: A simple pre-operative score to select patients for arthroscopic or open shoulder stabilisation. *J Bone Joint Surg Br* 2007;89(11):1470-1477.

6. Phadnis J, Arnold C, Elmorsy A, Flannery M: Utility of the Instability Severity Index Score in predicting failure after arthroscopic anterior stabilization of the shoulder. *Am J Sports Med* 2015;43(8):1983-1988.

7. Rowe CR: Prognosis in dislocations of the shoulder. *J Bone Joint Surg Am* 1956;38(5):957-977.

8. Waterman BR, Burns TC, McCriskin B, Kilcoyne K, Cameron KL, Owens BD: Outcomes after Bankart repair in a military population: Predictors for surgical revision and long-term disability. *Arthroscopy* 2014;30(2):172-177.

9. Li X, Ma R, Nielsen NM, Gulotta LV, Dines JS, Owens BD: Management of shoulder instability in the skeletally immature patient. *J Am Acad Orthop Surg* 2013;21(9):529-537.

10. Kirkley A, Griffin S, Richards C, Miniaci A, Mohtadi N: Prospective randomized clinical trial comparing the effectiveness of immediate arthroscopic stabilization versus immobilization and rehabilitation in first traumatic anterior dislocations of the shoulder. *Arthroscopy* 1999;15(5):507-514.

11. Jakobsen BW, Johannsen HV, Suder P, Søjbjerg JO: Primary repair versus conservative treatment of first-time traumatic anterior dislocation of the shoulder: A randomized study with 10-year follow-up. *Arthroscopy* 2007;23(2):118-123.

12. Cho NS, Yi JW, Lee BG, Rhee YG: Revision open Bankart surgery after arthroscopic repair for traumatic anterior shoulder instability. *Am J Sports Med* 2009;37(11):2158-2164.

13. Mologne TS, Zhao K, Hongo M, Romeo AA, An KN, Provencher MT: The addition of rotator interval closure after arthroscopic repair of either anterior or posterior shoulder instability: Effect on glenohumeral translation and range of motion. *Am J Sports Med* 2008;36(6):1123-1131.

14. Neer CS II, Foster CR: Inferior capsular shift for involuntary inferior and multidirectional instability of the shoulder: A preliminary report. *J Bone Joint Surg Am* 1980;62(6):897-908.

15. Provencher MT, Mologne TS, Hongo M, Zhao K, Tasto JP, An KN: Arthroscopic versus open rotator interval closure: Biomechanical evaluation of stability and motion. *Arthroscopy* 2007;23(6):583-592.

16. Cho NS, Hwang JC, Rhee YG: Arthroscopic stabilization in anterior shoulder instability: Collision athletes versus noncollision athletes. *Arthroscopy* 2006;22(9):947-953.

17. Rhee YG, Ha JH, Cho NS: Anterior shoulder stabilization in collision athletes: Arthroscopic versus open Bankart repair. *Am J Sports Med* 2006;34(6):979-985.

18. Burkhart SS, De Beer JF, Barth JR, Cresswell T, Roberts C, Richards DP: Results of modified Latarjet reconstruction in patients with anteroinferior instability and significant bone loss. *Arthroscopy* 2007;23(10):1033-1041.

19. Pagnani MJ: Open capsular repair without bone block for recurrent anterior shoulder instability in patients with and without bony defects of the glenoid and/or humeral head. *Am J Sports Med* 2008;36(9):1805-1812.

20. Shaha JS, Cook JB, Song DJ, et al: Redefining "critical" bone loss in shoulder instability: Functional outcomes worsen with "subcritical" bone loss. *Am J Sports Med* 2015;43(7):1719-1725.

21. Armitage MS, Faber KJ, Drosdowech DS, Litchfield RB, Athwal GS: Humeral head bone defects: Remplissage, allograft, and arthroplasty. *Orthop Clin North Am* 2010;41(3):417-425.

22. Bankart AS: Recurrent or habitual dislocation of the shoulder-joint. *Br Med J* 1923;2(3285):1132-1133.

23. Henry JH, Genung JA: Natural history of glenohumeral dislocation—revisited. *Am J Sports Med* 1982;10(3):135-137.

24. Rowe CR, Patel D, Southmayd WW: The Bankart procedure: A long-term end-result study. *J Bone Joint Surg Am* 1978;60(1):1-16.

25. Huijsmans PE, Haen PS, Kidd M, Dhert WJ, van der Hulst VP, Willems WJ: Quantification of a glenoid defect with three-dimensional computed tomography and magnetic resonance imaging: A cadaveric study. *J Shoulder Elbow Surg* 2007;16(6):803-809.

26. Sugaya H, Moriishi J, Dohi M, Kon Y, Tsuchiya A: Glenoid rim morphology in recurrent anterior glenohumeral instability. *J Bone Joint Surg Am* 2003;85(5):878-884.

27. Griffith JF, Antonio GE, Tong CW, Ming CK: Anterior shoulder dislocation: Quantification of glenoid bone loss with CT. *AJR Am J Roentgenol* 2003;180(5):1423-1430.

28. Singson RD, Feldman F, Bigliani L: CT arthrographic patterns in recurrent glenohumeral instability. *AJR Am J Roentgenol* 1987;149(4):749-753.

29. Boileau P, Villalba M, Héry JY, Balg F, Ahrens P, Neyton L: Risk factors for recurrence of shoulder instability after arthroscopic Bankart repair. *J Bone Joint Surg Am* 2006;88(8):1755-1763.

30. Richards RD, Sartoris DJ, Pathria MN, Resnick D: Hill-Sachs lesion and

normal humeral groove: MR imaging features allowing their differentiation. *Radiology* 1994;190(3):665-668.

31. Yamamoto N, Itoi E, Abe H, et al: Contact between the glenoid and the humeral head in abduction, external rotation, and horizontal extension: A new concept of glenoid track. *J Shoulder Elbow Surg* 2007;16(5):649-656.

32. Di Giacomo G, Itoi E, Burkhart SS: Evolving concept of bipolar bone loss and the Hill-Sachs lesion: From "engaging/non-engaging" lesion to "on-track/off-track" lesion. *Arthroscopy* 2014;30(1):90-98.

33. Trivedi S, Pomerantz ML, Gross D, Golijanan P, Provencher MT: Shoulder instability in the setting of bipolar (glenoid and humeral head) bone loss: The glenoid track concept. *Clin Orthop Relat Res* 2014;472(8):2352-2362.

34. Rowe CR, Zarins B, Ciullo JV: Recurrent anterior dislocation of the shoulder after surgical repair: Apparent causes of failure and treatment. *J Bone Joint Surg Am* 1984;66(2):159-168.

35. Cho SH, Cho NS, Rhee YG: Preoperative analysis of the Hill-Sachs lesion in anterior shoulder instability: How to predict engagement of the lesion. *Am J Sports Med* 2011;39(11):2389-2395.

36. Kaar SG, Fening SD, Jones MH, Colbrunn RW, Miniaci A: Effect of humeral head defect size on glenohumeral stability: A cadaveric study of simulated Hill-Sachs defects. *Am J Sports Med* 2010;38(3):594-599.

37. Sekiya JK, Wickwire AC, Stehle JH, Debski RE: Hill-Sachs defects and repair using osteoarticular allograft transplantation: Biomechanical analysis using a joint compression model. *Am J Sports Med* 2009;37(12):2459-2466.

38. Itoi E, Lee SB, Berglund LJ, Berge LL, An KN: The effect of a glenoid defect on anteroinferior stability of the shoulder after Bankart repair: A cadaveric study. *J Bone Joint Surg Am* 2000;82(1):35-46.

39. Greis PE, Scuderi MG, Mohr A, Bachus KN, Burks RT: Glenohumeral articular contact areas and pressures following labral and osseous injury to the anteroinferior quadrant of the glenoid. *J Shoulder Elbow Surg* 2002;11(5):442-451.

40. Cook JB, Shaha JS, Rowles DJ, Bottoni CR, Shaha S, Tokish JM: Paper No. 769. Clinical validation of the "on-track" vs. "off-track" concept in anterior glenohumeral instability. *AAOS 2015 Annual Meeting Proceedings*. Rosemont, IL, American Academy of Orthopaedic Surgeons, 2015.

41. Arciero RA, Parrino A, Diaz-Doran V, et al: Paper No. 607. Combined biomechanical assessment of combined glenoid and humeral head defects utilizing 3D modeling of 142 patients. *AAOS 2015 Annual Meeting Proceedings*. Rosemont, IL, American Academy of Orthopaedic Surgeons, 2015.

42. Blackman AJ, Krych AJ, Kuzma SA, Chow RM, Camp C, Dahm DL: Results of revision anterior shoulder stabilization surgery in adolescent athletes. *Arthroscopy* 2014;30(11):1400-1405.

43. McCabe MP, Weinberg D, Field LD, O'Brien MJ, Hobgood ER, Savoie FH III: Primary versus revision arthroscopic reconstruction with remplissage for shoulder instability with moderate bone loss. *Arthroscopy* 2014;30(4):444-450.

44. Arce G, Arcuri F, Ferro D, Pereira E: Is selective arthroscopic revision beneficial for treating recurrent anterior shoulder instability? *Clin Orthop Relat Res* 2012;470(4):965-971.

45. Friedman LG, Griesser MJ, Miniaci AA, Jones MH: Recurrent instability after revision anterior shoulder stabilization surgery. *Arthroscopy* 2014;30(3):372-381.

46. Ryu RK, Ryu JH: Arthroscopic revision Bankart repair: A preliminary evaluation. *Orthopedics* 2011;34(1):17.

47. Allain J, Goutallier D, Glorion C: Long-term results of the Latarjet procedure for the treatment of anterior instability of the shoulder. *J Bone Joint Surg Am* 1998;80(6):841-852.

48. Bessière C, Trojani C, Carles M, Mehta SS, Boileau P: The open Latarjet procedure is more reliable in terms of shoulder stability than arthroscopic Bankart repair. *Clin Orthop Relat Res* 2014;472(8):2345-2351.

49. Cerciello S, Edwards TB, Walch G: Chronic anterior glenohumeral instability in soccer players: Results for a series of 28 shoulders treated with the Latarjet procedure. *J Orthop Traumatol* 2012;13(4):197-202.

50. Hovelius L, Sandström B, Saebö M: One hundred eighteen Bristow-Latarjet repairs for recurrent anterior dislocation of the shoulder prospectively followed for fifteen years: Study II-the evolution of dislocation arthropathy. *J Shoulder Elbow Surg* 2006;15(3):279-289.

51. Shah AA, Butler RB, Romanowski J, Goel D, Karadagli D, Warner JJ: Short-term complications of the Latarjet procedure. *J Bone Joint Surg Am* 2012;94(6):495-501.

52. Delaney RA, Freehill MT, Janfaza DR, Vlassakov KV, Higgins LD, Warner JJ: 2014 Neer Award Paper: Neuromonitoring the Latarjet procedure. *J Shoulder Elbow Surg* 2014;23(10):1473-1480.

53. Lafosse L, Lejeune E, Bouchard A, Kakuda C, Gobezie R, Kochhar T: The arthroscopic Latarjet procedure for the treatment of anterior shoulder instability. *Arthroscopy* 2007;23(11):1242.e1-1242.e5.

54. Dumont GD, Fogerty S, Rosso C, Lafosse L: The arthroscopic Latarjet procedure for anterior shoulder instability: 5-year minimum follow-up. *Am J Sports Med* 2014;42(11):2560-2566.

55. Lafosse L, Boyle S: Arthroscopic Latarjet procedure. *J Shoulder Elbow Surg* 2010;19(2 suppl):2-12.

56. Warner JJ, Gill TJ, O'hollerhan JD, Pathare N, Millett PJ: Anatomical glenoid reconstruction for recurrent anterior glenohumeral instability with glenoid deficiency using an autogenous tricortical iliac crest bone graft. *Am J Sports Med* 2006;34(2):205-212.

57. Provencher MT, Ghodadra N, LeClere L, Solomon DJ, Romeo AA: Anatomic osteochondral glenoid reconstruction for recurrent glenohumeral instability with glenoid deficiency using a distal tibia allograft. *Arthroscopy* 2009;25(4):446-452.

58. Tokish JM, Fitzpatrick K, Cook JB, Mallon WJ: Arthroscopic distal clavicular autograft for treating shoulder

instability with glenoid bone loss. *Arthrosc Tech* 2014;3(4):e475-e481.

59. Purchase RJ, Wolf EM, Hobgood ER, Pollock ME, Smalley CC: Hill-Sachs "remplissage": An arthroscopic solution for the engaging hill-Sachs lesion. *Arthroscopy* 2008;24(6):723-726.

60. Connolly JF: Humeral head defects associated with shoulder dislocation: Their diagnostic and surgical significance. *Instr Course Lect* 1972;21:42-54.

61. Boileau P, O'Shea K, Vargas P, Pinedo M, Old J, Zumstein M: Anatomical and functional

results after arthroscopic Hill-Sachs remplissage. *J Bone Joint Surg Am* 2012;94(7):618-626.

62. Zhu YM, Lu Y, Zhang J, Shen JW, Jiang CY: Arthroscopic Bankart repair combined with remplissage technique for the treatment of anterior shoulder instability with engaging Hill-Sachs lesion: A report of 49 cases with a minimum 2-year follow-up. *Am J Sports Med* 2011;39(8):1640-1647.

63. Park MJ, Tjoumakaris FP, Garcia G, Patel A, Kelly JD IV: Arthroscopic remplissage with Bankart repair for the treatment of glenohumeral

instability with Hill-Sachs defects. *Arthroscopy* 2011;27(9):1187-1194.

64. Franceschi F, Papalia R, Rizzello G, et al: Remplissage repair—new frontiers in the prevention of recurrent shoulder instability: A 2-year follow-up comparative study. *Am J Sports Med* 2012;40(11):2462-2469.

65. Nourissat G, Kilinc AS, Werther JR, Doursounian L: A prospective, comparative, radiological, and clinical study of the influence of the "remplissage" procedure on shoulder range of motion after stabilization by arthroscopic Bankart repair. *Am J Sports Med* 2011;39(10):2147-2152.

Cubital Tunnel Syndrome

Claudius D. Jarrett, MD

Loukia K. Papatheodorou, MD, PhD

Dean G. Sotereanos, MD

Abstract

Cubital tunnel syndrome is the most common cause of symptomatic ulnar neuropathy. The unique anatomic course of the ulnar nerve around the elbow makes it particularly vulnerable at a location far from its terminal destination. The natural progression of cubital tunnel syndrome allows patients who have mild symptoms to be adequately treated nonsurgically. Minor changes in activity combined with appropriate splinting may acceptably alleviate symptoms. Surgical intervention is recommended for patients who have more severe symptoms. Current data confirm that in situ ulnar nerve decompression, partial medial epicondylectomy, and anterior transposition result in equal success rates; however, more invasive techniques may increase the risk for complications. If primary surgical intervention fails, revision surgery can provide good results. Modern techniques for revision surgery incorporate the placement of a protective circumferential barrier around the pathologic nerve to mitigate cicatrix formation. Although several attractive options are currently available for the management of cubital tunnel syndrome, further research is necessary to guide treatment.

Instr Course Lect 2017;66:91–101.

Cubital tunnel syndrome is one of the most common peripheral nerve compression disorders, second only to carpal tunnel syndrome. The unique anatomic course of the ulnar nerve around the elbow places it in a particularly vulnerable position. Patients with cubital tunnel syndrome are more likely to have later stages of nerve compression compared with patients who have carpal tunnel syndrome. Successful management of cubital tunnel syndrome requires an understanding and modulation of the inciting variables. Although cubital tunnel syndrome was originally described in the early 1900s, an ideal treatment algorithm remains elusive.[1] Surgeons should understand the etiology, diagnosis, and treatment options for primary and recurrent ulnar neuropathy at the elbow.

Anatomy and Pathophysiology

The motor and sensory axons of the ulnar nerve originate from the ventral rami of the C8 and T1 nerve roots before they incorporate into the lower trunk of the brachial plexus. The ulnar nerve exits the brachial plexus as a terminal branch of the medial cord and travels toward the anterior compartment of the upper arm. Approximately 8 cm above the medial epicondyle, the ulnar nerve passes into the posterior compartment through the arcade of Struthers. The ulnar nerve then travels behind the medial intermuscular septum to the cubital tunnel. Near the elbow, the ulnar nerve travels posterior to the medial epicondyle before it descends underneath the Osborne ligament. As the ulnar nerve leaves the cubital tunnel, it passes deep to the fascia of the two heads of the flexor carpi ulnaris (FCU) before it

Dr. Sotereanos or an immediate family member serves as a paid consultant to or is an employee of Arthrex, AxoGen, and Smith & Nephew. Neither of the following authors nor any immediate family member has received anything of value from or has stock or stock options held in a commercial company or institution related directly or indirectly to the subject of this chapter: Dr. Jarrett and Dr. Papatheodorou.

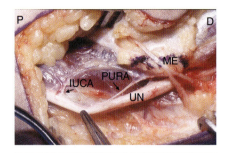

Figure 1 Intraoperative photograph of an elbow shows the blood supply of the ulnar nerve (UN) around the elbow. D = distal to the elbow, IUCA = inferior ulnar collateral artery, ME = medial epicondyle, P = proximal to the elbow, PURA = posterior ulnar recurrent artery.

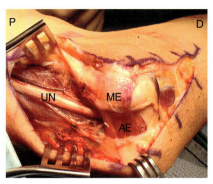

Figure 2 Intraoperative photograph of an elbow shows compression of the ulnar nerve (UN) by the anconeus epitrochlearis (AE). D = distal to the elbow, ME = medial epicondyle, P = proximal to the elbow.

descends down the forearm between the FCU and the flexor digitorum profundus muscle belly.[2]

Around the elbow, the ulnar nerve is perfused by three main arteries. The superior ulnar collateral, inferior ulnar collateral, and posterior ulnar recurrent arteries provide a consistent but segmental extraneural and intraneural vascular supply[3] (**Figure 1**). Only the inferior ulnar collateral artery provides direct vascularization to the ulnar nerve in the region just proximal to the cubital tunnel.[4] Often, this arterial branch can be easily identified approximately 25 mm proximal to the medial epicondyle and adjacent to the leading edge of the intermuscular septum.[4] Attempts should be made to preserve the blood supply to the ulnar nerve during its surgical dissection.

The size and number of nerve fascicles within the ulnar nerve change as the ulnar nerve approaches the cubital tunnel. Proximal to the cubital tunnel, the ulnar nerve is polyfascicular, containing numerous motor and sensory fascicles.[5] As the ulnar nerve enters the cubital tunnel, the motor and sensory

fascicles unite to form only a few large and small fascicles. Distal to the cubital tunnel, the ulnar nerve becomes polyfascicular again.[5,6] Topographically, the motor fibers of the flexor digitorum profundus to the little and ring fingers and the FCU are centrally located, and the sensory and intrinsic motor fibers are peripherally located. This spatial arrangement places the sensory and intrinsic motor fibers in a position that is more susceptible to injury.[6]

The medial antebrachial cutaneous nerve and several of its posterior branches travel superficial to the ulnar nerve at the elbow. The medial antebrachial cutaneous nerve travels down the anterior arm as a direct branch from the medial brachial plexus cord. The medial antebrachial cutaneous nerve innervates the skin along the anterior and medial forearm. The posterior branches of the medial antebrachial cutaneous nerve are present approximately 1.8 cm above the medial epicondyle in approximately 61% of elbows and are almost always present approximately 3.1 cm below the medial epicondyle.[7] Surgeons must remain attentive to the anatomic

variation of the posterior branches of the medial antebrachial cutaneous nerve to avoid iatrogenic injury.

The ulnar nerve can be compressed by several structures as it travels down the arm and across the elbow into the forearm. Classic locations for ulnar nerve compression include the arcade of Struthers; the medial intermuscular septum; the medial epicondyle; the deep flexor-pronator aponeurosis; and anomalous muscles, such as the anconeus epitrochlearis, which is present in approximately 11% of elbows[8] (**Figure 2**). The most common location for ulnar nerve compression is within the cubital tunnel (**Figure 3**).

The cubital tunnel is a dynamic fibro-osseous canal that is formed at the base of the elbow by the medial collateral ligament, the elbow joint capsule, and the olecranon and is covered by the Osborne ligament (ie, cubital tunnel aponeurosis). The shape of the cubital tunnel actively changes from a spacious oval shape to a narrow elliptical shape as the elbow moves from extension to flexion.[9] The cross-sectional area available for the ulnar nerve within the cubital tunnel decreases nearly 40% as the elbow moves from full extension to 135° of flexion.[10] As a result, the space available for the ulnar nerve decreases dramatically at higher angles of elbow flexion, which correlates with a substantial increase in extraneural pressure. As the elbow moves from full extension to 130° of flexion, extraneural pressure in the cubital tunnel increases from less than 7 mm Hg to approximately 30 mm Hg.[10]

The course of the ulnar nerve also submits it to frictional and tensile stresses that are sufficient to contribute to axonal injury. The ulnar nerve naturally slides proximally and distally to accommodate upper extremity activity. Approximately 5 mm of ulnar nerve excursion is required to allow the elbow to move from 10° to 90° of flexion. Approximately 22 mm of ulnar nerve excursion is required to allow for motion of the entire upper extremity (ie, shoulder, elbow, wrist, and hand).[11] The ulnar nerve also stretches and undergoes deformation with movement. Elbow flexion stretches the ulnar nerve and can lead to a 29% increase in ulnar nerve strain,[11] which is well above the threshold reported to substantially diminish neural blood flow and hinder peripheral nerve conduction.[12-14] Studies have reported that a 15% increase in ulnar nerve strain correlates with a more than 80% reduction in blood flow.[12,13] Other studies have reported complete blockage of nerve conduction with a 12% increase in ulnar nerve strain.[14] The deformation in the ulnar nerve with elbow motion correlates with an increase in the mean intraneural pressure of the ulnar nerve. As the elbow moves from full extension to 130° of flexion, the intraneural pressure of the ulnar nerve in the cubital tunnel increases from less than 8 mm Hg to more than 40 mm Hg.[10] An increase in the intraneural pressure of the ulnar nerve in the cubital tunnel supersedes an increase in extraneural pressure in the cubital tunnel, which highlights the contribution of traction to ulnar neuropathy in some patients.[10] The repetitive friction and strain experienced by the ulnar nerve can lead to inflammation and edema, which limits the ability of the ulnar nerve to accommodate further upper extremity motion and, thus, perpetuates the pathologic cycle.[15]

Diagnosis

Patients usually have painful numbness and tingling along the ulnar half of the

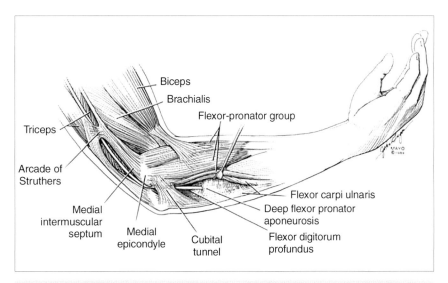

Figure 3 Illustration of an arm shows the five sites of potential ulnar nerve entrapment about the elbow: the arcade of Struthers, the medial intermuscular septum, the medial epicondyle, the cubital tunnel, and the deep flexor pronator aponeurosis. (Reproduced from Elhassan B, Steinmann SP: Entrapment neuropathy of the ulnar nerve. *J Am Acad Orthop Surg* 2007;15[11]:672-681.)

ring finger and the entire little finger. These symptoms often are exacerbated with activities or positions that require prolonged elbow hyperflexion. Many patients also may have weakness of grip. Intrinsic atrophy may be evident in patients who have advanced cubital tunnel syndrome. On physical examination, several provocative maneuvers can be used to assist with the diagnosis of cubital tunnel syndrome[16,17] (**Table 1**). A Tinel test, which involves the application of direct compression over the cubital tunnel, or the placement of the elbow in a position of hyperflexion can reproduce a patient's symptoms. A combination of elbow flexion with direct pressure, forearm supination, wrist extension, and/or shoulder abduction with internal rotation can increase the specificity and sensitivity of the physical examination in some patients. To determine the benefit of a modified elbow flexion and shoulder abduction/ internal rotation test for the diagnosis of cubital tunnel syndrome, Ochi et al[16]

evaluated 55 patients who had cubital tunnel syndrome and 123 control patients with the use of three provocative tests: the classic elbow flexion test, the elbow flexion and shoulder abduction/ internal rotation test, and the modified elbow flexion and shoulder abduction/ internal rotation test with the forearm supinated and the wrist extended. The authors reported that the combined elbow flexion and shoulder abduction/ internal rotation test with the forearm in supination and the wrist in extension increased the sensitivity and specificity for cubital tunnel syndrome to 87% and 98%, respectively. Performing these maneuvers, however, may increase the likelihood of a false-positive result.[18] Evidence of sensory changes in two-point discrimination and intrinsic strength should be documented. The elbow should be taken through a full range of motion to assess for signs of elbow subluxation or dislocation. Intrinsic weakness can be confirmed with an assessment for Wartenberg or Froment

Table 1
Provocative Maneuvers for the Diagnosis of Cubital Tunnel Syndrome

Test	Examination Maneuver	Sensitivity/Specificity (%)[a]
Tinel	4 to 6 taps on the ulnar nerve just proximal to the cubital tunnel	70/98
Elbow flexion	Elbow in maximum flexion with forearm supinated and wrist in neutral	75/99
Direct pressure	Using the index and middle fingers, an examiner places direct pressure on the patient's ulnar nerve proximal to the cubital tunnel with the elbow in 90° of flexion	89/98
Combined elbow flexion and direct pressure	An examiner places direct pressure on the patient's ulnar nerve just proximal to the cubital tunnel with the elbow in maximum flexion	98/95
Elbow flexion and shoulder abduction/internal rotation	Elbow in hyperflexion with shoulder abducted to 90° and in maximum internal rotation	58/100
Modified elbow flexion and shoulder abduction/internal rotation	Elbow in hyperflexion, shoulder abducted to 90° and internally rotated, forearm supinated, and wrist extended	87/98

[a]Sensitivity and specificity may vary depending on the amount of time the maneuver is held.
Data from Novak CB, Lee GW, Mackinnon SE, Lay L: Provocative testing for cubital tunnel syndrome. *J Hand Surg Am* 1994;19(5):817-820 and Ochi K, Horiuchi Y, Tanabe A, Waseda M, Kaneko Y, Koyanagi T: Shoulder internal rotation elbow flexion test for diagnosing cubital tunnel syndrome. *J Shoulder Elbow Surg* 2012;21(6):777-781.

signs. The ulnar nerve also should be evaluated for evidence of instability. The ulnar nerve is gently palpated within the cubital tunnel as the elbow is taken from full extension to flexion and back to extension. If unstable, the ulnar nerve will slide superficial and/or anterior to the medial epicondyle. The contralateral elbow should be assessed and compared with the injured elbow.

Although not required, electrodiagnostic testing may aid in a patient's clinical workup. An ulnar motor nerve conduction velocity across the elbow of less than 50 m/s or a conduction velocity across the elbow that is more than 10 m/s slower than that across the wrist suggests ulnar neuropathy at the elbow.[19] A heavy reliance on nerve conduction velocity studies for the diagnosis of cubital tunnel syndrome should be avoided because the likelihood of false-positive and false-negative results is high.[19] High-resolution ultrasonography is being investigated as an adjuvant diagnostic and prognostic tool for patients in whom cubital tunnel syndrome is suspected. Recent studies have reported enlargement of the ulnar nerve at the elbow in patients who have cubital tunnel syndrome. Zhong et al[20] performed preoperative and postoperative high-resolution ultrasonographic assessments of the ulnar nerve in 278 patients who had cubital tunnel syndrome and in 20 control patients. The authors reported that the patients with cubital tunnel syndrome had a substantially larger ulnar nerve cross-sectional area at the elbow compared with the control patients. In addition, the authors reported that the ulnar nerve cross-sectional area increased with advanced McGowan cubital tunnel syndrome grade and was inversely proportional with motor conduction velocity; however, further studies are necessary to standardize these findings. Ultrasonography also may be useful in the setting of trauma, tumor, or revision surgery to clarify alterations in anatomy before surgical management.

Radiographs of the elbow should be obtained in patients with a history of trauma, arthritis, and findings on physical examination that are consistent with abnormal elbow motion or an abnormal carrying angle. Radiographs should be assessed to rule out concomitant pathology, such as arthritic or posttraumatic changes (**Figure 4**). Several other pathologic processes that mimic cubital tunnel syndrome and that a surgeon should keep in mind for a differential diagnosis include ulnar nerve compression at the Guyon canal, radiculopathy, peripheral nerve tumor, diabetic neuropathy, multiple sclerosis, and thoracic outlet syndrome. Sensory changes along the distribution of the dorsal sensory branch of the ulnar nerve (ie, dorsum of the hand) can help confirm compression of the ulnar nerve proximal to the Guyon canal. In addition, ulnar nerve compression at the wrist is unlikely to lead to weakness of the ring and little finger flexor digitorum profundus. Evidence of vascular changes on physical examination, such as loss of radial pulse or edema, may indicate thoracic outlet syndrome.

Classification

The McGowan classification of cubital tunnel syndrome divides cubital tunnel syndrome into three grades based on the level of motor involvement.[21] Patients with grade I cubital tunnel syndrome have sensory weakness but no detectable motor weakness. Patients with grade II cubital tunnel syndrome have some objective motor weakness. Grade II cubital tunnel syndrome can be subdivided into grade IIA and grade IIB based on the presence of mild versus moderate intrinsic weakness (ie, strength of 3/5). Patients with grade III cubital tunnel syndrome have severe motor weakness with substantial muscle atrophy.[21] Dellon[22] modified the McGowan cubital tunnel syndrome classification system to include the presence and severity of sensory changes. According to Dellon,[22] patients with mild ulnar nerve compression at the elbow have intermittent paresthesia. Patients with moderate ulnar nerve compression may have a decrease in vibratory sensation. Patients with severe ulnar nerve compression may have abnormal two-point discrimination.[22]

Treatment

Nonsurgical Management

Patients who have mild cubital tunnel syndrome can often be treated nonsurgically. Because of the natural progression of cubital tunnel syndrome, nonsurgical management results in the alleviation of symptoms in almost one-half of patients who have cubital tunnel syndrome. Padua et al[23] followed 24 patients with both a clinical and neurophysiologic diagnosis of cubital tunnel

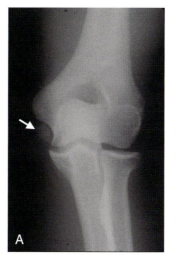 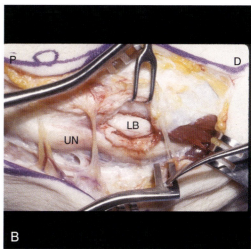

Figure 4   **A,** PA elbow radiograph demonstrates a large loose body (arrow). **B,** Intraoperative photograph of the elbow shown in panel **A** shows the large loose body (LB). D = distal to the elbow, P = proximal to the elbow, UN = ulnar nerve.

syndrome who did not undergo any formal treatment. At a mean follow-up of 13 months, 42% of the patients had complete or near-complete alleviation of their symptoms.[23] Providing patients with information about the pathologic process of cubital tunnel syndrome allows them to modify their activity to adequately address their symptoms.

If nonsurgical management is warranted and symptoms are mild, elbow extension splinting is fairly effective at alleviating symptoms. Often, elbow extension splinting is most effective at night. In a study of 22 patients who regularly wore a nighttime splint for 6 months, Seror[24] reported improvement in the symptoms of all of the patients at a mean follow-up of 11.3 months. Elbow extension splinting at approximately 45° from full extension keeps cubital tunnel pressure at a minimum. Gelberman et al[10] reported that the ulnar nerve is subject to the least amount of pressure in the cubital tunnel with the elbow positioned in 40° to 50° of flexion. Elbow pads can be

worn during the day and with activity to minimize direct trauma to the ulnar nerve. The current literature on cubital tunnel syndrome does not report a clear benefit with regard to cortisone injections or physical therapy. Ulnar nerve gliding exercises have failed to consistently show benefits in addition to those acquired from patient education. Svernlöv et al[25] randomized 70 patients who had mild or moderate cubital tunnel syndrome to receive either patient education only or patient education combined with nerve gliding exercises or a nighttime splint. The patients in the nerve gliding exercises and nighttime splint groups did not show improved outcomes compared with the patients in the education-only group.

Surgical Management

Patients who have moderate to severe cubital tunnel syndrome are less likely to be successfully treated nonsurgically. In a study of 128 patients who had cubital tunnel syndrome, Dellon et al[26] reported that 62% of the patients who

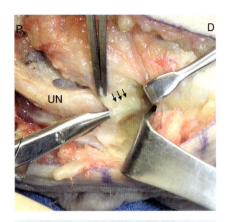

Figure 5 Intraoperative photograph of an elbow shows in situ ulnar nerve (UN) decompression with Osborne ligament (arrows) release. D = distal to the elbow, P = proximal to the elbow.

had severe cubital tunnel syndrome required surgery within 3 years, and 21% of the patients who had mild cubital tunnel syndrome required surgery within 6 years. Surgical treatment is recommended for patients in whom nonsurgical treatment fails and patients in whom symptoms of moderate to severe cubital tunnel syndrome are present. Several surgical options exist for cubital tunnel syndrome, none of which have been reported to be objectively superior to the other in the literature.

In Situ Ulnar Nerve Decompression

In situ ulnar nerve decompression can be performed with the use of an open or endoscopic technique.[27,28] In situ ulnar nerve decompression is the simplest and least invasive surgical option to address cubital tunnel syndrome. Advocates of in situ ulnar nerve decompression report that the technique is less likely to compromise the tenuous perineural blood supply to the ulnar nerve.[27] A relatively small incision is made, and the ulnar nerve is released from above the elbow through the Osborne ligament

distal to the two heads of the FCU (**Figure 5**). The ulnar nerve usually can be identified proximal to the medial epicondyle and adjacent to the medial intermuscular septum or can be relatively easily identified distal to the epicondyle by separating the natural raphe between the two heads of the FCU. Although a smaller incision is more attractive, concern remains with regard to the adequate decompression of all potential sites of ulnar nerve compression; therefore, the size of the incision for in situ ulnar nerve decompression should not limit complete decompression of the ulnar nerve. Ulnar nerve subluxation cannot be addressed with in situ ulnar nerve decompression alone; therefore, alternative surgical techniques must be implemented in patients who have ulnar nerve subluxation. Current available comparative studies report similar success rates in patients who undergo either open or endoscopic in situ decompression. In a study that compared the outcomes of 19 patients who underwent endoscopic in situ decompression with those of 15 patients who underwent open in situ decompression, Watts and Bain[29] reported that 79% of the patients in the endoscopic group and 60% of the patients in the open group were satisfied with their outcome 12 months postoperatively; however, the difference in satisfaction between the patients in the two groups was not statistically significant ($P = 0.229$).

Video 7.1: Cubital Tunnel Syndrome. Dean G. Sotereanos, MD (4 min)

Partial Medial Epicondylectomy

Partial medial epicondylectomy provides advantages similar to those of in situ ulnar nerve decompression.[30] A

12- to 16-cm incision centered over the medial epicondyle is made, and dissection is carried down through the skin and subcutaneous tissue. The ulnar nerve is identified and decompressed while preserving the branches of the medial antebrachial cutaneous nerve as well as the perineural blood supply. The flexor-pronator origin is incised over the medial epicondyle with the use of subperiosteal flaps (**Figure 6**). A partial bony resection (20%) of the medial epicondyle is performed with the use of a small osteotome while protecting the medial collateral ligament (**Figure 7**). This allows the ulnar nerve to freely glide anteriorly and posteriorly with elbow motion. Advocates of partial medial epicondylectomy report that the technique addresses the compressive and tensile forces on the ulnar nerve while minimizing injury to the blood supply to the ulnar nerve.[30] Excessive resection of the medial epicondyle should be avoided because damage to the medial collateral ligament may increase the risk for valgus instability.[31,32] O'Driscoll et al[31] reported that removal of more than 19% of the medial epicondyle can potentially injure the anterior band of the medial collateral ligament. In a study of 64 patients (66 elbows) with cubital tunnel syndrome who underwent partial medial epicondylectomy, Göbel et al[30] reported that 79% of the patients had good-to-excellent results at a mean follow-up of 27 months. The authors also reported that elbow instability was not observed in any of the patients.

Anterior Transposition

Anterior transposition attempts to address compressive and tensile forces on the ulnar nerve by decompressing and relocating the ulnar nerve anterior to the axis of elbow rotation.[27,28,33,34] Relative indications for anterior transposition include ulnar nerve subluxation, elbow deformity, and an unsuitable native bed for the ulnar nerve (ie, osteophyte, heterotopic bone, or fracture). The ulnar nerve can be transposed in front of the medial epicondyle subcutaneously, intramuscularly, or submuscularly.[27,28,33,34] All three anterior transposition techniques aim to remove compressive and tensile forces that are placed on the ulnar nerve in its native position.

Irrespective of the final position of the ulnar nerve, all three anterior transposition techniques begin in a similar manner. A 12- to 16-cm incision centered over the cubital tunnel is made. To provide adequate exposure, an anterior flap is raised by elevating the subcutaneous tissue directly off the flexor-pronator fascia. The ulnar nerve is identified and completely decompressed from the arcade of Struthers to the first motor branch of the FCU. Distal intramuscular neurolysis of the first motor branch of the FCU facilitates a tensionless anterior transposition because it prevents the ulnar nerve from being posteriorly tethered. The ulnar nerve is then circumferentially freed. The extrinsic blood supply to the ulnar nerve should be protected and transposed with the ulnar nerve as much as possible. A 3- to 4-cm segment of the distal aspect of the medial intermuscular septum should be resected to prevent secondary kinking of the ulnar nerve after it is transposed anterior to the medial epicondyle. The ulnar nerve can then be transposed anteriorly (**Figure 8**).

The final position of the ulnar nerve depends on the anterior transposition technique used. For a subcutaneous transposition, a flexor-pronator fascial

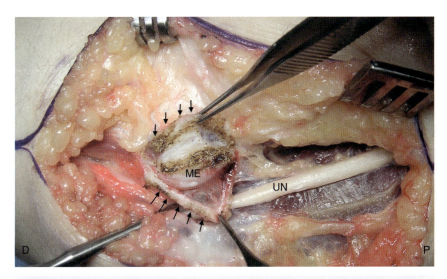

Figure 6   Intraoperative photograph of an elbow shows exposure of the medial epicondyle (ME) with subperiosteal flaps (arrows). D = distal to the elbow, P = proximal to the elbow, UN = ulnar nerve.

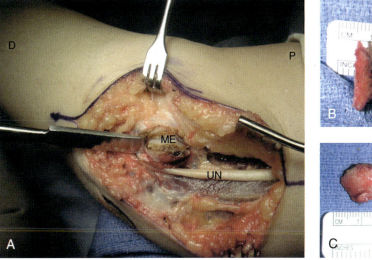
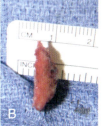
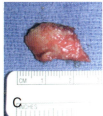

Figure 7   **A,** Intraoperative photograph of an elbow shows partial medial epicondylectomy with the use of a small osteotome. **B** and **C,** Clinical photographs show bony resection of the medial epicondyle (ME). D = distal to the elbow, P = proximal to the elbow, UN = ulnar nerve.

sling is created to maintain the ulnar nerve anteriorly through the full range of elbow motion. Typically, an approximately 2 × 2-cm ulnar-based flexor-pronator fascial flap is elevated. The ulnar nerve is then positioned anterior to the flexor-pronator fascial sling. The distal edge of the flexor-pronator fascial sling is sutured to the deep dermal tissue with the use of absorbable sutures to prevent posterior subluxation of the ulnar nerve. In thin patients, placement of the ulnar nerve subcutaneously may place it at risk for subsequent incidental trauma.

For an intramuscular transposition, a trough is created through the flexor-pronator mass along the new trajectory

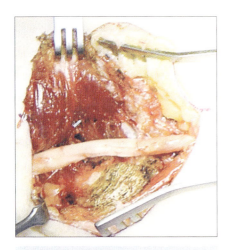

Figure 8 Intraoperative photograph of an elbow shows transposition of the ulnar nerve into a bed of muscle fibers and checked throughout its length for a smooth and unkinked course. Further careful evaluation is necessary to prevent iatrogenic compression as the muscular envelope is closed over the ulnar nerve. (Reproduced with permission from Henry M: Modified intramuscular transposition of the ulnar nerve. *J Hand Surg Am* 2006;31[9]:1535-1542.)

of the anteriorly transposed ulnar nerve. The ulnar nerve is then allowed to settle within the muscular bed. Although not required, sutures can be placed superficially through the overlying fascia to maintain the transposed position of the ulnar nerve.

A submuscular transposition is the most extensive of the three anterior transposition techniques.[35] For a submuscular transposition, the flexor-pronator mass is elevated from the medial epicondyle to allow access to its submuscular recess. The ulnar nerve is then placed beneath the common flexor-pronator muscle origin. The flexor-pronator mass is loosely repaired back to the medial epicondyle. Submuscular transposition of the ulnar nerve may lead to secondary ulnar nerve compression caused by the flexor-pronator

mass. Musculofascial lengthening or Z-lengthening of the flexor-pronator origin may help minimize the risk of secondary ulnar nerve compression.

Postoperative Management

Any of the surgical techniques for the management of cubital tunnel syndrome should allow for early elbow range of motion postoperatively, which facilitates gliding of the newly decompressed ulnar nerve and helps avoid perineural scar formation. Active range of motion is initiated immediately after surgery. A sling is used only for comfort. Often, heavy lifting is restricted for the first 6 weeks postoperatively.

Outcomes

Surgical management of cubital tunnel syndrome recalcitrant to nonsurgical management can reliably alleviate the symptoms of most patients.[36] Most patients can anticipate successful and durable results after adequate ulnar nerve decompression. Most studies report a 70% to 90% mean success rate after primary surgical management.[27,28,33,34,36] Currently, prospective comparative studies have failed to demonstrate the superiority of any one surgical technique.[27,28,33,34,36] In a prospective randomized controlled study of 152 patients with cubital tunnel syndrome who underwent either in situ decompression or anterior subcutaneous transposition, Bartels et al[28] reported a statistically similar success rate between the patients who underwent in situ decompression (65%) and the patients who underwent anterior subcutaneous transposition (70%). Similarly, in a prospective randomized study of 70 patients with cubital tunnel syndrome who underwent either in situ decompression or anterior submuscular

transposition, Gervasio et al[33] reported an 80% success rate in the patients who underwent in situ decompression and an 83% success rate in the patients who underwent submuscular transposition at a mean follow-up of 47 months; however, there was no statistically significant difference between the outcomes of the patients in the two groups.

More invasive procedures, however, appear to increase the risk for complications.[28,36] In a recent systematic review of six randomized controlled trials that included 430 patients who underwent treatment for cubital tunnel syndrome, Caliandro et al[36] reported that both simple decompression and decompression with transposition were equally effective at improving cubital tunnel syndrome symptoms. The authors reported that the patients who underwent transposition procedures had a higher incidence of complications. The authors of this chapter prefer to avoid anterior transposition in most patients who undergo primary surgical treatment for cubital tunnel syndrome and instead perform in situ ulnar nerve decompression with or without a partial medial epicondylectomy.

Recurrence

Most patients who undergo surgical treatment for cubital tunnel syndrome have good outcomes; however, a substantial number of patients may report recurrent or persistent symptoms.[37,38] Current data report that in up to approximately 30% of patients with cubital tunnel syndrome, primary surgical intervention fails or recurrent symptoms occur.[36] Recurrent symptoms likely stem from substantial perineural scarring (ie, cicatrix) that develops at the site of initial decompression.[39] The ideal approach to address recurrent compressive neuropathy has yet to be determined.[37,38]

In general, revision surgery for cubital tunnel syndrome has a good but lower success rate compared with primary surgical intervention for cubital tunnel syndrome.[37,38] Repeated in situ ulnar nerve decompression alone has a limited success rate. Although submuscular anterior transposition has been advocated for revision surgery for cubital tunnel syndrome, it may not always result in a good outcome, may exacerbate symptoms, and may not be superior compared with subcutaneous transposition.[37,38,40] In a study of 18 patients with cubital tunnel syndrome who underwent submuscular transposition for revision surgery, Vogel et al[37] reported that 78% of the patients were satisfied with their outcomes at final follow-up. In a study of 20 patients with cubital tunnel syndrome who underwent anterior subcutaneous transposition for revision surgery, Caputo and Watson[38] reported that 75% of the patients had good-to-excellent results at a minimum follow-up of 2 years. Revision surgery for patients who have perineural scarring must include meticulous external neurolysis and placement of a biologic soft-tissue barrier around the vulnerable nerve segment. Several techniques, ranging from nerve wraps to free tissue transfers, continue to be investigated in an attempt to prevent scar tissue from contacting the epineurium.[40-43] Studies have reported successful results with autologous vein wrapping.[41,42] In a study of four patients with refractory cubital tunnel syndrome who underwent autogenous vein wrapping after multiple failed prior surgical procedures, Varitimidis et al[41] reported that all four of the patients had improved pain and sensation postoperatively. In addition, both two-point discrimination and electromyographic findings in all four patients improved. Donor site complications and a limited amount of graft tissue, however, prevent the broad application of autologous vein wrapping.[41,42] Recent studies show promising results with porcine extracellular matrix nerve wrapping, which revascularizes the nerve, provides the nerve with a protective barrier that isolates it from the surrounding tissue and inflammatory response, and allows the nerve to glide within its chamber.[40,44]

Summary

Cubital tunnel syndrome is an important and perplexing peripheral nerve compression disorder. Patients with cubital tunnel syndrome have radiating, painful paresthesia in the ring and little fingers and/or severe intrinsic atrophy. Patients who have mild cubital tunnel syndrome can be treated with small activity modifications and splinting, both of which often minimize symptoms to an acceptable level. Surgical intervention is recommended for patients who have more substantial cubital tunnel syndrome symptoms. Complete in situ ulnar nerve decompression remains the preferred method of surgical intervention. The current literature reports equivalent success rates for patients who undergo in situ ulnar nerve decompression, partial medial epicondylectomy, or anterior transposition. Revision surgery can provide good results for patients in whom symptoms recur despite adequate initial ulnar nerve decompression. Recommended techniques for revision surgery include surrounding the nerve with a biologic soft-tissue barrier to prevent substantial scar formation. Further research is necessary to optimize management of cubital tunnel syndrome.

References

1. Buzzard EF: Some varieties of traumatic and toxic ulnar neuritis. *Lancet* 1922;199(5138):317-319.

2. O'Driscoll SW, Horii E, Carmichael SW, Morrey BF: The cubital tunnel and ulnar neuropathy. *J Bone Joint Surg Br* 1991;73(4):613-617.

3. Sunderland S: Blood supply of the nerves of the upper limb in man. *Arch Neurol Psychiatry* 1945;53(2):91-115.

4. Yamaguchi K, Sweet FA, Bindra R, Gelberman RH: The extraneural and intraneural arterial anatomy of the ulnar nerve at the elbow. *J Shoulder Elbow Surg* 1999;8(1):17-21.

5. Green JR Jr, Rayan GM: The cubital tunnel: Anatomic, histologic, and biomechanical study. *J Shoulder Elbow Surg* 1999;8(5):466-470.

6. Sunderland S: The intraneural topography of the radial, median and ulnar nerves. *Brain* 1945;68(4):243-299.

7. Lowe JB III, Maggi SP, Mackinnon SE: The position of crossing branches of the medial antebrachial cutaneous nerve during cubital tunnel surgery in humans. *Plast Reconstr Surg* 2004;114(3):692-696.

8. Dellon AL: Musculotendinous variations about the medial humeral epicondyle. *J Hand Surg Br* 1986;11(2):175-181.

9. Feindel W, Stratford J: The role of the cubital tunnel in tardy ulnar palsy. *Can J Surg* 1958;1(4):287-300.

10. Gelberman RH, Yamaguchi K, Hollstien SB, et al: Changes in interstitial pressure and cross-sectional area of the cubital tunnel and of the ulnar nerve with flexion of the elbow: An experimental study in human cadavera. *J Bone Joint Surg Am* 1998;80(4):492-501.

11. Wright TW, Glowczewskie F Jr, Cowin D, Wheeler DL: Ulnar nerve excursion and strain at the elbow and wrist associated with upper extremity motion. *J Hand Surg Am* 2001;26(4):655-662.

12. Ogata K, Naito M: Blood flow of peripheral nerve effects of dissection, stretching and compression. *J Hand Surg Br* 1986;11(1):10-14.

13. Clark WL, Trumble TE, Swiontkowski MF, Tencer AF: Nerve tension and blood flow in a rat model of immediate and delayed repairs. *J Hand Surg Am* 1992;17(4):677-687.

14. Wall EJ, Massie JB, Kwan MK, Rydevik BL, Myers RR, Garfin SR: Experimental stretch neuropathy: Changes in nerve conduction under tension. *J Bone Joint Surg Br* 1992;74(1):126-129.

15. Bozentka DJ: Cubital tunnel syndrome pathophysiology. *Clin Orthop Relat Res* 1998;351:90-94.

16. Ochi K, Horiuchi Y, Tanabe A, Waseda M, Kaneko Y, Koyanagi T: Shoulder internal rotation elbow flexion test for diagnosing cubital tunnel syndrome. *J Shoulder Elbow Surg* 2012;21(6):777-781.

17. Novak CB, Lee GW, Mackinnon SE, Lay L: Provocative testing for cubital tunnel syndrome. *J Hand Surg Am* 1994;19(5):817-820.

18. Rayan GM, Jensen C, Duke J: Elbow flexion test in the normal population. *J Hand Surg Am* 1992;17(1):86-89.

19. Campbell WW, Carroll DJ, Greenberg MK, et al: Literature review of the usefulness of nerve conduction studies and electromyography in the evaluation of patients with ulnar neuropathy at the elbow. *Muscle Nerve* 1999;22(8):S175-S205.

20. Zhong W, Zhang W, Zheng X, Li S, Shi J: The high-resolution ultrasonography and electrophysiological studies in nerve decompression for ulnar nerve entrapment at the elbow. *J Reconstr Microsurg* 2012;28(5):345-348.

21. McGowan AJ: The results of transposition of the ulnar nerve for traumatic ulnar neuritis. *J Bone Joint Surg Br* 1950;32(3):293-301.

22. Dellon AL: Review of treatment results for ulnar nerve entrapment at the elbow. *J Hand Surg Am* 1989;14(4):688-700.

23. Padua L, Aprile I, Caliandro P, Foschini M, Mazza S, Tonali P: Natural history of ulnar entrapment at elbow. *Clin Neurophysiol* 2002;113(12):1980-1984.

24. Seror P: Treatment of ulnar nerve palsy at the elbow with a night splint. *J Bone Joint Surg Br* 1993;75(2):322-327.

25. Svernlöv B, Larsson M, Rehn K, Adolfsson L: Conservative treatment of the cubital tunnel syndrome. *J Hand Surg Eur Vol* 2009;34(2):201-207.

26. Dellon AL, Hament W, Gittelshon A: Nonoperative management of cubital tunnel syndrome: An 8-year prospective study. *Neurology* 1993;43(9):1673-1677.

27. Nabhan A, Ahlhelm F, Kelm J, Reith W, Schwerdtfeger K, Steudel WI: Simple decompression or subcutaneous anterior transposition of the ulnar nerve for cubital tunnel syndrome. *J Hand Surg Br* 2005;30(5):521-524.

28. Bartels RH, Verhagen WI, van der Wilt GJ, Meulstee J, van Rossum LG, Grotenhuis JA: Prospective randomized controlled study comparing simple decompression versus anterior subcutaneous transposition for idiopathic neuropathy of the ulnar nerve at the elbow: Part 1. *Neurosurgery* 2005;56(3):522-530.

29. Watts AC, Bain GI: Patient-rated outcome of ulnar nerve decompression: A comparison of endoscopic and open in situ decompression. *J Hand Surg Am* 2009;34(8):1492-1498.

30. Göbel F, Musgrave DS, Vardakas DG, Vogt MT, Sotereanos DG: Minimal medial epicondylectomy and decompression for cubital tunnel syndrome. *Clin Orthop Relat Res* 2001;393:228-236.

31. O'Driscoll SW, Jaloszynski R, Morrey BF, An KN: Origin of the medial ulnar collateral ligament. *J Hand Surg Am* 1992;17(1):164-168.

32. Kaempffe FA, Farbach J: A modified surgical procedure for cubital tunnel syndrome: Partial medial epicondylectomy. *J Hand Surg Am* 1998;23(3):492-499.

33. Gervasio O, Gambardella G, Zaccone C, Branca D: Simple decompression versus anterior submuscular transposition of the ulnar nerve in severe cubital tunnel syndrome: A prospective randomized study. *Neurosurgery* 2005;56(1):108-117.

34. Biggs M, Curtis JA: Randomized, prospective study comparing ulnar neurolysis in situ with submuscular transposition. *Neurosurgery* 2006;58(2):296-304.

35. Fitzgerald BT, Dao KD, Shin AY: Functional outcomes in young, active duty, military personnel after submuscular ulnar nerve transposition. *J Hand Surg Am* 2004;29(4):619-624.

36. Caliandro P, La Torre G, Padua R, Giannini F, Padua L: Treatment for ulnar neuropathy at the elbow. *Cochrane Database Syst Rev* 2012;7(7):CD006839.

37. Vogel RB, Nossaman BC, Rayan GM: Revision anterior submuscular transposition of the ulnar nerve for failed subcutaneous transposition. *Br J Plast Surg* 2004;57(4):311-316.

38. Caputo AE, Watson HK: Subcutaneous anterior transposition of the ulnar nerve for failed decompression of cubital tunnel syndrome. *J Hand Surg Am* 2000;25(3):544-551.

39. Broudy AS, Leffert RD, Smith RJ: Technical problems with ulnar nerve transposition at the elbow: Findings and results of reoperation. *J Hand Surg Am* 1978;3(1):85-89.

40. Papatheodorou LK, Williams BG, Sotereanos DG: Preliminary results of recurrent cubital tunnel syndrome treated with neurolysis and porcine extracellular matrix nerve wrap. *J Hand Surg Am* 2015;40(5):987-992.

41. Varitimidis SE, Riano F, Sotereanos DG: Recalcitrant post-surgical neuropathy of the ulnar nerve at the elbow: Treatment with autogenous saphenous vein wrapping. *J Reconstr Microsurg* 2000;16(4):273-277.

42. Kokkalis ZT, Jain S, Sotereanos DG: Vein wrapping at cubital tunnel for ulnar nerve problems. *J Shoulder Elbow Surg* 2010;19(2 suppl):91-97.

43. Jones NF, Shaw WW, Katz RG, Angeles L: Circumferential wrapping of a flap around a scarred peripheral nerve for salvage of end-stage traction neuritis. *J Hand Surg Am* 1997;22(3):527-535.

44. Kokkalis ZT, Pu C, Small GA, Weiser RW, Venouziou AI, Sotereanos DG: Assessment of processed porcine extracellular matrix as a protective barrier in a rabbit nerve wrap model. *J Reconstr Microsurg* 2011;27(1):19-28.

Video Reference

7.1. Sotereanos DG: Video. *Cubital Tunnel Syndrome*. Pittsburgh, PA, 2016.

Thoracic Outlet Syndrome: Getting It Right So You Don't Have to Do It Again

Alan J. Micev, MD
Joshua M. Abzug, MD
A. Lee Osterman, MD

Abstract

Thoracic outlet syndrome is a disorder caused by thoracic outlet compression of the brachial plexus and/or the subclavian vessels. The characteristics of thoracic outlet syndrome are highly variable. Objective tests, such as electrodiagnostic studies, are often unreliable in characterizing thoracic outlet syndrome. The existence of thoracic outlet syndrome as a discrete entity is controversial. Surgeons who accept the existence of thoracic outlet syndrome acknowledge that diagnosis is clinical. The variability and complexity of thoracic outlet syndrome lends itself to mistakes in both diagnosis and surgical treatment.

Instr Course Lect 2017;66:103–113.

Thoracic outlet syndrome (TOS) is a condition in which important neurovascular structures, such as the subclavian vessels and the brachial plexus, may be compressed in the thoracic outlet region. The term was first used by Peet et al[1] in 1956 to define neurovascular symptoms of the upper extremity that were presumably caused by mechanical changes with narrowing of the spaces in the thoracic outlet. TOS describes a wide spectrum of clinical presentations with a variety of etiologies.

Anatomy

An understanding of the anatomy of the thoracic outlet is crucial to avoid errors in both diagnosis and surgical treatment. Variations in bony, muscular, vascular, and neural anatomy all contribute to the development of TOS. More than 30% of patients may demonstrate congenital anomalies that create additional challenges for surgeons.[2] A history of trauma or surgery about the thorax, neck, or shoulder should raise suspicion for anatomic alterations.[3]

The thoracic outlet extends from the outer edge of the first rib laterally to include the mediastinum medially and extends cranially in the neck to the level of the fifth cervical nerve root. The thoracic outlet space contains the anterior and middle scalene muscles; the five primary cervical nerves of the brachial plexus; the three trunks of the brachial plexus; the phrenic nerve; the long thoracic, suprascapular, and dorsal scapular nerves; the stellate ganglion; the subclavian artery and vein; the thoracic duct; the scalene lymph nodes; and the apex of the lung.[4]

The thoracic outlet region includes three common areas in which neurovascular compression can occur: the interscalene space, the costoclavicular space, and the retropectoralis minor space (**Figure 1**). The borders of the

Dr. Abzug or an immediate family member is a member of a speakers' bureau or has made paid presentations on behalf of Checkpoint Surgical and serves as a paid consultant to AxoGen. Dr. Osterman or an immediate family member has received royalties from Biomet and Skeletal Dynamics; is a member of a speakers' bureau or has made paid presentations on behalf of Auxilium and Biomet; serves as a paid consultant to A.M. Surgical, Arthrex, and Auxilium; has received research or institutional support from Auxilium and Skeletal Dynamics; and serves as a board member, owner, officer, or committee member of the American Association for Hand Surgery and the American Society for Surgery of the Hand. Neither Dr. Micev nor any immediate family member has received anything of value from or has stock or stock options held in a commercial company or institution related directly or indirectly to the subject of this chapter.

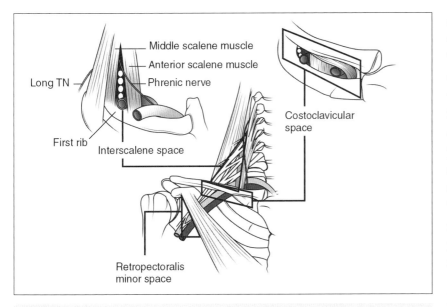

Figure 1 Illustration shows three potential sites of neurovascular compression: the interscalene triangle, the costoclavicular space, and the retropectoralis minor space. TN = thoracic nerve. (Reproduced from Kuhn JE, Lebus V GF, Bible JE: Thoracic outlet syndrome. *J Am Acad Orthop Surg* 2015;23[4]:222-232.)

interscalene triangle are formed anteriorly by the anterior scalene muscle, posteriorly by the middle scalene muscle, and inferiorly by the first rib. The costoclavicular space is a triangular area bordered anteriorly by the medial portion of the clavicle as well as the underlying subclavian muscle, its tendon, and the costocoracoid ligament. The costoclavicular space is bordered posteromedially by the first rib as well as the insertion of both the anterior and middle scalene muscles and posterolaterally by the upper border of the scapula. The retropectoralis minor space is less frequently encountered and located just below the coracoid process and under the pectoralis minor insertion to the coracoid process.

Etiology

Currently, the etiology of TOS is believed to be a combination of neck trauma and anatomic predisposition. A seemingly minor injury or repetitive stress usually is superimposed on the anatomic anomalies, which further compromises the thoracic outlet space. Anatomic variations may be either soft tissue or bony in nature.

Although neural compression usually generates the most obvious symptoms, arterial or venous compression may be predominant in any patient. If symptoms are localized to the subclavian artery, the subclavian vein, or a defined segment of the brachial plexus, the surgeon should suspect an anatomic variation.[5-7] If symptoms involve the entire contents of the thoracic outlet, the surgeon should suspect postural and scalene abnormalities. During surgery, all potential sites of compression must be examined systematically and thoroughly.

Soft-Tissue Causes

Anatomic variations in the scalene triangle from which the nerve roots of the brachial plexus emerge may play a substantial role in the predisposition of patients toward the development of TOS. Patients with TOS tend to have a narrower scalene triangle compared with the mean scalene triangle observed in cadaver models.[8] Congenital bands and ligaments are observed in many patients who have neurogenic TOS, and several types of congenital bands and ligaments have been recognized. These congenital bands and ligaments represent anatomic variations that can predispose a patient to TOS after a neck injury.

Bony Causes

Cervical ribs also are a predisposing factor for TOS in most patients in whom they are observed. Cervical ribs have been identified in 0.5% to 0.6% of the population. Occasionally, cervical ribs may cause symptoms of TOS without trauma or injury; however, in 80% of patients with cervical ribs, symptoms do not develop until after a neck injury.[9] Incomplete cervical ribs, which often are associated with fibrous bands, may be more of a predisposing factor for TOS. Other bony findings that predispose a patient to TOS include a prominent C7 transverse process, exostoses, or callus from prior trauma.

Clinical History and Presentation
General

Surgeons must obtain a meticulous patient history and perform a complete physical examination that includes the cervical spine, the shoulder, and the entire upper extremity bilaterally, even if symptoms are unilateral or relatively localized. Facial complaints, headaches, arm heaviness or swelling, and diffuse weakness are more frequent compared with the classic numbness or vascular

Table 1

Common Misdiagnoses of Thoracic Outlet Syndrome

Specialty	Misdiagnosis
Family doctor	Tendinitis
General orthopaedic surgeon	Rotator cuff syndrome
Rheumatologist	Fibromyalgia, Tietze syndrome
Neurosurgeon	Cervical disk disease
Physiatrist	Myofascial strain
Pain specialist	Complex regional pain syndrome
Hand surgeon	Carpal tunnel syndrome, cubital tunnel syndrome

symptoms that occur in an overhead elevated upper extremity. Medical specialists often misdiagnose patients who have TOS (**Table 1**). In addition, the diagnosis of TOS is more common in large urban centers.

TOS tends to occur in young and middle-aged adults and is three times more frequent in women than in men. Symptoms may develop spontaneously or after trauma to the neck or shoulder region. The most commonly reported symptoms are chronic pain involving the shoulder girdle, neck, or upper back in association with paresthesias in the upper extremity. The clinical presentation can be either neurogenic or vascular. Studies have estimated that more than 90% of all TOS cases are neurogenic in origin.[10]

Neurogenic

Sanders et al[10] reported that trapezius and/or arm pain; upper extremity paresthesia; and hand, arm, and shoulder weakness in addition to neck pain and occipital headaches were present in more than 80% of patients who had neurogenic TOS. Paresthesia most often involved all five fingers (58%); paresthesia of the ring and little fingers was less frequent (26%), and paresthesia of the thumb and the index and long fingers was rare (14%).[10] The authors reported that the Raynaud phenomenon, hand coldness, and color changes secondary to sympathetic trunk compression also were observed in patients who had neurogenic TOS.

Trauma or repetitive stress may precipitate neurologic TOS in susceptible individuals. Violinists, flutists, data entry personnel, and assembly line workers are particularly vulnerable to TOS. A motor vehicle accident with an associated whiplash injury that causes chronic muscle spasms or fibrosis in the scalene muscles may precipitate TOS. Cervical spine and shoulder symptoms often occur immediately; however, patients in whom these symptoms occur also may report arm pain and paresthesias, which may be delayed weeks or even months after trauma. Compression may involve either the upper or lower brachial plexus. Usually, upper brachial plexus TOS causes pain on either side of the neck that radiates upward to the ear and may include the mandible, the face, as well as the temporal and occipital regions. Alternatively, lower brachial plexus TOS usually causes discomfort of variable intensity in the anterior or posterior shoulder region that radiates down the arm to the medial aspect of the forearm and into the hand.

Paresthesias may principally affect the ring and little fingers. Neurogenic TOS must be differentiated from common peripheral compressive neuropathies and cervical radiculopathy.

Vascular

Venous obstruction at the thoracic outlet produces swelling, edema, and cyanosis of the arm that is aggravated with exercise. Primary subclavian vein thrombosis, which also is known as effort thrombosis or Paget-Schroetter syndrome, may occur at the level of the first rib, which may result in the sudden onset of edema, often with dusky cyanosis and limb discomfort. Physical findings of primary subclavian vein thrombosis include arm, forearm, and hand swelling as well as visible subcutaneous veins over the involved shoulder and chest wall. Arterial symptoms that arise from compression of the subclavian artery in the region of the first rib consist of coldness, pallor, and fatigue in the arm with exercise. Patients often experience vascular claudication of the arm with exercise, particularly with the arm elevated. A cervical rib or an elongated C7 transverse process often is present. The purely vascular forms of TOS are easily diagnosed but uncommon.

Differential Diagnosis

Compression of the neurovascular structures can cause a variety of symptoms in the upper extremity and neck, including deep pain, numbness, tingling, weakness, and vasomotor changes. Shoulder girdle pain and headaches also may occur, depending on the severity and duration of compression. Although the diagnosis of TOS must primarily be clinical, it also must be distinguished from other causes of

Table 2
Differential Diagnosis for Patients With Generalized Upper Extremity Pain

Cervical radiculopathy and/or degenerative disk disease

Brachial neuritis

Nerve injury about the shoulder (suprascapular, long thoracic, axillary)

Peripheral nerve compression (carpal tunnel syndrome, cubital tunnel syndrome)

Mechanical shoulder problems (rotator cuff impingement, dead arm syndrome)

Syringomyelia

Multiple sclerosis

Vascular syndromes (Raynaud, quadrilateral space compression)

Cardiac pathology

Tumors of the supraclavicular fossa or lung

Myofascial syndrome

Complex regional pain syndrome

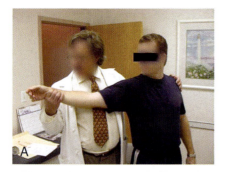 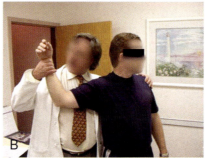

Figure 2 Clinical photographs show provocative tests for thoracic outlet syndrome. **A,** The Adson test is performed by bringing the patient's arm and shoulder into extension, turning the patient's head toward the affected side, and having the patient take a deep breath. **B,** The Wright test is performed by holding the patient's arm in hyperabduction and external rotation with the patient's head turned away from the affected side.

generalized upper extremity pain[11-24] (**Table 2**).

Physical Examination
General

The physical examination should focus on the diagnosis of all of a patient's maladies. Body habitus observations, such as the presence of a gazelle-like neck, asymmetric shoulder height, large breasts, or a slouching posture, should raise suspicion to the possibility of TOS.[25] The failure to identify subtle sensory changes that may be present on the medial aspect of the forearm or the ulnar hand is a common error in the physical examination. The medial antebrachial cutaneous nerve originates directly from the brachial plexus and can help define a site of brachial plexus irritation if such altered sensation is present. In some patients, weakness and atrophy may be difficult to distinguish from apprehension.

Neurogenic

Similar to peripheral nerve testing, a supraclavicular or infraclavicular Tinel sign is specific but not particularly sensitive for the diagnosis of TOS. The authors of this chapter note that direct thumb pressure over the brachial plexus that re-creates a patient's symptoms is a more common and rewarding diagnostic finding. The Gilliatt-Sumner hand, which was first described in 1970, is a characteristic finding of neurogenic TOS in which atrophy of the abductor pollicis brevis and, to a lesser extent, the hypothenar and interossei muscles has occurred in patients who have normal sensation in the median nerve distribution.[26,27]

Provocative maneuvers may have a relatively high sensitivity if performed correctly; however, their specificity is notably poor.[28,29] Simple obliteration of a patient's pulse with the Adson test or the Wright test should not be considered positive unless accompanied by a reproduction of the patient's symptoms (**Figure 2**). Many individuals without TOS may demonstrate pulse obliteration. The elevated arm stress test, which was believed to be pathognomonic by its describer, David Roos, has been reported to be equally positive in patients with isolated peripheral neuropathies, including cubital tunnel syndrome and carpal tunnel syndrome (**Figure 3**). Gillard et al[30] reported that the specificity of the Adson test and the elevated arm stress test for the diagnosis of TOS was 76% and 30%, respectively. Warrens and Heaton[28] reported that 58% of healthy volunteers had at least one positive provocative test; however, only 2% of healthy volunteers had more than two positive provocative tests, which indicates that the interpretation of multiple provocative tests in combination may increase the specificity for the diagnosis of TOS.

Vascular

In patients with vascular complaints, bruit auscultation over the brachial plexus area is important. In patients who have long-standing TOS, poststenotic dilatation of the subclavian artery may produce an audible bruit. Bruit auscultation can be enhanced if it is performed with the patient's arm in the symptomatic provocative position. A blood pressure difference between the two arms is significant if it is more than 20 mm Hg, which suggests insufficiency of the subclavian artery.[31] The upper extremity and chest wall may become congested and edematous with prominent superficial veins in venous TOS; in arterial TOS, the upper extremity may appear cold and pale. A failure to identify one of the previously mentioned causes of upper extremity pain may result in persistence or exacerbation of symptoms. TOS often occurs in conjunction with other diagnoses. The authors of this chapter have noted the frequent association of mechanical shoulder pathology and brachial plexopathy in the thoracic outlet region.

The surgeon must consider the possibility of a double crush phenomenon, in which a patient with TOS also may have a peripheral compression neuropathy, such as cubital, radial, or carpal tunnel syndrome.[32] In patients who have multiple areas of compression neuropathy, the surgeon should suspect a hereditary sensitivity to pressure palsy or an intrinsic neuropathy, such as diabetes mellitus.[33]

Diagnostic Studies
Imaging
Radiographs of the cervical spine are useful in the identification of a

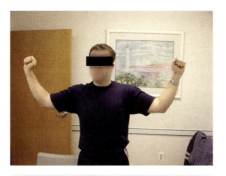

Figure 3   Clinical photograph shows the Roos test (also called the elevated arm stress test), which is performed by having the patient hold his or her arms in an abducted and externally rotated position with the elbows flexed to 90°. The patient pumps his or her hands open and closed quickly and repetitively for 3 minutes. A positive Roos test requires the reproduction of symptoms or rapid fatigue of the extremity.

prominent C7 transverse process or a cervical rib (**Figure 4**). If evidence of cervical spondylosis is present, an MRI of the cervical spine may help to assess root and/or disk involvement. The authors of this chapter have not found MRI of the brachial plexus to be helpful because its use in identifying congenital fibrous bands has not been well studied. The authors of this chapter use MRI only if concern for a possible tumor or other unusual mass exists. Sing et al[34] attempted to correlate MRI results with intraoperative findings; however, the authors were only able to successfully identify points of compression with the use of MRI in less than 50% of patients. Alternatively, CT is useful if a clavicular abnormality, such as a malunion or nonunion with abundant callous, exists because it details any bony deformity and its relationship to the thoracic outlet. Traditionally, ultrasonography has been considered unreliable in the diagnosis of TOS because the area of pathology

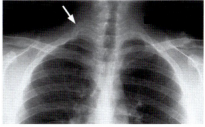

Figure 4   AP radiograph of the cervicothoracic junction. The arrow points to a cervical rib.

is obscured by the clavicle; however, duplex ultrasonography is able to identify stasis or thrombosis in patients who have venous TOS, and ultrasonography may demonstrate increased flow velocity through stenosis or aneurysmal dilatation distal to stenosis in patients who have arterial TOS.[35] Longley et al[36] reported that ultrasonography was 92% specific and 95% sensitive for the diagnosis of venous TOS.

Arteriography and Venography
Conventional arteriography is indicated in patients who have embolic disease, a palpable bruit, a suspected aneurysm, a blood pressure difference between the arms greater than 20 mm Hg, or a previous history of vascular surgery in the area. In these patients, conventional angiography may be both diagnostic and therapeutic (**Figure 5**). Alternatively, magnetic resonance angiography is a helpful noninvasive study that has been reported to have a diagnostic accuracy comparable with that of conventional arteriography.[37,38]

Venography is indicated in patients in whom venous TOS or Paget-Schroetter syndrome is suspected. Venography can be used to evaluate venous obstruction and collateralization. If an acute thrombosis is detected, early catheter-directed thrombolysis followed by early surgical

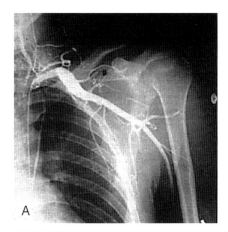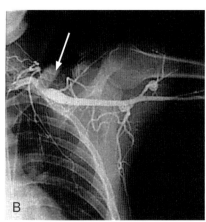

Figure 5 **A,** AP angiogram of a left upper extremity demonstrates the path of the subclavian artery with the arm in a dependent position. **B,** AP angiogram of a left upper extremity with the arm in the provocative position demonstrates obvious compression of the subclavian artery (arrow) at the level of the clavicle.

decompression can be performed to decrease the risk for recurrent thrombosis. Patients who have vascular TOS should undergo coagulation studies to rule out a coagulopathy.[31]

Neurophysiologic Studies

Neurophysiologic studies are notoriously unreliable and, often, are normal in patients who have TOS;[39] however, they may be useful to confirm the presence of cervical radiculopathy and other distal peripheral compression problems. In addition, studies of somatosensory-evoked potentials may help define brachial plexus irritation.[40,41] Tsao et al[42] reported that T1 sensory and motor nerve fibers were affected out of proportion to C8 sensory and motor nerve fibers in patients who had true neurogenic TOS, which manifested as a recognizable pattern of abnormal nerve conduction velocity studies of the medial antebrachial cutaneous nerve and the median motor nerve to the abductor pollicis brevis. Patients with a normal neurologic examination and no evidence of any neurologic involvement are generally advised that, despite their symptoms, no defined nerve damage exists and nonsurgical treatment is recommended.

Treatment

The management of TOS depends on the underlying etiology. Nonsurgical treatment is indicated as the initial treatment for most patients who have neurogenic TOS. Surgical treatment is indicated for patients who have arterial or venous TOS and patients with neurogenic TOS who have persistent symptoms, muscle atrophy, or progressive deficit.

Nonsurgical

Nonsurgical treatment is indicated as the initial treatment for patients who have disputed neurogenic TOS. The most common errors in the nonsurgical treatment of patients who have TOS include the failure to customize a treatment program for a particular patient and the failure to continue nonsurgical treatment for a sufficient duration to effectively alter a patient's symptoms.[1] Nonsurgical management should consist of an education program, activity modification, and physical therapy. Non-narcotic medications, such as amitriptyline or gabapentin, may help mitigate symptoms to a tolerable level.

A four-stage physical therapy program is typically prescribed. In the first stage, myofascial trigger points and local areas of spasm are identified. The second stage focuses on stretching, relaxation, breathing, and myofascial manipulation to restore normal mobility and a balanced posture. In the third stage, muscle strengthening is performed to increase endurance and restore patients to a presymptomatic level of function. In the final stage, patients are prescribed a home exercise program and a plan to return to the workplace. Novak et al[43] reported that 25 of 42 patients who had neurogenic TOS experienced symptomatic relief after 6 months of physical therapy. The authors reported that nonsurgical management was less successful in patients with obesity, workers' compensation patients, and patients who had double-crush pathology that involved the carpal or cubital tunnels.

Surgical Treatment

In general, most patients with TOS will have some response to an appropriate nerve-gliding program. A failure to respond to an appropriate nerve-gliding program should alert a surgeon to other possible nonsurgical entities and the potential for a poor surgical prognosis (**Figure 6**). Most importantly, a reproducible and valid clinical examination is essential to define a surgical candidate. Patients should be weaned from narcotic pain medications under the management of a pain control center.

Surgical management is indicated in patients with vascular TOS, TOS that was confirmed via electrodiagnostic

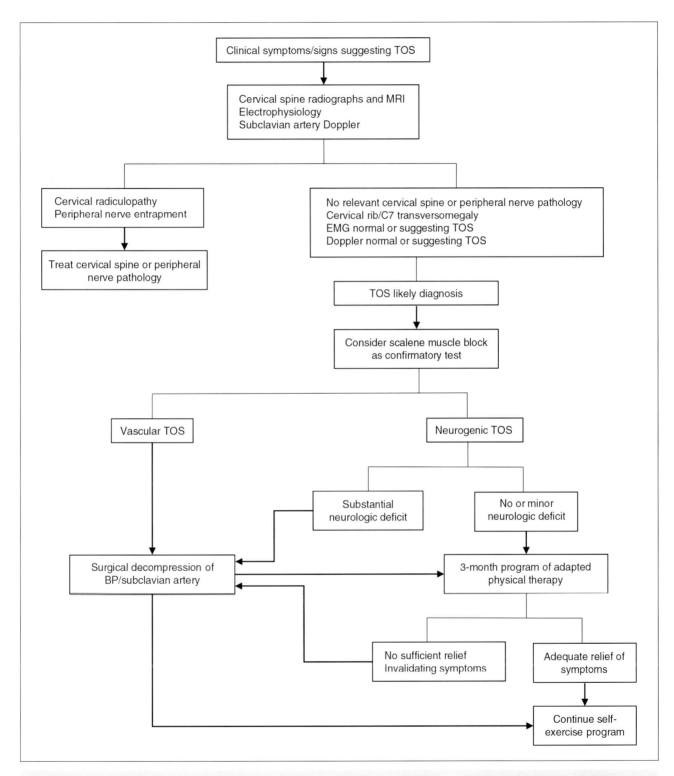

Figure 6   Treatment algorithm for a patient with suspected thoracic outlet syndrome (TOS). BP = brachial plexus, EMG = electromyography.

testing, and disputed neurogenic TOS in whom an adequate trial of nonsurgical treatment fails. Possible surgical treatment options for neurogenic TOS include cervical rib resection, first rib resection, the removal of anomalous bone or fibrous bands, scalenectomy, neurolysis, or claviculectomy in patients who have clavicle malunions or nonunions. Sanders et al[44] reported a 68% overall 5-year success rate for patients who underwent transaxillary first rib resection, anterior and middle scalenectomy, or combined scalenectomy and first rib resection. The authors reported that the patients who underwent combined scalenectomy and first rib resection had a slightly lower failure rate compared with the patients who underwent scalenectomy alone; however, the difference was not statistically significant. The first step in the surgical treatment of patients who have TOS involves communicating the goals and limitations of surgery to the patient. This discussion must include a delineation of the potential complications as well as the risk for the persistence of symptoms, the exacerbation of symptoms, and recurrence.

All types of complications, both minor and catastrophic, have been reported in patients with TOS who undergo surgical treatment. Potential major complications that should be discussed with patients include vascular injury, multiple transfusions, damage to the brachial plexus or phrenic nerve with transient or permanent paralysis, transient numbness of the hand, hemothorax, chylothorax, pneumothorax (possibly requiring a chest tube), and failure to adequately decompress the thoracic outlet. In a study of 280 patients with TOS who underwent first rib resection via the transaxillary

approach, Leffert et al[45] reported that pneumothorax was the most common complication. In a review of 3,914 patients who underwent primary thoracic outlet decompression, Urschel et al[46] reported no major arterial injuries; however, three patients had bleeding that required a second surgical procedure. The authors reported permanent nerve deficits in only four patients. Recurrent symptoms occurred in 1,221 of the patients, all of whom ultimately required a second surgical procedure.

A frank discussion of these complications is intended not to frighten a patient but to emphasize the potential risks of surgical treatment for TOS, which may cause a patient to reconsider the severity of his or her symptoms compared with the potential complications of surgical treatment. Surgeons also should explain to patients that thoracic outlet decompression will relieve only compressive symptoms and that neural symptoms that are related to intraneural scarring will not be affected.

Patients with TOS who have concomitant pathology that contributes to their symptoms must understand the specific symptoms being addressed in thoracic outlet decompression. Electrodiagnostic evidence of cervical radiculopathy or peripheral neuropathy may require additional treatment prior to or in conjunction with thoracic outlet decompression. Females who have excessively large breasts may benefit from mammoplasty prior to thoracic outlet decompression. Patients who have mechanical shoulder pathology may experience secondary relief from a less risky shoulder procedure. The failure to address concomitant pathology or, more importantly, the failure to communicate the goals and expected outcomes of surgical treatment with a

patient may adversely affect a patient's objective and subjective outcomes.

Intraoperative errors often result from a difficulty to recognize anatomic landmarks in patients who have anatomic variations. The key to avoid such errors involves obtaining both preoperative and intraoperative radiographs if doubt with regard to the rib level exists. Intraoperative nerve stimulation and monitoring is useful to actively map out the brachial plexus and identify the phrenic nerve as it crosses the anterior scalene muscle. Exposure must be sufficient to identify both normal and abnormal anatomy, including the offending structures, the structures being decompressed, and the structures at risk. Without an exposure large enough to visually inspect the structures of the thoracic outlet that are adjacent to the rib, it will be impossible to determine whether sufficient rib resection has been performed. Furthermore, damage to the pleura, the subclavian vessels, or the brachial plexus is far more likely if a surgeon is unable to visualize these structures.

Multiple approaches to the thoracic outlet, including transaxillary, supraclavicular, and posterior approaches, have been described. As with any procedure, the selection of the appropriate approach is paramount to avoid preventable complications.[47,48] The foremost consideration in the selection of the approach should be a surgeon's experience and comfort level with a particular approach.

Transaxillary first rib resection is an advantageous approach because the brachial plexus and subclavian vessels do not need to be manipulated. Transaxillary first rib resection should be performed with the patient placed in the lateral decubitus position, with an assistant available to control the upper extremity[49] (**Figure 7**). Use of a traction apparatus to hold the upper extremity may compromise exposure and may result in neurapraxic injury. Transaxillary first rib resection also requires complete skeletal muscle relaxation to allow full access to all of the necessary structures. The surgeon should be aware of the intercostobrachial nerve, which should be spared to prevent posterior arm numbness. The long thoracic nerve also may be at risk because it courses through or immediately posterior to the middle scalene muscle. The dome of the pleura may be damaged during transaxillary first rib resection because it is adherent to the first rib and the suprapleural membrane. Transaxillary first rib resection, if performed carefully, provides excellent access to the lower brachial plexus; however, it does not provide access to the upper, or supraclavicular, plexus.

The supraclavicular approach is technically easier compared with the transaxillary approach and provides the best access to the upper brachial plexus as well as visualization of fibrous bands (**Figure 8**). The supraclavicular approach is the preferred approach for isolated scalenectomy and removal of a cervical rib. In addition, the supraclavicular approach can be used for patients who have vascular TOS that requires arterial reconstruction.

The posterior approach violates the trapezius, levator scapulae, and rhomboid muscles;[50] therefore, it should not be used in patients who have trapezius weakness or ptotic scapulae or patients who plan to return to heavy labor after recovery. Surgeons must recognize that because the posterior approach does not use intermuscular planes, it often is bloody; therefore, meticulous hemostasis is required to maintain visualization

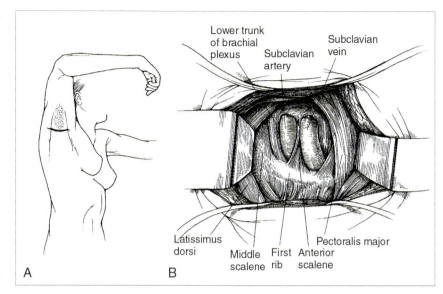

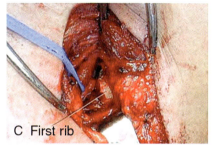

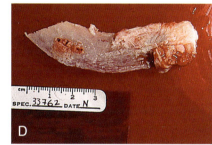

Figure 7   Images show transaxillary first rib resection for the treatment of thoracic outlet syndrome. Illustrations show the patient positioning and incision (**A**) as well as the exposure (**B**) for the transaxillary approach. **C,** Intraoperative photograph shows partial first rib resection. **D,** Clinical photograph shows a partially resected first rib. (Reproduced from Leffert RD: Thoracic outlet syndrome. *J Am Acad Orthop Surg* 1994;2[6]:317-325.)

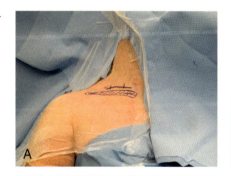

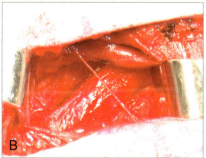

Figure 8   Photographs show the supraclavicular approach for the treatment of thoracic outlet syndrome. **A,** Preoperative photograph shows the landmarks and incision for the supraclavicular approach. **B,** Intraoperative photograph shows exposure of the upper brachial plexus.

as well as avoid excessive blood loss. The posterior approach also may result in postoperative shoulder stiffness and scapular winging.

Prior to wound closure, the surgeon must carefully inspect the field and attain meticulous hemostasis. A simple water seal approach should be used to assess the presence of a pneumothorax. If an air leak is detected, then an intraoperative chest radiograph is indicated; a chest tube should be placed if warranted.

Postoperative Care

A routine postoperative chest radiograph is obtained in the recovery room to identify any pneumothorax that may have been missed during wound closure. A small pneumothorax requires a repeat chest radiograph the next morning to identify whether its size has increased, whereas a large or symptomatic pneumothorax should be treated with a chest tube.

A shoulder immobilizer is worn for comfort. Gentle range-of-motion exercises are begun within the first postoperative week to avoid stiffness and atrophy about the shoulder girdle. Patients may gradually resume activities of daily living at approximately 1 month postoperatively. A nerve-gliding and stretching program is begun 1 week postoperatively. Patients should not perform any heavy lifting or extended arm work in the perioperative period for as many as 6 weeks postoperatively, at which time, if a patient is progressing as planned, a strengthening program is initiated. Some patients require permanent restrictions with regard to job activities.

Summary

Surgeons must be aware of the variability in the anatomy of, presentation of, and treatment options for TOS. A careful nonsurgical treatment regimen and the careful selection of candidates for surgical treatment enhance the likelihood of successful outcomes. The symptoms and signs of TOS vary drastically from patient to patient. Objective tests often are unreliable in characterizing TOS, and the diagnosis of TOS is primarily clinical. Consequently, the variability and complexity of TOS lends itself to mistakes in not only diagnosis but also surgical treatment. Even experienced surgeons must be vigilant and humble in the treatment of patients who have TOS.

References

1. Peet RM, Henriksen JD, Anderson TP, Martin GM: Thoracic-outlet syndrome: Evaluation of a therapeutic exercise program. *Proc Staff Meet Mayo Clin* 1956;31(9):281-287.

2. Roos DB: Congenital anomalies associated with thoracic outlet syndrome: Anatomy, symptoms, diagnosis, and treatment. *Am J Surg* 1976;132(6):771-778.

3. Mulder DS, Greenwood FA, Brooks CE: Posttraumatic thoracic outlet syndrome. *J Trauma* 1973;13(8):706-715.

4. Atasoy E: Thoracic outlet syndrome: Anatomy. *Hand Clin* 2004;20(1):7-14, v.

5. Cormier JM, Amrane M, Ward A, Laurian C, Gigou F: Arterial complications of the thoracic outlet syndrome: Fifty-five operative cases. *J Vasc Surg* 1989;9(6):778-787.

6. Judy KL, Heymann RL: Vascular complications of thoracic outlet syndrome. *Am J Surg* 1972;123(5):521-531.

7. Adson AW: Surgical treatment for symptoms produced by cervical ribs and the scalenus anticus muscle. *Surg Gynecol Obstet* 1947;85(6):687-700.

8. Sanders RJ, Roos DB: The surgical anatomy of the scalene triangle. *Contemp Surg* 1989;35:11-16.

9. Sanders RJ, Hammond SL: Management of cervical ribs and anomalous first ribs causing neurogenic thoracic outlet syndrome. *J Vasc Surg* 2002;36(1):51-56.

10. Sanders RJ, Hammond SL, Rao NM: Diagnosis of thoracic outlet syndrome. *J Vasc Surg* 2007;46(3):601-604.

11. Murphey F: Sources and patterns of pain in disc disease. *Clin Neurosurg* 1968;15:343-351.

12. McCarty EC, Tsairis P, Warren RF: Brachial neuritis. *Clin Orthop Relat Res* 1999;368:37-43.

13. Carroll RE, Hurst LC: The relationship of thoracic outlet syndrome and carpal tunnel syndrome. *Clin Orthop Relat Res* 1982;164:149-153.

14. Goslin KL, Krivickas LS: Proximal neuropathies of the upper extremity. *Neurol Clin* 1999;17(3):525-548, vii.

15. Singer GL, Brust JC, Challenor YB: Syringomyelia presenting as shoulder dysfunction. *Arch Phys Med Rehabil* 1992;73(3):285-288.

16. Melville ID: The differential diagnosis of nerve compression syndromes in the arm and hand: The neurologist's approach. *Hand* 1972;4(2):111-114.

17. Kutz JE, Rowland EB Jr: Vascular compression about the shoulder. *Hand Clin* 1993;9(1):131-138.

18. Cahill BR, Palmer RE: Quadrilateral space syndrome. *J Hand Surg Am* 1983;8(1):65-69.

19. Urschel HC Jr, Razzuk MA, Hyland JW, et al: Thoracic outlet syndrome masquerading as coronary artery disease (pseudoangina). *Ann Thorac Surg* 1973;16(3):239-248.

20. Boyle JJ: Is the pain and dysfunction of shoulder impingement lesion really second rib syndrome in disguise? Two case reports. *Man Ther* 1999;4(1):44-48.

21. Leffert RD, Gumley G: The relationship between dead arm syndrome and thoracic outlet syndrome. *Clin Orthop Relat Res* 1987;223:20-31.

22. Lauder TD: Musculoskeletal disorders that frequently mimic radiculopathy. *Phys Med Rehabil Clin N Am* 2002;13(3):469-485.

23. Detterbeck FC: Pancoast (superior sulcus) tumors. *Ann Thorac Surg* 1997;63(6):1810-1818.

24. Raja SN, Grabow TS: Complex regional pain syndrome I (reflex

sympathetic dystrophy). *Anesthesiology* 2002;96(5):1254-1260.

25. Kaye BL: Neurologic changes with excessively large breasts. *South Med J* 1972;65(2):177-180.

26. Huang JH, Zager EL: Thoracic outlet syndrome. *Neurosurgery* 2004;55(4):897-903.

27. Gilliatt RW, Le Quesne PM, Logue V, Sumner AJ: Wasting of the hand associated with a cervical rib or band. *J Neurol Neurosurg Psychiatry* 1970;33(5):615-624.

28. Warrens AN, Heaton JM: Thoracic outlet compression syndrome: The lack of reliability of its clinical assessment. *Ann R Coll Surg Engl* 1987;69(5):203-204.

29. Nord KM, Kapoor P, Fisher J, et al: False positive rate of thoracic outlet syndrome diagnostic maneuvers. *Electromyogr Clin Neurophysiol* 2008;48(2):67-74.

30. Gillard J, Pérez-Cousin M, Hachulla E, et al: Diagnosing thoracic outlet syndrome: Contribution of provocative tests, ultrasonography, electrophysiology, and helical computed tomography in 48 patients. *Joint Bone Spine* 2001;68(5):416-424.

31. Brantigan CO, Roos DB: Diagnosing thoracic outlet syndrome. *Hand Clin* 2004;20(1):27-36.

32. Wood VE, Biondi J: Double-crush nerve compression in thoracic-outlet syndrome. *J Bone Joint Surg Am* 1990;72(1):85-87.

33. Jaeger SH, Singer DI, Whitenack SH, Mandel S: Nerve injury complications: Management of neurogenic pain syndromes. *Hand Clin* 1986;2(1):217-234.

34. Singh VK, Jeyaseelan L, Kyriacou S, Ghosh S, Sinisi M, Fox M: Diagnostic value of magnetic resonance imaging in thoracic outlet syndrome. *J Orthop Surg (Hong Kong)* 2014;22(2):228-231.

35. Demondion X, Herbinet P, Van Sint Jan S, Boutry N, Chantelot C, Cotten A: Imaging assessment of thoracic outlet syndrome. *Radiographics* 2006;26(6):1735-1750.

36. Longley DG, Yedlicka JW, Molina EJ, Schwabacher S, Hunter DW, Letourneau JG: Thoracic outlet syndrome: Evaluation of the subclavian vessels by color duplex sonography. *AJR Am J Roentgenol* 1992;158(3):623-630.

37. Sällström J, Thulesius O: Non-invasive investigation of vascular compression in patients with thoracic outlet syndrome. *Clin Physiol* 1982;2(2):117-125.

38. Dymarkowski S, Bosmans H, Marchal G, Bogaert J: Three-dimensional MR angiography in the evaluation of thoracic outlet syndrome. *AJR Am J Roentgenol* 1999;173(4):1005-1008.

39. Urschel HC Jr, Razzuk MA, Wood RE, Parekh M, Paulson DL: Objective diagnosis (ulnar nerve conduction velocity) and current therapy of the thoracic outlet syndrome. *Ann Thorac Surg* 1971;12(6):608-620.

40. Veilleux M, Stevens JC, Campbell JK: Somatosensory evoked potentials: Lack of value for diagnosis of thoracic outlet syndrome. *Muscle Nerve* 1988;11(6):571-575.

41. Machleder HI, Moll F, Nuwer M, Jordan S: Somatosensory evoked potentials in the assessment of thoracic outlet compression syndrome. *J Vasc Surg* 1987;6(2):177-184.

42. Tsao BE, Ferrante MA, Wilbourn AJ, Shields RW: Electrodiagnostic features of true neurogenic thoracic outlet syndrome. *Muscle Nerve* 2014;49(5):724-727.

43. Novak CB, Collins ED, Mackinnon SE: Outcome following conservative management of thoracic outlet syndrome. *J Hand Surg Am* 1995;20(4):542-548.

44. Sanders RJ, Hammond SL: Supraclavicular first rib resection and total scalenectomy: Technique and results. *Hand Clin* 2004;20(1):61-70.

45. Leffert RD, Perlmutter GS: Thoracic outlet syndrome: Results of 282 transaxillary first rib resections. *Clin Orthop Relat Res* 1999;368:66-79.

46. Urschel HC Jr, Razzuk MA: Neurovascular compression in the thoracic outlet: Changing management over 50 years. *Ann Surg* 1998;228(4):609-617.

47. Sanders RJ, Pearce WH: The treatment of thoracic outlet syndrome: A comparison of different operations. *J Vasc Surg* 1989;10(6):626-634.

48. Kostic S, Kulka F: Reasons behind surgical failures in thoracic outlet syndrome. *Int Surg* 1990;75(3):159-161.

49. Roos DB: Transaxillary approach for first rib resection to relieve thoracic outlet syndrome. *Ann Surg* 1966;163(3):354-358.

50. Clagett OT: Research and prosearch. *J Thorac Cardiovasc Surg* 1962;44:153-166.

Hand and Wrist

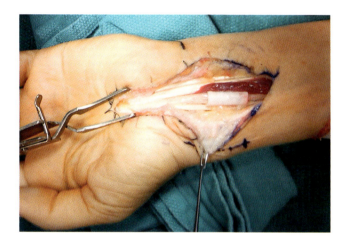

Management of Hand Fractures: Simple to Complex

Richard A. Bernstein, MD

Michael S. Bednar, MD

Craig S. Williams, MD

Randy Bindra, MD, FRACS

Abstract

Hand fractures are among the most common skeletal injuries. Approximately 150,000 hand fractures occur in the United States each year. The management of hand fractures consists of reduction, immobilization, and rehabilitation to return patients to their preinjury status. Hand fractures are managed by restoring articular congruity, reducing malrotation and angulation of the fracture, and maintaining the reduction, all of which should be accomplished with minimal surgical intervention. Surgeons must assess concomitant soft-tissue injuries and respect the soft tissues during the surgical management of hand fractures. Fractures through the metaphyseal bone at the base and neck will heal more quickly than fractures through the diaphyseal bone of the shaft, which makes provisional fixation of metaphyseal fractures more practical compared with provisional fixation of diaphyseal fractures. The fracture pattern determines the most practical type of fixation. Patterns of angulation should be anticipated and corrected during reduction. More rigid fixation is required if substantial comminution and bone loss are present. Bone loss also indicates a high-energy injury, which likely indicates more substantial soft-tissue injury. As the number of injured structures increases, the likelihood of full function after rehabilitation decreases.

Instr Course Lect 2017;66:117–139.

Fractures of the bones in the hand are a complex challenge for surgeons. The intimate association between the bones, tendons, and ligaments in the hand in combination with the complexity of digital motion requires surgeons to have an in-depth knowledge of hand anatomy and carefully consider treatment alternatives. Metacarpal fractures allow surgeons slightly greater flexibility in management. Conversely, little margin for error exists in patients with phalangeal fractures because even minimal angular or rotatory malalignment can result in substantial functional consequences. In patients with metacarpal fractures, the intermetacarpal ligaments provide inherent stability to the metacarpals and minimize angular and rotatory displacement, especially of the central digits. If surgical treatment is necessary for patients with metacarpal fractures, the distance between the flexor and extensor tendons and the bony architecture of the hand allow for greater flexibility in management and help reduce scarring. In patients with phalangeal fractures,

Dr. Bernstein or an immediate family member serves as a paid consultant to or is an employee of AM Surgical and serves as a board member, owner, officer, or committee member of American Society for Surgery of the Hand and the Shoreline Surgery Center. Dr. Bednar or an immediate family member serves as a paid consultant to or is an employee of Biomet and serves as a board member, owner, officer, or committee member of the American Board of Orthopaedic Surgery. Dr. Williams or an immediate family member has received royalties from Innomed. Dr. Bindra or an immediate family member has received royalties from Integra LifeSciences and is a member of a speakers' bureau or has made paid presentations on behalf of Acumed and Integra NeuroSciences.

the intimate association between the common extensor tendon, the intrinsic lateral bands and the central slip, and the terminal tendon that is located directly over the periosteum results in minimal space for hardware or callus. Similarly, the intimate association of the profundus and sublimis tendons on the flexor surface of the hand poses a great challenge for surgeons.

Phalangeal fractures and metacarpal fractures account for 23% and 18% of fractures, respectively, that occur below the elbow.[1] In a retrospective study of 36,518 patients who presented at the Accident and Emergency Department at the VU University Medical Center in Amsterdam, van Onselen et al[2] reported that hand fractures typically occurred in men aged 15 to 35 years, with the little finger being most commonly injured.

In the management of hand fractures, surgeons, especially orthopaedic surgeons, may be tempted to focus on the bony anatomy; however, the soft-tissue envelope of the hand should be considered as important as or more important than the bony injury. Superficially, the skin is a barrier between the body's internal tissue and the outside environment and protects underlying structures. Massive soft-tissue injuries that involve the flexor or extensor tendons affect the underlying bony architecture of the hand and make the decision-making process for fracture fixation complex. Ligaments are necessary for juxta-articular support, and the intrinsic muscles and periosteum are vital to the vascular supply of the bony architecture of the hand. Even the best-fixed hand fractures will result in poor outcomes if an adequate soft-tissue envelope is not present.

Fortunately, advances in flap coverage have resulted in exceptional soft-tissue coverage for patients with hand fractures. Occasionally, simple soft-tissue defects may be allowed to heal either via secondary intention or with the use of skin grafts. A plethora of local digital advancement and rotation flaps have been described for patients with more complex soft-tissue injuries; however, a description of these flaps is beyond the scope of this chapter. Advances in microsurgical techniques also have resulted in improved soft-tissue coverage for patients with hand fractures, either with the use of a posterior interosseous flap or a radial artery forearm flap regionally or with the use of a distal free tissue transfer flap. Furthermore, innervated myocutaneous free flaps, such as an innervated gracilis myocutaneous free flap, can be used in complex reconstructive procedures. Despite the ability of surgeons to reconstruct the soft-tissue envelope of the hand, certain complex hand fractures may be better managed via partial, full, or ray amputation.

The goal in the management of hand fractures is to return patients to their activities, vocations, and avocations as quickly as possible with the least amount of morbidity. The more quickly passive and active exercises are initiated, the more quickly ultimate range of motion and function can be achieved. Despite current osteosynthesis techniques, most hand fractures can be managed nonsurgically. In general, the surgical management of hand fractures, even with ideal conditions, generally results in higher complication rates compared with the nonsurgical management of hand fractures. Finite risks of anesthesia, infection, and hardware are associated with the surgical management of hand fractures; therefore, a clear role remains for the nonsurgical management of fractures and dislocations of the metacarpals and the phalanges.

Surgeons must ask the following questions with regard to a hand fracture: (1) Is the fracture stable? (2) Is the fracture reducible? (3) Is rotation acceptable? and (4) Are adequate methods of immobilization available? Closed reduction and cast or splint immobilization are viable options for the management of hand fractures; however, hand fractures managed in this manner require careful observation. If the answer to any of the aforementioned questions is no, the surgeon must consider the surgical treatment options. Percutaneous fracture fixation with the use of Kirschner wires (K-wires) or screws may help minimize soft-tissue damage; however patient factors, such as age, fracture comminution, and the need for early range of motion, must be considered. Formal open reduction and internal fixation (ORIF), especially of periarticular fractures, affords patients with hand fractures a stable fixation construct that allows for early physical therapy; however, this is more important in phalangeal fractures than metacarpal fractures. Because of the soft-tissue envelope of the hand, scar tissue develops quickly, especially over the extensor mechanism. Scar tissue and stiffness can easily occur if fracture stability cannot be restored via ORIF. **Figure 1** shows a treatment algorithm for the management of hand fractures.

Fractures of the Middle and Proximal Phalanges
Unique Features of the Phalanges

In response to injury, the middle and proximal phalanges behave in a manner similar to and exhibit fracture patterns

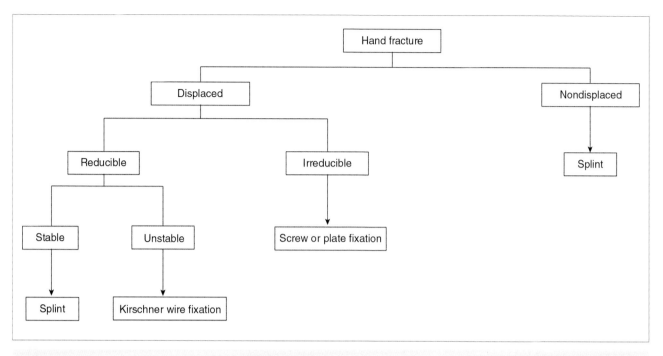

Figure 1 Treatment algorithm for the management of hand fractures. Surgical treatment may be considered as the primary intervention for patients with multiple fractures, patients with combined injuries, athletes, and patients with articular fractures.

that resemble those of the long bones of the extremities. Cortical fractures usually result in displacement, angulation, rotation, and shortening. Metaphyseal fractures usually result in impaction and angulation. The extensor mechanism drapes the phalanges dorsally, and the flexor tendons are closely held to bone by a pulley on the volar aspect of the digit, which increases the risk for tendon adhesions and stiffness with fracture displacement and leaves little room for bulky internal fixation. The pull of the interosseous insertion at the base of the proximal phalanx results in apex volar angulation of the proximal phalanx, whereas a middle phalanx fracture usually results in apex dorsal angulation because of the pull of the sublimis insertion on the distal phalanx.

Phalangeal fractures can be categorized as extra-articular or intra-articular injuries. Extra-articular phalanx

fractures include fractures of the neck, shaft, or base. Intra-articular phalanx fractures include condylar fractures; comminuted fractures (ie, bicondylar fractures); dorsal, volar, or lateral base fractures; fracture-dislocations; and shaft fractures that extend into the joint.

Extra-Articular Phalanx Fractures

A fractured phalanx is a soft-tissue injury with an associated fracture. The management of phalangeal fractures is similar to that for other soft-tissue injuries in the hand; the underlying skeleton is aligned and stabilized with the use of minimal hardware. Attention is then focused on rehabilitation of the soft tissues to promote tendon gliding and mobilization of the associated joints, especially the proximal interphalangeal (PIP) joint, which is critical to digital motion.

Decision Making

The management of a phalangeal fracture is based on a surgeon's ability to achieve satisfactory stability of the fracture after reduction. A stable phalanx fracture will not lose reduction spontaneously or with protected motion. The stability of a phalangeal fracture is determined based on initial displacement, configuration of the fracture, comminution or bone loss, and the extent of soft-tissue disruption. Most phalangeal fractures are stable and minimally displaced and can be managed with immobilization in a safe position for 3 weeks. The indications for reduction include angulation greater than 25° in the dorsopalmar plane, angulation greater than 15° in the coronal plane, shortening of more than 5 mm, and clinically apparent rotational deformity. The amount of deformity that a patient can tolerate

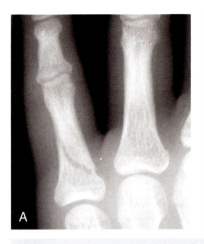 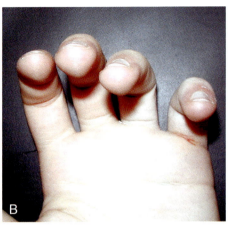

Figure 2 PA radiograph (**A**) and clinical photograph (**B**) of a hand show a minimally displaced proximal phalanx fracture of the little finger with malrotation.

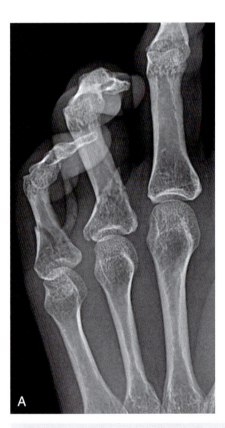 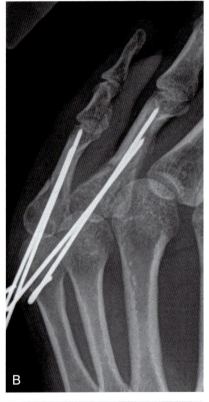

Figure 3 Oblique radiographs of a hand with comminuted and angulated proximal phalanx fractures of the ring and little fingers demonstrate reduction (**A**) and stabilization with the use of Kirschner wires that were passed through the metacarpal head (**B**).

Closed Reduction and Percutaneous Fixation

In general, closed reduction of most displaced phalanx fractures can be achieved under local anesthesia if patients are treated within 5 to 7 days of injury. Reduction is achieved via longitudinal traction with the metacarpophalangeal (MCP) joints flexed to 60°. While applying traction, angulation and rotation are corrected, and the fracture is stabilized via maximal flexion of the PIP joint. After reduction is achieved, the stability of the fracture is assessed by asking the patient to move his or her hand through a functional range of motion. If the fracture is unstable, fixation with K-wires is recommended. The K-wires may be placed percutaneously.

In proximal phalanx fractures, the wider base of the phalanx is an easy starting point for K-wire insertion. With the MCP joint flexed, the K-wires are passed on either side of the extensor tendon in an antegrade fashion through either the metacarpal head or the base of the proximal phalanx. One or two K-wires are passed and stopped short of the PIP joint. This technique is effective for the stabilization of fractures at the base and neck of the proximal phalanx. Pinning through the head of the metacarpal is especially helpful in elderly patients with osteoporosis who sustain angulated proximal phalanx fractures (**Figure 3**). The hand is immobilized in a cast for 3 weeks, after which the K-wires are removed in the clinic.

In patients with transverse mid-shaft phalanx fractures, the K-wires can be drawn out distally past the fracture to create a crossed-wire configuration that allows for limited mobility of the PIP and MCP joints. In patients with oblique or spiral phalangeal shaft

varies; therefore, the decision to intervene must be based on both clinical and radiographic findings. The rotation of a digit is accurately assessed clinically only by comparing it with the contralateral digit (**Figure 2**).

fractures, longitudinal K-wires are less effective. Oblique or spiral phalangeal shaft fractures are reduced with the use of traction and rotation and held in place with a percutaneously applied reduction clamp. Two or three K-wires are then percutaneously placed perpendicular to the fracture.

Open Reduction and Internal Fixation

In general, ORIF is indicated for phalangeal fractures that cannot be reduced via closed means and articular phalanx fractures in which anatomic reduction and stabilization are required for early movement. The proximal and middle phalanges can be approached dorsally by splitting the extensor tendon; this provides the surgeon with an extensive view of the phalangeal fracture and allows for the placement of implants on the dorsal or tension surface of the digit, which is biomechanically more favorable than lateral placement. A mid-lateral approach to the proximal or middle phalanx can be used by retracting or incising the lateral portion of the extensor tendon. A mid-lateral approach is not extensile and does not provide the surgeon with an extensive view of the phalangeal fracture; however, it is advantageous because it avoids an extensor tendon incision and scarring. The periosteum is elevated and is sewn over the implant, if possible, to minimize extensor tendon irritation. In patients with comminuted phalanx fractures, however, extraperiosteal bridge plating helps retain the vascularity of comminuted fragments. A volar approach to the proximal or middle phalanx rarely is used in patients with diaphyseal phalanx fractures, except in the case of replantation, in which ready access to the volar aspect of the phalanx

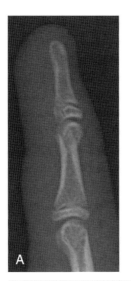
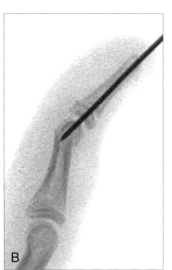
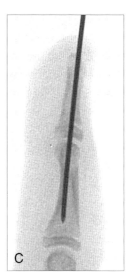

Figure 4   Lateral radiographs of a long finger with a hyperextension phalangeal neck fracture. **A,** Preoperative radiograph demonstrates a hyperextended distal fragment of the middle phalanx. **B,** Intraoperative radiograph demonstrates the placement of a Kirschner wire (K-wire) to engage the distal fragment; this was performed prior to correction of the deformity. **C,** Postoperative radiograph demonstrates final fixation, which was achieved after reduction was performed with the use of the K-wire by leveling the distal fragment into the corrected position and the K-wire was advanced past the fracture.

is possible. However, a mid-lateral approach for volar implant placement is useful in patients with articular fractures at the base of the phalanges.

Surgical Tactics

Neck Fractures

Neck fractures of the middle and proximal phalanges usually are observed in skeletally immature patients. Displaced neck fractures of the middle and proximal phalanges are inherently unstable. Neck fractures of the middle and proximal phalanges usually are angulated dorsally, and the metaphyseal spike forms a block to flexion. For neck fractures of the middle phalanx, a K-wire is percutaneously placed retrograde through the distal phalanx into the distal fragment, with the distal interphalangeal (DIP) joint hyperextended (**Figure 4**). The distal fragment is then manipulated into the corrected position, and the K-wire is advanced

into the medullary cavity of the middle phalanx. Proximal phalangeal neck fractures are stabilized with the use of antegrade K-wires placed through the metacarpal head or crossed K-wires.

Oblique Fractures

Oblique and spiral shaft fractures of the middle and proximal phalanges are prone to malrotation and are difficult to manage with the use of a cast or buddy taping. Reduction and compression of shaft fractures of the middle and proximal phalanges are achieved via the percutaneous application of pointed reduction clamps and stabilization of the fracture with the use of two or three K-wires placed perpendicular to the fracture. Alternatively, interfragmentary screws can be used for the fixation of shaft fractures of the middle and proximal phalanges. A shaft fracture of the middle or proximal phalanx can be approached by splitting

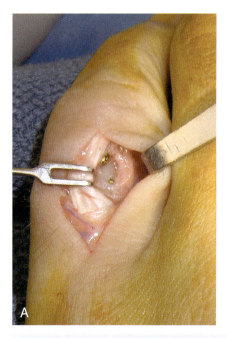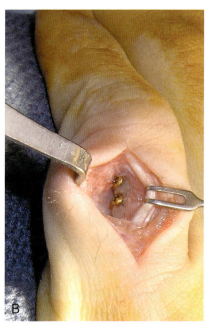

Figure 5 Intraoperative photographs of a little finger with a spiral oblique proximal phalangeal shaft fracture show that retraction of the extensor mechanism to the ulnar side (**A**) and the radial side (**B**) for the insertion of interfragmentary screws is possible via a midline dorsal incision.

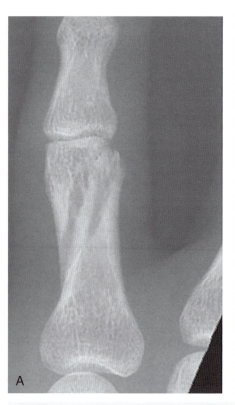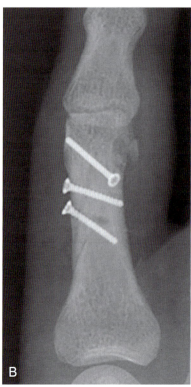

Figure 6 Preoperative (**A**) and postoperative (**B**) PA radiographs of the little finger shown in Figure 5 demonstrate fixation of the spiral oblique proximal phalangeal shaft fracture with the use of interfragmentary screws.

the extensor mechanism. In select patients, a midline dorsal incision can be used to retract the extensor mechanism for reduction and screw insertion (**Figure 5**). Surgeons must use appropriately sized mini-screws that, usually, are no larger than 1.5 mm in diameter. The screws must be placed at least two screw diameters from the fracture line (**Figure 6**). Overdrilling of the near cortex is essential to prevent fracture distraction, and countersinking the screw head minimizes the risk of near cortex failure and decreases screw prominence. A neutralizing plate may be necessary if comminution of the shaft extends into the articular surface.

Transverse Fractures

Because of their geometry, displaced transverse and short oblique fractures of the middle and proximal phalanges are unstable. Transverse and short oblique fractures of the middle and proximal phalanges are stabilized with the use of intramedullary or crossed K-wires. A dorsal or lateral plate with at least four screws provides enough stability to allow for early motion and may be considered in patients who have open fractures, patients who have fractures with associated soft-tissue injury in whom early motion is desired, and patients who have multiple fractures to facilitate rehabilitation. If plates and screws are used, patients must be counseled with regard to the possibility of additional surgery for implant removal and tenolysis.

Proximal Phalangeal Base Fractures

Patients with metaphyseal fractures at the base of the proximal phalanx usually have dorsal cortical comminution and apex volar angulation. Multiple adjacent fingers can fracture in this manner in elderly patients with osteoporosis who sustain a fall. Dorsal angulation of proximal phalangeal base fractures often is underappreciated on initial radiographs because of overlapping of the adjacent digits. Proximal phalangeal base fractures are reducible via digital flexion but are prone to late collapse with the use of cast immobilization. Antegrade crossed K-wires that are inserted at the periphery of the articular margin often are used to stabilize proximal phalangeal base fractures. Alternatively, these fractures can be stabilized with a longitudinal K-wire that is placed antegrade through the metacarpal head into the medullary cavity of the proximal phalanx. Additional pins may be inserted to provide rotational stability, especially in patients with more distal proximal phalangeal base fractures. If a proximal phalangeal base fracture is comminuted and extends into the joint, the use of a dorsal T-plate with the option of locking screws to support the articular surface is preferred (**Figure 7**).

Comminuted Fractures and Bone Loss

The availability of locking plates for hand fractures has facilitated the management of phalangeal fractures with comminution and bone loss. The application of a bridging plate with the periosteal envelope left intact allows for restoration of length, rotation, and alignment of the phalanx (**Figure 8**). Bone grafting may be considered in patients in whom no evidence of clinical or radiographic healing is present after 10 to 12 weeks.

Outcome Factors

The outcomes of phalangeal fracture management depend on several factors, most of which can be controlled by the surgeon. The severity of a patient's

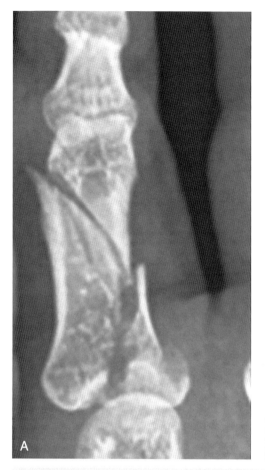
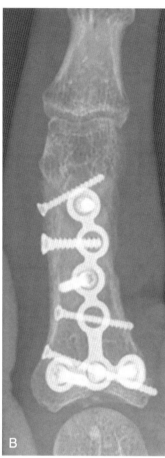

Figure 7   PA radiographs of an index finger with an extensively comminuted proximal phalangeal base fracture. The fracture, which extends into the metacarpophalangeal joint (**A**), was stabilized with the use of interfragmentary screws and a neutralizing plate (**B**).

injury has a direct effect on his or her outcome, with patients who have comminuted phalanx fractures and associated soft-tissue crush injuries having the worst outcomes. In general, patients with unstable phalanx fractures, bone loss, associated tendon injuries, and open phalanx fractures have poor outcomes. Among patient factors, age plays a major role in the outcomes of phalangeal fracture management. Restoration of approximately 90% mobility is expected in younger patients who undergo treatment for phalangeal fractures. Because of comorbidities and preexisting osteoarthritis, less than 60% of

active motion is expected in patients in their sixties and seventies who undergo treatment for phalangeal fractures.[3]

In a study of 100 consecutive proximal phalanx fractures, approximately one-half of which were oblique and spiral phalangeal shaft fractures, that were managed via closed reduction and percutaneous K-wire fixation, Belsky et al[4] reported 61 excellent results (pain-free union, no deformity, >100° of PIP motion, and >215° of total active motion) and 29 good results (pain-free union, minimal deformity, >80° of PIP motion, and >180° of total active motion). The authors

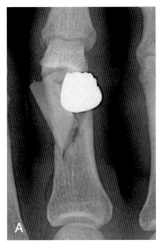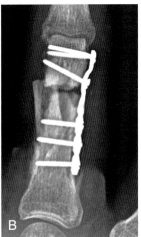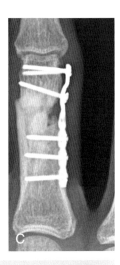

Figure 8   PA radiographs of the middle finger of a patient who sustained a gunshot wound. **A,** Radiograph demonstrates a proximal phalangeal fracture with comminution and bone loss. The bullet from the gunshot wound is observed as a white mass. **B,** Radiograph demonstrates a lateral plate applied to restore length and alignment of the phalanx. The intervening fragments were bridged without direct fixation. **C,** Radiograph taken 3 months postoperatively demonstrates fracture healing.

reported that 10 poor results occurred because of stiffness. In a prospective randomized study that compared the outcomes of 32 patients with oblique or spiral proximal phalangeal shaft fractures who underwent closed reduction and percutaneous K-wire fixation or open reduction and interfragmentary screw fixation, Horton et al[5] reported no significant differences between the patients in the two groups; however, three patients who were treated with the use of K-wire fixation underwent a second procedure for extensor tenolysis. In a large retrospective study of 105 metacarpal and/or phalangeal fractures that were managed with the use of minifragment implants, Page and Stern[6] reported major complications, including stiffness, nonunion, plate prominence, infection, and tendon rupture, in 36% of the fractures, especially in phalangeal and open fractures. Only 4 of the 37 phalangeal fractures achieved a final range of motion greater than 220° (11%). The authors believed that plates

were used for the management of more severe injuries, and that the outcomes of fracture management reflected the severity of injury. In a study that compared the outcomes of 43 patients with oblique or spiral metacarpal and/or proximal phalanx fractures who underwent internal fixation with the use of a plate and screws or screws alone, Başar et al[7] reported that the patients with proximal phalanx fractures in the screw-only fixation group appeared to have significantly better Quick Disabilities of the Arm, Shoulder and Hand questionnaire scores compared with the patients with proximal phalanx fractures who were treated with plate osteosynthesis. In the patients with metacarpal fractures, however, the use of plate-and-screw fixation allowed for earlier return of grasping strength and earlier return to work compared with the use of screws alone.

Patient compliance is critical to the outcomes of phalangeal fracture management, especially in patients with

complex injuries who undergo surgical treatment because the risk for stiffness may be higher as a result of additional surgical insult. The treatment and rehabilitation that are offered to a patient also may affect the outcomes of phalangeal fracture management. The factors that can be controlled by the surgeon in phalangeal fracture management include an appropriate initial evaluation, reduction and appropriate stabilization of the fracture, restoration of joint alignment, management of soft-tissue injuries and swelling, timely rehabilitation, and early detection and management of complications.

Intra-articular Fractures at the Base of the Middle Phalanx
Dorsal PIP Joint Fracture-Dislocations
Dorsal PIP joint fracture-dislocations are common and challenging injuries that require a careful clinical evaluation, critical radiographic evaluation, and, frequently, meticulous surgical management. These fracture-dislocations are caused by a combination of PIP joint hyperextension and varying degrees of axial load. Greater degrees of hyperextension can result in a simple volar avulsion fracture, whereas a greater axial load can result in an impaction fracture at the base of the middle phalanx.

Classification and Clinical Evaluation
Kiefhaber and Stern[8] classified dorsal PIP joint fracture-dislocations based on joint stability. Fractures are classified as stable, tenuous, or unstable patterns based on the percentage of the base of the middle phalanx that is involved (**Figure 9**). In general, stable dorsal PIP joint fracture-dislocations involve less than 30% of the volar portion of the base of the middle phalanx.

In patients with stable dorsal PIP joint fracture-dislocations, the intact dorsal joint tends to remain reduced. Tenuous or reducible dorsal PIP joint fracture-dislocations involve 30% to 50% of the volar base of the middle phalanx, which suggests that subluxation occurs at the time of injury; however, subluxation can be reduced via closed means. Unstable dorsal PIP joint fracture-dislocations involve more than 50% of the base of the middle phalanx. Subluxation, which occurs at the time of injury in unstable dorsal PIP joint fracture-dislocations, typically cannot be stably reduced via closed means.[8,9] Tyser et al[10] confirmed these degrees of stability in dorsal PIP joint fracture-dislocations in a cadaver model study.

Radiographic Evaluation

A radiographic evaluation of the congruency of the reduction of the intact dorsal portion of the base of the middle phalanx relative to the head of the proximal phalanx is necessary. If the joint surfaces are not concentric, then a V sign, which indicates that the joint space is larger at the dorsal portion of the intact base of the middle phalanx and narrower at the more volar portion of the articular surface, will be present (**Figure 10**). Fluoroscopy may aid in the evaluation of the reduction and the reducibility of dorsal PIP joint fracture-dislocations. This is especially true in patients with tenuous dorsal PIP joint fracture-dislocations, which may appear incongruous and unreduced in extension and congruous and reduced in progressive degrees of flexion. Further evaluation with the use of CT may help determine the percentage of the volar articular surface of the base of the middle phalanx that is involved and the extent of comminution.

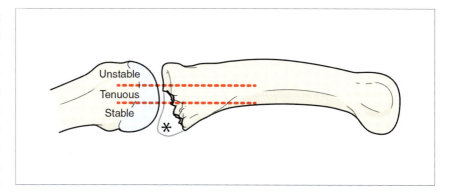

Figure 9   Illustration of a finger shows the Kiefhaber and Stern[8] classification of dorsal proximal interphalangeal (PIP) joint fracture-dislocations. Stable dorsal PIP joint fracture-dislocations involve less than 30% of the articular base of the middle phalanx. Tenuous dorsal PIP joint fracture-dislocations involve 30% to 50% of the articular base of the middle phalanx. Unstable dorsal PIP joint fracture-dislocations involve more than 50% of the articular base of the middle phalanx. The asterisk indicates the fracture zone.

Management

The classification of dorsal PIP joint fracture-dislocations described by Kiefhaber and Stern[8] can be used to guide the management of dorsal PIP joint fracture-dislocations, especially with regard to the decision to proceed with nonsurgical versus surgical management. In general, dorsal PIP joint fracture-dislocations that involve less than 15% of the volar articular surface of the base of the middle phalanx are managed nonsurgically with the use of buddy taping and early range of motion. If an associated dislocation is present, the finger should be splinted in slight flexion for 7 to 10 days to maintain stability, after which early range of motion should be initiated with the use of buddy taping to prevent hyperextension and redislocation. Although dorsal PIP joint fracture-dislocations that involve 15% to 30% of the joint surface generally are considered stable, they may occasionally demonstrate subtle subluxation in full extension, in which case they should be managed in the same manner as tenuous dorsal PIP joint fracture-dislocations. In general, a

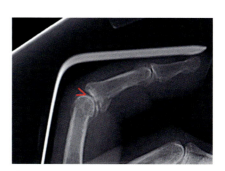

Figure 10   Lateral radiograph of a finger with a dorsal proximal interphalangeal joint fracture-subluxation demonstrates a dorsal V sign (red "V"), which suggests that the joint has not been congruously reduced and that persistent dorsal subluxation of the middle phalanx is present.

slightly less aggressive course of mobilization is advised for the management of stable dorsal PIP joint fracture-dislocations that involve 15% to 30% of the joint surface.

Tenuous dorsal PIP joint fracture-dislocations are unstable and incongruously reduced in full extension. However, concentric reduction and normal motion can be achieved with modest degrees of PIP joint flexion. The concept of extension block splinting was first introduced in 1972 by McElfresh et al.[11] Extension block splinting involves the use of a dorsal blocking splint across the PIP joint in a position that is 10° to 15° greater than the flexion necessary to achieve a congruous reduction. Active flexion away from the extension block is allowed because the PIP joint is stable in further flexion, but the extension block prevents extension of the PIP joint to an unstable position. Extension block splinting requires close follow-up on a weekly basis, with repeat radiographs and a gradual decrease of the extension block by approximately 10° each week. Tenuous dorsal PIP joint fracture-dislocations that require more than 50° of PIP joint flexion to achieve a congruous reduction will likely result in a residual flexion contracture.[12]

Alternative methods to achieve a block to extension have been proposed for the management of tenuous dorsal PIP joint fracture-dislocations. The concept of extension block pinning, which was first introduced in 1992 by Viegas,[13] involves the percutaneous placement of a K-wire through the central slip into the head of the proximal phalanx in a position that blocks extension beyond the position of a congruous reduction. The pin can be placed at any angle dorsal to the coronal plane of the proximal phalanx necessary to block extension. The maximum acceptable extension block involves an intramedullary pin that is placed in the coronal plane of the phalanx (**Figure 11, A** through **C**). Waris and Alanen[14] conducted a retrospective follow-up study of 16 patients with 18 dorsal PIP joint fracture-dislocations that were managed with extension block pinning. The authors used a second temporary intramedullary pin, which was directed from the head of the middle phalanx toward the base of the middle phalanx, as a tamp to improve reduction of the volar base of the middle phalanx if substantial incongruence occurred after placement of the extension block pin. This second temporary intramedullary pin was used for the reduction maneuver and then was removed. Passive flexion was performed at the PIP joint, and active motion was performed at the MCP and DIP joints. The authors removed the extension block pin after 3 to 4 weeks. The percentage of the base of the middle phalanx that was involved in the dorsal PIP joint fracture-dislocations ranged from 41% to 70%. The authors reported less than 15° of flexion contracture, a mean active PIP joint flexion of 86°, and congruous healing of the PIP joint in 9 of the 15 dorsal PIP joint fracture-dislocations that were examined at a mean follow-up of 5 years.[14] In a study of 12 patients with dorsal PIP joint fracture-dislocations (mean percentage of the base of the middle phalanx involved, 43%) who underwent extension block pinning, Bear et al[15] reported a mean active PIP range of motion of 7° to 91° at a mean follow-up of 35.5 months. The patients reported minimal pain; however, mild degenerative changes at the PIP joint were reported in four patients, and moderate degenerative changes at the PIP joint were reported in one patient.

Additional treatment considerations for patients with tenuous dorsal PIP joint fracture-dislocations include the use of an external fixation or dynamic traction device and, occasionally, ORIF. Various techniques for external fixation and dynamic traction exist. These techniques are discussed in more detail in the section on pilon fractures. Ideally, ORIF is most appropriate in the rare patient who has a large, single volar fragment and subluxation. Often, the amount of comminution of the volar fragment is greater than that observed on plain radiographs. If ORIF is considered for the management of tenuous dorsal PIP joint fracture-dislocations, the surgeon must have a backup plan if the volar fragment is not amenable to stable fixation.

Tenuous dorsal PIP joint fracture-dislocations also can be managed via volar plate arthroplasty. Described in 1980 by Eaton and Malerich,[16] volar plate arthroplasty, which involves the use of a volar approach to the PIP joint, allows for mobilization of the volar plate from its origin in the subcondylar fossa of the head of the proximal phalanx and advancement of the distal edge of the volar plate into the bony defect at the base of the middle phalanx. The volar plate is pulled into this interval, repaired, and fastened to the bone at the volar-most intact portion of the articular surface of the base of the middle phalanx with the use of a pullout suture (**Figure 11, D**). The vector pull of the volar plate counteracts the dorsal pull of the central slip and maintains reduction of the dorsal articular surface. After reduction of the dorsal articular surface is achieved, the PIP joint is temporarily pinned for 2 to 3 weeks, after which progressive motion is initiated. Patients who undergo volar plate arthroplasty less than 3 weeks postinjury have better outcomes compared with patients who undergo volar plate arthroplasty more than 3 weeks postinjury.[16,17] In a study of nine patients with an acute dorsal PIP fracture-dislocation who underwent volar plate arthroplasty, Dionysian and Eaton[18] reported a mean active PIP joint motion of 85° and a mean flexion contracture of 15° at a mean follow-up

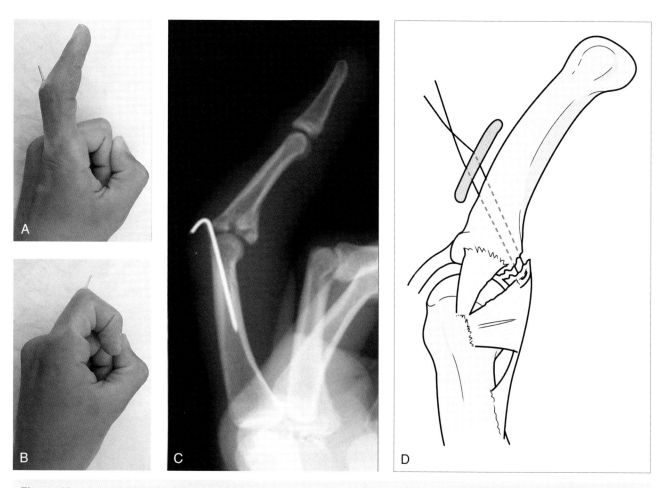

Figure 11 Images show the treatment options for a tenuous dorsal proximal interphalangeal joint fracture-dislocation. Clinical photographs of an index finger in extension (**A**) and flexion (**B**) and lateral radiograph of an index finger (**C**) show extension block pinning. **D,** Illustration of a finger shows volar plate arthroplasty. (Panels A, B, and C reproduced with permission from Bear DM, Weichbrodt MT, Huang C, Hagberg WC, Balk ML: Unstable dorsal proximal interphalangeal joint fracture-dislocations treated with extension-block pinning. *Am J Orthop [Belle Mead NJ]* 2015;44[3]:122-126.)

of 11.5 years. Degenerative changes at the PIP joint were reported in only two patients.

Treatment options are more limited for patients with unstable dorsal PIP fracture-dislocations that involve more than 50% of the joint surface. External fixation and dynamic distraction may be considered in patients with unstable dorsal PIP fracture-dislocations; however, recent studies have emphasized the use of hemicondylar hamate replacement arthroplasty for the management of unstable dorsal PIP fracture-dislocations, which was

first described in 1999 by Hastings et al.[19] The first clinical study on the use of hemicondylar hamate replacement arthroplasty for the management of unstable dorsal PIP fracture-dislocations was published in 2003 by Williams et al.[20] This technique attempts to replace the comminuted articular surface at the volar base of the middle phalanx with an osteoarticular autograft of a similar anatomic configuration. The dorsal distal articular surface of the hamate at the junction of the fourth and fifth carpometacarpal (CMC) joint is the donor site that provides a relatively

good match for the gull-winged contour of the articular surface of the base of the middle phalanx in the coronal plane and the concave contour of the articular surface of the base of the middle phalanx in the sagittal plane (**Figure 12**). Capo et al[21] evaluated and confirmed the suitability of the dorsal distal articular surface of the hamate at the junction of the fourth and fifth CMC joint as the donor site; however, the authors noted that, in the sagittal plane, the arc of curvature of the hamate is less than that of the base of the middle phalanx.

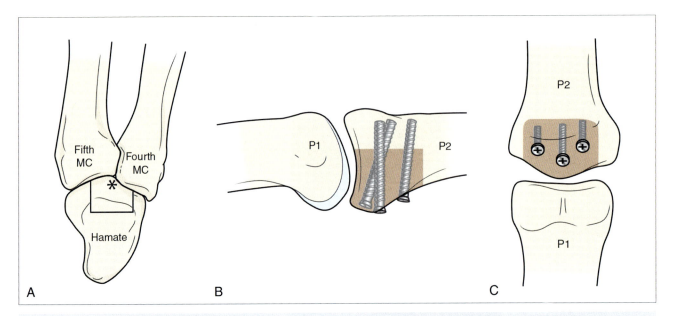

Figure 12 Illustrations of a finger with an unstable dorsal proximal interphalangeal (PIP) joint fracture-dislocation show hemicondylar hamate replacement arthroplasty. **A,** Dorsal view of the hamate, the fourth metacarpal (MC), and the fifth MC shows the donor site (black outlined area) on the dorsal hamate. Note the gull-winged contour of the distal articular surface of the hamate (asterisk). Lateral (**B**) and palmar (**C**) views of the PIP joint show final placement of the hemicondylar hamate graft. P1 = proximal phalanx, P2 = middle phalanx.

For hemicondylar hamate replacement arthroplasty, the PIP joint is approached via a volar incision, in which the tendon sheath between the second and fourth annular ligament pulleys is opened, and the flexor tendons are mobilized laterally. The collateral ligaments are released, and the PIP joint is hyperextended to expose the head of the proximal phalanx and the base of the middle phalanx (**Figure 13, A**). Excellent visualization of the base of the middle phalanx allows for removal of the fragments of the comminuted volar base of the middle phalanx, after which the size of the defect is measured in the transverse and vertical planes. An oscillating saw or rongeur is used to square off the defect in the coronal plane at the volar base of the intact dorsal articular surface and further distally in the axial plane at the base of the middle phalanx.[22-25] The coronal cut should be directed slightly volar to the longitudinal axis of the phalanx to facilitate reproduction of the normal concavity of the base of the middle phalanx.[25]

The hemicondylar hamate graft is harvested via a separate incision that is made on the dorsal aspect of the fourth and fifth CMC joint. Dissection is carried down to the joint, and the joint capsule is incised and elevated to expose the dorsal surface of the hamate. The dimensions of the hemicondylar hamate graft, which are centered about the articular ridge between the fourth and fifth metacarpal bases, are outlined on the dorsal hamate. The hemicondylar hamate graft is then cut with the use of an oscillating saw and harvested with the use of an osteotome. The donor graft is reversed so that the distal-facing articular surface of the hemicondylar hamate graft faces proximally and the cortical dorsal surface of the hemicondylar hamate graft faces volarly. The hemicondylar hamate graft is placed in the defect that was created at the base of the middle phalanx and is secured with the use of temporary K-wires (**Figure 13, B**).[20,22-25] Temporary reduction of the joint allows for clinical and radiographic assessment of stability. If necessary, a small amount of bone graft can be placed distally between the hemicondylar hamate graft and the native phalanx to increase the sagittal plane curvature of the volar aspect of the autograft.[22] After satisfactory reduction and good stability have been achieved, the hemicondylar hamate graft is fixed with the use of two or three screws that are 1 to 1.5 mm in diameter. The PIP joint is reduced, and the volar plate is repaired (**Figure 13, C**). Early active motion is initiated with the use of a figure-of-8 or dorsal blocking splint.

Complications of hemicondylar hamate replacement arthroplasty include recurrent subluxation, pain, stiffness, PIP flexion contracture, flexor tendon

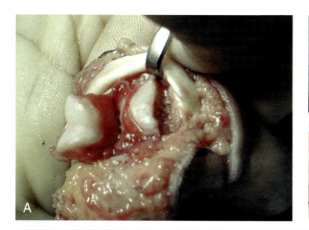
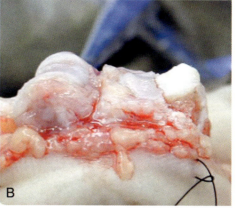
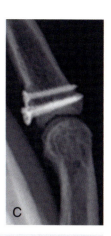

Figure 13   Images show hemicondylar hamate replacement arthroplasty to manage unstable dorsal proximal interphalangeal (PIP) joint fracture-dislocations. **A,** Intraoperative photograph of a finger shows exposure of the articular defect at the base of the middle phalanx. **B,** Intraoperative photograph of a finger shows placement of a hemicondylar hamate replacement arthroplasty graft. The sagittal contour of the joint has been restored. **C,** Lateral radiograph of a finger taken 5 years after hemicondylar hamate replacement arthroplasty demonstrates a healed graft, which was secured with screws, and stable reduction of the PIP joint. (Panel A reproduced with permission from McAuliffe JA: Hemi-hamate autograft for the treatment of unstable dorsal fracture dislocation of the proximal interphalangeal joint. *J Hand Surg Am* 2009;34[10]:1890-1894; panel B reproduced with permission from Williams RM, Kiefhaber TR, Sommerkamp TG, Stern PJ: Treatment of unstable dorsal proximal interphalangeal fracture/dislocations using a hemi-hamate autograft. *J Hand Surg Am* 2003;28[5]:856-865; and panel C reproduced with permission from Calfee RP, Kiefhaber TR, Sommerkamp TG, Stern PJ: Hemi-hamate arthroplasty provides functional reconstruction of acute and chronic proximal interphalangeal fracture-dislocations. *J Hand Surg Am* 2009;34[7]:1232-1241.)

adhesions, cold intolerance, and post-traumatic arthritis.[22,23,26,27] Donor site morbidity is rare. In a meta-analysis of 71 patients with dorsal PIP fracture-dislocations who underwent hemicondylar hamate replacement arthroplasty, Frueh et al[27] reported a mean PIP range of motion of 77° and a mean DIP range of motion of 59° at a mean follow-up of 36 months; however, posttraumatic arthritis was observed on the postoperative radiographs of 11 patients.

Volar PIP Joint Fracture-Dislocations

Volar PIP fracture-dislocations are uncommon. A volar PIP fracture-dislocation is equivalent to a central slip injury and requires critical radiographic evaluation after closed reduction. If the PIP joint is congruously reduced and good contact exists between the dorsal rim fragment and the base of the middle phalanx, a volar PIP fracture-dislocation can be managed by splinting the PIP joint in full extension until union occurs, after which progressive mobilization is initiated. If the dorsal rim fragment is displaced, a volar PIP fracture-dislocation will require surgical management. A small dorsal rim fragment can be managed as a central slip injury, with repair of the tendon and bone to the middle phalanx with the use of suture and/or suture anchor. In addition, the PIP joint should be pinned in extension. Larger dorsal rim fragments may be amenable to ORIF with the use of a screw or a pin. If substantial comminution is present at the base of the middle phalanx, a dynamic traction device may be required.[28]

Pilon Fractures of the Middle Phalangeal Base

Pilon fractures involve comminution, articular impaction, and disruption at the base of the middle phalanx. Often, pilon fractures result in volar or dorsal displacement of the shaft of the middle phalanx. The comminution and impaction present in patients with pilon fractures preclude treatment with ORIF, volar plate arthroplasty, or hemicondylar hamate replacement arthroplasty. Pilon fractures are primarily managed with the use of an external fixation or dynamic traction device.[29]

One of the most versatile and useful devices for the management of pilon fractures is a dynamic external fixator that is fabricated with the use of K-wires and rubber bands, which was described by Slade[30] in 1990 as dynamic distraction and by Suzuki et al[31] in 1994 as pins and rubbers traction. Dynamic distraction and pins and rubbers traction are similar techniques that involve the placement of 0.045-inch K-wires in three positions.

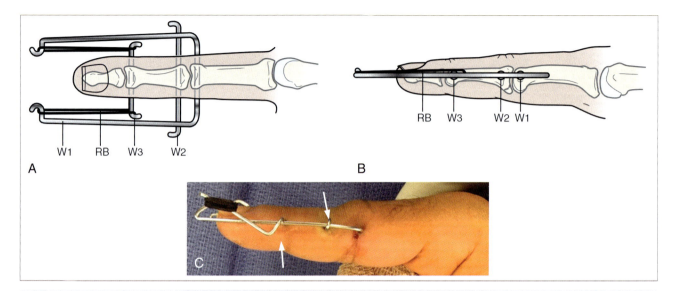

Figure 14   Images show dynamic external fixation of a pilon fracture of the base of the middle phalanx. Dorsal (**A**) and lateral (**B**) view illustrations of a finger show Kirschner wire (W) and rubber band (RB) placement for dynamic external fixation of a pilon fracture of the base of the middle phalanx. **C,** Clinical photograph of an index finger shows a dynamic external fixation device that was used to manage a pilon fracture of the base of the middle phalanx with dorsal subluxation. The arrows indicate the forces acting on the middle phalanx in combination with longitudinal traction.

The first K-wire is placed transversely through the central axis of rotation of the head of the proximal phalanx. Each end of the K-wire is bent 90° and directed distally. A second K-wire is placed through the base of the middle phalanx near the mid-axial line of the middle phalanx, such that when the two arms of the first K-wire are placed in the mid-axial line (above the second K-wire), a volarly directed vector on the base of the middle phalanx is generated, resulting in reduction of the dorsally subluxed PIP joint. A third K-wire is placed through the central axis of rotation of the head of the middle phalanx. The third K-wire is oriented transversely and lies dorsal to the longitudinal arms of the first K-wire. Dental rubber bands are then placed between the third K-wire and the longitudinal arms of the first K-wire to create traction (**Figure 14**). The placement of the K-wires and rubber bands in this manner results in longitudinal distraction of the comminuted articular surface at the base of the middle phalanx and a volarly directed force at the base of the middle phalanx. For patients with a pilon fracture that results in palmar displacement of the shaft of the middle phalanx, the relative positions of the second and third K-wires to the longitudinal arms of the first K-wire are reversed, which results in a dorsally directed force or translation at the base of the middle phalanx. Active range-of-motion therapy is initiated immediately postoperatively. The external fixation frame is left in place for 3 to 4 weeks, after which it is removed in the office. Studies of patients with pilon fractures who underwent dynamic external fixation have reported a mean PIP range of motion between 75° and 90° and a mean flexion contracture as great as 15°.[31-36] All of these studies had a short-term follow-up (<24 months), and the reported incidence of posttraumatic arthritis was relatively low.[31-36]

DIP Joint Dislocations and Fractures
Dislocation

Dislocation at the DIP joint is uncommon. The DIP joint typically dislocates dorsally, which usually is amenable to closed reduction. After closed reduction is achieved, the surgeon must confirm that flexor digitorum profundus (FDP) function is intact and that the FDP tendon has not been avulsed. After radiographic confirmation of reduction is obtained, the DIP joint is splinted in mild flexion to allow for healing of the volar plate, and early active flexion is initiated. Rarely, a DIP joint dislocation may be irreducible because of volar plate entrapment or buttonholing of the head of the middle phalanx around the FDP tendon. Patients in whom the DIP joint cannot be reduced in a closed manner require open reduction, and surgeons should strongly consider temporary pinning in these patients after satisfactory reduction has been achieved. Volar dislocation of the DIP joint is rare.[37]

Mallet Fracture

Mallet fractures are common injuries and result from forced hyperflexion of an extended DIP joint; often, this injury is accompanied by an axial force of differing severity. Mallet fractures result in avulsion of the terminal extensor tendon and involve a varying amount of bone, ranging from a small fleck of bone to more than 50% of the joint surface. Loss of the bony buttress of the phalangeal base may occur, and the unopposed pull of the FDP tendon may result in volar subluxation of the remaining intact volar joint in patients in whom a higher percentage of the dorsal articular surface of the base of the distal phalanx is involved. In a cadaver model study on the relationship between the percentage of the dorsal articular surface that is involved and DIP joint subluxation, Husain et al[38] reported no subluxation in the cadaver models in which less than 43% of the dorsal articular surface was involved. The authors reported that subluxation occurred in approximately one-half of the cadaver models in which 43% to 52% of the dorsal articular surface was involved and that subluxation consistently occurred in the cadaver models in which more than 52% of the dorsal articular surface was involved.

The management of mallet fractures is straightforward in patients in whom no subluxation is present. Simple extension splinting of the DIP joint in full extension with the use of a dorsal or volar splint of almost any configuration for 6 weeks will likely result in satisfactory healing, satisfactory function, minimal extensor lag, and minimal bony deformity. The management of mallet fractures in patients in whom subluxation is present is more controversial. Two studies with relatively short-term follow-up evaluated the outcomes of patients with mallet fractures in whom more than one-third of the dorsal articular surface was involved and/or in whom subluxation was present.[39,40] Both studies reported that the nonsurgical management of mallet fractures resulted in few complications and satisfactory motion and function with minimal pain complaints. Substantial bone remodeling was observed in the patients in both studies, and although degenerative changes were commonly observed on radiographs of the patients in both studies, these changes appeared to be well tolerated clinically.[39,40]

In 1984, Lubahn[41] compared the closed and open treatment of patients with mallet fractures in whom more than one-third of the dorsal articular surface was involved or in whom joint subluxation was present. Although the patients in both the closed and open treatment groups had satisfactory outcomes, the patients in the open treatment group demonstrated less dorsal bony prominence and improved extension compared with the patients in the closed treatment group; however, only short-term outcomes were reported (mean follow-up, <21 weeks).

Numerous techniques for the surgical management of bony mallet fractures, including closed reduction and pinning, closed extension block pinning, open repair and screw fixation, and open repair with pullout sutures and buttons, have been described.[42-45] Although the short-term outcomes of patients who undergo treatment for bony mallet fractures appear acceptable, the long-term outcomes, including the likelihood of degenerative changes, loss of motion, and pain, are unknown. With no clear literature to guide the management of bony mallet fractures, the authors of this chapter developed the following approach for the management bony mallet fractures. Patients who have small avulsion fractures without subluxation are treated with a volar splint of choice for 6 weeks, followed by 2 weeks of night splinting.

Patients who have larger bony fragments without subluxation are treated similarly; however, the surgeon should avoid splinting the DIP joint in hyperextension. After splinting, radiographs are obtained once or twice at 7- to 10-day intervals to monitor for late subluxation. Subluxation that is identified approximately at or before 3 weeks postinjury is considered reducible via closed means, but surgical management should be considered. Surgical management consists of closed pinning with the use of an axial pin to stabilize the DIP joint after the subluxation is reduced. Frequently, a dorsal pin is placed to stabilize the bony fragment (**Figure 15**). The pins are left in place for 6 weeks, after which the patient is treated with 2 weeks of night splinting and progressive mobilization.

In general, volar DIP joint fracture-subluxations that are identified more than 3 weeks postinjury are managed nonsurgically. Despite generally good outcomes after nonsurgical treatment, some patients may have persistent pain months after unrecognized or nonsurgically managed volar subluxation of a mallet fracture. Many of these cases may be associated with nonunion of the fracture fragment, and late management via open reduction can be performed to relieve pain. Open reduction requires débridement of the nonunion site and elevation of the dorsal fragment and the

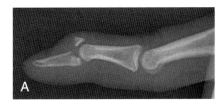
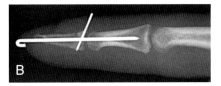

Figure 15 Lateral radiographs of a finger with an acute mallet fracture. **A,** Radiograph demonstrates a large dorsal fragment and volar subluxation. **B,** Radiograph demonstrates that the fracture was managed via closed reduction and pinning.

terminal tendon, followed by reduction and pinning of the DIP joint and repair of the bony dorsal fragment to the distal phalanx. Often, the small size of the bony dorsal fragment precludes stable fixation with the use of a screw or wire and requires repair with a tension-band suture or wire.[46]

Metacarpal Fractures

Anatomy of the Metacarpals

The anatomy of the metacarpals allows the hand to cup in two planes. Proximal to distal, the metacarpals curve concave palmar. The metacarpals of the index and long fingers are rigidly fixed at the CMC joints, and these CMC joints serve as the rigid central pillar of the hand. The metacarpals of the ring and little fingers are mobile, allowing for 15° and 30° of motion, respectively, at these CMC joints. The thumb CMC joint is a reciprocal, biconcave saddle joint, which allows for maximal motion.

Metacarpal Base Fractures

The most common location of a metacarpal base fracture-dislocation is the little finger CMC joint. A small palmar, radial articular fragment is left in place with the hamate, whereas the rest of the metacarpal is displaced dorsally and palmarly. The articular incongruity of the little finger metacarpal may appear subtle on AP radiographs. Shortening of the little finger metacarpal is best observed by drawing a line across the most distal aspect of the long, ring, and little finger metacarpals on an AP radiograph. A little finger metacarpal is proximally displaced if the metacarpal head does not touch this line. Dorsal displacement of the little finger metacarpal on the hamate is best observed on oblique radiographs. Lateral radiographs demonstrate increased palmar angulation of the little finger metacarpal compared with the rest of the metacarpals. Little finger CMC joint dislocations also may occur in combination with a fracture of the dorsal lip of the hamate, which is best observed on oblique and lateral radiographs. The goal of management for little finger CMC joint fracture-dislocations is to attain and maintain reduction of the dislocation as the fracture and soft tissues heal. Closed reduction is achieved via traction and palmar displacement of the metacarpal base. Smooth 0.45-inch K-wires are placed from the little finger metacarpal transversely into the ring finger metacarpal to maintain traction and into either the base of the ring finger metacarpal or the carpus to maintain palmar reduction at the base of the little finger metacarpal. If the fracture fragment is large enough, a headless compression screw can be used to maintain the reduction. Because little finger CMC joint fracture-dislocations occur in metaphyseal bone, healing can be expected within approximately 6 weeks.

Multiple CMC joint dislocations usually are associated with high-energy trauma. Often, multiple oblique radiographs and CT scans help surgeons assess the extent of injury in patients with multiple CMC joint dislocations. Open reduction is frequently required to remove interposed soft tissue. The reduction maneuvers and fixation for multiple CMC joint dislocations are the same as those for isolated little finger CMC joint fracture-dislocations. Because the rigid stability of the index and long finger CMC joints must be maintained, primary fusion should be considered in patients with highly comminuted fractures that remain unstable postoperatively. Arthrodesis also is the preferred treatment for patients with multiple CMC joint dislocations in whom painful posttraumatic arthritis develops.

Metacarpal Shaft Fractures

Metacarpal shaft fractures usually displace apex dorsal because the vector of the intrinsic muscles passes palmar to the axis of rotation of the MCP joints. Because of the rigid CMC joints, only 10° of angulation is accepted in the index and long fingers. In the ring and little fingers, up to 20° of angulation is accepted in the midshaft, with more angulation accepted if the location of the fracture is more distal. Palmar displacement of the distal metacarpal fragment leads to a disturbance in grip, with patient complaints that the metacarpal head is felt when objects are grasped. Shortening and palmar angulation of the metacarpal head leads to hyperextension of the MCP joint and loss of extension at the PIP joint, which is referred to as a pseudoclaw deformity. Metacarpal shortening of 3 to 5 mm is accepted without interfering with extensor tendon function. Less proximal migration often is present in patients with long and ring finger metacarpal shaft fractures because the deep interosseous ligaments prevent excessive shortening.[47]

Indications for the surgical management of metacarpal shaft fractures include open fractures, multiple fractures, unstable fractures, and malaligned fractures. Rotational malalignment may not be observed on radiographs. Rotational malalignment is best assessed by asking a patient to make a fist; the surgeon assesses the patient's fist for digital overlap, comparing it with that of the patient's contralateral hand. Rotational malalignment of 5° will result in a digital overlap of 1.5 cm.[48] The type of fixation used for the management of metacarpal shaft fractures depends on the direction of the fracture and the amount of comminution that is present. Plate-and–lag screw fixation is stronger than plate fixation alone, which is stronger than K-wire and interosseous wire fixation constructs, which are stronger than screw fixation, which is stronger than K-wire fixation alone.

For patients with a metacarpal shaft fracture that is managed with K-wire fixation, the K-wires can be placed transverse or longitudinal or in an intramedullary rod configuration. Little finger metacarpal shaft fractures are best managed with transverse K-wire fixation by pinning the reduced little finger metacarpal to the ring finger metacarpal. At least two K-wires must be placed distal to the fracture. A third K-wire may be placed proximal to the fracture if concern for motion of the proximal fragment at the fracture site distally and the CMC joint proximally exists. Longitudinal K-wires are used to manage transverse or short oblique metacarpal shaft fractures with minimal comminution. The K-wires may be placed either retrograde through the metacarpal head or antegrade via a short incision that is made at the base of the little finger metacarpal.[48] The K-wires are left outside the skin or buried underneath the skin proximally. The K-wires should not protrude distally because they may irritate the extensor hood mechanism. Intramedullary rodding involves the use of angled K-wires to reduce and maintain metacarpal shaft fractures.[49] The K-wires are left exposed proximally for later removal. Because longitudinal K-wires and intramedullary wires do not control the rotation of metacarpal shaft fractures as well as transverse K-wires, buddy taping is necessary to maintain the reduction.

Lag screw fixation is the best treatment option for patients with spiral and long oblique metacarpal shaft fractures if the length of the fracture is at least twice the diameter of the metacarpal at the fracture site.[7,50] Screws are placed in the plane that bisects the longitudinal axis of the metacarpal and the fracture plane. The screw hole should be at least two screw diameters from the fracture margin. At least two screws are required to maintain the reduction.

Interosseous wire techniques are the best treatment option for patients with metacarpal shaft fractures that are similar to amputations, in which the soft tissues are stripped circumferentially at the site of the fracture. Interosseous wire techniques help limit longitudinal stripping of the bone, which would be required for plate fixation. For the 90-90 wire technique, a 0.045-inch wire is used to make two perpendicular drill holes in each fragment; the holes should be located 5 to 10 mm from the edge of the fracture. A 20- or 22-gauge wire is placed through the drill holes. The metacarpal shaft fracture is reduced, and the wires are twisted.

Plate fixation is indicated for all metacarpal shaft fractures. Plates are better tolerated in the metacarpals than the phalanges because less intimate contact exists between the bone and the extensor mechanism, except over the neck of the metacarpal. Screw fixation of at least four cortices that are proximal and distal to the fracture site is required. Spanning plate fixation is the best fixation method to maintain length and allow for early active motion in patients with comminuted metacarpal shaft fractures.

Metacarpal Neck Fractures

Metacarpal neck fractures commonly result from striking a closed fist against a solid object. The amount of palmar angulation accepted in metacarpal neck fractures depends on the location of the fracture. Up to 10° of angulation is accepted in the index and long fingers, up to 30° of angulation is accepted in the ring finger, and up to 50° of angulation is accepted in the little finger. Metacarpal neck fractures are reduced with the use of the Jahss maneuver. The MCP joint is maximally flexed, and pressure is applied to the proximal phalanx and the proximal metacarpal. The proximal phalanx pushes dorsally on the metacarpal head to reduce the fracture. Most little finger metacarpal neck fractures can be managed in a closed manner.[51] Internal fixation is required for patients with metacarpal neck fractures in whom reduction cannot be maintained via closed means. Transverse pinning of the little finger metacarpal head to the ring finger metacarpal helps maintain the reduction and allows the patient to begin active range of motion within the first postoperative week. The K-wires are left in place for 5 to 6 weeks. An alternative method for fixation of metacarpal neck fractures involves the use of a headless compression screw that is placed from the metacarpal head into the isthmus of the metacarpal shaft.[52]

Metacarpal Head Fractures

Because most of the metacarpal head is covered with articular cartilage, osteonecrosis is likely to develop in patients with intra-articular metacarpal head fractures. If internal fixation of a metacarpal head fracture is required, the surgeon should limit soft-tissue dissection to prevent further stripping of the vascular supply to the fragments. Reduction is recommended if more than 25% of the MCP joint is involved and the fragment is displaced more than 1 mm. Open metacarpal head fractures that result from fight bites require formal surgical débridement to prevent infection. In patients with metacarpal head fractures that result from fight bites, a 1-cm transverse laceration will be present across the distal aspect of the MCP joint. Often, an extensor lag is present in patients with metacarpal head fractures caused by fight bites as a result of laceration of the extensor tendon.

Thumb Metacarpal Base Dislocations and Fractures

Dislocation

Dislocation of the thumb CMC joint is rare and results from a disruption of both the dorsoradial ligament and the anterior oblique ligament of the CMC joints. Traditionally, studies suggested that the anterior oblique ligament was the essential ligament that maintained thumb CMC joint stability; however, studies by D'Agostino

et al[53] and Strauch et al[54] reported that the dorsal radial ligament may be more structurally important to thumb CMC joint stability than the anterior oblique ligament.

No large studies have provided surgeons with guidance for the management of thumb CMC joint dislocations.[55-57] Typically, thumb CMC joint dislocations are reducible; however, stable congruous reduction is difficult to maintain with the use of cast immobilization. This difficulty in the maintenance of reduction may lead to persistent instability and poor outcomes. Surgeons should strongly consider closed reduction and percutaneous pinning of thumb CMC joint dislocations, which usually can be achieved easily via longitudinal traction with mild CMC joint flexion, slight pronation, and dorsally or palmarly directed pressure that is applied to the base of the thumb metacarpal. The thumb metacarpal should be pinned to the trapezium or the base of the index finger metacarpal. The role of open dorsoradial ligament repair or volar ligament reconstruction with the use of a tendon graft in patients with an acute thumb CMC joint dislocation is unknown. Open reduction of thumb CMC joint dislocations should be considered in patients in whom the thumb CMC joint is irreducible.[55]

Bennett and Rolando Fractures

A Bennett fracture results from an articular fracture that involves the base of thumb metacarpal, in which the minor volar fragment remains attached to the anterior oblique ligament and the major articular fragment subluxates dorsally and radially.[58] The deforming forces include the abductor pollicis longus, the extensor pollicis brevis, the extensor

pollicis longus, and the adductor pollicis. Closed reduction is performed in patients who have nondisplaced Bennett fractures with less than 1 mm of displacement; however, Livesley[59] advocated caution with regard to closed reduction. In a study of eight cadaver models with Bennett fractures that underwent closed reduction and pinning, Capo et al[60] reported substantial discrepancies between the radiographic evaluation of displacement, gapping, and stepoff after closed reduction and pinning and the actual reduction attained based on direct visual inspection.

In general, surgical management is indicated for Bennett fractures. Reduction of the major fragment (the base of the thumb metacarpal) to the trapezium is critical in the surgical management of Bennett fractures. Good bony contact between the minor volar fragment and the major dorsal articular fragment is necessary to restore ligamentous competency. Cullen et al[61] reported that articular stepoff of the minor volar fragment is less critical than thumb CMC joint reduction and good bony contact between the fragments. If the minor volar fragment involves a major portion of the thumb CMC joint, open reduction may be required because articular congruity and thumb CMC joint reduction are more critical if the minor volar fragment is large. In general, open reduction of a Bennett fracture is best approached via a Wagner incision. Fixation is achieved with the use of K-wires and screws. Few studies have evaluated the outcomes of patients who undergo treatment for Bennett fractures.[62-64] These studies suggested that, although the radiographic outcomes of Bennett fracture management correlate with the degree of satisfactory thumb CMC joint reduction, the clinical outcomes of Bennett fracture management do not correlate as closely with the degree of satisfactory thumb CMC joint reduction.[62-64]

A Rolando fracture is a comminuted fracture that involves the thumb metacarpal base and typically involves three or more fragments. Rolando fractures are relatively uncommon and generally are not amenable to closed reduction and percutaneous pinning. ORIF is the preferred treatment for patients with Rolando fractures; however, it may be a challenge. The treatment options for patients with Rolando fractures include plate fixation, tension-band wiring, and, in patients with severely comminuted fractures, external fixation and percutaneous pinning.[65]

MCP Joint Dislocations (Excluding the Thumb)

An MCP joint dislocation is an uncommon but interesting and controversial injury. MCP joint dislocations are most commonly observed in the index finger and are rarely observed in the little finger. Dorsal MCP joint dislocations are classified as simple or complex. A simple, dorsal MCP joint dislocation results from hyperextension of the MCP joint and rupture of the volar plate. Essentially, a marked hyperextension deformity exists at the MCP joint, and the base of the proximal phalanx may be perched on the dorsum of the metacarpal head. The reduction of simple, dorsal MCP joint dislocations is straightforward. Dorsal pressure is applied to the base of the proximal phalanx, which forces the proximal phalanx over the metacarpal head and into a reduced position. Subsequent management of simple, dorsal MCP joint dislocations includes dorsal splinting and active flexion, which allow

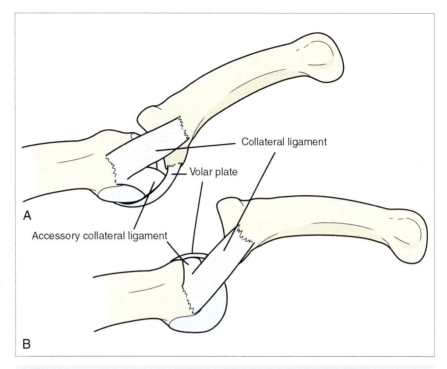

Figure 16   Illustrations show a finger with normal alignment (**A**) and a finger with a complex, irreducible, dorsal metacarpophalangeal (MCP) joint dislocation (**B**). Complex, dorsal MCP joint dislocations result from interposition of the volar plate, which is detached only from its proximal attachment to the metacarpal neck. Because the volar plate remains attached to the accessory collateral ligaments, it is tightly held against the dorsal metacarpal head. Attempts to force the proximal phalanx palmarly will increase tension on the volar plate, which will further resist reduction.

the volar plate to heal. In performing reduction of simple, dorsal MCP joint dislocations, surgeons must avoid any longitudinal traction that may allow the proximally detached volar plate to slide dorsally over the metacarpal head, which may result in a complex, irreducible dorsal MCP joint dislocation.[66]

Complex, dorsal MCP joint dislocations are characterized by puckering of the palmar skin, which results from interposition of the volar plate between the base of the proximal phalanx and the dorsum of the metacarpal head. Controversy exists with regard to the cause of irreducibility in patients with complex, dorsal MCP joint dislocations. Kaplan[67] reported that a noose, which consists of the index lumbrical displaced

radially on the metacarpal neck, the FDP tendon displaced ulnarly on the metacarpal neck, the natatory ligament displaced distally and dorsally, and the superficial transverse intermetacarpal ligament displaced proximally with the interposed volar plate, prevents reduction of complex, dorsal MCP joint dislocations. Other studies have reported that the volar plate is the true block to reduction of complex, dorsal MCP joint dislocations[68-70] (**Figure 16**). Afifi et al[71] subjected six cadaver model specimens to hyperextension impact loading of the index finger, which resulted in a complex, dorsal MCP joint dislocation of the index finger. The authors reported that the index lumbrical was displaced radially in five specimens, the flexor tendons were displaced ulnarly in all six specimens, the volar plate was entrapped dorsally in all six specimens, and the radial digital nerve was displaced radially in three specimens. The authors reported no involvement of the natatory ligament or the superficial transverse intermetacarpal ligament in any of the cadaver model specimens. In addition, the authors reported that release or division of the index lumbrical and the flexor tendons did not result in reduction of the complex, dorsal MCP joint dislocations, and that volar plate division was required for reduction.

The complex arrangement of the volar plate is responsible for the irreducibility of complex, dorsal MCP joint dislocations. A normal volar plate is attached proximally at the metacarpal neck, radially at the accessory collateral ligament, ulnarly at the accessory collateral ligament and the deep transverse intermetacarpal ligament, and distally at the volar phalangeal base. A complex, dorsal MCP joint dislocation involves disruption of the volar plate only from its proximal attachment at the metacarpal neck. The collateral ligament attachments to the metacarpal head, the proximal phalanx, and the volar plate remain largely intact in patients with complex, dorsal MCP joint dislocations. Severe hyperextension of the MCP joint to the maximal point of displacement allows the proximal free edge of the volar plate to ride up dorsally over the articular surface of the metacarpal head. As the axis of the metacarpal head decreases, the volar plate flips from concave to convex as it reaches the dorsal surface. Because the volar plate remains attached to the collateral ligaments, it is held taut against the dorsal metacarpal head. Attempts to force the proximal phalanx distally or volarly will increase

tension on the volar plate, which will further resist reduction.

Although a limited number of closed reduction attempts is reasonable in patients with complex, dorsal MCP joint dislocations, most complex, dorsal MCP joint dislocations require surgical management. Controversy exists with regard to the best approach for the open reduction of complex, dorsal MCP joint dislocations. A volar approach was advocated by Dinh et al,[66] Kaplan,[67] and Burman.[72] The advantages of the volar approach for open reduction of complex, dorsal MCP joint dislocations include access to and manipulation of the index lumbrical and flexor tendons and access to and repair of the volar plate. The disadvantages of this approach include the risk for injury to the digital nerve, which may be displaced from its normal location, and difficulty in accessing the volar plate from the volar wound on the volar side of the metacarpal head. The dorsal approach for open reduction of complex, dorsal MCP joint dislocations was first advocated in 1876 by Farabeuf[73] and was subsequently advocated in 1975 by Becton et al.[69] The advantages of the dorsal approach include easy access to the volar plate and no risk for nerve injury. The dorsal approach also allows for ORIF of an associated metacarpal head fracture. The disadvantages of this approach include longitudinal division of the volar plate and inability to repair the volar plate after reduction.

The authors of this chapter prefer to use a dorsal approach for open reduction of complex, dorsal MCP joint dislocations because it is relatively simple and safe. The dorsal approach is performed by splitting the extensor tendon, releasing a portion of the sagittal band, or retracting the extensor

mechanism distally and ulnarly.[70] The dorsal joint capsule is opened (if it is not already disrupted), and the volar plate is identified. The volar plate often is indistinguishable from the articular cartilage of the metacarpal head initially; however, a Freer elevator can be used to probe the white surface to help identify the volar plate. Occasionally, the proximal edge of the volar plate can be forced distally over the metacarpal head, which results in MCP joint reduction; however, longitudinal division of the volar plate in the midline often is necessary to release tension and allow the volar plate and, thus, the MCP joint to reduce. Postoperative management requires early mobilization with the use of a dorsal blocking finger splint for approximately 3 weeks. Immobilization often leads to stiffness and loss of motion, and a return to full activities with the use of buddy taping often occurs within 6 weeks postoperatively.

Volar MCP joint dislocations are rare and are primarily observed in the border digits. The literature contains few reports of volar MCP joint dislocations, which are described in small studies.[74-76] Volar MCP joint dislocations involve disruption of the joint capsule and at least one collateral ligament. Often, the extensor tendon or junctura is entrapped beneath the metacarpal head. Wood and Dobyns[74] hypothesized that hyperflexion, with a proximally directed force on the dorsal proximal phalanx, was the mechanism of injury responsible for volar MCP joint dislocations. Reducible, volar MCP joint dislocations are likely unstable and prone to volar resubluxation, and they should be splinted in extension. The close follow-up of patients with a reducible, volar MCP joint dislocation via radiographic reassessment, which may be difficult, is critical. Any evidence of resubluxation should prompt a change to surgical management, which involves repair of the collateral ligament and temporary pinning of the MCP joint in extension. Irreducible volar MCP joint dislocations can occur. Reduction of a volar MCP joint dislocation may be blocked by the dorsal joint capsule, the collateral ligaments, and/or an entrapped extensor mechanism. An open dorsal approach is advocated for the reduction of volar MCP joint dislocations because it allows for the removal of any entrapped capsular collateral ligament and the mobilization of any extensor elements that are entrapped beneath the metacarpal head. The collateral ligament and the dorsal capsule should be repaired, and pinning of the MCP joint in extension should be considered. Late complications of volar MCP joint dislocations include stiffness, resubluxation, and posttraumatic arthritis.[75]

Summary

Fractures of the bones in the hand are common injuries and are a treatment challenge. Surgeons must assess not only patient factors, such as age, hand dominance, vocation, and avocations, but also the amount of soft-tissue damage that is present and the specific characteristics of the fracture. Most hand fractures can be successfully managed nonsurgically. However, in patients in whom the surgical management of a hand fracture is warranted, the principles of soft-tissue management and anatomic reduction are imperative to afford stability and early range of motion.

References

1. Chung KC, Spilson SV: The frequency and epidemiology of hand and forearm fractures in the United States. *J Hand Surg Am* 2001;26(5):908-915.

2. van Onselen EB, Karim RB, Hage JJ, Ritt MJ: Prevalence and distribution of hand fractures. *J Hand Surg Br* 2003;28(5):491-495.

3. Strickland JW, Steichen JB, Kleinman WB, et al: Phalangeal fractures: Factors influencing digital performance. *Orthop Rev* 1982;11:39-50.

4. Belsky MR, Eaton RG, Lane LB: Closed reduction and internal fixation of proximal phalangeal fractures. *J Hand Surg Am* 1984;9(5):725-729.

5. Horton TC, Hatton M, Davis TR: A prospective randomized controlled study of fixation of long oblique and spiral shaft fractures of the proximal phalanx: Closed reduction and percutaneous Kirschner wiring versus open reduction and lag screw fixation. *J Hand Surg Br* 2003;28(1):5-9.

6. Page SM, Stern PJ: Complications and range of motion following plate fixation of metacarpal and phalangeal fractures. *J Hand Surg Am* 1998;23(5):827-832.

7. Başar H, Başar B, Başçı O, Topkar OM, Erol B, Tetik C: Comparison of treatment of oblique and spiral metacarpal and phalangeal fractures with mini plate plus screw or screw only. *Arch Orthop Trauma Surg* 2015;135(4):499-504.

8. Kiefhaber TR, Stern PJ: Fracture dislocations of the proximal interphalangeal joint. *J Hand Surg Am* 1998;23(3):368-380.

9. Barksfield RC, Bowden B, Chojnowski AJ: Hemi-hamate arthroplasty versus transarticular Kirschner wire fixation for unstable dorsal fracture-dislocation of the proximal interphalangeal joint in the hand. *Hand Surg* 2015;20(1):115-119.

10. Tyser AR, Tsai MA, Parks BG, Means KR Jr: Stability of acute dorsal fracture dislocations of the proximal interphalangeal joint: A biomechanical study. *J Hand Surg Am* 2014;39(1):13-18.

11. McElfresh EC, Dobyns JH, O'Brien ET: Management of fracture-dislocation of the proximal interphalangeal joints by extension-block splinting. *J Bone Joint Surg Am* 1972;54(8):1705-1711.

12. Dobyns JH, McElfresh EC: Extension block splinting. *Hand Clin* 1994;10(2):229-237.

13. Viegas SF: Extension block pinning for proximal interphalangeal joint fracture dislocations: Preliminary report of a new technique. *J Hand Surg Am* 1992;17(5):896-901.

14. Waris E, Alanen V: Percutaneous, intramedullary fracture reduction and extension block pinning for dorsal proximal interphalangeal fracture-dislocations. *J Hand Surg Am* 2010;35(12):2046-2052.

15. Bear DM, Weichbrodt MT, Huang C, Hagberg WC, Balk ML: Unstable dorsal proximal interphalangeal joint fracture-dislocations treated with extension-block pinning. *Am J Orthop (Belle Mead NJ)* 2015;44(3):122-126.

16. Eaton RG, Malerich MM: Volar plate arthroplasty of the proximal interphalangeal joint: A review of ten years' experience. *J Hand Surg Am* 1980;5(3):260-268.

17. Malerich MM, Eaton RG: The volar plate reconstruction for fracture-dislocation of the proximal interphalangeal joint. *Hand Clin* 1994;10(2):251-260.

18. Dionysian E, Eaton RG: The long-term outcome of volar plate arthroplasty of the proximal interphalangeal joint. *J Hand Surg Am* 2000;25(3):429-437.

19. Hastings H, Capo J, Steinberg B, et al: Abstract: Hemicondylar hamate replacement arthroplasty for proximal interphalangeal joint fracture-dislocations. *54th Annual Meeting of the American Society for Surgery of the Hand.* Boston, MA, September 3-5, 1999.

20. Williams RM, Kiefhaber TR, Sommerkamp TG, Stern PJ: Treatment of unstable dorsal proximal interphalangeal fracture/dislocations using a hemi-hamate autograft. *J Hand Surg Am* 2003;28(5):856-865.

21. Capo JT, Hastings H II, Choung E, Kinchelow T, Rossy W, Steinberg B: Hemicondylar hamate replacement arthroplasty for proximal interphalangeal joint fracture dislocations: An

assessment of graft suitability. *J Hand Surg Am* 2008;33(5):733-739.

22. Williams CS IV: Proximal interphalangeal joint fracture dislocations: Stable and unstable. *Hand Clin* 2012;28(3):409-416, xi.

23. Calfee RP, Kiefhaber TR, Sommerkamp TG, Stern PJ: Hemi-hamate arthroplasty provides functional reconstruction of acute and chronic proximal interphalangeal fracture-dislocations. *J Hand Surg Am* 2009;34(7):1232-1241.

24. Calfee RP, Sommerkamp TG: Fracture-dislocation about the finger joints. *J Hand Surg Am* 2009;34(6):1140-1147.

25. McAuliffe JA: Hemi-hamate autograft for the treatment of unstable dorsal fracture dislocation of the proximal interphalangeal joint. *J Hand Surg Am* 2009;34(10):1890-1894.

26. Afendras G, Abramo A, Mrkonjic A, Geijer M, Kopylov P, Tägil M: Hemi-hamate osteochondral transplantation in proximal interphalangeal dorsal fracture dislocations: A minimum 4 year follow-up in eight patients. *J Hand Surg Eur Vol* 2010;35(8):627-631.

27. Frueh FS, Calcagni M, Lindenblatt N: The hemi-hamate autograft arthroplasty in proximal interphalangeal joint reconstruction: A systematic review. *J Hand Surg Eur Vol* 2015;40(1):24-32.

28. Rosenstadt BE, Glickel SZ, Lane LB, Kaplan SJ: Palmar fracture dislocation of the proximal interphalangeal joint. *J Hand Surg Am* 1998;23(5):811-820.

29. Henn CM, Wolfe SW: Dynamic distraction fixation for proximal interphalangeal fracture dislocations, in Seitz W Jr, ed: *Fractures and Dislocations of the Hand and Fingers.* Chicago, IL, American Society for Surgery of the Hand, 2013, pp 150-165.

30. Slade JF: A dynamic distraction external fixation device for the proximal interphalangeal joint. *59th Annual Scientific Meeting of the American Society for Plastic and Reconstructive Surgeons.* Boston, MA, October 21-24, 1990.

31. Suzuki Y, Matsunaga T, Sato S, Yokoi T: The pins and rubbers traction system for treatment of comminuted intraarticular fractures and fracture-dislocations in the hand. *J Hand Surg Br* 1994;19(1):98-107.

32. Inanami H, Ninomiya S, Okutsu I, Tarui T: Dynamic external finger fixator for fracture dislocation of the proximal interphalangeal joint. *J Hand Surg Am* 1993;18(1):160-164.

33. De Smet L, Boone P: Treatment of fracture-dislocation of the proximal interphalangeal joint using the Suzuki external fixator. *J Orthop Trauma* 2002;16(9):668-671.

34. Duteille F, Pasquier P, Lim A, Dautel G: Treatment of complex interphalangeal joint fractures with dynamic external traction: A series of 20 cases. *Plast Reconstr Surg* 2003;111(5):1623-1629.

35. Badia A, Riano F, Ravikoff J, Khouri R, Gonzalez-Hernandez E, Orbay JL: Dynamic intradigital external fixation for proximal interphalangeal joint fracture dislocations. *J Hand Surg Am* 2005;30(1):154-160.

36. Ruland RT, Hogan CJ, Cannon DL, Slade JF: Use of dynamic distraction external fixation for unstable fracture-dislocations of the proximal interphalangeal joint. *J Hand Surg Am* 2008;33(1):19-25.

37. Rozmaryn LM: Distal phalangeal and fingertip injuries, in Seitz WH Jr, ed: *Fractures and Dislocations of the Hand and Fingers.* Chicago, IL, American Society for Surgery of the Hand, 2013, pp 56-57.

38. Husain SN, Dietz JF, Kalainov DM, Lautenschlager EP: A biomechanical study of distal interphalangeal joint subluxation after mallet fracture injury. *J Hand Surg Am* 2008;33(1):26-30.

39. Wehbé MA, Schneider LH: Mallet fractures. *J Bone Joint Surg Am* 1984;66(5):658-669.

40. Kalainov DM, Hoepfner PE, Hartigan BJ, Carroll C IV, Genuario J: Nonsurgical treatment of closed mallet finger fractures. *J Hand Surg Am* 2005;30(3):580-586.

41. Lubahn JD: Mallet finger fractures: A comparison of open and closed technique. *J Hand Surg Am* 1989; 14(2 pt 2):394-396.

42. Takami H, Takahashi S, Ando M: Operative treatment of mallet finger due to intra-articular fracture of the distal phalanx. *Arch Orthop Trauma Surg* 2000;120(1-2):9-13.

43. Hofmeister EP, Mazurek MT, Shin AY, Bishop AT: Extension block pinning for large mallet fractures. *J Hand Surg Am* 2003;28(3):453-459.

44. Zhang X, Meng H, Shao X, Wen S, Zhu H, Mi X: Pull-out wire fixation for acute mallet finger fractures with k-wire stabilization of the distal interphalangeal joint. *J Hand Surg Am* 2010;35(11):1864-1869.

45. Lee HJ, Jeon IH, Kim PT, Oh CW, Deslivia MF, Lee SJ: Transtendinous wiring of mallet finger fractures presenting late. *J Hand Surg Am* 2014;39(12):2383-2389.

46. Shah CM, Sommerkamp TG: Fracture dislocation of the finger joints. *J Hand Surg Am* 2014;39(4):792-802.

47. Khan A, Giddins G: The outcome of conservative treatment of spiral metacarpal fractures and the role of the deep transverse metacarpal ligaments in stabilizing these injuries. *J Hand Surg Eur Vol* 2015;40(1):59-62.

48. Kim JK, Kim DJ: Antegrade intramedullary pinning versus retrograde intramedullary pinning for displaced fifth metacarpal neck fractures. *Clin Orthop Relat Res* 2015;473(5):1747-1754.

49. Gonzalez MH, Hall RF Jr: Intramedullary fixation of metacarpal and proximal phalangeal fractures of the hand. *Clin Orthop Relat Res* 1996;327:47-54.

50. Firoozbakhsh KK, Moneim MS, Doherty W, Naraghi FF: Internal fixation of oblique metacarpal fractures: A biomechanical evaluation by impact loading. *Clin Orthop Relat Res* 1996;325:296-301.

51. Breddam M, Hansen TB: Subcapital fractures of the fourth and fifth metacarpals treated without splinting and reposition. *Scand J Plast Reconstr Surg Hand Surg* 1995;29(3):269-270.

52. Ruchelsman DE, Puri S, Feinberg-Zadek N, Leibman MI, Belsky MR: Clinical outcomes of limited-open retrograde intramedullary headless screw fixation of

metacarpal fractures. *J Hand Surg Am* 2014;39(12):2390-2395.

53. D'Agostino P, Kerkhof FD, Shahab-pour M, Moermans JP, Stockmans F, Vereecke EE: Comparison of the anatomical dimensions and mechanical properties of the dorsoradial and anterior oblique ligaments of the trapeziometacarpal joint. *J Hand Surg Am* 2014;39(6):1098-1107.

54. Strauch RJ, Behrman MJ, Rosenwasser MP: Acute dislocation of the carpometacarpal joint of the thumb: An anatomic and cadaver study. *J Hand Surg Am* 1994;19(1):93-98.

55. Bosmans B, Verhofstad MH, Gosens T: Traumatic thumb carpometacarpal joint dislocations. *J Hand Surg Am* 2008;33(3):438-441.

56. Alexander C, Abzug JM, Johnson AJ, Pensy RA, Eglseder WA, Paryavi E: Motorcyclist's thumb: Carpometacarpal injuries of the thumb sustained in motorcycle crashes. *J Hand Surg Eur Vol* 2016;41(7):707-709.

57. Lahiji F, Zandi R, Maleki A: First carpometacarpal joint dislocation and review of literatures. *Arch Bone Jt Surg* 2015;3(4):300-303.

58. Bennett EH: On fracture of the metacarpal bone of the thumb. *Br Med J* 1886;2(1331):12-13.

59. Livesley PJ: The conservative management of Bennett's fracture-dislocation: A 26-year follow-up. *J Hand Surg Br* 1990;15(3):291-294.

60. Capo JT, Kinchelow T, Orillaza NS, Rossy W: Accuracy of fluoroscopy in closed reduction and percutaneous fixation of simulated Bennett's fracture. *J Hand Surg Am* 2009;34(4):637-641.

61. Cullen JP, Parentis MA, Chinchilli VM, Pellegrini VD Jr: Simulated Bennett fracture treated with closed reduction and percutaneous pinning: A biomechanical analysis of residual incongruity of the joint. *J Bone Joint Surg Am* 1997;79(3):413-420.

62. Kjaer-Petersen K, Langhoff O, Andersen K: Bennett's fracture. *J Hand Surg Br* 1990;15(1):58-61.

63. Thurston AJ, Dempsey SM: Bennett's fracture: A medium to long-term review. *Aust N Z J Surg* 1993;63(2):120-123.

64. Oosterbos CJ, de Boer HH: Nonoperative treatment of Bennett's fracture: A 13-year follow-up. *J Orthop Trauma* 1995;9(1):23-27.

65. Carlsen BT, Moran SL: Thumb trauma: Bennett fractures, Rolando fractures, and ulnar collateral ligament injuries. *J Hand Surg Am* 2009;34(5):945-952.

66. Dinh P, Franklin A, Hutchinson B, Schnall SB, Fassola I: Metacarpophalangeal joint dislocation. *J Am Acad Orthop Surg* 2009;17(5):318-324.

67. Kaplan EB: Dorsal dislocation of the metacarpophalangeal joint of the index finger. *J Bone Joint Surg Am* 1957;39(5):1081-1086.

68. Green DP, Terry GC: Complex dislocation of the metacarpophalangeal joint: Correlative pathological anatomy. *J Bone Joint Surg Am* 1973;55(7):1480-1486.

69. Becton JL, Christian JD Jr, Goodwin HN, Jackson JG III: A simplified technique for treating the complex dislocation of the index metacarpophalangeal joint. *J Bone Joint Surg Am* 1975;57(5):698-700.

70. McGinnis MR, Green SM: Complex metacarpophalangeal joint dislocations. *Bull Hosp Jt Dis* 1993;53(2):7-10.

71. Afifi AM, Medoro A, Salas C, Taha MR, Cheema T: A cadaver model that investigates irreducible metacarpophalangeal joint dislocation. *J Hand Surg Am* 2009;34(8):1506-1511.

72. Burman M: Irreducible hyperextension dislocation of the metacarpophalangeal joint of a finger. *Bull Hosp Joint Dis* 1953;14(2):290-291.

73. Farabeuf LHF: De la luxation du ponce en arriè. *Bull Soc Chir* 1876;11:21-62.

74. Wood MB, Dobyns JH: Chronic, complex volar dislocation of the metacarpophalangeal joint. *J Hand Surg Am* 1981;6(1):73-76.

75. Patel MR, Bassini L: Irreducible palmar metacarpophalangeal joint dislocation due to junctura tendinum interposition: A case report and review of the literature. *J Hand Surg Am* 2000;25(1):166-172.

76. Hamada Y, Sairyo K, Tonogai I, Kasai T: Irreducible fracture dislocation of a finger metacarpophalangeal joint: A case report. *Hand (N Y)* 2008;3(1):76-78.

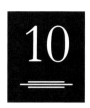

Carpal Tunnel Syndrome: Initial Management and the Treatment of Recalcitrant Patients

Karan Dua, MD
A. Lee Osterman, MD
Joshua M. Abzug, MD

Abstract

Carpal tunnel syndrome (CTS) is a focal compressive neuropathy of the median nerve at the level of the wrist. CTS is the most common type of compressive neuropathy that occurs in the upper extremity. Typically, patients with CTS have paresthesia, pain, and numbness in the radial three and one-half digits. Nighttime symptoms are more common earlier in the disease process, with daytime symptoms becoming more frequent as CTS progresses. Electrodiagnostic studies may be performed to confirm a diagnosis of CTS or to obtain a baseline before surgical treatment; however, electrodiagnostic studies may be normal in a subset of patients who have CTS. Patients who have mild CTS should undergo an initial trial of nonsurgical treatment that includes lifestyle modifications, nighttime splinting, and corticosteroid injections. Carpal tunnel release should be performed in patients in whom nonsurgical treatment fails and patients who have acute CTS secondary to infection or trauma or have advanced symptoms. Recalcitrant CTS, which may occur in as many as 25% of patients who undergo carpal tunnel release, most commonly results from an incomplete transverse carpal ligament release or an incorrect initial diagnosis. Patients with recurrent symptoms often have perineural fibrosis that tethers the median nerve.

Instr Course Lect 2017;66:141–152.

Epidemiology

Paget[1] first described median nerve compression in 1854 in the context of distal radius fractures. Subsequently, compressive neuropathy of the median nerve, which also is known as carpal tunnel syndrome (CTS), was established as a disease entity by Moersch[2] and Phalen.[3] CTS is a focal compression of the median nerve as it passes through the carpal tunnel deep to the transverse carpal ligament (TCL) at the level of the wrist. CTS is the most common type of compression neuropathy that occurs in the upper extremity, affecting an estimated 376 per 100,000 individuals in the United States.[4] The adjusted current annual incidence of CTS is approximately 65% higher than the incidence of CTS in the early 1980s. The incidence of CTS is significantly higher in women compared with men (491 versus 258, respectively, per 100,000), peaking in women aged 50 to 59 years and men aged 70 to 79 years.[4]

Dr. Osterman or an immediate family member has received royalties from Biomet and Skeletal Dynamics; is a member of a speakers' bureau or has made paid presentations on behalf of Auxilium Pharmaceuticals and Biomet; serves as a paid consultant to A M Surgical, Arthrex, and Auxilium Pharmaceuticals; has received research or institutional support from Auxilium Pharmaceuticals and Skeletal Dynamics; and serves as a board member, owner, officer, or committee member of the American Association for Hand Surgery and the American Society for Surgery of the Hand. Dr. Abzug or an immediate family member is a member of a speakers' bureau or has made paid presentations on behalf of Checkpoint Surgical and serves as a paid consultant to AxoGen. Neither Dr. Dua nor any immediate family member has received anything of value from or has stock or stock options held in a commercial company or institution related directly or indirectly to the subject of this chapter.

A recent epidemiologic study reported that the annual rate of carpal tunnel decompression surgery from 2000 to 2010 was significantly higher in women compared with men, with most procedures performed in patients who were in their seventies.[5] Approximately 500,000 carpal tunnel release (CTR) procedures are performed each year.[6]

The risk factors for CTS include diabetes mellitus; rheumatoid arthritis; systemic inflammatory conditions; pregnancy; and medical disorders that lead to generalized edema, acromegaly, hypothyroidism, obesity, uremia, gout, and vitamin B_6 (pyridoxine) deficiency.[7-11] CTS is more likely to develop in individuals who have occupations that include activities of repetition, exertion of force, and/or vibration.[12] Genetic variations in collagen and proteoglycan formation that increase the risk for CTS also have been identified.[13,14] The implications of CTS symptoms are multifold and negatively affect the mental health and occupational function of patients.[15] The cost of CTS management in the United States exceeds $2 billion each year.[16]

Pathoanatomy and Pathophysiology

The carpal tunnel is bordered volarly by the TCL and dorsally by the proximal carpal bones.[17] Ten structures are present in the carpal tunnel: four flexor digitorum superficialis tendons, four flexor digitorum profundus tendons, the flexor pollicis longus tendon, and the median nerve. The median nerve originates from the C5-T1 nerve roots of the brachial plexus and is the most superficial structure that runs through the carpal tunnel.[17,18] Numerous anatomic variations exist in the branching pattern of the median nerve about the

carpal tunnel. The Poisel[19] classification system identified three types of variations in the origin of the recurrent motor branch: extraligamentous (type I), subligamentous (type II), and transligamentous (type III). Lanz[20] adapted the Poisel classification system to include variations in median nerve anatomy with regard to the carpal tunnel. The Lanz[20] adaptation consists of variations in the origin of the recurrent motor branch according to the Poisel classification system (type I); accessory branches of the median nerve distal to the carpal tunnel (type II); high division of the median nerve, which usually is associated with a persistent median artery (type III); and accessory branches of the median nerve proximal to the carpal tunnel (type IV).[20] A recent meta-analysis reported that the origin of the recurrent motor branch is most often extraligamentous, branching distal to the TCL in 75% of patients.[18]

Compression of the median nerve results in a pathologic cascade that, ultimately, leads to irreversible nerve injury. Normal pressure in the carpal tunnel is approximately 2.5 mm Hg.[21] If pressure in the carpal tunnel is increased, the neural microvasculature and the blood flow dynamics of the median nerve are substantially altered.[22] Lower compression pressures lead to impaired venous outflow and venous stasis, which cause capillary leakage. Neural edema worsens, thus increasing intraneural pressure. Conversely, higher compression pressures lead to direct epineural arterial ischemia.[22] If pressures reach more than 30 mm Hg, decreased nerve conduction velocity occurs.[23] If compression persists, inflammation leads to fibrosis and demyelination, which, ultimately, result in axonal loss.[22]

Assessment of Injury
Signs and Symptoms

The clinical characteristics of CTS are predicated on disease progression. Typically, patients with CTS have pain, paresthesia, and numbness in the radial three and one-half digits; however, patients may describe their symptoms as affecting the entire hand. Pain is more prevalent in patients who have bilateral CTS and patients who smoke.[24] Symptoms may be exacerbated during wrist flexion and extension, and symptoms may be alleviated by shaking the hand or changing the position of the wrist. Nighttime symptoms that lead to frequent nighttime awakenings are more common earlier in the disease process. As the disease progresses, daytime symptoms, including morning wrist stiffness, occur more frequently, and patients become clumsier with activities that require finger dexterity. Typically, patients will report a history of dropping objects. Weakness of thumb abduction and eventual atrophy of the thenar musculature occur in the late stages of the disease process.[25] Bilateral CTS may be present in as many as 65% of patients; therefore, a thorough physical examination of both upper extremities is necessary. In addition to obtaining a patient's history with regard to why he or she visited the orthopaedic office, several additional components of a patient's history, including work and sport activity as well as history of the previously discussed risk factors for CTS, should be obtained.[25] Surgeons can ask patients to complete a Katz and Stirrat[26] hand symptom diagram to help localize the symptoms.

The physical examination should begin with a complete assessment of the cervical spine and upper extremities. The hands and limbs should be assessed for atrophy. Before a diagnosis of CTS is made, alternative causes of symptoms should be ruled out with the use of provocative tests. The Spurling test can be used to rule out cervical radiculopathy. A positive Hoffman test and an inverted brachioradialis reflex indicate cervical myelopathy. Surgeons should assess for more proximal sites of median nerve compression, including beneath the ligament of Struthers, the lacertus fibrosus, the pronator teres, and the arch of the flexor digitorum superficialis muscle. In addition, CTS may occur in 20% to 25% of patients who have cubital tunnel syndrome.[27,28]

Several provocative tests can be performed to support a diagnosis of CTS. These tests should be performed for 60 seconds and are considered positive if a patient's symptoms are reproduced. The Phalen test is performed by having a patient maximally flex both wrists, whereas the reverse Phalen test is performed by having a patient maximally extend both wrists; flexion and extension of the wrists increases pressure in the carpal tunnel. The Durkan compression test is the most sensitive and specific maneuver that can be performed to support a diagnosis of CTS.[29] The Durkan compression test is performed by compressing a patient's median nerve directly over his or her carpal tunnel. The Tinel sign is elicited by gently tapping the volar wrist over the carpal tunnel to determine if paresthesia occurs in the median nerve distribution.

Diagnostic Assessment

Often, a detailed history and physical examination are sufficient to make a clinical diagnosis of CTS. However, an electrodiagnostic study (EDS) may be performed to confirm a diagnosis

of CTS and rule out other etiologies of symptoms, such as cervical radiculopathy, brachial plexopathy, thoracic outlet syndrome, and nerve entrapment proximal to the carpal tunnel. An EDS consists of electromyography (EMG), which is performed by inserting a needle into muscles innervated by the nerve under investigation to measure electrical potential, and nerve conduction velocity studies, which are performed by stimulating a nerve at various locations along its course to locate any sites of entrapment. An EDS also may be performed to obtain a baseline, which can help determine the severity of CTS and if any muscle damage is present. Surgeons should be aware that an EDS may be normal in a subset of patients who have CTS.[30,31]

Double crush syndrome occurs if a peripheral nerve is compressed at multiple sites.[32] Studies have theorized that compression of the median nerve at one site increases the risk of symptomatic nerve compression at another site, which eventually results in disrupted axonal transport along the course of the nerve.[33] Typically, patients with double crush syndrome have CTS as well as cervical radiculopathy. Such patients are more likely to have proximal pain and less likely to have median nerve paresthesia compared with individuals who have only CTS.[34]

Typically, radiographs are not necessary to evaluate patients who have CTS. However, ultrasonography is an effective and noninvasive method that can be used to examine the carpal tunnel and has a sensitivity (82%) and specificity (87%) comparable with other diagnostic modalities.[35] The cross-sectional areas of the carpal tunnel and the median nerve are measured and compared with normative values. Multiple studies

report moderate to high intraobserver and interobserver reliability in measuring the cross-sectional area of the median nerve at the inlet of the carpal tunnel.[36,37] Other imaging studies, such as MRI, can be performed but are not necessary.[38]

No blood tests are currently available for the diagnosis of CTS. However, blood tests can help identify diagnoses that may lead to CTS, such as diabetes mellitus, hypothyroidism, rheumatoid arthritis, and pernicious anemia.

Treatment
Nonsurgical Treatment
A trial of nonsurgical management is warranted unless pronounced sensory and/or motor deficits or acute CTS secondary to infection or trauma are present.[25] However, patients with increased symptom duration, a positive Phalen test, and thenar muscle atrophy who undergo nonsurgical treatment are more likely to have poor outcomes.[39] Nonsurgical management includes lifestyle and activity modifications, wrist splinting in a neutral position, oral medications, and local corticosteroid injections.

Short-term wrist immobilization in a neutral position, especially at night, is beneficial for alleviating carpal tunnel symptoms.[40] Neutral positioning is optimal because carpal tunnel pressures are at a minimum with the wrist in $2° \pm 9°$ of extension and $2° \pm 6°$ of ulnar deviation.[41,42]

Oral medications used to manage CTS include NSAIDs, vitamin B_6 supplements, and diuretics. NSAIDs and diuretics are administered to decrease interstitial fluid pressure in the carpal tunnel. Early studies[43] reported that NSAIDs help relieve pain; however, subsequent studies did not find the use of NSAIDs beneficial.[44,45] Vitamin

B_6 is a cofactor necessary for protein synthesis. Vitamin B_6 supplementation is believed to prevent the alteration of normal protein metabolism, which is required for axonal regulation. Initially, support for vitamin B_6 supplementation was widespread;[46] however, oral vitamin B_6 supplements have not been reported to be beneficial.[47] A short course of medium-dose oral prednisone may improve symptoms for as many as 8 weeks.[48]

Steroid injections in the carpal tunnel have fewer systemic effects compared with oral medications. Steroid injections help reduce symptoms, albeit only for a limited time.[47] Blazar et al[49] reported that 79% and 31% of patients with CTS who were treated with the use of a steroid injection had symptom relief 6 weeks and 1 year, respectively, after injection. The authors also reported that 66% of patients did not require a repeat intervention 1 year after steroid injection. In addition, the authors reported that patients with CTS who have diabetes are 2.6 times more likely to have symptom recurrence.[49] Steroid injections also can be used to predict the success of surgical treatment. Patients who experience relief from steroid injections are more likely to have symptom resolution with definitive surgical treatment.[50] Bahrami et al[51] reported no significant differences in the therapeutic effects of steroid injections that consisted of triamcinolone acetonide versus 17-α hydroxyprogesterone. Steroid injections can increase fasting blood glucose levels for as many as 2 days after administration, especially in individuals who have type I diabetes;[52] therefore, patients who are administered steroid injections should closely monitor their blood glucose levels and temporarily adjust their insulin requirements accordingly.

Other nonsurgical modalities used to manage CTS include ultrasonography,[53,54] laser therapy or iontophoresis,[17,55,56] tendon gliding exercises,[57,58] and ergonomic lifestyle modifications,[17] all of which result in varying degrees of reported success.

Surgical Treatment

Indications and Techniques

Surgical treatment is indicated for patients who have persistent symptoms after a trial of nonsurgical treatment, acute CTS secondary to infection or trauma, and severe sensory or motor deficits at initial presentation. The objective of CTR is to decompress the median nerve by incising the TCL. Traditionally, a full open release was performed; however, concerns for incisional pain, poor cosmetic healing, pillar pain, flexor tendon bowstringing, and prolonged recovery times led to the development of numerous minimally invasive and endoscopic release techniques.[59,60]

Outcomes and Complications

Recent studies have reported the long-term outcomes of CTR in various patient populations. In a retrospective study of 211 patients who underwent open CTR, Louie et al[61] reported that the mean Levine-Katz symptom score and the mean Levine-Katz function score was 1.3 ± 0.5 points and 1.6 ± 0.8 points, respectively, at a mean follow-up of 13 years. Only 13% of the patients had a poor Levine-Katz symptom score, and 26% of the patients had a poor Levine-Katz function score. Approximately 74% of patients achieved complete symptom resolution, and only 1.8% of patients required revision surgery. The authors reported that the most common symptom-related

complaints were hand weakness, diurnal pain, numbness, and tingling.[61]

In a retrospective review of the EMG results of 115 patients that were obtained at a mean of 10.47 years after open CTR, Faour-Martín et al[62] reported a positive EMG diagnosis in 82% of the patients who were symptomatic and 58% of the patients who were asymptomatic.[62] In a prospective study that compared the 5-year clinical outcomes of 66 patients with or without diabetes mellitus who underwent open surgical decompression, Thomsen et al[63] reported no differences in sensory, motor, or functional outcomes between the patients with or without diabetes mellitus; however, the patients with diabetes mellitus had improved cold tolerance.

Although patients with metabolic syndromes often have delayed functional recovery after CTR, their hand function and symptom severity 1 year postoperatively is comparable with that of patients without metabolic syndromes.[64] Patient age, general medical comorbidities, and workers' compensation status have not been reported to influence symptom severity and hand function 1 year after open CTR.[65] Cha et al[66] reported that patients who underwent CTR without a delay had significantly improved Disabilities of the Arm, Shoulder and Hand questionnaire and Boston Carpal Tunnel Questionnaire scores as well as substantial increases in grip and pinch strength.

Studies also have compared the functional outcomes of patients with CTS who were treated via a variety of surgical techniques. In two separate randomized controlled trials that compared the outcomes of patients who underwent either open or endoscopic CTR, Atroshi et al[67,68] reported modestly lower postoperative pain in the patients who underwent endoscopic CTR; however, no differences in symptom and function scores were reported up to 5 years postoperatively between the patients who underwent either open or endoscopic CTR. In a recent follow-up study on the long-term outcomes of the patients who underwent either open or endoscopic CTR, Atroshi et al[69] reported no functional differences between the patients in the two treatment groups at 11 to 16 years postoperatively.[69] In a recent Cochrane Database review of 28 studies that included 2,586 hands with CTS that underwent either endoscopic or open CTR, Vasiliasdis et al[70] reported that low evidence supports the equal effectiveness of endoscopic versus open CTR with regard to symptom relief and improved functional status; however, the hands that were treated with endoscopic CTR had better grip strength compared with the hands that were treated with open CTR. The authors reported that the patients whose hands were treated with endoscopic CTR returned to work a mean 8 days earlier compared with the patients whose hands were treated with open CTR.[70] Studies that compared the outcomes of patients who underwent open versus mini-open CTR techniques did not report differences in patient-rated symptom severity or functional status outcomes.[71,72] In a recent systematic review and meta-analysis that compared the complications of patients who underwent open versus endoscopic CTR, Vasiliadis et al[73] reported that open CTR led to a higher rate of wound problems, whereas endoscopic CTR led to a higher rate of transient neurapraxia, numbness, and paresthesias.

Simultaneous bilateral CTR rather than a staged procedure may be beneficial in patients with bilateral CTS who are symptomatic. Osei et al[74] reported no differences with regard to a patient's ability to perform essential activities of daily living for personal hygiene or independence, such as bathing, dressing, eating, driving, or using the bathroom, after unilateral versus simultaneous bilateral CTR.

Recalcitrant CTS and Revision Strategies

Recalcitrant CTS is a substantial problem that occurs in as many as 25% of patients who undergo primary CTR.[75,76] Tung and Mackinnon[77] classified symptoms after primary CTR into three categories: (1) persistent (ongoing symptoms after CTR), (2) recurrent (relief of symptoms for a period of time before recurrence), and (3) new (increased pain or new symptoms after CTR). The most common causes of persistent symptoms are incomplete TCL release or an incorrect initial diagnosis.[78,79] All other possible disease etiologies that may be a cause of persistent symptoms, including more proximal locations of median nerve compression, double crush syndrome, and undiagnosed pronator syndrome, should be ruled out before the possibility of incomplete TCL release is considered.[79] Determining if the TCL was incompletely released or if the TCL reconstituted is difficult. Typically, full release of the TCL during revision CTR will yield favorable outcomes similar to those of primary CTR.[80] The mechanism for recurrent symptoms is not clearly understood but is likely related to perineural fibrosis that tethers the median nerve.[81] Typically, an ultrasonographic examination of patients with recurrent symptoms after primary CTR

will reveal median nerve swelling, incomplete TCL release, and perineural fibrosis.[82] New symptoms most commonly are associated with a nerve injury that occurred during CTR and usually affect the median nerve, the common digital nerves, the palmar cutaneous branch of the median nerve, and the ulnar nerve.[77,83,84]

In a retrospective study of 87 patients who underwent revision CTR during a 10-year period, Zieske et al[79] reported that incomplete release of the flexor retinaculum and scarring of the median nerve were the most common intraoperative findings in patients who had persistent, recurrent, and, even, new symptoms. The authors reported that most of the patients with recurrent symptoms had diabetes and were less likely to have pain symptoms.[79]

Typically, nonsurgical management is ineffective at relieving persistent or recurrent symptoms; therefore, revision CTR is warranted.[85] Critical principles associated with revision CTR include complete decompression of the median nerve and the prevention of scar formation. Revision CTR techniques include the use of neovascularization flaps to improve nerve regeneration and gliding and the interposition of materials that provide a mechanical barrier to prevent perineural scarring. Limited outcome data on revision CTR are available. Patients with intraneural fibrosis, severe preoperative sensory deficits, and sensory neuromas have been reported to have negative outcomes after revision CTR.[86] In a retrospective study of 78 patients who received a steroid injection before revision CTR, Beck et al[87] reported that symptom relief after the steroid injection had a high sensitivity and a positive predictive value

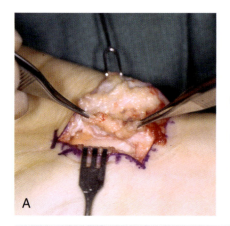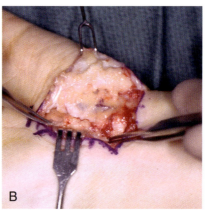

Figure 1 Intraoperative photographs of a wrist show a hypothenar fat pad procedure. **A,** Elevation of the hypothenar fat pad. **B,** Placement of the hypothenar fat pad over the median nerve.

for the surgical resolution of symptoms after revision CTR.

Neovascularization Flaps
Hypothenar Fat Pad

The hypothenar fat pad is mobilized on its pedicle and interposed between the median nerve and the remaining TCL. Ideally, an interposed hypothenar fat pad prevents median nerve adherence to the remnants of the TCL.[85] A hypothenar fat pad procedure is performed via a curvilinear incision that is made parallel to the hypothenar eminence. The palmar aponeurosis and the TCL are incised, after which external neurolysis of the median nerve is performed. The plane between the dermis of the hypothenar skin and adipose tissue is explored sharply. The dissection is continued ulnarly to the dermal insertion of the palmaris brevis. With the digital nerves distally protected and the ulnar nerve and artery proximally protected, the thick hypothenar fat pad is elevated, starting from the ulnar edge (**Figure 1, A**). The hypothenar fat pad is then flipped like a page of a book over the median nerve and sutured to the radial edge

of the flexor retinaculum of the carpal tunnel[88] (**Figure 1, B**).

In a study of 58 patients with recurrent symptoms after CTR who underwent revision CTR with the use of a hypothenar fat pad, Strickland et al[85] reported improved nocturnal symptoms, hypersensitivity, and proximally referred pain. The authors reported that 86% of the patients were able to return to work after revision CTR.[85] In a study of 20 patients with recalcitrant CTS who underwent revision CTR with the use of a hypothenar fat pad, Fusetti et al[89] reported that 18 of the patients had complete resolution of hyperesthesia and allodynia symptoms by 6 months postoperatively. In a study of 18 patients with recurrent symptoms after CTR who underwent revision CTR with the use of a hypothenar fat pad, Wichelhaus et al[88] reported that 15 of the patients reported improved symptoms and recovered 90% of their normal grip strength.

Arterial Fascial Flaps
Reverse Radial Artery Fascial Flap

Before a reverse radial artery fascial flap is considered, the Allen test should be

performed to ensure patency and dominance of the ulnar artery. A reverse radial artery fascial flap procedure is performed via a standard open CTR incision that is extended proximally to the proximal third of the forearm, anticipating that a point 4 cm proximal to the radial styloid will be the pivot point. Ideally, a reverse radial artery fascial flap should be at least 5 × 4 cm. Dissection is performed until just superficial to the antebrachial fascia, which is incised at the periphery and elevated superficially to the epimysium of the forearm muscles to ensure vascular continuity with the radial vessels. The radial artery and its venae comitantes are then divided proximally to adequately mobilize the fascial flap. The reverse radial artery fascial flap is turned distally deep to the flexor carpi radialis and wrapped loosely around the median nerve, after which it is sutured in place.[90]

Posterior Interosseous Artery Fascial Flap

A posterior interosseous artery fascial flap requires intact retrograde flow via a communicating artery between the anterior and posterior interosseous arteries proximal to the distal radioulnar joint. This communicating artery may be absent in as many as 5% of patients.[91] A posterior interosseous artery fascial flap procedure is performed with the use of a pivot point that is 2 cm proximal to the distal radioulnar joint along an axis between the lateral epicondyle and the distal radioulnar joint. Ideally, the middle perforator of the posterior interosseous artery should be included in a posterior interosseous artery fascial flap. The pedicle is explored by identifying the vessels on the interosseous membrane in the base of the septum between the fifth and sixth dorsal extensor compartments. If a communicating

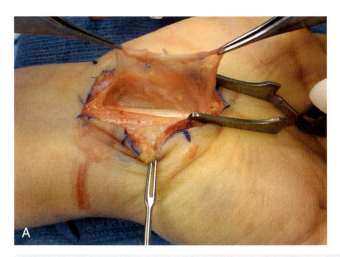
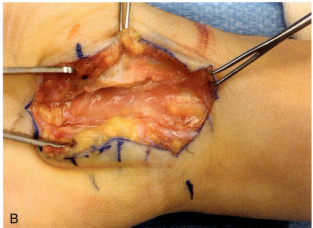

Figure 2   Intraoperative photographs of a wrist show a synovial flap procedure. **A,** Elevation of the tenosynovial flap, with the use of the ulnar aspect as the vascularized pedicle. **B,** Placement of the vascularized tenosynovial flap over the median nerve. (Courtesy of The Philadelphia Hand Center, Philadelphia, PA.)

artery is present, the pedicle is dissected in a distal-to-proximal direction, leaving a cuff of tissue to serve the venae comitantes. The ulnar edge of the fascia followed by the radial edge of the fascia are dissected, and the posterior interosseous artery fascial flap is elevated in a subfascial plane. The muscular arterial branches are ligated or cauterized until the septum is solely attached by the posterior interosseous artery. The posterior interosseous artery fascial flap is rotated over the carpal tunnel and sutured in place. Limited outcome data on posterior interosseous artery fascial flap procedures are available; however, preliminary data with regard to the alleviation of pain appear promising.[92]

Synovial Flaps

Synovial flaps also can be used for neovascularization. After median nerve neurolysis is performed, the tenosynovium deep to the median nerve is elevated in an ulnar direction (**Figure 2, A**). The synovial flap is placed superficial to the median nerve, and the radial aspect of the synovial flap is sutured to the wound bed (**Figure 2,**

B). Extensive dissection is not necessary for synovial flap procedures, which can be performed via the same incision that was used for median nerve neurolysis.[93,94] In a study of 45 patients with recalcitrant CTS who underwent revision CTR with the use of a tenosynovial flap, Murthy et al[93] reported that 96% of the patients had complete pain resolution postoperatively, and 80% of the patients had moderate to complete resolution of numbness and tingling postoperatively.

Interposition

Vein Wrapping

Autologous vein wrapping is performed via a standard open approach to the carpal tunnel. The median nerve is freed and débrided from the surrounding scar tissue. Typically, the great saphenous vein from the ipsilateral or contralateral leg is harvested. Alternatively, a superficial vein from a forearm can be used. If a vein from a leg is used, a longitudinal incision 1 cm anterior to the medial malleolus is made to identify the vein. A vein stripper is then used to harvest 25 to 30 cm of the vein. The vein is

subsequently incised in a longitudinal fashion, and the intimal portion of the vein is placed against the median nerve and sutured to the surrounding wound bed with the use of 7-0 or 8-0 nylon. The vein is then wrapped circumferentially around the median nerve, ensuring that no nerve constriction exists. After each circumferential wrap, the vein is loosely stabilized to the adjacent wrap with the use of 7-0 or 8-0 nylon until the proximal nerve bed is reached (**Figure 3**).

Sotereanos et al[95] first described the use of vein wrapping in a small case study of three patients who had recurrent CTS. All three patients demonstrated significant improvement on postoperative EMG, and two of the three patients had significant improvement in subjective and objective assessments. In a study of 15 patients with recurrent CTS who underwent vein wrapping, Varitimidis et al[96] reported that all of the patients had pain alleviation as well as improved nerve conduction velocity studies and two-point discrimination at a mean follow-up of 43 months.

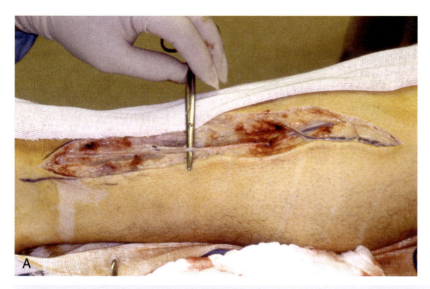
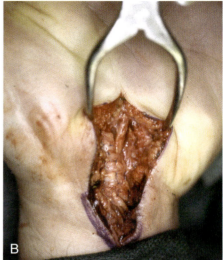

Figure 3 Intraoperative photographs show vein wrapping. **A,** A superficial vein is identified in a forearm. **B,** The superficial vein has been split longitudinally, and the intimal portion of the vein has been placed against the median nerve in a wrist. Subsequently, the superficial vein was wrapped around the median nerve multiple times.

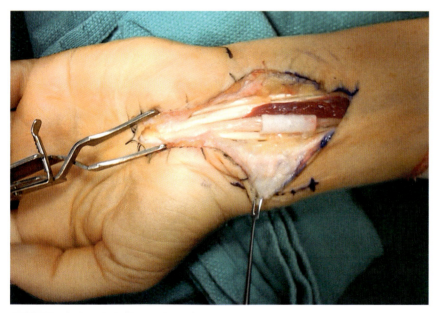

Figure 4 Intraoperative photograph of a wrist shows the placement of a synthetic device around the median nerve. (Courtesy of Joshua M. Abzug, MD, Baltimore, MD.)

Synthetic Devices

Synthetic devices, which were designed to prevent scar formation, have largely replaced vein wrapping. Synthetic tubes or wraps are made of a semipermeable collagen that is metabolically absorbed with time. The semipermeable membrane prevents fibroblast formation, which decreases the potential for perineural fibrosis.[97] The placement of a synthetic device around the median nerve, which is a technically straightforward procedure, is performed after median nerve neurolysis (**Figure 4**). In a retrospective study of 15 patients with recurrent or progressive cubital tunnel syndrome or CTS who underwent revision surgical decompression with the use of a collagen matrix wrap, Soltani et al[98] reported that 89% of the patients with CTS had subjective symptom resolution, with mean visual analog pain scale scores decreasing from 2.47 preoperatively to 0.47 postoperatively.

Summary

CTS is a focal compression of the median nerve as it passes through the carpal tunnel deep to the TCL. CTS most commonly affects females and individuals who have occupations that include activities of repetition, exertion of force, and/or vibration. Typically, patients with CTS have pain, paresthesia, and numbness in the radial three and one-half digits, with nighttime symptoms occurring earlier in the disease process and daytime symptoms becoming more frequent as CTS progresses.

A thorough history with regard to a patient's work and sport activity should be obtained. Provocative tests, including the Tinel sign, the Phalen test, and the Durkan test, are diagnostic for CTS if a patient's symptoms are reproduced. An EDS may be performed to confirm a diagnosis of CTS or to obtain a baseline before surgical treatment. Nonsurgical management, including lifestyle modifications, nighttime wrist splinting, and corticosteroid injections, should be attempted. CTR should be performed if CTS symptoms persist.

Recalcitrant or recurrent CTS can occur as a result of incomplete TCL release and/or perineural fibrosis. If the TCL was incompletely released, revision CTR should be performed, which will yield favorable outcomes. Scar formation can be prevented during revision CTR by either interposing a mechanical barrier or providing potential neovascularization to the median nerve.

References

1. Paget J: *Lectures on Surgical Pathology.* Philadelphia, PA, Lindsay and Blakiston, 1854.

2. Moersch FP: Median thenar neuritis. *Proc Staff Meet Mayo Clin* 1938;13:220 222.

3. Phalen GS: Spontaneous compression of the median nerve at the wrist. *J Am Med Assoc* 1951;145(15):1128-1133.

4. Gelfman R, Melton LJ III, Yawn BP, Wollan PC, Amadio PC, Stevens JC: Long-term trends in carpal tunnel syndrome. *Neurology* 2009;72(1):33-41.

5. English JH, Gwynne-Jones DP: Incidence of carpal tunnel syndrome requiring surgical decompression: A 10.5-year review of 2,309 patients. *J Hand Surg Am* 2015;40(12):2427-2434.

6. Fajardo M, Kim SH, Szabo RM: Incidence of carpal tunnel release: Trends and implications within the United States ambulatory care setting. *J Hand Surg Am* 2012;37(8):1599-1605.

7. Chen LH, Li CY, Kuo LC, et al: Risk of hand syndromes in patients with diabetes mellitus: A population-based cohort study in taiwan. *Medicine (Baltimore)* 2015;94(41):e1575.

8. Oktayoglu P, Nas K, Kilinç F, Tasdemir N, Bozkurt M, Yildiz I: Assessment of the presence of carpal tunnel syndrome in patients with diabetes mellitus, hypothyroidism and acromegaly. *J Clin Diagn Res* 2015;9(6):OC14-OC18.

9. Shiri R, Pourmemari MH, Falah-Hassani K, Viikari-Juntura E: The effect of excess body mass on the risk of carpal tunnel syndrome: A meta-analysis of 58 studies. *Obes Rev* 2015;16(12):1094-1104.

10. Solomon DH, Katz JN, Bohn R, Mogun H, Avorn J: Nonoccupational risk factors for carpal tunnel syndrome. *J Gen Intern Med* 1999;14(5):310-314.

11. Tseng CH, Liao CC, Kuo CM, Sung FC, Hsieh DP, Tsai CH: Medical and non-medical correlates of carpal tunnel syndrome in a Taiwan cohort of one million. *Eur J Neurol* 2012;19(1):91-97.

12. Kozak A, Schedlbauer G, Wirth T, Euler U, Westermann C, Nienhaus A: Association between work-related biomechanical risk factors and the occurrence of carpal tunnel syndrome: An overview of systematic reviews and a meta-analysis of current research. *BMC Musculoskelet Disord* 2015;16:231.

13. Burger MC, De Wet H, Collins M: The BGN and ACAN genes and carpal tunnel syndrome. *Gene* 2014;551(2):160-166.

14. Burger M, de Wet H, Collins M: The COL5A1 gene is associated with increased risk of carpal tunnel syndrome. *Clin Rheumatol* 2015;34(4):767-774.

15. Fernández-de-las-Peñas C, Fernández-Muñoz JJ, Palacios-Ceña M, Navarro-Pardo E, Ambite-Quesada S, Salom-Moreno J: Direct and indirect effects of function in associated variables such as depression and severity on pain intensity in women with carpal tunnel syndrome. *Pain Med* 2015;16(12):2405-2411.

16. Palmer DH, Hanrahan LP: Social and economic costs of carpal tunnel surgery. *Instr Course Lect* 1995;44:167-172.

17. Cranford CS, Ho JY, Kalainov DM, Hartigan BJ: Carpal tunnel syndrome. *J Am Acad Orthop Surg* 2007;15(9):537-548.

18. Henry BM, Zwinczewska H, Roy J, et al: The prevalence of anatomical variations of the median nerve in the carpal tunnel: A systematic review and meta-analysis. *PLoS One* 2015;10(8):e0136477.

19. Poisel S: Ursprung und verlauf des R. muscularis des nervus digitalis palmaris communis I (N. medianus). *Chir Prax* 1974;18:471-474.

20. Lanz U: Anatomical variations of the median nerve in the carpal tunnel. *J Hand Surg Am* 1977;2(1):44-53.

21. Gelberman RH, Hergenroeder PT, Hargens AR, Lundborg GN, Akeson WH: The carpal tunnel syndrome: A study of carpal canal pressures. *J Bone Joint Surg Am* 1981;63(3):380-383.

22. Tang DT, Barbour JR, Davidge KM, Yee A, Mackinnon SE: Nerve entrapment: Update. *Plast Reconstr Surg* 2015;135(1):199e-215e.

23. Rydevik B, Lundborg G, Bagge U: Effects of graded compression on intraneural blood blow: An in vivo study on rabbit tibial nerve. *J Hand Surg Am* 1981;6(1):3-12.

24. Duckworth AD, Jenkins PJ, Roddam P, Watts AC, Ring D, McEachan JE: Pain and carpal tunnel syndrome. *J Hand Surg Am* 2013;38(8):1540-1546.

25. Alfonso C, Jann S, Massa R, Torreggiani A: Diagnosis, treatment and follow-up of the carpal tunnel syndrome: A review. *Neurol Sci* 2010;31(3):243-252.

26. Katz JN, Stirrat CR: A self-administered hand diagram for the diagnosis of carpal tunnel syndrome. *J Hand Surg Am* 1990;15(2):360-363.

27. Cobb TK, Sterbank PT, Lemke JH: Endoscopic cubital tunnel recurrence rates. *Hand (N Y)* 2010;5(2):179-183.

28. Seradge H, Owen W: Cubital tunnel release with medial epicondylectomy factors influencing the outcome. *J Hand Surg Am* 1998;23(3):483-491.

29. Durkan JA: A new diagnostic test for carpal tunnel syndrome. *J Bone Joint Surg Am* 1991;73(4):535-538.

30. Grundberg AB: Carpal tunnel decompression in spite of normal electromyography. *J Hand Surg Am* 1983;8(3):348-349.

31. Taylor-Gjevre RM, Gjevre JA, Nair B: Suspected carpal tunnel syndrome: Do nerve conduction study results and symptoms match? *Can Fam Physician* 2010;56(7):e250-e254.

32. Kane PM, Daniels AH, Akelman E: Double crush syndrome. *J Am Acad Orthop Surg* 2015;23(9):558-562.

33. Upton AR, McComas AJ: The double crush in nerve entrapment syndromes. *Lancet* 1973;2(7825):359-362.

34. Osterman AL: The double crush syndrome. *Orthop Clin North Am* 1988;19(1):147-155.

35. Ziswiler HR, Reichenbach S, Vögelin E, Bachmann LM, Villiger PM, Jüni P: Diagnostic value of sonography in patients with suspected carpal tunnel syndrome: A prospective study. *Arthritis Rheum* 2005;52(1):304-311.

36. Fowler JR, Hirsch D, Kruse K: The reliability of ultrasound measurements of the median nerve at the carpal tunnel inlet. *J Hand Surg Am* 2015;40(10):1992-1995.

37. Junck AD, Escobedo EM, Lipa BM, et al: Reliability assessment of various sonographic techniques for evaluating carpal tunnel syndrome. *J Ultrasound Med* 2015;34(11):2077-2088.

38. Bordalo-Rodrigues M, Amin P, Rosenberg ZS: MR imaging of common entrapment neuropathies at the wrist. *Magn Reson Imaging Clin N Am* 2004;12(2):265-279, vi.

39. Burton CL, Chesterton LS, Chen Y, van der Windt DA: Clinical course and prognostic factors in conservatively managed carpal tunnel syndrome: A systematic review. *Arch Phys Med Rehabil* 2016;97(5):836-852.e1.

40. Levine DW, Simmons BP, Koris MJ, et al: A self-administered questionnaire for the assessment of severity of symptoms and functional status in carpal tunnel syndrome. *J Bone Joint Surg Am* 1993;75(11):1585-1592.

41. Burke DT, Burke MM, Stewart GW, Cambré A: Splinting for carpal tunnel syndrome: In search of the optimal angle. *Arch Phys Med Rehabil* 1994;75(11):1241-1244.

42. Weiss ND, Gordon L, Bloom T, So Y, Rempel DM: Position of the wrist associated with the lowest carpal-tunnel pressure: Implications for splint design. *J Bone Joint Surg Am* 1995;77(11):1695-1699.

43. Celiker R, Arslan S, Inanici F: Corticosteroid injection vs. nonsteroidal antiinflammatory drug and splinting in carpal tunnel syndrome. *Am J Phys Med Rehabil* 2002;81(3):182-186.

44. Chang MH, Chiang HT, Lee SS, Ger LP, Lo YK: Oral drug of choice in carpal tunnel syndrome. *Neurology* 1998;51(2):390-393.

45. Padua L, Padua R, Aprile I, Pasqualetti P, Tonali P; Italian CTS Study Group: Multiperspective follow-up of untreated carpal tunnel syndrome: A multicenter study. *Neurology* 2001;56(11):1459-1466.

46. Aufiero E, Stitik TP, Foye PM, Chen B: Pyridoxine hydrochloride treatment of carpal tunnel syndrome: A review. *Nutr Rev* 2004;62(3):96-104.

47. Gerritsen AA, de Krom MC, Struijs MA, Scholten RJ, de Vet HC, Bouter LM: Conservative treatment options for carpal tunnel syndrome: A systematic review of randomised controlled trials. *J Neurol* 2002;249(3):272-280.

48. O'Connor D, Marshall S, Massy-Westropp N: Non-surgical treatment (other than steroid injection) for carpal tunnel syndrome. *Cochrane Database Syst Rev* 2003;1:CD003219.

49. Blazar PE, Floyd WE IV, Han CH, Rozental TD, Earp BE: Prognostic indicators for recurrent symptoms after a single corticosteroid injection for carpal tunnel syndrome. *J Bone Joint Surg Am* 2015;97(19):1563-1570.

50. Edgell SE, McCabe SJ, Breidenbach WC, LaJoie AS, Abell TD: Predicting the outcome of carpal tunnel release. *J Hand Surg Am* 2003;28(2):255-261.

51. Bahrami MH, Shahraeeni S, Raeissadat SA: Comparison between the effects of progesterone versus corticosteroid local injections in mild and moderate carpal tunnel syndrome: A randomized clinical trial. *BMC Musculoskelet Disord* 2015;16:322.

52. Stepan JG, London DA, Boyer MI, Calfee RP: Blood glucose levels in diabetic patients following corticosteroid injections into the hand and wrist. *J Hand Surg Am* 2014;39(4):706-712.

53. Ebenbichler GR, Resch KL, Nicolakis P, et al: Ultrasound treatment for treating the carpal tunnel syndrome: Randomised "sham" controlled trial. *BMJ* 1998;316(7133):731-735.

54. Koren G, Pastuszak A, Ito S: Drugs in pregnancy. *N Engl J Med* 1998;338(16):1128-1137.

55. Banta CA: A prospective, nonrandomized study of iontophoresis, wrist splinting, and antiinflammatory medication in the treatment of early-mild carpal tunnel syndrome. *J Occup Med* 1994;36(2):166-168.

56. Irvine J, Chong SL, Amirjani N, Chan KM: Double-blind randomized controlled trial of low-level laser therapy in carpal tunnel syndrome. *Muscle Nerve* 2004;30(2):182-187.

57. Akalin E, El O, Peker O, et al: Treatment of carpal tunnel syndrome with nerve and tendon gliding exercises. *Am J Phys Med Rehabil* 2002;81(2):108-113.

58. Rozmaryn LM, Dovelle S, Rothman ER, Gorman K, Olvey KM, Bartko JJ: Nerve and tendon gliding exercises and the conservative management of carpal tunnel syndrome. *J Hand Ther* 1998;11(3):171-179.

59. Agee JM, McCarroll HR Jr, Tortosa RD, Berry DA, Szabo RM, Peimer CA: Endoscopic release of the carpal tunnel: A randomized prospective multicenter study. *J Hand Surg Am* 1992;17(6):987-995.

60. Vanni D, Sirabella FS, Galzio R, Salini V, Magliani V: The double tunnels technique: An alternative minimally invasive approach for carpal tunnel syndrome. *J Neurosurg* 2015;123(5):1230-1237.

61. Louie DL, Earp BE, Collins JE, et al: Outcomes of open carpal tunnel release at a minimum of ten years. *J Bone Joint Surg Am* 2013;95(12):1067-1073.

62. Faour-Martín O, Martín-Ferrero MA, Almaraz-Gómez A, Vega-Castrillo A: The long-term post-operative electromyographic evaluation of patients who have undergone carpal tunnel decompression. *J Bone Joint Surg Br* 2012;94(7):941-945.

63. Thomsen NO, Cederlund RI, Andersson GS, Rosén I, Björk J, Dahlin LB: Carpal tunnel release in patients with diabetes: A 5-year follow-up with matched controls. *J Hand Surg Am* 2014;39(4):713-720.

64. Roh YH, Lee BK, Noh JH, Oh JH, Gong HS, Baek GH: Effects of metabolic syndrome on the outcome of carpal tunnel release: A matched case-control study. *J Hand Surg Am* 2015;40(7):1303-1309.

65. Cagle PJ Jr, Reams M, Agel J, Bohn D: An outcomes protocol for carpal tunnel release: A comparison of outcomes in patients with and without medical comorbidities. *J Hand Surg Am* 2014;39(11):2175-2180.

66. Cha SM, Shin HD, Ahn JS, Beom JW, Kim DY: Differences in the postoperative outcomes according to the primary treatment options chosen by patients with carpal tunnel syndrome: Conservative versus operative treatment. *Ann Plast Surg* 2016;77(1):80-84.

67. Atroshi I, Larsson GU, Ornstein E, Hofer M, Johnsson R, Ranstam J: Outcomes of endoscopic surgery compared with open surgery for carpal tunnel syndrome among employed patients: Randomised controlled trial. *BMJ* 2006;332(7556):1473.

68. Atroshi I, Hofer M, Larsson GU, Ornstein E, Johnsson R, Ranstam J: Open compared with 2-portal endoscopic carpal tunnel release: A 5-year follow-up of a randomized controlled trial. *J Hand Surg Am* 2009;34(2):266-272.

69. Atroshi I, Hofer M, Larsson GU, Ranstam J: Extended follow-up of a randomized clinical trial of open vs endoscopic release surgery for carpal tunnel syndrome. *JAMA* 2015;314(13):1399-1401.

70. Vasiliadis HS, Georgoulas P, Shrier I, Salanti G, Scholten RJ: Endoscopic release for carpal tunnel

syndrome. *Cochrane Database Syst Rev* 2014;1:CD008265.

71. Cho YJ, Lee JH, Shin DJ, Park KH: Comparison of short wrist transverse open and limited open techniques for carpal tunnel release: A randomized controlled trial of two incisions. *J Hand Surg Eur Vol* 2016;41(2):143-147.

72. Murthy PG, Goljan P, Mendez G, Jacoby SM, Shin EK, Osterman AL: Mini-open versus extended open release for severe carpal tunnel syndrome. *Hand (N Y)* 2015;10(1):34-39.

73. Vasiliadis HS, Nikolakopoulou A, Shrier O, et al: Endoscopic and open release similarly safe for the treatment of carpal tunnel syndrome: A systematic review and meta-analysis. *PLoS One* 2015;10(12):e0143683.

74. Osei DA, Calfee RP, Stepan JG, Boyer MI, Goldfarb CA, Gelberman RH: Simultaneous bilateral or unilateral carpal tunnel release? A prospective cohort study of early outcomes and limitations. *J Bone Joint Surg Am* 2014;96(11):889-896.

75. Bloem JJ, Pradjarahardja MC, Vuursteen PJ: The post-carpal tunnel syndrome: Causes and prevention. *Neth J Surg* 1986;38(2):52-55.

76. Cseuz KA, Thomas JE, Lambert EH, Love JG, Lipscomb PR: Long-term results of operation for carpal tunnel syndrome. *Mayo Clin Proc* 1966;41(4):232-241.

77. Tung TH, Mackinnon SE: Secondary carpal tunnel surgery. *Plast Reconstr Surg* 2001;107(7):1830-1843, quiz 1844, 1933.

78. Langloh ND, Linscheid RL: Recurrent and unrelieved carpal-tunnel syndrome. *Clin Orthop Relat Res* 1972;83:41-47.

79. Zieske L, Ebersole GC, Davidge K, Fox I, Mackinnon SE: Revision carpal tunnel surgery: A 10-year review of intraoperative findings and outcomes. *J Hand Surg Am* 2013;38(8):1530-1539.

80. Cobb TK, Amadio PC, Leatherwood DF, Schleck CD, Ilstrup DM: Outcome of reoperation for carpal tunnel syndrome. *J Hand Surg Am* 1996;21(3):347-356.

81. Abzug JM, Jacoby SM, Osterman AL: Surgical options for recalcitrant carpal

tunnel syndrome with perineural fibrosis. *Hand (N Y)* 2012;7(1):23-29.

82. Karabay N, Toros T, Çetinkol E, Ada S: Correlations between ultrasonography findings and surgical findings in patients with refractory symptoms after primary surgical release for carpal tunnel syndrome. *Acta Orthop Traumatol Turc* 2015;49(2):126-132.

83. Jones NF, Ahn HC, Eo S: Revision surgery for persistent and recurrent carpal tunnel syndrome and for failed carpal tunnel release. *Plast Reconstr Surg* 2012;129(3):683-692.

84. Stütz N, Gohritz A, van Schoonhoven J, Lanz U: Revision surgery after carpal tunnel release—analysis of the pathology in 200 cases during a 2 year period. *J Hand Surg Br* 2006;31(1):68-71.

85. Strickland JW, Idler RS, Lourie GM, Plancher KD: The hypothenar fat pad flap for management of recalcitrant carpal tunnel syndrome. *J Hand Surg Am* 1996;21(5):840-848.

86. Djerbi I, César M, Lenoir H, Coulet B, Lazerges C, Chammas M: Revision surgery for recurrent and persistent carpal tunnel syndrome: Clinical results and factors affecting outcomes. *Chir Main* 2015;34(6):312-317.

87. Beck JD, Wingert NC, Rutter MR, Irgit KS, Tang X, Klena JC: Clinical outcomes of endoscopic carpal tunnel release in patients 65 and over. *J Hand Surg Am* 2013;38(8):1524-1529.

88. Wichelhaus A, Mittlmeier T, Gierer P, Beck M: Vascularized hypothenar fat pad flap in revision surgery for carpal tunnel syndrome. *J Neurol Surg A Cent Eur Neurosurg* 2015;76(6):438-442.

89. Fusetti C, Garavaglia G, Mathoulin C, Petri JG, Lucchina S: A reliable and simple solution for recalcitrant carpal tunnel syndrome: The hypothenar fat pad flap. *Am J Orthop (Belle Mead NJ)* 2009;38(4):181-186.

90. Tham SK, Ireland DC, Riccio M, Morrison WA: Reverse radial artery fascial flap: A treatment for the chronically scarred median nerve in recurrent carpal tunnel syndrome. *J Hand Surg Am* 1996;21(5):849-854.

91. Page R, Chang J: Reconstruction of hand soft-tissue defects:

Alternatives to the radial forearm fasciocutaneous flap. *J Hand Surg Am* 2006;31(5):847-856.

92. Vögelin E, Bignion D, Constantinescu M, Büchler U: Revision surgery after carpal tunnel release using a posterior interosseous artery island flap. *Handchir Mikrochir Plast Chir* 2008;40(2):122-127.

93. Murthy PG, Abzug JM, Jacoby SM, Culp RW: The tenosynovial flap for recalcitrant carpal tunnel syndrome. *Tech Hand Up Extrem Surg* 2013;17(2):84-86.

94. Wulle C: The synovial flap as treatment of the recurrent carpal tunnel syndrome. *Hand Clin* 1996;12(2):379-388.

95. Sotereanos DG, Giannakopoulos PN, Mitsionis GI, Xu J, Herndon JH: Vein-graft wrapping for the treatment of recurrent compression of the median nerve. *Microsurgery* 1995;16(11):752-756.

96. Varitimidis SE, Riano F, Vardakas DG, Sotereanos DG: Recurrent compressive neuropathy of the median nerve at the wrist: Treatment with autogenous saphenous vein wrapping. *J Hand Surg Br* 2000;25(3):271-275.

97. Archibald SJ, Krarup C, Shefner J, Li ST, Madison RD: A collagen-based nerve guide conduit for peripheral nerve repair: An electrophysiological study of nerve regeneration in rodents and nonhuman primates. *J Comp Neurol* 1991;306(4):685-696.

98. Soltani AM, Allan BJ, Best MJ, Mir HS, Panthaki ZJ: Revision decompression and collagen nerve wrap for recurrent and persistent compression neuropathies of the upper extremity. *Ann Plast Surg* 2014;72(5):572-578.

Ulnar Tunnel Syndrome, Radial Tunnel Syndrome, Anterior Interosseous Nerve Syndrome, and Pronator Syndrome

Adam B. Strohl, MD

David S. Zelouf, MD

Abstract

In addition to the more common carpal tunnel and cubital tunnel syndromes, orthopaedic surgeons must recognize and manage other potential sites of peripheral nerve compression. The distal ulnar nerve may become compressed as it travels through the wrist, which is known as ulnar tunnel or Guyon canal syndrome. The posterior interosseous nerve may become entrapped in the proximal forearm as it travels through the radial tunnel, which results in a pain syndrome without motor weakness. The median nerve may become entrapped in the proximal forearm, which can result in a variety of symptoms. Spontaneous neuropathy of the anterior interosseous nerve branch of the median nerve can be observed without external compression. Electrodiagnostic and imaging studies may aid surgeons in the diagnosis of these syndromes; however, a thorough physical examination is paramount to localize compressed segments of these nerves. An understanding of the anatomy of each of these nerve areas allows surgeons to appreciate a patient's clinical findings and helps guide surgical decompression.

Instr Course Lect 2017;66:153–162.

Peripheral nerves may become compressed at multiple anatomic locations in the upper extremity, which can lead to dysfunction such as motor weakness, sensory disturbance, and/or pain.

Median nerve compression at the wrist, which is known as carpal tunnel syndrome, followed by ulnar nerve compression at the elbow, which is known as cubital tunnel syndrome, are the most common compression neuropathies. In addition to carpal tunnel and cubital tunnel syndromes, orthopaedic surgeons must be familiar with less common compression neuropathies that may be encountered in the evaluation of patients with peripheral nerve entrapment. Surgeons should understand the patient complaints of, clinical findings of, and treatment options for compression and intraneural pathology of the ulnar, radial, and median nerves. An understanding of anatomy and nerve topography not only aids in the accurate diagnosis of peripheral nerve compression but also guides appropriate and effective management.

Ulnar Tunnel Syndrome

Although the ulnar nerve is most commonly compressed in the cubital tunnel region at the elbow, compression of the ulnar nerve also can occur distally at the wrist, which is known as ulnar tunnel syndrome. Similar to compression of the ulnar nerve in the cubital tunnel,

Dr. Zelouf or an immediate family member serves as a board member, owner, officer, or committee member of the Eastern Orthopaedic Association. Neither Dr. Strohl nor any immediate family member has received anything of value from or has stock or stock options held in a commercial company or institution related directly or indirectly to the subject of this chapter.

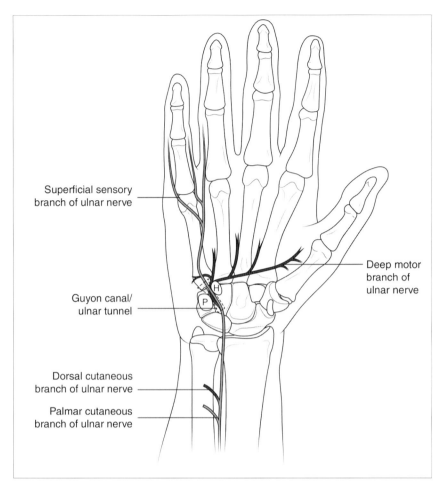

Figure 1 Illustration shows the anatomy of the ulnar tunnel at the wrist. H = hamate, P = pisiform. (Reproduced from Earp BE, Floyd WE, Louie D, Koris M, Protomastro P: Ulnar nerve entrapment at the wrist. *J Am Acad Orthop Surg* 2014;22[11]:699-706.)

distal compression of the ulnar nerve may lead to sensory and motor deficits in the hand and digits. Likewise, sensory paresthesias may affect the little finger and the ulnar half of the ring finger. Based on anatomic considerations, important clinical features of ulnar tunnel syndrome distinguish it from cubital tunnel syndrome. Because the palmar cutaneous and dorsal cutaneous branches of the ulnar nerve branch off the ulnar nerve before it enters the ulnar tunnel at the wrist, the ulnar palm and dorsum of the hand are spared.

In patients with advanced cubital tunnel syndrome at the elbow, intrinsic muscle atrophy and weakness can occur, which may lead to hand weakness, clumsiness, and/or dysfunction. However, in patients with only distal compression of the ulnar nerve, strength is preserved in the flexor carpi ulnaris and the flexor digitorum profundus (FDP) muscles of the ring and little fingers. Late clinical findings of ulnar claw deformity, which is referred to as ulnar paradox, are often more pronounced in patients with distal compression of the ulnar nerve. The preservation of proximally innervated FDP muscles allows for more flexion of the interphalangeal joints, which creates a more prominent

claw deformity. Ulnar nerve compression at the wrist can occur in isolation or in conjunction with compression of the ulnar nerve at more proximal locations. Furthermore, the physical examination findings of proximal ulnar nerve compression may mask concurrent pathology at the wrist.

Anatomy

In 1861, Jean Casimir Félix Guyon first described the course and division of the ulnar nerve through the hypothenar region. This space, which is the location at which Guyon first suggested potential pathologic constriction of the ulnar nerve, is currently referred to as the Guyon canal or the ulnar tunnel. Gross and Gelberman1 further described the unique space of the distal ulnar tunnel, which they divided into three zones based on the internal topography of the ulnar nerve as it courses through the ulnar tunnel. Characterization of the zones of the ulnar tunnel based on the presence of motor and sensory components within the ulnar nerve allows surgeons to localize the site of compression within the ulnar tunnel based on a patient's symptomatology and clinical findings. The distal ulnar tunnel is 4 to 4.5 cm long and begins at the proximal edge of the volar carpal ligament (**Figure 1**). The distal ulnar tunnel extends to the fibrous arch of the hypothenar muscles. The borders of the distal ulnar tunnel are not constant as the ulnar nerve courses between ulnar-sided wrist structures, most notably the pisiform and the hamate. In addition, the ulnar artery accompanies the ulnar nerve through the ulnar tunnel.

Zone 1 of the ulnar tunnel is slightly more than 3 cm in length and encompasses the portion of the ulnar tunnel that is proximal to the bifurcation of the ulnar nerve into its motor and sensory branches. Therefore, compression of the ulnar nerve in zone 1 results in both paresthesia and intrinsic muscle deficit. The ulnar nerve is first compressed between the volar carpal ligament palmarly and the transverse carpal ligament dorsally. More distally in zone 1, the floor of the ulnar tunnel is composed of the pisohamate and pisometacarpal ligaments. Ganglion cysts followed by hook of hamate fractures, traumatic adhesions, and anomalous muscles are the most common causes of compression of the ulnar nerve in zone 1 of the ulnar tunnel.[1,2] Zone 1 of the ulnar tunnel is the most commonly affected zone of the ulnar tunnel.

After the ulnar nerve bifurcates, the deep motor branch of the ulnar nerve pursues a dorsal and radial course around the hamate as it dives deep to the fibrous arch of the hypothenar muscles. This area comprises zone 2 of the ulnar tunnel. Pathology that is present within zone 2 of the ulnar tunnel leads to deficits in motor function only, without sensory disturbances. Similar to zone 1, ganglion cysts are the most common pathologic cause of compression of the ulnar nerve in zone 2 of the ulnar tunnel. Other causes of compression of the ulnar nerve in zone 2 of the ulnar tunnel include fractures and a thickened pisohamate ligament.[1,2]

Zone 3 of the ulnar tunnel encompasses the superficial sensory branch of the ulnar nerve as it courses palmar to the fascia of the hypothenar muscles. Pathology that is present within zone 3 of the ulnar tunnel leads to sensory disturbances only. Interestingly, connections between the ulnar and median nerves are identified in zone 3 of the ulnar tunnel. Ulnar artery thrombosis and ulnar artery aneurysm are the

most common causes of compression of the ulnar nerve in zone 3 of the ulnar tunnel.[1,2]

Surgeons should understand that the palmar cutaneous branch of the ulnar nerve, which is referred to as the nerve of Henle, is present in only 58% of individuals.[3] Therefore, the contribution of the palmar cutaneous branch of the ulnar nerve to palmar innervation is variable, dissimilar to the dorsal cutaneous branch of the ulnar nerve, which consistently arises approximately 5.5 cm proximal to the ulnar head. As a result, sensory examination for ulnar nerve function is more reliable in the little and ulnar ring fingers as well as the dorsal ulnar hand.

Clinical and Diagnostic Findings

A physical examination, which should include the Tinel test and sensory threshold testing, that suggests distal ulnar nerve compression at the wrist can be further supported with the use of electrodiagnostic studies. Multiple clinical findings, including the presence of interossei wasting, particularly over the first dorsal interosseous muscle; the inability to cross fingers; and abducted positioning of the little finger, which is known as the Wartenberg sign, suggest motor branch involvement. Ulnar claw deformity, which also is known as the Duchenne sign, may be observed secondary to lumbrical paralysis of the little and ring fingers. Intact extensor tendons may place the unopposed metacarpophalangeal joint in hyperextension, and the long flexors may place the proximal interphalangeal joint and distal interphalangeal joint in a flexed position. Attempted pinch between the thumb and the index finger may lead to compensatory thumb interphalangeal

flexion (Froment sign) and, occasionally, hyperextension of the thumb metacarpophalangeal joint (Jeanne sign), which occur secondary to paralysis of the adductor pollicis muscle.

Tenderness over the hamate or pisiform may suggest a fracture. A positive ulnar Allen test and/or ulceration of the ulnar fingertips supports a vascular etiology. As already mentioned, surgeons must recognize that ulnar nerve entrapment can occur at multiple locations as part of a double crush phenomenon. In patients without a history of trauma to the affected hand, surgeons should maintain high suspicion for ganglia, which account for 90% of pathology that is present within zone 1 and zone 2 of the ulnar tunnel.[4] Moreover, patients who have professional duties that require the use of repetitive blunt force, such as jackhammering, and patients who participate in hobbies such as racquet sports should be examined for possible related factors.

Electrodiagnostic studies can be performed to help support a diagnosis of ulnar tunnel syndrome and to differentiate the clinical findings of ulnar tunnel syndrome from other diagnoses, such as cubital tunnel, thoracic outlet, and cervical radiculopathy syndromes. Surgeons should expect prolonged motor and/or sensory latencies across the wrist but normal values from more proximal structures. Therefore, palmar and dorsal cutaneous nerves should have normal latencies, and electrodiagnostic studies should not detect abnormality in proximally innervated muscles, such as the flexor carpi ulnaris and/or the FDP of the little finger, which would suggest cubital tunnel syndrome. Similar to all peripheral compression neuropathies, paraspinal muscle findings suggest cervical radiculopathy.

Standard radiographs, including a carpal tunnel view, may help identify fractures. Advanced imaging, such as MRI or CT, can be performed to further evaluate fractures or to assess space-occupying lesions within the ulnar tunnel as well as vascular lesions of the ulnar artery.

Treatment

Patients with mild ulnar tunnel syndrome may be treated nonsurgically with protective splinting and anti-inflammatory medications. In addition, activity modification may help alleviate symptoms and prevent the progression of neuropathy. Aspiration of ganglion cysts, which has been used to successfully manage ulnar tunnel syndrome, should be performed with caution given the proximity of the neurovascular structures.

Surgical treatment should be reserved for patients with more severe ulnar tunnel syndrome, particularly those who have space-occupying lesions and those in whom nonsurgical treatment fails. The goals of the surgical management of ulnar tunnel syndrome include the removal of compressive masses and complete decompression of the ulnar tunnel. All three zones of the ulnar tunnel should be addressed, focusing on compressive structures, such as the antebrachial fascia, the volar carpal ligament, and the hypothenar fibrous arch (overlying the deep motor branch). The ulnar artery should be inspected, and any vascular lesions should be resected, with or without vessel reconstruction.

Radial Tunnel Syndrome

Located distal to the elbow, the radial nerve is composed of the superficial sensory branch, which provides innervation to the dorsoradial hand, and the posterior interosseous nerve (PIN), which provides motor input to the supinator and extensors of the wrist and digits. The terminal PIN provides sensory innervation and proprioception to the wrist joint. These nerves are subject to compression at the proximal forearm by various structures; however, clinical presentation may vary. Dissimilar to patients with PIN syndrome, patients with radial tunnel syndrome (RTS) lack clinical findings of motor weakness of the PIN-innervated digital extensors.[5] Patients with RTS have no paresthesias in the dorsoradial hand but, instead, have characteristic pain at the area of entrapment, which, typically, is located at the lateral forearm distal to the lateral epicondyle. Occasionally, vague wrist pain also may be associated with RTS.[6]

The diagnosis of RTS, and even the existence of the phenomenon, has been a subject of controversy for many years. The differential diagnosis for RTS includes lateral epicondylosis, an extensor carpi radialis brevis (ECRB) tear, osteoarthritis and/or synovitis of the radiocapitellar joint, and posterior plica impingement. Dissimilar to carpal tunnel and cubital tunnel syndromes, the pathophysiology of RTS is less straightforward. Many surgeons believe that radial nerve compression in patients with RTS is not severe enough to cause radial sensory or motor dysfunction, but that, instead, radial nerve irritation is perceived as pain.[6]

Anatomy

Anatomically, the radial tunnel is approximately 5 cm long and begins as the radial nerve courses past the radiocapitellar joint. The roof of the radial tunnel is formed by the brachioradialis muscle. Medially, the radial tunnel is bounded by the biceps tendon and the brachialis (**Figure 2**). Laterally, the radial tunnel is bounded by the ECRB and extensor carpi radialis longus muscles as well as the brachioradialis muscle. Distally, the radial tunnel is classically believed to end at the fibrous arch of the proximal edge of supinator muscle, which is referred to as the arcade of Frohse. Although constrictive, fibrous bands may exist at the distal end of the supinator muscle, the supinator fascia is the most common cause of compression of the radial nerve. Other causes of compression of the radial nerve include prominent recurrent radial vessels, a thickened edge of the ECRB, and schwannoma-like swelling of the radial nerve.[7]

Clinical and Diagnostic Findings

On clinical examination, a patient with RTS will report proximal lateral forearm or elbow pain that often worsens with rotational movements of the forearm. Pressure that is applied over a patient's lateral forearm approximately 3 to 5 cm distal to the elbow, more specifically over the supinator muscle, with the wrist in full supination should reproduce substantial pain. Pronation of the wrist during this maneuver, which moves the radial nerve away from the thumb-directed pressure, should relieve the pain.[6] Loh et al[8] proposed a Rule-of-Nine test, in which the volar, proximal forearm is divided into nine squares, to aid in the diagnosis of RTS. The authors reported that RTS pain is confined to squares one and two, which overlay the course of the radial nerve at the most radial, proximal portions of the forearm.[8] Other provocative maneuvers that can be used to aid in the diagnosis of RTS include pain with resisted active extension of the wrist or the long finger. Slight weakness of the extensors is believed to occur secondary to pain rather than motor nerve dysfunction. Often, the provocative maneuvers that can be used to aid in the diagnosis of RTS are positive in patients with lateral epicondylosis, which is a closely associated differential diagnosis.

Electrodiagnostic studies lack specific findings for RTS and often are normal in patients with RTS. Patients with conductive slowing of the radial nerve likely have associated motor findings, thereby precluding a diagnosis of RTS. However, abnormal findings on electrodiagnostic studies may elucidate other causes of pain, such as cervical radiculopathy. Sequential, selective lidocaine injections can help localize the source of pain and rule out other diagnoses, such as lateral epicondylosis. In addition, the scratch collapse test has been reported to be a useful adjunct for the diagnosis of RTS.[9]

Treatment

Nonsurgical treatment should be the first-line treatment for patients with RTS. Nonsurgical treatment may include the use of NSAIDs, wrist splinting, activity modification, and supervised physical therapy. Physical therapy may include nerve-gliding exercises, ultrasonographic therapy, and heat/cold modalities, which also may be used to manage associated symptoms of lateral epicondylosis. The use of counterforce or tennis elbow braces should be avoided because they apply external pressure on the radial nerve. Steroid injections also may play a role in the nonsurgical management of RTS.[10,11]

Surgical treatment may be considered to decompress the radial nerve within the radial tunnel in patients in whom nonsurgical treatment fails

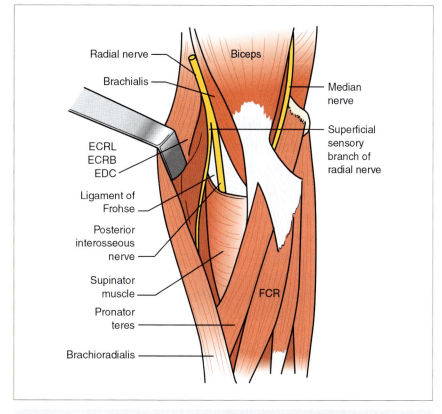

Figure 2   Illustration shows the course of the posterior interosseous nerve through the radial tunnel. ECRB = extensor carpi radialis brevis, ECRL = extensor carpi radialis longus, EDC = extensor digitorum communis, FCR = flexor carpi radialis.

to alleviate symptoms. The PIN can be accessed via multiple, different approaches, including the posterior and anterior approaches. Dorsal approaches include the following intervals: (1) between the ECRB and the extensor digitorum communis, which also is known as the dorsal (Henry) approach; (2) transmuscular via splitting of the brachioradialis; and (3) between the brachioradialis and the extensor carpi radialis longus. Regardless of the selected approach, the goal is complete decompression of the PIN within the radial tunnel. Areas of focus for decompression include the arcade of Froshe, the leading edge of the proximal ECRB, and the compressive fascia of the distal supinator. Occasionally, flattening or

congestion that is located proximal to the site of compression may appear as swelling or a pseudoneuroma.[10]

Reported outcomes of patients with RTS vary in the literature. Studies have suggested that patients with isolated RTS and no concurrent compressive neuropathy or tendinopathy have more favorable outcomes compared with patients with isolated RTS who have associated conditions. Lee et al[12] reported good outcomes in 86% of RTS-only patients compared with 43% of patients with concomitant lateral epicondylosis and 57% of patients with other compressive neuropathies. Other studies have reported that workers' compensation patients with RTS have poorer outcomes compared with non-workers' compensation patients with RTS.[10,13]

Anterior Interosseous Nerve Syndrome and Pronator Syndrome

Anterior interosseous nerve (AIN) syndrome and pronator syndrome are clinical entities of proximal median neuropathy in the forearm that have similar but uniquely different presentations and etiologies. Surgeons must have a thorough understanding of the anatomy of the median nerve to distinguish AIN syndrome from pronator syndrome.

Anatomy

Typically, no branches of the median nerve occur proximal to the elbow; however, a variable branch to the pronator teres may be observed in some patients (**Figure 3**). Distal to the elbow, the median nerve remains medial to the brachial artery and the biceps brachii tendon as well as anterior to the brachialis insertion. The median nerve provides motor innervation to the muscles of the superficial forearm compartment, which include the pronator teres, the palmaris longus, the flexor digitorum superficialis (FDS), and the flexor carpi radialis. The median nerve passes below the lacertus fibrosus, which is an ulnarly directed extension of the bicipital aponeurosis, to the antebrachial fascia, which also may have a deep component to the pronator teres fascia. The median nerve continues between the heads of the pronator teres before it dives deep to the fibrous arch of the FDS muscle origin. At this point, the AIN branches off, whereas the rest of the median nerve continues deep to the FDS muscle toward the carpal tunnel. The AIN provides motor innervation

to the flexor pollicis longus (FPL), the FDP of the index and long fingers, and the pronator quadratus. The AIN has no cutaneous sensory component, which is an important characteristic to keep in mind in the localization of median nerve dysfunction. The palmar cutaneous branch of the median nerve arises 6 to 7 cm proximal to the wrist crease on the ulnar side of the flexor carpi radialis and does not traverse through the carpal tunnel. The distal AIN is believed to provide capsular sensory innervation to the radiocarpal, intercarpal, carpometacarpal, and radioulnar joints.[14]

Pronator Syndrome Versus AIN Syndrome

First described by Seyffarth[15] in 1951, pronator syndrome originally referred to compression of the median nerve between the two heads of the pronator teres through which the median nerve passes in the proximal forearm. Other potential sites of median nerve entrapment include the lacertus fibrosus; the FDS aponeurotic arch; the aberrant radial artery; the variant muscles; and the ligament of Struthers, which is an anomalous extension from the supracondylar process of the humerus to the medial epicondyle. In addition to motor weakness, patients with pronator syndrome report paresthesias, most notably of the palm, secondary to involvement of the palmar cutaneous branch of the median nerve.

Because the AIN lacks cutaneous sensory fibers, patients with a true AIN palsy, similar to patients with pronator syndrome, will lack clinically relevant sensory deficits. Isolated palsy of the AIN often is spontaneous in nature and usually is self-limiting. Iatrogenic injury of the AIN can occur during surgical

procedures in the proximal forearm, and direct injury of the AIN can occur secondary to penetrating trauma. Rarely, entrapment of the AIN is attributed to an accessory FPL (ie, the Gantzer muscle). If not related to external forces, such as trauma or compression, the etiology and pathophysiology of a spontaneous AIN palsy, or AIN syndrome, is not entirely known; however, spontaneous AIN palsy is believed to be the result of an inflammatory neuritis. AIN syndrome often is associated with Parsonage-Turner syndrome, which is a brachial plexus neuritis that also is known as neuralgic amyotrophy. Triggers attributed to spontaneous AIN palsy include viral illness (25% to 55%), immunizations (15%), preoperative or peripartum periods (>14%), and strenuous exercise (8%).[16] A prodromal phase of flu-like symptoms may precede AIN syndrome, and patients with AIN syndrome may report vague forearm pain before weakness. Interestingly, Ochi et al[17] reported multiple patterns of fascicular constrictions (recessed, recessed-bulging, rotation, and rotation-bulging) of the median nerve in patients with spontaneous AIN palsy. Other studies also have recognized intraneural constrictions as a potential cause of median nerve dysfunction.[18]

Clinical and Diagnostic Findings

On physical examination, patients with proximal median neuropathy may have motor weakness in the muscles that correspond with the branches of the AIN and/or the median nerve distal to the area(s) of pathology. Manual motor testing should focus on the FPL (interphalangeal flexion of thumb), the FDP of the index and long fingers (distal interphalangeal flexion of the

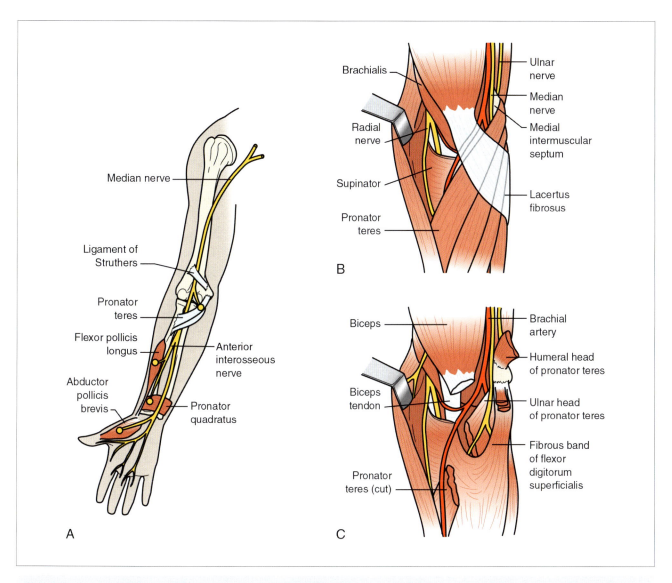

Figure 3   Illustrations show the course of the median nerve with potential compression points. **A,** Illustration shows the median-innervated muscles and potential sites of compression, which include the ligament of Struthers (if present) and the pronator teres. **B,** Illustration shows the median nerve passing beneath the lacertus fibrosus of the bicipital aponeurosis, which is another potential site of compression. **C,** Illustration shows the lacertus fibrosus and pronator teres divided and the median nerve passing deep to the fibrous arch of the flexor digitorum superficialis, which is another potential site of compression.

respective digits), and the pronator quadratus (wrist pronation with the elbow flexed). The pronator quadratus may be difficult to assess clinically in patients with a functioning pronator teres muscle. Patients with proximal median neuropathy will be unable to make the OK sign, which is known as the Kiloh-Nevin sign, whereby the tips of the thumb and the index finger

are brought together to form a circle shape.[16,19] The inability of a patient to grip a piece of paper with the tips of the index finger and the thumb is another indication of proximal median neuropathy. To compensate for this inability, patients with proximal median neuropathy will use a key pinch maneuver, relying on ulnar nerve-innervated function of thumb adduction against the index

finger. Variations in nerve innervation, in which an anastomosis between the ulnar and median nerves in the forearm may account for retained motor function despite AIN involvement, are very rare. Although similarly rare, intrinsic motor dysfunction may be observed in patients with AIN palsy if innervation is median nerve dominant. The FDP of the long finger also has been reported to be innervated by the ulnar nerve.[20] Other variations in nerve innervation include AIN innervation to the FDP muscles of all four fingers and AIN innervation to the FDS.[21]

As already mentioned, the presence of sensory deficits rules out an isolated AIN lesion but supports a diagnosis of pronator syndrome or similar entrapment of the median nerve proximal to the point at which the AIN branches off the median nerve. Palmar paresthesias may help surgeons distinguish carpal tunnel compression from compression at more proximal locations. In addition, patients with proximal median neuropathy commonly report vague pain in the proximal forearm. Provocative maneuvers that reproduce pain and/ or paresthesias may help surgeons localize common sites of median nerve compression. The lacertus fibrosus can be assessed via resisted elbow flexion with the forearm in a supinated position.[22] The pronator teres can be assessed via resisted forearm pronation. The FDS arch can be assessed via resisted finger flexion, particularly the proximal interphalangeal joint of the long finger. A positive Tinel sign and a positive scratch collapse test may be observed in patients with proximal median neuropathy.[23]

Surgeons must consider the differential diagnoses of proximal median neuropathy, such as Parsonage-Turner neuritis of the brachial plexus. Patients with partial lesions of the lateral cord may have clinical findings similar to those of patients with proximal median neuropathy. Mannerfelt syndrome, which refers to attritional rupture of the FPL secondary to a carpal osteophyte and is observed in patients with rheumatoid arthritis, may account for spontaneous loss of thumb interphalangeal flexion. Dissimilar to Mannerfelt syndrome, however, the tenodesis effect of the thumb interphalangeal joint is retained in patients with AIN palsy. Although uncommon, patients may have congenital absence of the FDP or the FPL, accounting for motor dysfunction without any median neuropathy.

In general, traditional imaging studies do not aid in the diagnosis of proximal median neuropathy, except in patients with space-occupying lesions or patients in whom the rare supracondylar process suggests the presence of the ligament of Struthers. If present, edema of AIN-innervated muscles or intraneural abnormalities of the AIN occasionally may be observed on MRI.[18,24] Electrodiagnostic studies may reveal sharp waves, fibrillations, and abnormal latencies in the affected muscles of patients with AIN syndrome. Similar findings and slowing of conduction across the elbow may be observed in patients with pronator syndrome; however, the electrodiagnostic study findings of patients with pronator syndrome may be normal or mimic those of patients with carpal tunnel syndrome.[22,25] Moreover, positive findings on electrodiagnostic studies/nerve conduction studies may suggest other sites of compression or disease, particularly in patients with brachial plexus involvement.

Management of Pronator Syndrome

Nonsurgical treatment is recommended as the initial treatment for patients with pronator syndrome. Nonsurgical treatment may include rest, activity modification, rotational immobilization, forearm flexor muscle stretching, nerve-gliding exercises, and the use of NSAIDs. Surgical treatment may be considered in patients in whom a 3- to 6-month trial of nonsurgical treatment fails to alleviate symptoms. The goal of surgical decompression is to relieve all potential sites of entrapment along the median nerve. In general, surgical decompression has been reported to be beneficial in patients with pronator syndrome.[16,22,26,27]

Management of AIN Syndrome

A more prolonged period of observation is warranted for patients in whom spontaneous AIN palsy of the neuritic variety is suspected. Patients in whom AIN syndrome is diagnosed early may be initially treated with high doses of corticosteroids and antiviral medications, such as acyclovir.[28] Spontaneous recovery of AIN function can occur; however, patients may require up to 1 year of observation. Despite lengthy expectant treatment, some patients may not recover AIN function. Earlier surgical treatment is acceptable in patients in whom a space-occupying lesion or local injury to the AIN is confirmed. Patients with AIN syndrome in whom no electrodiagnostic evidence of recovery is noted after 7 to 10 months of observation may be indicated for nerve exploration and neurolysis.[14]

Recent studies have reported improved outcomes in patients with AIN syndrome who undergo earlier surgical treatment that consists of epineurotomy and internal neurolysis based on the fascicular constriction theory, especially if more current MRI or ultrasonographic techniques suggest local swelling or constriction[17,18,24-26,29] (**Figure 4**). Wong and Dellon[30] reported that discrepancies in the treatment recommendations for patients with AIN syndrome exist in the literature. The authors reported that, prior to 1997, studies from the

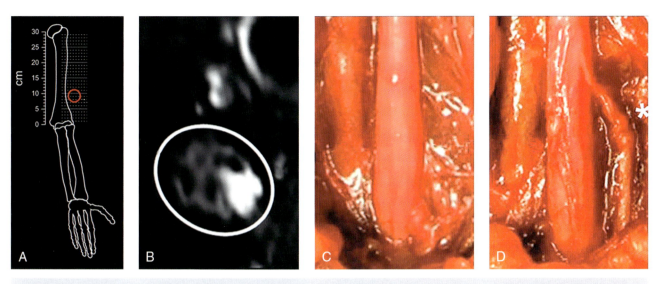

Figure 4   Images show targeted surgical epineurotomy of a lesion of the median nerve at the level of the upper arm. Illustration (**A**) and high-resolution T2-weighted MRI (**B**) demonstrate localization of the lesion 9.2 cm proximal to the humeroradial joint space (red circle in panel **A**). **C,** Intraoperative photograph taken before epineurotomy shows a subtle increase in nerve caliber. **D,** Intraoperative photograph taken after epineurotomy shows neurolysis and subsequent detorsion of the anterior interosseous nerve (asterisk), which was observed within the median nerve. (Reproduced with permission from Pham M, Bäumer P, Meinck HM, et al: Anterior interosseous nerve syndrome: Fascicular motor lesions of median nerve trunk. *Neurology* 2014;82[7]:598-606.)

surgical specialty literature reported exploration in 46 of 100 patients with AIN syndrome (46%), whereas studies from the medical specialty literature reported exploration in only 4 of 32 patients with AIN syndrome (12.5%).[30] Confusion and discrepancy with regard to the treatment of patients with AIN syndrome still exist; however, advances in imaging and additional studies that evaluate the outcomes of patients with AIN syndrome who undergo surgical treatment may provide surgeons with additional information with regard to which patients with AIN syndrome may benefit from surgical treatment rather than observation.

Summary

Ulnar neuropathy can be localized to the ulnar tunnel in a patient's wrist via a physical examination and/or electrodiagnostic studies. The unique anatomy of the ulnar tunnel allows surgeons to further localize pathology to one or more of the three zones of the ulnar tunnel based on the clinical findings and symptoms of a patient. Dissimilar to entrapment of the ulnar nerve in the cubital tunnel at the elbow, the ulnar nerve often is compressed within the ulnar tunnel at the wrist by external forces, such as masses, adhesions, or fractures.

RTS may be difficult to diagnose, especially in patients with other symptoms. The management of RTS remains controversial. A careful, clinical examination is paramount, and proper patient selection for the surgical management of RTS is important to achieve successful outcomes.

The median nerve is susceptible to entrapment in the proximal forearm as a result of various neuropathic etiologies. Lesions of the median nerve must be localized proximal or distal to the point at which the AIN and the palmar cutaneous branches of the median nerve branch off the median nerve. Median nerve entrapment before these divisions usually will result in distal sensory deficits and motor weakness in particular muscles. Pronator syndrome originally referred to compression of the median nerve between the two heads of the pronator teres; however, other potential sites of median nerve compression include the lacertus fibrosus and the FDS aponeurotic arch. Isolated anterior interosseous neuropathy, if not related to external forces or a direct injury, may be spontaneous and neuritic in nature. Patients with spontaneous AIN palsy may have profound motor weakness, with cutaneous sensory function spared. Surgeons must be able to differentiate between pronator syndrome and AIN syndrome because the type and time course of treatment for patients with pronator syndrome differs from that of patients with AIN syndrome.

References

1. Gross MS, Gelberman RH: The anatomy of the distal ulnar tunnel. *Clin Orthop Relat Res* 1985;196:238-247.

2. Murata K, Shih JT, Tsai TM: Causes of ulnar tunnel syndrome: A retrospective study of 31 subjects. *J Hand Surg Am* 2003;28(4):647-651.

3. Balogh B, Valencak J, Vesely M, Flammer M, Gruber H, Piza-Katzer H: The nerve of Henle: An anatomic and immunohistochemical study. *J Hand Surg Am* 1999;24(5):1103-1108.

4. Bachoura A, Jacoby SM: Ulnar tunnel syndrome. *Orthop Clin North Am* 2012;43(4):467-474.

5. Moradi A, Ebrahimzadeh MH, Jupiter JB: Radial tunnel syndrome, diagnostic and treatment dilemma. *Arch Bone Jt Surg* 2015;3(3):156-162.

6. Stanley J: Radial tunnel syndrome: A surgeon's perspective. *J Hand Ther* 2006;19(2):180-184.

7. Ferdinand BD, Rosenberg ZS, Schweitzer ME, et al: MR imaging features of radial tunnel syndrome: Initial experience. *Radiology* 2006;240(1):161-168.

8. Loh YC, Lam WL, Stanley JK, Soames RW: A new clinical test for radial tunnel syndrome—the Rule-of-Nine test: A cadaveric study. *J Orthop Surg (Hong Kong)* 2004;12(1):83-86.

9. Hagert E, Hagert C-G: Upper extremity nerve entrapments: The axillary and radial nerves—clinical diagnosis and surgical treatment. *Plast Reconstr Surg* 2014;134(1):71-80.

10. Naam NH, Nemani S: Radial tunnel syndrome. *Orthop Clin North Am* 2012;43(4):529-536.

11. van den Ende KI, Steinmann SP: Radial tunnel syndrome. *J Hand Surg Am* 2010;35(6):1004-1006.

12. Lee JT, Azari K, Jones NF: Long term results of radial tunnel release—the effect of co-existing tennis elbow, multiple compression syndromes and workers' compensation. *J Plast Reconstr Aesthet Surg* 2008;61(9):1095-1099.

13. Jebson PJ, Engber WD: Radial tunnel syndrome: Long-term results of surgical decompression. *J Hand Surg Am* 1997;22(5):889-896.

14. Mackinnon SE, Novak CB: Compression neuropathies, in Wolfe SW, Hotchkiss RN, Pederson WC, Kozin SH, eds: *Green's Operative Hand Surgery*, ed 6. Philadelphia, PA, Elsevier, 2011, pp 977-1014.

15. Seyffarth H: Primary myoses in the M. pronator teres as cause of lesion of the N. medianus (the pronator syndrome). *Acta Psychiatr Neurol Scand, Suppl* 1951;74:251-254.

16. Rodner CM, Tinsley BA, O'Malley MP: Pronator syndrome and anterior interosseous nerve syndrome. *J Am Acad Orthop Surg* 2013;21(5):268-275.

17. Ochi K, Horiuchi Y, Tazaki K, Takayama S, Matsumura T: Fascicular constrictions in patients with spontaneous palsy of the anterior interosseous nerve and the posterior interosseous nerve. *J Plast Surg Hand Surg* 2012;46(1):19-24.

18. Pham M, Bäumer P, Meinck HM, et al: Anterior interosseous nerve syndrome: Fascicular motor lesions of median nerve trunk. *Neurology* 2014;82(7):598-606.

19. Kiloh LG, Nevin S: Isolated neuritis of the anterior interosseous nerve. *Br Med J* 1952;1(4763):850-851.

20. Rodriguez-Niedenführ M, Vazquez T, Ferreira B, Parkin I, Nearn L, Sañudo JR: Intramuscular Martin-Gruber anastomosis. *Clin Anat* 2002;15(2):135-138.

21. Spinner M: The anterior interosseous-nerve syndrome, with special attention to its variations. *J Bone Joint Surg Am* 1970;52(1):84-94.

22. Hagert E: Clinical diagnosis and wide-awake surgical treatment of proximal median nerve entrapment at the elbow: A prospective study. *Hand (N Y)* 2013;8(1):41-46.

23. Davidge KM, Sammer DM: Median nerve entrapment and injury, in Mackinnon SE, Yee A, eds: *Nerve Surgery*. New York, NY, Thieme, 2015, 207-250.

24. Dunn AJ, Salonen DC, Anastakis DJ: MR imaging findings of anterior interosseous nerve lesions. *Skeletal Radiol* 2007;36(12):1155-1162.

25. Bridgeman C, Naidu S, Kothari MJ: Clinical and electrophysiological presentation of pronator syndrome. *Electromyogr Clin Neurophysiol* 2007;47(2):89-92.

26. Ulrich D, Piatkowski A, Pallua N: Anterior interosseous nerve syndrome: Retrospective analysis of 14 patients. *Arch Orthop Trauma Surg* 2011;131(11):1561-1565.

27. Tulwa N, Limb D, Brown RF: Median nerve compression within the humeral head of pronator teres. *J Hand Surg Br* 1994;19(6):709-710.

28. MacKinnon SE, Novak CB: Compression neuropathies, in Wolfe SW, Hotchkiss RN, Pederson WC, Kozin SH, eds: *Green's Operative Hand Surgery: Expert Consult. Online and Print*, ed 6. Philadelphia, PA, Elsevier, 2010, pp 977-1014.

29. Aljawder A, Faqi MK, Mohamed A, Alkhalifa F: Anterior interosseous nerve syndrome diagnosis and intraoperative findings: A case report. *Int J Surg Case Rep* 2016;21:44-47.

30. Wong L, Dellon AL: Brachial neuritis presenting as anterior interosseous nerve compression—implications for diagnosis and treatment: A case report. *J Hand Surg Am* 1997;22(3):536-539.

Adult Reconstruction: Hip and Knee

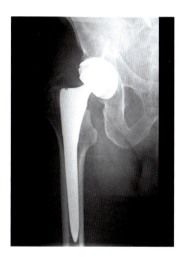

Primary Total Hip Arthroplasty: Everything You Need to Know

Jay R. Lieberman, MD
William Pannell, MD
Robert T. Trousdale, MD
J. Bohannon Mason, MD
John J. Callaghan, MD

Abstract

Total hip arthroplasty is an extremely successful procedure that relieves pain and improves function. Orthopaedic surgeons should understand how to improve outcomes of patients who undergo primary total hip arthroplasty. Orthopaedic surgeons can enhance the outcomes of total hip arthroplasty by optimizing preoperative and perioperative management, improving surgical techniques, and selecting an appropriate femoral component and bearing surface.

Instr Course Lect 2017;66:165–179.

Total hip arthroplasty (THA) is an extremely successful procedure that relieves pain and improves function. The outcomes of patients who undergo primary THA must be improved given the current environment of bundled payments. The outcomes of THA can be improved by optimizing preoperative and perioperative management, improving surgical techniques, and selecting an appropriate femoral component and bearing surface for primary THA.

Perioperative Management
Reduction of Surgical Site Infection

A number of steps have been identified to help reduce surgical site infections that are associated with THA. These steps include the use of prophylactic antibiotics; appropriate skin preparation, including preoperative shower, hair removal, and skin antisepsis; and preoperative screening for bacterial colonization.

The standard antibiotic prophylaxis protocol for THA consists of either cefazolin or cefuroxime, which is administered less than 1 hour before THA. Patients who are allergic to cefazolin or cefuroxime can be administered either vancomycin or clindamycin for antibiotic prophylaxis. Recently, the use of

Dr. Lieberman or an immediate family member has received royalties from DePuy; serves as a paid consultant to or is an employee of DePuy; has stock or stock options held in Hip Innovation Technology; and serves as a board member, owner, officer, or committee member of the American Academy of Orthopaedic Surgeons and the Western Orthopaedic Association. Dr. Trousdale or an immediate family member has received royalties from DePuy and Medtronic; serves as a paid consultant to or is an employee of DePuy; and serves as a board member, owner, officer, or committee member of the American Association of Hip and Knee Surgeons, the Hip Society, and the Knee Society. Dr. Bohannon Mason or an immediate family member has received royalties from DePuy; serves as a paid consultant to or is an employee of DePuy; has received nonincome support (such as equipment or services), commercially derived honoraria, or other non-research–related funding (such as paid travel) from DePuy; and serves as a board member, owner, officer, or committee member of the American Association of Hip and Knee Surgeons. Dr. Callaghan or an immediate family member has received royalties from DePuy; serves as a paid consultant to or is an employee DePuy, Wolters Kluwer Health–Lippincott, Williams & Wilkins, and the Journal of Arthroplasty; and serves as a board member, owner, officer, or committee member of the International Hip Society, the Knee Society, and the Orthopaedic Research and Education Foundation. Neither Dr. Pannell nor any immediate family member has received anything of value from or has stock or stock options held in a commercial company or institution related directly or indirectly to the subject of this chapter.

vancomycin for antibiotic prophylaxis has increased, particularly in patients who have a lactam allergy, in patients with known methicillin-resistant *Staphylococcus aureus* (MRSA) colonization, and at institutions at which recent MRSA outbreaks have occurred. Surgeons, with the help of an infectious disease consultant, should determine the microbiologic environment at their institution to determine if vancomycin should be administered as part of the standard antibiotic prophylaxis regimen. Some orthopaedic surgeons are concerned about routinely administering vancomycin because of the potential for vancomycin-resistant organisms.[1]

Recently, skin antisepsis for the prevention of surgical site infection has received increased attention.[2] Most studies have assessed the effectiveness of a preoperative shower or bath in general surgery patients. However, Johnson et al[3] assessed the efficacy of a 2% chlorhexidine gluconate-impregnated cloth that was used by 954 patients the night before and the morning of THA. The authors compared the infection rate of the 157 patients who completed the chlorhexidine gluconate-impregnated cloth protocol with that of 897 patients who received only a standard perioperative skin preparation of iodine povacrylex with alcohol. No surgical site infections occurred in the patients who used a chlorhexidine gluconate-impregnated cloth, whereas infections occurred in 1.6% of the patients who underwent only the standard perioperative skin preparation.

Limited data exist with regard to the influence of hair removal on surgical site infection.[4] Data are insufficient to determine if a difference exists between shaving and the use hair removal creams. In general, most surgeons recommend that hair be removed with the use of clippers as close to a THA procedure as possible.

A number of different skin antiseptic options can be used before THA.[5] Povidone-iodine; iodine povacrylex, which is iodine with long-lasting alcohol; and chlorhexidine gluconate are the skin antiseptic agents most frequently used before THA. Currently, no skin antiseptic agent has been identified as superior to another. Chlorhexidine gluconate has been reported to disrupt cellular membranes, has long-lasting activity against gram-positive and gram-negative organisms, and is not inactivated by blood or serum proteins. Iodophors are active against skin floras but are short-acting and inactivated by blood and serum proteins.[6] Most studies have assessed the effectiveness of skin antiseptic agents in patients who undergo clean-contaminated general surgery; however, studies on the effectiveness of skin antiseptic agents in THA patients are lacking.[7]

Nasal decolonization with the use of mupirocin has received increased attention because of concerns for methicillin-sensitive *S aureus* infection and MRSA infection and the interest in eliminating the nasal carriage of methicillin-sensitive *S aureus* and MRSA preoperatively. In a single-center, prospective study of 7,019 patients who underwent elective orthopaedic surgery, Kim et al[8] reported that surgical site infections could be reduced with the use of a prescreening program. The authors reported that the surgical site infection rate in patients who underwent a prescreening program was 0.19%, whereas the infection rate in a group of historical control patients was 0.45% ($P = 0.009$). Currently, some orthopaedic surgeons treat the nares of all patients rather than screen all patients and treat only those with positive cultures; however, studies are necessary to determine if this nasal decolonization protocol is cost effective.

Venous Thromboembolic Prophylaxis

Orthopaedic surgeons are concerned about the prevention of fatal pulmonary embolism, symptomatic pulmonary embolism, and deep vein thrombosis in patients who undergo THA because such complications are associated with considerable morbidity and even death. The selection of an appropriate venous thromboembolic prophylactic agent involves a balance between bleeding and efficacy. Patients should receive sufficient venous thromboembolic prophylaxis to reduce the risk for symptomatic deep vein thrombosis and pulmonary embolism; however, concurrent concern exists with regard to the overcoagulation of patients, which may lead to bleeding and other wound problems.

Both the American Academy of Orthopaedic Surgeons and the American College of Chest Physicians (ACCP) have published clinical practice guidelines (CPGs) to help orthopaedic surgeons select appropriate venous thromboembolic prophylactic agents.[9,10] The ACCP has been publishing CPGs for more than 25 years. The orthopaedic community had concerns about the original ACCP CPG on venous thromboembolic prophylaxis because of the belief that the CPG placed an increased focus on efficacy but insufficient focus on concerns with regard to bleeding. The original ACCP CPG on venous thromboembolic prophylaxis strongly recommended against the use of aspirin for venous thromboembolic prophylaxis. The most recent ACCP

CPG on venous thromboembolic prophylaxis was published in 2012, and the ACCP CPG Committee should be commended for listening to the concerns of the orthopaedic community.[11] The most recent ACCP CPG on venous thromboembolic prophylaxis recommended (grade 1B recommendation) the use of one of many available chemoprophylactic agents or an intermittent pneumatic compression device (grade 1C recommendation) for 10 to 14 days for venous thromboembolic prophylaxis in orthopaedic surgery patients[11] (**Table 1**). The most recent American Academy of Orthopaedic Surgeons CPG on venous thromboembolic prophylaxis was published in 2011. The American Academy of Orthopaedic Surgeons CPG on venous thromboembolic prophylaxis did not make recommendations for the specific venous thromboembolic prophylactic regimen that should be used or the duration of venous thromboembolic prophylaxis because of insufficient data.[9]

Surgeons must understand the CPGs on venous thromboembolic prophylaxis to be able to adapt them in practice.[12] The ACCP CPG on venous thromboembolic prophylaxis recommended the use of one of many available chemoprophylactic agents or an intermittent pneumatic compression device rather than no venous thromboembolic prophylaxis[11] (**Table 1**). The AACP CPG on venous thromboembolic prophylaxis did not recommend one venous thromboembolic prophylactic agent more than another; however, based on the available data, low-molecular-weight heparin, rivaroxaban, and apixaban appear to be the most potent venous thromboembolic prophylactic agents, but they are associated with a higher

rate of bleeding. Warfarin may be considered an intermediate anticoagulant. Warfarin is advantageous because it is an oral agent that can be titrated to the desired level of anticoagulation; however, warfarin requires frequent patient monitoring and interacts with various drugs and food products. Aspirin may be a less effective anticoagulant compared with the already discussed venous thromboembolic prophylactic agents; however, it appears to be associated with less bleeding. In addition, aspirin is an oral agent that has good patient compliance.[10] Some studies have reported promising data with regard to the efficacy of intermittent pneumatic compression devices;[13] however, concerns exist with regard to both patient compliance with as well as the cost of intermittent pneumatic compression devices, and more data from multicenter randomized trials are necessary to determine the true efficacy of intermittent pneumatic compression devices. The ACCP CPG on venous thromboembolic prophylaxis recommended that chemoprophylaxis be combined with the use of an intermittent pneumatic compression device during a patient's

hospital stay. The addition of an intermittent pneumatic compression device is particularly important if chemoprophylaxis is delayed until 18 to 24 hours postoperatively to reduce bleeding.

Surgical Approaches

THA involves multiple steps, the first of which is determining the appropriate surgical approach. Surgeons must understand the anatomy involved in as well as the advantages and disadvantages of different THA approaches. A number of approaches, including anterior, posterior, lateral, and two-incision approaches, have been described for THA. This chapter will discuss the posterior and anterior approaches for THA. Most surgeons select a THA approach based on their experience and training. Surgeons must be familiar with multiple exposures. Less invasive THA has gained popularity because it results in less muscle damage, faster recovery, and improved clinical outcomes. Recently, a variety of direct anterior approaches have received increased attention; however, little evidence exists to support the superiority of one THA approach more than another.

Table 1

American College of Chest Physicians (ACCP) Evidence-Based Clinical Practice Guideline on the Prevention of Venous Thromboembolism (VTE) in Orthopaedic Surgery Patients

ACCP Recommendation	VTE Prophylaxis
Grade 1B	Low-molecular-weight heparin
	Fondaparinux
	Apixaban
	Dabigatran
	Rivaroxaban
	Low-dose unfractionated heparin
	Adjusted-dose vitamin K antagonist
	Aspirin
Grade 1C	Intermittent pneumatic compression device

Posterior Approach

The posterior approach to the hip is a versatile approach that allows hemiarthroplasty, THA, hip resurfacing, open reduction and internal fixation of various acetabular fractures, and arthrotomy drainage of the hip joint to manage infection to be performed.

Anatomy

The muscular anatomy of the posterolateral aspect of the hip is divided into superficial and deep layers. Henry[14] described the outer surface as the deltoid muscle of the hip, which is similar to the deltoid muscle of the shoulder. This layer consists of the gluteus maximus and the tensor fascia lata, both of which form the outer sheath of the hip musculature. The deep muscular layer of the hip that is encountered during the posterior approach for THA consists of the short external rotators, including the piriformis, gemelli, obturator internus, obturator externus, and quadratus femoris. The musculotendinous insertions of the gluteus medius and minimus insert at the tip of the greater trochanter and should not be disturbed during the posterior approach for THA.

Surgeons must be aware of the location of the neurovascular structures about the hip during the posterior approach for THA. The piriformis tendon defines the pathway of the sciatic nerve. Multiple neurovascular structures enter the hip through the sciatic notch, passing superior and inferior to the piriformis tendon to supply the given muscles. Typically, the superior gluteal nerve and the superior gluteal artery are located above the piriformis muscle. Typically, the inferior gluteal nerve, inferior gluteal artery, inferior pudendal nerve, inferior pudendal artery, obturator internus nerve, sciatic

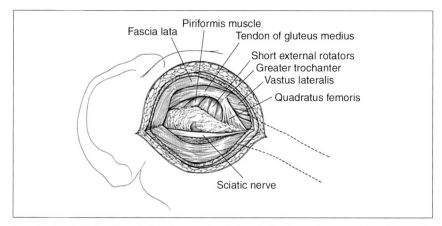

Figure 1   Illustration of a deeply dissected hip shows important muscular and neurovascular structures encountered during the posterior approach for total hip arthroplasty. (Reproduced from Vail TP, Callaghan JJ: Minimal incision total hip arthroplasty. *J Am Acad Orthop* 2007;15[12]:707-715.)

nerve, posterior femoral cutaneous nerve, and quadratus femoris nerve are located below the piriformis muscle (**Figure 1**). Damage to the superior gluteal nerve can lead to dysfunction of the abductor muscles, and damage to the superior gluteal artery can lead to brisk pelvic bleeding, which may be difficult to control because the superior gluteal artery can retract into the pelvis. Typically, the sciatic nerve enters the hip below the piriformis muscle and traverses between the gluteus maximus and the short external rotators of the hip. In general, the sciatic nerve is protected by the short external rotators during the posterior approach for THA; however, the sciatic nerve may injured during errant posterior retractor placement or excessive leg lengthening.

Advantages and Disadvantages

The posterior approach for THA is advantageous because it allows the surgeon to readily extend the exposure both proximally and distally. A surgeon can attain full access to the posterior column of the acetabulum during the posterior approach for THA and can attain distal femoral exposure via a classic trochanteric osteotomy, trochanteric slide osteotomy, or posterior-based trochanteric osteotomy. No consensus exists on the optimal THA approach for every patient; however, because the posterior approach for THA is versatile, it can be used to treat most patients who undergo primary or revision THA. The ability to easily convert the posterior approach for THA to an extensile exposure makes it an essential approach for arthroplasty surgeons.

The main concern with regard to the posterior approach for THA is its association with a higher rate of dislocation compared with other surgical approaches. A 0.2% to 9.5% dislocation rate has been reported in patients who undergo primary THA via the posterior approach.[15] A number of factors influence the risk for dislocation after THA, one of which is the THA approach that is used. Preservation and repair of the posterior hip capsule have been reported to decrease the rate of posterior instability. Reduced dislocation rates have been reported in patients who undergo primary THA via the posterior approach and in whom capsular repair is performed. The posterior approach for THA is advantageous because it is versatile, allows for extensile exposure, and preserves the abductor mechanism.

Technique

Typically, the patient is placed in the lateral decubitus position. The contralateral leg should be padded to ensure minimal pressure on the peroneal nerve at the knee. Various positioners are available to help stabilize the pelvis for THA. Adequate exposure of the hip joint for the posterior approach to THA requires an appropriately placed incision. Typically, the authors of this chapter make a laterally-based incision that curves slightly posterior at the tip of the greater trochanter (**Figure 2, A**). The authors of this chapter use an incision that is long enough to perform THA, which varies depending on a patient's body habitus.[16] Currently, no prospective randomized trials have reported that the length of the incision for THA has any effect on a patient's recovery or surgical outcome. After the skin incision has been made, dissection is carried down through the deep subcutaneous tissue to expose the deep fascia of the thigh (**Figure 2, B**). The deep fascia is split in line with the skin incision, extending proximally to the tip of the greater trochanter, after which the fibers of the gluteus maximus are split. The fascia is retracted, which exposes the deep muscular layers of the hip joint and the trochanteric bursa on the short external rotators (**Figure 2, C**). The posterior approach for THA has no true internervous plane because the gluteus maximus, which is supplied by the inferior gluteal nerve, is split along its fibers. Typically, the authors of this chapter place a retractor just

posterior to the tendinous insertion of the gluteus medius tendon near the greater trochanter to expose the posterior structures of the hip. The authors of this chapter tag the short external rotators with a suture, ensuring that the sciatic nerve is positioned well posterior to the tag with the use of gentle retraction (**Figure 2, D**). After the short external rotators have been tagged, the thick posterior hip capsule that runs from the posterior wall of the acetabulum to the femoral neck should be exposed. The short external rotators are incised just above the piriformis tendon with the hip capsule in either a single layer or two separate layers, which are then reflected posteriorly to protect the sciatic nerve. The femoral head, neck, and posterior wall are then visualized. The authors of this chapter perform an inferior capsule release, after which the hip is easily dislocated. After the hip has been dislocated, the authors of this chapter resect the femoral head above the lesser trochanter per the preoperative plan (**Figure 2, E**). Patients who have severe hip stiffness may require an in situ femoral neck osteotomy before hip dislocation to allow for dislocation of the femur without creating undue stress that may increase the risk for femoral shaft fracture

The posterior approach allows for excellent exposure of the acetabulum but requires anterior translation of the femur in front of the acetabulum. Typically, anterior translation of the femur in front of the acetabulum is achieved with the use of Hohmann retractors that are placed at the level of the anterior inferior iliac spine (**Figure 2, F**). Care should be taken during the placement of the Hohmann retractors to ensure that they remain flush against the bone and are not placed too anteriorly, which

may put the femoral artery, vein, and nerve at risk for injury. Slight hip flexion after rotation of the hip allows for anterior translation of the femur. After the Hohmann retractors have been placed, circumferential exposure of the acetabulum should be attained. The surgeon should be able to visualize the transverse ligament, anterior wall, posterior wall, ischium, and acetabular teardrop without difficulty. After the acetabulum has been prepared and placed, femoral exposure is easily attained with the use of minimal retraction. The authors of this chapter place a Hohmann retractor along the femoral neck as an assistant positions the patient's leg in flexion and rotation so that the lower portion of the leg is perpendicular to the floor; this allows for the unhindered placement of the femoral stem and allows the surgeon to accurately assess for femoral anteversion. A retractor can be placed anteriorly to subluxate the femur laterally out of the hip wound, which is especially helpful in patients who have a high body mass index (**Figure 2, G**). After the THA has been completed, the authors of this chapter repair the posterior hip capsule and the short external rotators with the use of nonabsorbable sutures (**Figure 2, H**).

Anterior Approach
Advantages and Disadvantages
The anterior approach to the hip, which was first described by Smith-Peterson,[17,18] has gained increased attention in the past few years, and is currently the fastest growing approach used for primary THA.[19] This increased attention has resulted from unproven claims of faster patient recovery, reduced dislocation risk, and increased component accuracy as well as from a number of economic and marketing

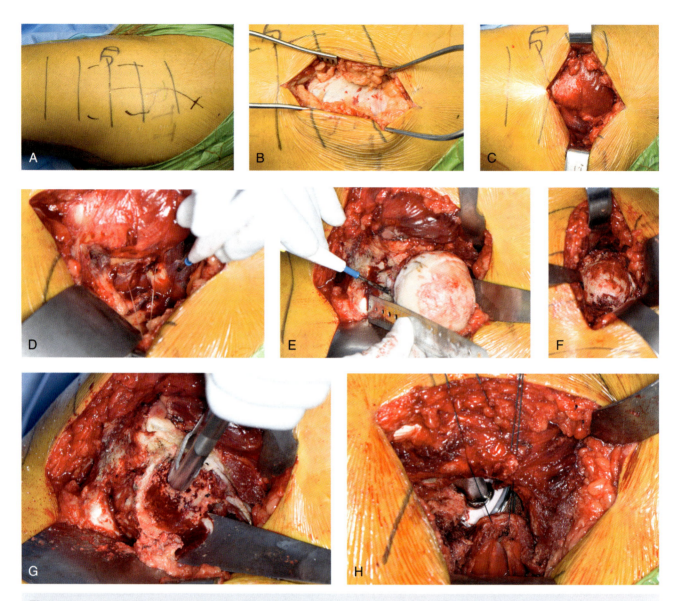

Figure 2 Intraoperative photographs of the left hip of a patient show the posterior approach for total hip arthroplasty. **A,** A laterally based incision (curved line) that curves slightly posterior at the tip of the greater trochanter is made. The patient's head is to the right, and the patient's foot is to the left. The deep fascia is exposed (**B**) and split (**C**). The gluteus medius is to the right, and the vastus lateralis is to the left. **D,** The short external rotators are tagged, ensuring that the sciatic nerve is positioned posterior to the tag. **E,** The hip is dislocated, after which the femoral head is resected above the lesser trochanter per the preoperative plan. **F,** Circumferential exposure of the acetabulum is achieved with the use of Hohmann retractors that are placed in the ischium and the anterior column. **G,** The hip is adducted and internally rotated, after which a retractor is used to lift the femur out of the wound, and the entry hole is made in the proximal aspect of the femur in anticipation of femoral canal preparation. **H,** The short external rotators are repaired after total hip arthroplasty is complete.

pressures, which have influenced some surgeons to examine their THA approach.[20] Although no approach is ideal for all surgeons or for all patients, the literature is beginning to offer some insights on the advantages and disadvantages of the anterior approach for THA.

The direct anterior approach represents a number of different anterior surgical exposures to the hip that may be performed with the use of a fracture table and fluoroscopy. Some surgeons perform the direct anterior approach without the use of a fracture table or fluoroscopy. The most frequently used direct anterior approach involves the intermuscular internervous plane of the hip joint between the sartorius and tensor muscles (superficial) and the rectus femoris muscle and tensor muscle (deep), which does not disrupt the abductor or deltoid muscles of the hip.[21]

Disadvantages of the direct anterior approach include the learning curve associated with the approach, which may be a problem for some surgeons; the increased risk for lateral femoral cutaneous nerve injury; increased blood loss and length of surgery, particularly for surgeons in the early stages of their learning curve; difficult access to the femur; and increased risk for trochanteric injury. Although no absolute indications exist for the direct anterior approach for THA, many surgeons consider the direct anterior approach for THA in patients who have a high-risk for dislocation, such as those with dementia, neuromuscular disorders, or alcoholism, and in patients without major deformity who are undergoing bilateral THA. Current studies of joint registries have reported that the risk for dislocation is diminished in most patients who undergo THA with the use of larger femoral heads and in whom capsular repair is performed.[22] However, in a recent large study of more than 22,000 hips that underwent THA, Sheth et al[23] reported that the hips that underwent THA via anterior or anterolateral approaches had a lower risk for dislocation without an increased risk for revision compared with the hips that underwent THA via the posterior approach ($P = 0.017$).

Several studies have reported faster functional recovery after THA via the direct anterior approach;[24-26] however, in most studies, functional gains attributed to the direct anterior approach for THA diminish after 6 weeks. In a clinical cohort study of 182 patients who underwent THA via either the direct anterior approach or a mini-posterior approach, Nakata et al[24] reported that the patients in the direct anterior approach group had improved functional parameters that reached significance at 3 weeks postoperatively compared with the patients in the mini-posterior approach group. In a study of 120 patients who underwent THA via either the direct anterior approach or the posterior approach, Rodriguez et al[25] reported that the patients in the direct anterior approach group had a faster functional recovery at 2 weeks postoperatively compared with the patients in the posterior approach group; however, no differences were observed between the patients in the two groups after 6 weeks postoperatively, and the general health outcomes of, surgical times for, and complications in the patients in both groups were similar. In a consecutive case series of 150 patients who underwent THA via either the mini-posterior approach or the direct anterior approach, Zawadsky et al[26] reported that the patients in the direct anterior approach group had a decreased length of hospitalization, an increased discharge to home versus a skilled facility, and diminished use of walking aids at 6 weeks postoperatively compared with the patients in the mini-posterior group. Conversely, in a retrospective review of 222 patients who underwent THA via either the direct anterior approach or the mini-posterior approach, Poehling-Monaghan et al[27] reported no differences in length of hospital stay, the number of complications, or the timing of discharge to home between the patients in the two groups.

In a prospective randomized clinical trial of 100 patients who underwent THA via either the direct anterior approach or the direct lateral approach, Restrepo et al[28] reported that the patients in the direct anterior approach group had significantly better Medical Outcomes Study 36-Item Short Form, Western Ontario and McMasters Universities Osteoarthritis Index, and Linear Analog Scale Assessment scores that remained significant for as long as 1 year postoperatively compared with the patients who underwent THA via the direct lateral approach. Three recent prospective randomized trials reported that the direct anterior approach for THA resulted in improved functional results, including significantly improved walking distance,[29] faster cessation of walking aids,[30,31] and shorter length of hospital stay, compared with the posterior approach.[31] However, these three studies were underpowered, and the authors of the studies were not blinded to the THA approach that was used for each patient. Based on the current available literature, the best THA approach cannot be determined.

Often, the direct anterior approach is performed with the use of a specialized surgical table. Specialized surgical tables are advantageous because fluoroscopy can be easily incorporated into the surgical workflow. The use of fluoroscopy during THA via the direct anterior approach results in improved acetabular component accuracy but has not yet demonstrated a defined clinical benefit.[25,32,33] In addition, the surgeon and other personnel in the operating room must wear leaded vests. Often, the learning curve that is associated with the direct anterior approach for THA is cited as a reason for complications, including fracture, that occur in patients who undergo THA via the direct anterior approach early in a case series. de Steiger et al[34] reported that the cumulative revision rate was higher for surgeons who performed 50 or fewer THAs via the direct anterior approach; however, the influence of the learning curve that is associated with the direct anterior approach for THA was absent in surgeons who performed more than 100 THAs via the direct anterior approach. Although Masonis et al[35] reported safe adoption of the direct anterior approach for THA, some studies have reported increased complication rates in patients who undergo THA via the direct anterior approach, which underscores the effect of the learning curve that is associated with the direct anterior approach for THA on patient outcomes; therefore, caution should be exercised by surgeons who begin using the direct anterior approach for THA.[36,37]

The direct anterior approach for THA is a safe surgical approach. The learning curve for the direct anterior approach requires consideration but can be mastered. Some single-center prospective clinical trials have reported that the direct anterior approach for THA may result in earlier functional recovery and decreased length of hospital stay; however, any functional advantages that result from THA via the direct anterior approach compared with other approaches diminish after 4 to 6 weeks postoperatively. An increased risk for femoral fracture and an increased risk for wound healing problems in the early postoperative period are concerns for patients who undergo THA via the direct anterior approach.[31,38] Long-term studies are necessary to determine if the direct anterior approach for THA results in superior long-term outcomes compared with THA performed via other approaches. Careful preoperative planning, rapid recovery regimens,

innovative pain management protocols, and meticulous surgical technique may be more important in determining both the short-term and long-term outcomes of THA compared with the THA approach that is used.

Technique

The patient is positioned supine on a surgical table. A specialized surgical table can be used to allow for extension and rotation of the surgical extremity. If a specialized surgical table is not used, both extremities are prepared and draped to allow for manipulation of the surgical leg in a figure-of-4 position via external rotation and adduction. If a specialized surgical table is not used, a small bolster typically is placed under the surgical hip to assist in elevation of the femur. Typically, the incision is made 2 cm distal and 2 cm lateral to the anterior superior iliac spine over the anterior margin of the tensor fasciae lata muscle and is extended obliquely for 10 to 12 cm toward the Gerdy tubercle at the knee (**Figure 3, A**). The incision is carried down to the level of the deep fascia; the incision should be lateral to the lateral femoral cutaneous nerve, which arborizes at the level of the fascia. The surgeon should avoid overdissection of the perifascial fat to prevent postoperative seroma formation. The fascia of the tensor muscle is incised in line with the tensor muscle, the tensor muscle is gently swept laterally, and a retractor is placed around the superior femoral neck (**Figure 3, B**). A double layer of fascia exists at the dorsal aspect of the tensor fascia between the tensor muscle and the rectus muscle through which the ascending branches of the femoral circumflex artery course. The ascending branches of the femoral circumflex vessels should be cauterized

or ligated before the inferior hip capsule is exposed (**Figure 3, C**). A retractor is placed under the rectus femoris muscle and around the inferior aspect of the hip capsule to allow for visualization of the anterior hip capsule.

The hip capsule is incised from the reflected rectus femoris muscle, lateral to the inferior iliac spine, to the anterolateral aspect of the insertion of the hip capsule on the femur. The anterior hip capsule is released off of the intertrochanteric line of the femur anteriorly just proximal to the vastus intermedius muscle origin and is tagged, after which a curved retractor is placed intracapsularly to expose the femoral neck. A second retractor is placed in the hip capsule around the superior femoral neck, and the superior leaf of the hip capsule is slightly released from the femoral attachment. The lateral reflection of the femoral neck and the greater trochanter are used as points of orientation for femoral neck resection, which is referenced against the preoperative plan (**Figure 3, D**). A napkin ring resection may aid in removal of the femoral head. Typically, a corkscrew is used to remove the femoral head from the acetabulum.

External rotation of the femur 50° to 60° before the placement of acetabular retractors may improve visualization of the acetabulum from the anterolateral wound. Retractors are placed over the anterior and posterior columns between the sulcus of the hip capsule and the labrum, after which the labrum and pulvinar are excised. Acetabular reaming may be performed under fluoroscopic guidance, if desired; minimization of the number of retractors that are in the wound during reaming assists in passing the reamer in and out of the wound. An offset reamer handle may be beneficial (**Figure 3, E**). In addition,

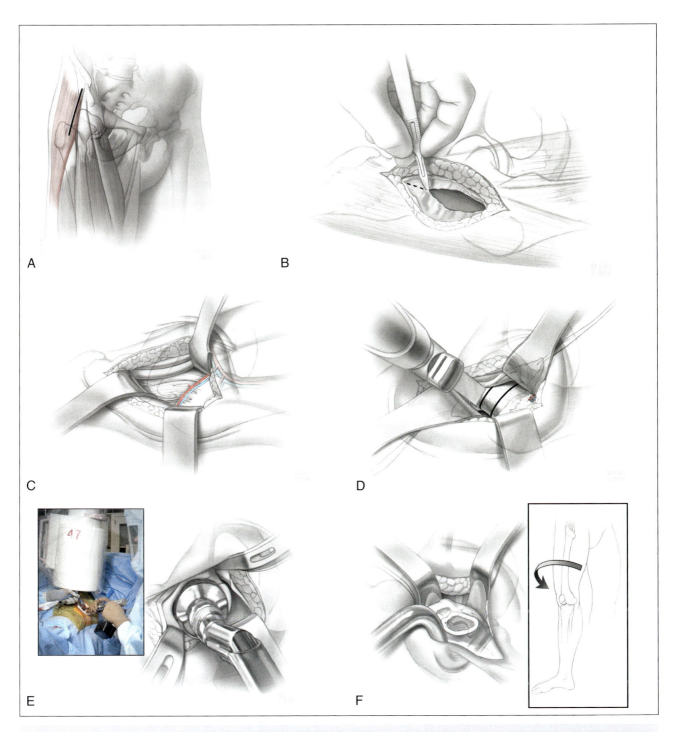

Figure 3   Illustrations of a hip show the direct anterior approach for total hip arthroplasty. **A,** The incision (line) is oriented over the tensor muscle and is extended obliquely for 10 to 12 cm toward the lateral knee. **B,** The fascial sheath of the tensor muscle is incised (dashed line), and the tensor muscle is swept laterally. **C,** The ascending branches of the femoral circumflex vessels are identified and ligated or cauterized. **D,** Neck resection (area between the two black lines) is performed with the aid of blunt retractors that are placed around the superior and inferior femoral neck. **E,** Acetabular reaming is performed with the use of an offset shaft reamer. Inset, Intraoperative photograph shows acetabular reaming under fluoroscopic guidance. **F,** A femoral lift hook is used as a fulcrum to attain adequate exposure. Inset, Illustration of a leg shows that femoral exposure is enhanced with external rotation, extension, and adduction of the leg. (Panels A through F reproduced with permisssion from the Mayo Foundation for Education and Research, Rochester, MN, and panel E inset reproduced with permission from Mason JB, Taunton M: Anterior approach total hip arthroplasty, in Berry DJ, Maloney WJ, eds: *Master Techniques in Orthopaedic Surgery: The Hip*, ed 3. Philadelphia, PA, Wolters Kluwer, 2015, pp 1-11.)

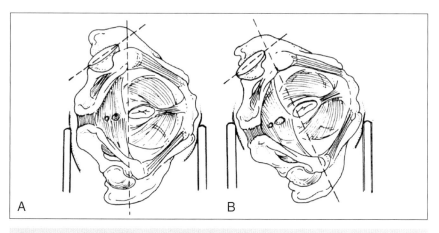

Figure 4 Illustrations of a pelvis in a neutral position (**A**) and tilted anteriorly (**B**) show the mechanism by which pelvic rotation may lead to retroversion of the acetabular component during total hip arthroplasty. (Reproduced with permission from Woo RY, Morrey BF: Dislocations after total hip arthroplasty. *J Bone Joint Surg Am* 1982;64[9]:1295-1306.)

surgeons should maintain the integrity of the inferior hip capsule.

After preparation and implantation of the acetabular component is complete, attention should be directed to the femur. A femoral lift hook, which is passed under the tensor and gluteus maximus muscles and supports the proximal lateral aspect of the femur, can help elevate the proximal femur into the surgical field. The patient's leg is externally rotated and extended to facilitate exposure of the proximal femur (**Figure 3, F**). The superior hip capsule is released from its insertion on the reflection between the femoral neck and the greater trochanter, which allows for both the elevation of the femur and access to the lateral proximal femur for broaching. Further exposure can be attained with the use of a retractor that is placed over the tip of the greater trochanter proximally and via release of the conjoint tendon at the posterior proximal femur. The posterior hip capsule is not disturbed. The piriformis tendon may be released in patients in whom exposure is difficult.

The obturator externus tendon is not disturbed.

After the proximal femur has been opened with the use of either a rongeur or box osteotome, broaching is performed with the use of an offset broach handle. Again, fluoroscopy may be used to confirm the orientation of the femoral trial. Trial components are assessed for stability before final implant placement. The hip capsule is reapproximated with the use of absorbable sutures, and the thin tensor fascia is closed with the use of a running suture. Subcutaneous closure of the skin is recommended. The skin is then sealed with the use of an adhesive cyanoacrylate tape, which allows the patient to shower postoperatively.

Acetabular Component Preparation and Implantation

Currently, cementless acetabular components are used for most patients who undergo THA in the United States and in many other countries. Excellent fixation and durability have been reported in patients who undergo THA with

the use of contemporary cementless porous-coated acetabular components with or without screw augmentation.[39,40] The goal of acetabular component preparation and implantation is to achieve a well-positioned, stable acetabular component that allows bone ingrowth fixation but prevents impingement and dislocation. This goal can be consistently achieved via proper patient positioning, acetabular exposure, bony acetabular preparation, and acetabular component insertion.

If a patient is placed in the lateral decubitus position, the patient's pelvis must be secured with the device that is used for patient positioning. If the pelvis is allowed to tilt forward, especially during anterior femur retraction, the surgeon may inadvertently place the acetabular component in less anteversion[41] (**Figure 4**). Incorrect acetabular component positioning also may occur in patients who have excessive lumbar lordosis or a flat lumbar spine if they are positioned in the supine position.

Proper acetabular exposure, especially with the use of smaller incisions, cannot be compromised at the risk of improper acetabular preparation and component insertion. Removal of the acetabular labrum ensures adequate visualization of the bony landmarks of the acetabulum. The placement of a retractor inferior to the transverse acetabular ligament, usually in the obturator foramen, helps the surgeon identify the inferior aspect of the acetabulum and allows the transverse acetabular ligament to be used as a guide for proper anteversion of the acetabular component.[42] The surgeon must be able to identify the ischium, ilium, and pelvis via palpation, if not via visualization, to determine the relationship of the normal anatomy of the acetabulum to any osteophytes and to the position selected for acetabular component placement (**Figure 5**).

If maximum acetabular exposure is attained, bony acetabular preparation requires little guidance. In most patients, a large or small medial osteophyte that covers the underlying medial acetabular pulvinar fat is present. Medial acetabular reaming should proceed until the pulvinar fat has been removed. Aggressive medial reaming should be avoided in patients who have osteopenic bone and medialized acetabular anatomy (medial acetabular wall that is observed medial to the Kohler line on AP radiographs). In patients in whom one-half of the acetabulum is osteoporotic and one-half of the acetabulum is osteosclerotic, surgeons should ream the osteosclerotic bone to avoid excessive removal of osteoporotic bone. To prevent oblong acetabular reaming, surgeons should begin acetabular reaming with the use of a reamer that is 2 or 4 mm smaller than the size of the templated acetabular component. After medial acetabular reaming is complete, reaming should be directed parallel to the transverse acetabular ligament. Adequate reaming is achieved after the acetabular reamer engages the anterior and posterior acetabular walls and an acetabular reamer that is 1 mm larger in diameter than the previous reamer fits securely in the reamed surface (with contact medially and with ability to only be removed forcefully with the use of a robust towel clip).

The final step in achieving a well-positioned acetabular component, which will provide durable fixation, is proper insertion of the acetabular component. Proper acetabular component insertion includes appropriate orientation of the acetabular component, with

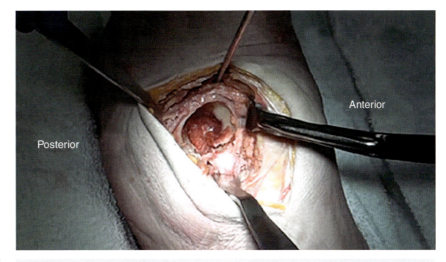

Figure 5   Intraoperative photograph of the right hip of a patient in the lateral decubitus position shows acetabular retractor positioning to allow for maximum acetabular exposure.

maximal bone contact and stability of the component in the acetabulum to ensure short-term fixation (to allow for ingrowth and prevent dislocation) and long-term durability. Underreaming of the acetabulum by 1 or 2 mm with respect to the outer diameter of the acetabular component provides excellent stability; however, excessive under-reaming of the acetabulum may result in acetabular fractures, which most commonly occur in the greater sciatic notch.[43,44] Positioning the acetabular component parallel to the transverse acetabular ligament allows for appropriate anteversion in most patients; aligning the anteroinferior acetabular cup flush with or just medial to the cortical bone of the pubis is another manner in which adequate anteversion can be achieved.[45] The acetabular cup should be tilted 10° less than vertical to an acetabular component positioner that is set at 45° to ensure acetabular cup insertion in less than 45° of abduction. Impaction of the acetabular cup requires a force of at least 200 N to ensure that the acetabular component

contacts the medial acetabular wall. Screws, if used, should be placed posterior to a line that extends from the anterior superior iliac spine to the ischial tuberosity.[46]

Femoral Component Selection and Implantation

Both cementless and cemented femoral fixation are associated with excellent long-term outcomes after THA. This chapter will discuss cementless femoral fixation. A number of different femoral component designs are associated with durable cementless femoral fixation.[47] The surgical technique used for femoral component insertion is determined by the overall geometry of the femoral stem and the location of femoral fixation.

In general, cementless femoral stems are divided into those for proximal femoral fixation, those for distal femoral fixation, and modular femoral stems. Newer femoral stem designs include both standard and high-offset options, which allow surgeons to maintain a patient's leg length yet restore offset. A number of proximally coated femoral

Table 2
Femoral Component Designs for Cementless Fixation

Design	Description	Location of Fixation
Single wedge[48-51]	Thin in anteroposterior plane Engages medial-lateral cortices Proximally coated	Metaphyseal
Double-wedge metaphyseal filling[52,53]	Engages anteroposterior cortices Engages medial-lateral cortices Proximally coated	Metaphyseal
Tapered stem[54]	Extensive porous coating	Metaphyseal-diaphyseal junction

stem designs are available for THA. The most commonly used femoral stems include single-wedge prostheses, double-wedge metaphyseal-filling prostheses, and tapered femoral stems. Single-wedge prostheses, which are flat and thin in the anteroposterior plane, engage the metaphyseal cortical bone in the medial to lateral plane. Double-wedge metaphyseal filling prostheses allow for fixation in both the anteroposterior and medial-lateral planes. Typically, fixation with the use of double-wedge metaphyseal-filling prostheses is attained at the metadiaphyseal junction rather than just the metaphysis. Tapered femoral stems allow for fixation at the metaphyseal-diaphyseal junction. Distal femoral fixation with the use of extensively porous-coated femoral stems is associated with durable fixation; however, extensively porous-coated femoral stems are used less frequently for routine THA compared with proximally coated femoral stems because they are more difficult to insert. In addition, more proximal stress shielding and less bone preservation for revision THA are associated with extensively porous-coated femoral stems[48-54] (Table 2).

Surgeons must understand the location at which femoral fixation will occur and the technique necessary to implant a femoral stem to achieve stable fixation and avoid femoral fracture. A number of general principles for femoral implantation must be followed. First, the surgeon must have adequate visualization of the proximal femur. Second, the broach must be lateralized to avoid placement of the femoral stem in a varus position. Third, the femoral stem must be rotationally stable in the femoral canal on implantation. The long-term results of THA with the use of cementless tapered femoral stems include excellent fixation, low loosening rates, and minimal thigh pain[55-58] (Table 3).

Bearing Surface Selection
Because cementless femoral fixation is reliable, wear and subsequently osteolysis lead to revision THA. Currently, the most popular bearing surface options for THA include a metal (cobalt-chromium) femoral head that is mated with a highly cross-linked polyethylene (XLPE) acetabular liner, a ceramic femoral head that is mated with a highly XLPE acetabular liner, and a ceramic femoral head that is mated with a ceramic acetabular liner. Either a metal or ceramic femoral head can be mated with a highly XLPE acetabular liner. Recent concerns with regard to trunnion corrosion have resulted in an increase in the use of ceramic femoral heads that are mated with highly XLPE acetabular liners.[59]

A highly XLPE acetabular liner is advantageous because no potential for fracture of the femoral head or squeaking exists. Compared with a ceramic-on-ceramic bearing surface, a highly XLPE acetabular liner is able to tolerate more variation in component positioning and, in general, allows for easier restoration of anatomy. In addition, more femoral head sizes and, if appropriate, elevated rims, protrusio liners, and face changing liners, are available for use with a highly XLPE acetabular liner. The major concern associated with highly XLPE acetabular liners is reduced mechanical properties compared with conventional polyethylene acetabular liners. The cross-linking of polyethylene leads to better wear resistance but also leads to diminished mechanical properties. Therefore, interest exists with regard to the placement of antioxidants, such as vitamin E, in polyethylene to limit polyethylene oxidation.[60]

In general, highly XLPE acetabular liners that are mated with either a metal or ceramic femoral head and ceramic-on-ceramic bearing surfaces result in excellent THA outcomes. A review of data from the Australian Orthopaedic Association National Joint Replacement Registry revealed that, at a follow-up of 13 years, the cumulative percent revision for patients who underwent THA with a metal femoral head that was mated with a highly XLPE acetabular liner (4.7%) was slightly better compared with that for patients who underwent THA with a ceramic-on-ceramic bearing surface (6.3%).[61] The data also revealed that, regardless of femoral head

Table 3
Long-Term Results of Total Hip Arthroplasty With Cementless Tapered Femoral Stems

Authors (Year)	No. of Hips	Implant Type	Mean Patient Age in Years (Range)	Mean Follow-up in Years (Range)	Thigh Pain (%)	Revision (%)
Cameron et al[57] (2006)	795	SROM (DePuy)	55 (22–71)	11.5 (2–17)	1.8	0.25
Epinette and Manley[55] (2008)	571	HA-coated	NA	17 (NA)	NA	0.7
McLaughlin and Lee[58] (2008)	65	Taperloc (Biomet)	50 (20–75)	20 (18–22.6)	3	1%
Suckel et al[56] (2009)	320	Alloclassic Zweymuller (Zimmer)	67 (29–99)	15 (15–17)	NA	0.7

HA = hydroxyapatite, NA = not available.

size, the cumulative percent revision for patients who underwent THA with a highly XLPE acetabular liner was superior compared with that for patients who underwent THA with a conventional polyethylene acetabular liner.

In a study on the effect of femoral head size with regard to wear, Bragdon et al[62] reported that minimal femoral head penetration existed in patients who underwent THA with a 36-mm femoral head that was mated with a highly XLPE acetabular liner. Based on the current data, the authors of this chapter recommend the use of either a highly XLPE acetabular liner that is mated with a ceramic femoral head or a ceramic-on-ceramic bearing surface in younger patients who undergo THA. The authors of this chapter tend to use a highly XLPE acetabular liner that is mated with a ceramic femoral head in younger, active patients who undergo THA; however, more research is necessary to determine the extent of metal femoral head corrosion. In general, a highly XLPE acetabular liner that is mated with a metal femoral head should be used in elderly patients who undergo THA.

Summary
Careful perioperative management and meticulous surgical technique in patients who undergo THA can lead to improved function and excellent outcomes. Given the current environment of bundled payments, careful perioperative management of patients who undergo primary THA is essential to reduce associated costs. The authors of this chapter believe that, in the past few years, too much focus has been placed on the surgical approach for THA, and that an optimal surgical approach for THA has yet to be identified. Surgeons should concentrate on obtaining rigid fixation of the prosthetic components, which will lead to a durable THA.

References
1. Ponce B, Raines BT, Reed RD, Vick C, Richman J, Hawn M: Surgical site infection after arthroplasty: Comparative effectiveness of prophylactic antibiotics, Do surgical care improvement project guidelines need to be updated? *J Bone Joint Surg Am* 2014;96(12):970-977.

2. Webster J, Osborne S: Preoperative bathing or showering with skin antiseptics to prevent surgical site infection. *Cochrane Database Syst Rev* 2006;2(2):CD004985.

3. Johnson AJ, Daley JA, Zywiel MG, Delanois RE, Mont MA: Preoperative chlorhexidine preparation and the incidence of surgical site infections after hip arthroplasty. *J Arthroplasty* 2010;25(6 suppl):98-102.

4. Tanner J, Woodings D, Moncaster K: Preoperative hair removal to reduce surgical site infection. *Cochrane Database Syst Rev* 2006;3(3):CD004122.

5. Kapadia BH, Johnson AJ, Daley JA, Issa K, Mont MA: Pre-admission cutaneous chlorhexidine preparation reduces surgical site infections in total hip arthroplasty. *J Arthroplasty* 2013;28(3):490-493.

6. Anderson MJ, Horn ME, Lin YC, Parks PJ, Peterson ML: Efficacy of concurrent application of chlorhexidine gluconate and povidone iodine against six nosocomial pathogens. *Am J Infect Control* 2010;38(10):826-831.

7. Morrison TN, Chen AF, Taneja M, Küçükdurmaz F, Rothman RH, Parvizi J: Single vs repeat surgical skin preparations for reducing surgical site infection after total joint arthroplasty: A prospective, randomized, double-blinded study. *J Arthroplasty* 2016;31(6):1289-1294.

8. Kim DH, Spencer M, Davidson SM, et al: Institutional prescreening for detection and eradication of methicillin-resistant Staphylococcus

aureus in patients undergoing elective orthopaedic surgery. *J Bone Joint Surg Am* 2010;92(9):1820-1826.

9. Mont MA, Jacobs JJ, Boggio LN, et al: Preventing venous thromboembolic disease in patients undergoing elective hip and knee arthroplasty. *J Am Acad Orthop Surg* 2011;19(12):768-776.

10. Lieberman JR, Pensak MJ: Prevention of venous thromboembolic disease after total hip and knee arthroplasty. *J Bone Joint Surg Am* 2013;95(19):1801-1811.

11. Falck-Ytter Y, Francis CW, Johanson NA, et al: Prevention of VTE in orthopedic surgery patients: Antithrombotic Therapy and Prevention of Thrombosis, 9th ed: American College of Chest Physicians Evidence-Based Clinical Practice Guidelines. *Chest* 2012;141(2 suppl):e278S-e325S.

12. Lieberman JR: The new AAOS clinical practice guidelines on venous thromboembolic prophylaxis: How to adapt them to your practice. *J Am Acad Orthop Surg* 2011;19(12):717-721.

13. Colwell CW Jr, Froimson MI, Mont MA, et al: Thrombosis prevention after total hip arthroplasty: A prospective, randomized trial comparing a mobile compression device with low-molecular-weight heparin. *J Bone Joint Surg Am* 2010;92(3):527-535.

14. Henry AK: *Extensile Exposure,* ed 2. Edinburgh, Scotland, Livingstone, 1966, pp 180-197.

15. Springer BP: Posterior approaches to the hip, in Berry DJ, Lieberman JR, eds: *Surgery of the Hip.* Philadelphia, PA, Elsevier, 2013, pp 249-256.

16. Vail TP, Callaghan JJ: Minimal incision total hip arthroplasty. *J Am Acad Orthop Surg* 2007;15(12):707-715.

17. Smith-Petersen MN: A new supra-articular subperiosteal approach to the hip joint. *Am J Orthop Surg* 1917;15:592.

18. Smith-Petersen MN: Approach to and exposure of the hip joint for mold arthroplasty. *J Bone Joint Surg Am* 1949;31(1):40-46.

19. Berry DJ, Bozic KJ: Current practice patterns in primary hip and knee arthroplasty among members of the American Association of Hip and Knee Surgeons. *J Arthroplasty* 2010;25(6 suppl):2-4.

20. Mohan R, Yi PH, Hansen EN: Evaluating online information regarding the direct anterior approach for total hip arthroplasty. *J Arthroplasty* 2015;30(5):803-807.

21. Bhandari M, Matta JM, Dodgin D, et al: Outcomes following the single-incision anterior approach to total hip arthroplasty: A multicenter observational study. *Orthop Clin North Am* 2009;40(3):329-342.

22. Jameson SS, Mason J, Baker P, et al: A comparison of surgical approaches for primary hip arthroplasty: A cohort study of patient reported outcome measures (PROMs) and early revision using linked national databases. *J Arthroplasty* 2014;29(6):1248-1255.e1.

23. Sheth D, Cafri G, Inacio MC, Paxton EW, Namba RS: Anterior and anterolateral approaches for THA are associated with lower dislocation risk without higher revision risk. *Clin Orthop Relat Res* 2015;473(11):3401-3408.

24. Nakata K, Nishikawa M, Yamamoto K, Hirota S, Yoshikawa H: A clinical comparative study of the direct anterior with mini-posterior approach: Two consecutive series. *J Arthroplasty* 2009;24(5):698-704.

25. Rodriguez JA, Deshmukh AJ, Rathod PA, et al: Does the direct anterior approach in THA offer faster rehabilitation and comparable safety to the posterior approach? *Clin Orthop Relat Res* 2014;472(2):455-463.

26. Zawadsky MW, Paulus MC, Murray PJ, Johansen MA: Early outcome comparison between the direct anterior approach and the mini-incision posterior approach for primary total hip arthroplasty: 150 consecutive cases. *J Arthroplasty* 2014;29(6):1256-1260.

27. Poehling-Monaghan KL, Kamath AF, Taunton MJ, Pagnano MW: Direct anterior versus miniposterior THA with the same advanced perioperative protocols: Surprising early clinical results. *Clin Orthop Relat Res* 2015;473(2):623-631.

28. Restrepo C, Parvizi J, Pour AE, Hozack WJ: Prospective randomized study of two surgical approaches for total hip arthroplasty. *J Arthroplasty* 2010;25(5):671-9.e1.

29. Barrett WP, Turner SE, Leopold JP: Prospective randomized study of direct anterior vs postero-lateral approach for total hip arthroplasty. *J Arthroplasty* 2013;28(9):1634-1638.

30. Taunton MJ, Mason JB, Odum SM, Springer BD: Direct anterior total hip arthroplasty yields more rapid voluntary cessation of all walking aids: A prospective, randomized clinical trial. *J Arthroplasty* 2014;29(9 suppl):169-172.

31. Christensen CP, Jacobs CA: Comparison of patient function during the first six weeks after direct anterior or posterior total hip arthroplasty (THA): A randomized study. *J Arthroplasty* 2015;30(9 suppl):94-97.

32. Rathod PA, Bhalla S, Deshmukh AJ, Rodriguez JA: Does fluoroscopy with anterior hip arthroplasty decrease acetabular cup variability compared with a nonguided posterior approach? *Clin Orthop Relat Res* 2014;472(6):1877-1885.

33. Slotkin EM, Patel PD, Suarez JC: Accuracy of fluoroscopic guided acetabular component positioning during direct anterior total hip arthroplasty. *J Arthroplasty* 2015; 30(9 suppl):102-106.

34. de Steiger RN, Lorimer M, Solomon M: What is the learning curve for the anterior approach for total hip arthroplasty? *Clin Orthop Relat Res* 2015;473(12):3860-3866.

35. Masonis J, Thompson C, Odum S: Safe and accurate: Learning the direct anterior total hip arthroplasty. *Orthopedics* 2008;31(12 suppl 2).

36. Woolson ST, Pouliot MA, Huddleston JI: Primary total hip arthroplasty using an anterior approach and a fracture table: Short-term results from a community hospital. *J Arthroplasty* 2009;24(7):999-1005.

37. Jewett BA, Collis DK: High complication rate with anterior total hip arthroplasties on a fracture table. *Clin Orthop Relat Res* 2011;469(2):503-507.

38. Christensen CP, Karthikeyan T, Jacobs CA: Greater prevalence of wound complications requiring reoperation with direct anterior approach

total hip arthroplasty. *J Arthroplasty* 2014;29(9):1839-1841.

39. Bedard NA, Callaghan JJ, Stefl MD, Willman TJ, Liu SS, Goetz DD: Fixation and wear with a contemporary acetabular component and cross-linked polyethylene at minimum 10-year follow-up. *J Arthroplasty* 2014;29(10):1961-1969.

40. Poultsides LA, Sioros V, Anderson JA, Bruni D, Beksac B, Sculco TP: Ten- to 15-year clinical and radiographic results for a compression molded monoblock elliptical acetabular component. *J Arthroplasty* 2012;27(10):1850-1856.

41. Woo RY, Morrey BF: Dislocations after total hip arthroplasty. *J Bone Joint Surg Am* 1982;64(9):1295-1306.

42. Archbold HA, Mockford B, Molloy D, McConway J, Ogonda L, Beverland D: The transverse acetabular ligament: An aid to orientation of the acetabular component during primary total hip replacement. A preliminary study of 1000 cases investigating postoperative stability. *J Bone Joint Surg Br* 2006;88(7):883-886.

43. Kim YS, Callaghan JJ, Ahn PB, Brown TD: Fracture of the acetabulum during insertion of an oversized hemispherical component. *J Bone Joint Surg Am* 1995;77(1):111-117.

44. MacKenzie JR, Callaghan JJ, Pedersen DR, Brown TD: Areas of contact and extent of gaps with implantation of oversized acetabular components in total hip arthroplasty. *Clin Orthop Relat Res* 1994;298:127-136.

45. Hill JC, Gibson DP, Pagoti R, Beverland DE: Photographic measurement of the inclination of the acetabular component in total hip replacement using the posterior approach. *J Bone Joint Surg Br* 2010;92(9):1209-1214.

46. Wasielewski RC, Cooperstein LA, Kruger MP, Rubash HE: Acetabular anatomy and the transacetabular fixation of screws in total hip

arthroplasty. *J Bone Joint Surg Am* 1990;72(4):501-508.

47. Khanuja HS, Vakil JJ, Goddard MS, Mont MA: Cementless femoral fixation in total hip arthroplasty. *J Bone Joint Surg Am* 2011;93(5):500-509.

48. Burt CF, Garvin KL, Otterberg ET, Jardon OM: A femoral component inserted without cement in total hip arthroplasty: A study of the Tri-Lock component with an average ten-year duration of follow-up. *J Bone Joint Surg Am* 1998;80(7):952-960.

49. Sharkey PF, Albert TJ, Hume EL, Rothman RH: Initial stability of a collarless wedge-shaped prosthesis in the femoral canal. *Semin Arthroplasty* 1990;1(1):87-90.

50. Hozack WJ, Booth RE Jr: Clinical and radiographic results with the Trilock femoral component—a wedge-fit porous ingrowth stem design. *Semin Arthroplasty* 1990;1(1):64-69.

51. Vresilovic EJ, Hozack WJ, Rothman RH: Radiographic assessment of cementless femoral components: Correlation with intraoperative mechanical stability. *J Arthroplasty* 1994;9(2):137-141.

52. Sinha RK, Dungy DS, Yeon HB: Primary total hip arthroplasty with a proximally porous-coated femoral stem. *J Bone Joint Surg Am* 2004;86(6):1254-1261.

53. Luites JW, Spruit M, Hellemondt GG, Horstmann WG, Valstar ER: Failure of the uncoated titanium ProxiLock femoral hip prosthesis. *Clin Orthop Relat Res* 2006;448:79-86.

54. Engh CA, Hooten JP Jr, Zettl-Schaffer KF, Ghaffarpour M, McGovern TF, Bobyn JD: Evaluation of bone ingrowth in proximally and extensively porous-coated anatomic medullary locking prostheses retrieved at autopsy. *J Bone Joint Surg Am* 1995;77(6):903-910.

55. Epinette JA, Manley MT: Uncemented stems in hip

replacement—hydroxyapatite or plain porous: Does it matter? Based on a prospective study of HA Omnifit stems at 15-years minimum follow-up. *Hip Int* 2008;18(2):69-74.

56. Suckel A, Geiger F, Kinzl L, Wulker N, Garbrecht M: Long-term results for the uncemented Zweymuller/Alloclassic hip endoprosthesis: A 15-year minimum follow-up of 320 hip operations. *J Arthroplasty* 2009;24(6):846-853.

57. Cameron HU, Keppler L, McTighe T: The role of modularity in primary total hip arthroplasty. *J Arthroplasty* 2006;21(4 suppl 1):89-92.

58. McLaughlin JR, Lee KR: Total hip arthroplasty with an uncemented tapered femoral component. *J Bone Joint Surg Am* 2008;90(6):1290-1296.

59. Cooper HJ, Urban RM, Wixson RL, Meneghini RM, Jacobs JJ: Adverse local tissue reaction arising from corrosion at the femoral neck-body junction in a dual-taper stem with a cobalt-chromium modular neck. *J Bone Joint Surg Am* 2013;95(10):865-872.

60. Nebergall AK, Troelsen A, Rubash HE, Malchau H, Rolfson O, Greene ME: Five-year experience of vitamin e–diffused highly cross-linked polyethylene wear in total hip arthroplasty assessed by radiostereometric analysis. *J Arthroplasty* 2016;31(6):1251-1255.

61. Australian Orthopaedic Association National Joint Replacement Registry: 2015 Annual Report. Adelaide, South Australia, Australia, Australian Orthopaedic Association, 2015. Available at: https://aoanjrr.sahmri.com. Accessed May 3, 2016.

62. Bragdon CR, Doerner M, Martell J, et al: The 2012 John Charnley Award: Clinical multicenter studies of the wear performance of highly crosslinked remelted polyethylene in THA. *Clin Orthop Relat Res* 2013;471(2):393-402.

Arthroplasty for Unreconstructable Acute Fractures and Failed Fracture Fixation About the Hip and Knee in the Active Elderly: A New Paradigm

Richard F. Kyle, MD

Paul J. Duwelius, MD

George J. Haidukewych, MD

Andrew H. Schmidt, MD

Abstract

The techniques, materials, and designs for total joint arthroplasty underwent major improvements in the past 30 years. During this time, trauma surgeons classified the severity of fractures as well as identified certain articular fractures that do not have good outcomes and have a high rate of failure after internal fixation. Advanced improvements in arthroplasty have increased its reliability and longevity. Total joint arthroplasty is becoming a standard of care for some acute articular fractures, particularly displaced femoral neck fractures in the active elderly. Total joint arthroplasty also has become the standard of care after failed internal fixation in patients who have very complicated fractures about the knee, hip, and shoulder. As the population ages, fractures worldwide continue to rapidly increase. Elderly patients have a high risk for fractures that result from falls because of their poor bone quality. The current active elderly population participates in higher risk activities than previous elderly populations, which places them at risk for more injuries. This has become both a worldwide healthcare problem and an economic problem. Surgeons need to manage fractures in the active elderly with the latest advancements in technology and patient selection to ensure rapid recovery and the reduction of complications.

Instr Course Lect 2017;66:181–192.

Total joint arthroplasty has become the standard of care for articular fractures in active elderly patients who have a high failure rate after open reduction and internal fixation (ORIF). Surgeons should understand how to select fractures that will benefit from early arthroplasty as well as the appropriate total joint arthroplasty technique. Surgeons also should understand the techniques that are necessary to perform total joint arthroplasty in patients in whom ORIF fails.

Diagnosis and Prevention of Infection

Arthroplasty is increasingly being used to manage periarticular fractures in the elderly. Deep infection is one of the most severe complications after arthroplasty; therefore, surgeons who are contemplating total joint arthroplasty for the management of a fracture in a trauma patient must be adept at prevention and early diagnosis of infection to minimize associated morbidity.

Infection also is a problem in patients who undergo arthroplasty to salvage a fracture after previous surgery has failed. The risk of infection is more than double in patients who undergo revision joint arthroplasty compared with patients who undergo primary joint arthroplasty.[1] Likewise, the risk of infection is higher in patients who undergo total hip arthroplasty (THA) for the management of failed internal fixation of a femoral neck fracture compared with patients who undergo primary THA for the same diagnosis.[2] Infection is more common in joints in which previous surgery has failed because of bacterial biofilms on the surface of implants that were placed in the wound.

A surgeon should consider many factors in the evaluation of a patient who underwent prior surgery at the same site, including the appearance of prior incisions, the history of the patient's prior treatment, and the results of imaging and laboratory studies, to determine if ongoing sepsis is possible. Physical examination findings that indicate infection include pain, joint effusion, erythema, and wound drainage. Imaging findings that indicate infection are absent in patients who have acute infections; however, periostitis or lucencies may be observed on the imaging studies of patients who have chronic infections. CT scans or MRIs may demonstrate abscesses. C-reactive protein levels can be very helpful, especially if multiple values

that were obtained at different times are available.[3,4] Joint aspiration can be performed; however, both false-positive and false-negative results may occur. Specimens obtained during surgery can be sent for culture, histopathology, and molecular diagnostics.

Bachoura et al[5] reported that the strongest predictor for infection after fracture surgery was the number of prior surgeries. In a study that evaluated whether prior infection altered the outcome of knee arthroplasty after tibial plateau fracture, Larson et al[6] reported that 53% of previously infected patients sustained complications, and 26% of previously infected patients sustained recurrent infections. Previously infected knees were 4.1 times more likely to require additional procedures than knees with no previous infection.[6]

Methods are available to predict the risk of infection in patients who undergo total joint arthroplasty. Berbari et al[7] described the Mayo Prosthetic Joint Infection Risk Score, which incorporates multiple variables that are believed to affect a patient's risk of infection, including body mass index, prior surgery on the index joint, prior arthroplasty, immunosuppression, the American Society of Anesthesiologists Physical Classification score, and

procedure duration;[7] however, the Mayo Prosthetic Joint Infection Risk Score has not been validated.

It is easier to prevent infections than to manage them. Patients should undergo a thorough metabolic evaluation, including an assessment of their nutritional status (albumin levels, total protein levels, transferrin levels, and white blood cell count), endocrine state (vitamin D levels, thyroid function, parathyroid function, and glucose metabolism), tobacco use, and social circumstances, before any elective surgery. Adherence to surgical principles, including débridement, skeletal stability, and perioperative antibiotics, is critical. Local antibiotics can be added to bone cement and used with the so-called "bead-pouch" technique.[8] Free antibiotic powder can be placed in open wounds. A recent animal study reported that the use of antibiotic powder can reduce the risk of surgical site infection.[9] Perioperative wound care also is important. Newer perioperative wound care approaches that appear to decrease the risk of wound infections include the use of silver-impregnated dressings[10] and negative-pressure wound therapy.[11]

Salvage After Failed Management of Hip Fractures

Although most proximal femur fractures will heal after well-performed internal fixation, failure of fixation occasionally occurs. Effective salvage options are important to help restore function and minimize complications. In general, salvage options should be separated into those for the failed management of fractures of the femoral neck and fractures of the intertrochanteric region. Patient age and remaining bone stock also should be considered.

Dr. Kyle or an immediate family member has received royalties from DJ Orthopaedics, Smith & Nephew, and Zimmer; has stock or stock options held in Circle Biologics; and serves as a board member, owner, officer, or committee member of the Orthopaedic Research and Education Foundation and Excelen. Dr. Duwelius or an immediate family member has received royalties from Zimmer; is a member of a speakers' bureau or has made paid presentations on behalf of Signature HealthCARE; serves as a paid consultant to or is an employee of Zimmer; has stock or stock options held in UniteOR; has received research or institutional support from Providence Orthopedic Foundation, Providence Orthopedic Institute, and Zimmer; and serves as a board member, owner, officer, or committee member of the American Academy of Orthopaedic Surgeons and Operation Walk–Freedom to Move. Dr. Haidukewych or an immediate family member has received royalties from DePuy and Biomet; serves as a paid consultant to or is an employee of Biomet, DePuy, and Synthes; has stock or stock options held in OrthoPediatrics and the Institute for Better Bone Health; has received nonincome support (such as equipment or services), commercially derived honoraria, or other non–research-related funding (such as paid travel) from Synthes; and serves as a board member, owner, officer, or committee member of the American Academy of Orthopaedic Surgeons. Dr. Schmidt or an immediate family member serves as a paid consultant to or is an employee of Acumed, Bone Support AB, and St. Jude Medical; serves as an unpaid consultant to Twin Star Medical and Conventus Orthopaedics; has stock or stock options held in Conventus Orthopaedics, Epien Medical, Epix VAN, the International Spine and Orthopedic Institute, and Twin Star Medical; and serves as a board member, owner, officer, or committee member of the Orthopaedic Trauma Association.

Salvage for Failed Femoral Neck Fixation

Young Patients

In general, all salvage efforts for younger patients should focus on preservation of the native femoral neck. Nonunion of the femoral neck is typically the result of shear forces from a vertical femoral neck fracture that were not neutralized by the fixation device. A valgus osteotomy is typically indicated and can be successful, even in patients who have small patches of osteonecrosis. Valgus osteotomies convert shear stresses into compressive forces, which helps facilitate fracture union. In general, function after successful salvage is good; however, a persistent limp is common. The authors of this chapter generally reserve valgus osteotomy for patients younger than 40 years who do not have evidence of osteonecrosis. Various vascularized pedicle grafts have been used for the management of femoral neck nonunion in young patients; however, the authors of this chapter do not have experience with these techniques.

Older Patients

In general, THA is the most predictable reconstructive strategy for older patients in whom femoral neck fixation fails. Hemiarthroplasty may be reasonable in lower demand patients who have normal acetabular cartilage; however, THA offers more predictable pain relief and eliminates concerns for acetabular erosion. The surgeon should be prepared for very poor bone quality as a result of disuse osteopenia and osteoporosis. Surgeons should supplement uncemented acetabular component fixation with multiple screws and be prepared to cement the femoral component, if necessary. The authors of this chapter prefer to prepare the femur for an uncemented component, if possible. If poor broach stability as a result of a capacious femoral canal or severe osteopenia is noted, then cemented femoral component fixation should be selected. The surgeon should consider approaches that optimize hip stability, such as the anterolateral or anterior approach. The surgeon should use large-diameter femoral heads. The available literature reports good functional outcomes for patients who undergo THA for the management of failed femoral neck fixation.[2,12-20]

Salvage for Failed Intertrochanteric Fixation

Young Patients

Failed intertrochanteric fixation is rarely encountered in young patients; however, repeat internal fixation attempts with fixed angle devices (such as a 95° blade plate) and bone grafting are preferred. It is important to avoid varus of the proximal fragment and target the inferior femoral head bone, which usually has not been violated by prior fixation devices.

Older Patients

THA is the preferred reconstructive strategy for older patients in whom intertrochanteric fixation fails. The decision of whether to perform hemiarthroplasty or THA depends on a patient's activity level, the condition of the remaining acetabular cartilage, and whether the acetabulum was damaged after the previous fixation device was removed. In general, the authors of this chapter prefer THA because it offers more predictable pain relief. The surgeon should dislocate the hip before removing hardware to avoid fracture of the femoral shaft. Because of bone defects, long stems to bypass femoral shaft stress risers and calcar replacement stems or modular stems may be necessary. The surgeon should bypass the most distal femoral stress riser by two diaphyseal diameters (approximately 6 cm). Deformity of the proximal femur may require an extended trochanteric osteotomy to allow access to the femoral canal. A high-speed burr can be used to remove sclerotic hardware tracts, which can deflect reamers as well as broaches and lead to femoral perforation. The use of intraoperative fluoroscopy may be beneficial. Greater trochanteric fixation must be stable. The results of arthroplasty for the management of failed intertrochanteric fixation are generally good; however, trochanteric complaints are common.[12-14,21]

Total Knee Replacement for Failed Tibial Plateau Fixation

The rate of degenerative joint disease in patients who undergo treatment for tibial plateau fractures is high. At a 7.6-year follow-up, Honkonen[22] reported a 44% rate of posttraumatic arthritis in 131 tibial plateau fractures. Higher rates of degenerative changes in patients who have tibial plateau fractures are correlated with advanced age, meniscal resection, and residual deformity (**Figure 1**).

Preoperative planning is essential. The surgeon must obtain a patient's C-reactive protein levels and erythrocyte sedimentation rate to rule out infection. The surgeon should perform a knee aspiration because a low white blood cell count can be used to rule out infection. A white blood cell count greater than 1,100 cells/µL for fluid leukocyte count and greater than 64% for neutrophil differential indicates an ongoing infection.[23] Preoperative planning also includes identification

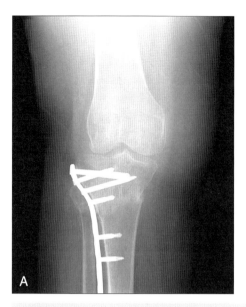
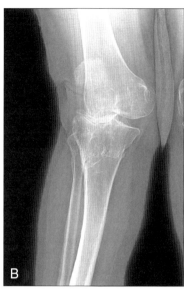

Figure 1 Radiographs of the knee of a patient who had a tibial plateau fracture. **A,** AP view demonstrates treatment of the tibial plateau fracture with a locked plate. **B,** Lateral view taken after healing and plate removal at 6-year follow-up demonstrates posttraumatic arthritis.

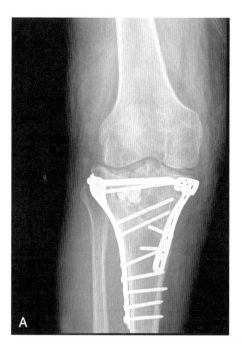
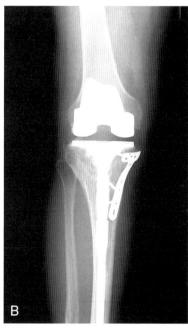

Figure 2 AP radiographs of the knee of a patient who had a severely displaced comminuted tibial plateau fracture. **A,** Radiograph taken after open reduction and internal fixation of the tibial plateau fracture demonstrates failed reconstruction and grafting. **B,** Radiograph taken after total knee replacement with partial hardware removal and the use of a long tibial stem demonstrates stabilization of the tibial component despite bone deficiency.

previous hardware is removed. Augments should be available to address bone loss. Revision stems should be available to bypass stress risers left after previous hardware removal (**Figure 2**). Deformity may require tissue balancing. A posterior stabilized knee is necessary in patients who have loss of the posterior cruciate ligament. The authors of this chapter recommend hardware removal only if absolutely necessary. The equipment required for hardware removal must be specific to the implant being removed. If only a screw tip or a small piece of hardware is present, a high-speed pneumatic drill should be available to facilitate removal.

The technique should use the previous incision, if possible. If use of the previous incision is not possible, care must be taken during placement of a new incision near the densely scarred area to prevent vascular compromise of the skin, which can cause skin necrosis. The surgeon should attain wide exposure of the knee by extending the quadriceps-splitting incision proximally as necessary. The surgeon will encounter scar tissue, particularly on the capsule and the ligaments, which may be scarred against the injured tibial plateau. For this reason, the patellar ligament must be protected with a retractor during tibial resection. Care must be taken to preserve the entire extensor mechanism during surgery. Antibiotic-impregnated cement is used during insertion of the total knee implant to decrease the risk of infection.

Few clinical studies are available on the outcomes of total knee arthroplasty (TKA) for the management of failed tibial plateau fixation. Wound complications, extensor mechanism disruption, and infection rates are much higher in patients who undergo TKA for the

of the equipment necessary to remove previous hardware. The surgeon must evaluate bone defects, deformity, and stress risers that may be left after management of failed tibial plateau fixation compared with patients who undergo primary knee replacement. In a study of 62 patients who underwent TKA for the management of failed tibial plateau fixation, Weiss et al[24] reported complications, including stiffness, wound problems (three patients), infection (superficial, two patients; deep, two patients), patellar subluxation, hematoma, reflex sympathetic dystrophy, deep vein thrombosis, and medial collateral ligament deficiency, in 16 patients (**Figure 3**). The authors reported extensor mechanism disruption in five patients, all of whom required manipulation. The mean range of motion improved from 99.2° to 102.5°. In a study of 15 patients who underwent TKA for the management of failed tibial plateau fixation, Saleh et al[25] reported infection in three patients, extensor mechanism disruption in two patients, and wound problems in four patients. Manipulation was required in three patients. The mean range of motion improved from 87° to 105°. All of Saleh et al's[25] TKAs had undergone previous surgery, and only one-half of Weiss et al's[24] TKAs had undergone previous surgery.

Total knee replacement for the management of failed tibial plateau fixation is difficult and comparable with revision TKA. Preoperative planning is essential to ensure that proper equipment, including augments as well as long stems to fill defects and bypass stress risers, is available. Exposure is difficult because of previous scarring and should be extensile. Complications are higher in patients who undergo total knee replacement for the management of failed tibial plateau fixation compared with patients who undergo primary knee replacement and can be minimized by removing only the hardware necessary

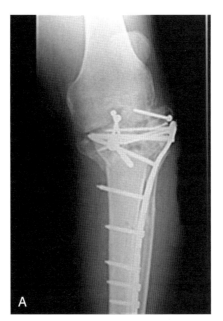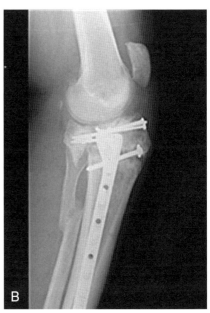

Figure 3   AP (**A**) and lateral (**B**) radiographs of a knee with a comminuted tibial plateau fracture that was converted to total knee arthroplasty after failed open reduction and internal fixation demonstrate posttraumatic arthritis.

to allow for placement of the new implant components. Overall, the results of total knee replacement for the management of failed tibial plateau fixation can be satisfactory if the surgeon pays attention to detail.

Cases in Which Arthroplasty Alone Should Not Be an Option

Patients who have undergone THA may be more at risk for fracture because of their age, sex, and preexisting conditions. The risk for osteolysis, loosening, and the progression of osteoporosis rise as a patient ages, which not only increases the likelihood of fracture but also complicates the management of periprosthetic fractures if they occur.[26] A total hip replacement that has been implanted for an extended period of time inevitably leads to polyethylene wear and the possibility of subsequent osteolysis, which can be compounded by osteoporosis. Patients with total hip

replacements may have impaired cellular function at the osteoblast level and impaired cytokine function. All these factors may increase a patient's risk for periprosthetic fracture and complicate treatment. Berry[27] reported that 9.5% of revision surgeries after THA were attributed to periprosthetic hip (PPH) fracture. The author also reported that surgically managed PPH fractures were associated with a 1-year mortality rate of 11%.[27]

The management of PPH fractures requires a basic understanding of PPH fracture classification.[28-37] The Vancouver classification system was developed to assist surgeons in the successful management of PPH fractures.[28] Typically, more proximal femur fractures are Vancouver type B2 fractures. In a study of PPH fractures from the Swedish National Hip Arthroplasty Register, Lindahl et al[34] reported that 53% of the PPH fractures were Vancouver type B2 fractures, and 4% of

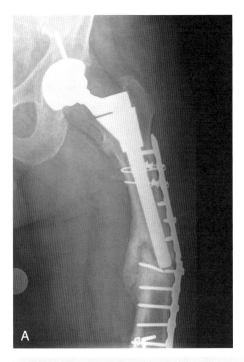
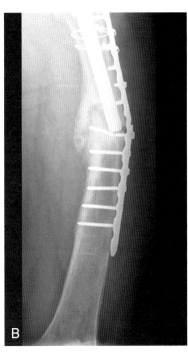

Figure 4 AP radiographs of the hip (**A**) and femur (**B**) of a patient who had a transverse periprosthetic hip fracture pattern that was fixed with a stable implant interface demonstrate nonunion at the tip of the fracture and plate breakage.

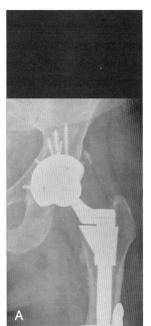
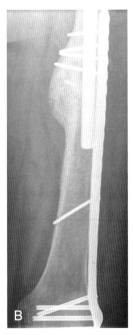
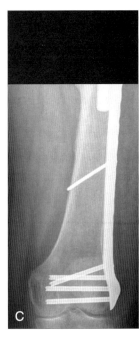

Figure 5 AP radiographs of the hip (**A**), femur (**B**), and knee (**C**) of the same patient shown in Figure 4 demonstrate revision of the prosthesis to a longer stem implant that extends past the fracture and replating of the nonunion with a longer supracondylar plate to eliminate transition zones.

the PPH fractures were Vancouver type B3 fractures. Bhattacharyya et al[38] reviewed PPH fractures from trauma and surgical registries and reported similar results: 1% of the PPH fractures were Vancouver type A fractures, 21% of the PPH fractures were Vancouver type B1 fractures, 41% of the PPH fractures were Vancouver type B2 fractures, 8% of the PPH fractures were Vancouver type B3 fractures, and 30% of the PPH fractures were Vancouver type C fractures. Seventy percent of patients with PPH fractures have a loose prosthesis, which is discovered either on preoperative radiographs or at the time of surgery.[35] If the stem is unstable, then the prosthesis needs to be revised to an implant with a longer stem.[26] If the implant interface is stable and the implant is well fixed at the bone-cement or implant-bone interface, then the fracture needs to be managed with a plate device.[39] Mulay et al[36] reviewed Vancouver type B2 and type B3 PPH fractures that were revised to a tapered, fluted, long-stem femoral implant. A transverse fracture at the stem tip is extremely unstable biomechanically and can lead to nonunion.[33,40] Regardless of whether an implant is stable or unstable, the risk for subsequent failure with the use of plate fixation alone is high. An example of successful management of a PPH fracture with nonunion is illustrated in **Figures 4**, **5**, and **6**. The initial stem was stable; however, the transverse fracture pattern at the stem tip required revision of the stem sleeve and replating because of initial plate fixation failure.

It is important for surgeons to correctly assess whether an implant is stable or unstable. Unstable implant interface fractures require revision for a successful treatment outcome. Stable fractures can be managed with plate fixation because the preexisting implant precludes intramedullary nail fixation. The management of PPH fractures requires surgeons to have expertise in both fracture management and revision THA. Surgeons may expect PPH fractures to change if osteolysis rates decline as a result of highly cross-linked polyethylene components. Future demand for the management of PPH fractures necessitates that they be emphasized in total joint adult reconstruction and trauma residency and fellowship programs.

Acetabular Fractures

The Role of Arthroplasty

In general, acetabular fractures are managed using ORIF, with the goals of anatomic reduction and preservation of the native hip joint. THA plays a role in the management of acetabular fractures in two general situations: for an acute fracture in an elderly patient with joint impaction in whom internal fixation attempts are likely to fail and for sequelae of an acetabular fracture, namely posttraumatic arthritis and osteonecrosis. Acute THA can provide effective, durable reconstruction in select patients. Three-dimensional CT reconstruction can help guide decision making. Patients who have acetabular dome impaction may exhibit the so-called "gull sign," which is predictive of early failure of internal fixation. Acute THA is the preferred reconstructive strategy for an elderly patient in whom acetabular dome impaction or severe femoral head impaction is noted. Preoperative medical optimization is recommended because acute THA can be a lengthy surgical procedure that involves extensive blood loss. Restoration of columnar continuity, typically with the use of posterior column plates

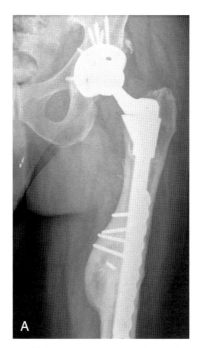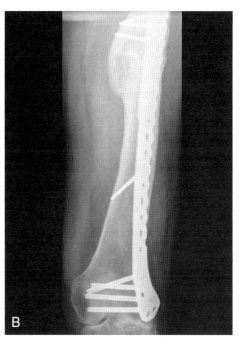

Figure 6   AP radiographs of the hip (**A**) and femur (**B**) of the same patient shown in Figures 4 and 5 that were taken 1.5 years postoperatively demonstrate successful union and healing of the periprosthetic hip fracture.

and uncemented acetabular components with screw fixation, remains the preferred surgical strategy. Enhanced metals (trabecular tantalum or titanium) may be considered because cavitary and segmental bony deficiency are commonly present. Liberal autograft from the resected femoral head is applied to any bony defects. Typically, low anterior column fractures can be ignored. Fixation should prioritize stabilization of the ilium to the ischium via posterior columnar plate fixation. Anterior column fixation is rarely necessary. Femoral reconstruction is typically routine. The authors of this chapter prefer that patients undergo 6 to 8 weeks of protected weight bearing postoperatively.

THA also plays a role in the management of sequelae of acetabular fractures, namely posttraumatic arthritis and osteonecrosis. Surgeons must be prepared to manage heterotopic bone, scars, bony defects, and retained hardware in the

management of sequelae of acetabular fractures. Preoperative CT can assist in locating heterotopic bone and hardware, which may influence the surgical approach. Typically, hardware can be left in situ. The authors of this chapter prefer to leave hardware in situ and remove screws only if they are encountered during reaming. A high-speed burr can be used to cut away screws within the acetabulum, after which reaming can continue to the desired size. Enhanced metal acetabular components and multiple screws are generally recommended to improve fixation in challenging patients. Femoral reconstruction is routine. Careful attention to detail is required to improve outcomes and avoid complications. The available literature reports excellent results in patients who undergo THA for the management of sequelae of acetabular fractures; however, surgeons should expect a higher rate of complications.[41-43]

THA for Failed Fixation of Acetabular Fractures

Several studies have reported improved survivorship in patients who undergo ORIF for the management of acetabular fractures.[44-49] However, because of the severity of acetabular fractures, it is not uncommon for patients who undergo ORIF for the management of acetabular fractures to eventually require THA. Patients who undergo THA for previously managed acetabular fractures tend to have higher complication rates compared with patients who undergo primary THA.[42,49-59]

Studies have described the use of a variety of components in patients who undergo THA for previously managed acetabular fractures. Cemented acetabular cups are associated with a higher complication rate in patients who undergo THA for previously managed acetabular fractures, with a reported failure rate of up to 40% as a result of aseptic loosening, which is especially relevant for younger patients.[54,60] Currently, there is debate on the outcome variance between one-stage and two-stage surgery as well as the protocol for hardware removal.

The available literature allows for a review of the treatment guidelines for patients who undergo THA for previously managed acetabular fractures. In a study of patients who underwent THA for the management of osteoarthritis that developed after ORIF of an acetabular fracture, Weber et al[60] reported that uncemented acetabular cups were superior to cemented acetabular cups. In a 20-year follow-up study, von Roth et al[55] reported that uncemented acetabular cups were successful in patients who underwent THA for the management of posttraumatic arthritis that developed after ORIF of an acetabular

fracture; however, the rates of polyethylene wear and osteolysis were less than satisfactory. The authors speculated that the results of THA for patients in whom posttraumatic arthritis developed after ORIF of an acetabular fracture would improve with the use of newer bearing surfaces and remodeled metal surfaces.[55] Bellabarba et al[42] compared the outcomes of patients who underwent single-stage THA with uncemented acetabular cups for the management of posttraumatic arthritis that developed after ORIF of an acetabular fracture with the outcomes of patients who underwent the same procedure for the management of nontraumatic arthritis that developed after closed management of an acetabular fracture. The authors reported that surgical time, blood loss, transfusion requirements, hip instability, and complications were higher in the posttraumatic arthritis group compared with the nontraumatic arthritis group. Fifty percent of the patients in the posttraumatic arthritis group required a nontraditional polyethylene acetabular liner. Harris hip scores improved dramatically in both groups, and 90% of the patients in the posttraumatic arthritis group had an excellent or good outcome.

Determination of a best-practice surgical technique for THA in patients with a previously managed acetabular fracture requires a thorough review of the orthopaedic literature. Routine assessment of patients for complications via radiographic imaging and infection identification improves preoperative planning. Surgical techniques include careful avoidance of hardware and selective removal of hardware that precludes accurate reaming or acetabular cup placement. Staged THA is not necessary for the successful treatment

of patients with a previously managed acetabular fracture and involves risks associated with secondary surgery. Additional screw fixation of the acetabular cup decreases the likelihood of aseptic loosening. The use of highly porous acetabular cups and highly cross-linked polyethylene may improve long-term outcomes.

The outcomes of patients who undergo THA for a previously managed acetabular fracture may not be as successful compared with those of patients who undergo primary THA. Patients with a previously managed acetabular fracture can undergo single-stage THA that is performed via a single incision. Hardware should be removed as necessary. The current standard of care for patients who undergo THA for a previously managed acetabular fracture involves the use of uncemented acetabular components. The use of highly porous uncemented acetabular components that are supplemented with multiple screw fixation, highly cross-linked polyethylene liners, and single-stage surgery with selective hardware removal can help improve the outcomes of patients who undergo THA for a previously managed acetabular fracture.

THA for Acute Displaced Femoral Neck Fractures

Hip fractures worldwide are increasing exponentially. The management of femoral neck fractures with ORIF has led to an overall failure rate of 30%, which has not changed since 1937 when Speed[61] reported his results of ORIF in patients who had hip fractures.

To properly manage femoral neck fractures, surgeons must decide if a fracture should be fixed or if a prosthesis is required (**Figure 7**). At the time that the type of prosthesis is selected, surgeons also must determine if hemiarthroplasty or THA should be performed. THA has become a viable option for the management of femoral neck fractures in the active elderly as a result of advances made in THA techniques, materials, and designs, all of which have increased the reliability and longevity of THA.

The literature supports internal fixation in patients who have nondisplaced femoral neck fractures and in physiologically young patients.[16-18] The current literature has shown that ORIF of displaced femoral neck fractures results in failure and revision surgery in 30% of elderly patients.[16,19,20] Performing arthroplasty instead of internal fixation in patients with femoral neck fractures who have comorbidities, including renal disease, diabetes mellitus, rheumatoid arthritis, and severe osteoporosis, can substantially reduce the rate of revision surgery. The physiologic age and activity level of a patient are important considerations in selection of the appropriate surgical procedure. Anatomic reduction is the single most important factor that prevents failure after ORIF.[62] Patients with a femoral neck fracture that is left in varus have a high failure rate and will require revision surgery regardless of age or comorbidities.

A prosthesis should be used to treat most patients physiologically older than 65 years who have displaced femoral neck fractures.[15-18] THA should be considered in patients who are active and healthy,[15,16,19,20] which includes older patients who are physiologically younger than their chronologic age (**Figure 8**). A hemiprosthesis should be considered in elderly patients who have multiple comorbidities and are relatively inactive or lower level community ambulators. Yu et al[20] reported that THA should

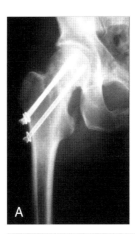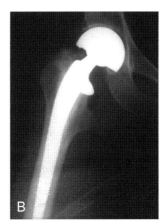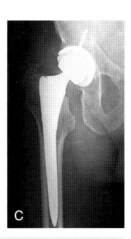

Figure 7   AP hip radiographs demonstrate options for the successful treatment of femoral neck fractures. **A,** Radiograph demonstrates successful open reduction and internal fixation of a displaced femoral neck fracture. **B,** Radiograph demonstrates successful hemiarthroplasty in an elderly patient who had a displaced femoral neck fracture. **C,** Radiograph demonstrates successful total joint arthroplasty in a patient who had a displaced femoral neck fracture.

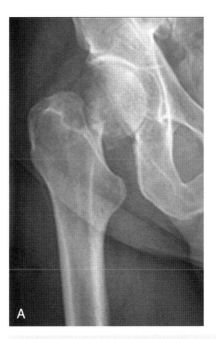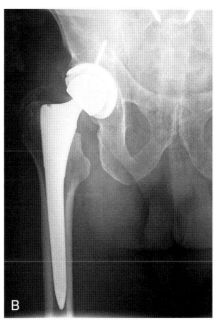

Figure 8   **A,** AP radiograph of the hip of an 82-year-old-man who is very active and has no comorbidities demonstrates a displaced femoral neck fracture. **B,** AP radiograph taken 6 months after total hip arthroplasty demonstrates that the procedure was successful. The patient is able to ambulate without a limp or pain.

be the surgery of choice for active elderly patients because it allows for better function and lower revision surgery rates compared with hemiarthroplasty. Despite these conclusions, surgeons

should always involve the patient in the decision-making process.

The technique for THA in elderly patients who have a displaced femoral neck fracture is important. Care must

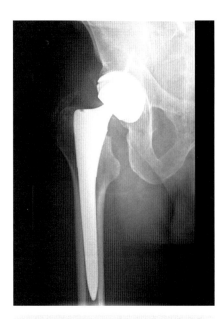

Figure 9 AP radiograph of the hip of an elderly patient in whom a press-fit implant was successfully fixed with the use of a large femoral head and capsular repair. The anterolateral approach was used in this patient to reduce the incidence of dislocation.

be taken avoid using excessive force and overreaming of the acetabulum. A base of bleeding subchondral bone may be left in patients who have severe osteoporosis to ensure sufficient stability of the acetabular shell. The surgeon should use the largest femoral head that matches the size of the shell to prevent dislocation. Care must be taken to not use excessive force when rasping the femur, which may result in fracture of the proximal femur. A cemented rather than a press-fit prosthesis may be preferred for fixation in patients who have severe osteoporosis. The choice of a cemented versus press-fit prosthesis for fixation of the femoral component depends, to a large extent, on the skill set and experience of the surgeon as well as the bone quality of the proximal femur. Many surgeons prefer to use the anterior or anterolateral approach to reduce dislocation. Some surgeons may prefer to use the posterior approach because it is more familiar; however, care must be taken to repair the capsule, which helps prevent dislocation. Current studies have reported that the use of a large femoral head in combination with capsular repair as well as selection of an approach with which a surgeon is familiar have reduced the dislocation rate to 1% to 2%.[63-66]

Low-level nursing home or community ambulators who are not expected to live longer than 6 to 7 years are candidates for hemiarthroplasty. Ravikumar and Marsh[18] reported a 24% revision surgery rate at a 13-year follow-up of patients who underwent hemiarthroplasty for the management of displaced femur fractures. Most patients underwent revision surgery within 7 years postoperatively. THA should be considered in active elderly patients with displaced femur fractures who have few comorbidities because it not only is cost effective but also provides the best pain relief, best function, and fastest rehabilitation of all the management options for displaced femoral neck fractures[19] (**Figure 9**). The management of femoral neck fractures remains a challenge, and surgeons must select the appropriate treatment based on fracture displacement as well as the physiologic age and comorbidities of the patient. THA is the best option for active elderly patients who have displaced femur fractures.

Summary

Total joint arthroplasty has become the standard of care after failed ORIF of select fractures in active elderly patients. Improvements in the techniques, materials, and designs for total joint arthroplasty in the past 30 years have increased its reliability and longevity. In addition, studies have identified that high-risk fractures, most of which frequently occur about the hip, knee, and shoulder, have a high rate of failure, particularly in the elderly. Patients with select fractures who undergo early total joint arthroplasty have better outcomes and a faster rehabilitation compared with patients who undergo ORIF. Special techniques and equipment are necessary to manage most fractures in which ORIF fails.

References

1. Hanssen AD, Rand JA: Evaluation and treatment of infection at the site of a total hip or knee arthroplasty. *Instr Course Lect* 1999;48:111-122.

2. McKinley JC, Robinson CM: Treatment of displaced intracapsular hip fractures with total hip arthroplasty: Comparison of primary arthroplasty with early salvage arthroplasty after failed internal fixation. *J Bone Joint Surg Am* 2002;84(11):2010-2015.

3. Alijanipour P, Bakhshi H, Parvizi J: Diagnosis of periprosthetic joint infection: The threshold for serological markers. *Clin Orthop Relat Res* 2013;471(10):3186-3195.

4. Neumaier M, Scherer MA: C-reactive protein levels for early detection of postoperative infection after fracture surgery in 787 patients. *Acta Orthop* 2008;79(3):428-432.

5. Bachoura A, Guitton TG, Smith RM, Vrahas MS, Zurakowski D, Ring D: Infirmity and injury complexity are risk factors for surgical-site infection after operative fracture care. *Clin Orthop Relat Res* 2011;469(9):2621-2630.

6. Larson AN, Hanssen AD, Cass JR: Does prior infection alter the outcome of TKA after tibial plateau fracture? *Clin Orthop Relat Res* 2009;467(7):1793-1799.

7. Berbari EF, Osmon DR, Lahr B, et al: The Mayo prosthetic joint infection risk score: Implication for surgical site infection reporting and risk stratification. *Infect Control Hosp Epidemiol* 2012;33(8):774-781.

8. Henry SL, Ostermann PA, Seligson D: The antibiotic bead pouch technique: The management of severe compound fractures. *Clin Orthop Relat Res* 1993;295:54-62.

9. Zebala LP, Chuntarapas T, Kelly MP, Talcott M, Greco S, Riew KD: Intrawound vancomycin powder eradicates surgical wound contamination: An in vivo rabbit study. *J Bone Joint Surg Am* 2014;96(1):46-51.

10. Jones SA, Bowler PG, Walker M, Parsons D: Controlling wound bioburden with a novel silver-containing Hydrofiber dressing. *Wound Repair Regen* 2004;12(3):288-294.

11. Schlatterer DR, Hirschfeld AG, Webb LX: Negative pressure wound therapy in grade IIIB tibial fractures: Fewer infections and fewer flap procedures? *Clin Orthop Relat Res* 2015;473(5):1802-1811.

12. Haidukewych GJ, Berry DJ: Salvage of failed treatment of hip fractures. *J Am Acad Orthop Surg* 2005;13(2):101-109.

13. Haidukewych GJ, Berry DJ: Salvage of failed internal fixation of intertrochanteric hip fractures. *Clin Orthop Relat Res* 2003;412:184-188.

14. Haidukewych GJ, Berry DJ: Hip arthroplasty for salvage of failed treatment of intertrochanteric hip fractures. *J Bone Joint Surg Am* 2003;85(5):899-904.

15. Keating JF, Grant A, Masson M, Scott NW, Forbes JF: Randomized comparison of reduction and fixation, bipolar hemiarthroplasty, and total hip arthroplasty: Treatment of displaced intracapsular hip fractures in healthy older patients. *J Bone Joint Surg Am* 2006;88(2):249-260.

16. Bhandari M, Devereaux PJ, Swiontkowski MF, et al: Internal fixation compared with arthroplasty for displaced fractures of the femoral neck: A meta-analysis. *J Bone Joint Surg Am* 2003;85(9):1673-1681.

17. Lu-Yao GL, Keller RB, Littenberg B, Wennberg JE: Outcomes after displaced fractures of the femoral neck: A meta-analysis of one hundred and six published reports. *J Bone Joint Surg Am* 1994;76(1):15-25.

18. Ravikumar KJ, Marsh G: Internal fixation versus hemiarthroplasty versus total hip arthroplasty for displaced subcapital fractures of femur—13 year results of a prospective randomised study. *Injury* 2000;31(10):793-797.

19. Iorio R, Healy WL, Lemos DW, Appleby D, Lucchesi CA, Saleh KJ: Displaced femoral neck fractures in the elderly: Outcomes and cost effectiveness. *Clin Orthop Relat Res* 2001;383:229-242.

20. Yu L, Wang Y, Chen J: Total hip arthroplasty versus hemiarthroplasty for displaced femoral neck fractures: Meta-analysis of randomized trials. *Clin Orthop Relat Res* 2012;470(8):2235-2243.

21. Mabry TM, Prpa B, Haidukewych GJ, Harmsen WS, Berry DJ: Long-term results of total hip arthroplasty for femoral neck fracture nonunion. *J Bone Joint Surg Am* 2004;86(10):2263-2267.

22. Honkonen SE: Degenerative arthritis after tibial plateau fractures. *J Orthop Trauma* 1995;9(4):273-277.

23. Parvizi J, Ghanem E, Sharkey P, Aggarwal A, Burnett RS, Barrack RL: Diagnosis of infected total knee: Findings of a multicenter database. *Clin Orthop Relat Res* 2008;466(11):2628-2633.

24. Weiss NG, Parvizi J, Trousdale RT, Bryce RD, Lewallen DG: Total knee arthroplasty in patients with a prior fracture of the tibial plateau. *J Bone Joint Surg Am* 2003;85(2):218-221.

25. Saleh KJ, Sherman P, Katkin P, et al: Total knee arthroplasty after open reduction and internal fixation of fractures of the tibial plateau: A minimum five-year follow-up study. *J Bone Joint Surg Am* 2001;83(8):1144-1148.

26. Shah RP, Sheth NP, Gray C, Alosh H, Garino JP: Periprosthetic fractures around loose femoral components. *J Am Acad Orthop Surg* 2014;22(8):482-490.

27. Berry DJ: Periprosthetic fractures associated with osteolysis: A problem on the rise. *J Arthroplasty* 2003;18(3, suppl 1):107-111.

28. Garbuz DS, Masri BA, Duncan CP: Periprosthetic fractures of the femur: Principles of prevention and management. *Instr Course Lect* 1998;47:237-242.

29. Beals RK, Tower SS: Periprosthetic fractures of the femur: An analysis of 93 fractures. *Clin Orthop Relat Res* 1996;327:238-246.

30. Duwelius PJ, Schmidt AH, Kyle RF, Talbott V, Ellis TJ, Butler JB: A prospective, modernized treatment protocol for periprosthetic femur fractures. *Orthop Clin North Am* 2004;35(4):485-492, vi.

31. Kelley SS: Periprosthetic femoral fractures. *J Am Acad Orthop Surg* 1994;2(3):164-172.

32. Moran MC: Treatment of periprosthetic fractures around total hip arthroplasty with an extensively coated femoral component. *J Arthroplasty* 1996;11(8):981-988.

33. Lewallen DG, Berry DJ: Periprosthetic fracture of the femur after total hip arthroplasty: Treatment and results to date. *Instr Course Lect* 1998;47:243-249.

34. Lindahl H, Garellick G, Regnér H, Herberts P, Malchau H: Three hundred and twenty-one periprosthetic femoral fractures. *J Bone Joint Surg Am* 2006;88(6):1215-1222.

35. Pike J, Davidson D, Garbuz D, Duncan CP, O'Brien PJ, Masri BA: Principles of treatment for periprosthetic femoral shaft fractures around well-fixed total hip arthroplasty. *J Am Acad Orthop Surg* 2009;17(11):677-688.

36. Mulay S, Hassan T, Birtwistle S, Power R: Management of types B2 and B3 femoral periprosthetic fractures by a tapered, fluted, and distally fixed stem. *J Arthroplasty* 2005;20(6):751-756.

37. Lindahl H, Malchau H, Herberts P, Garellick G: Periprosthetic femoral fractures classification and demographics of 1049 periprosthetic femoral fractures from the Swedish National Hip Arthroplasty Register. *J Arthroplasty* 2005;20(7):857-865.

38. Bhattacharyya T, Chang D, Meigs JB, Estok DM II, Malchau H: Mortality after periprosthetic fracture of the femur. *J Bone Joint Surg Am* 2007;89(12):2658-2662.

39. Crockarell JR Jr, Berry DJ, Lewallen DG: Nonunion after periprosthetic femoral fracture associated with total

hip arthroplasty. *J Bone Joint Surg Am* 1999;81(8):1073-1079.

40. Cook RE, Jenkins PJ, Walmsley PJ, Patton JT, Robinson CM: Risk factors for periprosthetic fractures of the hip: A survivorship analysis. *Clin Orthop Relat Res* 2008;466(7):1652-1656.

41. Anglen JO, Burd TA, Hendricks KJ, Harrison P: The "Gull Sign": A harbinger of failure for internal fixation of geriatric acetabular fractures. *J Orthop Trauma* 2003;17(9):625-634.

42. Bellabarba C, Berger RA, Bentley CD, et al: Cementless acetabular reconstruction after acetabular fracture. *J Bone Joint Surg Am* 2001;83(6):868-876.

43. Pagenkopf E, Grose A, Partal G, Helfet DL: Acetabular fractures in the elderly: Treatment recommendations. *HSS J* 2006;2(2):161-171.

44. Matta JM: Fractures of the acetabulum: Accuracy of reduction and clinical results in patients managed operatively within three weeks after the injury. *J Bone Joint Surg Am* 1996;78(11):1632-1645.

45. Matta JM, Merritt PO: Displaced acetabular fractures. *Clin Orthop Relat Res* 1988;230:83-97.

46. Letournel E: Acetabulum fractures: Classification and management. *Clin Orthop Relat Res* 1980;151:81-106.

47. Letournel E, Lytle JO: Open reduction internal fixation of acetabulum fractures: Long-term results and analysis of 960 cases. *Presented at the Annual Meeting of the American Academy of Orthopaedic Surgeons*, San Francisco, CA, February 19, 1993.

48. Mayo KA: Open reduction and internal fixation of fractures of the acetabulum: Results in 163 fractures. *Clin Orthop Relat Res* 1994;305:31-37.

49. Carnesale PG, Stewart MJ, Barnes SN: Acetabular disruption and central fracture-dislocation of the hip: A long-term study. *J Bone Joint Surg Am* 1975;57(8):1054-1059.

50. Boardman KP, Charnley J: Low-friction arthroplasty after fracture-dislocations of the hip. *J Bone Joint Surg Br* 1978;60(4):495-497.

51. Harris WH: Traumatic arthritis of the hip after dislocation and acetabular fractures: Treatment by mold arthroplasty. An end-result study using a new method of result evaluation. *J Bone Joint Surg Am* 1969;51(4):737-755.

52. Karpos PA, Christie MJ, Chenger JD: Total hip arthroplasty following acetabular fracture: The effect of prior open reduction, internal fixation. *Orthop Trans* 1993;17:589.

53. Rogan IM, Weber FA, Solomon L: Total hip replacement following fracture dislocation of the acetabulum: From the Proceedings of the South African Orthopaedic Association. *J Bone Joint Surg Br* 1979;61(2):252.

54. Romness DW, Lewallen DG: Total hip arthroplasty after fracture of the acetabulum: Long-term results. *J Bone Joint Surg Br* 1990;72(5):761-764.

55. von Roth P, Abdel MP, Harmsen WS, Berry DJ: Total hip arthroplasty after operatively treated acetabular fracture: A concise follow-up, at a mean of twenty years, of a previous report. *J Bone Joint Surg Am* 2015;97(4):288-291.

56. Berger RA, Kull LR, Rosenberg AG, Galante JO: Hybrid total hip arthroplasty: 7- to 10-year results. *Clin Orthop Relat Res* 1996;333:134-146.

57. Mohler CG, Kull LR, Martell JM, Rosenberg AG, Galante JO: Total hip replacement with insertion of an acetabular component without cement and a femoral component with cement: Four to seven-year results. *J Bone Joint Surg Am* 1995;77(1):86-96.

58. Stauffer RN: Ten-year follow-up study of total hip replacement. *J Bone Joint Surg Am* 1982;64(7):983-990.

59. Tompkins GS, Jacobs JJ, Kull LR, Rosenberg AG, Galante JO: Primary total hip arthroplasty with a porous-coated acetabular component: Seven-to-ten-year results. *J Bone Joint Surg Am* 1997;79(2):169-176.

60. Weber M, Berry DJ, Harmsen WS: Total hip arthroplasty after operative treatment of an acetabular fracture. *J Bone Joint Surg Am* 1998;80(9):1295-1305.

61. Speed K: Untoward results in the treatment of fractures. *N Engl J Med* 1937;217(23):908-909.

62. Weinrobe M, Stankewich CJ, Mueller B, Tencer AF: Predicting the mechanical outcome of femoral neck fractures fixed with cancellous screws: An in vivo study. *J Orthop Trauma* 1998;12(1):27-37.

63. White RE Jr, Forness TJ, Allman JK, Junick DW: Effect of posterior capsular repair on early dislocation in primary total hip replacement. *Clin Orthop Relat Res* 2001;393:163-167.

64. Berry DJ, von Knock M, Schleck CD, Harmsen WS: Effect of femoral head diameter and operative approach on risk of dislocation after primary total hip arthroplasty. *J Bone Joint Surg Am* 2005;87(11):2456-2463.

65. Peters CL, McPherson E, Jackson JD, Erickson JA: Reduction in early dislocation rate with large-diameter femoral heads in primary total hip arthroplasty. *J Arthroplasty* 2007;22(6 suppl 2):140-144.

66. Jameson SS, Lees D, James P, et al: Lower rates of dislocation with increased femoral head size after primary total hip replacement: A five-year analysis of NHS patients in England. *J Bone Joint Surg Br* 2011;93(7):876-880.

Bicompartmental Knee Arthroplasty

Nirav H. Amin, MD
Travis Scudday, MD
Fred D. Cushner, MD

Abstract

Knee arthritis is one of the leading causes of disability and functional limitations in the United States and worldwide. Total knee arthroplasty results in good functional outcomes and high survival rates in patients who have tricompartmental arthritis. Bicompartmental knee arthroplasty is being used more often in patients who have arthritis that is isolated to two compartments: the patellofemoral compartment and either the medial or the lateral compartment. Bicompartmental knee arthroplasty preserves the kinematics, ligaments, and bone stock of the knee and is a good option for younger, active, high-demand patients who wish to return to their previous level of activity.

Instr Course Lect 2017;66:193–199.

Knee arthritis is the most common type of arthritis in the elderly and is one of the leading causes of disability and functional limitations in the United States and worldwide.[1] Total knee arthroplasty (TKA) results in good functional outcomes and high survival rates in patients who have tricompartmental arthritis.[2] Isolated bicompartmental knee arthroplasty (BiKA) is being used more often in patients who have arthritis that does not involve all three compartments: medial, lateral, and patellofemoral. BiKA preserves the kinematics, ligaments, and bone stock of the knee and is a good option for high-demand patients who have a higher risk for revision surgery.[3-6]

Bicompartmental knee arthritis is a loss of native cartilage and a narrowing of the joint space that involves the patellofemoral compartment and either the medial or the lateral compartment. BiKA most commonly involves the medial tibiofemoral and the patellofemoral compartments.[7] Miller et al[8] reported that knee cartilage degeneration typically progresses from the medial condyle to the patellofemoral compartment. Tibesku et al[9] reported similar radiographic findings, with knee cartilage degeneration progressing from the medial compartment to the patellofemoral compartment. BiKA is gaining appeal because of improved clinical data, changes in prosthetic design, and evolving surgical techniques.[7,10-12]

Similar to unicompartmental knee arthroplasty (UKA), which has gained popularity since being introduced in 1972, BiKA has undergone modifications and alterations in implant design, fixation methods, and surgical techniques and has reliable outcomes and high survival rates.[13-16] The primary goals of BiKA are to preserve the cruciate ligaments as well as bone stock and allow the knee to function

Dr. Cushner or an immediate family member has received royalties from Smith & Nephew; is a member of a speakers' bureau or has made paid presentations on behalf of Chemed, Pacira Pharmaceuticals, and Smith & Nephew; serves as a paid consultant to or is an employee of Pacira Pharmaceuticals and Smith & Nephew; has stock or stock options held in Aperion Biologics and AlterG; has received research or institutional support from Pacira Pharmaceuticals; and serves as a board member, owner, officer, or committee member of the Knee Society. Neither of the following authors nor any immediate family member has received anything of value from or has stock or stock options held in a commercial company or institution related directly or indirectly to the subject of this chapter: Dr. Amin and Dr. Scudday.

with nearly normal kinematics, both of which result in good functional outcomes and a high likelihood of return to normal functional activities.[3,4,6,17-19] Theoretically, UKA is advantageous in younger, fit patients who have a desire to return to an active lifestyle; however, UKA is not the best option for patients in whom arthritis of the patellofemoral compartment is identified on a skyline radiograph. In a study of 600 patients, Rolston et al[19] reported that skyline radiographs revealed patellofemoral osteoarthritis (OA) in 73% of the patients who had medial-sided arthritis. Walker et al[20,21] reported that as many as 24% of women and 11% of men who are older than 55 years have symptomatic OA of the knee that involves the patellofemoral joint.

In the early days of BiKA, two separate implants were used to address patellofemoral arthritis and either medial or lateral arthritis. To reduce the amount of bone loss and complexity of surgery, two monolithic BiKA implants were commercially available in the United States. The Journey Deuce (Smith & Nephew) allowed for resurfacing of the medial compartment and the patellofemoral compartment, and the iDuo (ConforMIS) offered resurfacing options for the medial and lateral compartments as well as the patellofemoral compartment. The Journey Deuce is no longer commercially available in the United States. Recent studies have reported better long-term outcomes in patients who underwent BiKA with modular unlinked components compared with patients who underwent BiKA with modern monolithic femoral components, which is associated with a higher rate of revision surgery.[22,23]

Clinical Evaluation
History
BiKA is a favorable alternative to TKA for patients who have degenerative disease that is limited to two compartments. The symptoms of patellofemoral and either medial or lateral compartment disease must be discerned to ensure an optimal outcome after BiKA. Patients should be able to localize pain to the medial or lateral compartment with one finger rather than use an entire hand to demonstrate global knee pain.[24] Anterior knee pain, which is exacerbated with ascending or descending stairs, squatting, or kneeling, is often associated with patellofemoral pathology.[25]

Physical Examination
The physical examination should confirm a patient's symptoms of medial or lateral joint line tenderness and patellofemoral crepitus. Patients should have an arc of motion of at least 90° and a flexion contracture of less than 15°. A positive J-sign, which occurs if the patella subluxates laterally with the knee near full extension, indicates patellar maltracking.[26] Further workup for patellar maltracking is critical before BiKA is performed. Because stability after BiKA relies on functional cruciate and collateral ligaments, a determination of ligamentous integrity is another important component of the physical examination. The lack of an anterior cruciate ligament (ACL) has been reported to accelerate component wear in certain implants that are used for UKA; therefore, ligamentous stability is a theoretical factor that predicts the longevity of BiKA.[27] Although a subset of older patients with a nonfunctioning ACL reported no instability after UKA, no studies are currently available on the outcomes of BiKA in patients who have deficient anterior and posterior cruciate ligaments.

Imaging
Radiographs are critical to help determine suitable candidates for BiKA. Radiographs should include weight-bearing AP, 45° flexed-knee PA, lateral, and Merchant views of the patella (**Figure 1**). Varus/valgus alignment should be assessed on AP radiographs, and posterior condylar wear and isolated tibiofemoral compartment involvement should be assessed on PA radiographs. Merchant radiographs should be obtained to assess for patellofemoral arthritis (**Figure 2**).

Surgical Technique
Given the technical challenges associated with assessing optimal coronal and sagittal alignment for BiKA, a 10-cm midline incision allows for sufficient access for instrumentation and final implantation and results in minimal soft-tissue damage. The authors of this chapter prefer to use a midvastus approach, if possible; however, a medial arthrotomy is a good option for patients who are large or muscular. Based on the tibiofemoral compartment involved, either a medial or a lateral parapatellar arthrotomy is performed.

The next steps depend on the type of implant selected; however, balancing principles should be used throughout the procedure to ensure that both coronal and sagittal alignment are maintained (**Figure 3**). The senior author of this chapter (F.D.C.) prefers to address the tibia first. The tibial plateau is removed with the use of a series of oscillating and reciprocating saws. Caution should be used to avoid resection of the cruciate ligaments and/or, based on the depth of the bony resection, the creation of a future tibial plateau fracture. It is important to avoid undercutting the tibia; therefore, the senior author of this chapter prefers to make the sagittal cut adjacent to the ACL but not in line with the edge of the trochlea, which allows for maximum sizing of the tibial component. Using the medial one-third of the patellar tendon as a reference point, an extramedullary alignment rod is used to check the anatomic axis of the knee in relationship to the tibia and ensure appropriate sizing with a reproduced anatomic tibial slope. The flexion and extension gaps are assessed before the femur is addressed.

After the flexion and extension gaps are balanced, the femur is prepared with an intramedullary alignment rod in a manner similar to that for TKA. Newer implant systems allow the distal femoral cut to be based off a jig that is linked to the tibial cut. Although these implant systems avoid the intramedullary hole, the surgeon must ensure that the limb is in full extension before the distal femoral cut is made. Errors in obtaining full extension can result in flexion or extension of the femoral component. The anterior femur is resected, and varus/valgus alignment is assessed in relationship to a reference line that is perpendicular to the epicondylar axis along the intercondylar notch and the anterior cut surface. The femoral cuts are completed, and the trial components are assessed in flexion, extension, varus, and valgus. Sizing is important, and care should be taken to avoid impingement on the already selected UKA.

After the UKA is complete, attention is then focused on the patellofemoral joint. A small intramedullary alignment hole is used to create the anterior femoral cut for the patellofemoral

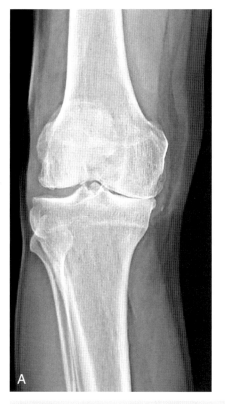 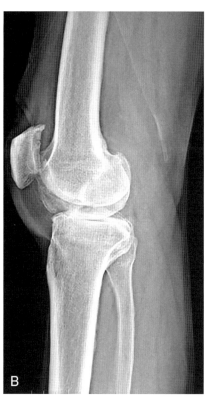

Figure 1   Preoperative AP (**A**) and lateral (**B**) weight-bearing knee radiographs demonstrate severe medial compartment degeneration with posteromedial wear and substantial patellofemoral arthritis.

joint. The goals are to add some external rotation, which improves patellar tracking, and create a cut that is as low to the anterior femur as possible without notching the femoral shaft, which helps unload the patellofemoral joint. A stylus is used to ensure adequate bony resection of the anterior femur for the trochlear component. Rotation is assessed based on the anterior/posterior axis or the transepicondylar axis. The pins are set, and the anterior femoral cut is made. The femoral trochlea is sized to confirm anterior bone coverage and intercondylar notch clearance. The surgeon should avoid medial or lateral overhang, which can result in soft-tissue impingement. The patella is resurfaced in a standard fashion. Care should be taken to avoid overstuffing the patellofemoral joint. Although it is common

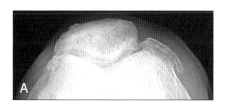
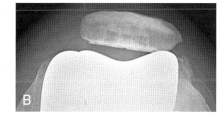

Figure 2   Preoperative (**A**) and postoperative (**B**) Merchant radiographs of a patellofemoral joint.

for surgeons to attempt to reproduce preoperative patellar thickness, it may not always be possible because of severe patellar wear. Anatomic landmarks

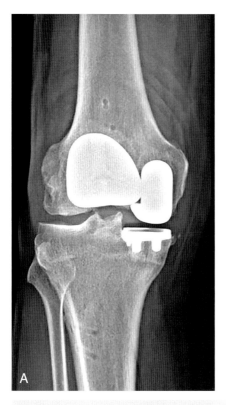 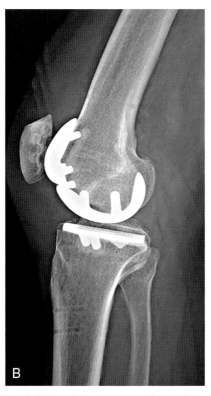

Figure 3 AP (**A**) and lateral (**B**) weight-bearing knee radiographs taken after bicompartmental knee arthroplasty demonstrate improved alignment.

that are located just above the origin of the patellar tendon are a better starting point if the free-hand technique will be used. All the trials are placed, and the knee is taken through a range of motion to assess soft-tissue balancing throughout the arc of motion. Some implant systems allow for the exchange of femoral component sizes without the redrilling of lug holes, which allows the femoral component to be adjusted without much difficulty.

The postoperative protocol after BiKA is similar to that after TKA or UKA. The goal is progressive range of motion until maximum intraoperative knee flexion and extension are attained.

Clinical Results

Historically, literature on BiKA outcomes was limited; however, the recent increase in the use of BiKA implants

has led to studies on the short-term and midterm outcomes of unlinked BiKA components. In a study of 95 patients who underwent monoblock BiKA with the Journey Deuce prosthesis, Rolston et al[19] reported that, at a follow-up of more than 33 months, patients had a mean range of motion of 117° and did not demonstrate lateral joint line tenderness or ongoing patellofemoral pain. The authors reported that postoperative patient satisfaction was high, and blood transfusion was not necessary. In a study of 137 patients who underwent monoblock BiKA, 77 of whom had substantial varus mechanical axis deviation preoperatively, Rolston and Siewert[28] reported that 130 patients had a neutral mechanical axis postoperatively and concluded that monoblock BiKA is an effective procedure for the restoration of proper knee alignment.

In a study of 36 knees in 32 patients who underwent monoblock BiKA with the Journey Deuce prosthesis, Palumbo et al[23] reported that, at a mean follow-up of 21 months, 31% of the patients were unsatisfied with the surgery, and 53% of the patients stated that they would not repeat the surgery. The authors reported a mean Knee Society functional survey score of 65.4 and a high rate of conversion to TKA because of persistent knee pain and reduced knee function. Morrison et al[29] reported a 14% rate of conversion from monoblock BiKA to TKA at 1 year postoperatively and an increased trend for conversion from monoblock BiKA to TKA at 2 years postoperatively. In a study on biomechanical changes of the knee, Heyse et al[30] reported that modular BiKA leads to an increased dorsal tibial contact point, a medial femoral condyle that is located more posteriorly, and more medial collateral ligament strain. Müller et al[31] reported that positional guidance and insufficient implant sizes led to malalignment and instability in patients who underwent BiKA with the Journey Deuce prosthesis, which resulted in a higher rate of conversion to TKA.

Lonner[32] reported improvements in modular BiKA component alignment with the use of robotic arm assistance, which may be effective in the treatment of younger patients who undergo UKA or patellofemoral arthroplasty and in whom arthritis develops in the unresurfaced compartment. In a study on the retrospective clinical and radiologic outcomes of robotic-assisted BiKA, Tamam et al[33] reported that 83% of the patients had good or excellent results at a minimum follow-up of 1 year (range, 12 to 54 months). The authors expanded the indications for BiKA beyond those described by Kozinn and Scott[34] to include patients who had correctible varus deformity up to 15°, valgus deformity up to 17°, flexion contracture up to 15°, a range of motion of at least 90°, and a mean body mass index of 34.7 kg/m^2, with no upper age restriction.

The authors of this chapter think that newer surgical techniques, such as the use of preoperative CT or MRI to create customized implants, should be used at a surgeon's discretion. Minas et al[35] reported the outcomes of 34 knees in 31 patients (mean age, 47 years) who underwent BiKA with a customized, individually made, monolithic, bicompartmental component (26 medial-patellofemoral iDuo implants and eight lateral-patellofemoral iDuo implants). At a mean follow-up of 30 months, no revision surgeries had been performed, 97% of the patients reported that they would undergo the procedure again, and 82% of the patients reported a visual analog pain scale score between 0 and 3.[35] In a kinematic study, Park et al[36] reported that patients who undergo BiKA with a monoblock component have the potential to retain more natural knee function during weight-bearing activities, such as kneeling, lunging, and stair stepping. Wang et al[37] compared the in vivo kinematics of four patients who underwent BiKA with the iDuo component and seven patients who underwent TKA with the Persona component (Zimmer) with the in vivo kinematics of 12 patients in a control group. Because of patient-specific imaging, which led to customized implants, the authors reported that the patients who underwent BiKA had similar knee strength, walking speeds, and biomechanics compared with the patients in the control group.

The midterm and long-term outcomes of monoblock BiKA components are limited; however, recent studies have reported that a bone- and ligament-sparing BiKA component preserves knee proprioception and kinematics and may be advantageous in the management of bicompartmental arthritis. In a prospective study of 29 patients who underwent modular unlinked BiKA for the management of patellofemoral arthritis and either medial or lateral arthritis, Kamath et al[10] reported statistically significant improvement in Knee Society knee and functional survey scores, Knee Injury and Osteoarthritis Outcome Scores, Medical Outcomes Study 12-Item Short Form scores, and Western Ontario and McMaster Universities Osteoarthritis Index scores at a mean follow-up of 31 months (range, 24 to 46 months). The authors reported that one patient underwent conversion to TKA at 3 years postoperatively for the management of knee instability. In a study that compared the outcomes of patients who underwent modular BiKA with those of patients who underwent TKA, Shah et al[38] reported that the patients who underwent BiKA had a significantly greater range of motion at all points in time for a 24-month follow-up period, and concluded that modular BiKA is a viable option for patients who have arthritis of the patellofemoral and medial compartments. In a study of nine patients who underwent UKA combined with patellofemoral replacement, Heyse et al[7] reported that, at a mean follow-up of 12 years, all patients reported satisfactory outcomes, and no conversions to TKA were required. To the knowledge of the authors of this chapter, Heyse et al[7] is the longest follow-up study of BiKA that reported promising

results. Similar results were reported by Tan et al[39] in a study that compared the outcomes of 27 patients with grade 2 to grade 4 (minimal to severe) OA of the medial and patellofemoral compartments and an intact ACL who underwent either BiKA or TKA. The patients in the BiKA group had longer surgical times, less blood loss, shorter length of hospital stays, and increased range of motion compared with the patients in the TKA group. The authors reported that no patients had complications at a follow-up of 24 months.

In a prospective matched case-control study that compared the outcomes of patients who underwent contemporary modular BiKA with those of patients who underwent TKA, Parratte et al[40] reported that, at a minimum follow-up of 2 years, the patients who underwent unlinked BiKA had higher mean Knee Society knee and functional survey scores, Timed Up-and-Go scores, and University of California–Los Angeles Activity scores compared with the patients who underwent TKA. In a separate study, Parratte et al[41] followed 77 knees in 71 patients for a longer period of time (range, 5 to 23 years). These patients underwent UKA of the medial compartment combined with patellofemoral arthroplasty. The authors reported mean Knee Society knee and functional survey scores of 84 and 79, respectively; however, 35% of the knees required revision surgery. In a separate study on the long-term outcomes of BiKA, Parratte et al[42] reported that the disappointing long-term outcomes of bicompartmental implants may have been caused by implant design and fixation issues.

In a study of patients who underwent either TKA or BiKA, Chung and Min[43] reported no differences in knee muscle strength and physical performance between the patients in the two groups at 1-year follow-up. In one of the first prospective randomized studies that compared the outcomes of patients who underwent unlinked modular BiKA with those of patients who underwent TKA, Yeo et al[44] randomized 48 patients with arthritis of the medial and patellofemoral components into either a BiKA group (26 patients) or a TKA group (22 patients). At a 5-year follow-up, the patients who underwent BiKA had similar functional outcomes compared with the patients who underwent TKA; however, decreased intraoperative blood loss was noted in the patients who underwent BiKA. In general, more long-term prospective, randomized studies that compare the outcomes of patients who undergo BiKA with those of patients who undergo TKA are necessary to develop more definitive treatment recommendations. Heekin et al[45] reported that 28% of patients who undergo TKA may be candidates for BiKA, and BiKA may be a suitable treatment option for patients with OA of the knee who have ideal clinical and radiographic findings because it preserves both cruciate ligaments as well as bone stock, minimizes soft-tissue surgical trauma, and allows for a faster recovery.

Summary

BiKA is a favorable alternative to TKA for patients who have arthritis that is isolated to two compartments. Bone- and ligament-sparing BiKA preserves knee proprioception and kinematics, which allows younger, active, high-demand patients who have advanced OA of the patellofemoral compartment and either the medial or lateral compartment to return to an active lifestyle.

Acknowledgment

The authors of this chapter would like to thank Dr. Jess Lonner for preparing the radiographs.

References

1. Misra D, Felson DT, Silliman RA, et al: Knee osteoarthritis and frailty: Findings from the Multicenter Osteoarthritis Study and Osteoarthritis Initiative. *J Gerontol A Biol Sci Med Sci* 2015;70(3):339-344.

2. Rand JA, Ilstrup DM: Survivorship analysis of total knee arthroplasty: Cumulative rates of survival of 9200 total knee arthroplasties. *J Bone Joint Surg Am* 1991;73(3):397-409.

3. Fuchs S, Tibesku CO, Genkinger M, Volmer M, Laass H, Rosenbaum D: Clinical and functional comparison of bicondylar sledge prostheses retaining all ligaments and constrained total knee replacement. *Clin Biomech (Bristol, Avon)* 2004;19(3):263-269.

4. Fuchs S, Tibesku CO, Genkinger M, Laass H, Rosenbaum D: Proprioception with bicondylar sledge prostheses retaining cruciate ligaments. *Clin Orthop Relat Res* 2003;406:148-154.

5. Berger RA, Meneghini RM, Sheinkop MB, et al: The progression of patellofemoral arthrosis after medial unicompartmental replacement: Results at 11 to 15 years. *Clin Orthop Relat Res* 2004;428:92-99.

6. Fuchs S, Tibesku CO, Frisse D, Genkinger M, Laass H, Rosenbaum D: Clinical and functional comparison of uni- and bicondylar sledge prostheses. *Knee Surg Sports Traumatol Arthrosc* 2005;13(3):197-202.

7. Heyse TJ, Khefacha A, Cartier P: UKA in combination with PFR at average 12-year follow-up. *Arch Orthop Trauma Surg* 2010;130(10):1227-1230.

8. Miller R, Kettelkamp DB, Laubenthal KN, Karagiorgos A, Smidt GL: Quantitative correlations in degenerative arthritis of the knee. *J Bone Joint Surg Am* 1973;55(5):956-962.

9. Tibesku CO, Innocenti B, Wong P, Salehi A, Labey L: Can CT-based patient-matched instrumentation achieve consistent rotational alignment in knee arthroplasty? *Arch Orthop Trauma Surg* 2012;132(2):171-177.

10. Kamath AF, Levack A, John T, Thomas BS, Lonner JH: Minimum two-year outcomes of modular bicompartmental knee arthroplasty. *J Arthroplasty* 2014;29(1):75-79.

11. Argenson JN, Parratte S, Bertani A, et al: The new arthritic patient and arthroplasty treatment options. *J Bone Joint Surg Am* 2009;91(suppl 5):43-48.

12. Argenson JN, Flecher X, Parratte S, Aubaniac JM: Patellofemoral arthroplasty: An update. *Clin Orthop Relat Res* 2005;440:50-53.

13. Repicci JA, Hartman JF: Minimally invasive unicondylar knee arthroplasty for the treatment of unicompartmental osteoarthritis: An outpatient arthritic bypass procedure. *Orthop Clin North Am* 2004;35(2):201-216.

14. Berger RA, Meneghini RM, Jacobs JJ, et al: Results of unicompartmental knee arthroplasty at a minimum of ten years of follow-up. *J Bone Joint Surg Am* 2005;87(5):999-1006.

15. Squire MW, Callaghan JJ, Goetz DD, Sullivan PM, Johnston RC: Unicompartmental knee replacement: A minimum 15 year followup study. *Clin Orthop Relat Res* 1999;367:61-72.

16. O'Rourke MR, Gardner JJ, Callaghan JJ, et al: The John Insall Award: Unicompartmental knee replacement. A minimum twenty-one-year followup, end-result study. *Clin Orthop Relat Res* 2005;440:27-37.

17. Saccomanni B: Unicompartmental knee arthroplasty: A review of literature. *Clin Rheumatol* 2010;29(4):339-346.

18. Labek G, Sekyra K, Pawelka W, Janda W, Stöckl B: Outcome and reproducibility of data concerning the Oxford unicompartmental knee arthroplasty: A structured literature review including arthroplasty registry data. *Acta Orthop* 2011;82(2):131-135.

19. Rolston L, Bresch J, Engh G, et al: Bicompartmental knee arthroplasty: A bone-sparing, ligament-sparing, and minimally invasive alternative for active patients. *Orthopedics* 2007;30(8 suppl):70-73.

20. Walker T, Perkinson B, Mihalko WM: Patellofemoral arthroplasty: The other unicompartmental knee replacement. *J Bone Joint Surg Am* 2012;94(18):1712-1720.

21. Walker T, Perkinson B, Mihalko WM: Patellofemoral arthroplasty: The other unicompartmental knee replacement. *Instr Course Lect* 2013;62:363-371.

22. Thienpont E, Price A: Bicompartmental knee arthroplasty of the patellofemoral and medial compartments. *Knee Surg Sports Traumatol Arthrosc* 2013;21(11):2523-2531.

23. Palumbo BT, Henderson ER, Edwards PK, Burris RB, Gutiérrez S, Raterman SJ: Initial experience of the Journey-Deuce bicompartmental knee prosthesis: A review of 36 cases. *J Arthroplasty* 2011;26(6 suppl):40-45.

24. Lester JD, Watson JN, Hutchinson MR: Physical examination of the patellofemoral joint. *Clin Sports Med* 2014;33(3):403-412.

25. Lonner JH: Patellofemoral arthroplasty. *J Am Acad Orthop Surg* 2007;15(8):495-506.

26. Shelbourne KD, Urch SE, Gray T: Results of medial retinacular imbrication in patients with unilateral patellar dislocation. *J Knee Surg* 2012;25(5):391-396.

27. Engh GA, Ammeen D: Is an intact anterior cruciate ligament needed in order to have a well-functioning unicondylar knee replacement? *Clin Orthop Relat Res* 2004;428:170-173.

28. Rolston L, Siewert K: Assessment of knee alignment after bicompartmental knee arthroplasty. *J Arthroplasty* 2009;24(7):1111-1114.

29. Morrison TA, Nyce JD, Macaulay WB, Geller JA: Early adverse results with bicompartmental knee arthroplasty: A prospective cohort comparison to total knee arthroplasty. *J Arthroplasty* 2011;26(6 suppl):35-39.

30. Heyse TJ, El-Zayat BF, De Corte R, et al: Biomechanics of medial unicondylar in combination with patellofemoral knee arthroplasty. *Knee* 2014;21(suppl 1):S3-S9.

31. Müller M, Matziolis G, Falk R, Hommel H: The bicompartmental knee joint prosthesis Journey Deuce: Failure analysis and optimization strategies. *Orthopade* 2012;41(11):894-904.

32. Lonner JH: Modular bicompartmental knee arthroplasty with robotic arm assistance. *Am J Orthop (Belle Mead NJ)* 2009;38(2 suppl):28-31.

33. Tamam C, Plate JF, Augart M, Poehling GG, Jinnah RH: Retrospective clinical and radiological outcomes after robotic assisted bicompartmental knee arthroplasty. *Adv Orthop* 2015;2015:747309.

34. Kozinn SC, Scott R: Unicondylar knee arthroplasty. *J Bone Joint Surg Am* 1989;71(1):145-150.

35. Minas T, Bryant T, Gomoll AH: Abstract No. 152. Bi-compartmental arthroplasty with a one-pieced customized device: Early experience and patient outcomes. *British Association of the Knee Annual Spring Meeting.* Telford, United Kingdom, March 10-11, 2015.

36. Park BH, Leffler J, Franz A, Dunbar NJ, Banks SA: Kinematics of monoblock bicompartmental knee arthroplasty during weight-bearing activities. *Knee Surg Sports Traumatol Arthrosc* 2015;23(6):1756-1762.

37. Wang H, Foster J, Francksen N, Estes J, Rolston L: Lunging after knee replacement surgeries. *2015 World Arthroplasty Congress.* Paris, France, April 16-18, 2015.

38. Shah SM, Dutton AQ, Liang S, Dasde S: Bicompartmental versus total knee arthroplasty for medio-patellofemoral osteoarthritis: A comparison of early clinical and functional outcomes. *J Knee Surg* 2013;26(6):411-416.

39. Tan SM, Dutton AQ, Bea KC, Kumar VP: Bicompartmental versus total knee arthroplasty for medial and patellofemoral osteoarthritis. *J Orthop Surg (Hong Kong)* 2013;21(3):281-284.

40. Parratte S, Ollivier M, Opsomer G, Lunebourg A, Argenson JN, Thienpont E: Is knee function better with contemporary modular bicompartmental arthroplasty compared to total knee arthroplasty? Short-term outcomes of a prospective matched study including 68 cases. *Orthop Traumatol Surg Res* 2015;101(5):547-552.

41. Parratte S, Pauly V, Aubaniac JM, Argenson JN: Survival of bicompartmental knee arthroplasty at 5 to 23 years. *Clin Orthop Relat Res* 2010;468(1):64-72.

42. Parratte S, Ollivier M, Lunebourg A, Abdel MP, Argenson JN: Long-term results of compartmental arthroplasties of the knee: Long term results of partial knee arthroplasty. *Bone Joint J* 2015;97(10 suppl A):9-15.

43. Chung JY, Min BH: Is bicompartmental knee arthroplasty more favourable to knee muscle strength and physical performance compared to total knee arthroplasty? *Knee Surg Sports Traumatol Arthrosc* 2013;21(11):2532-2541.

44. Yeo NE, Chen JY, Yew A, Chia SL, Lo NN, Yeo SJ: Prospective randomised trial comparing unlinked, modular bicompartmental knee arthroplasty and total knee arthroplasty: A five years follow-up. *Knee* 2015;22(4):321-327.

45. Heekin RD, Fokin AA: Incidence of bicompartmental osteoarthritis in patients undergoing total and unicompartmental knee arthroplasty: Is the time ripe for a less radical treatment? *J Knee Surg* 2014;27(1):77-81.

Medial Unicompartmental Knee Arthroplasty

Andrew Barrister Richardson, MD

Michael J. Morris, MD

Abstract

Unicompartmental knee arthroplasty (UKA) has substantial benefits, including lower perioperative morbidity and earlier recovery, compared with total knee arthroplasty. The traditionally strict indications for UKA have been challenged by studies that expanded the indications based on a diagnosis of anteromedial osteoarthritis of the knee and demonstrated successful outcomes. The Nuffield criteria no longer prohibit patients from UKA based on age, obesity, anterior knee pain, or involvement of the patellofemoral joint. UKA implant designs have evolved substantially in the past three decades, and both fixed- and mobile-bearing UKA implants are currently available. Both fixed- and mobile-bearing UKA implants demonstrate excellent clinical outcomes at more than 10 years postoperatively but continue to have different modes of long-term implant failure. Proper patient selection and execution of surgical technique are critical to optimize patient outcomes.

Instr Course Lect 2017;66:201–209.

Osteoarthritis (OA) of the knee is one of the most common causes of pain and loss of motion in the aging population. Total knee arthroplasty (TKA) is the current preferred treatment method for tricompartmental OA of the knee; however, surgeons have long recognized that knee OA often involves only a single knee compartment. Compared with TKA, unicompartmental knee arthroplasty (UKA), which is known as partial knee replacement, in particular medial UKA, offers patients with unicompartmental knee OA several substantial benefits. Compared with patients who undergo TKA, patients who undergo UKA are half as likely to have a major complication, such as myocardial infarction, venous thromboembolism, or deep infection; three time less likely to have a stroke; and four times less likely to die in the first 30 days postoperatively. Patients who undergo UKA also have a substantially lower mortality rate within 8 years postoperatively compared with patients who undergo TKA.[1,2] In addition, patients who undergo UKA have a faster recovery, more normal knee kinematics, increased range of motion (ROM), and better patient-reported outcome measures compared with patients who undergo TKA.[3]

Because of the increased interest in minimally invasive techniques and emphasis on rapid postoperative recovery as well as recent studies that have demonstrated the long-term success of UKA versus TKA, interest in medial UKA has gained substantial popularity in the past two decades. Surgeons should understand the history of UKA, surgical indications for medial UKA, proper patient evaluation and selection for UKA, technical considerations for UKA, and outcomes of UKA.

History

The first generation of modern UKA implants, which included the Marmor (Smith & Nephew) and St. George SLED (Waldemar LINK) knee

Dr. Morris or an immediate family member has received research or institutional support from OrthoSensor, Pacira Pharmaceuticals, SPR Therapeutics, and Zimmer; and serves as a paid consultant to Zimmer. Neither Dr. Richardson nor any immediate family member has received anything of value from or has stock or stock options held in a commercial company or institution related directly or indirectly to the subject of this chapter.

implants, were introduced in the 1970s. These first-generation UKA implants had a metallic femoral component that articulated with an all-polyethylene, fixed-bearing cemented tibia. Patients who underwent UKA with first-generation implants were plagued by problems such as progression of arthritis, aseptic loosening, subsidence, and high rates of component wear. Improper prosthesis design, poor patient selection, and a steep learning curve for implantation were attributed to the failure of first-generation UKA implants.[4-7]

The second generation of UKA implants attempted to rectify the problems of first-generation UKA implants by introducing metal-backed tibial components. Metal-backed tibial components had increased rigidity; this allowed for greater distribution of forces, which decreased the risk for subsidence, and polyethylene exchange, which addressed component wear. Unfortunately, patients who underwent UKA with second-generation implants were plagued by substantial problems with component loosening and polyethylene wear. The greater amount of tibial resection that was required by the metal baseplates and the lack of congruency between the polyethylene insert and femoral component, which resulted in a decreased contact area and increased contact stresses on the polyethylene component, were attributed to the failure of second-generation UKA implants.[7,8]

In 1974, Goodfellow et al[9] introduced the concept of a fully congruent mobile bearing for knee prostheses. Originally designed for bicondylar total knee replacement, the Oxford Total Knee implant (Zimmer Biomet) was adapted for UKA in the 1980s. The Oxford Partial Knee implant (Zimmer

Biomet) has a metal femoral component with a spherical articular surface, a flat metal tibial component, and a polyethylene mobile bearing, which is spherically concave above and flat below, that is interposed between the femoral and tibial components. The polyethylene mobile bearing is fully congruent at both interfaces and fully unconstrained throughout knee ROM, which allows for a greater distribution of contact stresses during weight bearing and results in decreased polyethylene wear.

Both fixed- and mobile-bearing UKA implants are currently available for use. The superiority of one UKA implant design over the other continues to be a subject of debate. The potential advantages of mobile-bearing UKA implants include a larger contact area and decreased contact stresses, which decrease polyethylene wear and, theoretically, allow for more normal knee kinematics.[10] Despite these potential advantages, several studies that directly compared fixed- and mobile-bearing UKA implants failed to find a substantial advantage of one UKA implant design over the other.[11-15] The survivorship and specific causes of failure for each UKA implant design will be discussed later in this chapter.

Indications and Contraindications

The original indications for UKA, which were described by Kozinn and Scott[16] in 1989, included patients with a diagnosis of OA or osteonecrosis in either the medial or lateral knee compartment who were older than 60 years, had low physical demands, weighed less than 82 kg (181 lb), had minimal pain at rest, had a ROM arc greater than 90° with less than 5° of flexion contracture, and had an angular deformity less than

15° that was passively correctable to neutral. Specific contraindications to UKA included patients with a diagnosis of inflammatory arthritis, patients younger than 60 years, patients with high physical demands, patients who had pain at rest, and patients who had patellofemoral pain or exposed bone in the patellofemoral joint or opposite compartment. Successful UKA results were reported if surgeons strictly adhered to these stringent indications and contraindications; however, only 2% to 15% of patients with knee OA were candidates for UKA with strict adherence to these stringent indications and contraindications.[17,18]

Several studies have reported that more liberal indications than those described by Kozinn and Scott[16] may be used to achieve successful UKA results.[17,19-24] The Nuffield criteria describe a more liberal set of indications for UKA, in which eligibility for UKA is based on the diagnoses of anteromedial OA (AMOA) of the knee or spontaneous osteonecrosis of the knee. White et al[25] defined AMOA of the knee as a specific pathognomonic osteoarthritic condition in which bone-on-bone arthritis is present in the medial knee compartment, but the joint space in the lateral knee compartment is fully preserved. In addition, the medial collateral ligament and the anterior cruciate ligament (ACL) in patients with AMOA of the knee should be functionally normal; this is best evaluated on a valgus stress radiograph, which allows a surgeon to determine if intra-articular varus is fully correctable without loss of lateral joint space. Berend et al[26] reported that AMOA of the knee and a correctable deformity are present if mechanical knee alignment is less than or equal to 10° of varus and if flexion contracture is less than 15°. Although the degree of deformity is not an absolute contraindication for UKA, a deformity greater than 10° in the coronal plane with more than 15° of fixed flexion is routinely associated with ACL deficiency rather than AMOA of the knee. Patients with AMOA of the knee who undergo UKA have long-term implant survivorship greater than 90%.[22,24] These more liberal indications for UKA allow 30% to 50% of patients with knee OA to be candidates for the procedure.

Contraindications to UKA are limited to active infection, inflammatory arthropathy, ligamentous instability or contracture of the medial collateral ligament, a functionally absent ACL, and previous high tibial osteotomy. Patient factors, including age, activity level, and weight, which were previously believed to be contraindications to UKA, are no longer contraindicated. Patients younger than 60 years and patients who had high physical demands were contraindicated because of concerns for early implant failure that resulted from polyethylene wear in traditional fixed-bearing UKA implants. Recent data have demonstrated that patients younger than 60 years with high physical demands who undergo either fixed- or mobile-bearing UKA have excellent midterm to long-term outcomes.[27,28] Ali et al[29] reported that patients with high physical demands who underwent UKA had better 12-year implant survival rates compared with patients with low physical demands who underwent UKA. Berend et al[30] reported no increased risk of implant failure in patients younger than 60 years who underwent UKA; however, slightly lower clinical scores were reported in younger patients who underwent UKA, which may have been the result of increased demands on the

implant and/or higher expectations in this younger, more active patient population.

Obesity and increased body mass index (BMI) have remained of concern for many surgeons contemplating UKA candidacy. Fixed-bearing, all-polyethylene UKA implants have poor implant survival rates in patients with a BMI greater than 32 kg/m²;[30] however, multiple studies have reported that patients with obesity who undergo either fixed- or mobile-bearing UKA with the use of metal-backed tibial components have excellent UKA implant survivorship that may be equivalent to or better compared with nonobese patients who undergo UKA. Cavaignac et al[31] reported similar 10-year implant survival rates in patients with a BMI greater than or equal to 30 kg/m² and in patients with a BMI less than or equal to 30 kg/m² (92% and 94%, respectively). In a study of 2,438 patients who underwent UKA with the Oxford Partial Knee implant, Murray et al[32] reported no difference in implant survival at a mean follow-up of 5 years between patients with obesity and nonobese patients. Furthermore, the authors reported that, although the overall outcome scores of the patients with obesity were lower compared with those of the nonobese patients, the patients with obesity had greater improvement in outcome scores compared with the nonobese patients. Therefore, obesity and increased BMI are not considered contraindications to UKA with metal-backed tibial components.

The most debated contraindication for UKA is the preoperative status of a patient's patellofemoral joint. Substantial involvement of the patellofemoral joint was considered a contraindication to fixed-bearing UKA; however, the

clinical results of mobile-bearing UKA have been outstanding, and progression of disease in the patellofemoral joint has not been a clinical problem. Beard et al[33] reported the survival of the Oxford Partial Knee implant in 100 knees in which the preoperative radiologic status of the patellofemoral joint was defined. The authors reported that clinical outcome was independent of the presence or absence of preoperative patellofemoral joint disease. Berend et al[34] reported similar results with the use of Kaplan-Meier analysis, which predicted 97.9% implant survival in knees with patellofemoral joint disease and 93.8% implant survival in knees without patellofemoral joint disease 70 months after UKA. Munk et al[35] reported that involvement of the lateral facet and/or lateral subluxation of the patella was highly predictive of implant failure in patients who underwent UKA with a mobile-bearing implant. Similar successful results have not been observed in patients with patellofemoral joint disease who underwent UKA with a fixed-bearing implant, and progression of patellofemoral joint disease was a substantial cause of implant failure in the second postoperative decade for patients who underwent UKA with certain fixed-bearing implants.[36] This variation in outcomes between fixed- and mobile-bearing implants has been attributed to the abnormal biomechanics of fixed-bearing UKA implants. Argensen et al[10] reported that patients who underwent UKA with the Miller/Galante Unicompartmental Knee implant (Zimmer Biomet) had postoperative knee function similar to that of patients with ACL-deficient knees, which led to increased contact stresses on the patellofemoral joint. Conversely, in a study of patients who underwent

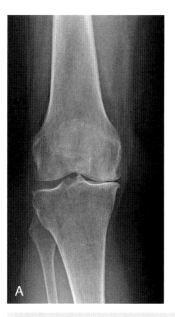
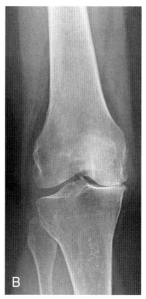
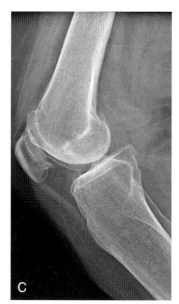
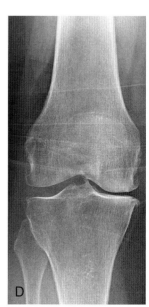

Figure 1 Preoperative radiographs of a knee demonstrate anteromedial osteoarthritis. **A,** AP view demonstrates full-thickness cartilage loss in the medial knee compartment. **B,** PA view confirms full-thickness cartilage loss and demonstrates severe osteoarthritis, which may not be seen on the AP view. **C,** Lateral view demonstrates anterior osteoarthritis with the bone preserved posteriorly. **D,** Valgus stress view demonstrates correction of the intra-articular varus deformity with preservation of the lateral joint space, which indicates maintenance of full-thickness cartilage in the lateral knee compartment.

UKA with the Oxford Partial Knee implant, Price et al[37] reported virtually normal knee kinematics without abnormal loading of the patellofemoral joint 10 years postoperatively. Consequently, surgeons think that loss of ACL function with subsequent increased contact stresses on the patellofemoral joint is the primary reason why patients who undergo UKA with fixed-bearing implants have a higher incidence of progression of patellofemoral joint disease compared with patients who undergo UKA with mobile-bearing implants. The Nuffield Orthopaedic Centre currently recommends that the status of the patellofemoral joint may be safely ignored in patients in whom medial UKA with a mobile-bearing implant is being considered unless substantial lateral facet involvement or lateral subluxation of the patella exists. Stricter adherence to the Kozinn and Scott[16] indications for UKA with regard to the preoperative status of the patellofemoral joint may be necessary in patients in whom fixed-bearing UKA is being considered.

Patient Evaluation

The preoperative assessment for UKA includes a detailed patient history, physical examination, and radiographic imaging. Pain is often localized along the medial joint line; however, the localization of pain has been reported to be unreliable, and anterior, posterior, lateral, or even global pain may be present in patients who have isolated AMOA of the knee.[38] Pain localized to areas other than the medial joint line is thought to be caused by reactive synovitis in response to the involvement of the medial compartment and should not preclude the possibility of UKA if the patient meets all other preoperative indications. Typically, varus deformity is present; however, the deformity should be correctable in 90° of flexion and with the application of valgus stress in 20° of flexion. Evaluation of the cruciate ligaments with the Lachman test, pivot shift test, and anterior drawer test is often difficult to interpret in patients who have an arthritic knee; however, gross ligamentous stability should be present.

Standing AP, 45° flexed-knee PA, lateral, and patellar radiographs are routinely obtained in all patients (**Figure 1, A** through **C**). Lateral radiographs should be examined for maintenance of the posterior tibial cortex, with wear isolated to the anteromedial tibial plateau. Valgus stress radiographs should be obtained in patients who have isolated AMOA of the knee (**Figure 1, D**). Valgus stress radiographs are used to ensure that a deformity is correctable and the lateral joint space is maintained. Valgus stress radiographs should be obtained with the patient positioned supine on a radiographic table. The knee is flexed to 20° on a foam support, and, with the patella pointed upward, a valgus force is applied across the joint. The x-ray should be directed 10° cephalad to vertical. The valgus stress can be applied manually or with a patient-directed force as described by Mauerhan et al.[39] The presence of AMOA of the knee on radiographic imaging indicates a functionally intact ACL. MRI and arthroscopy have not been validated as imaging modalities that help determine appropriate candidates for medial UKA; therefore, they are not routinely recommended. In patients who have spontaneous osteonecrosis of the knee, MRI is useful to evaluate the extent of the disease and to evaluate for lateral compartment involvement.

Surgical Considerations

Patients can be positioned in several ways for UKA. The authors of this chapter prefer to place the patient in the semi-lithotomy position. A thigh tourniquet is used, and the surgical extremity is placed in a thigh support with the hip flexed to approximately 40° and abducted, which allows the leg to hang freely. The knee must be able to flex to at least 135°, and care should be taken to keep the thigh support out of the popliteal fossa to minimize the risk of injury to the popliteal neurovascular structures. Typically, the incision is made via a paramedial approach that extends from just above the medial pole of the patella to a point distal to the joint line just medial to the tibial tubercle. Surgeons who are performing UKA in the early stages of their learning curve may extend this incision to the superior pole of the patella as necessary.

Resection of the proximal tibia should be conservative, typically resecting 1 to 2 mm below the arthritic surface. Resection of the proximal tibial should be performed perpendicular to the long axis of the tibia in the coronal plane and should match the native slope of the tibia. Proper depth and alignment of the resection will dictate the size of the flexion gap and, subsequently, the extension gap. Care should be taken to prevent breaching of the posterior tibial cortex during sagittal resection because it can compromise the structural stability of the tibia and increase the risk for tibial plateau fracture. In addition, the tibial component should be sized to maximize coverage of the tibial plateau because under sizing of the tibia results in increased stresses on the tibia and can increase the risk for tibial stress fracture and/or component subsidence. The femoral component should be placed in the center of the femoral condyle. If necessary, biasing the femoral component laterally (into the notch) is preferred because it will provide better congruency with the tibial component in extension.

At the end of the surgery, the gaps should be balanced in flexion and extension. The varus deformity should not be overcorrected because doing so may result in persistent postoperative tenderness along the medial tibia as well as the medial collateral ligament and will lead to increased stresses on the lateral compartment, which promote early arthritic changes in the lateral compartment. Most surgeons recommend 1 to 2 mm of laxity in both flexion and extension to prevent overcorrection.

Perioperative Management and Rehabilitation

Most UKA procedures can be performed as outpatient or 23-hour observation procedures. Several rapid recovery models for both TKA and UKA have been described in the literature.[40,41] For patients who undergo UKA at the institution of the authors of this chapter, an adductor canal block is used in conjunction with a general anesthetic agent. In addition, a local anesthetic agent is injected into the pericapsular tissues at the end of the procedure. Although able to bear weight as tolerated in the immediate postoperative period, patients are encouraged to use a walker and be weaned to a cane as tolerated in the first 1 to 2 weeks postoperatively. Most patients who undergo UKA require outpatient physical therapy; however, the duration of physical therapy for patients who undergo UKA typically is not as long as that of a typical patient who undergoes TKA. Although the incidence of deep vein thrombosis and pulmonary embolism after UKA is low compared with that after TKA, surgeons should use the same prophylaxis strategy for patients who undergo UKA as that for patients who undergo TKA.[42]

Outcomes

The results of UKA have improved substantially in the past two decades, with several studies reporting more than 90% 5- to 10-year survivorship for both fixed- and mobile-bearing UKA implants. In a study on the outcomes of 818 patients who underwent UKA with the Oxford Partial Knee implant, Pandit et al[22] reported a 94% 10-year implant survival rate and a 91% 15-year implant survival rate. In a study on the outcomes of 62 patients who underwent UKA with the Miller/Galante Unicompartmental Knee implant, Berger et al[19] reported a 96% overall implant survival rate at a minimum follow-up of 10 years (mean follow-up, 12 years). The authors reported that 92% of the patients had an excellent or good outcome at final follow-up.

The timing of revision surgery varies in the literature. Pandit et al[22] reported a 5.5-year mean time to revision surgery (range, 0.2 to 14.7 years) in patients who underwent UKA with the Oxford Partial Knee implant. The authors reported that the most common reasons for revision surgery were progression of lateral compartment arthritis, bearing dislocation, and unexplained pain. In a retrospective review of 18 patients (22 knees) in whom fixed-bearing UKA failed, Springer et al[43] reported an 8.3-year mean time to revision surgery. The authors reported that the most common reasons for implant failure were polyethylene wear and component loosening.

Several studies have directly compared the clinical results of patients who underwent UKA with a mobile-bearing implant with those of patients who underwent UKA with a fixed-bearing implant. Emerson et al[13] reported a 99% and 93% 11-year implant survival rate in 20 patients who underwent UKA with either a mobile- or fixed-bearing implant, respectively. Parratte et al[44] reported comparable implant survivorship at a minimum 15-year follow-up of 75 patients who underwent UKA with either the Miller/Galante Unicompartmental Knee implant or the Oxford Partial Knee implant, with revision surgery rates of 12% and 15%, respectively. Furthermore, the authors reported that patients in both groups had equivalent outcome scores for pain and function. The most prominent difference observed between the two UKA implants was the mechanism of implant failure. Fixed-bearing UKA implants were more commonly associated with polyethylene wear and the progression of patellofemoral arthritis, and mobile-bearing UKA implants were associated with bearing dislocation and the progression of lateral compartment arthritis.

Complications

Despite reports of good long-term survivorship for patients who undergo UKA, common important causes of implant failure include progression of adjacent compartment arthritis, bearing dislocation, and polyethylene wear. Although less common, aseptic loosening, tibial component subsidence, periprosthetic tibial fracture, and infection are other important causes of implant failure. Other complications include synovial impingement, metallosis, and meniscal injury.

Progression of adjacent compartment arthritis remains one of the most commonly reported complications after UKA. The sites of progression differ between patients who undergo UKA with a fixed-bearing implant and patients who undergo UKA with a mobile-bearing implant. Progression of patellofemoral arthritis is common in the second postoperative decade for patients who undergo UKA with a fixed-bearing implant;[36] however, as discussed previously, this has not been observed in patients who undergo UKA with a mobile-bearing implant. Although progression of lateral compartment arthritis is prevalent in patients who undergo UKA with either a fixed- or mobile-bearing implant, it appears to be more prevalent in patients who undergo UKA with a mobile-bearing implant. Progression of lateral compartment arthritis has been hypothesized to occur secondary to overcorrection, with concerns for bearing dislocation as the primary reason for the increased prevalence in patients who undergo UKA with a mobile-bearing implant. Therefore, most surgeons recommend 1 to 2 mm of laxity in both flexion and extension to prevent overcorrection.

Polyethylene insert dislocation is a complication that is unique to patients who undergo UKA with a mobile-bearing implant. Traditionally, polyethylene insert dislocation rates as high as 3.5% to 4.1% were reported.[45,46] In a study of 818 patients who underwent UKA with the Oxford Partial Knee implant, Pandit et al[22] reported a 0.7% rate of bearing dislocation at a follow-up of 15 years. Surgeon experience with the Oxford Partial Knee implant has shown that implant malpositioning and intra-articular impingement increase the risk for bearing dislocation.[46] Recent improvements to Microplasty Instrumentation (Zimmer Biomet) for the Oxford Partial Knee implant have improved the accuracy and reproducibility of intraoperative implant placement and decreased the risk of bearing dislocation.[47,48]

Polyethylene wear is a complication that occurs in patients who undergo UKA with either a fixed- or mobile-bearing implant; however, polyethylene wear is substantially lower in patients who undergo UKA with a mobile-bearing implant. Price et al[37] used radiostereometric analysis to measure the wear rate of seven patients who underwent medial UKA with the Oxford Partial Knee implant and reported a mean linear wear rate of 0.02 mm/year at 10 years postoperatively. Similarly, Kendrick et al[49] used radiostereometric analysis to measure the wear rate of 13 knees that underwent medial UKA with the Oxford Partial Knee implant and reported a mean wear rate of 0.045 mm/year at a mean follow-up of 21 years. Retrieval studies also have reported low rates of polyethylene wear in patients who underwent UKA with a mobile-bearing implant. In a retrieval study of 47 Oxford Partial Knee implants, Kendrick et al[50] reported a mean linear penetration rate of 0.07 mm/year. Conversely, in a retrieval study of 19 fixed-bearing UKA implants, Ashraf et al[51] reported a mean linear penetration rate of 0.15 mm/year.

The incidence of aseptic loosening after UKA is currently a subject of debate. National registry data have suggested that aseptic loosening is extremely prevalent after UKA, with reported rates of aseptic loosening as high as 47%.[52] Conversely, data from the Nuffield Orthopaedic Centre suggested a 0.2% rate of aseptic loosening at the most recent follow-up of patients who underwent UKA with the Oxford Partial Knee implant. This remarkable difference in the incidence of aseptic loosening has been attributed to the misinterpretation of normal physiologic radiolucencies. Radiolucent lines, which are commonly observed under the tibial component, have been reported in patients who undergo UKA with either a fixed- or mobile-bearing implant. The cause of physiologic radiolucency remains unknown; however, physiologic radiolucencies have been reported to form and consolidate during the first 2 years postoperatively, after which they remain stable with no proven correlation with component loosening or implant failure.[53] Although the true incidence of aseptic loosening is likely extremely low in patients who undergo UKA with modern UKA implants, it is an important cause of implant failure after any arthroplasty. Therefore, surgeons should pay strict attention to

the surgical and cementation techniques used during UKA to minimize the risk of aseptic loosening.

Proximal tibial component subsidence and periprosthetic tibial fracture are rare but serious complications of UKA that typically occur in the early postoperative period. Yoshida et al[54] reported a 1.0% rate of tibial component subsidence at 10 years postoperatively. Of the 12 patients with tibial component subsidence, tibial component subsidence developed in eight patients within the first 2 years postoperatively. Similarly, in a study of three patients who underwent UKA, Van Loon et al[55] reported periprosthetic tibial fracture in all three patients, two in whom periprosthetic tibial fracture occurred intraoperatively and one in whom periprosthetic tibial fracture occurred 6 days postoperatively. The risk of tibial component subsidence and periprosthetic tibial fracture has been associated with component positioning and surgical technique. Suboptimal tibial component slope, overresection of the proximal tibia, medial positioning of the tibial component, malrotation, and violation of the posterior cortex have been correlated with early revision surgery. Maintenance of proper tibial component slope, minimal distal resection, proper sizing of the tibial component with the most lateral positioning possible, neutral component rotation, and posterior cortex integrity have been reported to minimize the risk of tibial component subsidence and periprosthetic tibial fracture.[56]

Infection is a serious concern after any arthroplasty. Fortunately, the incidence of deep infection after UKA is relatively low. Multiple studies have reported a substantially lower risk for

deep infection after UKA compared with TKA. Bolognesi et al[57] reported that the 1-year postoperative deep infection rate for Medicare beneficiaries after UKA versus TKA was 1.4% and 2.1%, respectively. Similarly, Brown et al[2] reported a 0.8% and 0.2% deep infection rate in patients who underwent TKA versus UKA, respectively.

Summary

UKA has evolved substantially in the past several decades. The current literature demonstrates that, compared with TKA, UKA is an inherently safe and effective treatment option. Current surgical indications for UKA are based on a diagnosis of AMOA of the knee; obesity, age, the location of pain, and a high activity level are no longer considered contraindications to UKA. The preoperative status of a patient's patellofemoral joint remains a topic of debate with regard to UKA; however, the status of the patellofemoral joint may be safely ignored in most patients in whom UKA with a mobile-bearing implant is being considered given that no lateral subluxation or lateral grooving is present.

Although more long-term prospective randomized trials are necessary to definitively demonstrate any substantial difference between fixed- and mobile-bearing UKA implants, the authors of this chapter prefer to use the Oxford Partial Knee implant for UKA. This preference is based on improved wear characteristics demonstrated by retrieval and radiostereometric analysis data, improved clinical outcomes with regard to the patellofemoral joint, and improved instrumentation, which allows for improved accuracy of component positioning.

References

1. Liddle AD, Judge A, Pandit H, Murray DW: Adverse outcomes after total and unicompartmental knee replacement in 101,330 matched patients: A study of data from the National Joint Registry for England and Wales. *Lancet* 2014;384(9952):1437-1445.

2. Brown NM, Sheth NP, Davis K, et al: Total knee arthroplasty has higher postoperative morbidity than unicompartmental knee arthroplasty: A multicenter analysis. *J Arthroplasty* 2012;27(8 suppl):86-90.

3. Lombardi AV Jr, Berend KR, Walter CA, Aziz-Jacobo J, Cheney NA: Is recovery faster for mobile-bearing unicompartmental than total knee arthroplasty? *Clin Orthop Relat Res* 2009;467(6):1450-1457.

4. Laskin RS: Unicompartmental tibiofemoral resurfacing arthroplasty. *J Bone Joint Surg Am* 1978;60(2):182-185.

5. Mallory TH, Danyi J: Unicompartmental total knee arthroplasty: A five- to nine-year follow-up study of 42 procedures. *Clin Orthop Relat Res* 1983;175:135-138.

6. Marmor L: The Marmor knee replacement. *Orthop Clin North Am* 1982;13(1):55-64.

7. Squire MW, Callaghan JJ, Goetz DD, Sullivan PM, Johnston RC: Unicompartmental knee replacement: A minimum 15 year followup study. *Clin Orthop Relat Res* 1999;367:61-72.

8. Palmer SH, Morrison PJ, Ross AC: Early catastrophic tibial component wear after unicompartmental knee arthroplasty. *Clin Orthop Relat Res* 1998;350:143-148.

9. Goodfellow JW, O'Connor J, Pandit H, Dodd C, Murray D: *Unicompartmental Arthroplasty with the Oxford Knee*, ed 2. Oxford, United Kingdom, Goodfellow Publishers, 2015, pp 1-14.

10. Argenson JN, Komistek RD, Aubaniac JM, et al: In vivo determination of knee kinematics for subjects implanted with a unicompartmental arthroplasty. *J Arthroplasty* 2002;17(8):1049-1054.

11. Parratte S, Ollivier M, Lunebourg A, Abdel MP, Argenson JN: Long-term results of compartmental arthroplasties of the knee: Long term results of partial knee arthroplasty. *Bone Joint J* 2015;97(10 suppl A):9-15.

12. Ko YB, Gujarathi MR, Oh KJ: Outcome of unicompartmental knee arthroplasty: A systematic review of comparative studies between fixed and mobile bearings focusing on complications. *Knee Surg Relat Res* 2015;27(3):141-148.

13. Emerson RH Jr, Hansborough T, Reitman RD, Rosenfeldt W, Higgins LL: Comparison of a mobile with a fixed-bearing unicompartmental knee implant. *Clin Orthop Relat Res* 2002;404:62-70.

14. Confalonieri N, Manzotti A, Pullen C: Comparison of a mobile with a fixed tibial bearing unicompartmental knee prosthesis: A prospective randomized trial using a dedicated outcome score. *Knee* 2004;11(5):357-362.

15. Li MG, Yao F, Joss B, Ioppolo J, Nivbrant B, Wood D: Mobile vs. fixed bearing unicondylar knee arthroplasty: A randomized study on short term clinical outcomes and knee kinematics. *Knee* 2006;13(5):365-370.

16. Kozinn SC, Scott R: Unicondylar knee arthroplasty. *J Bone Joint Surg Am* 1989;71(1):145-150.

17. Berend KR, Lombardi AV Jr, Adams JB: Obesity, young age, patellofemoral disease, and anterior knee pain: Identifying the unicondylar arthroplasty patient in the United States. *Orthopedics* 2007;30(5 suppl):19-23.

18. Ritter MA, Faris PM, Thong AE, Davis KE, Meding JB, Berend ME: Intra-operative findings in varus osteoarthritis of the knee: An analysis of pre-operative alignment in potential candidates for unicompartmental arthroplasty. *J Bone Joint Surg Br* 2004;86(1):43-47.

19. Berger RA, Meneghini RM, Jacobs JJ, et al: Results of unicompartmental knee arthroplasty at a minimum of ten years of follow-up. *J Bone Joint Surg Am* 2005;87(5):999-1006.

20. Goodfellow JW, Kershaw CJ, Benson MK, O'Connor JJ: The Oxford Knee for unicompartmental osteoarthritis: The first 103 cases. *J Bone Joint Surg Br* 1988;70(5):692-701.

21. Price AJ, Waite JC, Svard U: Long-term clinical results of the medial Oxford unicompartmental knee arthroplasty. *Clin Orthop Relat Res* 2005;435:171-180.

22. Pandit H, Hamilton TW, Jenkins C, Mellon SJ, Dodd CA, Murray DW: The clinical outcome of minimally invasive Phase 3 Oxford unicompartmental knee arthroplasty: A 15-year follow-up of 1000 UKAs. *Bone Joint J* 2015;97(11):1493-1500.

23. Pennington DW, Swienckowski JJ, Lutes WB, Drake GN: Unicompartmental knee arthroplasty in patients sixty years of age or younger. *J Bone Joint Surg Am* 2003;85(10):1968-1973.

24. Price AJ, Short A, Kellett C, et al: Ten-year in vivo wear measurement of a fully congruent mobile bearing unicompartmental knee arthroplasty. *J Bone Joint Surg Br* 2005;87(11):1493-1497.

25. White SH, Ludkowski PF, Goodfellow JW: Anteromedial osteoarthritis of the knee. *J Bone Joint Surg Br* 1991;73(4):582-586.

26. Berend KR, Berend ME, Dalury DF, Argenson JN, Dodd CA, Scott RD: Consensus Statement on Indications and Contraindications for Medial Unicompartmental Knee Arthroplasty. *J Surg Orthop Adv* 2015;24(4):252-256.

27. Heyse TJ, Khefacha A, Peersman G, Cartier P: Survivorship of UKA in the middle-aged. *Knee* 2012;19(5):585-591.

28. Tabor OB Jr, Tabor OB, Bernard M, Wan JY: Unicompartmental knee arthroplasty: Long-term success in middle-age and obese patients. *J Surg Orthop Adv* 2005;14(2):59-63.

29. Ali AM, Pandit H, Liddle AD, et al: Does activity affect the outcome of the Oxford unicompartmental knee replacement? *Knee* 2016;23(2):327-330.

30. Berend KR, Lombardi AV Jr, Mallory TH, Adams JB, Groseth KL: Early failure of minimally invasive unicompartmental knee arthroplasty is associated with obesity. *Clin Orthop Relat Res* 2005;440:60-66.

31. Cavaignac E, Lafontan V, Reina N, et al: Obesity has no adverse effect on the outcome of unicompartmental knee replacement at a minimum

follow-up of seven years. *Bone Joint J* 2013;95(8):1064-1068.

32. Murray DW, Pandit H, Weston-Simons JS, et al: Does body mass index affect the outcome of unicompartmental knee replacement? *Knee* 2013;20(6):461-465.

33. Beard DJ, Pandit H, Gill HS, Hollinghurst D, Dodd CA, Murray DW: The influence of the presence and severity of pre-existing patellofemoral degenerative changes on the outcome of the Oxford medial unicompartmental knee replacement. *J Bone Joint Surg Br* 2007;89(12):1597-1601.

34. Berend KR, Lombardi AV Jr, Morris MJ, Hurst JM, Kavolus JJ: Does preoperative patellofemoral joint state affect medial unicompartmental arthroplasty survival? *Orthopedics* 2011;34(9):e494-e496.

35. Munk S, Odgaard A, Madsen F, et al: Preoperative lateral subluxation of the patella is a predictor of poor early outcome of Oxford phase-III medial unicompartmental knee arthroplasty. *Acta Orthop* 2011;82(5):582-588.

36. Berger RA, Meneghini RM, Sheinkop MB, et al: The progression of patellofemoral arthrosis after medial unicompartmental replacement: Results at 11 to 15 years. *Clin Orthop Relat Res* 2004;428:92-99.

37. Price AJ, Rees JL, Beard DJ, Gill RH, Dodd CA, Murray DM: Sagittal plane kinematics of a mobile-bearing unicompartmental knee arthroplasty at 10 years: A comparative in vivo fluoroscopic analysis. *J Arthroplasty* 2004;19(5):590-597.

38. Inaba Y, Numazaki S, Koshino T, Saito T: Provoked anterior knee pain in medial osteoarthritis of the knee. *Knee* 2003;10(4):351-355.

39. Mauerhan DR, Cook KD, Botts TD, Williams ST: Patient-directed valgus stress radiograph of the knee: A new and novel technique. *Am J Orthop (Belle Mead NJ)* 2016;45(1):44-46.

40. Lombardi AV, Berend KR, Adams JB: A rapid recovery program: Early home and pain free. *Orthopedics* 2010;33(9):656.

41. Cross MB, Berger R: Feasibility and safety of performing outpatient unicompartmental knee arthroplasty. *Int Orthop* 2014;38(2):443-447.

42. Morris MJ, Molli RG, Berend KR, Lombardi AV Jr: Mortality and perioperative complications after unicompartmental knee arthroplasty. *Knee* 2013;20(3):218-220.

43. Springer BD, Scott RD, Thornhill TS: Conversion of failed unicompartmental knee arthroplasty to TKA. *Clin Orthop Relat Res* 2006;446:214-220.

44. Parratte S, Pauly V, Aubaniac JM, Argenson JN: No long-term difference between fixed and mobile medial unicompartmental arthroplasty. *Clin Orthop Relat Res* 2012;470(1):61-68.

45. Verdonk R, Cottenie D, Almqvist KF, Vorlat P: The Oxford unicompartmental knee prosthesis: A 2-14 year follow-up. *Knee Surg Sports Traumatol Arthrosc* 2005;13(3):163-166.

46. Lee SY, Bae JH, Kim JG, et al: The influence of surgical factors on dislocation of the meniscal bearing after Oxford medial unicompartmental knee replacement: A case-control study. *Bone Joint J* 2014;96(7):914-922.

47. Koh IJ, Kim JH, Jang SW, Kim MS, Kim C, In Y: Are the Oxford(®) medial unicompartmental knee arthroplasty new instruments reducing the bearing dislocation risk while improving components relationships? A case control study. *Orthop Traumatol Surg Res* 2016;102(2):183-187.

48. Price AJ, Webb J, Topf H, et al: Rapid recovery after oxford unicompartmental arthroplasty through a short incision. *J Arthroplasty* 2001;16(8):970-976.

49. Kendrick BJ, Simpson DJ, Kaptein BL, et al: Polyethylene wear of mobile-bearing unicompartmental knee

replacement at 20 years. *J Bone Joint Surg Br* 2011;93(4):470-475.

50. Kendrick BJ, Longino D, Pandit H, et al: Polyethylene wear in Oxford unicompartmental knee replacement: A retrieval study of 47 bearings. *J Bone Joint Surg Br* 2010;92(3):367-373.

51. Ashraf T, Newman JH, Desai VV, Beard D, Nevelos JE: Polyethylene wear in a non-congruous unicompartmental knee replacement: A retrieval analysis. *Knee* 2004;11(3):177-181.

52. Niinimäki T, Eskelinen A, Mäkelä K, Ohtonen P, Puhto AP, Remes V: Unicompartmental knee arthroplasty survivorship is lower than TKA survivorship: A 27-year Finnish registry study. *Clin Orthop Relat Res* 2014;472(5):1496-1501.

53. Hooper N, Snell D, Hooper G, Maxwell R, Frampton C: The five-year radiological results of the uncemented Oxford medial compartment knee arthroplasty. *Bone Joint J* 2015; 97(10):1358-1363.

54. Yoshida K, Tada M, Yoshida H, Takei S, Fukuoka S, Nakamura H: Oxford phase 3 unicompartmental knee arthroplasty in Japan—clinical results in greater than one thousand cases over ten years. *J Arthroplasty* 2013; 28(9 suppl):168-171.

55. Van Loon P, de Munnynck B, Bellemans J: Periprosthetic fracture of the tibial plateau after unicompartmental knee arthroplasty. *Acta Orthop Belg* 2006;72(3):369-374.

56. Small SR, Berend ME, Rogge RD, Archer DB, Kingman AL, Ritter MA: Tibial loading after UKA: Evaluation of tibial slope, resection depth, medial shift and component rotation. *J Arthroplasty* 2013;28(9 suppl):179-183.

57. Bolognesi MP, Greiner MA, Attarian DE, et al: Unicompartmental knee arthroplasty and total knee arthroplasty among Medicare beneficiaries, 2000 to 2009. *J Bone Joint Surg Am* 2013;95(22):e174.

Patellofemoral Arthroplasty: An Evolving Science

Jess H. Lonner, MD

Abstract

Patellofemoral arthroplasty (PFA) has long been a clinical option for patients with isolated patellofemoral arthritis. However, a high rate of failure as a result of patellar instability related to component malposition, soft-tissue imbalance, errant surgical techniques, and poor trochlear implant designs contributed to the underutilization of PFA. The evolution of surgical indications, trochlear implant design, component positioning, and soft-tissue balance has led to improved patellar tracking, fewer failures related to patellar instability, and improved functional outcomes. The development and broad adoption of onlay-style trochlear components, which can be positioned perpendicular to the AP axis of the femur, has substantially improved patellar tracking and, thus, improved the durability of PFA. In addition, favorable data showing success after secondary surgery or revision to total knee arthroplasty after PFA have emerged, which has led to increased use of PFA in appropriately selected patients.

Instr Course Lect 2017;66:211–221.

Epidemiologic studies indicate that isolated patellofemoral arthritis affects approximately 10% of the population older than 40 years.[1] Females are more than twice as likely as males to have isolated anterior compartment degeneration (24% versus 11%, respectively),[2] which is likely related to subtle dysplasia and malalignment.[3] As the population ages and the burden of arthritis increases,[4] more patients will likely seek treatment for patellofemoral arthritis. In addition, conservative surgical treatments, such as patellofemoral arthroplasty (PFA), will remain important alternatives to total knee arthroplasty (TKA) in younger patients (aged 30 to 59 years) with patellofemoral arthritis in whom nonsurgical treatment is ineffective. The challenge of effectively managing patellofemoral arthritis is immense given the high rate of failure of biologic treatments, such as grafting and unloading procedures, and the limited enthusiasm for performing TKA in patients who have localized grade IV chondromalacia or frank arthritis because these patients tend to be young.

Since the 1970s, PFA has been a clinical option for patients who have isolated patellofemoral arthritis.[5,6] For decades, a high rate of failure as a result of patellar instability secondary to component malposition, soft-tissue imbalance, errant surgical techniques, and poor trochlear implant designs have tarnished the reputation of PFA.[7-12] The various elements necessary to optimize PFA outcomes, including patient evaluation and selection, trochlear implant design, component positioning, and soft-tissue balance, have evolved, which has led to improved patellar tracking, fewer patellofemoral-related failures, and a decreased need for secondary surgery.[8,13-27] In addition, favorable data showing success after secondary surgery or revision to TKA after PFA have emerged, which has led to increased use of PFA in appropriately selected patients.[28-30]

Dr. Lonner or an immediate family member has received royalties from Zimmer Biomet and Blue Belt Technologies; is a member of a speakers' bureau or has made paid presentations on behalf of Blue Belt Technologies and Zimmer Biomet; serves as a paid consultant to Blue Belt Technologies, CD Diagnostics, and Zimmer Biomet; has stock or stock options held in Blue Belt Technologies, CD Diagnostics, and HealthpointCapital; has received research or institutional support from Zimmer Biomet; and serves as a board member, owner, officer, or committee member of the Knee Society.

Patient Selection

A key to the increased success of PFA has been an improved understanding of the ideal candidate for PFA. PFA outcomes are optimized in patients who have isolated patellofemoral osteoarthritis, posttraumatic arthritis, or diffuse Outerbridge grade IV chondromalacia of either the patellar or trochlear surfaces. In addition, PFA is best reserved for patients who have isolated retropatellar and/or peripatellar pain. Functional limitations and pain should worsen with provocative activities that specifically load the patellofemoral compartment, such as stair or hill ambulation, squatting, or prolonged sitting. Pain should be negligible with ambulation on level surfaces. PFA should not be performed in patients who have inflammatory arthritis or chondrocalcinosis that involves the menisci or tibiofemoral chondral surfaces, and PFA should not be offered to patients who have unrealistic postoperative expectations.[31-33] Medial or lateral joint line pain suggests more diffuse chondral disease and should be considered a contraindication to isolated patellofemoral resurfacing. Patients who have alternative etiologies of anterior knee pain, such as patellar tendinitis, synovitis, patellar instability, sympathetic mediated pain, or pain referred from the back or ipsilateral hip, should not be considered for PFA.

Although PFA can be effectively used to manage patellofemoral dysplasia,[26,27,34] it should not be used in patients who have considerable patellar maltracking or malalignment unless patellar maltracking or malalignment are corrected. However, PFA may be contraindicated in patients who have moderate patellar tilt that is observed on preoperative tangential radiographs or when arthrotomy is performed and in patients who have trochlear dysplasia. A lateral retinacular recession or release may be necessary at the time of PFA in these patients.[35] Persistent patellar subluxation may cause pain and snapping and, potentially, polyethylene wear of the prosthesis. In patients with excessive Q angles, tibial tubercle realignment should be performed before or at the same time as PFA; however, some trochlear prostheses may accommodate a slightly increased Q angle. In addition, the presence of tibiofemoral arthrosis should discourage isolated PFA. Even the presence of focal grade III tibiofemoral chondromalacia can compromise PFA outcomes; however, patients who have focal grade III tibiofemoral chondromalacia will experience resolution of the most prominent component of pain after PFA. Performing PFA in combination with medial or lateral unicompartmental knee arthroplasty or autologous osteochondral grafting is reasonable for patients who have focal grade III tibiofemoral chondromalacia.[36-38]

Although intuitive concerns exist, no data are available on whether obesity or cruciate ligament insufficiency increases the risk for failure in patients who undergo PFA. Strict age criteria do not apply for PFA given that the other criteria are met; however, PFA is uncommonly performed in patients younger than 30 years. If selected appropriately, elderly patients who undergo PFA have good outcomes. Patients who require narcotics for patellofemoral arthritis are not good candidates for PFA because their pain tends to persist postoperatively, and their postoperative satisfaction is low. Efforts should be taken to wean patients off narcotics before PFA is offered as a treatment option.

Some studies have suggested that the mental health status of patients be determined before PFA is performed. Kazarian et al[21] reported that, despite significant functional improvements after PFA with an onlay-style prosthesis, patients who had significantly lower Mental Health scores were more likely to be dissatisfied with their outcomes. Dahm et al[39] reported that 42% of patients who underwent PFA had preexisting psychiatric conditions (anxiety or depression), which may, in part, explain the tendency for lingering pain or dissatisfaction after PFA.

Clinical Evaluation

The evaluation of a patient in whom PFA is being considered should confirm that pain is localized to the anterior compartment of the knee and is attributed to the patellofemoral chondral surfaces and not soft tissues. Obtaining a detailed history of the problem, performing a meticulous physical examination, and obtaining appropriate imaging studies will confirm the source of the pain.

History

The key elements of a patient's history include previous trauma to the knee, a history of patellar dislocation, and prior patellofemoral problems. A history of recurrent atraumatic patellar dislocations may indicate the presence of considerable malalignment that may require correction before PFA. The location of the pain should be clearly described; PFA will not relieve discomfort in any location other than directly retropatellar or just lateral or medial to the patella. Often, patellofemoral pain is exacerbated by activities such as stair or hill ambulation, standing from a seated position, sitting with the knee flexed, and squatting. Pain should be negligible with ambulation on level surfaces. A description of anterior crepitus is common. After the location and quality of pain have been established, the surgeon should ascertain whether previous interventions, such as physical therapy, weight reduction, medications, injections, or surgery, were undertaken.

Physical Examination

Pain elicited via patellar inhibition testing as well as patellofemoral crepitus and retropatellar knee pain that occurs with squatting are typical findings of the physical examination. Any associated medial or lateral tibiofemoral joint line tenderness should alert the surgeon to the possibility of more diffuse chondral disease, even if radiographs are relatively normal, and may be considered a contraindication to isolated PFA. Other potential sources of anterior knee pain, such as pes anserinus bursitis, patellar tendinitis, prepatellar bursitis, instability, or pain referred from the ipsilateral hip or back, must be ruled out. Surgeons must carefully assess patellar tracking and the Q angle. As previously discussed, even subtle patellar tracking abnormalities and malalignment may predispose patients to inferior outcomes, particularly with the use of certain PFA prostheses. For patients who have high Q angles, a tibial tubercle realignment procedure (anteromedialization) should be performed before or at the same time as PFA. Anterior or posterior cruciate ligament insufficiency may be a contraindication to PFA if subtle tibiofemoral articular cartilage damage is present.

Imaging

In general, AP and midflexion PA radiographs must be weight bearing to determine the presence of tibiofemoral arthritis. Mild squaring of the femoral condyles and even small marginal osteophytes may be acceptable, given that a patient does not have tibiofemoral pain during functional activities and during the physical examination and that minimal chondral degeneration is noted during arthroscopy or arthrotomy. Occasionally, lateral radiographs may demonstrate patellofemoral osteophytes; however, lateral radiographs usually are more useful in identifying if patella alta or baja is present. Axial radiographs show the position of the patella in the trochlear groove and the extent of arthritis; however, occasionally, relative radiographic patellofemoral joint space preservation with minimal or no osteophytes will be present despite substantial cartilage loss (**Figure 1**).

Currently, MRI is used to evaluate for patellofemoral arthritis but, more importantly, is used to assess for evidence of chondral wear of the medial and lateral compartments. Images from prior arthroscopic treatment provide surgeons with valuable information on the extent of anterior compartment arthritis and the status of the tibiofemoral articular cartilage and menisci. Surgeons who are committed to performing PFA in patients with diffuse degeneration or focal condylar cartilage defects should consider concomitant autologous osteochondral grafting for the management of associated focal condylar defects or unicompartmental knee arthroplasty (as part of modular bicompartmental knee arthroplasty).[36-38]

Trochlear Morphology, Component Positioning and Design, and Clinical Outcomes

Surgeons' understanding of how the variability in native trochlear morphology and orientation affect the positioning of the trochlear component of inlay-style implants as well as, ultimately, patellar tracking and the outcomes of PFA has improved.[17,22,32,33,40-42] This improved understanding has led to a broad shift in implant designs and a trend toward the selection of onlay-style trochlear designs rather than inlay-style implants.

Two general categories of trochlear designs exist: inlay-style designs and onlay-style designs[17,32,33] (**Table 1**). Inlay-style components require the removal of very little trochlear bone and, therefore, are a conservative method for bone preparation. Using a curet or a motorized burr, the trochlear bed is prepared by removing a small volume of bone to accommodate the prosthesis, which is inlayed so that its edges are flush with the surrounding trochlear and condylar cartilage surfaces. In this method of bone preparation, regardless of whether the component is off the shelf or customized, the axial rotational alignment of the trochlear prosthesis is parallel with the patient's native trochlear inclination. Typically, an inlay-style component ends at the proximal cartilage edge of the native trochlea, does not extend further up the femur, and is relatively narrow so that its edges can be inset in the surrounding cartilage without extension to the edges of the trochlea. Unless an inlay-style prosthesis is customized, a relatively poor fit with the native trochlea may exist as a result of considerable morphologic variability. In addition, the position and rotational alignment of an inlay-style prosthesis will depend on the shape of a patient's trochlear surfaces (**Figure 2**).

Onlay-style components generally tend to be wider, have more favorable sagittal radii of curvature, and extend

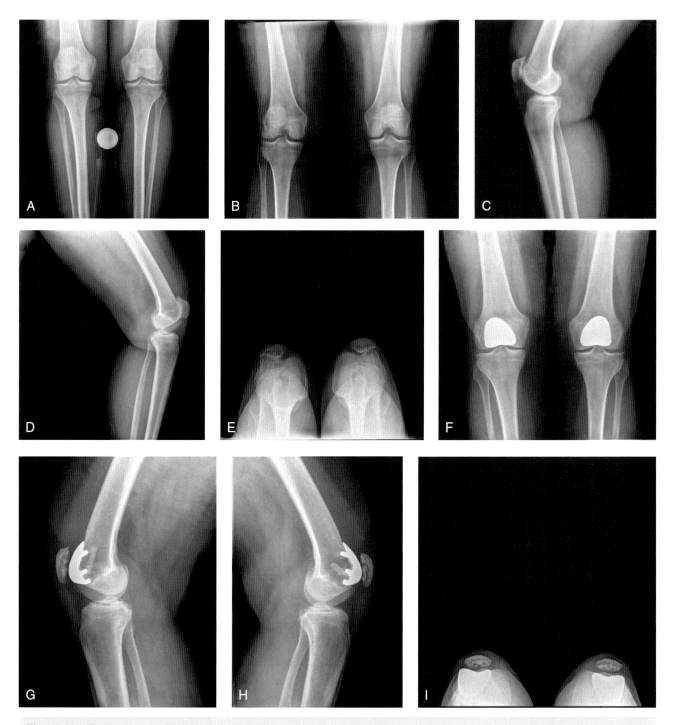

Figure 1   Radiographs of the knees of a 59-year-old woman. Weight-bearing bilateral AP (**A**) and weight-bearing bilateral midflexion PA (**B**) radiographs demonstrate preservation of the tibiofemoral spaces. Lateral radiographs of the right (**C**) and left (**D**) knees and bilateral sunrise radiograph (**E**) demonstrate patellofemoral arthritis with slight patellar subluxation. Weight-bearing bilateral AP radiograph (**F**), lateral radiographs of the right (**G**) and left (**H**) knees, and bilateral sunrise radiograph (**I**) taken after bilateral patellofemoral arthroplasty demonstrate appropriate component positioning and normalized patellar position relative to the trochlear component.

more proximally up the femur compared with inlay-style designs.[7,17] The method of bone preparation for onlay-style prostheses involves anterior trochlear resection perpendicular to the Whiteside (AP) axis or parallel to the transepicondylar axis and flush with the anterior femoral cortex (**Figure 3**). Both the trochlear design features of and the method of bone preparation for onlay-style prostheses contribute to the superior clinical outcomes and optimized patellar tracking observed in patients who undergo PFA with an onlay-style trochlear implant.[7,17,22]

Given the shape, morphology, and rotational alignment of the trochlear surfaces of the human knee, it is clear why PFA with an inlay-style prosthesis results in a higher incidence of patellar component maltracking and instability. In a study of 200 trochlear resection specimens (100 from women and 100 from men) that were obtained when TKA was performed, Lonner et al[41] reported that the mean lateral and medial trochlear flange heights in women were 10.47 mm (range, 2.0 to 19.0 mm) and 6.95 mm (range, 2.0 to 18.0 mm), respectively. The authors reported that the mean lateral and medial trochlear flange heights in men were 11.95 mm (range, 6.5 to 20.5 mm) and 7.71 mm (range, 1.0 to 18.0 mm), respectively.[41] The differences in the mean heights between the lateral and medial trochlear flanges, which were approximately 3.5 to 4 mm in both the men and the women, have implications for trochlear implant positioning in PFA with an inlay-style prosthesis. These data were corroborated in a study by Biedert et al,[42] which reported that, in a nondysplastic trochlea, the anterior-most aspect of the lateral trochlear condyle is higher than the anterior-most aspect of the medial trochlear condyle.

Typically, these differences in the anterior-most heights of the lateral and medial trochlear peaks result in internal rotation of the anterior trochlear surface relative to the Whiteside axis or the transepicondylar axis, even in patients who have trochlear dysplasia[40] (**Figure 4**). In a review of MRI studies of the knees of more than 300 patients, which had been obtained to evaluate for a variety of random pathologic conditions, Kamath et al[40] reported that the mean anterior trochlear inclination angle (the angle from the lateral to medial peaks of the trochlear articular cartilage relative to the AP axis of the femur) was internally rotated 11.3°; no significant differences were reported between the

Table 1

General Design Characteristics of Inlay- and Onlay-Style Patellofemoral Prostheses

Characteristic	Inlay-Style Prosthesis	Onlay-Style Prosthesis
Positioning	Inset flush with the native trochlea	Replaces entire trochlea; perpendicular to the AP axis
Rotation	Determined by the native trochlea	Set by surgeon; perpendicular to the AP axis
Width	Narrower	Wider
Proximal extension	No further than the native trochlear surface	Extends further proximal than the native trochlea

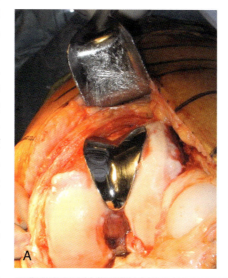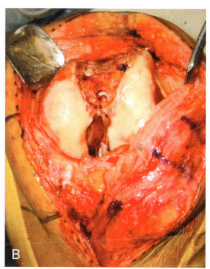

Figure 2   Intraoperative photographs of a knee show an inlay-style trochlear prosthesis. **A,** The component appears to be internally rotated, which can result in lateral patellar instability and catching. **B,** Bone preparation common with an inlay-style trochlear prosthesis demonstrates conservative removal of bone that is tangential to the articular surfaces. In this knee, a previous inlay style trochlear prosthesis was removed during revision to an onlay-style prosthesis. (Reproduced from Lombardi AV Jr, Berend KR, Berend ME, et al: Current controversies in partial knee arthroplasty. *Instr Course Lect* 2012;61:347-381.)

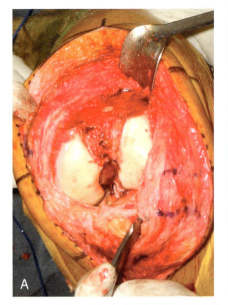 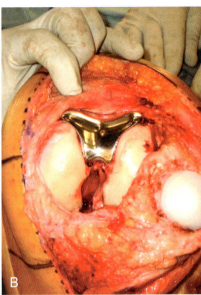

Figure 3 **A,** Intraoperative photograph of a knee shows anterior bone resection perpendicular to the AP axis (or parallel to the transepicondylar axis) for an onlay-style trochlear prosthesis. **B,** Intraoperative photograph of a knee shows the position of an onlay-style trochlear prosthesis that is appropriately externally rotated relative to the AP axis of the femur. (Reproduced from Lombardi AV Jr, Berend KR, Berend ME, et al: Current controversies in partial knee arthroplasty. *Instr Course Lect* 2012;61:347-381.)

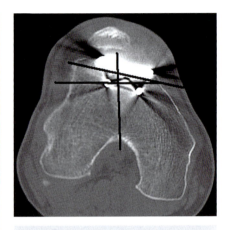

Figure 4 Axial CT scan of a knee with an inlay-style trochlear component that was implanted tangential to the anterior trochlear surfaces, which can result in component internal rotation and predisposes the knee to lateral patellar subluxation. The black lines represent the AP and transepicondylar axes of the femur as well as the extent of internal rotation of the trochlear component relative to those axes. (Reproduced from Lombardi AV Jr, Berend KR, Berend ME, et al: Current controversies in partial knee arthroplasty. *Instr Course Lect* 2012;61:347-381.)

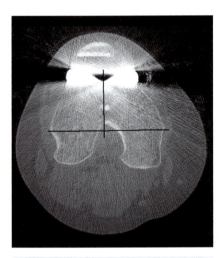

Figure 5 Axial CT scan of a knee with an onlay-style trochlear component demonstrates improved positioning perpendicular to the AP axis and parallel to the transepicondylar axis (indicated by the black lines) and improved patellar tracking. (Reproduced from Lombardi AV Jr, Berend KR, Berend ME, et al: Current controversies in partial knee arthroplasty. *Instr Course Lect* 2012;61:347-381.)

anterior trochlear inclination angles of women and men. Even in patients who had trochlear dysplasia, the mean anterior trochlear inclination angle was internally rotated 8.2°.

The aforementioned studies elucidate why inlay-style trochlear designs tend to be internally rotated. Similar to malrotated femoral components in TKA, which are implanted in internal rotation relative to the transepicondylar or Whiteside axes, internal rotation of the trochlear component in PFA medializes the trochlear groove, increases the Q angle, and places tension on the lateral retinaculum; these factors predispose patients to patellar maltracking and instability.[43] Conversely, onlay-style trochlear designs, which are implanted perpendicular to the AP axis of the femur or parallel to the transepicondylar axis, help minimize these factors.[17,35] (**Figure 5**).

An analysis of PFA outcomes revealed a disparity in the early and midterm failures that occur as a result of patellar instability and maltracking, depending on whether an inlay-style or onlay-style component was used.[5-27,44] If patellar tracking is satisfactory after PFA, progressive tibiofemoral arthritis will be the primary mode of failure, irrespective of the type of trochlear prosthesis used. Unfortunately, inlay-style components have a higher tendency for patellar maltracking compared with onlay-style components; more often, inlay-style components require early secondary surgery to realign the extensor mechanism, revision PFA, or conversion to TKA.[22] That is the major evolution in PFA—recognition that the improved design features of

Table 2
Results of Patellofemoral Arthroplasty With Inlay-Style Implants

Authors(s) (Year)	Implant Type	No. of Knees	Mean Patient Age in Years (Range)	Mean Follow-up in Years (Range)	Good or Excellent Results (%)	Revised (%)
Blazina et al[5] (1979)	Richards I and II (Smith & Nephew)	57	39 (19–81)	2 (0.6–3.5)	NA	35
Arciero and Toomey[9] (1988)	Richards II and CFS (Wright Medical Technology)	25	62 (33–86)	5.3 (3–9)	85	28
Cartier et al[24] (1990)	Richards II and III (Smith & Nephew)	72	65 (23–89)	4 (2–12)	85	7
Argenson et al[26] (1995)	Autocentric (DePuy)	66	57 (19–82)	5.5 (2–10)	84	15
de Winter et al[12] (2001)	Richards II	26	59 (22–90)	11 (1–20)	76	19
Tauro et al[11] (2001)	Lubinus (Waldermar Link)	62	66 (50–87)	7.5 (5–10)	45	28
Smith et al[10] (2002)	Lubinus	45	72 (42–86)	4 (0.5–7.5)	69	19
Kooijman et al[23] (2003)	Richards II	45	50 (20–77)	17 (15–21)	86	22
Lonner[7] (2004)	Lubinus	30	38 (34–51)	4 (2–6)	84	33
Argenson et al[27] (2005)	Autocentric	66	57 (21–82)	16.2 (12–20)	NA	42
Cartier et al[25] (2005)	Richards II and III	79	60 (36–81)	10 (6–16)	77	25
Charalambous et al[45] (2011)	LCS (DePuy)	51	64 (47–84)	2.1 (0.4–5)	33	33

NA = not available.

onlay-style trochlear components has led to improved component positioning and, thus, improved patellar tracking and improved PFA outcomes.

Studies have reported a 17% to 44% incidence of patellar maltracking and the need for secondary surgery in patients who underwent PFA with an inlay-style implant.[5,7,10-12] In these studies, the components likely were positioned flush with some but not all of the articular surfaces (because of morphologic mismatch between the surface anatomy and the trochlear implant) and internally rotated as a result of the native trochlear inclination, both of which predispose patients to patellar catching and subluxation. Alternatively, studies

have reported a considerably lower incidence of patellar maltracking (typically, less than 1%) in patients who underwent PFA with an onlay-style trochlear implant.[7,14-19,21,22] In a recent study of 70 knees that underwent PFA with an onlay-style implant, Kazarian et al[21] reported that, at a minimum follow-up of 2 years (mean, 4.9 years), mean range of motion and Knee Society knee and functional scores improved significantly ($P < 0.0001$), and less than 4% of the patients required revision arthroplasty for progressive tibiofemoral arthritis. The authors reported no radiographic evidence of component loosening or wear, and no clinical or radiographic evidence of patellar

instability was present. The dichotomy between inlay-style and onlay-style designs is highlighted in the Australian Orthopaedic Association National Joint Replacement Registry,[44] which shows that the 5-year cumulative revision surgery rate was more than 20% for PFA with inlay-style prostheses and less than 10% for PFA with onlay-style prostheses[5,7,9-12,14-16,18-21,23-27,45] (**Tables 2** and **3**).

In an analysis of treatment strategies for patellofemoral arthritis, surgeons should compare the outcomes of PFA with those of TKA. In a retrospective study of the outcomes of 45 patients with isolated patellofemoral arthritis who underwent either PFA or TKA, Dahm et al[39] reported similar Knee

Table 3

Results of Patellofemoral Arthroplasty With Onlay-Style Implants

Authors (Year)	Implant Type	No. of Knees	Mean Patient Age in Years (Range)	Mean Follow-up in Years (Range)	Good or Excellent Results (%)	Revised (%)
Ackroyd et al[14] (2007)	Avon (Stryker)	109	68 (46–86)	5.2 (5–8)	80	4
Leadbetter et al[16] (2009)	Avon	79	58 (34–77)	3 (2–6)	84	6
Starks et al[15] (2009)	Avon	37	66 (30–82)	2 (NA)	86	Zero
Odumenya et al[18] (2010)	Avon	50	66 (42–88)	5.3 (2.1–10.2)	NA	4
Mont et al[19] (2012)	Avon	43	49 (27–67)	7 (4–8)	NA	12
Beitzel et al[20] (2013)	Journey PFJ (Smith & Nephew)	22	46 (26–67)	2 (NA)	NA	5
Kazarian et al[21] (2016)	Zimmer Gender Solutions PFJ (Zimmer)	70	51 (36–80)	4.9 (2.3–7.4)	NA	4

NA = not available.

Society Clinical Rating System and pain scores between the patients in the two groups at a mean follow-up of 2.5 years; however, the patients in the PFA group had significantly higher activity scores. In a recent meta-analysis of 28 studies that compared the complications of patients with isolated patellofemoral arthritis who underwent either PFA or TKA, Dy et al[22] reported an eightfold higher likelihood of additional procedures and revision surgery for the patients who underwent PFA compared with the patients who underwent TKA. However, in a comparison of the complications of the patients who underwent either PFA with a second-generation onlay-style prosthesis or TKA, the authors reported no significant differences with regard to additional procedures, revision surgery, pain, or mechanical complications, which indicates the important effects of implant design and rotational positioning of the trochlear component on PFA outcomes. A subgroup analysis performed by the authors revealed that significant complications were more than four times more likely to develop in patients who underwent PFA with a first-generation inlay-style prosthesis compared with patients who underwent PFA with a second-generation onlay-style prosthesis, which likely created a bias in the overall results of the study. The authors concluded that patients who undergo PFA with an onlay-style implant likely have similar rates of complications compared with patients who undergo TKA.

Revision Surgery After PFA

Patients in whom PFA with an inlay-style implant fails as a result of patellar instability secondary to internal rotation of the trochlear component can be effectively treated with revision PFA with an onlay-style trochlear component. Patellar prostheses that are well fixed, unworn, and positioned appropriately should be retained. Hendrix et al[28] revised 14 knees with failed first-generation inlay-style prostheses to second-generation onlay-style implants.

Standard off-the-shelf implants were used, and no compromise in bone support was noted. The modes of primary implant failure included component malposition, patellar subluxation and catching, polyethylene wear, and overstuffing. At a mean follow-up of 5 years (range, 3 to 7 years), the authors reported significant improvements in mean Bristol Knee Scores as well as mean Bristol Knee pain and functional subscores. Two of the five patients who had evidence of mild tibiofemoral arthritis at the time of revision, which predicted poorer outcomes, underwent revision to TKA by final follow-up.

The uncertainty of how PFA may affect surgical complexity and outcomes if conversion to TKA is required was a concern for some surgeons and another barrier to the broad appeal of PFA. Recent studies have addressed these concerns and further improved surgeons' understanding of PFA. Although early failures as a result of patellar instability have been mitigated by the use of more onlay-style trochlear implants, failure primarily as a result of progressive tibiofemoral arthritis may occur in 20% to 25% of knees 15 years after PFA.[23,25,27] Incidentally, disease progression is more likely in patients with primary patellofemoral arthritis and less likely in patients with secondary patellofemoral arthritis that is related to patellar instability, patellofemoral dysplasia, or posttraumatic arthritis.[26,27,34] In most studies,[23,25,27] loosening is an infrequent cause of late revision unless noncemented implants were used.[26,27]

A paucity of studies on the revision of PFA to TKA exist in the literature. Lonner et al[29] revised 12 knees in which PFA failed to TKA to manage the progression of tibiofemoral arthritis alone or in combination with patellar maltracking and catching. The authors performed revision to TKA at a mean of 4 years (range, 1 to 9.7 years) after PFA. A posterior-stabilized implant was used in each knee, without a need for stems, augments, or structural bone graft. The authors reported significant improvements in mean Knee Society scores ($P < 0.001$) at a mean follow-up of 3.1 years (range, 2 to 5.2 years) after revision to TKA. Mean Knee Society clinical and functional scores increased from 57 points and 51 points, respectively, preoperatively to 96 points and 91 points, respectively, postoperatively. At the most recent follow-up, no clinical or radiographic evidence of patellofemoral maltracking, loosening, or wear was present. In that study, the outcomes of conversion from PFA to TKA were similar compared with those after primary TKA; however, the authors only revised the trochlear components. The outcomes of revision from PFA to TKA may not have been as optimal if the patellar components also required revision.[29] More recently,

Parratte et al[30] reported that revision from PFA to TKA is comparable to primary TKA with regard to surgical characteristics, such as blood loss and postoperative clinical outcomes (including knee scores and range of motion). The authors also reported that the outcomes of both revision from PFA to TKA and primary TKA are superior to revision TKA; however, the frequency of complications in patients who undergo revision from PFA to TKA is higher compared with those of patients who undergo primary TKA.

Summary

PFA has evolved in the past 30 years. Surgeons have learned more about appropriate patient selection and evaluation as well as the interplay between the anatomic features of the anterior trochlear surface and how it may influence trochlear component positioning and PFA outcomes. Perhaps, the most important development in PFA is the recognition that outcomes will vary depending on whether an inlay-style or onlay-style trochlear prosthesis is used, with the former resulting in a high-rate of early failure as a result of internal rotation of the component, which predisposes patients to patellar instability. PFA outcomes have been optimized and patellar tracking complications have been minimized with the use of onlay-style prostheses, which are positioned perpendicular to the AP axis of the femur. Performing PFA with an onlay-style prosthesis has minimized the risk for patellar instability, which has enhanced the midterm and long-term outcomes of patients who undergo PFA and shifted the risk for progressive tibiofemoral arthritis as a primary mode of implant failure to more than 10 to 15 years after PFA; this is a reasonable

outcome, given the young age of many patients who require PFA.

References

1. Davies AP, Vince AS, Shepstone L, Donell ST, Glasgow MM: The radiologic prevalence of patellofemoral osteoarthritis. *Clin Orthop Relat Res* 2002;402:206-212.

2. McAlindon TE, Snow S, Cooper C, Dieppe PA: Radiographic patterns of osteoarthritis of the knee joint in the community: The importance of the patellofemoral joint. *Ann Rheum Dis* 1992;51(7):844-849.

3. Grelsamer RP, Dejour D, Gould J: The pathophysiology of patellofemoral arthritis. *Orthop Clin North Am* 2008;39(3):269-274, v.

4. Kurtz S, Ong K, Lau E, Mowat F, Halpern M: Projections of primary and revision hip and knee arthroplasty in the United States from 2005 to 2030. *J Bone Joint Surg Am* 2007;89(4):780-785.

5. Blazina ME, Fox JM, Del Pizzo W, Broukhim B, Ivey FM: Patellofemoral replacement. *Clin Orthop Relat Res* 1979;144:98-102.

6. Lubinus HH: Patella glide bearing total replacement. *Orthopedics* 1979;2(2):119-127.

7. Lonner JH: Patellofemoral arthroplasty: Pros, cons, and design considerations. *Clin Orthop Relat Res* 2004;428:158-165.

8. Lonner JH: Patellofemoral arthroplasty. *J Am Acad Orthop Surg* 2007;15(8):495-506.

9. Arciero RA, Toomey HE: Patellofemoral arthroplasty: A three- to nine-year follow-up study. *Clin Orthop Relat Res* 1988;236:60-71.

10. Smith AM, Peckett WR, Butler-Manuel PA, Venu KM, d'Arcy JC: Treatment of patello-femoral arthritis using the Lubinus patello-femoral arthroplasty: A retrospective review. *Knee* 2002;9(1):27-30.

11. Tauro B, Ackroyd CE, Newman JH, Shah NA: The Lubinus patellofemoral arthroplasty: A five- to ten-year prospective study. *J Bone Joint Surg Br* 2001;83(5):696-701.

12. de Winter WE, Feith R, van Loon CJ: The Richards type II patellofemoral arthroplasty: 26 cases followed for 1-20 years. *Acta Orthop Scand* 2001;72(5):487-490.

13. Sisto DJ, Sarin VK: Custom patellofemoral arthroplasty of the knee. *J Bone Joint Surg Am* 2006;88(7):1475-1480.

14. Ackroyd CE, Newman JH, Evans R, Eldridge JD, Joslin CC: The Avon patellofemoral arthroplasty: Five-year survivorship and functional results. *J Bone Joint Surg Br* 2007;89(3):310-315.

15. Starks I, Roberts S, White SH: The Avon patellofemoral joint replacement: Independent assessment of early functional outcomes. *J Bone Joint Surg Br* 2009;91(12):1579-1582.

16. Leadbetter WB, Kolisek FR, Levitt RL, et al: Patellofemoral arthroplasty: A multi-centre study with minimum 2-year follow-up. *Int Orthop* 2009;33(6):1597-1601.

17. Lonner JH: Patellofemoral arthroplasty: The impact of design on outcomes. *Orthop Clin North Am* 2008;39(3):347-354, vi.

18. Odumenya M, Costa ML, Parsons N, Achten J, Dhillon M, Krikler SJ: The Avon patellofemoral joint replacement: Five-year results from an independent centre. *J Bone Joint Surg Br* 2010;92(1):56-60.

19. Mont MA, Johnson AJ, Naziri Q, Kolisek FR, Leadbetter WB: Patellofemoral arthroplasty: 7-year mean follow-up. *J Arthroplasty* 2012;27(3):358-361.

20. Beitzel K, Schöttle PB, Cotic M, Dharmesh V, Imhoff AB: Prospective clinical and radiological two-year results after patellofemoral arthroplasty using an implant with an asymmetric trochlea design. *Knee Surg Sports Traumatol Arthrosc* 2013;21(2):332-339.

21. Kazarian GS, Tarity TD, Hansen EN, Cai J, Lonner JH: Significant functional improvement at 2 years after isolated patellofemoral arthroplasty with an onlay trochlear implant, but low mental health scores predispose to dissatisfaction. *J Arthroplasty* 2016;31(2):389-394.

22. Dy CJ, Franco N, Ma Y, Mazumdar M, McCarthy MM, Gonzalez Della Valle A: Complications after patellofemoral versus total knee replacement in the treatment of isolated patellofemoral osteoarthritis: A meta-analysis. *Knee Surg Sports Traumatol Arthrosc* 2012;20(11):2174-2190.

23. Kooijman HJ, Driessen AP, van Horn JR: Long-term results of patellofemoral arthroplasty: A report of 56 arthroplasties with 17 years of follow-up. *J Bone Joint Surg Br* 2003;85(6):836-840.

24. Cartier P, Sanouiller JL, Grelsamer R: Patellofemoral arthroplasty: 2-12-year follow-up study. *J Arthroplasty* 1990;5(1):49-55.

25. Cartier P, Sanouiller JL, Khefacha A: Long-term results with the first patellofemoral prosthesis. *Clin Orthop Relat Res* 2005;436:47-54.

26. Argenson JN, Guillaume JM, Aubaniac JM: Is there a place for patellofemoral arthroplasty? *Clin Orthop Relat Res* 1995;321:162-167.

27. Argenson JN, Flecher X, Parratte S, Aubaniac JM: Patellofemoral arthroplasty: An update. *Clin Orthop Relat Res* 2005;440:50-53.

28. Hendrix MR, Ackroyd CE, Lonner JH: Revision patellofemoral arthroplasty: Three- to seven-year follow-up. *J Arthroplasty* 2008;23(7):977-983.

29. Lonner JH, Jasko JG, Booth RE Jr: Revision of a failed patellofemoral arthroplasty to a total knee arthroplasty. *J Bone Joint Surg Am* 2006;88(11):2337-2342.

30. Parratte S, Lunebourg A, Ollivier M, Abdel MP, Argenson JN: Are revisions of patellofemoral arthroplasties more like primary or revision TKAs. *Clin Orthop Relat Res* 2015;473(1):213-219.

31. Leadbetter WB, Seyler TM, Ragland PS, Mont MA: Indications, contraindications, and pitfalls of patellofemoral arthroplasty. *J Bone Joint Surg Am* 2006;88(suppl 4):122-137.

32. Lonner JH: Patellofemoral arthroplasty. *Instr Course Lect* 2010;59:67-84.

33. Lombardi AV Jr, Berend KR, Berend ME, et al: Current controversies in partial knee arthroplasty. *Instr Course Lect* 2012;61:347-381.

34. Nicol SG, Loveridge JM, Weale AE, Ackroyd CE, Newman JH: Arthritis progression after patellofemoral joint replacement. *Knee* 2006;13(4):290-295.

35. Lonner JH: Patellofemoral arthroplasty, in Lotke PA, Lonner JH, eds: *Master Techniques in Orthopaedic Surgery: Knee Arthroplasty*, ed 3. Philadelphia, PA, Lippincott, Williams and Wilkins, 2009, 343-360.

36. Lonner JH, Mehta S, Booth RE Jr: Ipsilateral patellofemoral arthroplasty and autogenous osteochondral femoral condylar transplantation. *J Arthroplasty* 2007;22(8):1130-1136.

37. Kamath AF, Levack A, John T, Thomas BS, Lonner JH: Minimum two-year outcomes of modular bicompartmental knee arthroplasty. *J Arthroplasty* 2014;29(1):75-79.

38. Argenson JN, Parratte S, Bertani A, et al: The new arthritic patient and arthroplasty treatment options. *J Bone Joint Surg Am* 2009;91(suppl 5):43-48.

39. Dahm DL, Al-Rayashi W, Dajani K, Shah JP, Levy BA, Stuart MJ: Patellofemoral arthroplasty versus total knee arthroplasty in patients with isolated patellofemoral osteoarthritis. *Am J Orthop (Belle Mead NJ)* 2010;39(10):487-491.

40. Kamath AF, Slattery TR, Levack AE, Wu CH, Kneeland JB, Lonner JH: Trochlear inclination angles in normal and dysplastic knees. *J Arthroplasty* 2013;28(2):214-219.

41. Lonner JH, Jasko JG, Thomas BS: Anthropomorphic differences between the distal femora of men and women. *Clin Orthop Relat Res* 2008;466(11):2724-2729.

42. Biedert R, Sigg A, Gal I, Gerber H: 3D representation of the surface topography of normal and dysplastic trochlea using MRI. *Knee* 2011;18(5):340-346

43. Berger RA, Crossett LS, Jacobs JJ, Rubash HE: Malrotation causing patellofemoral complications after total knee arthroplasty. *Clin Orthop Relat Res* 1998;356:144-153.

44. Australian Orthopaedic Association
     National Joint Replacement Registry.
     Adelaide, South Australia, Australia,
     Australian Orthopaedic Association.
     Available at: https://aoanjrr.sahmri.
     com. Accessed July 5, 2016.

45. Charalambous CP, Abiddin Z, Mills
     SP, Rogers S, Sutton P, Parkinson R:
     The low contact stress patellofemoral
     replacement: High early failure rate.
     J Bone Joint Surg Br 2011;93(4):484-489.

Prevention and Diagnosis of Periprosthetic Knee Infection

Bilal Mahmood, MD
Mouhanad M. El-Othmani, MD
William M. Mihalko, MD, PhD
William A. Jiranek, MD, FACS
Wayne G. Paprosky, MD, FACS
Khaled J. Saleh, MD, MSc, FACSC, MHCM, CPE

Abstract

Total knee arthroplasty (TKA) has become an increasingly common treatment option for patients who have debilitating knee arthritis. TKA is a relatively safe and efficient procedure that results in promising outcomes and has a positive effect on a patient's quality of life. More TKAs are being performed annually because the procedure substantially reduces pain and improves functionality; however, as the number of TKAs continues to rise, there is concern for potential complications that may result in prosthetic joint failure. Primary TKA failure may result in revision procedures that have high costs and an increased risk for additional complications. Infection is the second most common cause of primary TKA failure and the single most common cause of revision TKA failure. Surgeons who have a better understanding of the epidemiology, risk factors, and diagnostic modalities associated with periprosthetic knee infection will be able to implement preventive measures and treat patients in whom such a complication occurs.

Instr Course Lect 2017;66:223–233.

Epidemiology

Total knee arthroplasty (TKA) is quickly becoming one of the most common surgical procedures performed in the United States. An estimated 3,823,167 TKAs were performed in the United States between 1998 and 2007.[1] During this time span, almost twice as many TKAs were performed compared with total hip arthroplasties.[1] Between 1991 and 2010, the number of TKAs performed in US Medicare patients increased 161.5% from 93,230 TKAs to 243,802 TKAs.[2] The number of TKAs performed continues to rise, and, currently, an estimated 600,000 TKAs are performed annually in the United States.[2] In the next few decades, the demand for TKA will increase in conjunction with the expected rise in the prevalence of arthritis from 12.9% to 20%.[3]

In addition to notable success rates, the lack of strict indications and contraindications for TKA are two of the most important factors responsible for the rising number of TKAs. A recent study reported that pain that is not responsive to medical therapy was the only indication for TKA that gained consensus among orthopaedic surgeons, rheumatologists, and primary care physicians. The study reported that major psychiatric disorder, including dementia, was the only contraindication for TKA that gained consensus among orthopaedic surgeons, rheumatologists, and primary care physicians.[3]

Revision TKA is often performed to correct a failed primary TKA. Therefore, it is expected that as the number of primary TKAs increase, the number of revision TKAs also will increase.

Table 1

Definition of Periprosthetic Knee Infection (PKI) According to the International Consensus Group on Periprosthetic Joint Infection[a]

Criteria	Definition
Major criteria	1. Two positive periprosthetic cultures with phenotypically identical organisms, **OR**
	2. A sinus tract communicating with the joint, **OR**
Minor criteria	1. Elevated C-reactive protein level **AND** erythrocyte sedimentation rate
	2. Elevated synovial white blood cell count **OR** ++ change on leukocyte esterase test strip
	3. Elevated synovial polymorphonuclear neutrophil percentage
	4. Positive histologic analysis of periprosthetic tissue
	5. A single positive culture

[a]The International Consensus Group on Periprosthetic Joint Infection states that PKI may be present without a patient meeting these criteria, specifically in the case of less virulent organisms (eg, *Propionibacterium acnes*). Therefore, clinicians are urged to exercise their judgment and clinical acumen in reaching a diagnosis of PKI.

Adapted from Parvizi J, Gehrke T; International Consensus Group on Periprosthetic Joint Infection: Definition of periprosthetic joint infection. *J Arthroplasty* 2014;29(7):1331.

Between 1991 and 2010, the number of revision TKAs performed in US Medicare patients increased 105.9% from 9,650 revision TKAs to 19,871 revision TKAs.[2]

Periprosthetic knee infection (PKI) occurs in 1.1% of patients who undergo primary TKA and is the second most common factor, after aseptic joint loosening, that is responsible for implant failure and the need for revision surgery.[4,5] Approximately one in every five revision TKAs is performed because of a periprosthetic knee infection.[5]

Dr. Mihalko or an immediate family member has received royalties from Aesculap/B. Braun; is a member of a speakers' bureau or has made paid presentations on behalf of Aesculap/B. Braun; is an employee of Aesculap/B. Braun, Medtronic, and Panoramic Healthcare; has received research or institutional support from Aesculap/B. Braun, MicroPort, Smith & Nephew, and Stryker; and serves as a board member, owner, officer, or committee member of the American Board of Orthopaedic Surgery, the American Orthopaedic Association, and ASTM International. Dr. Jiranek or an immediate family member has received royalties from DePuy; serves as a paid consultant to Cayenne Medical and DePuy; has stock or stock options held in Johnson & Johnson; has received research or institutional support from DePuy and Stryker; and serves as a board member, owner, officer, or committee member of the American Association of Hip and Knee Surgeons, LifeNet Health, and the Orthopaedic Learning Center. Dr. Paprosky or an immediate family member has received royalties from Intellijoint Surgical, Stryker, and Zimmer; serves as a paid consultant to DePuy, Medtronic, Stryker, and Zimmer; has stock or stock options held in Intellijoint Surgical; has received nonincome support (such as equipment or services), commercially derived honoraria, or other non-research–related funding (such as paid travel) from Cadence Health; and serves as a board member, owner, officer, or committee member of the Hip Society. Dr. Saleh or an immediate family member has received royalties from Aesculap/B. Braun; is a member of a speakers' bureau or has made paid presentations on behalf of Aesculap/B. Braun; is an employee of the Southern Illinois University School of Medicine, Division of Orthopaedics; serves as a paid consultant to Aesculap/B. Braun, the Memorial Medical Center Co-management Orthopaedic Board, and Watermark; has received research or institutional support from Smith & Nephew, the Orthopaedic Research and Education Foundation, and the National Institutes of Health (NIAMS); and serves as a board member, owner, officer, or committee member of the American Academy of Orthopaedic Surgeons, the American Orthopaedic Association, the American Orthopaedic Association Finance Committee, the Orthopaedic Research and Education Foundation Industry Relations Committee, the Orthopaedic Research and Education Foundation Clinical Research Awards Committee, the American Board of Orthopaedic Surgeons Oral Examiner, the Board of Specialty Societies, Notify, and the American Academy of Orthopaedic Surgeons Performance Measures Committee. Neither of the following authors nor any immediate family member has received anything of value from or has stock or stock options held in a commercial company or institution related directly or indirectly to the subject of this chapter: Mr. Mahmood and Dr. El-Othmani.

Infection also is the single most common reason for failure after revision TKA, accounting for 44% of revision TKA failures.[5] The most common infecting organisms isolated in both primary and revision TKA infections are *Staphylococcus aureus* and *Staphylococcus epidermidis*.[4,5]

The cost of health care in the United States accounts for approximately 16% of the gross domestic product, with totals nearing $2 trillion annually.[6] The cumulative annual cost of septic revision TKA is more than $566 million and is projected to surpass $1.6 billion by 2020.[7] An uncomplicated primary TKA costs an estimated $28,249, whereas the mean cost of an infected TKA is $116,383.[7] Much of this cost discrepancy is attributed to the increased readmission rate, longer hospitalization time, and more frequent clinic visits for patients in whom an infection occurs after TKA.[7] Surgeons who have a better understanding of the pathophysiology, risk factors, and diagnostic modalities associated with infected TKA will be able to implement preventive measures and alternative treatment methods to help improve TKA outcomes.

Periprosthetic Knee Infection Diagnosis

The diagnosis of PKI remains a challenge because there is no preferred method for diagnosis. An international consensus group that was endorsed by the Musculoskeletal Infection Society reported that PKI is present in patients in whom one major infection criterion or three of five minor infection criteria that are listed in **Table 1** exist.[8] After a PKI has been diagnosed, the infection can be classified by the duration of the symptoms (**Table 2**) or by the duration of the infection in combination with the seeding source (hematogenous versus direct)[8] (**Table 3**). The classification of PKI is essential because it is correlated with a patient's prognosis and guides treatment (**Table 3**).

Risk Factors

A preoperative assessment of patient- and healthcare-related factors that may play a role in PKI is important in reducing the prevalence of infected TKA. Preoperative patient-related risk factors for PKI include male sex, diabetes mellitus, a body mass index greater than 40 kg/m^2, and an American Society of Anesthesiologists Physical Status Score higher than 2.[4,9] Important healthcare-related risk factors for PKI include postoperative myocardial infarction, atrial fibrillation, and urinary tract infection.[4] In addition, patients who receive allogeneic transfusions and those who require longer hospital stays have an increased risk for PKI.[4,10]

Reducing the Risk for PKI
Preoperative Medical Optimization

The overall medical health status of TKA candidates should be assessed and optimized in the preoperative planning period. Medical comorbidities that increase the risk for postoperative complications (both in general and for PKI,

specifically) should be addressed and optimized. Obesity and morbid obesity are correlated with PKI, and the risk for PKI exponentially increases as body mass index increases.[11,12] Lifestyle modifications, bariatric surgery, and other weight loss methods as well as adjusted antibiotic dosing help reduce the risk of PKI in patients with obesity and are recommended before elective TKA.[13] Nutritional status optimization is recommended for all TKA candidates because it may help reduce the risk for postoperative infection. Poor nutritional status is often indicated by

a low serum albumin level and a low lymphocyte count, both of which may lead to a delay in wound healing and an increased risk for wound complications, including infection.[13,14] Patients who have a lymphocyte count less than or equal to 1,500 cells/mm^3 and a serum albumin level less than 3.5 g/dL have a greater risk for major wound complications.[14] In addition, appropriate management of a patient's medical comorbidities, whether caused by the disease process or pharmacotherapy, may help reduce the risk for PKI. Patients who are being treated with chronic

Table 2
Minor Diagnostic Threshold Criteria for the Classification of Periprosthetic Knee Infection (PKI)

Criterion	Acute PKI (<90 days)	Chronic PKI (>90 days)
Erythrocyte sedimentation rate (mm/h)	Not helpful. No threshold was determined.	30
C-reactive protein level (mg/L)	100	10
Synovial white blood cell count (cells/μL)	10,000	3,000
Synovial polymorphonuclear neutrophil (%)	90	80
Leukocyte esterase test strip	+ or ++	+ or ++
Histologic analysis of tissue	>5 neutrophils per high-power field in five high-power fields (×400)	Same as acute

Adapted from Parvizi J, Gehrke T; International Consensus Group on Periprosthetic Joint Infection: Definition of periprosthetic joint infection. *J Arthroplasty* 2014;29(7):1331.

Table 3
Classification of Periprosthetic Knee Infection by Duration and Seeding Source

Variable	Type I	Type II	Type III	Type IV
Timing	Positive intraoperative cultures	Early postoperative infection	Acute hematogenous infection	Late chronic infection
Definition	2 or more positive cultures	4 weeks after index surgery	Hematogenous seeding of a well-functioning arthroplasty	Chronic infection present >1 month
Treatment	Antibiotics	Attempt débridement with prosthesis salvage	Attempt débridement with prosthesis salvage	Prosthesis removal

immunosuppressive therapy for systemic or localized disease processes, such as rheumatoid arthritis and systemic lupus erythematosus, have a particularly high risk for postoperative infection.[14,15] Glycemic control in patients who have diabetes mellitus reduces the risk for infection as well as other intraoperative and postoperative complications.[13,16]

Preoperative optimization that includes patient empowerment and patient education has been correlated with improved postoperative outcomes. Although not specific to orthopaedics or PKI, patient activation has been reported to improve patient satisfaction as well as decrease healthcare-associated costs.[17,18] Therefore, patient activation should be incorporated as a crucial component in the preoperative medical clearance process.

Smoking and alcohol cessation that begins 6 to 8 weeks before surgery has been reported to simultaneously reduce the risk for PKI and improve wound healing potential.[13,16] Patients who have prolonged wound drainage, longer surgical times, longer hospital stays, or urinary tract infections have a considerable risk for PKI; therefore, these conditions must be diagnosed and managed preoperatively.[4] In addition, minimization of intraoperative blood loss and preoperative correction of chronic anemia in TKA candidates helps reduce unnecessary allogeneic transfusions, which substantially reduces the risk for PKI.[13]

Preoperative Infection Screening

Preoperative screening of patients for methicillin-resistant *S aureus* (MRSA) followed by prophylactic decolonization of patients who are MRSA carriers may help reduce a patient's overall risk for infection and prevent disease

transmission.[19] Screening and decolonization of MRSA-colonized patients with mupirocin and chlorhexidine baths have been reported to effectively reduce the risk for surgical site infection (SSI).[20] Preoperative treatment with mupirocin may effectively reduce the risk of SSI regardless of a patient's MRSA colonization status.[13,21] Furthermore, perioperative antibiotic therapy with first- or second-generation cephalosporin or vancomycin may help prevent PKI.[13] Prophylactic vancomycin should be used in high-risk patients and those who have known drug allergies to cephalosporin to prevent antimicrobial-resistant bacteria and avoid adverse pharmacologic side effects, respectively.[13,22]

Intraoperative Draping and Sterilization Techniques

Surgical draping and preparation play a key role in infection prevention. The use of plastic, disposable, nonwoven draping creates a successful barrier against microorganisms.[13,16] Administration of at-home chlorhexidine the night before and the morning of surgery may effectively reduce the risk for infection after TKA.[23,24] The administration of chlorhexidine is not only an effective method for potential source disinfection but also an inexpensive and simple measure that makes patient noncompliance less of a concern.[23] In addition, preoperative skin preparation with chlorhexidine-alcohol is more effective in the prevention of SSI and deep incisional infection compared with povidone-iodine.[25] No sufficient evidence proves that surgical site hair removal has any benefit in reducing the risk of infection; however, if hair is to be removed, lower SSI rates have been reported with the use of electric clippers compared with razor-shaving.[26] The use

of a sterile stockinette on an unprepared foot may contribute to local bacterial contamination of the surgical field and increase the risk for infection.[27] Infection can be prevented by preparing the foot with an antiseptic, such as chlorhexidine, before a sterile stockinette is used.[27] Traditionally, members of the surgical team scrub their arms and forearms before they are dressed in sterile gloves and gowns; however, data suggest that the use of an alcohol-based hand rub is as effective as traditional scrubbing techniques but is better tolerated, which increases surgical staff compliance.[28]

Surgical glove perforation occurs in more than one-half of joint arthroplasties and substantially increases the risk of SSI; however, no convincing data indicate that double gloving reduces the risk of infection.[16] Historically, the use of body exhaust suits has been advocated as a method to reduce the risk for PKI; however, the literature does not support or refute the use of body exhaust suits.[16] Operating rooms with laminar airflow systems and less human traffic have been reported to effectively reduce infection rates.[16] With respect to surgical wound closure after an orthopaedic procedure, higher infection rates have been reported with the use of staples compared with sutures.[29] Furthermore, barbed sutures are associated with faster wound closure but have not been reported to reduce the number of complications after TKA.[30]

Prophylactic Antibiotic Therapies

Prophylactic antibiotics are very effective at reducing the risk of PKI. Antibiotic therapy should be directed toward controlling *S aureus* and *S epidermidis*, which are the most common organisms responsible for PKI.[22] Other organisms, such as *Streptococcus* and gram-negative bacteria, also may be responsible for PKI but are far less common. The use of cephalosporins, such as cefazolin or cefuroxime, is preferred because these antibiotics provide good joint penetration; provide excellent coverage of gram-positive bacteria, such as methicillin-sensitive *S aureus* (MSSA) and *S epidermidis*; and are effective against some gram-negative bacteria and anaerobes.[22,31] In addition, cephalosporins have excellent osteogenic and soft-tissue penetration, which makes them particularly effective for the prevention and treatment of PKI.

Antibiotic prophylaxis should be initiated within 1 hour of incision and discontinued within 24 hours after surgery. Intraoperative antibiotic levels should be maintained above the minimum inhibitory concentration.[13,22] Continuation of antibiotic prophylaxis more than 24 hours postoperatively increases a patient's risk for bacterial resistance and has not been reported to reduce the risk for PKI.[22]

Polymethyl methacrylate (PMMA) bone cement that is loaded with antibiotics may provide further antimicrobial protection in patients who undergo TKA; however, the efficacy of prophylactic antibiotic-impregnated bone cement in patients who undergo primary TKA has not been determined. Some studies suggest that antibiotic-impregnated bone cement may decrease deep infection rates but has little or no effect on SSI in patients who undergo TKA.[16,32] Furthermore, infection rates remain unchanged in patients who undergo revision TKA with the use of antibiotic-impregnated bone cement compared with those who undergo revision TKA with the use of bone cement without antibiotic impregnation.[16] Currently, there are no evidence-based guidelines on the amount and type of antibiotic that should be blended into PMMA bone cement.[31-34] Gentamicin is commonly loaded into bone cement because it has favorable elution characteristics and has antimicrobial activity against MSSA, coagulase-negative staphylococci, *Pseudomonas aeruginosa*, and *Escherichia coli*. Gentamicin-loaded bone cement is superior compared with several other broad-spectrum antibiotics that can be loaded into bone cement because gentamicin does not affect the biomechanical properties of PMMA cement.[34] Oxacillin-loaded bone cement provides protection against MSSA, and vancomycin-loaded bone cement provides protection against MRSA.[31] Furthermore, systemic antibiotic prophylaxis can be used in combination with antibiotic-loaded bone cement to enhance antimicrobial activity in patients who undergo TKA.[31]

Diagnosis of PKI

Currently, there is no preferred laboratory test used to diagnose PKI. Diagnostic criteria used to identify PKI include the presence of a sinus tract in connection with the prosthesis, positive fluid and tissue cultures, elevated C-reactive protein (CRP) level, elevated erythrocyte sedimentation rate (ESR), elevated synovial white blood cell (WBC) count, elevated polymorphonuclear (PMN) neutrophil percentage, and the presence of neutrophils on histologic examination.[35,36] Diagnosis of a PKI begins with obtaining a patient's clinical history and performing a physical examination. Patients who have a PKI commonly report localized pain, which often is the only presenting symptom.[35] The surgeon should assess whether the pain is localized or radiating to differentiate pain that is referred from the lumbar spine or the hip.[36] Often, pain that is noticeable at rest may occur within several months after TKA.[37] Signs of inflammation, such as fistulas, sinus tracts, tenderness on palpation, erythema, and swelling, may be present in some but not all patients.[35-38] In addition, a fever higher than or equal to 102.2°F for consecutive days after TKA raises suspicion of a postoperative PKI.[39]

Serologic Testing

Surgeons who suspect a PKI after obtaining a patient's clinical history and performing a physical examination should perform serologic testing to diagnose or rule out PKI. Unfortunately, no single test is 100% specific for the diagnosis of an infection.[36] An elevated CRP level and ESR indicate the likelihood of a PKI;[37,40] however, although these markers are sensitive for infection, they lack specificity because any inflammatory process can cause their elevation.[10,14,41] A patient's ESR peaks 5 to 7 days after surgery and returns to baseline within 3 to 12 months postoperatively.[42] An elevated ESR is greater than 30 mm/h at 3 to 12 months postoperatively.[42] An elevated ESR is 87% sensitive and 83% specific for the diagnosis of a PKI.[42] CRP is an acute phase reactant that is produced by hepatocytes and responds to infection, acute injury, and inflammation.[42] A patient's serum CRP level peaks 2 to 3 days after surgery and returns to baseline within 14 to 21 days postoperatively.[42] An elevated CRP level is 10 mg/L at 14 to 21 days postoperatively.[42] An elevated CRP level is 93% sensitive and 83% specific for the diagnosis of a PKI.[42]

Although not included in the International Consensus Group on Periprosthetic Joint Infection's criteria for the classification of PKI, blood cultures may help identify offending organisms and guide therapy in patients in whom hematogenous infection from a vegetative valve or other source of bacteremia is suspected.[37] The use of a serum WBC count for the diagnosis of PKI has not been established because evidence is inconsistent, with many patients having a normal serum WBC count and signs of infection.[36,43] Serum interleukin-6 (IL-6) levels, which also may be elevated in patients who have a PKI, provide robust specificity, sensitivity, and negative predictive value that aids in a patient's preoperative evaluation.[43] In addition, an elevated IL-6 level in combination with an elevated CRP level are very useful in the identification of a PKI;[43] however, IL-6 assays are not commonly available in many clinical settings.[36] Other markers, such as lipopolysaccharide-binding protein levels, also have been reported to be elevated in patients who have a PKI; however, the usefulness of lipopolysaccharide-binding protein levels are not clear because they have not been reported to be more accurate at identifying a PKI compared with CRP levels.[44]

Imaging Modalities

Several imaging modalities may aid in the diagnosis of a PKI. Radiographs are the first imaging study indicated for patients who have lower extremity pain. Radiographs are primarily used to assess joint space and bony structures; however, they also may reveal various late signs of infection, including periosteal bone formations, scattered foci of osteolysis, and subchondral bone resorption. Serial radiographs,

if available, may help rule out aseptic loosening, hardware failure, osteolysis, and fracture.[45] Nuclear medicine imaging (NMI) is recommended only for patients in whom continued suspicion for infection exists without adequate confirmation.

NMI is indicated for patients in whom suspicion for PKI is high but infection criteria have not been met.[46,47] NMI is not affected by metallic hardware; therefore, it is the current imaging modality of choice for patients in whom a PKI is suspected. Bone scintigraphy is an affordable, widely available NMI technique that is sensitive for the detection of bone remodeling; however, increased periprosthetic bone activity in the first year after TKA may be caused by several conditions other than infection, which makes the sensitivity, specificity, and accuracy of bone scintigraphy poor for the diagnosis of a PKI.[48,49] Three-phase bone scintigraphy is moderately more accurate for the diagnosis of a PKI compared with bone scintigraphy (62% and 50%, respectively); however, it is primarily used as a screening test.[50]

Gallium-67 citrate scintigraphy, another NMI technique, uses gallium-67 citrate, which is an isotope that preferentially localizes to marrow as well as areas of high bone turnover, infection, and inflammation. Gallium-67 citrate scintigraphy lacks specificity (15%) if used alone; however, its diagnostic accuracy improves (67% to 81%) if used in combination with bone scintigraphy.[50-55]

Indium-111–labeled leukocyte scanning, another NMI technique, is well suited for the diagnosis of PKI because leukocytes frequently accumulate at sites of infection. Studies have repeatedly reported that indium-111–labeled leukocyte scans have a high sensitivity

(100%) and a low specificity (<50%) for the diagnosis of a PKI.[56-58] Although many studies have attempted to interpret this discrepancy, the use of indium-111–labeled leukocyte scans for the detection of inflammatory processes is well established.[59] Studies have reported that indium-111–labeled leukocyte imaging combined with bone scintigraphy has greater diagnostic accuracy compared with either imaging technique alone; however, these studies also reported varying results.[56,57]

Leukocyte-marrow scintigraphy, which combines indium-111–labeled leukocyte imaging and bone marrow imaging, measures radiotracer accumulation in bone marrow. Several recent studies have reported that leukocyte-marrow scintigraphy demonstrates encouraging results for the diagnosis of a PKI, with a sensitivity ranging from 92% to 100%, a specificity ranging from 91% to 100%, and an accuracy of 95%.[50,58,60] In a study that compared the results of other NMI techniques with those of leukocyte-marrow scintigraphy, Love et al[50] reported that leukocyte-marrow scintigraphy was more accurate for the diagnosis of a PKI compared with bone scintigraphy (50%), gallium-67 citrate scintigraphy (66%), and indium-111–labeled leukocyte scanning (70%). The results of this study support the efficacy and superiority of leukocyte-marrow scintigraphy for the diagnosis of a PKI compared with other NMI techniques.

Leukocyte-marrow scintigraphy, although effective, has several disadvantages, including cost, exposure to blood products, and the labor-intensive leukocyte labeling process. Consequently, interest in fluorine-18 fluorodeoxyglucose positron emission tomography ([18]FDG-PET) is rising. [18]FDG-PET is a NMI technique that labels deoxyglucose, which is a glucose analogue, to a radionuclide. Inflammatory cells are metabolically more active compared with surrounding tissue, which results in an accumulation of deoxyglucose and fluorine-18 at sites of infection. Zhuang et al[61] reported that [18]FDG-PET is 91% sensitive, 72% specific, and 78% accurate for the diagnosis of a PKI. Chacko et al[62] reported that the presence of activity at the bone prosthesis interface was 92% sensitive and 97% specific for infection. Both Zhuang et al[61] and Chacko et al[62] noted that the intensity of fluorodeoxyglucose uptake was not important in the differentiation of infection from aseptic processes.[62] Love et al[50] reported that, although [18]FDG-PET was fairly accurate for the diagnosis of a PKI (71%), it was not a suitable replacement for leukocyte-marrow scintigraphy.

Joint Fluid Analysis

Arthrocentesis that is guided by aseptic technique is recommended for patients in whom a PKI is suspected. The synovial fluid obtained from arthrocentesis should be sent for cultures, crystal analysis, a WBC count, and a differential count. Antibiotic use before knee aspiration may lead to false-negative results and should be avoided. Recent studies suggest that a synovial WBC count higher than 1,100 cells/μL is 91% sensitive and 88% specific for the diagnosis of a PKI.[10] In addition, a synovial PMN neutrophil percentage greater than 64% is 95% sensitive and 94% specific for the diagnosis of a PKI.[10] If both a patient's synovial WBC count and PMN neutrophil percentage are elevated, the likelihood of infection is 98.6%.[10] Conversely, if both a patient's synovial WBC count and PMN neutrophil

percentage are within normal levels, the negative predictive value for infection is 98.2%.[46,63,64]

Synovial inflammatory markers, such as CRP and IL-6 levels, are more accurate for the diagnosis of PKI compared with serum inflammatory markers.[65,66] The leukocyte esterase test strip is a rapid, inexpensive test that can detect the presence of leukocyte esterase within synovial fluid.[35,65] The leukocyte esterase test strip is a very promising test for the diagnosis of PKI because it has a high positive predictive value and a high negative predictive value; however, additional studies are necessary to establish its true diagnostic use.[35,65] Synovial cultures are very useful to confirm a diagnosis of a PKI and identify the infecting organism; however, synovial cultures are often negative in patients who have a PKI, which results in a large number of false negatives.[35,40] Polymerase chain reaction (PCR) and fluorescence in situ hybridization (FISH) may help detect and identify bacteria within synovial fluid in patients in whom other methods fail to identify the causative bacteria and in patients who do not have classic symptoms of infection.[67,68]

α-Defensin, an antimicrobial peptide that is released by neutrophils and kills pathogens via disruption of the cellular membrane, is gaining interest as a biologic marker for the diagnosis of PKI.[69] In a prospective study of 149 patients who underwent synovial fluid aspiration, Deirmengian et al[70] reported that synovial α-defensin levels at a cutoff value of 5.2 mg/L were 95.5% specific and 97.3% sensitive for the detection of infection. The authors reported that synovial α-defensin levels at a cutoff value of 5.2 mg/L combined with synovial CRP levels at a cutoff value of

3 mg/L were 100% specific and 97.3% sensitive for the detection of infection.[70] The authors noted that the results of the combined measurement of synovial α-defensin and synovial CRP levels were not affected by the inclusion of patients who had systemic inflammatory disease and those who were being treated with antibiotics at the time of testing.[70] In addition, the measurement of α-defensin levels provides consistent results regardless of the offending pathogen type, virulence, or species or whether the pathogen is gram-positive or gram-negative.[71] Therefore, the combined measurement of synovial α-defensin and synovial CRP levels should be considered a robust diagnostic tool; however, further studies are necessary to assess its application in various clinical settings.

Frozen Sections

Intraoperative frozen sections are very useful in the diagnosis of a PKI, especially for patients who are undergoing revision TKA and in whom infection has not been confirmed or ruled out.[36] Frozen samples are analyzed under magnification to determine the number of neutrophils present per high-power field.[35,37,72] At least 5 neutrophils per high-power field at 400 times magnification is very predictive of acute inflammation secondary to infection.[35,37,72] Intraoperative Gram stains are not very sensitive or reliable for the identification of infection and are not recommended to rule out an infection.[36] Cultures from removed implants and tissue cultures can be used to establish a diagnosis and identify the infecting organisms of a PKI. Cultures obtained from removed implants are more sensitive for the identification of bacteria compared with tissue cultures.[73]

Sonication is a technique that exposes implants to ultrasound waves, which break away bacterial biofilms and allow an enhanced sample collection to be cultured.[37,74] Cultures obtained via sonication are more sensitive to growth compared with those obtained via traditional culturing techniques.[73,74]

Molecular Diagnostic Tests

Many advances in molecular biology have occurred in the past decade, which has improved the ability of investigators to isolate infective organisms with the use of biomarkers and biochemical technology. Biomarkers are biologic byproducts of infecting organisms or immunologic cells that are activated after infection. Recent studies have described the use of the colorimetric leukocyte esterase test strips for the detection of PKI.[75] Leukocyte esterase test strips are easy to use, inexpensive, and accurate.[76] The limitations of biomarkers include the inability to identify an infecting pathogen and antibiotic susceptibility.

PCR is a biochemical technology that is designed to amplify specific DNA and RNA sequences. Although PCR-based technologies have streamlined the diagnosis of PKI, the practical use of PCR is limited by cost, specialized equipment, and a high rate of false-positive cultures.[77,78] DNA-based PCR protocols amplify circular bacterial DNA, which frequently exist long after cell death, and result in a high rate of false-positive results.[79] Consequently, investigators have developed PCR techniques that amplify more labile genomic sequences, including messenger RNA and ribosomal RNA; ribosomal RNA-based PCR techniques are of particular interest to investigators because of the high ribosomal activity present in bacteria.[79,80]

FISH is a molecular diagnostic modality that provides spatial resolution to bacterial groups that are removed from the involved tissue or prosthesis. FISH uses samples that are fixed and permeable, which allow fluorescent DNA probes or nucleic acid probes to hybridize to their target. FISH can be used in patients who have culture-negative PKI because the fluorescent probes are able to hybridize with biofilm-encapsulated bacteria.[81-85]

A DNA microarray, or DNA chip, which is a technique that is similar to FISH, is gaining interest for the diagnosis of PKI. Microarrays consist of thousands of unique microscopic DNA probes that are complementary to taxonomy-specific or antibiotic-resistant gene sequences.[86] Hybridization of nucleic acid samples with microarray probes indicates a match. A combination of matches for unique gene sequences may help identify the infecting organism. A drawback of DNA microarrays is that their accuracy depends on the specificity and number of DNA probes incorporated in the array.[86,87] Therefore, surgeons must be attentive to the latest trends in biomarkers and biochemical technology that continue to advance the capabilities of molecular testing for the detection of PKI.

Summary

As the number of TKAs performed in the United States continues to rise and the total cost of health care continues to be a major concern, the diagnosis and prevention of infection after TKA will become increasingly important. PKIs cause substantial morbidity and can affect the quality of life of patients who undergo TKA. Identification of risk factors, optimization of patients,

and implementation of effective preoperative and intraoperative prophylactic techniques play a crucial role in the prevention of PKIs. Newer techniques, such as the use of antibiotic-impregnated bone cement, show great potential for prevention against PKI; however, additional studies are necessary to optimize the effectiveness of these techniques. Surgeons must recognize the signs and symptoms as well as make an early and definitive diagnosis of PKIs to prevent morbidity in and avoid unnecessary financial burden for patients who undergo TKA. No single preferred test for the diagnosis of PKI exists. Therefore, surgeons should understand the role and reliability that various serum and joint aspirate findings as well as newer diagnostic techniques play in confirming or ruling out a diagnosis of infection after TKA.

Acknowledgment

The authors of this chapter wish to thank Dr. Afshin Anoushiravani and Mr. Zain Sayeed for their help in writing this chapter.

References

1. Poultsides LA, Ma Y, Della Valle AG, Chiu YL, Sculco TP, Memtsoudis SG: In-hospital surgical site infections after primary hip and knee arthroplasty—incidence and risk factors. *J Arthroplasty* 2013;28(3):385-389.

2. Cram P, Lu X, Kates SL, Singh JA, Li Y, Wolf BR: Total knee arthroplasty volume, utilization, and outcomes among Medicare beneficiaries, 1991-2010. *JAMA* 2012;308(12):1227-1236.

3. Cross WW III, Saleh KJ, Wilt TJ, Kane RL: Agreement about indications for total knee arthroplasty. *Clin Orthop Relat Res* 2006;446:34-39.

4. Pulido L, Ghanem E, Joshi A, Purtill JJ, Parvizi J: Periprosthetic joint infection: The incidence, timing, and

predisposing factors. *Clin Orthop Relat Res* 2008;466(7):1710-1715.

5. Mortazavi SM, Molligan J, Austin MS, Purtill JJ, Hozack WJ, Parvizi J: Failure following revision total knee arthroplasty: Infection is the major cause. *Int Orthop* 2011;35(8):1157-1164.

6. Healy WL, Iorio R: Implant selection and cost for total joint arthroplasty: Conflict between surgeons and hospitals. *Clin Orthop Relat Res* 2007;457:57-63.

7. Kapadia BH, McElroy MJ, Issa K, Johnson AJ, Bozic KJ, Mont MA: The economic impact of periprosthetic infections following total knee arthroplasty at a specialized tertiary-care center. *J Arthroplasty* 2014;29(5):929-932.

8. Parvizi J, Gehrke T; International Consensus Group on Periprosthetic Joint Infection: Definition of periprosthetic joint infection. *J Arthroplasty* 2014;29(7):1331.

9. Dowsey MM, Choong PF: Obese diabetic patients are at substantial risk for deep infection after primary TKA. *Clin Orthop Relat Res* 2009;467(6):1577-1581.

10. Kheir MM, Clement RC, Derman PB, et al: Are there identifiable risk factors and causes associated with unplanned readmissions following total knee arthroplasty? *J Arthroplasty* 2014;29(11):2192-2196.

11. Chen J, Cui Y, Li X, et al: Risk factors for deep infection after total knee arthroplasty: A meta-analysis. *Arch Orthop Trauma Surg* 2013;133(5):675-687.

12. Malinzak RA, Ritter MA, Berend ME, Meding JB, Olberding EM, Davis KE: Morbidly obese, diabetic, younger, and unilateral joint arthroplasty patients have elevated total joint arthroplasty infection rates. *J Arthroplasty* 2009;24(6 suppl):84-88.

13. Alijanipour P, Heller S, Parvizi J: Prevention of periprosthetic joint infection: What are the effective strategies? *J Knee Surg* 2014;27(4):251-258.

14. Greene KA, Wilde AH, Stulberg BN: Preoperative nutritional status of total joint patients: Relationship to postoperative wound complications. *J Arthroplasty* 1991;6(4):321-325.

15. Tyllianakis ME, Karageorgos ACh, Marangos MN, Saridis AG, Lambiris EE: Antibiotic prophylaxis in primary hip and knee arthroplasty: Comparison between cefuroxime and two specific antistaphylococcal agents. *J Arthroplasty* 2010;25(7):1078-1082.

16. Kapadia BH, Pivec R, Johnson AJ, et al: Infection prevention methodologies for lower extremity total joint arthroplasty. *Expert Rev Med Devices* 2013;10(2):215-224.

17. Hibbard JH, Greene J: What the evidence shows about patient activation: Better health outcomes and care experiences; fewer data on costs. *Health Aff (Millwood)* 2013;32(2):207-214.

18. Jerofke T, Weiss M, Yakusheva O: Patient perceptions of patient-empowering nurse behaviours, patient activation and functional health status in postsurgical patients with life-threatening long-term illnesses. *J Adv Nurs* 2014;70(6):1310-1322.

19. Buehlmann M, Frei R, Fenner L, Dangel M, Fluckiger U, Widmer AF: Highly effective regimen for decolonization of methicillin-resistant Staphylococcus aureus carriers. *Infect Control Hosp Epidemiol* 2008;29(6):510-516.

20. Goyal N, Miller A, Tripathi M, Parvizi J: Methicillin-resistant Staphylococcus aureus (MRSA): Colonisation and pre-operative screening. *Bone Joint J* 2013;95(1):4-9.

21. Rao N, Cannella BA, Crossett LS, Yates AJ Jr, McGough RL III, Hamilton CW: Preoperative screening/decolonization for Staphylococcus aureus to prevent orthopedic surgical site infection: Prospective cohort study with 2-year follow-up. *J Arthroplasty* 2011;26(8):1501-1507.

22. Meehan J, Jamali AA, Nguyen H: Prophylactic antibiotics in hip and knee arthroplasty. *J Bone Joint Surg Am* 2009;91(10):2480-2490.

23. Johnson AJ, Kapadia BH, Daley JA, Molina CB, Mont MA: Chlorhexidine reduces infections in knee arthroplasty. *J Knee Surg* 2013;26(3):213-218.

24. Zywiel MG, Daley JA, Delanois RE, Naziri Q, Johnson AJ, Mont MA: Advance pre-operative chlorhexidine reduces the incidence of surgical site infections in knee arthroplasty. *Int Orthop* 2011;35(7):1001-1006.

25. Darouiche RO, Wall MJ Jr, Itani KM, et al: Chlorhexidine-alcohol versus povidone-iodine for surgical-site antisepsis. *N Engl J Med* 2010;362(1):18-26.

26. Tanner J, Norrie P, Melen K: Preoperative hair removal to reduce surgical site infection. *Cochrane Database Syst Rev* 2011;11:CD004122.

27. Boekel P, Blackshaw R, Van Bavel D, Riazi A, Hau R: Sterile stockinette in orthopaedic surgery: A possible pathway for infection. *ANZ J Surg* 2012;82(11):838-843.

28. Parienti JJ, Thibon P, Heller R, et al: Hand-rubbing with an aqueous alcoholic solution vs traditional surgical hand-scrubbing and 30-day surgical site infection rates: A randomized equivalence study. *JAMA* 2002;288(6):722-727.

29. Smith TO, Sexton D, Mann C, Donell S: Sutures versus staples for skin closure in orthopaedic surgery: Meta-analysis. *BMJ* 2010;340:c1199.

30. Gililland JM, Anderson LA, Sun G, Erickson JA, Peters CL: Perioperative closure-related complication rates and cost analysis of barbed suture for closure in TKA. *Clin Orthop Relat Res* 2012;470(1):125-129.

31. Ueng SW, Hsieh PH, Shih HN, Chan YS, Lee MS, Chang Y: Antibacterial activity of joint fluid in cemented total-knee arthroplasty: An in vivo comparative study of polymethylmethacrylate with and without antibiotic loading. *Antimicrob Agents Chemother* 2012;56(11):5541-5546.

32. Wang J, Zhu C, Cheng T, et al: A systematic review and meta-analysis of antibiotic-impregnated bone cement use in primary total hip or knee arthroplasty. *PLoS One* 2013;8(12):e82745.

33. Lewis G, Brooks JL, Courtney HS, Li Y, Haggard WO: An approach for determining antibiotic loading for a physician-directed antibiotic-loaded PMMA bone cement formulation. *Clin Orthop Relat Res* 2010;468(8):2092-2100.

34. Chang Y, Tai CL, Hsieh PH, Ueng SW: Gentamicin in bone cement: A potentially more effective prophylactic measure of infection in joint arthroplasty. *Bone Joint Res* 2013;2(10):220-226.

35. Del Arco A, Bertrand ML: The diagnosis of periprosthetic infection. *Open Orthop J* 2013;7:178-183.

36. Springer BD, Scuderi GR: Evaluation and management of the infected total knee arthroplasty. *Instr Course Lect* 2013;62:349-361.

37. Konigsberg BS, Hartman CW, Hewlett AL, Garvin KL: Current and future trends in the diagnosis of periprosthetic hip infection. *Orthop Clin North Am* 2014;45(3):287-293.

38. Patel R, Osmon DR, Hanssen AD: The diagnosis of prosthetic joint infection: Current techniques and emerging technologies. *Clin Orthop Relat Res* 2005;437:55-58.

39. Lu X, Jin J, Lin J, Qian W, Weng X: Course of fever and potential infection after total joint replacement. *Knee Surg Sports Traumatol Arthrosc* 2015;23(6):1870-1876.

40. Parvizi J, Ghanem E, Sharkey P, Aggarwal A, Burnett RS, Barrack RL: Diagnosis of infected total knee: Findings of a multicenter database. *Clin Orthop Relat Res* 2008;466(11):2628-2633.

41. Bauer TW, Parvizi J, Kobayashi N, Krebs V: Diagnosis of periprosthetic infection. *J Bone Joint Surg Am* 2006;88(4):869-882.

42. Greidanus NV, Masri BA, Garbuz DS, et al: Use of erythrocyte sedimentation rate and C-reactive protein level to diagnose infection before revision total knee arthroplasty: A prospective evaluation. *J Bone Joint Surg Am* 2007;89(7):1409-1416.

43. Abou El-Khier NT, El Ganainy Ael-R, Elgeidy A, Rakha SA: Assessment of interleukin-6 and other inflammatory markers in the diagnosis of Egyptian patients with periprosthetic joint infection. *Egypt J Immunol* 2013;20(2):93-99.

44. Friedrich MJ, Randau TM, Wimmer MD, et al: Lipopolysaccharide-binding protein: A valuable biomarker in the differentiation between periprosthetic joint infection and aseptic loosening? *Int Orthop* 2014;38(10):2201-2207.

45. Abdul-Karim FW, McGinnis MG, Kraay M, Emancipator SN, Goldberg V: Frozen section biopsy assessment for the presence of polymorphonuclear leukocytes in patients undergoing revision of arthroplasties. *Mod Pathol* 1998;11(5):427-431.

46. Ghanem E, Parvizi J, Burnett RS, et al: Cell count and differential of aspirated fluid in the diagnosis of infection at the site of total knee arthroplasty. *J Bone Joint Surg Am* 2008;90(8):1637-1643.

47. Parvizi J, Adeli B, Zmistowski B, Restrepo C, Greenwald AS: Management of periprosthetic joint infection: The current knowledge. AAOS exhibit selection. *J Bone Joint Surg Am* 2012;94(14):e104.

48. Love C, Tronco GG, Palestro CJ: Imaging of infection and inflammation with 99mTc-Fanolesomab. *Q J Nucl Med Mol Imaging* 2006;50(2):113-120.

49. Palestro CJ, Swyer AJ, Kim CK, Goldsmith SJ: Infected knee prosthesis: Diagnosis with In-111 leukocyte, Tc-99m sulfur colloid, and Tc-99m MDP imaging. *Radiology* 1991;179(3):645-648.

50. Love C, Marwin SE, Tomas MB, et al: Diagnosing infection in the failed joint replacement: A comparison of coincidence detection 18F-FDG and 111In-labeled leukocyte/99mTc-sulfur colloid marrow imaging. *J Nucl Med* 2004;45(11):1864-1871.

51. Merkel KD, Fitzgerald RH Jr, Brown ML: Scintigraphic examination of total hip arthroplasty: Comparison of indium with technetium-gallium in the loose and infected canine arthroplasty. *Hip* 1984;163-192.

52. Merkel KD, Brown ML, Fitzgerald RH Jr: Sequential technetium-99m HMDP-gallium-67 citrate imaging for the evaluation of infection in the painful prosthesis. *J Nucl Med* 1986;27(9):1413-1417.

53. Gómez-Luzuriaga MA, Galán V, Villar JM: Scintigraphy with Tc, Ga and In in painful total hip prostheses. *Int Orthop* 1988;12(2):163-167.

54. Kraemer WJ, Saplys R, Waddell JP, Morton J: Bone scan, gallium scan, and hip aspiration in the diagnosis of infected total hip arthroplasty. *J Arthroplasty* 1993;8(6):611-616.

55. Reing CM, Richin PF, Kenmore PI: Differential bone-scanning in the evaluation of a painful total joint replacement. *J Bone Joint Surg Am* 1979;61(6A):933-936.

56. Wukich DK, Abreu SH, Callaghan JJ, et al: Diagnosis of infection by preoperative scintigraphy with indium-labeled white blood cells. *J Bone Joint Surg Am* 1987;69(9):1353-1360.

57. Johnson JA, Christie MJ, Sandler MP, Parks PF Jr, Homra L, Kaye JJ: Detection of occult infection following total joint arthroplasty using sequential technetium-99m HDP bone scintigraphy and indium-111 WBC imaging. *J Nucl Med* 1988;29(8):1347-1353.

58. Palestro CJ, Kim CK, Swyer AJ, Capozzi JD, Solomon RW, Goldsmith SJ: Total-hip arthroplasty: Periprosthetic indium-111-labeled leukocyte activity and complementary technetium-99m-sulfur colloid imaging in suspected infection. *J Nucl Med* 1990;31(12):1950-1955.

59. Fineman DS, Palestro CJ, Kim CK, et al: Detection of abnormalities in febrile AIDS patients with In-111-labeled leukocyte and Ga-67 scintigraphy. *Radiology* 1989;170(3 pt 1):677-680.

60. Mulamba L, Ferrant A, Leners N, de Nayer P, Rombouts JJ, Vincent A: Indium-111 leucocyte scanning in the evaluation of painful hip arthroplasty. *Acta Orthop Scand* 1983;54(5):695-697.

61. Zhuang H, Duarte PS, Pourdehnad M, et al: The promising role of 18F-FDG PET in detecting infected lower limb prosthesis implants. *J Nucl Med* 2001;42(1):44-48.

62. Chacko TK, Zhuang H, Stevenson K, Moussavian B, Alavi A: The importance of the location of fluorodeoxyglucose uptake in periprosthetic infection in painful hip prostheses. *Nucl Med Commun* 2002;23(9):851-855.

63. Della Valle C, Parvizi J, Bauer TW, et al: Diagnosis of periprosthetic joint infections of the hip and knee. *J Am Acad Orthop Surg* 2010;18(12):760-770.

64. Trampuz A, Hanssen AD, Osmon DR, Mandrekar J, Steckelberg JM, Patel R: Synovial fluid leukocyte count and differential for the diagnosis of prosthetic knee infection. *Am J Med* 2004;117(8):556-562.

65. Parvizi J, Walinchus L, Adeli B: Molecular diagnostics in periprosthetic joint infection. *Int J Artif Organs* 2011;34(9):847-855.

66. Randau TM, Friedrich MJ, Wimmer MD, et al: Interleukin-6 in serum and in synovial fluid enhances the differentiation between periprosthetic joint infection and aseptic loosening. *PLoS One* 2014;9(2):e89045.

67. Høgdall D, Hvolris JJ, Christensen L: Improved detection methods for infected hip joint prostheses. *APMIS* 2010;118(11):815-823.

68. Bereza PL, Ekiel A, Auguściak-Duma A, et al: Identification of silent prosthetic joint infection: Preliminary report of a prospective controlled study. *Int Orthop* 2013;37(10):2037-2043.

69. Ganz T, Selsted ME, Szklarek D, et al: Defensins: Natural peptide antibiotics of human neutrophils. *J Clin Invest* 1985;76(4):1427-1435.

70. Deirmengian C, Kardos K, Kilmartin P, Cameron A, Schiller K, Parvizi J: Combined measurement of synovial fluid α-Defensin and C-reactive protein levels: Highly accurate for diagnosing periprosthetic joint infection. *J Bone Joint Surg Am* 2014;96(17):1439-1445.

71. Deirmengian C, Kardos K, Kilmartin P, Gulati S, Citrano P, Booth RE Jr: The alpha-defensin test for periprosthetic joint infection responds to a wide spectrum of organisms. *Clin Orthop Relat Res* 2015;473(7):2229-2235.

72. Tsaras G, Maduka-Ezeh A, Inwards CY, et al: Utility of intraoperative frozen section histopathology in the diagnosis of periprosthetic joint infection: A systematic review and meta-analysis. *J Bone Joint Surg Am* 2012;94(18):1700-1711.

73. Trampuz A, Piper KE, Jacobson MJ, et al: Sonication of removed hip and knee prostheses for diagnosis of infection. *N Engl J Med* 2007;357(7):654-663.

74. Holinka J, Pilz M, Hirschl AM, Graninger W, Windhager R, Presterl E: Differential bacterial load on components of total knee prosthesis in patients with prosthetic joint infection. *Int J Artif Organs* 2012;35(10):735-741.

75. Aggarwal VK, Tischler E, Ghanem E, Parvizi J: Leukocyte esterase from synovial fluid aspirate: A technical note. *J Arthroplasty* 2013;28(1):193-195.

76. Wetters NG, Berend KR, Lombardi AV, Morris MJ, Tucker TL, Della Valle CJ: Leukocyte esterase reagent strips for the rapid diagnosis of periprosthetic joint infection. *J Arthroplasty* 2012;27(8 suppl):8-11.

77. Panousis K, Grigoris P, Butcher I, Rana B, Reilly JH, Hamblen DL: Poor predictive value of broad-range PCR for the detection of arthroplasty infection in 92 cases. *Acta Orthop* 2005;76(3):341-346.

78. Borst A, Box AT, Fluit AC: False-positive results and contamination in nucleic acid amplification assays: Suggestions for a prevent and destroy strategy. *Eur J Clin Microbiol Infect Dis* 2004;23(4):289-299.

79. Bergin PF, Doppelt JD, Hamilton WG, et al: Detection of periprosthetic infections with use of ribosomal RNA-based polymerase chain reaction. *J Bone Joint Surg Am* 2010;92(3):654-663.

80. Birmingham P, Helm JM, Manner PA, Tuan RS: Simulated joint infection assessment by rapid detection of live bacteria with real-time reverse transcription polymerase chain reaction. *J Bone Joint Surg Am* 2008;90(3):602-608.

81. Costerton JW, Post JC, Ehrlich GD, et al: New methods for the detection of orthopedic and other biofilm infections. *FEMS Immunol Med Microbiol* 2011;61(2):133-140.

82. Krimmer V, Merkert H, von Eiff C, et al: Detection of Staphylococcus aureus and Staphylococcus epidermidis in clinical samples by 16S rRNA-directed in situ hybridization. *J Clin Microbiol* 1999;37(8):2667-2673.

83. Nistico L, Gieseke A, Stoodley P, Hall-Stoodley L, Kerschner JE, Ehrlich GD: Fluorescence "in situ" hybridization for the detection of biofilm in the middle ear and upper respiratory tract mucosa. *Methods Mol Biol* 2009;493:191-213.

84. Stoodley P, Ehrlich GD, Sedghizadeh PP, et al: Orthopaedic biofilm infections. *Curr Orthop Pract* 2011;22(6):558-563.

85. Xu Y, Rudkjøbing VB, Simonsen O, et al: Bacterial diversity in suspected prosthetic joint infections: An exploratory study using 16S rRNA gene analysis. *FEMS Immunol Med Microbiol* 2012;65(2):291-304.

86. Hamady M, Knight R: Microbial community profiling for human microbiome projects: Tools, techniques, and challenges. *Genome Res* 2009;19(7):1141-1152.

87. DeSantis TZ, Brodie EL, Moberg JP, Zubieta IX, Piceno YM, Andersen GL: High-density universal 16S rRNA microarray analysis reveals broader diversity than typical clone library when sampling the environment. *Microb Ecol* 2007;53(3):371-383.

Single-Stage Revision Total Knee Arthroplasty in the Setting of Periprosthetic Knee Infection: Indications, Contraindications, and Postoperative Outcomes

Afshin A. Anoushiravani, MD

Zain Sayeed, MSc, MHA

Mouhanad M. El-Othmani, MD

Monique C. Chambers, MD, MSL

William M. Mihalko, MD, PhD

William A. Jiranek, MD, FACS

Wayne G. Paprosky, MD, FACS

Khaled J. Saleh, MD, MSc, FACSC, MHCM, CPE

Abstract

Single-stage revision total knee arthroplasty has become an increasingly common treatment option for patients with failed knee prostheses. Periprosthetic knee infection is the leading and most devastating cause of revision total knee arthroplasty. Although periprosthetic knee infection has been extensively studied in the orthopaedic literature, the role of single-stage revision total knee arthroplasty for the treatment of periprosthetic knee infection warrants further research. As healthcare reform shifts from a volume-based to a value-based system, it is imperative that orthopaedic surgeons understand the procedural indications, risks, and benefits of single-stage revision total knee arthroplasty.

Instr Course Lect 2017;66:235–247.

Total knee arthroplasty (TKA) is a successful treatment option for patients who have end-stage knee arthritis because it reliably reduces pain and improves quality of life.[1] In 2011, 718,000 TKAs were performed in the United States, accounting for 4.6% of all surgical procedures.[2,3] Studies have projected that 3.5 million primary TKAs will be performed annually by 2030.[4] TKA, although a common procedure, includes risk for surgical candidates, the most serious of which is periprosthetic knee infection (PKI). PKI has a postoperative prevalence of 1% to 3%,[5-8] and studies have estimated that approximately $1.62 billion will be spent revising 121,000 septic TKAs by 2020.[4,6] The definition of a PKI remains controversial; however, the American Academy of Orthopaedic Surgcons' (AAOS) clinical practice guideline on periprosthetic joint infections of the hip and knee provides direction for the diagnosis of PKI,[9] which may be defined as meeting one of three criteria highlighted in **Table 1**.[10,11]

The goals for the treatment of PKI are eradication of infection, alleviation of pain, and maintenance of the functional extremity. Seven options are currently available for the treatment of PKI: (1) chronic antibiotic suppression, (2) open débridement, (3) single-stage revision TKA, (4) two-stage revision TKA, (5) resection arthroplasty,

Table 1

Criteria Required for the Diagnosis of Periprosthetic Knee Infection (PKI)

A PKI exists if:

1. There is a sinus tract communicating with the prosthesis; **OR**

2. The same pathogen is isolated by culture from two or more separate tissue or fluid samples obtained from the affected prosthetic joint; **OR**

3. **THREE** of the following five criteria exist:

   a. Elevated erythrocyte sedimentation rate **AND** serum C-reactive protein level

   b. Elevated synovial fluid white blood cell count **OR** ++ change on leukocyte esterase test strips

   c. Elevated synovial polymorphonuclear neutrophil percentage

   d. Isolation of a microorganism in one culture of periprosthetic tissue or fluid

   e. Positive histologic analysis of periprosthetic tissue

Data from Zmistowski B, Della Valle C, Bauer TW, et al: Diagnosis of periprosthetic joint infection. *J Arthroplasty* 2014; 29(2 suppl):77-83.

(6) arthrodesis, and (7) amputation. The indications and contraindications for each procedure are primarily determined by the infecting pathogen and the timing of postoperative infection. In the United States, the preferred definitive treatment for PKI remains two-stage revision TKA;[12] however, single-stage revision TKA is a treatment option for PKI that is underutilized by the orthopaedic community.

Periprosthetic Knee Infection

A PKI after TKA is a life-threatening complication that is associated with a 32-fold increase in mortality.[13] The pathophysiology of PKI is complex and poorly understood; however, PKIs can be effectively categorized by the duration of infection, the infecting pathogen, and the bacterial growth pattern. Categorization of a PKI guides management and determines if single-stage revision TKA is an appropriate treatment option.

Duration of Infection

The duration of PKI has been defined by the Musculoskeletal Infection Society and adopted by the Centers for Disease Control and Prevention as either acute (<90 days) or chronic (>90 days).[14] Acute PKIs are often associated with direct infection of a prosthesis that was contracted during implantation. Typically, patients with an acute PKI have passive joint pain, tenderness, erythema, fever, and, in patients who have severe PKI, fistula formation. The organisms responsible for acute PKIs include highly virulent bacteria, such as *Staphylococcus aureus* and gram-negative rods.[15] Chronic PKIs are acquired hematogenously and are associated with cellulitis, urinary tract infection, respiratory infection, and oral infections.[16] Patients with chronic PKIs have subtle findings, such as persistent joint pain or implant loosening. Furthermore, the onset and progression of a chronic PKI is more subtle compared with an acute PKI. Coagulase-negative staphylococci are frequently associated with chronic PKIs.[15] The nonspecific signs and symptoms of a chronic PKI make its diagnosis difficult to differentiate from aseptic loosening, which results in a poorer prognosis.

Infecting Pathogen

In accordance with the AAOS clinical practice guideline on periprosthetic joint infections of the hip and knee, special care should be taken to identify the infecting organism of a PKI before

Dr. Mihalko or an immediate family member has received royalties from Aesculap/B. Braun; is a member of a speakers' bureau or has made paid presentations on behalf of Aesculap/B. Braun; is an employee of Aesculap/B. Braun, Medtronic, and Panoramic Healthcare; has received research or institutional support from Aesculap/B. Braun, MicroPort, Smith & Nephew, and Stryker; and serves as a board member, owner, officer, or committee member of the American Board of Orthopaedic Surgery, the American Orthopaedic Association, and ASTM International. Dr. Jiranek or an immediate family member has received royalties from DePuy; serves as a paid consultant to Cayenne Medical and DePuy; has stock or stock options held in Johnson & Johnson; has received research or institutional support from DePuy and Stryker; and serves as a board member, owner, officer, or committee member of the American Association of Hip and Knee Surgeons, LifeNet Health, and the Orthopaedic Learning Center. Dr. Paprosky or an immediate family member has received royalties from Intellijoint Surgical, Stryker, and Zimmer; serves as a paid consultant to DePuy, Medtronic, Stryker, and Zimmer; has stock or stock options held in Intellijoint Surgical; has received nonincome support (such as equipment or services), commercially derived honoraria, or other non-research–related funding (such as paid travel) from Cadence Health; and serves as a board member, owner, officer, or committee member of the Hip Society. Dr. Saleh or an immediate family member has received royalties from Aesculap/B. Braun; is a member of a speakers' bureau or has made paid presentations on behalf of Aesculap/B. Braun; is an employee of the Southern Illinois University School of Medicine, Division of Orthopaedics; serves as a paid consultant to Aesculap/B. Braun, the Memorial Medical Center Co-management Orthopaedic Board, and Watermark; has received research or institutional support from Smith & Nephew, the Orthopaedic Research and Education Foundation, and the National Institutes of Health (NIAMS); and serves as a board member, owner, officer, or committee member of the American Academy of Orthopaedic Surgeons, the American Orthopaedic Association, the American Orthopaedic Association Finance Committee, the Orthopaedic Research and Education Foundation Industry Relations Committee, the Orthopaedic Research and Education Foundation Clinical Research Awards Committee, the American Board of Orthopaedic Surgeons Oral Examiner, the Board of Specialty Societies, Notify, and the American Academy of Orthopaedic Surgeons Performance Measures Committee. None of the following authors nor any immediate family member has received anything of value from or has stock or stock options held in a commercial company or institution related directly or indirectly to the subject of this chapter: Dr. Anoushiravani, Dr. Sayeed, Dr. El-Othmani, and Dr. Chambers.

Table 2

Reported Incidence of Infecting Organisms After Total Knee Arthroplasty

Organism	Incidence (%)
Coagulase-negative staphylococci	30–43
Staphylococcus aureus	12–23
Streptococci	9–10
Enterococci	3–7
Gram-negative bacteria	3–6
Anaerobes	2–4

Data from Pandey R, Berendt AR, Athanasou NA; The OSIRIS Collaborative Study Group; Oxford Skeletal Infection Research and Intervention Service: Histological and microbiological findings in non-infected and infected revision arthroplasty tissues. *Arch Orthop Trauma Surg* 2000;120(10):570-574.

medical or surgical management is initiated.[9] The organisms most frequently associated with PKI are *S aureus* and *Staphylococcus epidermidis*[15,17] (**Table 2**); however, small-colony variants within these bacterial genera may exhibit multidrug resistance tendencies.[18] Infections caused by small-colony variants are more difficult to manage and less amenable to irrigation and débridement, polyexchange, and single-stage revision TKA.[19-24] In addition, polymicrobial and fungal infections are frequently more resilient and require two-stage TKA or salvage procedures. Failure to identify the infecting pathogen before treatment is initiated may result in refractory infections, which increases patient morbidity and mortality.[13] Consequently, it is critical that surgeons identify the microorganism and obtain antibiotic sensitivities before pharmacologic and surgical intervention is initiated.

Bacterial Growth Pattern

Bacterial infections can be categorized into two physiologic states: infections that consist of sessile or immobile bacteria and infections that consist of planktonic or free-floating microbes.[25] Sessile infections are more likely to exhibit quorum sensing, which is a chemo-induced mechanism for the regulation of gene expression.[26] Sessile bacteria frequently induce quorum sensing in the presence of abiotic devices, such as knee prostheses; this results in the formation of biofilms, which better equips bacteria to establish localized infections.[25] Conversely, planktonic bacteria demonstrate more virulent characteristics compared with sessile bacteria but are more susceptible to a patient's immune system and antibiotic therapies.[25] The classification of whether a bacterial infection is primarily caused by planktonic or sessile bacteria helps determine a patient's prognosis and guides treatment. Planktonic infections can be effectively managed with irrigation and débridement, polyexchange, and antibiotic therapies, whereas sessile infections frequently require single- or two-stage revision TKA.

Biofilm is an extracellular polysaccharide matrix that is composed of nucleic acids, polypeptides, and carbohydrates, all of which aid in the survival of resident microorganisms.[27,28] Biofilms are not static entities that encapsulate bacteria but are complex microbial matrices of defined architecture that form stable bacterial communities.[22,29] The widespread presence of biofilm is evidence of the survival benefits afforded to bacteria by bacterial matrices. Bacterial biofilm phenotypically optimizes microbial communities in a manner similar to multicellular organisms. In addition

to providing an exocapsular structure that protects resident microbes from the bactericidal effects of antibiotics and a patient's immune system,[30] biofilms are capable of reducing metabolic cellular activity and the upregulation of genes that are responsible for antibiotic resistance by 1,000-fold.[22,31-33] Although not all bacteria have the same threshold for the development of biofilm, studies estimate that approximately 99% of bacteria are capable of synthesizing biofilm, with most bacteria forming a lattice structure between 36 hours and 3 weeks.[34-36] The rapid synthesis of biofilm as well as its ability to phenotypically optimize bacterial communities complicates the management of PKIs.

Culture-Negative PKI

Despite laboratory, radiologic, and molecular tests that aid in the diagnosis of PKI, approximately 7% to 12% of patients with periprosthetic infections have negative cultures.[17,20,37-40] The most common cause of culture-negative PKI is antibiotic administration before aspiration and tissue sampling.[41] Berbari et al[20] reported that 53% of patients who had culture-negative PKIs were administered antibiotics before joint culture. Trampuz et al[21] reported that antibiotic therapy within 2 weeks of joint culture increased the rate of false-negative results. Therefore, antibiotic therapy should be discontinued for a minimum of 2 weeks before fluid or tissue culture, particularly if fastidious organisms are suspected.[20,21]

Infectious disease consultation is recommended for all patients who have a periprosthetic infection because it may help streamline diagnosis and treatment. Conventional tissue sampling techniques may fail to isolate sufficient infectious inoculum, which may result

Table 3

Inclusion and Exclusion Criteria for Single-Stage Revision Total Knee Arthroplasty (TKA)

Inclusion Criteria	Exclusion Criteria
Aseptic	Sepsis with substantial systemic manifestations
Early periprosthetic infection (≤12 weeks)	Delayed or late infection (>12 weeks)
Known bacteriology and antibiotic sensitivity	Culture-negative periprosthetic knee infection
Susceptible monomicrobial infection	Multidrug-resistant infection
Adequate soft-tissue coverage with no sinus tract communicating with the joint	Sinus tract communicating with the joint
Immunocompetent state	Infection involving neurovascular bundles
	Lack of adequate soft-tissue coverage
	Immunocompromised state
	Fungal infection
	Two or more single-stage revision TKA failures

in culture-negative PKI.[30,34] Furthermore, poor sample collection may hinder microbial isolation; therefore, surgeons must be aware of the diluting effects of local anesthetics and irrigation fluids.[42-44] Improper use of culture media and inadequate growth time also may result in culture-negative PKI, particularly for organisms such as *Propionibacterium acnes* and some coagulase-negative staphylococci, both of which often require more than 2 weeks to isolate.[43] In addition, fungi, mycobacteria, and other atypical microbes will not grow on standard media.[45-47] Finally, all collected synovial fluid and hematologic samples should be sent to the laboratory without delay to prevent false-negative results.[48]

Despite the implementation of appropriate sample and culture protocols, culture-negative PKIs continue to occur. Sonication and enzyme-linked immunosorbent assay (ELISA) are two promising laboratory techniques that may help reduce the incidence of culture-negative PKIs. Sonication uses ultrasound waves to mechanically disrupt the biofilm on tissue samples, which increases the number of infectious particles collected for polymerase chain reaction and ELISA analysis.[21] ELISA is a highly sensitive and specific analytical immunoassay that can be used to aid in the diagnosis of infection via the identification of specific bacterial antigens.[49] The number of infectious particles may be amplified with sonication and ELISA, which allows for a more robust analysis of the infecting pathogen.[21,50]

Management

The proper management of a PKI is individualized based on patient- and infection-specific variables. The orthopaedic literature contains many studies on the outcomes of two-stage revision TKA for the treatment of PKI; however, single-stage revision TKA is a treatment option for PKI that has been underutilized in the United States.[51-53] US surgeons are beginning to reassess PKI treatment algorithms as more

European studies report the advantages of single-stage revision TKA.[52,53]

Indications

Wroblewski[54] first demonstrated single-stage revision in 1986 with the revision of an infected total hip arthroplasty. More than three decades later, single-stage revision total hip arthroplasty has become common practice, and studies have reported adequate infection control as well as reduced morbidity and mortality in patients who undergo single-stage revision total hip arthroplasty.[55-57] Although single-stage revision was quickly implemented for septic total hip arthroplasties, until recently, it was rarely considered a treatment option for PKIs. An international group of orthopaedic surgeons and researchers were not able to reach a consensus on the contraindications for single-stage revision TKA until 2014.[14,51,53,58-61] The AAOS clinical practice guideline on periprosthetic joint infections of the hip and knee and the recommendations made by an international consensus group on periprosthetic joint infection were used to develop the inclusion and exclusion criteria for single-stage revision TKA that are listed in **Table 3**.[9,14]

Preoperative Considerations

All candidates for single-stage revision TKA require preoperative microbial identification and antimicrobial sensitivity testing. The diagnosis of a PKI requires sampling and analysis of synovial fluid for aerobic, anaerobic, fungi, and mycobacterial cultures.[11] Two-stage revision TKA is recommended for patients in whom synovial fluid cultures identify a polymicrobial infection and those in whom sensitivities indicate the presence of resistant organisms because these infections have higher rates of reoccurrence.[62,63] Furthermore, the AAOS clinical practice guideline on periprosthetic joint infections of the hip and knee states that patients who have a suspected PKI should not receive antibiotics until the diagnosis of a PKI is confirmed or ruled out.[9] If antibiotic therapy is initiated, aspiration of the knee should be delayed until 2 weeks after the last antibiotic dose.[20,21] Failure to follow these recommendations may increase a patient's risk for a culture-negative PKI.

Surgical Technique

Single-stage revision TKA is a viable alternative to two-stage revision TKA for patients who meet the inclusion criteria listed in **Table 3**. Single-stage revision TKA is split into two separate stages. The first portion of the surgery begins with an elliptical incision that incorporates the scar from the index procedure. The periarticular tissues are aggressively débrided, and the component is resected to reduce the pathogenic bioburden, which improves the efficacy of the entire procedure. All efforts should be made to minimize bone loss, and any interfacing tissue should be excised and sent for microbiologic and histologic analysis.[64-66] Surgeons may consider obtaining CT scans with three-dimensional reconstruction before performing single-stage revision TKA to estimate the amount of expected bone loss. The use of a tourniquet is generally not recommended during débridement because the absence of bleeding aids in the identification of both necrotic soft-tissue and osseous tissue. A minimum of three to six tissue samples should be obtained from the femur, tibia, and posterior capsule before joint lavage is performed.[9,67,68]

The débrided joint is then washed with copious amounts of saline (15 L) and soaked with povidone-iodine swabs.[64,65] The wound edges are reapproximated with sutures, and a temporary compressive dressing is applied.[64] Appropriate antibiotics based on patient sensitivities that were established preoperatively are administered intravenously.[64]

At this time, the entire surgical team re-scrubs, the patient is re-draped, and new instruments are used for the second portion of the surgery.[64,65] A tourniquet is inflated, and the compressive dressing and sutures are removed.[64] The joint is copiously irrigated with normal saline, and culture swabs of the bone surface are obtained.[64] The new implant is fitted and stabilized with antibiotic-impregnated cement.[64] After successful hardware implantation, two suction drains are placed in the joint, and the deep incision is closed in layers with interrupted sutures.[64] The wound edges are reapproximated and stapled.[64] The incision is bandaged, and the patient is allowed to bear weight as tolerated.[64]

Intraoperative Considerations

Proper intraoperative management during single-stage revision TKA includes meticulous surgical technique, intraoperative biopsies, and rigorous joint lavage. In addition, the design and composition of the prosthesis and cement may affect a patient's long-term postoperative outcomes. The AAOS clinical practice guideline on periprosthetic joint infections of the hip and knee strongly recommends that surgeons obtain multiple intraoperative tissue biopsies for culture and microbiologic analysis.[9] A patient's intraoperative tissue cultures and sensitivities should agree with his or her preoperative cultures. If these cultures

differ, appropriate antibiotic therapy should be initiated immediately.[64] Currently, most surgeons use copious amounts of normal saline to lavage the infected joint; however, chlorhexidine gluconate, which is an antiseptic that is used for preoperative skin preparation, may be superior compared with pulsed saline.[69] The development of biofilm-disrupting materials, such as cationic steroid antimicrobial-13, is underway for patients who have a higher susceptibility to infection.[70] Cationic steroid antimicrobial-13 can be combined with medical grade polydimethylsiloxane to create an antiseptic coating agent that shields the prosthesis from re-inoculation.[70] Advancements in antiseptic biomaterials may broaden the indications for single-stage revision TKA.

Prosthesis selection must account for patient variables, including age, weight, activity level, and bone stock.[71] A constrained-hinge knee prosthesis is frequently used for revision TKA in patients who have extensive bone loss, altered knee anatomy, joint instability, and soft-tissue laxity. Surgeons may elect to use larger, more invasive, modular implants in patients who have severe bone loss to help reconstruct the distal femur and proximal tibia. Furthermore, to help achieve adequate fixation, revision TKA prostheses generally have a noticeably longer stem compared with primary implants.

The composition of the implant also has been reported to affect outcomes after revision TKA. Cordero et al[72] reported that cobalt-chromium was more resistant to bacterial colonization compared with titanium. Other studies have reported that polished surfaces require greater inoculum compared with porous surfaces.[73,74] Tokarski et al[75] reported lower recurrent infection rates

Table 4

Indications and Unique Properties of Antibiotics Used to Impregnate Bone Cement

Antibiotic	Indications	Unique Properties
Aminoglycosides (gentamicin, tobramycin)	Gram negative Pseudomonas	First-line therapy
Vancomycin	Gram-positive cocci: MRSA	First-line therapy Less effective against MSSA
Macrolide (erythromycin)	Gram positive Atypicals	No MRSA coverage
Clindamycin	Gram-positive cocci: MRSA Gram-negative rods Anaerobic	
Daptomycin	Gram-positive cocci: MRSA	
Ciprofloxacin	Gram negative Anaerobic Pseudomonas	
Cephalosporins (first through second generation, second through fourth generation)	Gram positive Gram negative	Fourth generation covers pseudomonas

MRSA = methicillin-resistant *Staphylococcus aureus*, MSSA = methicillin-susceptible *Staphylococcus aureus*.

in patients who underwent revision TKA with a tantalum implant compared with those who underwent revision TKA with a titanium prosthesis. The findings of Tokarski et al[75] are in concordance with those of a study by Schildhauer et al[74] on the bacterial adhesion characteristics of tantalum, titanium, and stainless steel. Schildhauer et al[74] reported that pure tantalum implants had superior antimicrobial adhesive properties compared with titanium composites. The scientific rationale for these observations may be the result of the higher osseointegration potential of tantalum compared with titanium.[76] In addition, studies have hypothesized that the three-dimensional structure and pore size of tantalum prostheses prohibit bacterial

growth and biofilm formation.[75] To the knowledge of the authors of this chapter, no study has comparatively assessed cobalt-chromium and tantalum implants. Therefore, the authors of this chapter can only conclude that cobalt-chromium and tantalum implants are superior compared with titanium prostheses,[72,74,75] and that polished stems require a greater microbial load compared with porous stems.[73,74]

Regardless of implant composition and surface properties, antibiotic-impregnated cement should be used to achieve definitive fixation.[77] The use of antibiotic-impregnated cement is associated with improved postoperative outcomes after single-stage revision TKA.[78] Two major types of bone cement exist for patients who undergo revision

TKA for the treatment of PKI: acrylic-based polymer cement (ie, polymethyl methacrylate) and calcium phosphate/sulfate cement. Acrylic-based polymer cements are nonabsorbable bone cements that have high-strain force resistance and burst antibiotic elution properties.[79,80] Calcium sulfate/phosphate cements are absorbable bone cements that have improved elution of a wider range of antibiotics; however, there are limited data on the antimicrobial and antibiofilm efficacy of calcium sulfate/phosphate cements.[81] Although acrylic-based polymer cements may provide a nidus for future infection after antibiotic elution,[81] the current consensus among orthopaedic surgeons is that antibiotic-impregnated acrylic bone cement should be used in the treatment of periprosthetic infections.[77,82]

The use of antibiotic-impregnated bone cement has become increasingly common and is essential for the eradication of infection. Aminoglycosides and vancomycin are considered first-line antibiotics because of their thermal properties, water solubility, broad-spectrum coverage, favorable pharmacokinetics, low allergy profile, and availability in a crystalline form.[83] Alternative antibiotics that can be used to impregnate bone cement are listed in **Table 4**. These antibiotics can be used alone or in combination to provide improved coverage and biphasic antibiotic elution profiles, with inhibitory concentrations that are maintained for up to 4 to 6 weeks.[79,80]

Surgeons also must be cognizant of the biomechanical properties of bone cement, particularly if adding crystalline antibiotics. In single-stage revision TKA, the amount of antibiotic added to the cement should not exceed 10% of the total mass of the cement because its mechanical strength may be compromised.[84,85] Numerous studies have compared antibiotic elution properties in relation to atmospheric hand-mixing versus vacuum-mixing. To the knowledge of the authors of this chapter, neither mixing technique is inferior. Hand-mixing results in a porous cement that has improved antibiotic elution properties; however, elution characteristics at the cement surface are difficult to predict because of cement heterogeneity.[86] Conversely, vacuum-mixing results in a homogenous cement that has superior mechanical properties but reduced antibiotic elution properties.[85] In a study of six commercially available antibiotic-impregnated cements, Meyer et al[87] reported that vacuum-mixing had a deleterious effect on antibiotic elution for low-viscosity cements and a beneficial effect on antibiotic elution for high-viscosity cements. The authors reported that vacuum-mixing had an unpredictable effect on antibiotic elution for intermediate-viscosity cements, which demonstrates that neither hand- nor vacuum-mixing is universally superior, but that both techniques have unique indications.

Postoperative Considerations

The selection of an antibiotic regimen is based on a patient's preoperative bacterial susceptibilities; the antibiotic regimen can be altered, if necessary, after a patient's intraoperative cultures and sensitivities are available.[64] The first antibiotic dose is administered intravenously after irrigation and débridement of the septic joint.[64] In general, intravenous antibiotics are continued for 2 weeks postoperatively, after which they are converted to an oral antibiotic regimen for 4 to 6 weeks postoperatively.[64,85]

Although the optimal antibiotic regimen for patients who undergo single-stage revision TKA is unclear, postoperative antibiotics are indicated for all patients who undergo single-stage revision TKA. The devascularized nature of implants and the tendency of microbes to form biofilms make the eradication of even the most susceptible organisms a challenge.[47] Although not evidence-based, 6 months of antibiotic therapy that includes an initial 2 to 4 weeks of parenteral antibiotics is common after single-stage revision TKA.[47,88,89] The administration of parenteral antibiotics should be curtailed and transitioned to an oral antibiotic regimen to effectively use healthcare resources and minimize patient morbidity.[90] Such measures reduce catheter- and antibiotic-related complications in approximately 33% of patients who have a PKI.[91]

Bernard et al[85] comparatively assessed the infection eradication rates of oral and parenteral antibiotics as well as the effects of 6 and 12 weeks of antibiotic therapy in a cohort of 144 patients with periprosthetic joint infections who underwent various surgical interventions (single and two stage revision TKAs as well as irrigation and débridement with implant retention). The authors reported that the inciting infection was eradicated in 80% of the patients.[85] Interestingly, the eradication rate was not affected by the duration of antibiotic therapy or the route of antibiotic administration, which suggests that long-term antibiotic therapy and parenteral antibiotic administration may be less beneficial than previously thought.[85] Although not statistically significant, the authors reported that the patients who underwent irrigation and débridement with implant retention

had a tendency for lower eradication rates.[85] In a study of 118 patients who had osteogenic infections, 52% of whom had periprosthetic infections, Farhad et al[92] reported an infection eradication rate of 91.5% after 6 weeks of antibiotic therapy, which suggests that 6 weeks of antibiotic therapy is effective for the treatment of most patients who have osteogenic infections regardless of the pathophysiology,[92] and that extending antibiotic therapy may postpone treatment failure rather than prevent its onset.[93]

The selection of antibiotics with bone- and soft-tissue penetrance is essential to eradicate infection after single-stage revision TKA. Several antibiotics, such as quinolones and linezolid alone or in combination with rifampin or clindamycin, are particularly effective because they have a high bone penetration and an oral bioavailability greater than 90%.[88,89,92,94] Other intravenous and oral antibiotics frequently used to treat osteogenic infections are vancomycin, third- and fourth-generation cephalosporins, and carbapenem.[92] Several studies have reported the use of unconventional routes of antibiotic delivery, including high-dose intra-articular antibiotic administration after single-stage revision TKA.[95-97] In a study of 57 patients with periprosthetic joint infection who were treated with intra-articular antibiotics after single-stage revision TKA, Antony et al[95] reported a 100% eradication rate and an 89% cure rate at a follow-up of 11 months. Regardless of the method of antibiotic administration, infectious disease consultation is recommended for all patients who have a periprosthetic infection because proper antibiotic selection is essential to achieve optimal outcomes.[85]

Advantages of Single-Stage Revision TKA

In 1991, von Foerster et al[61] published the first study on single-stage revision TKA as a treatment option for PKI. This landmark study reported an infection eradication rate of 73% with single-stage revision TKA and antibiotic-impregnated cement; however, postoperative systemic antibiotics were not used[61] (**Table 5**). Conversely, in a study of 22 consecutive patients with PKIs who were treated with single-stage revision TKA, antibiotic-impregnated cement, and 4 to 6 weeks of postoperative intravenous antibiotics, Buechel et al[59] reported a 90.9% eradication rate at a mean follow-up of 10.2 years. In addition, the authors reported good or excellent Knee Society knee scores in 85.7% of the patients[59] (**Table 5**). In a recent study of 102 patients who were treated for PKI, 28 (27%) of whom underwent single-stage revision TKA and 74 (73%) of whom underwent two-stage revision TKA, Haddad et al[53] reported that the patients who underwent single-stage TKA had an infection eradication rate of 100%, and the patients who underwent two-stage revision TKA had an infection eradication rate of 93%.[53] It should be noted that the indications for single-stage revision TKA were stringent, including only immunocompetent patients with minimal to moderate bone loss, healthy soft tissues, and susceptible pathogens. There were no specific inclusion or exclusion criteria for the patients who underwent two-stage revision TKA[53] (**Table 5**).

Other studies have evaluated the outcomes of patients with chronic PKIs who underwent single-stage revision TKA with less stringent inclusion criteria.[52,64] Tibrewal et al[64] studied the outcomes of 50 consecutive patients who underwent single-stage revision TKA over a 30-year period (**Table 5**). The indications for single-stage revision TKA included patients who had an infection with proven bacteriology, available cultures and sensitivities, and a knee with sufficient soft-tissue coverage.[64] The authors reported a 98% eradication rate, with only one patient who required further surgical intervention.[64] Jenny et al[52] followed 47 patients for 24 months after single-stage revision TKA that was used to treat PKI. The authors reported that the only contraindications for single-stage revision TKA were fungal infection and repeated treatment failure.[52] At a follow-up of 2 years, the authors reported that 91% of the patients were free from the index infection, and 87% of the patients were free from any infection.[52] To the knowledge of the authors of this chapter, there are no well-designed studies that compare the postoperative outcomes of single- and two-stage revision TKA for the treatment of PKI; however, the results of the studies previously discussed suggest that single-stage revision TKA can result in infection eradication rates and Knee Society knee scores comparable with those of two-stage revision TKA[51-53,59,61,64,98-100] (**Table 5**).

Reduced Patient Morbidity

Patients who undergo revision TKA are frequently older and have a greater number of comorbidities compared with patients who undergo primary TKA, which increases the risk for intra-operative and postoperative complications.[101-103] Studies have reported that the use of general anesthesia in older patients may lead to postoperative cognitive dysfunction, which results in increased patient morbidity and prolonged hospital stay.[104,105] Single-stage revision TKA is advantageous because it combines two surgical procedures into one, which minimizes the likelihood of an adverse reaction from exposure to anesthesia. Extended periods of immobilization after two-stage revision TKA have led to concern for decreased Knee Society functional scores. Studies have reported that the Knee Society functional scores of patients who undergo single-stage revision TKA are equal or superior compared with those of patients who undergo two-stage revision TKA.[98,106] Conversely, Jenny et al[52] reported no difference in Knee Society functional scores among patients who underwent either single- or two-stage revision TKA. Jämsen et al[58] reported no statistically significant difference in Knee Society functional scores among patients who underwent either single- or two-stage revision TKA.

Reduced Healthcare Costs

With the passage of the Affordable Care Act, treatment options for PKI must be both clinically and financially sound before they are implemented. Kapadia et al[107] reported that the mean annual cost associated with patients who underwent two-stage revision TKA for the treatment of an infectious etiology was significantly higher ($116,383) compared with that of patients who underwent two-stage revision TKA for the treatment of a noninfectious etiology ($28,249).[107,108] The authors also noted that the patients in the infectious etiology cohort had longer hospitalization stays (5.3 days versus 3.0 days), more readmissions (3.6 versus 0.1), and more clinic visits (6.5 versus 1.3) compared with the patients in the noninfectious etiology cohort.[107] This

Table 5

Results of Single-Stage Revision Total Knee Arthroplasty (TKA)

Study (Year)	Number of Patients	Procedure	Mean Patient Age in Years (Range)	Mean Follow-up (Range)	Infection Eradication Rate (%)	Mean Postoperative Knee Society Knee Score
von Foerster et al[61] (1991)	118 (104 available for follow-up)	Single-stage revision TKA with antibiotic-impregnated cement	NA	NA (5–15 yr)	73	NA
Göksan and Freeman[51] (1992)	18	Single-stage revision TKA with antibiotic-impregnated cement and systemic antibiotics	61.4 (42–74)	5 yr (1–10 yr)	94.4	NA
Scott et al[99] (1993)	17 (single-stage, 10; two-stage, 7)	Single- and two-stage revision TKA with antibiotic-impregnated cement and systemic antibiotics until removal of drain	Single-stage: 71.5 (55–88) Two-stage: 66.9 (55–83)	NA	57	NA
Buechel et al[59] (2004)	22	Single-stage revision TKA with antibiotic-impregnated cement and systemic antibiotics	NA	10.2 yr (1.4–19.6 yr)	90.9	79.5
Bauer et al[100] (2006)	107 (single-stage, 30; two-stage, 77)	Single- and two-stage revision TKA	NA	52 mo (NA)	67	Single-stage: 75.5 Two-stage: 74.8
Singer et al[98] (2012)	63	Single-stage revision TKA	70.7 (31–89)	36 mo (24–70 mo)	95	72
Jenny et al[52] (2013)	47	Single-stage revision TKA with antibiotic-impregnated cement and systemic antibiotics	NA (45–93)	NA (5–76 mo)	Free of any infection: 87 Free of index infection: 91	85
Tibrewal et al[64] (2014)	50	Single-stage revision TKA with antibiotic-impregnated cement and systemic antibiotics	66.8 (42–84)	10.5 yr (2–24 yr)	98	NA
Haddad et al[53] (2015)	102 (single-stage, 28; two-stage, 74)	Single- and two-stage revision TKA with antibiotic-impregnated cement and systemic antibiotics	65 (45–87)	6.5 yr (3–9 yr)	Single-stage: 100 Two-stage: 93	Single-stage: 88 Two-stage: 76

NA = not available.

fourfold increase in cost has been at least partially attributed to higher readmission rates, extended hospital stays, and the prolonged use of pharmacotherapy.[109] Studies on the cost savings of single-stage revision total hip arthroplasty have reported a decrease in the use of healthcare resources;[65,110] however, to the knowledge of the authors of this chapter, there are no studies in the literature on the cost savings of single-stage revision TKA compared with two-stage revision TKA.

Summary

In the appropriate patient population, single-stage revision TKA effectively eradicates PKIs at a rate similar to, if not exceeding that of, two-stage revision TKA. Furthermore, single-stage revision TKA reduces patient morbidity and may result in improved functional outcomes. Single-stage revision TKA is associated with fewer surgical procedures and a shorter duration of pharmacotherapy, which minimizes resource utilization. Although single-stage revision TKA is a promising alternative to two-stage revision TKA, randomized controlled trials that compare single-stage revision TKA with two-stage revision TKA are necessary to better elucidate the rate of infection eradication and resource utilization associated with each procedure.

References

1. NIH Consensus Statement on total knee replacement. *NIH Consens State Sci Statements* 2003;20(1):1-34.

2. Weiss AJ, Elixhauser A, Andrews RM: Statistical brief #170: Characteristics of operating room procedures in U.S. hospitals, 2011. Rockville, MD, Agency for Healthcare Research and Quality, February 2014. Available at: www.hcup-us.ahrq.gov/reports/statbriefs/sb170-Operating-Room-Procedures-United-States-2011.pdf.

3. Pfuntner A, Wier LM, Stocks C: Statistical brief #149: Most frequent procedures performed in U.S. hospitals, 2010. Rockville, MD, Agency for Healthcare Research and Quality, February 2014. Available at: www.hcup-us.ahrq.gov/reports/statbriefs/sb149.pdf.

4. Kurtz S, Ong K, Lau E, Mowat F, Halpern M: Projections of primary and revision hip and knee arthroplasty in the United States from 2005 to 2030. *J Bone Joint Surg Am* 2007;89(4):780-785.

5. Harris WH, Sledge CB: Total hip and total knee replacement (1). *N Engl J Med* 1990;323(11):725-731.

6. Kurtz SM, Lau E, Schmier J, Ong KL, Zhao K, Parvizi J: Infection burden for hip and knee arthroplasty in the United States. *J Arthroplasty* 2008;23(7):984-991.

7. Vessely MB, Whaley AL, Harmsen WS, Schleck CD, Berry DJ: The Chitranjan Ranawat Award: Long-term survivorship and failure modes of 1000 cemented condylar total knee arthroplasties. *Clin Orthop Relat Res* 2006;452:28-34.

8. Fehring TK, Odum S, Griffin WL, Mason JB, Nadaud M: Early failures in total knee arthroplasty. *Clin Orthop Relat Res* 2001;392:315-318.

9. American Academy of Orthopaedic Surgeons: *Clinical Practice Guideline on The Diagnosis of Periprosthetic Joint Infections of the Hip and Knee*. Rosemont, IL, American Academy of Orthopaedic Surgeons, June 2010. www.aaos.org/research/guidelines/PJIsummary.pdf.

10. Ghanem E, Parvizi J, Burnett RS, et al: Cell count and differential of aspirated fluid in the diagnosis of infection at the site of total knee arthroplasty. *J Bone Joint Surg Am* 2008;90(8):1637-1643.

11. Parvizi J, Adeli B, Zmistowski B, Restrepo C, Greenwald AS: Management of periprosthetic joint infection: the current knowledge: AAOS exhibit selection. *J Bone Joint Surg Am* 2012;94(14):e104.

12. Wongworawat MD: Clinical faceoff: One- versus two-stage exchange arthroplasty for prosthetic joint infections. *Clin Orthop Relat Res* 2013;471(6):1750-1753.

13. Vogel TR, Dombrovskiy VY, Carson JL, Graham AM, Lowry SF: Postoperative sepsis in the United States. *Ann Surg* 2010;252(6):1065-1071.

14. Parvizi J, Gehrke T: International consensus on periprosthetic joint infection: Let cumulative wisdom be a guide. *J Bone Joint Surg Am* 2014;96(6):441.

15. Willenegger H, Roth B: Treatment tactics and late results in early infection following osteosynthesis. *Unfallchirurgie* 1986;12(5):241-246.

16. Maderazo EG, Judson S, Pasternak H: Late infections of total joint prostheses: A review and recommendations for prevention. *Clin Orthop Relat Res* 1988;229:131-142.

17. Pandey R, Berendt AR, Athanasou NA; The OSIRIS Collaborative Study Group; Oxford Skeletal Infection Research and Intervention Service: Histological and microbiological findings in non-infected and infected revision arthroplasty tissues. *Arch Orthop Trauma Surg* 2000;120(10):570-574.

18. Neut D, van der Mei HC, Bulstra SK, Busscher HJ: The role of small-colony variants in failure to diagnose and treat biofilm infections in orthopedics. *Acta Orthop* 2007;78(3):299-308.

19. Stoodley P, Ehrlich GD, Sedghizadeh PP, et al: Orthopaedic biofilm infections. *Curr Orthop Pract* 2011;22(6):558-563.

20. Berbari EF, Marculescu C, Sia I, et al: Culture-negative prosthetic joint infection. *Clin Infect Dis* 2007;45(9):1113-1119.

21. Trampuz A, Piper KE, Jacobson MJ, et al: Sonication of removed hip and knee prostheses for diagnosis of infection. *N Engl J Med* 2007;357(7):654-663.

22. Bjarnsholt T, Ciofu O, Molin S, Givskov M, Høiby N: Applying insights from biofilm biology to drug development - can a new approach be developed? *Nat Rev Drug Discov* 2013;12(10):791-808.

23. Khoury AE, Lam K, Ellis B, Costerton JW: Prevention and control of bacterial infections associated with medical devices. *ASAIO J* 1992;38(3):M174-M178.

24. Osmon DR, Berbari EF, Berendt AR, et al: Diagnosis and management of prosthetic joint infection: Clinical practice guidelines by the Infectious Diseases Society of America. *Clin Infect Dis* 2013;56(1):e1-e25.

25. Oggioni MR, Trappetti C, Kadioglu A, et al: Switch from planktonic to sessile life: A major event in pneumococcal pathogenesis. *Mol Microbiol* 2006;61(5):1196-1210.

26. Miller MB, Bassler BL: Quorum sensing in bacteria. *Annu Rev Microbiol* 2001;55:165-199.

27. Zimmerli W, Waldvogel FA, Vaudaux P, Nydegger UE: Pathogenesis of foreign body infection: Description and characteristics of an animal model. *J Infect Dis* 1982;146(4):487-497.

28. Zimmerli W, Lew PD, Waldvogel FA: Pathogenesis of foreign body infection: Evidence for a local granulocyte defect. *J Clin Invest* 1984;73(4):1191-1200.

29. Wolcott RD, Ehrlich GD: Biofilms and chronic infections. *JAMA* 2008;299(22):2682-2684.

30. Cerca N, Jefferson KK, Oliveira R, Pier GB, Azeredo J: Comparative

antibody-mediated phagocytosis of Staphylococcus epidermidis cells grown in a biofilm or in the planktonic state. *Infect Immun* 2006;74(8):4849-4855.

31. Costerton JW, Lewandowski Z, Caldwell DE, Korber DR, Lappin-Scott HM: Microbial biofilms. *Annu Rev Microbiol* 1995;49:711-745.

32. Stewart PS, Costerton JW: Antibiotic resistance of bacteria in biofilms. *Lancet* 2001;358(9276):135-138.

33. Donlan RM: Biofilms: Microbial life on surfaces. *Emerg Infect Dis* 2002;8(9):881-890.

34. Costerton JW: Biofilm theory can guide the treatment of device-related orthopaedic infections. *Clin Orthop Relat Res* 2005;437:7-11.

35. Parvizi J, Zmistowski B, Adeli B: Periprosthetic joint infection: Treatment options. *Orthopedics* 2010;33(9):659.

36. Choong PF, Dowsey MM, Carr D, Daffy J, Stanley P: Risk factors associated with acute hip prosthetic joint infections and outcome of treatment with a rifampin-based regimen. *Acta Orthop* 2007;78(6):755-765.

37. Parvizi J, Ghanem E, Menashe S, Barrack RL, Bauer TW: Periprosthetic infection: What are the diagnostic challenges? *J Bone Joint Surg Am* 2006;88(suppl 4):138-147.

38. Font-Vizcarra L, García S, Martínez-Pastor JC, Sierra JM, Soriano A: Blood culture flasks for culturing synovial fluid in prosthetic joint infections. *Clin Orthop Relat Res* 2010;468(8):2238-2243.

39. Duff GP, Lachiewicz PF, Kelley SS: Aspiration of the knee joint before revision arthroplasty. *Clin Orthop Relat Res* 1996;331:132-139.

40. Ghanem E, Parvizi J, Clohisy J, Burnett S, Sharkey PF, Barrack R: Perioperative antibiotics should not be withheld in proven cases of periprosthetic infection. *Clin Orthop Relat Res* 2007;461:44-47.

41. Trampuz A, Piper KE, Hanssen AD, et al: Sonication of explanted prosthetic components in bags for diagnosis of prosthetic joint infection is associated with risk of contamination. *J Clin Microbiol* 2006;44(2):628-631.

42. Patel R, Osmon DR, Hanssen AD: The diagnosis of prosthetic joint infection: Current techniques and emerging technologies. *Clin Orthop Relat Res* 2005;437:55-58.

43. Hughes JG, Vetter EA, Patel R, et al: Culture with BACTEC Peds Plus/F bottle compared with conventional methods for detection of bacteria in synovial fluid. *J Clin Microbiol* 2001;39(12):4468-4471.

44. Powles JW, Spencer RF, Lovering AM: Gentamicin release from old cement during revision hip arthroplasty. *J Bone Joint Surg Br* 1998;80(4):607-610.

45. Neogi DS, Kumar A, Yadav CS, Singh S: Delayed periprosthetic tuberculosis after total knee replacement: Is conservative treatment possible? *Acta Orthop Belg* 2009;75(1):136-140.

46. Zappe B, Graf S, Ochsner PE, Zimmerli W, Sendi P: Propionibacterium spp. in prosthetic joint infections: A diagnostic challenge. *Arch Orthop Trauma Surg* 2008;128(10):1039-1046.

47. Zimmerli W, Trampuz A, Ochsner PE: Prosthetic-joint infections. *N Engl J Med* 2004;351(16):1645-1654.

48. Meermans G, Haddad FS: Is there a role for tissue biopsy in the diagnosis of periprosthetic infection? *Clin Orthop Relat Res* 2010;468(5):1410-1417.

49. Selan L, Passariello C, Rizzo L, et al: Diagnosis of vascular graft infections with antibodies against staphylococcal slime antigens. *Lancet* 2002;359(9324):2166-2168.

50. Trampuz A, Osmon DR, Hanssen AD, Steckelberg JM, Patel R: Molecular and antibiofilm approaches to prosthetic joint infection. *Clin Orthop Relat Res* 2003;414:69-88.

51. Göksan SB, Freeman MA: One-stage reimplantation for infected total knee arthroplasty. *J Bone Joint Surg Br* 1992;74(1):78-82.

52. Jenny JY, Barbe B, Gaudias J, Boeri C, Argenson JN: High infection control rate and function after routine one-stage exchange for chronically infected TKA. *Clin Orthop Relat Res* 2013;471(1):238-243.

53. Haddad FS, Sukeik M, Alazzawi S: Is single-stage revision according to a strict protocol effective in treatment of chronic knee arthroplasty infections? *Clin Orthop Relat Res* 2015;473(1):8-14.

54. Wroblewski BM: One-stage revision of infected cemented total hip arthroplasty. *Clin Orthop Relat Res* 1986;211:103-107.

55. Callaghan JJ, Katz RP, Johnston RC: One-stage revision surgery of the infected hip: A minimum 10-year followup study. *Clin Orthop Relat Res* 1999;369:139-143.

56. Rudelli S, Uip D, Honda E, Lima AL: One-stage revision of infected total hip arthroplasty with bone graft. *J Arthroplasty* 2008;23(8):1165-1177.

57. Gehrke T, Kendoff D: Peri-prosthetic hip infections: In favour of one-stage. *Hip Int* 2012;22(suppl 8):S40-S45.

58. Jämsen E, Stogiannidis I, Malmivaara A, Pajamäki J, Puolakka T, Konttinen YT: Outcome of prosthesis exchange for infected knee arthroplasty: The effect of treatment approach. *Acta Orthop* 2009;80(1):67-77.

59. Buechel FF, Femino FP, D'Alessio J: Primary exchange revision arthroplasty for infected total knee replacement: A long-term study. *Am J Orthop (Belle Mead NJ)* 2004;33(4):190-198.

60. Lu H, Kou B, Lin J: One-stage reimplantation for the salvage of total knee arthroplasty complicated by infection. *Zhonghua Wai Ke Za Zhi* 1997;35(8):456-458.

61. von Foerster G, Klüber D, Käbler U: Mid- to long-term results after treatment of 118 cases of periprosthetic infections after knee joint replacement using one-stage exchange surgery. *Orthopade* 1991;20(3):244-252.

62. Zmistowski B, Fedorka CJ, Sheehan E, Deirmengian G, Austin MS, Parvizi J: Prosthetic joint infection caused by gram-negative organisms. *J Arthroplasty* 2011;26(6 suppl):104-108.

63. Pelt CE, Grijalva R, Anderson L, Anderson MB, Erickson J, Peters CL: Two-stage revision TKA is associated with high complication and failure rates. *Adv Orthop* 2014;2014:659047.

64. Tibrewal S, Malagelada F, Jeyaseelan L, Posch F, Scott G: Single-stage revision for the infected total knee

replacement: Results from a single centre. *Bone Joint J* 2014;96(6):759-764.

65. Gulhane S, Vanhegan IS, Haddad FS: Single stage revision: Regaining momentum. *J Bone Joint Surg Br* 2012;94(11 suppl A):120-122.

66. Mirra JM, Marder RA, Amstutz HC: The pathology of failed total joint arthroplasty. *Clin Orthop Relat Res* 1982;170:175-183.

67. Fink B, Makowiak C, Fuerst M, Berger I, Schäfer P, Frommelt L: The value of synovial biopsy, joint aspiration and C-reactive protein in the diagnosis of late peri-prosthetic infection of total knee replacements. *J Bone Joint Surg Br* 2008;90(7):874-878.

68. Schäfer P, Fink B, Sandow D, Margull A, Berger I, Frommelt L: Prolonged bacterial culture to identify late periprosthetic joint infection: A promising strategy. *Clin Infect Dis* 2008;47(11):1403-1409.

69. Darouiche RO, Wall MJ Jr, Itani KM, et al: Chlorhexidine-alcohol versus povidone-iodine for surgical-site antisepsis. *N Engl J Med* 2010;362(1):18-26.

70. Williams DL, Sinclair KD, Jeyapalina S, Bloebaum RD: Characterization of a novel active release coating to prevent biofilm implant-related infections. *J Biomed Mater Res B Appl Biomater* 2013;101(6):1078-1089.

71. Iorio R, Healy WL, Kirven FM, Patch DA, Pfeifer BA: Knee implant standardization: An implant selection and cost reduction program. *Am J Knee Surg* 1998;11(2):73-79.

72. Cordero J, Munuera L, Folgueira MD: The influence of the chemical composition and surface of the implant on infection. *Injury* 1996;27(suppl 3):SC34-SC37.

73. Cordero J, Munuera L, Folgueira MD: Influence of metal implants on infection: An experimental study in rabbits. *J Bone Joint Surg Br* 1994;76(5):717-720.

74. Schildhauer TA, Robie B, Muhr G, Köller M: Bacterial adherence to tantalum versus commonly used orthopedic metallic implant materials. *J Orthop Trauma* 2006;20(7):476-484.

75. Tokarski AT, Novack TA, Parvizi J: Is tantalum protective against infection

in revision total hip arthroplasty? *Bone Joint J* 2015;97(1):45-49.

76. Brown NM, Bell JA, Jung EK, Sporer SM, Paprosky WG, Levine BR: The use of trabecular metal cones in complex primary and revision total knee arthroplasty. *J Arthroplasty* 2015; 30(9 suppl):90-93.

77. Chiu FY, Lin CF: Antibiotic-impregnated cement in revision total knee arthroplasty: A prospective cohort study of one hundred and eighty-three knees. *J Bone Joint Surg Am* 2009;91(3):628-633.

78. Buchholz HW, Elson RA, Engelbrecht E, Lodenkämper H, Röttger J, Siegel A: Management of deep infection of total hip replacement. *J Bone Joint Surg Br* 1981;63(3):342-353.

79. Masri BA, Duncan CP, Beauchamp CP: Long-term elution of antibiotics from bone-cement: An in vivo study using the prosthesis of antibiotic-loaded acrylic cement (PROSTALAC) system. *J Arthroplasty* 1998;13(3):331-338.

80. Klemm K: The use of antibiotic-containing bead chains in the treatment of chronic bone infections. *Clin Microbiol Infect* 2001;7(1):28-31.

81. Howlin RP, Brayford MJ, Webb JS, Cooper JJ, Aiken SS, Stoodley P: Antibiotic-loaded synthetic calcium sulfate beads for prevention of bacterial colonization and biofilm formation in periprosthetic infections. *Antimicrob Agents Chemother* 2015;59(1):111-120.

82. Parvizi J, Saleh KJ, Ragland PS, Pour AE, Mont MA: Efficacy of antibiotic-impregnated cement in total hip replacement. *Acta Orthop* 2008;79(3):335-341.

83. Kalore NV, Gioe TJ, Singh JA: Diagnosis and management of infected total knee arthroplasty. *Open Orthop J* 2011;5:86-91.

84. Wahlig H, Dingeldein E, Buchholz HW, Buchholz M, Bachmann F: Pharmacokinetic study of gentamicin-loaded cement in total hip replacements: Comparative effects of varying dosage. *J Bone Joint Surg Br* 1984;66(2):175-179.

85. Bernard L, Legout L, Zürcher-Pfund L, et al: Six weeks of antibiotic treatment is sufficient following surgery for septic arthroplasty. *J Infect* 2010;61(2):125-132.

86. Neut D, van de Belt H, van Horn JR, van der Mei HC, Busscher HJ: The effect of mixing on gentamicin release from polymethylmethacrylate bone cements. *Acta Orthop Scand* 2003;74(6):670-676.

87. Meyer J, Philler G, Spiegel CA, Hetzel S, Squire M: Vacuum-mixing significantly changes antibiotic elution characteristics of commercially available antibiotic-impregnated bone cements. *J Bone Joint Surg Am* 2011;93(22):2049-2056.

88. Zimmerli W, Widmer AF, Blatter M, Frei R, Ochsner PE; Foreign-Body Infection (FBI) Study Group: Role of rifampin for treatment of orthopedic implant-related staphylococcal infections: A randomized controlled trial. *JAMA* 1998;279(19):1537-1541.

89. Trampuz A, Zimmerli W: Antimicrobial agents in orthopaedic surgery: Prophylaxis and treatment. *Drugs* 2006;66(8):1089-1105.

90. Mermel LA, Farr BM, Sherertz RJ, et al: Guidelines for the management of intravascular catheter-related infections. *Clin Infect Dis* 2001;32(9):1249-1272.

91. Pulcini C, Couadau T, Bernard E, et al: Adverse effects of parenteral antimicrobial therapy for chronic bone infections. *Eur J Clin Microbiol Infect Dis* 2008;27(12):1227-1232.

92. Farhad R, Roger PM, Albert C, et al: Six weeks antibiotic therapy for all bone infections: Results of a cohort study. *Eur J Clin Microbiol Infect Dis* 2010;29(2):217-222.

93. Byren I, Bejon P, Atkins BL, et al: One hundred and twelve infected arthroplasties treated with 'DAIR' (debridement, antibiotics and implant retention): Antibiotic duration and outcome. *J Antimicrob Chemother* 2009;63(6):1264-1271.

94. Bernard L, Hoffmeyer P, Assal M, Vaudaux P, Schrenzel J, Lew D: Trends in the treatment of orthopaedic prosthetic infections. *J Antimicrob Chemother* 2004;53(2):127-129.

95. Antony SJ, Westbrook RS, Jackson JS, Heydemann JS, Nelson JL: Efficacy of single-stage revision with aggressive debridement using intra-articular antibiotics in the treatment of infected joint prosthesis. *Infect Dis (Auckl)* 2015;8:17-23.

96. Whiteside LA, Nayfeh TA, LaZear R, Roy ME: Reinfected revised TKA resolves with an aggressive protocol and antibiotic infusion. *Clin Orthop Relat Res* 2012;470(1):236-243.

97. Whiteside LA, Peppers M, Nayfeh TA, Roy ME: Methicillin-resistant Staphylococcus aureus in TKA treated with revision and direct intra-articular antibiotic infusion. *Clin Orthop Relat Res* 2011;469(1):26-33.

98. Singer J, Merz A, Frommelt L, Fink B: High rate of infection control with one-stage revision of septic knee prostheses excluding MRSA and MRSE. *Clin Orthop Relat Res* 2012;470(5):1461-1471.

99. Scott IR, Stockley I, Getty CJ: Exchange arthroplasty for infected knee replacements: A new two-stage method. *J Bone Joint Surg Br* 1993;75(1):28-31.

100. Bauer T, Piriou P, Lhotellier L, Leclerc P, Mamoudy P, Lortat-Jacob A: Results of reimplantation for infected total knee arthroplasty: 107 cases. *Rev Chir Orthop Reparatrice Appar Mot* 2006;92(7):692-700.

101. Manku K, Bacchetti P, Leung JM: Prognostic significance of postoperative in-hospital complications in elderly patients: I. Long-term survival. *Anesth Analg* 2003;96(2):583-589.

102. Turrentine FE, Wang H, Simpson VB, Jones RS: Surgical risk factors, morbidity, and mortality in elderly patients. *J Am Coll Surg* 2006;203(6):865-877.

103. Bentrem DJ, Cohen ME, Hynes DM, Ko CY, Bilimoria KY: Identification of specific quality improvement opportunities for the elderly undergoing gastrointestinal surgery. *Arch Surg* 2009;144(11):1013-1020.

104. Deiner S, Silverstein JH: Postoperative delirium and cognitive dysfunction. *Br J Anaesth* 2009;103(suppl 1):i41-i46.

105. Youngblom E, DePalma G, Sands L, Leung J: The temporal relationship between early postoperative delirium and postoperative cognitive dysfunction in older patients: A prospective cohort study. *Can J Anaesth* 2014;61(12):1084-1092.

106. Sofer D, Regenbrecht B, Pfeil J: Early results of one-stage septic revision arthroplasties with antibiotic-laden cement: A clinical and statistical analysis. *Orthopade* 2005;34(6):592-602.

107. Kapadia BH, McElroy MJ, Issa K, Johnson AJ, Bozic KJ, Mont MA: The economic impact of periprosthetic infections following total knee arthroplasty at a specialized tertiary-care center. *J Arthroplasty* 2014;29(5):929-932.

108. Bengtson S: Prosthetic osteomyelitis with special reference to the knee: Risks, treatment and costs. *Ann Med* 1993;25(6):523-529.

109. Hebert CK, Williams RE, Levy RS, Barrack RL: Cost of treating an infected total knee replacement. *Clin Orthop Relat Res* 1996;331:140-145.

110. Oussedik S, Gould K, Stockley I, Haddad FS: Defining peri-prosthetic infection: Do we have a workable gold standard? *J Bone Joint Surg Br* 2012;94(11):1455-1456.

Two-Stage Revision Total Knee Arthroplasty in the Setting of Periprosthetic Knee Infection

Zain Sayeed, MSc, MHA
Afshin A. Anoushiravani, MD
Mouhanad M. El-Othmani, MD
Monique C. Chambers, MD, MSL
William M. Mihalko, MD, PhD
William A. Jiranek, MD, FACS
Wayne G. Paprosky, MD, FACS
Khaled J. Saleh, MD, MSc, FACSC, MHCM, CPE

Abstract

Two-stage revision total knee arthroplasty (TKA) is the standard of care for patients who require a revision procedure for the mangement of a late or chronic periprosthetic knee infection. A careful examination of two-stage revision TKA is warranted as the number of patients who require revision TKA in the United States continues to rise. Surgeons should understand the intricacies involved in two-stage revision TKA, including the indications, procedural variations, and current deliberations on two-stage revision TKA in the literature. Surgeons also should understand the alternative treatments for periprosthetic knee infections.

Instr Course Lect 2017;66:249–262.

Total knee arthroplasty (TKA) is one of the most effective surgical procedures in the United States.[1] Despite the clinical success of TKA, the number of revision TKAs continues to rise.[2,3] The exponential growth in the number of primary TKAs, patient-specific factors, and broader indications for TKA to include younger, more active patients all contribute to the rising rate of revision TKA.[3] The most common reason for revision TKA is infection.[3] Reported rates of infection after primary TKA range from 0.5% to 1.9%.[4,5] For the past several decades, two-stage revision TKA has been the standard of care for the management of late or chronic periprosthetic knee infections (PKIs).

Classification and Diagnosis of PKI

PKI is a type of periprosthetic joint infection (PJI). The International Consensus Group on Periprosthetic Joint Infection reported that a PJI is present in patients in whom either two positive periprosthetic cultures with phenotypically identical organisms are obtained, a sinus tract is communicating with the joint, or three of the following five criteria are met: (1) elevated C-reactive protein (CRP) level and erythrocyte sedimentation rate (ESR); (2) elevated synovial white blood cell (WBC) count or positive change on leukocyte esterase test strip; (3) elevated synovial fluid polymorphonuclear (PMN) neutrophil percentage; (4) positive histologic analysis of periprosthetic tissue; and (5) a single positive culture.

The Musculoskeletal Infection Society classifies PJIs as either acute (<90 days) or chronic (>90 days; **Table 1**). Different treatment options exist within the spectrum of infection depending on whether a PKI is acute or chronic. Acute PKIs are often manged with antibiotics, irrigation

Table 1

Minor Diagnostic Threshold Criteria for the Classification of Periprosthetic Knee Infection (PKI)

Criterion	Acute PKI (<90 days)	Chronic PKI (>90 days)
Erythrocyte sedimentation rate	Not helpful. No threshold was determined.	30 mm/h
C-reactive protein level (mg/L)	100	10
Synovial white blood cell count (cells/μL)	10,000	3,000
Synovial polymorpho-nuclear neutrophil (%)	90	80
Leukocyte esterase test strip	+ or ++	+ or ++
Histologic analysis of tissue	>5 neutrophils per high-power field in five high-power fields (×400)	Same as acute

Adapted from Parvizi J, Gehrke T; International Consensus Group on Periprosthetic Joint Infection: Definition of periprosthetic joint infection. *J Arthroplasty* 2014;29(7):1331.

and débridement, modular exchange, and mechanical component retention. Conversely, chronic PKIs require resection of mechanical components and reimplantation. Although the timing of infection is typically used to classify PKIs, this infection classification system was originally based on the time it takes for biofilm to form on prosthesis surfaces.[6] Newer studies have reported that biofilms may form on prosthesis surfaces within hours to days;[7,8] therefore, surgeons have recommended that the current classification system be modified.[9,10]

In the clinical setting, surgeons often consider a painful TKA as infected until proven otherwise. Classically, patients with a PKI have cardinal signs of inflammation, including redness, swelling, pain, and, possibly, a low-grade fever. Surgeons must understand that use of systemic antibiotics may affect a patient's levels of serologic and synovial diagnostic markers.[11] Furthermore, a repeat arthrocentesis should be considered for patients in whom a marked distinction between their clinical examination and synovial fluid analysis exists.

Two-Stage Revision TKA
Indications

First advocated by Insall et al,[12] two-stage revision TKA is considered the preferred treatment for patients who have a chronic PKI.[13,14] In 1988, Cohen et al[15] enhanced two-stage revision TKA with use of antibiotic-impregnated cement after the contaminated prosthesis was débrided and removed. The first stage of two-stage revision TKA includes extensive débridement of soft tissue and cement, resection arthroplasty, and the introduction of a spacer.[16,17] The spacer remains in a patient's joint space for 4 to 6 weeks or until the infection is eradicated. The indications for two-stage revision TKA include chronic PKI, failed irrigation and débridement, and acute periprosthetic infection that is present in an immunocompromised patient or in whom the organism is virulent.[17] Surgeons must thoroughly understand the inclusion criteria for two-stage revision TKA to ensure optimal patient outcomes.

Dr. Mihalko or an immediate family member has received royalties from Aesculap/B. Braun; is a member of a speakers' bureau or has made paid presentations on behalf of Aesculap/B. Braun; is an employee of Aesculap/B. Braun, Medtronic, and Panoramic Healthcare; has received research or institutional support from Aesculap/B. Braun, MicroPort, Smith & Nephew, and Stryker; and serves as a board member, owner, officer, or committee member of the American Board of Orthopaedic Surgery, the American Orthopaedic Association, and ASTM International. Dr. Jiranek or an immediate family member has received royalties from DePuy; serves as a paid consultant to Cayenne Medical and DePuy; has stock or stock options held in Johnson & Johnson; has received research or institutional support from DePuy and Stryker; and serves as a board member, owner, officer, or committee member of the American Association of Hip and Knee Surgeons, LifeNet Health, and the Orthopaedic Learning Center. Dr. Paprosky or an immediate family member has received royalties from Intellijoint Surgical, Stryker, and Zimmer; serves as a paid consultant to DePuy, Medtronic, Stryker, and Zimmer; has stock or stock options held in Intellijoint Surgical; has received nonincome support (such as equipment or services), commercially derived honoraria, or other non-research–related funding (such as paid travel) from Cadence Health; and serves as a board member, owner, officer, or committee member of the Hip Society. Dr. Saleh or an immediate family member has received royalties from Aesculap/B. Braun; is a member of a speakers' bureau or has made paid presentations on behalf of Aesculap/B. Braun; is an employee of the Southern Illinois University School of Medicine, Division of Orthopaedics; serves as a paid consultant to Aesculap/B. Braun, the Memorial Medical Center Co-management Orthopaedic Board, and Watermark; has received research or institutional support from Smith & Nephew, the Orthopaedic Research and Education Foundation, and the National Institutes of Health (NIAMS); and serves as a board member, owner, officer, or committee member of the American Academy of Orthopaedic Surgeons, the American Orthopaedic Association, the American Orthopaedic Association Finance Committee, the Orthopaedic Research and Education Foundation Industry Relations Committee, the Orthopaedic Research and Education Foundation Clinical Research Awards Committee, the American Board of Orthopaedic Surgeons Oral Examiner, the Board of Specialty Societies, Notify, and the American Academy of Orthopaedic Surgeons Performance Measures Committee. None of the following authors nor any immediate family member has received anything of value from or has stock or stock options held in a commercial company or institution related directly or indirectly to the subject of this chapter: Mr. Sayeed, Dr. Anoushiravani, Dr. El-Othmani, and Dr. Chambers.

Candidacy

Preoperative planning is an essential component of two-stage revision TKA because two-stage revision TKA is both physically demanding and invasive. To predict postoperative outcomes, patients should be risk-stratified by the duration of infection, medical comorbidities, and the ability to heal.[18,19] Cierny et al[20] classified patient healing ability as either type A, type B, or type C. Type A healing ability suggests no evidence of healing compromise. Type B healing ability indicates local compromise, systemic compromise, or combined compromise. Type C healing ability indicates substantial compromising factors, poor prognosis, and an increased risk of lasting morbidity.[20] **Table 2** lists the local and systemic factors that surgeons should consider to help determine the healing capacity of patients who undergo two-stage revision TKA. Patients with type B or type C healing ability may require extensive preoperative optimization to improve their healing ability. A patient's nutritional status, which can be assessed by obtaining a total WBC count and a serum albumin level, may help predict wound healing insufficiency.[21] Preoperative oral or parenteral antibiotic supplementation may enhance a patient's healing response.[22]

Technique

A patient is deemed medically fit to undergo revision TKA after completion of a thorough preoperative evaluation. The first stage of revision TKA begins with resection arthroplasty, which encompasses excision of all infected tissue, foreign material, and implant hardware, followed by installation of a static or articulating antibiotic-impregnated spacer.[23-29]

An elliptical incision is made on the hyperemic portion of the scar from the index procedure and, if possible, should include any sinus tracts. Sinus tracts that cannot be included in the incision must still be thoroughly débrided and addressed intraoperatively. Débridement includes arthrotomy, synovectomy, and excision of all infected tissues.[23-29] Débridement is followed by implantation of a new polyethylene liner. Gherke et al[9] reported that meticulous débridement is a necessary component of two-stage revision TKA because poor débridement may result in reinfection. The removal of all implant components (tibial, femoral, and patellar), bone cement, bone restrictors, screws, and wires may result in unavoidable bone loss. The polyethylene insert is removed first, followed by femoral and tibial trays as well as any remaining cement. Cultures should be obtained from multiple sites, including the femoral and tibial canal. The femoral and tibial canals should be opened and reamed to remove pseudomembranes. Cortical windows can be made with curved saws and high-speed burrs to aid in component removal. Surgeons must patiently work around the cement-component interface to maintain bone stock and ensure removal of all infected material.

Spacers

After extensive irrigation and débridement of a PKI, antibiotic-impregnated cement spacers (AICSs) are used to deliver high local concentrations of antibiotics.[30] In addition, AICSs help maintain leg length, minimize soft-tissue contractures, and reduce bone loss, all of which facilitate reimplantation.[31] Cement spacers vary considerably in design and are either commercially manufactured[32] or can be customized

intraoperatively.[33,34] Cement spacers are either static (non-articulating or block) or dynamic (articulating or mobile).[35-37] Cement spacers are typically composed entirely of polymethyl methacrylate (PMMA) or a metal prosthesis with an outer antibiotic-coated cement layer.[33,34] Some surgeons avoid the use of spacers and instead use antibiotic-impregnated cement pelts.

Antibiotic-Impregnated Cement Spacers

Antibiotic-impregnated cement is frequently used to eradicate any residual organisms that may remain after irrigation and débridement.[31] The antibiotics that are available for the impregnation of cement are limited by several intrinsic antibiotic properties. Antibiotics that are used to impregnate cement must be thermodynamically stable at high temperatures (>202°F) because PMMA polymerization is an exothermic reaction.[38] Antibiotics that are used to impregnate cement also must

Table 2
Factors That Help Determine Patient Healing Capacity

Systemic Factors	Local Factors
Diabetes	Extensive scarring
Rheumatic diseases	Lymphedema
Renal or liver disease	Poor vascular perfusion
Steroid use	Excessive local adipose tissue
Poor nutritional status	
Immunocompromised state	
Tobacco use	

Data from Cierny G III, Mader JT, Penninck JJ: A clinical staging system for adult osteomyelitis. *Clin Orthop Relat Res* 2003; 414:7-24.

Table 3

Antibiotic-Impregnated Cement Regimens for Various Pathogens

Offending Pathogen	Antibiotic-Impregnated Regimen
Gram-positive (*Staphylococcus aureus*, *Staphylococcus epidermidis*)	Penicillinase-sensitive and penicillinase-resistant penicillins, vancomycin
Gram-negative	Aminoglycosides, clindamycin
Polymicrobial	Vancomycin, gentamicin
Methicillin-resistant *S aureus*/methicillin-resistant *S epidermidis*	Vancomycin
Enterobacteriaceae	Gentamicin, cefotaxime
Pseudomonas aeruginosa	Antipseudomonal aminoglycosides, gentamicin, cefotaxime
Fungi (*Candida*)	Fluconazole, amphotericin B

be hydrophilic and bactericidal to allow for antibiotic diffusion and eradication of organisms within the knee joint.[39] In addition, antibiotics that are used to impregnate cement must be available in crystalline form. Liquid antibiotics should be avoided because of the increased polymerization time and decreased cement strength associated with their use.[39-41] Seldes et al[40] reported that compressive and tensile strength decreased by 49% and 46%, respectively, if liquid gentamicin was added to antibiotic-free cement; however, the authors reported that a similar dose of crystalline tobramycin resulted in no measurable biomechanical changes.

Antibiotics selected for cement impregnation must agree with the sensitivity profile of the infecting organism(s) (**Table 3**).[42] Vancomycin, aminoglycosides (tobramycin and gentamicin), and cephalosporins are frequently used independently or in combination, particularly if broad microbial coverage and improved antibiotic elution properties are necessary.[39,43] Most PKIs are caused by gram-positive organisms (*Staphylococcus aureus*, *Staphylococcus epidermidis*), which make the use of vancomycin and cephalosporins par-

ticularly effective. Moreover, vancomycin is active against methicillin-resistant *S aureus*, and gentamicin is active against Enterobacteriaceae and *Pseudomonas aeruginosa*. Cefotaxime can be used for infecting pathogens that are resistant to gentamicin. In addition, if prophylactic antibiotic-impregnated cement was used in the index procedure, it is recommended that the surgeon avoid using the same antibiotics in two-stage revision TKA because the infecting pathogen may exhibit antibiotic resistance.[44]

Fungal infections require special consideration because of their recalcitrant nature and poor prognosis.[45] Surgeons must educate their patients on the nature of fungal PKIs and emphasize the outcomes of two-stage revision TKA as well as alternative treatments. In a systematic review of 45 fungal PKIs, Jakobs et al[45] reported that 80% of the PKIs were caused by *Candida*. Furthermore, the authors reported that two-stage revision TKA failed in approximately one-half of the patients.[45] Although the management of fungal PKIs is difficult, studies have reported effective antibiotic elution of fluconazole and amphotericin B from cement;[42,46-48] however, optimal

pharmacologic concentrations necessary for the management of fungal PJIs require further investigation.[49]

Antibiotic Elution

The elution of antibiotics from bone cement depends on the cement type, porosity, and surface area as well as the type, number, and respective concentrations of the antibiotics administered.[50-52] Masri et al[52] observed antibiotic elution for 4 months in 49 patients who underwent two-stage revision TJA. The authors reported that vancomycin in combination with tobramycin had superior antibiotic elution properties compared with vancomycin alone.[52] These findings were consistent with those of an in vitro study conducted by Penner et al[53] that described the process of passive opportunism, in which the elution of one antibiotic (tobramycin) resulted in increased cement porosity, thereby enabling increased elution of the second antibiotic (vancomycin). More recent studies, however, have questioned the synergistic elution properties of vancomycin and tobramycin.[54] Duey et al[54] evaluated the elution properties of tobramycin and vancomycin, both in combination and separately, and reported that combination therapy did not have the expected synergistic effect. The discrepancy in predicted antibiotic elution properties within bone cement demonstrates the poor understanding of in vivo antibiotic kinetics.

Mixing Antibiotic-Impregnated Cement

Antibiotic-impregnated cement is mixed within a vacuum-sealed container or mixed atmospherically, both of which result in bone cement that has different biomechanical properties. Surgeons should understand that the clinical goals of antibiotic-impregnated bone cement for spacers and for definitive implant fixation are different. AICSs are used to stabilize the joint and eradicate any remaining infection; therefore, antibiotic doses that constitute up to 20% of the cement mass may be used.[9] Hanssen and Spangehl[43] proposed mixing PMMA monomers (accelerator) and prepolymerized PMMA (initiator) atmospherically to introduce air bubbles and increase cement porosity. The authors recommended adding antibiotic crystalline (and preserving large antibiotic crystals if possible) after the bone cement had begun the polymerization processes.[43] However, the authors reported that, during the second stage, the crystalline antibiotic dose should not constitute more than 10% of the bone cement's mass or it may compromise prosthesis fixation.[55] Most surgeons atmospherically mix bone cement for two-stage revision TKA; however, this practice is not entirely evidence-based and may be deleterious if high-viscosity cements are used.[56] Therefore, future in vivo studies on the antibiotic elution and biomechanical properties of antibiotic-impregnated bone cement are necessary.

Static Versus Articulating Spacers

Static AICSs consist of PMMA bone cement mixed with crystalline antibiotics and are shaped to fit osteogenic defects after resection arthroplasty. Although static AICSs maintain joint space integrity in conjunction with the delivery of high doses of antibiotics, studies have reported concern for the knee's limited range of motion (ROM), which results in shortening of the quadriceps, contracture formation, and bone loss. Conversely, articulating AICSs are well-fitted spacers that are designed to

preserve soft- and bony-tissue tension and allow for greater ROM. Recent studies have reported improved knee scores, improved ROM, and reduced bone loss in patients who undergo two-stage revision TKA with articulating knee spacers.[57,58] In a study of 48 patients who were treated with AICSs (26 static knee spacers and 22 articulating knee spacers), Emerson et al[35] reported that the patients who were treated with articulating spacers had significantly better knee ROM compared with those who were treated with static spacers; however, there was no benefit between static spacers and articulating spacers with regard to the eradication of infection. Several other studies, namely Fehring et al[36] and Johnson et al,[59] have reported comparable reinfection rates, Knee Society Scores, and ROM in patients who undergo two-stage revision TKA with either articulating knee spacers or static knee spacers.

Guild et al[60] reported no significant difference between static spacers and articulating spacers with regard to Hospital for Special Surgery Scores, Knee Society Scores, and ROM;[60] however, articulating spacers were superior with regard to infection eradication, particularly in complex patients who had resistant organisms, bone loss, or draining sinus tracts; the prevention of bone loss between the two stages of two-stage revision TKA; and reduced soft-tissue manipulation during reimplantation.[60] Although articulating AICSs are gaining popularity among orthopaedic surgeons, it is unclear whether articulating spacers improve clinical outcomes.

Postoperative Antibiotic Treatment

After irrigation and débridement, component removal, and spacer placement

are complete, the incision is closed. The patient is then prescribed an antibiotic regimen based on intraoperative microbial findings.[61] Insall et al[12] first described the timing of systemic antibiotics for two-stage revision TKA. The authors' antibiotic protocol consisted of 6 to 8 weeks of intravenous (IV) antibiotics that were administered between the two stages of two-stage revision TKA, several hospital visits, parenteral antibiotic infusion, and a home-health consultation.[12] The type of antibiotic depends on the results of intraoperative cultures, and an infectious disease consultation is recommended to help determine the type and the duration of antibiotic treatment.[62] Several studies on two-stage revision TKA have reported long-term use of IV antibiotics between the two stages of surgery.[63,64] Osmon et al[65] recommended that antibiotic treatment for periprosthetic joint infection be individualized based on a patient's needs. Two-stage revision TKA may compromise blood supply to the periarticular tissues, which prevents the hematogenous distribution of antibiotics at the site of infection and further prolongs antibiotic regimens. Kilgus et al[66] reported that only 2 weeks of IV-administered antibiotics are necessary, after which oral antibiotics may be appropriate depending on a patient's bacterial resistance profile. Studies on prolonged antibiotic therapy for two-stage revision TKA continue to be conducted because chronic antibiotic therapy and multiple hospital visits are associated with substantial costs for patients and healthcare systems.[67]

Hoad-Reddick et al[68] evaluated 38 patients who did not receive a prolonged course of antibiotics between the two stages of two-stage revision TKA. The authors administered a broad-spectrum IV antibiotic, typically cefuroxime (1.5 g at induction and 750 mg at 8 and 16 hours postoperatively), without additional oral or IV antibiotics.[68] Recurrent or persistent infection did not develop in approximately 89% of the patients. The authors reported that, compared with prolonged IV antibiotic therapy, meticulous débridement that is performed in the initial stage of two-stage revision TKA, the use of antibiotic cement, and the use of custom-made antibiotic beads may result in more cost-effective outcomes in patients who undergo two-stage revision TKA.[68] A shorter course of IV antibiotic therapy may be beneficial to patients because it reduces the likelihood of systemic complications and future microbial resistance.

Hart and Jones[69] reported the outcomes of 48 patients who underwent two-stage revision TKA with use of articulating cement spacers and were treated with short-term parenteral antibiotics postoperatively. In the initial stage of revision two-stage TKA, patients were treated with prefashioned spacers that used cement mixed with gentamicin and vancomycin. IV vancomycin was administered for 14 days postoperatively, and adjustments were made depending on microbial cultures. The authors reported an infection eradication rate of approximately 88%, which they suggested was comparable with that reported by Hoad-Reddick et al,[68] and reported that prolonged antibiotic therapy may not be essential to successfully eradicate infection. Future studies on antibiotic timing are necessary to determine the optimal postoperative antibiotic regimen for patients who undergo two-stage revision TKA.

Reimplantation

The timing of reimplantation depends on several patient-specific factors and the results of laboratory tests that aid in clinical decision-making. No preferred tests or measurements to determine the optimal timing of the second stage of two-stage revision TKA exist. Proceeding with the second stage of two-stage revision TKA in patients who have persistent infection may result in further complications that can lead to resection arthroplasty, arthrodesis, and, potentially, amputation.[70,71] Testing for the presence of infection should occur no less than 2 weeks after antibiotic cessation. A patient's ESR and CRP level are two major serologic markers that are commonly assessed to determine the presence of infection. Using an aseptic technique, a joint fluid analysis of the knee can be obtained and then sent for fungal, aerobic, and anaerobic culture as well as a WBC count and a differential of PMN neutrophils.

Greidanus et al[72] used receiver operating characteristic curve analysis to demonstrate that ESR and CRP level are robust diagnostic tools that help establish the presence of infection before two-stage revision TKA. However, few studies in the literature demonstrate the efficacy of routine serologic testing and joint fluid analysis between the first and second stages of two-stage revision TKA; therefore, they are not recommended.[73] Studies have reported conflicting results on the applicability of ESR and CRP level as indicators for reimplantation.[72-74] In a retrospective study of 109 patients who underwent two-stage revision TKA, Ghanem et al[73] reported that ESR and CRP level were not effective indicators that differentiated infected and noninfected knees for reimplantation. Using receiver

operating characteristic curve analysis, the authors were not able to identify a specific ESR or CRP level that discriminated between persistent and eradicated PKI. Kusuma et al[74] studied the records of 76 patients who underwent two-stage revision TKA to determine the role of ESR, CRP level, and synovial WBC count with differential. The authors reported a substantial decline in all four laboratory values between the first and second stages of two-stage revision TKA; however, it was concluded that none of the four laboratory tests were independent predictors of persistent infection and recommended that surgeons proceed with reimplantation if tissues appear noninfected, intraoperative frozen sections are consistent with controlled infection, and synovial WBC count and PMN neutrophil percentage are within normal limits.[74]

In the past decade, the use of serum cytokines as indicators for reimplantation has gained popularity in the orthopaedic literature. Serum interleukin-6 (IL-6), specifically, has shown promise to be a robust marker of PKI.[75,76] Hoell et al[75] used receiver operating characteristic curve analysis as well as classification and regression tree analyses to assess the prognostic value of serum IL-6 level as an indicator for reimplantation in 55 patients who underwent revision joint arthroplasty. Although limited by sample size, the authors reported that a serum IL-6 level greater than or equal to 13 pg/mL may indicate persistent infection.[62] Patients with gram-negative bacteremia tend to have a higher serum IL-6 level compared with patients with gram-positive bacteremia,[77] which should raise a surgeon's index of suspicion for infection.

After eradication of infection is confirmed via serologic testing and joint fluid analysis, the patient is prepared for reimplantation. For the second stage of two-stage revision TKA, an elliptical incision that incorporates the hyperemic portion of the scar from the index procedure is made. Further meticulous débridement should be performed, after which the antibiotic spacer is removed. Three to six sets of intraoperative cultures are obtained, and synovial tissues are sent for frozen section and histopathologic analysis. Orthopaedists should obtain tissue samples from the synovium, intramedullary material, bone fragments, granulation tissue, and other areas suggestive of infection as determined intraoperatively.[78] Assessment of the surgical field is critical in the decision of whether to implant a new prosthesis. Surgeons must evaluate for an absence of exuberant granulation tissue, necrotic debris, and purulent fluid collection. If there is any evidence of persistent infection at the time of the second stage of revision TKA, the procedure should be aborted, repeat débridement should be performed, and a new antibiotic spacer should be placed in the joint space.

Many studies have investigated the efficacy of frozen section analysis as an adjuvant indicator for reimplantation. Charoski et al[79] first recommended that intraoperative frozen section analysis be used to guide the management of revision total joint arthroplasty. The requirements for frozen section analysis are listed in **Table 4**. Feldman et al[80] reported that frozen sections with more than 5 PMN neutrophils per high-power field had a 100% sensitivity and 96% specificity for the detection of infection. Della Valle et al[78] compared the results of 33 frozen section analyses with the results of analyses of permanent histologic sections of the same tissues.

Table 4

Frozen Section Analysis Requirements

1. Granulation tissue is obtained and analyzed
2. At least two samples of tissue are used
3. At least five high-power cellular fields (assessed by number of PMN neutrophils) are used in diagnostic analysis
4. PMN neutrophil counts are performed at ×40 magnification (high power) in selected fields
5. Only PMN neutrophils within tissue, not fibrin, are included in count
   a. Nuclear fragmentation of cells warrant exclusion

PMN = polymorphonuclear.

The authors reported that persistent infection was present if patients had two positive intraoperative cultures or they met two of the following three criteria: (1) histopathology was consistent with infection (10 PMN neutrophils in five high-power fields); (2) at least one positive intraoperative culture; and (3) tissues with visually apparent infection at time of revision surgery.[78,81,82] In contrast to Feldman et al,[80] the stricter criteria for persistent infection reported by Della Valle et al[78] resulted in a sensitivity of 25% and specificity of 98% for the detection of infection. Cho et al[83] examined the outcomes of 15 patients who underwent two-stage revision TKA in the presence of 5 to 20 PMN neutrophils per high-power field at time of reimplantation. The authors reported a 100% infection eradication rate at a minimum follow-up of 2 years despite the reimplantation of prostheses in seven patients who had an intraoperative PMN neutrophil count greater than or equal to 10 PMN neutrophils per high-power field. Thus, frozen section analysis remains an adjuvant indicator for reimplantation.

Assessment of Bone Stock

The reconstructive efforts of two-stage revision TKA may be severely impeded in patients who have depleted bone stock. Surgeons often use the Anderson Orthopaedic Research Institute's bone loss classification system to separately determine the adequacy of a patient's femoral and tibial bone stock[84] (**Table 5**). Femoral bone defects are classified as either F1, F2a, F2b, or F3. Tibial bone defects are classified as either T1, T2a, T2b, or T3.[85] The classification of bone defects helps surgeons select the technique and implant most suitable for two-stage revision TKA. AP radiographs of the lower limb, AP and lateral radiographs of the knee, and axial radiographs of the patella taken at a 45° angle are recommended to assess bone stock.[86,87] In addition, radiographs must be obtained under axial loading and compared with the contralateral knee.[86,87] CT with three-dimensional reconstruction is recommended because standard radiographs often underestimate bone loss.

Although preoperative imaging may help surgeons prepare for surgical obstacles, only an intraoperative evaluation after implant and cement removal will reveal the true extent of bone loss. Nonetheless, surgeons must be cognizant that the long-term goals of two-stage revision TKA are to restore the joint line, attain optimal ligament

Table 5

Anderson Orthopaedic Research Institute Classification of Bone Loss

Bone Defect	Type 1	Type 2A	Type 2B	Type 3
Femoral	Small amount of bone loss that does not compromise component stability (contained)	Unicondylar structural damage to bone (noncontained)	Bicondylar structural damage to bone (noncontained)	Substantial bone loss with ligamentous instability (noncontained)
Tibial	Small amount of bone loss that does not compromise component stability; metaphyseal bone intact (contained)	Unilateral metaphyseal bone defect that necessitates augmentation (noncontained)	Bilateral metaphyseal bone defect that necessitates augmentation (noncontained)	Substantial bone loss; may involve detachment of the patellar tendon (noncontained)

Data from Panegrossi G, Ceretti M, Papalia M, Casella F, Favetti F, Falez F: Bone loss management in total knee revision surgery. *Int Orthop* 2014;38(2):419-427.

balance, and optimize joint kinematics.[84] Type 2 and type 3 Anderson Orthopaedic Research Institute classified bone defects usually require adequate bone reconstruction to ensure the stability of a new prosthesis.[84] It is critical that surgeons implement indicated procedures, such as bone grafting or modular metal augmentation,[88,89] for the management of both femoral and/or tibial defects.[90] Exciting preliminary research on the use of alternative methods to build patient-specific scaffolds, such as three-dimensional printing, have shown promise for the management of bone defects.[91] Three-dimensional scaffolds with osteoinductive properties are currently used to restore bone structures with an optimal fit.[92] Patients in whom two-stage revision TKA is unable to overcome sizable bone defects may require alternative treatment modalities.

Outcomes

The reinfection rate after two-stage revision TKA has been reported to be as high as 28%.[93] Such a variation in success rates often correlates with variations in surgeon practice, which include but are not limited to the duration of antibiotic therapy between the two stages of two-stage revision TKA, varying antibiotic cement mixtures, the use of static versus articulating spacers, and postresection serologic and synovial fluid analyses. The protocol for two-stage revision TKA is constantly being refined by the orthopaedic community, and an analysis of the current outcomes reported in the literature is warranted. Most outcome analyses of two-stage revision TKA tend to be low-powered and usually include fewer than 60 patients.[14] **Table 6** summarizes the recent results of two-stage revision TKA.[59,94-97]

Alternative Treatments to Two-Stage Revision TKA

The reconstructive efforts of two-stage revision TKA may be impeded in patients who have persistent infection, severe bone defects, or ligament instability. In these patients, alternative treatments, including chronic antibiotic suppression, arthrodesis, and amputation, may be considered to alleviate symptoms. Each alternative treatment has procedure-specific indications, techniques, and outcomes. The indications and contraindications for alternative treatments to two-stage revision TKA are listed in **Table 7**.

Antibiotic Suppression

The goal of chronic antibiotic suppression, which is defined as the management of an infection with oral antibiotics for a minimum of 6 months, is to control rather than eradicate infection.[98] Chronic antibiotic suppression is commonly indicated in elderly or frail patients who may be unable to tolerate surgical procedures. Five-year success rates as high as 86% have been reported for patients treated with chronic antibiotic suppression; however, proper patient selection is necessary.[99] Siqueira et al[98] compared the outcomes of 92 patients who were treated with chronic antibiotic suppression with those of a matched cohort of 276 patients who were not treated with chronic antibiotic suppression. The authors reported a 57.4% 5-year success rate for the patients who were treated with chronic antibiotic suppression. Although both Siqueira et al[98] and Rao et al[99] reported favorable results for patients who were treated with chronic antibiotic suppression, successful treatment relied heavily on patient selection. The failure to follow strict patient selection criteria results in poor outcomes, with some studies reporting positive outcomes in only 18% to 24% of patients who

Table 6

Results of Two-Stage Revision Total Knee Arthroplasty (TKA)

Authors (Year)	Number of Patients (Knees)	Procedure or Approach	Mean Patient Age in Years (Range)	Mean Follow-up (Range)	Reinfection Rate	Mean Functional Scores
Johnson et al[59] (2012)	111 (115)	Two-stage revision TKA with dynamic (34 knees) or static (81 knees) spacers	Dynamic: 62 (59–65) Static: 61 (58–64)	Dynamic: 27 mo (12–72 mo) Static: 66 mo (12–121 mo)	Dynamic: 6 patients (17%; 95% CI, 8%–34%) Static: 14 patients (17%; 95% CI, 10%–27%)	**Objective Knee** Dynamic: Pre, 62; Post, 83 Static: Pre, 73; Post, 84
Kalore et al[95] (2012)	53 (NA)	Two-stage revision TKA with articulating spacers via AOC (15 patients), NFC (16 patients), or SMC (22 patients)	64 (NA) AOC: 67.3 (NA) NFC: 63.6 (NA) SMC: 61.1 (NA)	39 mo (12–105 mo)	15 patients (28%) AOC: 5 patients (33%) NFC: 2 patients (12.5%) SMC: 8 patients (36%)	NA
Mahmud et al[94] (2012)	239 (253)	Two-stage revision TKA	70 (NA)	NA (12–276 mo)	16 patients (7%)	**WOMAC** Pre: 48 (±21) Post: 60 (±21) **Clinical Knee** Pre: 64 (±31) Post: 129 (±41)
Puhto et al[96] (2014)	46 (NA)	Two-stage revision TKA	69.4 (NA)	NA (6–86 mo)	5 patients (10.9%)	NA
Matsumoto et al[97] (2015)	50 (NA)	Prosthesis retention (13 patients with acute early infections and 4 patients with acute hematogenous infections) or two-stage revision TKA (33 patients with late chronic infections)	71.1 (NA)	4.7 yr (NA)	22 patients (44%) Acute early: 7 patients (54%) Acute hematogenous: 3 patients (75%) Late chronic: 12 patients (36%)	NA

AOC = autoclaved original femoral component, CI = confidence interval, Clinical Knee = Knee Society clinical score, NA = not available, NFC = new femoral component, Objective Knee = Knee Society objective score, Post = postoperative, Pre = preoperative, SMC = silicon mold component, WOMAC = Western Ontario and McMaster Universities Osteoarthritis Index.

were treated with chronic antibiotic suppression.[100,101]

Arthrodesis

Arthrodesis is a surgical procedure in which a joint is immobilized via fusion of the surrounding bones. Surgeons may use intramedullary nailing, external fixation, or compression plates to achieve arthrodesis. Surgeons generally prefer to use intramedullary nailing to achieve arthrodesis because it results in a superior fusion, with several studies reporting fusion rates of 100%;[102,103] however, residual hardware may be detrimental to the outcomes of patients who have active or recurrent infection. The presence of infection and the type of implant previously used are two major factors that affect the success rate of knee arthrodesis.[104] External fixation with a circular, biplanar, or uniplanar fixator is associated with lower rates of infection compared with intramedullary nailing; however, external fixation also is associated with a comparatively decreased rate of union.[105] The use of compression plates is reserved for patients in whom intramedullary nailing or external fixation fails.[106] Dual plating

Table 7
Alternative Treatments to Two-Stage Revision Total Knee Arthroplasty

Treatment	Indications	Contraindications
Chronic antibiotic suppression	Patient is unable to tolerate surgical procedure Well-fixed implant Nonvirulent pathogen Oral antibiotics are available for the management of the organism Elderly, frail patient	Presence of other implants that are not infected by organism Presence of artificial heart valve
Arthrodesis	Young, active patient Multiple failed reconstructions Loss of extensor mechanism Compromised bone stock Multiresistant pathogens	Bilateral knee disease Ipsilateral hip or ankle disease Segmental bone loss Contralateral lower extremity amputation
Amputation	Infection displays extensive soft-tissue involvement Massive bone loss that precludes ability to perform arthrodesis Persistent infection after multiple failed attempts to control infection	Inability to tolerate larger systemic resistance

offers more rigid fixation compared with single plating.[106] The ideal position for arthrodesis of the knee is 15° of flexion and 5° to 7° of valgus with mild external rotation of the extremity.

Amputation

Patients in whom multiple attempts at two-stage revision TKA or arthrodesis fail may qualify for above-the-knee amputation. In the United States, the prevalence of amputation after two-stage revision TKA remains low.[107] If an amputation is necessary, the surgeon should preserve as much of the healthy extremity as possible and ensure sufficient prosthetic function. The authors of this chapter suggest patients undergo a thorough cardiac evaluation before any amputation because the loss of an extremity increases systemic resistance and, consequently, cardiac load. Walking after an above-the-knee amputation

requires higher energy expenditure compared with normal gait, which may be intolerable for patients with obesity or elderly patients.[107] Postoperative ambulation may be severely limited in select patient populations. In a study of 25 patients who underwent above-the-knee amputation, Sierra et al[107] reported that only 20% of patients were able to walk at final follow-up. Because the literature suggests poor patient function after amputation,[108] the authors of this chapter recommend thorough patient education before amputation is pursued.

Summary

Two-stage revision TKA is the preferred treatment for patients who have PJI. Orthopaedic surgeons must discuss the risks and benefits of two-stage revision TKA with patients before treatment is initiated. Surgeons must meticulously evaluate a surgical candidate's medical

comorbidities, determine the duration of infection, and isolate the pathogen responsible for infection. These patient- and infection-specific variables will help guide the type and duration of treatment. Chronic antibiotic suppression, arthrodesis, and amputation are viable options for patients with recalcitrant infection.

References

1. Losina E, Walensky RP, Kessler CL, et al: Cost-effectiveness of total knee arthroplasty in the United States: Patient risk and hospital volume. *Arch Intern Med* 2009;169(12):1113-1122.

2. Kurtz S, Ong K, Lau E, Mowat F, Halpern M: Projections of primary and revision hip and knee arthroplasty in the United States from 2005 to 2030. *J Bone Joint Surg Am* 2007;89(4):780-785.

3. Bozic KJ, Kamath AF, Ong K, et al: Comparative epidemiology of revision arthroplasty: Failed THA poses greater clinical and economic burdens than failed TKA. *Clin Orthop Relat Res* 2015;473(6):2131-2138.

4. Kurtz SM, Ong KL, Lau E, Bozic KJ, Berry D, Parvizi J: Prosthetic joint infection risk after TKA in the Medicare population. *Clin Orthop Relat Res* 2010;468(1):52-56.

5. Bozic KJ, Kurtz SM, Lau E, et al: The epidemiology of revision total knee arthroplasty in the United States. *Clin Orthop Relat Res* 2010;468(1):45-51.

6. Donlan RM: Biofilms: Microbial life on surfaces. *Emerg Infect Dis* 2002;8(9):881-890.

7. Ramage G, Tunney MM, Patrick S, Gorman SP, Nixon JR: Formation of Propionibacterium acnes biofilms on orthopaedic biomaterials and their susceptibility to antimicrobials. *Biomaterials* 2003;24(19):3221-3227.

8. Sakimura T, Kajiyama S, Adachi S, et al: Biofilm-forming Staphylococcus epidermidis expressing vancomycin resistance early after adhesion to a metal surface. *Biomed Res Int* 2015;2015:943056.

9. Gehrke T, Alijanipour P, Parvizi J: The management of an infected total knee arthroplasty. *Bone Joint J* 2015;97(10 suppl A):20-29.

10. Parvizi J, Adeli B, Zmistowski B, Restrepo C, Greenwald AS: Management of periprosthetic joint infection: The current knowledge. AAOS exhibit selection. *J Bone Joint Surg Am* 2012;94(14):e104.

11. Shahi A, Deirmengian C, Higuera C, et al: Premature therapeutic antimicrobial treatments can compromise the diagnosis of late periprosthetic joint infection. *Clin Orthop Relat Res* 2015;473(7):2244-2249.

12. Insall JN, Thompson FM, Brause BD: Two-stage reimplantation for the salvage of infected total knee arthroplasty. *J Bone Joint Surg Am* 1983;65(8):1087-1098.

13. Volin SJ, Hinrichs SH, Garvin KL: Two-stage reimplantation of total joint infections: A comparison of resistant and non-resistant organisms. *Clin Orthop Relat Res* 2004;427:94-100.

14. Jämsen E, Stogiannidis I, Malmivaara A, Pajamäki J, Puolakka T, Konttinen YT: Outcome of prosthesis exchange for infected knee arthroplasty: The effect of treatment approach. *Acta Orthop* 2009;80(1):67-77.

15. Cohen JC, Hozack WJ, Cuckler JM, Booth RE Jr: Two-stage reimplantation of septic total knee arthroplasty: Report of three cases using an antibiotic-PMMA spacer block. *J Arthroplasty* 1988;3(4):369-377.

16. Singer J, Merz A, Frommelt L, Fink B: High rate of infection control with one-stage revision of septic knee prostheses excluding MRSA and MRSE. *Clin Orthop Relat Res* 2012;470(5):1461-1471.

17. Parvizi J, Kerr GJ, Glynn A, Higuera CA, Hansen EN: *Periprosthetic Joint Infection: Practical Management Guide.* New Delhi, India, Jaypee Brothers Medical Publishers, 2013.

18. Tigani D, Trisolino G, Fosco M, Ben Ayad R, Costigliola P: Two-stage reimplantation for periprosthetic knee infection: Influence of host health status and infecting microorganism. *Knee* 2013;20(1):9-18.

19. Holmberg A, Thórhallsdóttir VG, Robertsson O, W-Dahl A, Stefánsdóttir A: 75% success rate after open debridement, exchange of tibial insert, and antibiotics in knee prosthetic joint infections. *Acta Orthop* 2015;86(4):457-462.

20. Cierny G III, Mader JT, Penninck JJ: A clinical staging system for adult osteomyelitis. *Clin Orthop Relat Res* 2003;414:7-24.

21. Rai J, Gill SS, Kumar BR: The influence of preoperative nutritional status in wound healing after replacement arthroplasty. *Orthopedics* 2002;25(4):417-421.

22. Jones RE: Wound healing in total joint arthroplasty. *Orthopedics* 2010;33(9):660.

23. Brimmo O, Ramanathan D, Schiltz NK, Pillai AL, Klika AK, Barsoum WK: Irrigation and debridement before a 2-stage revision total knee arthroplasty does not increase risk of failure. *J Arthroplasty* 2016;31(2):461-464.

24. Sherrell JC, Fehring TK, Odum S, et al: The Chitranjan Ranawat Award: Fate of two-stage reimplantation after failed irrigation and débridement for periprosthetic knee infection. *Clin Orthop Relat Res* 2011;469(1):18-25.

25. Wang KH, Yu SW, Iorio R, Marcantonio AJ, Kain MS: Long term treatment results for deep infections of total knee arthroplasty. *J Arthroplasty* 2015;30(9):1623-1628.

26. Chung JY, Ha CW, Park YB, Song YJ, Yu KS: Arthroscopic debridement for acutely infected prosthetic knee: Any role for infection control and prosthesis salvage? *Arthroscopy* 2014;30(5):599-606.

27. Waldman BJ, Hostin E, Mont MA, Hungerford DS: Infected total knee arthroplasty treated by arthroscopic irrigation and débridement. *J Arthroplasty* 2000;15(4):430-436.

28. Kalore NV, Gioe TJ, Singh JA: Diagnosis and management of infected total knee arthroplasty. *Open Orthop J* 2011;5:86-91.

29. Bradbury T, Fehring TK, Taunton M, et al: The fate of acute methicillin-resistant Staphylococcus aureus

periprosthetic knee infections treated by open debridement and retention of components. *J Arthroplasty* 2009; 24(6 suppl):101-104.

30. Jämsen E, Sheng P, Halonen P, et al: Spacer prostheses in two-stage revision of infected knee arthroplasty. *Int Orthop* 2006;30(4):257-261.

31. Springer BD, Lee GC, Osmon D, Haidukewych GJ, Hanssen AD, Jacofsky DJ: Systemic safety of high-dose antibiotic-loaded cement spacers after resection of an infected total knee arthroplasty. *Clin Orthop Relat Res* 2004;427:47-51.

32. Haddad FS, Masri BA, Campbell D, McGraw RW, Beauchamp CP, Duncan CP: The PROSTALAC functional spacer in two-stage revision for infected knee replacements: Prosthesis of antibiotic-loaded acrylic cement. *J Bone Joint Surg Br* 2000;82(6):807-812.

33. Tsukayama DT, Goldberg VM, Kyle R: Diagnosis and management of infection after total knee arthroplasty. *J Bone Joint Surg Am* 2003;85(suppl 1):S75-S80.

34. Hofmann AA, Goldberg T, Tanner AM, Kurtin SM: Treatment of infected total knee arthroplasty using an articulating spacer: 2- to 12-year experience. *Clin Orthop Relat Res* 2005;430:125-131.

35. Emerson RH Jr, Muncie M, Tarbox TR, Higgins LL: Comparison of a static with a mobile spacer in total knee infection. *Clin Orthop Relat Res* 2002;404:132-138.

36. Fehring TK, Odum S, Calton TF, Mason JB: Articulating versus static spacers in revision total knee arthroplasty for sepsis: The Ranawat Award. *Clin Orthop Relat Res* 2000;380:9-16.

37. Freeman MG, Fehring TK, Odum SM, Fehring K, Griffin WL, Mason JB: Functional advantage of articulating versus static spacers in 2-stage revision for total knee arthroplasty infection. *J Arthroplasty* 2007;22(8):1116-1121.

38. Koo KH, Yang JW, Cho SH, et al: Impregnation of vancomycin, gentamicin, and cefotaxime in a cement spacer for two-stage cementless reconstruction in infected

total hip arthroplasty. *J Arthroplasty* 2001;16(7):882-892.

39. Joseph TN, Chen AL, Di Cesare PE: Use of antibiotic-impregnated cement in total joint arthroplasty. *J Am Acad Orthop Surg* 2003;11(1):38-47.

40. Seldes RM, Winiarsky R, Jordan LC, et al: Liquid gentamicin in bone cement: A laboratory study of a potentially more cost-effective cement spacer. *J Bone Joint Surg Am* 2005;87(2):268-272.

41. Armstrong MS, Spencer RF, Cunningham JL, Gheduzzi S, Miles AW, Learmonth ID: Mechanical characteristics of antibiotic-laden bone cement. *Acta Orthop Scand* 2002;73(6):688-690.

42. Silverberg D, Kodali P, Dipersio J, Acus R, Askew M: In vitro analysis of antifungal impregnated polymethylmethacrylate bone cement. *Clin Orthop Relat Res* 2002;403:228-231.

43. Hanssen AD, Spangehl MJ: Practical applications of antibiotic-loaded bone cement for treatment of infected joint replacements. *Clin Orthop Relat Res* 2004;427:79-85.

44. Hendriks JG, Neut D, van Horn JR, van der Mei HC, Busscher HJ: Bacterial survival in the interfacial gap in gentamicin-loaded acrylic bone cements. *J Bone Joint Surg Br* 2005;87(2):272-276.

45. Jakobs O, Schoof B, Klatte TO, et al: Fungal periprosthetic joint infection in total knee arthroplasty: A systematic review. *Orthop Rev (Pavia)* 2015;7(1):5623.

46. Sealy PI, Nguyen C, Tucci M, Benghuzzi H, Cleary JD: Delivery of antifungal agents using bioactive and nonbioactive bone cements. *Ann Pharmacother* 2009;43(10):1606-1615.

47. Marra F, Robbins GM, Masri BA, et al: Amphotericin B-loaded bone cement to treat osteomyelitis caused by Candida albicans. *Can J Surg* 2001;44(5):383-386.

48. Buranapanitkit B, Oungbho K, Ingviya N: The efficacy of hydroxyapatite composite impregnated with amphotericin B. *Clin Orthop Relat Res* 2005;437:236-241.

49. Coad BR, Kidd SE, Ellis DH, Griesser HJ: Biomaterials surfaces capable of resisting fungal attachment and biofilm formation. *Biotechnol Adv* 2014;32(2):296-307.

50. Durbhakula SM, Czajka J, Fuchs MD, Uhl RL: Spacer endoprosthesis for the treatment of infected total hip arthroplasty. *J Arthroplasty* 2004;19(6):760-767.

51. Hanssen AD, Rand JA, Osmon DR: Treatment of the infected total knee arthroplasty with insertion of another prosthesis: The effect of antibiotic-impregnated bone cement. *Clin Orthop Relat Res* 1994;309:44-55.

52. Masri BA, Duncan CP, Beauchamp CP: Long-term elution of antibiotics from bone-cement: An in vivo study using the prosthesis of antibiotic-loaded acrylic cement (PROSTALAC) system. *J Arthroplasty* 1998;13(3):331-338.

53. Penner MJ, Masri BA, Duncan CP: Elution characteristics of vancomycin and tobramycin combined in acrylic bone-cement. *J Arthroplasty* 1996;11(8):939-944.

54. Duey RE, Chong AC, McQueen DA, et al: Mechanical properties and elution characteristics of polymethylmethacrylate bone cement impregnated with antibiotics for various surface area and volume constructs. *Iowa Orthop J* 2012;32:104-115.

55. Duncan CP, Masri BA: The role of antibiotic-loaded cement in the treatment of an infection after a hip replacement. *Instr Course Lect* 1995;44:305-313.

56. Meyer J, Piller G, Spiegel CA, Hetzel S, Squire M: Vacuum-mixing significantly changes antibiotic elution characteristics of commercially available antibiotic-impregnated bone cements. *J Bone Joint Surg Am* 2011;93(22):2049-2056.

57. Park SJ, Song EK, Seon JK, Yoon TR, Park GH: Comparison of static and mobile antibiotic-impregnated cement spacers for the treatment of infected total knee arthroplasty. *Int Orthop* 2010;34(8):1181-1186.

58. Hsu YC, Cheng HC, Ng TP, Chiu KY: Antibiotic-loaded cement articulating spacer for 2-stage reimplantation in infected total knee arthroplasty: A simple and economic method. *J Arthroplasty* 2007;22(7):1060-1066.

59. Johnson AJ, Sayeed SA, Naziri Q, Khanuja HS, Mont MA: Minimizing dynamic knee spacer complications in infected revision arthroplasty. *Clin Orthop Relat Res* 2012;470(1):220-227.

60. Guild GN III, Wu B, Scuderi GR: Articulating vs. Static antibiotic impregnated spacers in revision total knee arthroplasty for sepsis: A systematic review. *J Arthroplasty* 2014;29(3):558-563.

61. Moyad TF, Thornhill T, Estok D: Evaluation and management of the infected total hip and knee. *Orthopedics* 2008;31(6):581-590.

62. Frommelt L: Principles of systemic antimicrobial therapy in foreign material associated infection in bone tissue, with special focus on periprosthetic infection. *Injury* 2006;37(suppl 2):S87-S94.

63. Hanssen AD: Managing the infected knee: As good as it gets. *J Arthroplasty* 2002;17(4 suppl 1):98-101.

64. Whiteside LA: Treatment of infected total knee arthroplasty. *Clin Orthop Relat Res* 1994;299:169-172.

65. Osmon DR, Berbari EF, Berendt AR, et al: Executive summary: Diagnosis and management of prosthetic joint infection. Clinical practice guidelines by the Infectious Diseases Society of America. *Clin Infect Dis* 2013;56(1):1-10.

66. Kilgus DJ, Howe DJ, Strang A: Results of periprosthetic hip and knee infections caused by resistant bacteria. *Clin Orthop Relat Res* 2002;404:116-124.

67. Barrack RL: Economics of the infected total knee replacement. *Orthopedics* 1996;19(9):780-782.

68. Hoad-Reddick DA, Evans CR, Norman P, Stockley I: Is there a role for extended antibiotic therapy in a two-stage revision of the infected knee arthroplasty? *J Bone Joint Surg Br* 2005;87(2):171-174.

69. Hart WJ, Jones RS: Two-stage revision of infected total knee replacements using articulating cement spacers and short-term antibiotic therapy. *J Bone Joint Surg Br* 2006;88(8):1011-1015.

70. Mont MA, Waldman BJ, Hungerford DS: Evaluation of preoperative cultures before second-stage reimplantation of a total knee prosthesis complicated by infection: A comparison-group study. *J Bone Joint Surg Am* 2000;82(11):1552-1557.

71. Wolff LH III, Parvizi J, Trousdale RT, et al: Results of treatment of infection in both knees after bilateral total knee arthroplasty. *J Bone Joint Surg Am* 2003;85(10):1952-1955.

72. Greidanus NV, Masri BA, Garbuz DS, et al: Use of erythrocyte sedimentation rate and C-reactive protein level to diagnose infection before revision total knee arthroplasty: A prospective evaluation. *J Bone Joint Surg Am* 2007;89(7):1409-1416.

73. Ghanem E, Azzam K, Seeley M, Joshi A, Parvizi J: Staged revision for knee arthroplasty infection: What is the role of serologic tests before reimplantation? *Clin Orthop Relat Res* 2009;467(7):1699-1705.

74. Kusuma SK, Ward J, Jacofsky M, Sporer SM, Della Valle CJ: What is the role of serological testing between stages of two-stage reconstruction of the infected prosthetic knee? *Clin Orthop Relat Res* 2011;469(4):1002-1008.

75. Hoell S, Borgers L, Gosheger G, et al: Interleukin-6 in two-stage revision arthroplasty: What is the threshold value to exclude persistent infection before re-implanatation? *Bone Joint J* 2015;97(1):71-75.

76. Bottner F, Wegner A, Winkelmann W, Becker K, Erren M, Götze C: Interleukin-6, procalcitonin and TNF-alpha: Markers of periprosthetic infection following total joint replacement. *J Bone Joint Surg Br* 2007;89(1):94-99.

77. Abe R, Oda S, Sadahiro T, et al: Gram-negative bacteremia induces greater magnitude of inflammatory response than Gram-positive bacteremia. *Crit Care* 2010;14(2):R27.

78. Della Valle CJ, Bogner E, Desai P, et al: Analysis of frozen sections of intraoperative specimens obtained at the time of reoperation after hip or knee resection arthroplasty for the treatment of infection. *J Bone Joint Surg Am* 1999;81(5):684-689.

79. Charosky CB, Bullough PG, Wilson PD Jr: Total hip replacement failures: A histological evaluation. *J Bone Joint Surg Am* 1973;55(1):49-58.

80. Feldman DS, Lonner JH, Desai P, Zuckerman JD: The role of intraoperative frozen sections in revision total joint arthroplasty. *J Bone Joint Surg Am* 1995;77(12):1807-1813.

81. Austin MS, Ghanem E, Joshi A, Lindsay A, Parvizi J: A simple, cost-effective screening protocol to rule out periprosthetic infection. *J Arthroplasty* 2008;23(1):65-68.

82. Wasson JH, Walsh TB, LaBrecque MC, Sox HC, Pantell R: *The Common Symptom Guide: A Guide to the Evaluation of Common Adult and Pediatric Symptoms*, ed 5. New York, NY, McGraw-Hill, 2002.

83. Cho WS, Byun SE, Cho WJ, Yoon YS, Dhurve K: Polymorphonuclear cell count on frozen section is not an absolute index of reimplantation in infected total knee arthroplasty. *J Arthroplasty* 2013;28(10):1874-1877.

84. Panegrossi G, Ceretti M, Papalia M, Casella F, Favetti F, Falez F: Bone loss management in total knee revision surgery. *Int Orthop* 2014;38(2):419-427.

85. Engh GA, Ammeen DJ: Bone loss with revision total knee arthroplasty: Defect classification and alternatives for reconstruction. *Instr Course Lect* 1999;48:167-175.

86. Merchant AC, Mercer RL, Jacobsen RH, Cool CR: Roentgenographic analysis of patellofemoral congruence. *J Bone Joint Surg Am* 1974;56(7):1391-1396.

87. Engh GA, Ammeen DJ: Classification and preoperative radiographic evaluation: Knee. *Orthop Clin North Am* 1998;29(2):205-217.

88. Radnay CS, Scuderi GR: Management of bone loss: Augments, cones, offset stems. *Clin Orthop Relat Res* 2006;446:83-92.

89. Brand MG, Daley RJ, Ewald FC, Scott RD: Tibial tray augmentation with modular metal wedges for tibial bone stock deficiency. *Clin Orthop Relat Res* 1989;248:71-79.

90. Sassoon AA, Nelms NJ, Trousdale RT: Intraoperative fracture during staged total knee reimplantation in the treatment of periprosthetic infection. *J Arthroplasty* 2014;29(7):1435-1438.

91. Eltorai AE, Nguyen E, Daniels AH: Three-dimensional printing in orthopedic surgery. *Orthopedics* 2015;38(11):684-687.

92. Meseguer-Olmo L, Vicente-Ortega V, Alcaraz-Baños M, et al: In-vivo behavior of Si-hydroxyapatite/polycaprolactone/DMB scaffolds fabricated by 3D printing. *J Biomed Mater Res A* 2013;101(7):2038-2048.

93. Mortazavi SM, Vegari D, Ho A, Zmistowski B, Parvizi J: Two-stage exchange arthroplasty for infected total knee arthroplasty: Predictors of failure. *Clin Orthop Relat Res* 2011;469(11):3049-3054.

94. Mahmud T, Lyons MC, Naudie DD, Macdonald SJ, McCalden RW: Assessing the gold standard: A review of 253 two-stage revisions for infected TKA. *Clin Orthop Relat Res* 2012;470(10):2730-2736.

95. Kalore NV, Maheshwari A, Sharma A, Cheng E, Gioe TJ: Is there a preferred articulating spacer technique for infected knee arthroplasty? A preliminary study. *Clin Orthop Relat Res* 2012;470(1):228-235.

96. Puhto AP, Puhto TM, Niinimäki TT, Leppilahti JI, Syrjälä HP: Two-stage revision for prosthetic joint infection: Outcome and role of reimplantation microbiology in 107 cases. *J Arthroplasty* 2014;29(6):1101-1104.

97. Matsumoto T, Ishida K, Tsumura N, et al: Treatment of 50 deep infections after total knee arthroplasty. *Orthopedics* 2015;38(6):e529-e535.

98. Siqueira MB, Saleh A, Klika AK, et al: Chronic suppression of periprosthetic joint infections with oral antibiotics increases infection-free survivorship. *J Bone Joint Surg Am* 2015;97(15):1220-1232.

99. Rao N, Crossett LS, Sinha RK, Le Frock JL: Long-term suppression of infection in total joint arthroplasty. *Clin Orthop Relat Res* 2003;414:55-60.

100. Bengtson S, Knutson K: The infected knee arthroplasty: A 6-year follow-up of 357 cases. *Acta Orthop Scand* 1991;62(4):301-311.

101. Hanssen AD, Rand JA: Evaluation and treatment of infection at the site of a total hip or knee arthroplasty. *Instr Course Lect* 1999;48:111-122.

102. Incavo SJ, Lilly JW, Bartlett CS, Churchill DL: Arthrodesis of the knee: Experience with intramedullary nailing. *J Arthroplasty* 2000;15(7):871-876.

103. Christie MJ, DeBoer DK, McQueen DA, Cooke FW, Hahn DL: Salvage procedures for failed total knee arthroplasty. *J Bone Joint Surg Am* 2003;85(suppl 1):S58-S62.

104. Knutson K, Hovelius L, Lindstrand A, Lidgren L: Arthrodesis after failed knee arthroplasty: A nationwide multicenter investigation of 91 cases. *Clin Orthop Relat Res* 1984;191:202-211.

105. Mabry TM, Jacofsky DJ, Haidukewych GJ, Hanssen AD: Comparison of intramedullary nailing and external fixation knee arthrodesis for the infected knee replacement. *Clin Orthop Relat Res* 2007;464:11-15.

106. Nichols SJ, Landon GC, Tullos HS: Arthrodesis with dual plates after failed total knee arthroplasty. *J Bone Joint Surg Am* 1991;73(7):1020-1024.

107. Sierra RJ, Trousdale RT, Pagnano MW: Above-the-knee amputation after a total knee replacement: Prevalence, etiology, and functional outcome. *J Bone Joint Surg Am* 2003;85(6):1000-1004.

108. Pring DJ, Marks L, Angel JC: Mobility after amputation for failed knee replacement. *J Bone Joint Surg Br* 1988;70(5):770-771.

Foot and Ankle

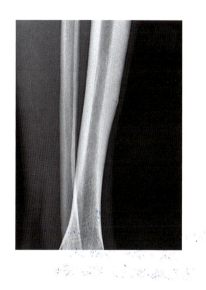

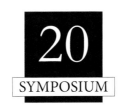

Achilles Tendon Rupture in Elite Athletes

Michael Isiah Sandlin, MD

Cyrus E. Taghavi, MD

Timothy P. Charlton, MD

Abstract

The management of acute Achilles tendon rupture in elite athletes is a current area of clinical controversy. Recent studies have reported near-equivocal outcomes in patients who undergo either nonsurgical or surgical treatment of Achilles tendon rupture; however, similar functional outcomes may not be observed in elite athletes who are at the highest levels of athletic performance and undergo nonsurgical or surgical treatment of Achilles tendon rupture. Surgeons should understand the risks and benefits of nonsurgical and surgical management of acute Achilles tendon rupture. Surgeons also should understand the accelerated rehabilitation protocols; functional nonsurgical and postoperative rehabilitation protocols; as well as the standard open, percutaneous, and minimally invasive surgical techniques for the management of Achilles tendon rupture from the perspective of a sports medicine foot and ankle specialist.

Instr Course Lect 2017;66:265–274.

The Achilles tendon is the thickest and strongest tendon in the human body. The Achilles tendon also is the most commonly injured tendon in the human body, with an estimated incidence of 18 to 37 ruptures per 100,000 individuals per year.[1-3] The Achilles tendon injury rate continues to increase as adults stay active and participate in sports and athletics for longer periods.[4-6] Recent studies have reported that major functional deficits occur and often persist after Achilles tendon rupture.[7-10] Current treatment recommendations for elite athletes who have acute Achilles tendon rupture are controversial. Advances in the nonsurgical rehabilitation of Achilles tendon rupture have resulted in near-equivalent outcomes and a lower rate of complications compared with the surgical management of Achilles tendon rupture; however, surgical intervention may provide patients who have Achilles tendon rupture, especially those who are at the highest levels of athletic performance, with functional benefits beyond those that are able to be achieved with nonsurgical management. Newer surgical techniques, including minimally invasive and percutaneous approaches, in combination with accelerated postoperative rehabilitation protocols may help optimize functional outcomes as well as patient satisfaction and limit complications in patients who elect to undergo surgical treatment for Achilles tendon rupture.

Anatomy and Biomechanics

The Achilles tendon consists of fibers from the soleus and the two heads of the gastrocnemius muscles. The plantaris tendon, which exists in 92% to 98% of the population, is located medial to and, in most patients, is distinct from the Achilles tendon. The gastrocnemius-soleus musculotendinous unit, which spans the knee, ankle, and subtalar joints, contributes

Dr. Charlton or an immediate family member has stock or stock options held in the Green Bay Packers Football Club and the Manchester United Football Club. Neither of the following authors nor any immediate family member has received anything of value from or has stock or stock options held in a commercial company or institution related directly or indirectly to the subject of this chapter: Dr. Sandlin and Dr. Taghavi.

Table 1

Common Factors That Contribute to Achilles Tendon Rupture

Poorly conditioned gastrocnemius-soleus musculotendinous unit

Alterations in activity level or sporting demands

Patients aged in their thirties or forties

Male sex

Previous injury

Poor tendon blood supply

Overpronating foot mechanics

Poor shoe wear

Attritional injuries

Fluoroquinolone use

to knee flexion, ankle plantar flexion, and subtalar inversion (via the medially prominent calcaneal pull of the Achilles tendon). The Achilles tendon internally rotates 90° during its course with the more posterior gastrocnemius contribution and the more anterior soleus contribution, inserting laterally and medially, respectively, on the calcaneal tuberosity. A normal Achilles tendon is composed of 95% type I collagen.[11] In a ruptured Achilles tendon, the proportion of type III collagen, which is inferior in tensile strength, durability, and elasticity, is substantially increased.[12] The Achilles tendon lacks a true synovial sheath and is instead enveloped in a bilayer of paratenon, which is richly vascularized and allows for 1.5 cm of tendon glide.[13] The superficial layer of paratenon is adherent to the fascia cruris of the lower leg, which covers the posterior aspect of the tendon complex.[14] The sural nerve invests the area of the Achilles tendon, crossing approximately 11 cm proximal to the calcaneal tuberosity and 3.5 cm distal to the musculotendinous junction. A vascular watershed area that is

approximately 2 to 6 cm proximal to the Achilles tendon insertion into the calcaneus is the most common site of Achilles tendon rupture. Poor vascularity likely plays a role in the pathogenesis of Achilles tendon rupture.[15]

No consensus on the process by which the Achilles tendon ruptures exists. Multiple factors, including alterations in activity level or sporting demands, patients aged in their thirties or forties, male sex, previous injury, or a poorly conditioned gastrocnemius-soleus unit may contribute to Achilles tendon rupture. **Table 1** lists the most common factors that contribute to Achilles tendon rupture. Two nonexclusive theories inform the process by which the Achilles tendon ruptures.[16] The degenerative theory suggests that chronic low-grade trauma from repetitive activity and maladaptive repair mechanisms weaken the tendon microstructure, eventually resulting in tendon rupture without excessive loading. The mechanical theory suggests that Achilles tendon rupture may occur, even in patients with healthy tendons, if the coordination of muscle contractions or lower leg mechanics is suboptimal. The mechanical theory of Achilles tendon rupture is particularly noteworthy in athletes who return to high-demand sporting activity after a long period of inactivity or with eccentric loading of the Achilles tendon in a fatigued state.[17,18] Fluoroquinolones and anabolic steroids are known to induce dystrophic changes in collagen and may predispose patients to tendon rupture via weakening of the tendon microstructure.[19]

Acute Achilles tendon ruptures in athletes typically occur as a result of dynamic loading of the Achilles tendon during sport-related forefoot push-off

with an extended knee,[20] which is the most common mechanism of injury in patients who perform sprinting, cutting, or jumping activities. A second mechanism of injury involves rapid ankle dorsiflexion as a result of a sudden, unexpected eccentric load that is placed on the foot, which typically occurs after stepping into an unseen hole or missing a stair. The third and least common mechanism of injury occurs in patients who are subject to forced dorsiflexion of an actively plantarflexed foot, such as that which occurs as a result of floorboard intrusion while the foot is on the brake pedal during a motor vehicle collision or as a result of a fall from a height.

Clinical Evaluation

The evaluation of a patient with a suspected Achilles tendon injury should consist of a detailed history that includes an assessment of the mechanism of injury; prior foot, ankle, or Achilles tendon injuries; medical conditions (especially diabetes mellitus or renal disease); medications (particularly steroid injections or fluoroquinolone use); and social activity (tobacco or anabolic steroid use). A high degree of suspicion for Achilles tendon injury may be required in patients who have an elevated risk for delayed diagnosis, including patients older than 55 years, patients with obesity, and patients who were injured in non–sports-related activities.[21] A high level of suspicion for Achilles tendon rupture is necessary because a reported 20% to 25% of acute Achilles tendon ruptures are not diagnosed by the initial examining physician.[22-24]

Most patients who have Achilles tendon injury report a history of acute-onset posterior ankle or lower leg pain and the sensation of being kicked or hit in the back of the ankle. The physical examination should include a general examination of the lower extremity, including the knee, ankle, and subtalar joints. Typically, patients with Achilles tendon injury are unable to bear weight or have severely antalgic gait patterns. The specific evaluation of the Achilles tendon should include an assessment for swelling and ecchymosis as well as palpation for gaps in tendon continuity, which are most frequently found 2 cm to 6 cm from the calcaneal insertion in patients with Achilles tendon rupture. In some patients, edema may obscure any appreciable gap. The resting position of the injured foot should be compared with the contralateral foot. Active plantar flexion may be partially present as a result of contributions from the flexor hallucis longus (FHL) and flexor digitorum longus tendons, and passive dorsiflexion may be increased. The Thompson test is performed with the patient placed in the prone position with the knee flexed to 90°; alternatively, the test can be performed with the patient placed in the prone position with the ankles hanging off the end of the examination table. The examiner squeezes the patient's calf to assess corresponding plantar flexion, which typically is absent in patients who have complete Achilles tendon rupture; however, some degree of plantar flexion may occur as a result of contributions from the FHL and flexor digitorum longus tendons. A false-positive result may occur in patients who have a soleus or gastrocnemius tear. The stand and maintain plantar flexion test will be positive in patients with acute Achilles tendon rupture who are unable to maintain a plantarflexed foot position during attempted heel raise.[25]

Imaging studies are not required for a patient with a history, physical examination, and mechanism of injury that are consistent with acute Achilles tendon rupture; however, imaging studies may be considered in patients in whom concern for delayed diagnosis, bony avulsion, or preexisting calcific tendinosis, all of which may alter treatment protocols, exists. Plain radiographs may show loss of the Kager triangle, which is the radiolucent triangle observed posteriorly between an intact Achilles tendon, the superior border of the calcaneus, and the soft-tissue density of the FHL muscle and tendon that is just posterior to the tibia on a lateral radiograph.

Ultrasonography may be considered to help evaluate Achilles tendon continuity and estimate gap size. Ultrasonography also can help assess for loss of the normal paradoxical motion of the FHL tendon that is observed during dynamic Thompson testing if concern for a complete versus partial Achilles tendon rupture exists. MRI is not routinely required but can be useful in the evaluation of Achilles tendon gap size and tear distance from the calcaneal insertion. In addition, MRI can help identify muscle atrophy or fatty infiltration in patients with chronic Achilles tendon rupture. Care should be taken with regard to partial Achilles tendon ruptures observed on MRI because these injuries often are clinically complete Achilles tendon ruptures.

Treatment

Traditionally, surgical intervention has been the preferred treatment option for athletes with acute Achilles tendon rupture. Multiple studies have reported decreased re-rupture rates, improved strength, improved early functional outcomes, and earlier return to work in patients with Achilles tendon rupture who undergo surgical treatment;[26,27] however, surgical treatment also is associated with an increased risk for complications, including infection, wound dehiscence, scar irritation, and sural nerve injury. Advances in nonsurgical rehabilitation protocols, including early range of motion, functional bracing, and early weight bearing, have resulted in improved outcomes compared with previous immobilization-focused nonsurgical rehabilitation protocols. Recent meta-analyses have reported that, compared with patients who undergo surgical treatment for Achilles tendon rupture, patients who undergo nonsurgical treatment for Achilles tendon rupture with accelerated nonsurgical rehabilitation may have noninferior outcomes with respect to re-rupture rates without the complications associated with surgical treatment.[3,28] Given these findings, European studies have reported a recent downtrend in the surgical treatment of patients who have Achilles tendon tears despite the increased incidence of Achilles tendon rupture;[29,30] this has been attributed to advances in the nonsurgical management of Achilles tendon rupture reported in the literature. This downtrend in the surgical treatment of European patients with Achilles tendon ruptures has not been mirrored in the United States.[31]

Nonsurgical Treatment

Traditionally, nonsurgical management of acute Achilles tendon rupture was reserved for elderly patients with low physical demands or patients who had a high risk for surgical complications, such as those with diabetes mellitus or who were smokers. Until recently, nonsurgical management of acute Achilles tendon rupture consisted of prolonged non–weight-bearing cast immobilization in equinus, with graded dorsiflexion and progression to weight bearing over a period of 6 to 8 weeks or longer. Risks of surgical treatment were avoided; however, nonsurgical management resulted in severe calf atrophy, diminished early strength and function, as well as delayed return to work. Re-rupture was the most concerning complication after nonsurgical management, with re-rupture rates ranging from 11% to 35%.[32,33] Multiple recent studies have reported improved outcomes in patients with Achilles tendon rupture who undergo accelerated nonsurgical rehabilitation and early weight-bearing protocols. Khan et al[3] reported a decreased re-rupture rate in patients with Achilles tendon rupture who underwent accelerated nonsurgical rehabilitation protocols and functional bracing (2.4%) compared with patients with Achilles tendon rupture who underwent cast immobilization (12.2%). Similarly, Jones et al[28] reported re-rupture rates of 3.3% and 11.4% in patients with Achilles tendon rupture who underwent accelerated nonsurgical rehabilitation versus cast immobilization, respectively.

Patients with Achilles tendon rupture who undergo nonsurgical functional rehabilitation have outcomes comparable with those of patients with Achilles tendon rupture who undergo surgical treatment. In a study of 144 patients with Achilles tendon rupture who underwent either surgical treatment or nonsurgical treatment with an accelerated nonsurgical rehabilitation protocol, Willits et al[10] reported no significant difference in the re-rupture rate between the patients in the surgical and nonsurgical groups (2.8% versus 4.2%, respectively) at 2 years postinjury; however, the authors reported an increased risk for infection (6.9%) and wound dehiscence (2.8%) in the surgical group. In a study of 50 patients with Achilles tendon rupture who underwent either surgical treatment or nonsurgical treatment with an early motion protocol that began 10 days postinjury, Twaddle and Poon[34] reported no differences in functional outcomes, the re-rupture rate, or complications between the patients in the two groups. In a meta-analysis of 10 studies that included 418 patients with Achilles tendon rupture who underwent either surgical treatment or nonsurgical treatment with functional rehabilitation and early motion, Soroceanu et al[35] reported no statistically significant difference in the re-rupture rate between the patients in the two groups (risk difference, 1.7% in favor of surgical treatment). Furthermore, the authors reported that surgical treatment was associated with a 15.8% absolute risk increase for complications other than re-rupture.

As observed in the studies already mentioned, the successful management of Achilles tendon rupture has often been measured by a decreased risk for re-rupture and other serious complications. Large-scale reviews and meta-analyses have reported re-rupture rates of approximately 3% to 4% after surgical treatment and 2% to 7% after nonsurgical treatment with functional rehabilitation.[3,10,36-38] Despite these relatively low re-rupture rates, many patients who undergo treatment for Achilles tendon rupture remain symptomatic and fail to achieve complete recovery. A complete recovery that takes a full year or longer is not uncommon. Given the relatively long recovery period, the focus of current Achilles tendon rupture management has shifted from an emphasis on re-rupture and wound complications to a focus on functional outcomes, which is a topic of particular relevance to performance-oriented athletes.[21,39] However, differences in functional scores and performance after the management of Achilles tendon rupture have been inconsistent across the limited number of studies in the literature. In a study of 100 patients with Achilles tendon rupture who underwent either surgical or nonsurgical treatment, Olsson et al[39] reported that hopping ability and the drop countermovement jump (a one-footed drop from a height of 20 cm followed by a rapid maximal vertical jump) were the primary functional benefits of surgical treatment. The authors reported no differences in strength testing, muscular endurance, and heel-raise height between the patients in the surgical and nonsurgical groups. Other studies, however, have reported improved plantar flexion strength at both 1 year and 2 years postinjury in patients who underwent surgical treatment for Achilles tendon rupture.[10] In a questionnaire-based follow-up study of 487 patients with Achilles tendon rupture who underwent either surgical or nonsurgical treatment, Bergkvist et al[40] reported that the patients who underwent surgical treatment had superior heel-raise endurance at a mean follow-up of 3.6 years. In a study of 111 patients with acute Achilles tendon rupture who underwent either surgical or nonsurgical treatment, Cetti et al[41] reported that the patients who underwent surgical treatment had a significantly higher rate of return to sports activity at their preinjury level, a lesser degree of calf atrophy, better ankle movement, and fewer complaints at 1 year postinjury compared with the patients who underwent nonsurgical treatment. In a recent meta-analysis of 10 studies that included 418 patients with Achilles tendon rupture who underwent either surgical or nonsurgical treatment, Soroceanu et al[35] reported that, despite no differences in functional scores, calf strength, or calf circumference, the patients who underwent surgical treatment returned to work nearly 3 weeks earlier compared with the patients who underwent nonsurgical treatment.

Preclinical studies have helped inform the process of Achilles tendon healing. Animal models have demonstrated that Achilles tendon repair mechanisms depend on a balance of tissue loading and unloading.[42] The treatment of Achilles tendon rupture with complete immobilization results in decreased healing callus size, diminished mechanical strength, and increased adhesions. Some degree of Achilles tendon loading appears to be good for healing, leading to a stronger Achilles tendon with better excursion.[43-46] A human roentgen stereophotogrammetric analysis demonstrated that tension loading of a repaired Achilles tendon leads to a higher tendon elastic modulus; this analysis suggests that controlled early mobilization can improve the mechanical properties of a healing Achilles tendon, which may lead to improved functional outcomes.[47] Some studies report that both early weight bearing and early mobilization of the ankle and the Achilles tendon are necessary to achieve optimal Achilles tendon healing;[39] however, excessive early motion may induce gap formation at the sites of Achilles tendon repair, which can lead to alterations in the ultimate functional capacity of the Achilles tendon.[48] These findings have informed Achilles tendon

rupture management strategies and suggest that, regardless whether surgical or nonsurgical management is selected, early, functional rehabilitation and tendon gap prevention are likely the keys to maximizing the functional outcomes of patients with Achilles tendon rupture.

Video 20.1: Achilles Tendon Rupture in Athletes. Timothy P. Charlton, MD (3 min)

Surgical Treatment

Despite the noted risks, surgical management of Achilles tendon rupture has been the standard of care for athletes, younger patients, and patients in whom delayed rupture is present primarily because the risk for re-rupture after surgical treatment is lower compared with that after traditional immobilization-oriented nonsurgical treatment protocols.[49] In a meta-analysis of six studies that compared surgical management versus nonsurgical management of acute Achilles tendon ruptures, Bhandari et al[37] reported a 3% re-rupture rate in patients who underwent surgical treatment and a 13% re-rupture rate in patients who underwent nonsurgical treatment with varying periods of immobilization.

Several techniques, including open, percutaneous, and minimally invasive procedures, are commonly used for the surgical management of Achilles tendon rupture. Open repair, which has been the classic technique for the surgical management of Achilles tendon rupture, allows for direct visualization, end-to-end approximation, and potentially superior repair strength; however, it is associated with the highest rate of complications.[45,49,50] In a study of 10 fresh frozen cadaver models that underwent either open or percutaneous

Achilles tendon rupture repair, Hockenbury and Johns[51] reported that, compared with the cadaver models in the percutaneous repair group, the cadaver models in the open repair group were able to resist almost twice the amount of ankle dorsiflexion before repair site gapping occurred, which suggested a stronger repair. Conversely, after finding no difference in the strength of Achilles tendon repair between patients who underwent either open or minimally invasive Achilles tendon rupture repair, Ismail et al[52] reported that the strength of an Achilles tendon repair was related more to the diameter of the Achilles tendon than to the technique used to repair the Achilles tendon rupture.

Percutaneous and minimally invasive Achilles tendon rupture repair techniques were developed to minimize the risk for wound complications and infection but maintain the benefits of surgical Achilles tendon rupture repair.[3,53,54] Percutaneous Achilles tendon rupture repair, which was originally described by Ma and Griffith,[53] has demonstrated improved outcomes compared with traditional nonsurgical management of Achilles tendon rupture.[55] In a study that compared the outcomes of 14 patients with Achilles tendon rupture who underwent nonsurgical treatment with cast immobilization in equinus with those of 10 patients with Achilles tendon rupture who underwent percutaneous Achilles tendon rupture repair, Rowleley and Scotland[56] reported that the patients in the percutaneous group achieved normal plantar flexion strength and returned to activity earlier compared with the patients in the nonsurgical group. In a recent meta-analysis of four studies that included

174 patients who underwent either open or percutaneous Achilles tendon rupture repair, Jones et al[28] reported fewer total and major complications in the patients who underwent percutaneous Achilles tendon rupture repair. Open Achilles tendon rupture repair was associated with an 18.2% infection rate, and percutaneous Achilles tendon rupture repair was not associated with infection; however, the authors reported no differences in functional scores, return to sport, or the rerupture rate between the patients in the open and the percutaneous groups. The most commonly reported complication of percutaneous Achilles tendon rupture repair is sural nerve entrapment. Klein et al[55] reported sural nerve injury in 13% of 38 patients who underwent percutaneous Achilles tendon rupture repair. In a study of five cadaver models that underwent percutaneous Achilles tendon rupture repair using the technique that was originally described by Ma and Griffith,[53] Hockenbury and Johns et al[51] reported sural nerve entrapment in three of the cadaver models and Achilles tendon stump malalignment in four of the cadaver models.

Modified percutaneous and minimally invasive Achilles tendon rupture repair techniques have been developed to improve the strength of Achilles tendon repair and minimize sural nerve entrapment.[45,57-59] Majewski et al[60] reported no sural nerve symptoms in a study of 35 patients who underwent percutaneous Achilles tendon rupture repair with the use of a modified technique. Jones et al[28] reported sural nerve symptoms in 1.1% of 88 patients who underwent percutaneous Achilles tendon rupture repair. A minimally invasive technique that uses a small, vertical

midline incision and allows sutures to be placed completely inside the paratenon may decrease the risk for sural nerve injury.[43,61] In a study of 87 patients who underwent minimally invasive Achilles tendon rupture repair, Assal et al[44] reported no sural nerve injuries. In a recent review of six studies that compared the outcomes of 375 patients who underwent open Achilles tendon rupture repair with those of 406 patients who underwent minimally invasive Achilles tendon rupture repair, Del Buono et al[46] reported no deep infections in the patients in the minimally invasive repair group and a 2.4% rate of deep infection in the patients in the open repair group. Wound necrosis also was higher in the open repair group compared with the minimally invasive repair group (4.5% versus 0.2%, respectively). In addition to a lower complication rate, minimally invasive Achilles tendon rupture repair also appears to provide functional outcomes equivalent with those of open Achilles tendon rupture repair. Several studies have reported no differences in functional scores, range of motion, calf circumference, plantar flexion torque strength, or heel raises between patients who underwent either open or minimally invasive Achilles tendon rupture repair.[45,60]

Compared with direct Achilles tendon rupture repair techniques, improved outcomes have not been reported in patients who undergo augmentation of Achilles tendon rupture repair with primary tendon transfers, fascial turndowns, or tendon weaves.[27,61] Heikkinen et al[27] reported no advantage of FHL tendon augmentation in the repair of acute Achilles tendon rupture. Adjuvant treatments, such as platelet-rich plasma injections, also have been used to augment

Achilles tendon healing; however, such adjuvant treatments have not been reported to be beneficial in patients with Achilles tendon rupture.[62,63]

Postoperative Rehabilitation

Postoperative rehabilitation protocols for patients who undergo surgical treatment for Achilles tendon rupture continue to evolve. Studies have reported improved outcomes in patients who undergo functional rehabilitation, including early protected motion and weight bearing, compared with patients who undergo prolonged immobilization. Compared with progressive cast immobilization, early motion with mobile cast immobilization allows patients to return to sport activities and work sooner as well as results in fewer cutaneous adhesions, a decreased need for rehabilitation, and higher rates of satisfaction.[36,64] Suchak et al[36] reported better early functional outcomes in patients who underwent weight bearing 2 weeks after surgical treatment compared with patients who underwent delayed weight bearing after surgical treatment. Maffulli et al[65] reported no detrimental effects in patients who were allowed to fully bear weight 2 weeks postoperatively, with patients no longer using crutches at a mean of 2.5 weeks postoperatively. Some studies have expressed concern for Achilles tendon elongation and Achilles tendon gapping in patients with Achilles tendon rupture who undergo a postoperative rehabilitation protocol that includes early motion; however, Kangas et al[66] reported no difference in postoperative Achilles tendon lengthening between patients who underwent either postoperative immobilization or postoperative functional bracing that allowed for early motion.

Current evidence suggests that major functional deficits may exist and persist after acute Achilles tendon rupture regardless of treatment type. Accelerated postoperative rehabilitation protocols that include early weight bearing are not detrimental postoperatively and are likely superior compared with nonsurgical management with cast immobilization. In addition, compared with patients who undergo traditional surgical treatment for Achilles tendon rupture, patients who undergo nonsurgical functional rehabilitation protocols for Achilles tendon rupture may have noninferior outcomes with respect to re-rupture rates without the risk for wound complications or infection. The results of the surgical management of Achilles tendon rupture have demonstrated trends toward decreased re-rupture rates and improved functional outcomes; however, these results have not been fully elucidated and may only affect athletic performance at the highest levels of activity. Compared with open Achilles tendon rupture repair, percutaneous and minimally invasive Achilles tendon rupture repair are associated with a substantially decreased risk for infection but maintain the low re-rupture rate and repair strength that are associated with open Achilles tendon rupture repair. The limitations of current studies on the treatment of Achilles tendon rupture include difficulties in drawing conclusions based on nonstandardized treatment protocols for separate treatment groups and the small number of studies that compare various Achilles tendon rupture repair techniques. Questions about the tendon gapping that may persist despite maximal ankle plantar flexion after nonsurgical management also exist.

Additional treatment concerns for patients who have Achilles tendon rupture include the consideration of prophylaxis for deep vein thrombosis (DVT) and pulmonary embolism. Symptomatic DVT and pulmonary embolism have been reported to be as high as 6.3% and 1.4%, respectively, in patients with Achilles tendon rupture.[67] Nilsson-Helander et al[68] reported that color duplex ultrasonography demonstrated a 34% overall rate of DVT in 95 patients who underwent treatment for Achilles tendon rupture. The authors reported no difference in the rate of DVT between patients who underwent surgical or nonsurgical treatment. Despite the concern for DVT and pulmonary embolism in patients who have Achilles tendon rupture, the current recommendations for anticoagulation after acute Achilles tendon rupture lack consensus. Two recent large healthcare database reviews of patients who had Achilles tendon rupture revealed lower rates of DVT and pulmonary embolism compared with those that were previously reported.[31,69] The studies reported a 0.4% to 1.1% risk for DVT and an approximately 0.3% risk for pulmonary embolism, with no identifiable difference in the risk for DVT or pulmonary embolism in patients who underwent surgical or nonsurgical treatment.[31,69]

The approach of the authors of this chapter for the management of acute Achilles tendon rupture in an athlete begins with a discussion on the expectations of injury, surgical treatment, and postoperative rehabilitation. The authors of this chapter establish the expectation of a return to effective sporting activity by 1 year postinjury. The treatment algorithm of the authors of this chapter is based on the time from

the diagnosis of Achilles tendon rupture. For patients in whom a diagnosis of Achilles tendon rupture is made less than 3 weeks postinjury, the authors of this chapter typically recommend minimally invasive or closed treatment based on patient preference. For patients in whom a diagnosis of Achilles tendon rupture is made more than 3 weeks postinjury, the authors of this chapter are more likely to recommend open, direct tendon repair. Postoperative management for all patients who undergo surgical treatment consists of 2 weeks in a soft, well-padded splint followed by a transition to an adjustable equinus-positioned controlled ankle motion boot at 4 weeks postoperatively. The authors of this chapter also begin rehabilitation at 4 weeks postoperatively. Ankle dorsiflexion in the controlled ankle motion boot is advanced by 10° each postoperative week, and ankle resting tension is reassessed on a monthly basis. The target of the authors of this chapter is a symmetric resting position at 4 months postoperatively. Dynamic sport-related rehabilitation begins at 6 months postoperatively, with an expectation of return to competition and preinjury level of function by at least 1 year postoperatively. Prophylactic anticoagulation may be considered in patients with known risk factors for DVT or pulmonary embolism.

Summary

The management of acute Achilles tendon rupture is controversial. Compared with patients who undergo traditional surgical treatment for Achilles tendon rupture, patients who undergo accelerated nonsurgical rehabilitation protocols with functional bracing, early motion, and early weight bearing for Achilles tendon rupture appear to have noninferior re-rupture rates and substantially lower combined complication rates. Although open surgical treatment has been the standard of care for athletes who have Achilles tendon rupture, recent advances in percutaneous and minimally invasive Achilles tendon rupture repair have shown promise, substantially decreasing the risk for complications but maintaining the repair strength and the potential functional benefits associated with open Achilles tendon rupture repair. Given these considerations, the authors of this chapter recommend percutaneous or minimally invasive surgical repair techniques and accelerated rehabilitation for elite athletes who have Achilles tendon rupture.

References

1. Ames PR, Longo UG, Denaro V, Maffulli N: Achilles tendon problems: Not just an orthopaedic issue. *Disabil Rehabil* 2008;30(20-22):1646-1650.

2. Maffulli N, Waterston SW, Squair J, Reaper J, Douglas AS: Changing incidence of Achilles tendon rupture in Scotland: A 15-year study. *Clin J Sport Med* 1999;9(3):157-160.

3. Khan RJ, Fick D, Keogh A, Crawford J, Brammar T, Parker M: Treatment of acute achilles tendon ruptures: A meta-analysis of randomized, controlled trials. *J Bone Joint Surg Am* 2005;87(10):2202-2210.

4. Möller A, Astron M, Westlin N: Increasing incidence of Achilles tendon rupture. *Acta Orthop Scand* 1996;67(5):479-481.

5. Józsa L, Kvist M, Bálint BJ, et al: The role of recreational sport activity in Achilles tendon rupture: A clinical, pathoanatomical, and sociological study of 292 cases. *Am J Sports Med* 1989;17(3):338-343.

6. Leppilahti J, Puranen J, Orava S: Incidence of Achilles tendon rupture. *Acta Orthop Scand* 1996;67(3):277-279.

7. Bostick GP, Jomha NM, Suchak AA, Beaupré LA: Factors associated with calf muscle endurance recovery 1 year after achilles tendon rupture repair. *J Orthop Sports Phys Ther* 2010;40(6):345-351.

8. Möller M, Lind K, Movin T, Karlsson J: Calf muscle function after Achilles tendon rupture: A prospective, randomised study comparing surgical and non-surgical treatment. *Scand J Med Sci Sports* 2002;12(1):9-16.

9. Olsson N, Nilsson-Helander K, Karlsson J, et al: Major functional deficits persist 2 years after acute Achilles tendon rupture. *Knee Surg Sports Traumatol Arthrosc* 2011;19(8):1385-1393.

10. Willits K, Amendola A, Bryant D, et al: Operative versus nonoperative treatment of acute Achilles tendon ruptures: A multicenter randomized trial using accelerated functional rehabilitation. *J Bone Joint Surg Am* 2010;92(17):2767-2775.

11. Kader D, Saxena A, Movin T, Maffulli N: Achilles tendinopathy: Some aspects of basic science and clinical management. *Br J Sports Med* 2002;36(4):239-249.

12. Maffulli N, Ewen SW, Waterston SW, Reaper J, Barrass V: Tenocytes from ruptured and tendinopathic achilles tendons produce greater quantities of type III collagen than tenocytes from normal achilles tendons: An in vitro model of human tendon healing. *Am J Sports Med* 2000;28(4):499-505.

13. Saltzman CL, Tearse DS: Achilles tendon injuries. *J Am Acad Orthop Surg* 1998;6(5):316-325.

14. Kvist H, Kvist M: The operative treatment of chronic calcaneal paratenonitis. *J Bone Joint Surg Br* 1980;62(3):353-357.

15. Aström M, Westlin N: Blood flow in chronic Achilles tendinopathy. *Clin Orthop Relat Res* 1994;308:166-172.

16. Longo UG, Petrillo S, Maffulli N, Denaro V: Acute achilles tendon rupture in athletes. *Foot Ankle Clin* 2013;18(2):319-338.

17. Clement DB, Taunton JE, Smart GW: Achilles tendinitis and peritendinitis: Etiology and treatment. *Am J Sports Med* 1984;12(3):179-184.

18. Knörzer E, Folkhard W, Geercken W, et al: New aspects of the etiology of tendon rupture: An analysis of time-resolved dynamic-mechanical measurements using synchrotron radiation. *Arch Orthop Trauma Surg* 1986;105(2):113-120.

19. Charlton T, Sakowski CM, Mulvihill J, Cohen JR, Wang JC, Hatch III GF: Paper No. 743. Achilles tendonopathy and ruptures: Analysis of a large private insurance database. *AAOS 2016 Annual Meeting Proceedings*. Rosemont, IL, American Academy of Orthopaedic Surgeons, 2015.

20. Arner O, Lindholm A: Subcutaneous rupture of the Achilles tendon; a study of 92 cases. *Acta Chir Scand Suppl* 1959;116(suppl 239):1-51.

21. Guss D, Smith JT, Chiodo CP: Acute Achilles tendon rupture. *JBJS Rev* 2015;3(4):e2.

22. Maffulli N: Rupture of the Achilles tendon: A critical analysis review. *J Bone Joint Surg Am* 1999;81(7):1019-1036.

23. Maffulli N: The clinical diagnosis of subcutaneous tear of the Achilles tendon: A prospective study in 174 patients. *Am J Sports Med* 1998;26(2):266-270.

24. O'Brien T: The needle test for complete rupture of the Achilles tendon. *J Bone Joint Surg Am* 1984;66(7):1099-1101.

25. Kaplan J, Lundergan W, Charlton T: The STAMP Test: A novel clinical test in diagnosing Achilles tendon ruptures. Presented at the American Orthopaedic Foot and Ankle Society Annual Meeting. Long Beach, CA, July 14-18, 2015.

26. Möller M, Movin T, Granhed H, Lind K, Faxén E, Karlsson J: Acute rupture of tendon Achillis: A prospective randomised study of comparison between surgical and non-surgical treatment. *J Bone Joint Surg Br* 2001;83(6):843-848.

27. Heikkinen J, Lantto I, Flinkkilä T, et al: Augmented compared with nonaugmented surgical repair after total Achilles rupture: Results of a prospective randomized trial with thirteen or more years of follow-up. *J Bone Joint Surg Am* 2016;98(2):85-92.

28. Jones MP, Khan RJ, Carey Smith RL: Surgical interventions for treating acute achilles tendon rupture: Key findings from a recent co-chrane review. *J Bone Joint Surg Am* 2012;94(12):e88.

29. Mattila VM, Huttunen TT, Haapasalo H, Sillanpää P, Malmivaara A, Pihlajamäki H: Declining incidence of surgery for Achilles tendon rupture follows publication of major RCTs: Evidence-influenced change evident using the Finnish registry study. *Br J Sports Med* 2015;49(16):1084-1086.

30. Huttunen TT, Kannus P, Rolf C, Felländer-Tsai L, Mattila VM: Acute achilles tendon ruptures: Incidence of injury and surgery in Sweden between 2001 and 2012. *Am J Sports Med* 2014;42(10):2419-2423.

31. Wang D, Sandlin MI, Cohen JR, Lord EL, Petrigliano FA, SooHoo NF: Operative versus nonoperative treatment of acute Achilles tendon rupture: An analysis of 12,570 patients in a large healthcare database. *Foot Ankle Surg* 2015;21(4):250-253.

32. Wong J, Barrass V, Maffulli N: Quantitative review of operative and nonoperative management of achilles tendon ruptures. *Am J Sports Med* 2002;30(4):565-575.

33. Persson A, Wredmark T: The treatment of total ruptures of the Achilles tendon by plaster immobilisation. *Int Orthop* 1979;3(2):149-152.

34. Twaddle BC, Poon P: Early motion for Achilles tendon ruptures: Is surgery important? A randomized, prospective study. *Am J Sports Med* 2007;35(12):2033-2038.

35. Soroceanu A, Sidhwa F, Aarabi S, Kaufman A, Glazebrook M: Surgical versus nonsurgical treatment of acute Achilles tendon rupture: A meta-analysis of randomized trials. *J Bone Joint Surg Am* 2012;94(23):2136-2143.

36. Suchak AA, Bostick GP, Beaupré LA, Durand DC, Jomha NM: The influence of early weight-bearing compared with non-weight-bearing after surgical repair of the Achilles tendon. *J Bone Joint Surg Am* 2008;90(9):1876-1883.

37. Bhandari M, Guyatt GH, Siddiqui F, et al: Treatment of acute Achilles tendon ruptures: A systematic overview and metaanalysis. *Clin Orthop Relat Res* 2002;400:190-200.

38. Ingvar J, Tägil M, Eneroth M: Non-operative treatment of Achilles tendon rupture: 196 consecutive patients with a 7% re-rupture rate. *Acta Orthop* 2005;76(4):597-601.

39. Olsson N, Silbernagel KG, Eriksson BI, et al: Stable surgical repair with accelerated rehabilitation versus nonsurgical treatment for acute Achilles tendon ruptures: A randomized controlled study. *Am J Sports Med* 2013;41(12):2867-2876.

40. Bergkvist D, Åström I, Josefsson PO, Dahlberg LE: Acute Achilles tendon rupture: A questionnaire follow-up of 487 patients. *J Bone Joint Surg Am* 2012;94(13):1229-1233.

41. Cetti R, Christensen SE, Ejsted R, Jensen NM, Jorgensen U: Operative versus nonoperative treatment of Achilles tendon rupture: A prospective randomized study and review of the literature. *Am J Sports Med* 1993;21(6):791-799.

42. Killian ML, Cavinatto L, Galatz LM, Thomopoulos S: The role of mechanobiology in tendon healing. *J Shoulder Elbow Surg* 2012;21(2):228-237.

43. Kakiuchi M: A combined open and percutaneous technique for repair of tendo Achillis: Comparison with open repair. *J Bone Joint Surg Br* 1995;77(1):60-63.

44. Assal M, Jung M, Stern R, Rippstein P, Delmi M, Hoffmeyer P: Limited open repair of Achilles tendon ruptures: A technique with a new instrument and findings of a prospective multicenter study. *J Bone Joint Surg Am* 2002;84(2):161-170.

45. Čretnik A, Kosanović M, Smrkolj V: Percutaneous versus open repair of the ruptured Achilles tendon: A comparative study. *Am J Sports Med* 2005;33(9):1369-1379.

46. Del Buono A, Volpin A, Maffulli N: Minimally invasive versus open surgery for acute Achilles tendon rupture: A systematic review. *Br Med Bull* 2014;109:45-54.

47. Schepull T, Aspenberg P: Early controlled tension improves the material properties of healing human achilles tendons after ruptures: A randomized trial. *Am J Sports Med* 2013;41(11):2550-2557.

48. James R, Kesturu G, Balian G, Chhabra AB: Tendon: Biology, biomechanics, repair, growth factors, and evolving treatment options. *J Hand Surg Am* 2008;33(1):102-112.

49. Leppilahti J: *Achilles Tendon Rupture, With Special Reference to Epidemiology and Results of Surgery, Thesis.* Oulu, Finland, University of Oulu, 1996.

50. Carter TR, Fowler PJ, Blokker C: Functional postoperative treatment of Achilles tendon repair. *Am J Sports Med* 1992;20(4):459-462.

51. Hockenbury RT, Johns JC: A biomechanical in vitro comparison of open versus percutaneous repair of tendon Achilles. *Foot Ankle* 1990;11(2):67-72.

52. Ismail M, Karim A, Shulman R, Amis A, Calder J: The Achillon achilles tendon repair: Is it strong enough? *Foot Ankle Int* 2008;29(8):808-813.

53. Ma GW, Griffith TG: Percutaneous repair of acute closed ruptured achilles tendon: A new technique. *Clin Orthop Relat Res* 1977;128:247-255.

54. FitzGibbons RE, Hefferon J, Hill J: Percutaneous Achilles tendon repair. *Am J Sports Med* 1993;21(5):724-727.

55. Klein W, Lang DM, Saleh M: The use of the Ma-Griffith technique for percutaneous repair of fresh ruptured tendo Achillis. *Chir Organi Mov* 1991;76(3):223-228.

56. Rowley DI, Scotland TR: Rupture of the Achilles tendon treated by a simple operative procedure. *Injury* 1982;14(3):252-254.

57. Webb JM, Bannister GC: Percutaneous repair of the ruptured tendo Achillis. *J Bone Joint Surg Br* 1999;81(5):877-880.

58. McClelland D, Maffulli N: Percutaneous repair of ruptured Achilles tendon. *J R Coll Surg Edinb* 2002;47(4):613-618.

59. Carmont MR, Maffulli N: Modified percutaneous repair of ruptured Achilles tendon. *Knee Surg Sports Traumatol Arthrosc* 2008;16(2):199-203.

60. Majewski M, Rohrbach M, Czaja S, Ochsner P: Avoiding sural nerve injuries during percutaneous Achilles tendon repair. *Am J Sports Med* 2006;34(5):793-798.

61. Aktas S, Kocaoglu B, Nalbantoglu U, Seyhan M, Guven O: End-to-end versus augmented repair in the treatment of acute Achilles tendon ruptures. *J Foot Ankle Surg* 2007;46(5):336-340.

62. de Vos RJ, Weir A, van Schie HT, et al: Platelet-rich plasma injection for chronic Achilles tendinopathy: A randomized controlled trial. *JAMA* 2010;303(2):144-149.

63. Schepull T, Kvist J, Norrman H, Trinks M, Berlin G, Aspenberg P: Autologous platelets have no effect on the healing of human achilles tendon ruptures: A randomized

single-blind study. *Am J Sports Med* 2011;39(1):38-47.

64. Mortensen HM, Skov O, Jensen PE: Early motion of the ankle after operative treatment of a rupture of the Achilles tendon: A prospective, randomized clinical and radiographic study. *J Bone Joint Surg Am* 1999;81(7):983-990.

65. Maffulli N, Tallon C, Wong J, Lim KP, Bleakney R: Early weightbearing and ankle mobilization after open repair of acute midsubstance tears of the achilles tendon. *Am J Sports Med* 2003;31(5):692-700.

66. Kangas J, Pajala A, Ohtonen P, Leppilahti J: Achilles tendon elongation after rupture repair: A randomized comparison of 2 postoperative regimens. *Am J Sports Med* 2007;35(1):59-64.

67. Healy B, Beasley R, Weatherall M: Venous thromboembolism following prolonged cast immobilisation for injury to the tendo Achillis. *J Bone Joint Surg Br* 2010;92(5):646-650.

68. Nilsson-Helander K, Thurin A, Karlsson J, Eriksson BI: High incidence of deep venous thrombosis after Achilles tendon rupture: A prospective study. *Knee Surg Sports Traumatol Arthrosc* 2009;17(10):1234-1238.

69. Patel A, Ogawa B, Charlton T, Thordarson D: Incidence of deep vein thrombosis and pulmonary embolism after Achilles tendon rupture. *Clin Orthop Relat Res* 2012;470(1):270-274.

Video Reference

20.1: Charlton TP: Video. *Achilles Tendon Rupture in Athletes*. Los Angeles, CA, 2016.

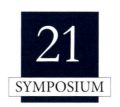

Lisfranc Injuries in the Elite Athlete

Michael Isiah Sandlin, MD
Cyrus E. Taghavi, MD
Timothy P. Charlton, MD
Robert B. Anderson, MD

Abstract

The management of sports-related Lisfranc injuries is optimized by a detailed understanding of the relevant anatomy, mechanisms of injury, clinical diagnostic maneuvers, imaging, and treatment options for patients with this disabling injury. A lower energy ligamentous variant Lisfranc injury, which was first observed in professional football players, has recently been described. The treatment options for patients with a Lisfranc injury include nonsurgical management, open reduction and internal fixation, suture-button fixation techniques, and arthrodesis.

Instr Course Lect 2017;66:275–280.

Injuries to the Lisfranc joint complex have classically been associated with high-energy trauma, such as that which occurs during motor vehicle collisions, falls from a height, and industrial accidents.[1,2] Recently, there has been increased identification of a spectrum of Lisfranc injuries that result from lower-energy trauma, such as that which occurs in sports. Foot injuries represent approximately 16% of all sports-related injuries, with midfoot sprains occurring in 4% of collegiate football players each year.[3] Offensive linemen (29%) are the collegiate football players who most commonly sustain midfoot sprains, and the mechanism of injury for midfoot sprain in collegiate football players more commonly involves a twisting injury (50%) rather than axial loading (37%).[4] In a study of 15 patients who had subtle injuries of the Lisfranc joint,

Faciszewski et al[5] reported that nine of the patients (60%) sustained injury via low-energy twisting mechanisms of injury, five of whom sustained injury while playing sports. Subtle Lisfranc injuries can have variable injury patterns and may be a challenge to diagnose, with delays in appropriate management resulting in persistent pain and disability. Treatment recommendations for patients who have a subtle ligamentous Lisfranc injury are based on joint diastasis and the instability pattern, with surgery performed to reduce the risk of joint degeneration and improve functional outcomes. Subtle ligamentous Lisfranc injuries are particularly relevant given the high demands an elite athlete places on the foot.

Video 21.1: Lisfranc Injuries in the Elite Athlete. Robert B. Anderson, MD (9 min)

Anatomy and Mechanism of Injury

Injuries to the Lisfranc joint complex may include disruption of the bony

Dr. Charlton or an immediate family member has stock or stock options held in the Green Bay Packers Football Club and the Manchester United Football Club. Dr. Anderson or an immediate family member has received royalties from Arthrex, DJ Orthopaedics, and Wright Medical Technology; and serves as a paid consultant to Amniox Medical, Wright Medical Technology, and Arthrex. Neither of the following authors nor any immediate family member has received anything of value from or has stock or stock options held in a commercial company or institution related directly or indirectly to the subject of this chapter: Dr. Sandlin and Dr. Taghavi.

and/or soft-tissue structures of the midfoot, including the tarsometatarsal (TMT), intercuneiform, cubocuneiform, and naviculocuneiform joints. In an uninjured foot, the combination of osseous architecture and stout capsuloligamentous support allows the midfoot to function as a rigid lever arm during gait. The keystone configuration of the recessed second metatarsal base within the mortise of the cuneiforms forms the classic Roman arch structure, which provides maximal bony stability. Capsuloligamentous support provides secondary, indirect stability via the plantar and dorsal bridging ligaments and the transverse intermetatarsal ligaments.[6] The plantar midfoot ligaments are three times stronger than the dorsal ligaments, which likely accounts for the typical dorsal dislocation pattern observed in patients who have a Lisfranc injury. Only the first and second metatarsals are without intermetatarsal ligamentous connection. The Lisfranc ligament is located plantarly between the medial cuneiform and second metatarsal base. The Lisfranc ligament in conjunction with two stout Y-shaped plantar ligaments that connect the medial cuneiform and the second and third metatarsal bases form the Lisfranc ligament complex, which is key to the overall stability of the Lisfranc joint. Injury to both the two plantar ligaments and the Lisfranc ligament is required before transverse instability is observed, whereas disruption of the interosseous ligaments between the medial and middle cuneiforms results in longitudinal instability.[7,8] Injuries to the Lisfranc joint complex range from mild sprains with no displacement to severe fracture-dislocations.

Sports-related Lisfranc injuries may involve two separate mechanisms of injury, which result in a spectrum of injury patterns. The classic mechanism of injury involves direct axial loading of the midfoot combined with a twisting or bending moment, such as that which occurs when an athlete, whose foot is plantarflexed and in contact with the ground, has another athlete fall on his or her heel. This mechanism of injury may result in intermetatarsal or first intercuneiform diastasis with or without fractures of the metatarsals or tarsal bones. A less common mechanism of injury involves a noncontact injury that typically is associated with cleated footwear and the increased torsional forces that occur with the use of high-friction spikes on turf surfaces.[9,10] In this mechanism of injury, an athlete generates an axial force via his or her plantarflexed and slightly rotated foot. When the athlete's cleated foot engages with the turf, his or her midfoot is subject to forceful abduction and/or twisting, such as that which occurs with dynamic push-off or a sudden change of direction. These sports-related Lisfranc injuries, which include proximal or medial column instability patterns that extend through the first intercuneiform articulation and naviculocuneiform joint, were first described in professional football players.[9,10]

Clinical Evaluation
Physical Examination
Low-energy Lisfranc injuries may be difficult to diagnose and are commonly missed on initial physical examination.[11-13] The clinical evaluation of an athlete is informed by a detailed history that includes activity type and a description of the foot position at the time of injury. In patients who have a more subtle Lisfranc injury, midfoot swelling and an inability to bear weight may be the only initial findings. Additional findings may include tenderness of the dorsal midfoot, TMT joints, and medial naviculocuneiform joint. Midfoot pain may be substantially increased with attempted weight bearing. Gentle stressing of the forefoot into plantar flexion and abduction also may elicit pain. Patients with proximal Lisfranc injury variants may have an unstable first ray and difficulty with toe push-off. Comparison of the injured foot with the contralateral foot may reveal subtle first ray hypermobility. Plantar ecchymosis may be a late finding.

Imaging
Imaging should include standard AP, oblique, and lateral foot radiographs. Weight-bearing radiographs are strongly recommended because subtle joint diastasis is missed on initial non–weight-bearing radiographs in as many as 20% of athletes who have a Lisfranc injury.[14] Comparison radiographs of the injured foot with the contralateral foot may be helpful to assess consistent anatomic relationships. Single-limb standing radiographs are recommended as tolerated by the patient. Radiographs should be evaluated for joint diastasis, malalignment, and loss of longitudinal arch height. Fleck cortical avulsion fractures also may be present. Foster and Foster[15] reported that the most consistent radiographic finding in patients who had Lisfranc injuries was loss of alignment of the medial border of the second metatarsal and the medial border of the middle cuneiform. If initial imaging findings are negative but a high suspicion for midfoot injury exists, repeat radiographs may be obtained in 7 to 14 days; however, plain radiographs may not reliably detect malalignment of 1 to 2 mm.[16] Stress radiographs

under fluoroscopic guidance may be obtained but should not be considered sufficient to rule out midfoot injury. Stress radiographs are obtained by stabilizing the hindfoot and applying alternating supination/pronation as well as abduction/adduction stresses to the forefoot. Displacement of 2 mm or more is commonly reported as suggestive of instability, whereas cadaver model studies have reported that joint diastasis of as little as 1.3 mm may differentiate between an intact and a torn Lisfranc ligament.[17]

Both CT and MRI provide superior anatomic detail; however, because CT and MRI typically are static, non–weight-bearing imaging modalities, they may not identify subtle force-dependent joint diastasis. Despite these limitations, CT can be used to evaluate fracture comminution and displacement, and MRI can help identify ligamentous injury.[18,19] In a study on the utility of MRI for the diagnosis of subtle Lisfranc injury, Raikin et al[19] reported that, compared with intraoperative stress assessment, disruption of the Lisfranc ligament complex on MRI was the strongest predictor of instability, reliably identifying disruption in 90% of Lisfranc ligament complex injuries.

Treatment

The management of Lisfranc injury in athletes is based on the goal of attaining and maintaining anatomic alignment, which provides the best long-term outcomes.[14] According to Nunley and Vertullo,[14] nonsurgical treatment should be reserved for patients who have a nondisplaced stable Lisfranc injury. The authors proposed a classification system for Lisfranc injuries in athletes based on clinical examination findings, weight-bearing radiographic evaluation,

and bone scintigraphy results. Stage I Lisfranc injuries are considered stable injuries, demonstrating no joint diastasis on radiographs and positive bone scintigraphy results. Stage II Lisfranc injuries involve rupture of the Lisfranc ligament, with 1 to 5 mm of joint diastasis and no longitudinal arch height loss. Stage III Lisfranc injuries involve 1 to 5 mm or more of joint diastasis and loss of longitudinal arch height. Nunley and Vertullo[14] recommended nonsurgical treatment for patients who had stage I Lisfranc injuries and surgical fixation for patients who had stage II or stage III Lisfranc injuries.

Surgical indications for sports-related Lisfranc injury do not include a specific threshold for joint diastasis and are based on instability as much as the amount of displacement. The stability of the TMT, intermetatarsal, intercuneiform, and naviculocuneiform joints should be assessed and addressed surgically if they are unstable. Lisfranc injuries, even those with a seemingly stable injury pattern, that fail to improve with nonsurgical treatment should raise concern for subtle instability that may require intraoperative assessment.

Nonsurgical Treatment

Nonsurgical management of Lisfranc injury in athletes is controversial. Curtis et al[20] recommended surgical intervention for all athletes and active patients; however, nonsurgical management has been successful in athletes who are returning to high-level sports activity.[4,14,21] Ideally, nonsurgical treatment in athletes is reserved for those with stage I Lisfranc injuries in whom minimal to no displacement is observed on CT. Nonsurgical treatment of 6 weeks of non–weight-bearing in a cast has shown excellent results.[14]

In minimally symptomatic patients with a Lisfranc injury that appears stable, some studies have recommended 2 weeks of protected weight bearing in a cast or boot followed by a repeat physical examination and repeat weight-bearing radiographs. In these patients, if stability is maintained and the repeat physical examination is asymptomatic, then a graded return to activity with or without the use of an orthotic support for several months is allowed as tolerated.[14,22] Despite reported successes in the nonsurgical management of Lisfranc injuries, multiple studies have reported poor results in both athletic and nonathletic patients who underwent nonsurgical treatment for Lisfranc injuries that were unstable or in whom joint diastasis was present.[23-26]

Surgical Treatment

Surgery, if undertaken, should be performed as soon after injury as the soft tissues allow. In patients with severe Lisfranc injury, Trevino and Kodros[26] as well as Arntz et al[27] recommended performing surgery within the first 24 hours postinjury. A 1- to 2-week delay of surgery to allow for swelling to subside may be appropriate and does not appear to alter long-term outcomes;[18] however, surgical correction that is performed 6 weeks or more postinjury generally results in poorer outcomes.[18]

Regardless of which surgical treatment option is selected, the goal is to attain a stable, anatomic reduction of the Lisfranc injury. Closed reduction may be possible in some patients; however, several studies have reported that restoration of anatomic reduction and joint congruency is best achieved via open reduction.[28,29] Kirschner wire (K-wire) fixation has been described for the definitive fixation of minimally displaced Lisfranc injuries;[30-32] however, because of the biomechanical superiority of screw fixation and the higher rate of complications after K-wire fixation, including loss of reduction, pin migration, and pin site infection, K-wire fixation has been largely abandoned.[23,28,32]

Current recommendations for the surgical management of Lisfranc injury support screw fixation after open reduction.[33] Surgical techniques for screw fixation and open reduction vary; however, many surgeons who perform Lisfranc fixation with isolated 3.5-mm, 4.0-mm, or 4.5-mm screws report excellent results.[22,27,34,35] Despite reported successes of screw fixation and open reduction, concern for chondral injury exists. Alberta et al[33] reported that a 3.5-mm screw can damage 2% to 3.6% of the articular surface of the TMT joint. However, Gaines et al[36] reported that a 4.0-mm cannulated screw can damage 3.2% to 5.3% of the articular surface of the TMT joint. The authors reported that more than one guidewire passage attempt led to fractures of the metatarsal base and cuneiform in more than 40% of the cadaver models in the study. Fixation with extra-articular plate constructs is advantageous because it avoids articular cartilage damage. Dorsal plating techniques have been reported to be at least as stable as transarticular screw constructs, and plantar plating techniques have been reported to provide even more stability, albeit at the cost of additional soft-tissue dissection and difficulty with hardware removal.[33,37] Locking plate technology has helped advance dorsal plating techniques and improved construct strength.[37] Although newer-generation plate and screw constructs are lower

profile, dorsal plates increase the risk for hardware irritation and, therefore, delayed hardware removal. Hardware removal, if undertaken, typically occurs no earlier than 4 to 6 months after fixation.

Suture button fixation of Lisfranc injury has been performed in an attempt to provide a more physiologic fixation and decrease the need for delayed screw removal. However, in a recent cadaver model study, Ahmed et al[38] reported that, compared with 4.0-mm cannulated screw fixation, suture button fixation resulted in increased intermetatarsal stress widening; therefore, the authors recommended the continued use of screw fixation for the management of Lisfranc injuries. Fourth or fifth TMT joint injury, although less common in patients who have a low-energy Lisfranc injury, if unstable, may require percutaneous K-wire fixation for 6 weeks followed by hardware removal.

The role of primary arthrodesis in the management of Lisfranc injury is controversial. Ly and Coetzee[24] reported that arthrodesis resulted in lower complication and revision surgery rates compared with open reduction and internal fixation (ORIF). Conversely, Mulier et al[39] reported that, at a follow-up of 30 months, patients who underwent ORIF or partial arthrodesis had decreased rates of pain, forefoot stiffness, metatarsal arch loss, and complex regional pain syndrome without an increased risk for revision surgery compared with patients who underwent complete arthrodesis. Interestingly, degenerative joint changes were observed on the plain radiographs of 94% of the patients who underwent ORIF; because a substantial portion of these patients required eventual arthrodesis, the authors reported that partial arthrodesis

may be the preferred surgical treatment option for patients with a Lisfranc injury in whom fracture comminution or substantially displaced ligamentous injuries are present. Although arthrodesis may result in improved pain and function in patients in whom Lisfranc injury is missed and in patients who have posttraumatic arthritis, the authors of this chapter do not prefer to use arthrodesis for the management of acute athletic Lisfranc injuries. Despite reports of professional athletes returning to a high of level play after arthrodesis of a Lisfranc injury, the authors of this chapter do not recommend arthrodesis for the treatment of elite athletes who have a Lisfranc injury, and believe that primary ORIF results in better overall pain and functional outcomes.[14,28]

The treatment recommendation of the authors of this chapter for elite athletes who have a Lisfranc injury includes a low threshold for an open, intraoperative evaluation of stability. The authors of this chapter perform internal fixation of all unstable segments, with dorsal bridge plating of the TMT joints to preserve joint surfaces. Care is taken to evaluate for subtle ligamentous injuries that extend to the proximal midfoot; fixation of these injuries includes intercuneiform stabilization with one or two screws. The authors of this chapter have reported that naviculocuneiform fixation is rarely necessary after fixation of the adjacent midfoot joints; however, they recommend observation of the medial naviculocuneiform column for collapse because it can deteriorate rapidly. The authors of this chapter avoid arthrodesis for the treatment of athletes who have a Lisfranc injury because of the risks previously discussed as well as the potential for symptomatic malunion or nonunion.

Postoperative Management

Postoperative management for patients with Lisfranc injuries includes 2 weeks of splint immobilization followed by the transition to a boot and initiation of a non–weight-bearing rehabilitation program. Weight bearing in a walking boot is begun at 6 weeks postoperatively. At 3 months postoperatively, patients are transitioned to normal shoe wear with molded orthotic support. Because of the prolonged healing time for ligaments, the authors of this chapter routinely retain fixation hardware for a minimum of 4 months. Despite lower profile plate and screw technology, the authors of this chapter have found that dorsal bridge plates can still become symptomatic and may require removal; however, plates or screws are less likely to become symptomatic if they break before removal. Intercuneiform screws are kept in situ indefinitely because of the concern for late joint diastasis. The authors of this chapter counsel patients on the relatively long postoperative recovery for Lisfranc injuries. In a study of 170 patients who underwent surgical treatment for a Lisfranc injury, Brunet and Wiley[40] reported an ongoing improvement in symptoms until 1.3 years postoperatively, with 80% of patients being pain free and most patients returning to their preinjury level of activity and sport. Although chronic discomfort and stiffness may occur in some patients, it rarely limits function.

Complications

Posttraumatic joint degeneration is the most common complication of Lisfranc injury. Delayed diagnosis of a Lisfranc injury and malunion increases the risk for posttraumatic arthritis. In a retrospective study of 92 patients with a Lisfranc injury who underwent ORIF, Kuo et al[23] reported that arthritis developed in 25% of the patients, 50% of whom required arthrodesis. Limited evidence on the long-term outcomes of athletes who undergo treatment for Lisfranc injury exists. Typically, sports-related midfoot injuries are low-energy injuries that include a higher rate of stage I and stage II Lisfranc injuries, in which substantially better outcomes are reported. In a study of 17 professional soccer and rugby athletes with a Lisfranc injury who underwent surgical treatment, Deol et al[41] reported that only one athlete retired as a result of injury. All of the other athletes had a mean time of return to sport training and full competition of 20.1 weeks and 25.3 weeks, respectively. The patients with ligamentous injuries had a slightly earlier mean time of return to competition compared with the patients who had bony injuries (22.5 weeks versus 26.9 weeks, respectively).

Summary

Lisfranc injuries in athletes are typically low-energy injuries that include variable instability patterns, which may add to the challenges of diagnosis and treatment. A high level of suspicion for Lisfranc injury as well as a careful physical examination, a thorough evaluation of imaging, and prompt treatment may allow athletes to return to a high level of competition and maximize functional outcomes. Typically, nonsurgical treatment is reserved for patients who have a stable stage I Lisfranc injury. Surgical treatment, which is recommended for patients who have displaced or unstable injury patterns, involves attaining a stable anatomic articular reduction of the Lisfranc injury without causing iatrogenic chondral injury. Arthrodesis should be reserved for patients who have complex high-energy fracture patterns with chondral injury and is rarely indicated in athletes who have a Lisfranc injury. Despite optimal treatment, elite athletes with a Lisfranc injury may have a prolonged postoperative recovery; therefore, athletes, sports teams, and athletic trainers should be aware of the severity of Lisfranc injury.

References

1. Hardcastle PH, Reschauer R, Kutscha-Lissberg E, Schoffmann W: Injuries to the tarsometatarsal joint: Incidence, classification and treatment. *J Bone Joint Surg Br* 1982;64(3):349-356.

2. Myerson MS, Fisher RT, Burgess AR, Kenzora JE: Fracture dislocations of the tarsometatarsal joints: End results correlated with pathology and treatment. *Foot Ankle* 1986;6(5):225-242.

3. Garrick JG, Requa RK: The epidemiology of foot and ankle injuries in sports. *Clin Sports Med* 1988;7(1):29-36.

4. Meyer SA, Callaghan JJ, Albright JP, Crowley ET, Powell JW: Midfoot sprains in collegiate football players. *Am J Sports Med* 1994;22(3):392-401.

5. Faciszewski T, Burks RT, Manaster BJ: Subtle injuries of the Lisfranc joint. *J Bone Joint Surg Am* 1990;72(10):1519-1522.

6. Peicha G, Labovitz J, Seibert FJ, et al: The anatomy of the joint as a risk factor for Lisfranc dislocation and fracture-dislocation. An anatomical and radiological case control study. *J Bone Joint Surg Br* 2002;84(7):981-985.

7. Kaar S, Femino J, Morag Y: Lisfranc joint displacement following sequential ligament sectioning. *J Bone Joint Surg Am* 2007;89(10):2225-2232.

8. Pearce CJ, Calder JD: Surgical anatomy of the midfoot. *Knee Surg Sports Traumatol Arthrosc* 2010;18(5):581-586.

9. Anderson RB, Hammit MD: Recognizing and treating the subtle Lisfranc injury. Presented at the 20th Annual Summer Meeting of the American Orthopaedic Foot and Ankle Society, Seattle, WA, July 29-31, 2004.

10. Ardoin GT, Anderson RB: Subtle Lisfranc injury. *Tech Foot Ankle Surg* 2010;9(3):100-106.

11. Burroughs KE, Reimer CD, Fields KB: Lisfranc injury of the foot: A commonly missed diagnosis. *Am Fam Physician* 1998;58(1):118-124.

12. Englanoff G, Anglin D, Hutson HR: Lisfranc fracture-dislocation: A frequently missed diagnosis in the emergency department. *Ann Emerg Med* 1995;26(2):229-233.

13. Perron AD, Brady WJ, Keats TE: Orthopedic pitfalls in the ED: Lisfranc fracture-dislocation. *Am J Emerg Med* 2001;19(1):71-75.

14. Nunley JA, Vertullo CJ: Classification, investigation, and management of midfoot sprains: Lisfranc injuries in the athlete. *Am J Sports Med* 2002;30(6):871-878.

15. Foster SC, Foster RR: Lisfranc's tarsometatarsal fracture-dislocation. *Radiology* 1976;120(1):79-83.

16. Lu J, Ebraheim NA, Skie M, Porshinsky B, Yeasting RA: Radiographic and computed tomographic evaluation of Lisfranc dislocation: A cadaver study. *Foot Ankle Int* 1997;18(6):351-355.

17. Panchbhavi VK, Andersen CR, Vallurupalli S, Yang J: A minimally disruptive model and three-dimensional evaluation of Lisfranc joint diastasis. *J Bone Joint Surg Am* 2008;90(12):2707-2713.

18. Buzzard BM, Briggs PJ: Surgical management of acute tarsometatarsal fracture dislocation in the adult. *Clin Orthop Relat Res* 1998;353:125-133.

19. Raikin SM, Elias I, Dheer S, Besser MP, Morrison WB, Zoga AC: Prediction of midfoot instability in the subtle Lisfranc injury: Comparison of magnetic resonance imaging with intraoperative findings. *J Bone Joint Surg Am* 2009;91(4):892-899.

20. Curtis MJ, Myerson M, Szura B: Tarsometatarsal joint injuries in the athlete. *Am J Sports Med* 1993;21(4):497-502.

21. Shapiro MS, Wascher DC, Finerman GA: Rupture of Lisfranc's ligament in athletes. *Am J Sports Med* 1994;22(5):687-691.

22. Eleftheriou KI, Rosenfeld PF: Lisfranc injury in the athlete: Evidence supporting management from sprain to fracture dislocation. *Foot Ankle Clin* 2013;18(2):219-236.

23. Kuo RS, Tejwani NC, Digiovanni CW, et al: Outcome after open reduction and internal fixation of Lisfranc joint injuries. *J Bone Joint Surg Am* 2000;82(11):1609-1618.

24. Ly TV, Coetzee JC: Treatment of primarily ligamentous Lisfranc joint injuries: Primary arthrodesis compared with open reduction and internal fixation. A prospective, randomized study. *J Bone Joint Surg Am* 2006;88(3):514-520.

25. Rajapakse B, Edwards A, Hong T: A single surgeon's experience of treatment of Lisfranc joint injuries. *Injury* 2006;37(9):914-921.

26. Trevino SG, Kodros S: Controversies in tarsometatarsal injuries. *Orthop Clin North Am* 1995;26(2):229-238.

27. Arntz CT, Veith RG, Hansen ST Jr: Fractures and fracture-dislocations of the tarsometatarsal joint. *J Bone Joint Surg Am* 1988;70(2):173-181.

28. Rammelt S, Schneiders W, Schikore H, Holch M, Heineck J, Zwipp H: Primary open reduction and fixation compared with delayed corrective arthrodesis in the treatment of tarsometatarsal (Lisfranc) fracture dislocation. *J Bone Joint Surg Br* 2008;90(11):1499-1506.

29. Pérez Blanco R, Rodríguez Merchán C, Canosa Sevillano R, Munuera Martínez L: Tarsometatarsal fractures and dislocations. *J Orthop Trauma* 1988;2(3):188-194.

30. Tan YH, Chin TW, Mitra AK, Tan SK: Tarsometatarsal (Lisfranc's) injuries— results of open reduction and internal fixation. *Ann Acad Med Singapore* 1995;24(6):816-819.

31. Lee CA, Birkedal JP, Dickerson EA, Vieta PA Jr, Webb LX, Teasdall RD: Stabilization of Lisfranc joint injuries: A biomechanical study. *Foot Ankle Int* 2004;25(5):365-370.

32. Stavlas P, Roberts CS, Xypnitos FN, Giannoudis PV: The role of reduction and internal fixation of Lisfranc fracture-dislocations: A systematic review of the literature. *Int Orthop* 2010;34(8):1083-1091.

33. Alberta FG, Aronow MS, Barrero M, Diaz-Doran V, Sullivan RJ, Adams DJ: Ligamentous Lisfranc joint injuries: A biomechanical comparison of dorsal plate and transarticular screw fixation. *Foot Ankle Int* 2005;26(6):462-473.

34. DeOrio M, Erickson M, Usuelli FG, Easley M: Lisfranc injuries in sport. *Foot Ankle Clin* 2009;14(2):169-186.

35. Sangeorzan BJ, Hansen ST Jr: Early and late posttraumatic foot reconstruction. *Clin Orthop Relat Res* 1989;243:86-91.

36. Gaines RJ, Wright G, Stewart J: Injury to the tarsometatarsal joint complex during fixation of Lisfranc fracture dislocations: An anatomic study. *J Trauma* 2009;66(4):1125-1128.

37. Cantu RV, Koval KJ: The use of locking plates in fracture care. *J Am Acad Orthop Surg* 2006;14(3):183-190.

38. Ahmed S, Bolt B, McBryde A: Comparison of standard screw fixation versus suture button fixation in Lisfranc ligament injuries. *Foot Ankle Int* 2010;31(10):892-896.

39. Mulier T, Reynders P, Dereymaeker G, Broos P: Severe Lisfrancs injuries: Primary arthrodesis or ORIF? *Foot Ankle Int* 2002;23(10):902-905.

40. Brunet JA, Wiley JJ: The late results of tarsometatarsal joint injuries. *J Bone Joint Surg Br* 1987;69(3):437-440.

41. Deol RS, Roche A, Calder JD: Return to training and playing after acute Lisfranc injury in elite professional soccer and rugby players. *Am J Sports Med* 2016;44(1):166-170.

Video Reference

21.1: Anderson RB: Video. *Lisfranc Injuries in the Elite Athlete*. Charlotte, NC, 2016.

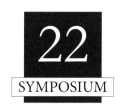

High-Risk Stress Fractures in Elite Athletes

Michael Isiah Sandlin, MD
Andrew J. Rosenbaum, MD
Cyrus E. Taghavi, MD
Timothy P. Charlton, MD
Martin J. O'Malley, MD

Abstract

Surgeons should understand common factors that predispose high-level athletes to stress injuries as well as the importance of vitamin D and specifics related to vascular supply, location of injury, biomechanics, and susceptibility factors in high-level athletes who have stress injuries. Surgeons should be aware of diagnostic- and management-based recommendations for and the outcomes of anterior tibia, medial malleolus, tarsal navicular, and proximal fifth metatarsal stress fractures in professional athletes.

Instr Course Lect 2017;66:281–292.

Stress fractures and stress reactions are conditions that exist on a spectrum that ranges from maladaptive bone response to strain. Under normal circumstances, increased strain leads to coordinated resorption and remodeling, which results in stronger bone. If adaptive mechanisms are overloaded by increased duration or intensity of activity or an athlete is not getting sufficient rest or nutrition, the imbalance leads to fatigue failure. A stress reaction, which precedes a stress fracture, is observed as periosteal thickening and bone marrow edema on MRI.[1] As repetitive strain accumulates and overwhelms the regenerative potential of a bone, a stress fracture occurs.

Stress fractures are relatively rare in the general adult population, occurring in 0.5% of individuals annually.[2] The incidence of stress fractures in the athletic population is much higher, accounting for approximately 15% to 20% of overuse injuries in athletes, with an estimated annual incidence that ranges from 2% to 21%.[3-5] Armstrong et al[6] reported that approximately 5% of US Navy military recruits sustained stress fractures during training. Retrospective studies have reported a higher incidence of bone stress injuries in female runners and track and field athletes compared with male runners and track and field athletes.[5,7,8] More than 95% of stress fractures occur in the lower extremity.[3,6,9] The primary location of stress fracture is the tibia (49%) followed by the tarsal bones (25%), metatarsals (9%), femur (7%), fibula (7%), pelvis (2%), hallux sesamoids (1%), and spine (0.6%).[3]

Stress fractures are categorized as high risk or low risk based on the risk for progression to completion, delayed union, nonunion, and refracture.[10-12] Low-risk stress fractures include posteromedial tibia, femoral diaphysis, rib, ulnar shaft, calcaneal,

Dr. Rosenbaum or an immediate family member serves as a board member, owner, officer, or committee member of the American Orthopaedic Foot and Ankle Society. Dr. Charlton or an immediate family member has stock or stock options held in the Green Bay Packers Football Club and the Manchester United Football Club. Dr. O'Malley or an immediate family member serves as a paid consultant to CurveBeam. Neither of the following authors nor any immediate family member has received anything of value from or has stock or stock options held in a commercial company or institution related directly or indirectly to the subject of this chapter: Dr. Sandlin and Dr. Taghavi.

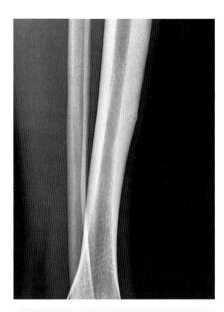

Figure 1 Lateral radiograph of the tibia of a 20-year-old man who is a professional basketball player with a 2-month history of pretibial discomfort in his left lower extremity demonstrates an anterior tibia stress fracture.

and first through fourth metatarsal fractures.[11] High-risk stress fractures include tension-sided femoral neck, patellar, anterior tibial cortex, medial malleolus, talar, tarsal navicular, fifth metatarsal, and hallux sesamoid fractures. High-risk stress fractures are believed to be the result of tensile forces and vascular insufficiency at the site of injury.[10] Low-risk stress fractures rarely require surgical intervention and can be managed symptomatically with respect to return to play. Typically, high-risk stress fractures that are managed nonsurgically result in delayed healing, which can substantially increase loss of time from sport. Surgical management options include percutaneous fixation or open fixation, with possible bone marrow augmentation techniques at the fracture site.

Intrinsic factors in athletes that contribute to the risk for stress fractures include general metabolic state, muscle size and endurance, hormone function, foot type, lower limb structural patterns (ie, Q angle, limb-length discrepancy, pes planus, or pes cavus), body habitus, female sex, menstrual patterns, and the female athlete triad.[7] Women who meet the criteria for the female athlete triad (low-energy availability [disordered eating], amenorrhea, and osteoporosis) have a 50% increased risk for stress fractures.[13] Extrinsic factors in athletes that contribute to the risk for stress fractures include training regimen; playing surface; footwear; and dietary habits, including nutrient or caloric deficiencies. Ogan and Pritchett[14] reported that approximately 77% of the general adult population is vitamin D insufficient. Vitamin D insufficiency is particularly relevant for athletes because vitamin D levels can affect physical performance, including muscle strength, pain signaling, and balance, as well as bone health. Lappe et al[15] reported a 20% lower incidence of stress fractures in female US Navy military recruits who received 800 IU of vitamin D per day for 8 weeks. In a prospective study of 800 Finnish male military recruits, Ruohola et al[16] reported that vitamin D status was a determinant of peak bone mass, and that vitamin D levels that were below the reported median vitamin D level were significantly associated with an increased risk for stress fracture. Recommendations for patients who have a high risk for stress fractures include a minimum intake of 1,000 mg of calcium and 1,000 to 2,000 IU of vitamin D_3 per day.[17] In female athletes, cyclical therapy with conjugated estrogens and progesterone also may be considered.[9]

Tibial Stress Fractures

Tibial stress fractures are fairly common. Matheson et al[3] reported that nearly one-half of all stress fractures (49.1%) occur in the tibia. Tibial stress fractures typically result in lower limb pain that begins at the onset of activity. The pain may be localized to the shin area or radiate to the ankle or knee and can result from any number of sporting activities. Distance running is the most common sport in which these injuries occur; however, tibial stress fractures have been reported to occur in athletes who participate in ballet, volleyball, basketball, gymnastics, or rowing.[18-24] The location of these stress fractures determine management options and prognosis.[25] Posteromedial tibia stress fractures occur on the compression side of the bone and, therefore, respond more readily to rest and activity modifications. Anterior tibia stress fractures are less common and more difficult to manage. Anterior tibia stress fractures occur on the tension side of the bone and have a hypovascular environment with limited soft-tissue attachments and supporting structures (**Figure 1**). Runners may have a higher risk for posteromedial tibia stress fractures, whereas athletes who perform repetitive leaping and jumping activities may have a higher risk for anterior tibia stress fractures.[26]

Physical Examination

Because the complaints of patients who have a suspected tibial stress fracture are often vague, the physical examination findings will vary depending on the degree of symptoms. Often, patients will have an antalgic gait. Swelling is variably present. Because of the subcutaneous position of the anterior tibia, tenderness to palpation can help identify the area of maximal discomfort. Athletes may have slightly different locations of maximal tenderness on physical examination. Maximal tenderness is likely to be localized to the middle third of the tibia in ballet dancers, the proximal third of the tibia in military recruits, and the junction of the middle and distal thirds of the tibia in runners.[27,28]

Imaging

Radiographs, which are the first step in imaging studies, may reveal periosteal reaction, cortical thickening, early callus formation, or radiolucent lines. The dreaded black line that is observed on the radiographs of patients who have high-risk anterior tibial cortex fractures may predict poor results if nonsurgical management is undertaken.[26] Radiographs obtained 1 week postinjury will reveal changes in only 10% of patients who have tibial stress fractures; peak radiographic changes can be observed at 6 weeks postinjury.[3,29] Previously, technetium bone scanning was the imaging modality of choice for the evaluation of stress reactions and early stress fractures; however, technetium bone scanning has been largely replaced by MRI. Similar to technetium bone scanning, MRI has a high sensitivity for stress reactions and stress fractures;[30] however, it also provides surgeons with anatomic detail of the surrounding soft tissues.

Treatment

Usually, surgical management is reserved for patients with tibial stress fractures in whom nonsurgical management of rest and graded rehabilitation fails. Some studies, however, recommend early surgical treatment for elite athletes with tibial stress fractures to decrease loss of time from sport.[31] In a study of eight basketball players with anterior cortex stress fractures who underwent nonsurgical treatment that consisted of rest and electrical stimulation, Rettig et al[32] reported that a mean of 8.7 months of nonsurgical treatment was required before the basketball players returned to activity.

Surgical management of tibial stress fractures typically involves intramedullary nail fixation with or without reaming and with or without bone grafting. Some surgeons suggest that chronic stress fractures function similar to pseudoarthroses; therefore, excision of interfragmentary fibrous material via additional drilling of the injury site and bone grafting are recommended to stimulate healing.[33] Reamed intramedullary fixation delivers local bone graft to the fracture site via deposition of reamings and stabilizes the tibial fracture site with the use of a load-sharing implant.[34,35] In a study of 11 college-level athletes with chronic anterior tibia stress fractures who underwent reamed intramedullary nail fixation, Varner et al[25] reported that all of the fractures had healed by 3 months postoperatively, and that the mean return to play was 4 months postoperatively. Surgeons who perform intramedullary rod fixation in athletes should consider a parapatellar approach and avoid proximal nail prominence to limit potential injury to the patellar tendon. Attaining a good cortical fit with intramedullary fixation may obviate the need for distal interlocking screws and, thus, eliminate the risk for potential hardware irritation.

Complications of intramedullary nail fixation, which primarily are reported in the orthopaedic trauma literature, include chronic anterior knee pain and muscular atrophy. In a study of 50 patients with tibial shaft fractures who underwent intramedullary nail fixation, Väistö et al[36] reported chronic anterior knee pain in 29% of the patients at a follow-up of 8 years, regardless of whether a parapatellar or transpatellar tendon insertion technique was used. In a study of 56 patients with tibia fractures who underwent intramedullary tibial nail fixation, Lefaivre et al[37] reported knee pain in 73.2% of the patients and quadriceps and calf atrophy in 27.3% of the patients.

These complications may be less likely in athletes who undergo treatment for chronic stress injuries. Chang and Harris[38] retrospectively analyzed the records of five active-duty military patients with chronic anterior tibial stress fractures who underwent intramedullary nailing. All of the patients had undergone a minimum of 1 year of nonsurgical treatment before they underwent intramedullary nailing. The authors reported that two of the patients had excellent outcomes, with no residual symptoms and unlimited pain-free running, and three of the patients had good outcomes, with occasional pain during high-level activity and limited pain-free running. In a study of a competitive athlete with a stress fracture who underwent bilateral tibial nailing, Gardiner et al[39] reported no fracture or knee pain at 4 weeks postoperatively and return to competition without restriction by 6 months postoperatively. In a study of a college football player with an anterior tibial stress fracture who underwent intramedullary nailing and aggressive rehabilitation, Kelly et al[40] reported symmetric thigh girth at 4 weeks postoperatively, quadriceps and hamstring strength at 5 weeks postoperatively, and a return to competitive sport at 4 months postoperatively.

However, the surgical management of tibial stress fractures in athletes is not without risk. In a case study of a patient with a chronic tibial stress fracture who underwent intramedullary nailing, Pandya et al[41] reported a recurrent stress fracture that required revision intramedullary nailing and open bone grafting. In a study of three female collegiate athletes with chronic tibial stress fractures who underwent intramedullary nailing, Yamada and Kahanov[42] reported distal tibia peri-implant stress reactions that required additional surgical management.

Anterior tension band plating techniques also have been described for the management of tibial stress fractures. In a study of four high-level female athletes with anterior tibial cortex stress fractures who underwent anterior tension band plating, Borens et al[33] reported complete fracture healing in all four of the patients, a mean return to activity of 10 weeks postoperatively, and no complications. In a study of 12 professional or college athletes who underwent anterior tension band plating for the management of 13 chronic anterior tibial stress fractures in which a trial of nonsurgical management failed, Zbeda et al[43] reported that 92% of the patients returned to their prior level of competition at a mean follow-up of 11.1 weeks; however, 38% of the patients required an additional procedure to remove prominent hardware.

Medial Malleolus Stress Fractures

Medial malleolus stress fractures are relatively rare, accounting for 1% to 4% of lower extremity stress fractures.[44,45] Often, medial malleolus stress fractures occur in high-level athletes who participate in running and jumping activities. In a study of eight patients who had medial malleolus stress fractures, Orava et al[46] reported that seven of the patients were high-level or internationally competitive athletes who participated in sprinting, jumping, hurdling, and middle-distance running, and one of the patients was a recreational athlete who reportedly walked a substantial amount on uneven ground. Several studies[26,46,47] have reported that patients with specific anatomic findings, including narrow tibial canals, leg-length discrepancy, pes cavus, forefoot or subtalar varus, increased external hip rotation, and tibial varus, are predisposed to medial malleolus stress fractures. Biomechanically, loads across the ankle in patients who have varus alignment of the foot, ankle, or distal tibia subject the medial malleolus to increased shear and rotational stresses; however, this malalignment may not be clinically significant or require specific treatment. In a study of seven patients with medial malleolus stress fractures, Schils et al[48] reported malalignment (bilateral tibial varus) in only one of the patients; the patient was successfully treated nonsurgically. Okada et al[49] reported that distal tibial varus was an important etiologic factor of a medial malleolus stress fracture in a Kendo fencing athlete; the athlete was successfully treated nonsurgically. Realignment procedures in high-level athletes should be carefully considered because they may result in complications, such as postoperative stiffness, residual deformity, delayed union, or nonunion. To the knowledge of the authors of this chapter, the use of osteotomies to correct malalignment in elite athletes who have medial malleolus stress fractures has not been reported in the literature.

Physical Examination

Initial symptoms of medial malleolus stress fractures tend to be poorly localized medial ankle or distal leg pain. As the injury progresses, focal tenderness at the medial malleolus may occur. Similar to other stress fractures, activity aggravates the injury and rest relieves pain. Often, the physical examination will reveal an antalgic gait, normal ankle range of motion, and, in patients who have advanced injuries, joint or soft-tissue swelling. Varus ankle malalignment should be assessed because it has been reported to be a risk factor for medial malleolus stress fractures.[48]

Imaging

Typically, radiographs of patients who have medial malleolus stress fractures will appear negative for up to 6 to 8 weeks postinjury, after which an oblique or vertically oriented fracture line may be observed. Anteromedial distal tibial spurring also may be present.[50] MRI is a useful adjunct and can provide surgeons with detail of the fracture pattern (**Figure 2, A**). Although fine-cut CT is less sensitive in the diagnosis of stress fractures compared with MRI, it may provide surgeons with additional bony details, including possible anteromedial distal tibial spurring.[50]

Treatment

Medial malleolus stress fractures can be successfully managed nonsurgically. In a study of eight patients with a medial malleolus fracture, Orava et al[46] reported that five patients were successfully treated nonsurgically. Of the three patients who were treated surgically, one patient required screw fixation because of high-risk vertical fracture orientation, and two patients required drilling for delayed healing after several months of initial nonsurgical treatment. Nonsurgical management of medial malleolus stress fractures includes immobilization and rest for 3 to 8 weeks; patients are transitioned to a walking boot after they are pain free. Symptoms may take 4 to 5 months or more to resolve with nonsurgical management.

Indications for the surgical management of medial malleolus stress fractures include displaced fractures or, in high-level athletes, a fracture line, a perilucency cyst, or local osteopenia that is observed on plain radiographs.[51] Compared with nonsurgical management, surgical management is associated with a faster rate of fracture healing (6.7 months versus 4.2 months, respectively), a faster return to sports (7 weeks versus 4.5 weeks, respectively), and a potentially lower probability of nonunion.[50,52] Mean return to sport after the surgical management of medial malleolus stress fractures has been reported to be 4.2 months postoperatively.[4] Although some studies have advocated for the arthroscopic removal of any impinging osteophyte lesions,[50] the literature on the management of these lesions is limited.

Timing with regard to sporting season may be a factor for athletes who attempt nonsurgical treatment. Treatment considerations include parallel screw techniques versus medial plating constructs. Plate-screw constructs are biomechanically superior if they are placed perpendicular to a vertically oriented fracture line (**Figure 2, B**). Percutaneous screw fixation requires less exposure and allows for a faster recovery; however, poor healing has been reported in some high-level athletes who underwent percutaneous screw fixation with isolated screws. Drilling of the fracture site may be considered in

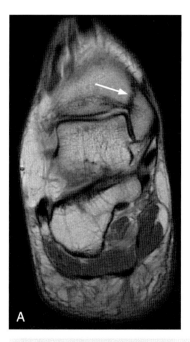 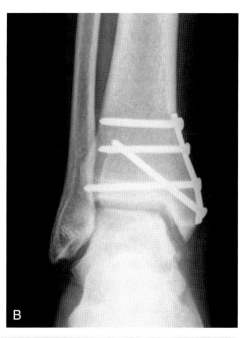

Figure 2   Images of the medial malleolus of a 22-year-old man who is a professional basketball player. **A,** Coronal T1-weighted MRI shows a medial malleolus stress fracture (arrow). **B,** AP radiograph taken 6 weeks after open reduction and internal fixation demonstrates union of the medial malleolus stress fracture. The patient was able to return to sport at this time.

patients in whom nonsurgical management results in delayed union.[46]

Tarsal Navicular Stress Fractures

Traditionally, tarsal navicular stress fractures were considered uncommon, with a reported incidence that ranged from 0.7% to 2.4%.[53,54] Current estimates suggest that tarsal navicular stress fractures are more common than previously believed, accounting for 14% to 35% of all foot and ankle stress fractures.[5,44,55] An increase in surgeon awareness and the increased use of advanced imaging modalities may partially explain this increase in tarsal navicular stress fractures.[56] Athletes with highest risk for tarsal navicular stress fractures include those who participate in sprinting, jumping, or explosive forefoot push-off activities. These athletes often report dorsal midfoot or

ankle pain that is worse with weight bearing, particularly at the onset of activity.

The tarsal navicular, which is located in the medial midfoot, forms part of the structural link between the hindfoot and forefoot, allowing for force transmission and push-off during ambulation. The navicular, via its robust ligamentous attachments and bony articulations, lends stability to the longitudinal and transverse arches of the foot. The tarsal navicular bone articulates with the three cuneiforms distally and the talar head proximally. The articulations with the cuneiforms allow for minimal motion and maximal stability, whereas the articulation with the talar head allows for a high degree of rotation and multiplanar translation. Motion allowed by these articulations allows for hindfoot inversion/eversion and midfoot abduction/adduction. Fusion of the talonavicular joint diminishes normal hindfoot eversion and inversion by more than 80%.[57]

The vascular anatomy of the tarsal navicular is important in the development of tarsal navicular stress fractures. The blood supply of the tarsal navicular arises from the dorsal tarsal navicular branch of the dorsalis pedis artery and the plantar tarsal navicular branch of the posterior tibial artery. Torg et al[58] reported that the anastomosis of these vessels allows for adequate intraosseous blood supply laterally and medially; however, blood supply to the dorsal central third of the tarsal navicular, which is the area that is most often associated with tarsal navicular stress fractures, is diminished. This classic finding that was described by Torg et al[58] was somewhat questioned in a cadaver model study that was conducted by McKeon et al,[59] which reported a central avascular zone in 41.2% of the tarsal navicular specimens; however, the central avascular zone extended to the dorsal central border, which is the location at which most tarsal navicular stress fractures occur, in only 11.8% of the cadaver models.

Biomechanically, the location of the tarsal navicular in the midfoot predisposes it to compression and shear stresses during ambulation.[60] Kitaoka et al[60] reported that compressive forces were highest in the dorsal central zone of the tarsal navicular with axial loading. Although no morphologic or anatomic structural pattern has been definitively associated with tarsal navicular stress fractures, Lee and Anderson[61] reported that a cavus or cavovarus foot with some degree of metatarsus adductus morphology tends to be stiffer and allows for less force dissipation, which may result in elevated pressure across the navicular. Fitch et al[62] reported that the lateral portion of the tarsal navicular was subject to high stress in patients who had a short first metatarsal and a long second metatarsal, which may increase susceptibility to tarsal navicular stress fractures. Pavlov et al[63] reported that metatarsus adductus was an additional contributor to increased tarsal navicular loading. Athletes who have the highest risk for tarsal navicular stress fractures include those who participate in activities that require repetitive loading of the forefoot, such as sprinting, jumping, or dynamic push-off sports including basketball, football, track and field, and rugby.[51,55,58,62] Although endurance athletes, such as distance runners or military recruits, appear to have a lesser risk for tarsal navicular stress fractures, such injuries also have been reported in this athletic popuation.[53,64,65]

Physical Examination

Often, initial symptoms of tarsal navicular stress fractures are incremental and may include vague pain or discomfort in the midfoot or ankle at the onset and conclusion of activity. As increased stress persists, symptoms may become more intense and occur earlier in activity or persist after activity and between activities. Eventually, symptoms progress to the point at which participation in activity is completely limited. The diagnosis of a tarsal navicular stress fracture can be a challenge, and many athletes who have tarsal navicular stress fractures are initially misdiagnosed with midfoot sprains, anterior or posterior tibial tendinitis, or even plantar fasciitis. Often, the location of discomfort is ambiguous, and patients may report nonspecific midfoot or ankle pain because of the proximity of the tarsal navicular to the tibiotalar and talonavicular joints. Khan et al[55] reported that the N spot, which is an area of tenderness localized over the dorsal central tarsal navicular, correlates with navicular injury. Single leg hopping may be used as a provocative test to assess for tarsal navicular stress fracture.[62] Typically, strength testing and the appearance of the foot are normal. Because of the vague nature of symptoms in patients who have tarsal navicular stress fractures, diagnosis of tarsal navicular stress fractures often is delayed by a mean of 4 to 7 months from the onset of symptoms.[58,61]

Imaging

Often, initial radiographs of patients who have tarsal navicular stress fractures appear normal. In a retrospective review of bone scans that were positive for tarsal navicular stress fracture, Pavlov et al[63] reported that plain radiographs identified only 39% of the known complete tarsal navicular stress fractures, 22% of which were diagnosed prospectively. None of the incomplete tarsal navicular stress fractures in the study were identified with the use of plain radiographs. In a study on navicular stress fracture diagnosis and imaging, Khan et al[55] reported that only 24% of incomplete tarsal navicular stress fractures and 81% of complete tarsal navicular stress fractures were diagnosed with the use of radiographs. A careful examination of radiographs may reveal talar neck spurring or a dorsal avulsion fragment from the talonavicular capsule.

Currently, MRI is the preferred imaging modality for patients who have a suspected tarsal navicular stress fracture because it may be positive for a tarsal navicular stress fracture before the fracture is apparent on either

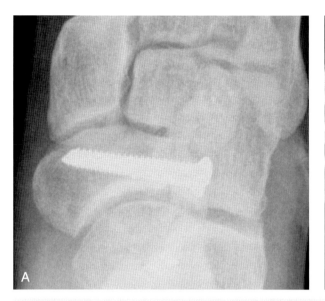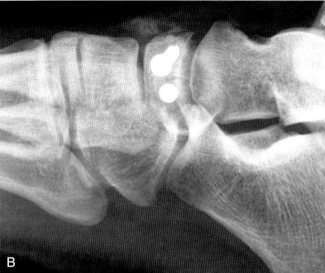

Figure 3   AP (**A**) and lateral (**B**) radiographs of the left foot of a 21-year-old woman who is a college volleyball player taken 2 weeks after percutaneous screw fixation of a type III tarsal navicular stress fracture demonstrate good fracture reduction.

radiographs or CT scans. MRI has a high sensitivity for stress reactions and provides surgeons with good anatomic detail of stress fracture patterns. CT can aid in preoperative planning, identifying if a tarsal navicular stress fracture is complete or incomplete, and determining the orientation of a fracture line.

Typically, tarsal navicular stress fractures are identified as an incomplete fracture line that begins at the proximal dorsal cortex of the central third of the navicular. As a stress fracture progresses to completion, the fracture line typically propagates in a distal plantar direction.[55] Saxena et al[66] proposed a CT-based classification of tarsal navicular stress fractures, which are divided into three types, each of which is associated with a specific management plan. Type I tarsal navicular stress fractures involve a dorsal cortical break, type II tarsal navicular stress fractures involve fracture extension into the tarsal navicular body, and type III tarsal navicular stress fractures involve fracture

extension into another cortex. The authors reported a mean return to activity of 3.0 months for type I tarsal navicular stress fractures, 3.6 months for type II tarsal navicular stress fractures, and 6.8 months for type III tarsal navicular stress fractures. Type I tarsal navicular stress fractures most often were managed nonsurgically unless they occurred in an athlete. Type II tarsal navicular stress fractures were managed either nonsurgically or, in active patients, surgically. Type III tarsal navicular stress fractures most often were managed surgically. Any patients who had a tarsal navicular stress fracture with osteonecrosis, cystic degeneration, or sclerotic fracture lines were more likely to undergo surgical treatment with possible bone grafting regardless of tarsal navicular stress fracture type.

Treatment
Currently, high-level athletes who have tarsal navicular stress fractures are primarily treated surgically (**Figure 3**).

Typically, nonsurgical treatment is reserved for low-demand patients who have incomplete or nondisplaced tarsal navicular stress fractures. Often, nonsurgical management consists of 6 to 8 weeks of non–weight bearing in a cast followed by the advancement to functional rehabilitation after tenderness has resolved.[55,58,62] In some patients, tarsal navicular stress fractures that are managed nonsurgically may take up to 8 months to heal.[62] In high-demand athletes, the potential 6- to 8-month healing period that is associated with nonsurgical treatment is unacceptable. Saxena et al[66] reported a significant difference in return to activity between patients with tarsal navicular stress fractures who underwent surgical versus nonsurgical treatment (12.4 versus 17.2 weeks, respectively). Mallee et al[67] also reported an expedited return to activity in patients with tarsal navicular stress fractures who underwent surgical treatment. The authors reported that the surgical management of tarsal navicular stress fractures resulted in a mean return to activity of 16 weeks, whereas the nonsurgical management of tarsal navicular stress fractures with the use of a non–weight-bearing cast resulted in a mean return to activity of 22 weeks.

Using the current evidence, the authors of this chapter have established a treatment algorithm for athletes who have tarsal navicular stress fractures. Saxena type I tarsal navicular stress fractures should be managed with percutaneous screw fixation using one to two screws. Saxena type II tarsal navicular stress fractures often require screw fixation as well as bone marrow aspirate via a percutaneous or open approach. Type III tarsal navicular stress fractures should be managed with open reduction and internal fixation as well as bone graft and bone marrow aspirate. Postoperative protocols vary; however, typical postoperative recommendations include 6 weeks of non–weight bearing and, based on symptoms, an additional 2 to 6 weeks of protected weight bearing in a surgical boot, at which point functional rehabilitation that consists of weight-bearing activity in a walker boot and cycling or pool-based, low-impact rehabilitation begins. In general, return to play is delayed until 6 to 12 months postoperatively, depending on patient recovery and the demands of a particular sport.

Proximal Fifth Metatarsal Stress Fractures

Proximal fifth metatarsal stress fractures, which are among the most common foot injuries in young athletes, can be particularly problematic in elite-level athletes. Controversy exists with regard to the decision to manage proximal fifth metatarsal stress fractures surgically or nonsurgically, the decision to use intramedullary screws or other implant types, the role of bone grafting or other osteogenic material, and management of acute, chronic, and recurrent proximal fifth metatarsal stress fractures.

Typically, proximal fifth metatarsal stress fractures occur in athletes who participate in repetitive running, jumping, and cutting activities. The anatomy about the region of the proximal fifth metatarsal creates an area for stress concentration. The mobile fourth and fifth metatarsals are stabilized by strong ligamentous attachments that connect their bases and the cuboid. These ligaments terminate at the metaphyseal-diaphyseal junction, and forces of the mobile forefoot are translated proximally and act as a fulcrum, which focuses stress about the region of the proximal fifth metatarsal. The proximal fifth metatarsal also has diminished vascular supply, which may impede healing.[68,69] The main nutrient artery of the proximal fifth metatarsal enters medially at the junction of the proximal and middle thirds of the fifth metatarsal and then splits, flowing in both a proximal and distal direction. Therefore, any injury to the proximal fifth metatarsal may compromise blood supply to the proximal diaphysis or metaphyseal-diaphyseal junction.

Proximal fifth metatarsal fractures were originally described by Dr. Robert Jones in a 1902 study of six patients, one of whom was himself, with proximal fifth metatarsal fractures.[70] Recognition of anatomic differences in fracture location, mechanism of injury, and management have made proximal fifth metatarsal stress fractures less ambiguous. The proximal fifth metatarsal is divided into three anatomic zones: the tuberosity (zone 1), the metaphyseal-diaphyseal junction (zone 2), and the proximal diaphysis (zone 3).[71]

Zone 1 Injuries

Zone 1 injuries, which are proximal fifth metatarsal tuberosity avulsion injuries, typically are acute injuries rather than chronic stress fractures. Zone 1 injuries are briefly discussed in this chapter for completeness. Typically, zone 1 fractures are caused by an inversion injury to the foot, which results in avulsion of the attachment of the lateral band of the plantar fascia and, less commonly, the peroneus brevis tendon. Proximal fifth metatarsal tuberosity fractures occur in cancellous bone with good vascular supply. Therefore, proximal fifth metatarsal tuberosity fractures that are managed nonsurgically heal reliably well.[72,73] Interestingly, radiographic union in patients who undergo nonsurgical treatment for proximal fifth metatarsal tuberosity fractures lags behind clinical union and pain resolution, even in athletes. Surgery may be recommended for patients who have substantial articular step-off (>2 mm) or large fragments, including those of the articular surface, with or without rotational abnormality.[73,74]

Zone 2 Injuries

Zone 2 injuries, which are located at the metaphyseal-diaphyseal junction, are true Jones fractures (**Figure 4, A**). Typically, Jones fractures are transversely oriented, emerging laterally, with medial propagation into the articulation of the fourth and fifth metatarsals.[74] Jones fractures are notoriously difficult to successfully manage nonsurgically with the use of non–weight-bearing immobilization techniques, particularly because of the demands of athletic patients and their increased rate of refracture, delayed union, and nonunion (4% to 12%).[70,75-78]

In a study of 37 athletes with Jones fractures that were randomized to early screw fixation or cast immobilization, Mologne et al[79] reported that the patients in the screw fixation group had an improved union rate (94% versus 67%, respectively) and an earlier return to sport (8 weeks versus 15 weeks, respectively) compared with the patients in the cast immobilization group. In a study of 83 elite college football players with Jones fractures (86 fractures) who participated in the National Football League (NFL) Combine and underwent either surgical or nonsurgical treatment, Low et al[80] reported a 94% union rate in the patients who were treated surgically and an 80% union rate in the patients who were treated nonsurgically. Kerkhoffs et al[81] reported that the surgical management of Jones fractures resulted in shorter time to union and decreased delayed unions and nonunions compared with the nonsurgical management of Jones fractures.

Two recent studies evaluated return to play in NFL players and National Basketball Association (NBA) players who underwent surgical treatment for proximal fifth metatarsal stress fractures. In a study of 25 NFL players with zone 2 or zone 3 proximal fifth metatarsal stress fractures who underwent surgical treatment, which consisted of Jones-specific intramedullary screw fixation, bone marrow aspirate and demineralized bone matrix injection, as well as the use of noninvasive bone stimulators, Lareau et al[82] reported a mean return to NFL play of 8.7 weeks and a 12% re-fracture rate (**Figure 4, B**). In a study of 10 NBA players with zone 2 or zone 3 proximal fifth metatarsal stress fractures who underwent surgical treatment, which consisted of either standard percutaneous screw fixation

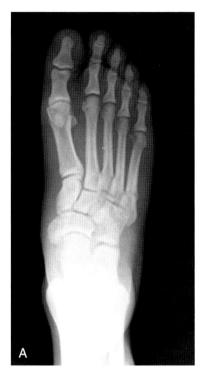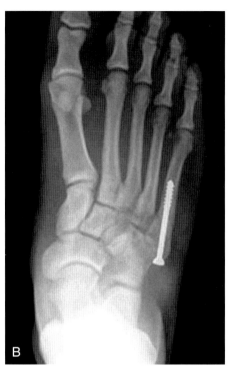

Figure 4 Images of the right foot of a 25-year-old man who is a professional football player. **A,** AP radiograph demonstrates a Jones fracture. **B,** AP radiograph taken 7 weeks after intramedullary screw fixation demonstrates healing.

with bone marrow aspirate concentrate (seven NBA players) or primary open bone grafting in addition to percutaneous screw fixation with bone marrow aspirate concentrate (three NBA players who were deemed to have the highest risk for re-fracture), O'Malley et al[83] reported radiographic union at a mean of 7.5 weeks postoperatively, a mean return to NBA play at 9.8 weeks postoperatively, and a 30% re-fracture rate. The authors hypothesized that the size of the NBA players, increased body mass index, and a unique foot type that is associated with an increased risk for proximal fifth metatarsal stress fractures led to the high re-fracture rate.

Zone 3 Injuries

Zone 3 stress fractures occur in the proximal diaphyseal region of the fifth metatarsal. High-level athletes who have zone 3 injuries should be treated surgically via limited-incision solid intramedullary screw fixation, with autologous bone marrow adjuncts considered in patients who have a high risk for re-fracture or nonunion.[75,84,85] Chuckpaiwong et al[86] reported that patients with zone 2 injuries and patients with zone 3 injuries have similar prognoses, and that distinguishing between these two zones of injury is unnecessary. The authors reported that competitive athletes with zone 3 injuries who underwent surgical treatment had a rate of return to sport that was nearly one-half that of competitive athletes with zone 3 injuries who underwent nonsurgical treatment (15.2 weeks versus 26.3 weeks, respectively).

Summary

Stress fractures in athletes are caused by an imbalanced combination of bone stress and repair mechanisms. Multiple factors, including vitamin D deficiency, caloric deficiency, and lack of rest, may place an athlete at risk for stress fractures. The management of lower extremity stress fractures varies based on the site of the stress fracture as well as athlete- and sport-specific demands.

References

1. Arendt EA, Griffiths HJ: The use of MR imaging in the assessment and clinical management of stress reactions of bone in high-performance athletes. *Clin Sports Med* 1997;16(2):291-306.

2. Court-Brown CM, Caesar BC: The epidemiology of fractures, part 1: Overview of epidemiology, in Buchloz RW, Heckman JD, Court-Brown CM, Tornetta P III, eds: *Rockwood and Green's Fractures in Adults*, ed 6. Philadelphia, PA, Lippincott Williams and Wilkins, 2006, pp 95-113.

3. Matheson GO, Clement DB, McKenzie DC, Taunton JE, Lloyd-Smith DR, MacIntyre JG: Stress fractures in athletes: A study of 320 cases. *Am J Sports Med* 1987;15(1):46-58.

4. Anderson RB, Hunt KJ, McCormick JJ: Management of common sports-related injuries about the foot and ankle. *J Am Acad Orthop Surg* 2010;18(9):546-556.

5. Bennell KL, Malcolm SA, Thomas SA, Wark JD, Brukner PD: The incidence and distribution of stress fractures in competitive track and field athletes: A twelve-month prospective study. *Am J Sports Med* 1996;24(2):211-217.

6. Armstrong DW III, Rue JP, Wilckens JH, Frassica FJ: Stress fracture injury in young military men and women. *Bone* 2004;35(3):806-816.

7. Fredericson M, Jennings F, Beaulieu C, Matheson GO: Stress fractures in athletes. *Top Magn Reson Imaging* 2006;17(5):309-325.

8. Nattiv A: Stress fractures and bone health in track and field athletes. *J Sci Med Sport* 2000;3(3):268-279.

9. Sallis RE, Jones K: Stress fractures in athletes: How to spot this underdiagnosed injury. *Postgrad Med* 1991;89(6):191-192.

10. Boden BP, Osbahr DC: High-risk stress fractures: Evaluation and treatment. *J Am Acad Orthop Surg* 2000;8(6):344-353.

11. Boden BP, Osbahr DC, Jimenez C: Low-risk stress fractures. *Am J Sports Med* 2001;29(1):100-111.

12. Brukner P, Bradshaw C, Bennell K: Managing common stress fractures: Let risk level guide treatment. *Phys Sportsmed* 1998;26(8):39-47.

13. Barrack MT, Gibbs JC, De Souza MJ, et al: Higher incidence of bone stress injuries with increasing female athlete triad-related risk factors: A prospective multisite study of exercising girls and women. *Am J Sports Med* 2014;42(4):949-958.

14. Ogan D, Pritchett K: Vitamin D and the athlete: Risks, recommendations, and benefits. *Nutrients* 2013;5(6):1856-1868.

15. Lappe J, Cullen D, Haynatzki G, Recker R, Ahlf R, Thompson K: Calcium and vitamin d supplementation decreases incidence of stress fractures in female navy recruits. *J Bone Miner Res* 2008;23(5):741-749.

16. Ruohola JP, Laaksi I, Ylikomi T, et al: Association between serum 25(OH)D concentrations and bone stress fractures in Finnish young men. *J Bone Miner Res* 2006;21(9):1483-1488.

17. McCabe MP, Smyth MP, Richardson DR: Current concept review: Vitamin D and stress fractures. *Foot Ankle Int* 2012;33(6):526-533.

18. Martinez SF, Murphy GA: Tibial stress fracture in a male ballet dancer: A case report. *Am J Sports Med* 2005;33(1):124-130.

19. Tejwani SG, Motamedi AR: Stress fracture of the tibial tubercle in a collegiate volleyball player. *Orthopedics* 2004;27(2):219-222.

20. Losito JM, Laird RC, Alexis MR, Mora J: Tibial and proximal fibular stress fracture in a rower. *J Am Podiatr Med Assoc* 2003;93(4):340-343.

21. Israeli A, Ganel A, Blankstein A, Horoszowski H: Stress fracture of the tibial tuberosity in a high jumper: Case report. *Int J Sports Med* 1984;5(6):299-300.

22. Khan K, Brown J, Way S, et al: Overuse injuries in classical ballet. *Sports Med* 1995;19(5):341-357.

23. Larson CM, Traina SM, Fischer DA, Arendt EA: Recurrent complete proximal tibial stress fracture in a basketball player. *Am J Sports Med* 2005;33(12):1914-1917.

24. Jensen JE: Stress fracture in the world class athlete: A case study. *Med Sci Sports Exerc* 1998;30(6):783-787.

25. Varner KE, Younas SA, Lintner DM, Marymont JV: Chronic anterior midtibial stress fractures in athletes treated with reamed intramedullary nailing. *Am J Sports Med* 2005;33(7):1071-1076.

26. Caesar BC, McCollum GA, Elliot R, Williams A, Calder JD: Stress fractures of the tibia and medial malleolus. *Foot Ankle Clin* 2013;18(2):339-355.

27. Hershman EB, Mailly T: Stress fractures. *Clin Sports Med* 1990;9(1):183-214.

28. Meyer SA, Saltzman CL, Albright JP: Stress fractures of the foot and leg. *Clin Sports Med* 1993;12(2):395-413.

29. Knapp TP, Garrett WE Jr: Stress fractures: General concepts. *Clin Sports Med* 1997;16(2):339-356.

30. Niva MH, Sormaala MJ, Kiuru MJ, Haataja R, Ahovuo JA, Pihlajamaki HK: Bone stress injuries of the ankle and foot: An 86-month magnetic resonance imaging-based study of physically active young adults. *Am J Sports Med* 2007;35(4):643-649.

31. Brockwell J, Yeung Y, Griffith JF: Stress fractures of the foot and ankle. *Sports Med Arthrosc* 2009;17(3):149-159.

32. Rettig AC, Shelbourne KD, McCarroll JR, Bisesi M, Watts J: The natural history and treatment of delayed union stress fractures of the anterior cortex of the tibia. *Am J Sports Med* 1988;16(3):250-255.

33. Borens O, Sen MK, Huang RC, et al: Anterior tension band plating for anterior tibial stress fractures in high-performance female athletes: A report of 4 cases. *J Orthop Trauma* 2006;20(6):425-430.

34. Pecina M, Bojanic I, Smoljanovic T, Ivkovic A, Mirkovic M, Jelic M: Surgical treatment of diaphyseal stress fractures of the fifth metatarsal in competitive athletes: Long-term follow-up and computerized pedobarographic analysis. *J Am Podiatr Med Assoc* 2011;101(6):517-522.

35. Weinfeld SB, Haddad SL, Myerson MS: Metatarsal stress fractures. *Clin Sports Med* 1997;16(2):319-338.

36. Väistö O, Toivanen J, Kannus P, Järvinen M: Anterior knee pain after intramedullary nailing of fractures of the tibial shaft: An eight-year follow-up of a prospective, randomized study comparing two different nail-insertion techniques. *J Trauma* 2008;64(6):1511-1516.

37. Lefaivre KA, Guy P, Chan H, Blachut PA: Long-term follow-up of tibial shaft fractures treated with intramedullary nailing. *J Orthop Trauma* 2008;22(8):525-529.

38. Chang PS, Harris RM: Intramedullary nailing for chronic tibial stress fractures: A review of five cases. *Am J Sports Med* 1996;24(5):688-692.

39. Gardiner JR, Isbell WM, Johnson DL: Bilateral anterior tibial stress fractures treated with dynamic intramedullary nailing. *Orthopedics* 2003;26(7):720-722.

40. Kelly JJ, Johnson DL, Uhl TL, Madaleno JA, Blackport RM: Intramedullary nailing of an anterior tibial stress fracture in a football player. *Athletic Therapy Today* 2005;10(6):42-45.

41. Pandya NK, Webner D, Sennett B, Huffman GR: Recurrent fracture after operative treatment for a tibial stress fracture. *Clin Orthop Relat Res* 2007;456:254-258.

42. Yamada T, Kahanov L: Complications of intramedullary rodding for chronic tibial stress fractures in female athletes: Three case reports. *Res Sports Med* 2004;12(1):1-13.

43. Zbeda RM, Sculco PK, Urch EY, et al: Tension band plating for chronic anterior tibial stress fractures in high-performance athletes. *Am J Sports Med* 2015;43(7):1712-1718.

44. Brukner P, Bradshaw C, Khan KM, White S, Crossley K: Stress fractures: A review of 180 cases. *Clin J Sport Med* 1996;6(2):85-89.

45. Iwamoto J, Takeda T: Stress fractures in athletes: Review of 196 cases. *J Orthop Sci* 2003;8(3):273-278.

46. Orava S, Karpakka J, Taimela S, Hulkko A, Permi J, Kujala U: Stress fracture of the medial malleolus. *J Bone Joint Surg Am* 1995;77(3):362-365.

47. Giladi M, Milgrom C, Simkin A, Danon Y: Stress fractures: Identifiable risk factors. *Am J Sports Med* 1991;19(6):647-652.

48. Schils JP, Andrish JT, Piraino DW, Belhobek GH, Richmond BJ, Bergfeld JA: Medial malleolar stress fractures in seven patients: Review of the clinical and imaging features. *Radiology* 1992;185(1):219-221.

49. Okada K, Senma S, Abe E, Sato K, Minato S: Stress fractures of the medial malleolus: A case report. *Foot Ankle Int* 1995;16(1):49-52.

50. Jowett AJ, Birks CL, Blackney MC: Medial malleolar stress fracture secondary to chronic ankle impingement. *Foot Ankle Int* 2008;29(7):716-721.

51. Shelbourne KD, Fisher DA, Rettig AC, McCarroll JR: Stress fractures of the medial malleolus. *Am J Sports Med* 1988;16(1):60-63.

52. Shabat S, Sampson KB, Mann G, et al: Stress fractures of the medial malleolus—review of the literature and report of a 15-year-old elite gymnast. *Foot Ankle Int* 2002;23(7):647-650.

53. Goergen TG, Venn-Watson EA, Rossman DJ, Resnick D, Gerber KH: Tarsal navicular stress fractures in runners. *AJR Am J Roentgenol* 1981;136(1):201-203.

54. Orava S, Puranen J, Ala-Ketola L: Stress fractures caused by physical exercise. *Acta Orthop Scand* 1978;49(1):19-27.

55. Khan KM, Brukner PD, Kearney C, Fuller PJ, Bradshaw CJ, Kiss ZS: Tarsal navicular stress fracture in athletes. *Sports Med* 1994;17(1):65-76.

56. Gross CE, Nunley JA II: Navicular stress fractures. *Foot Ankle Int* 2015;36(9):1117-1122.

57. Astion DJ, Deland JT, Otis JC, Kenneally S: Motion of the hindfoot after simulated arthrodesis. *J Bone Joint Surg Am* 1997;79(2):241-246.

58. Torg JS, Pavlov H, Cooley LH, et al: Stress fractures of the tarsal navicular: A retrospective review of twenty-one cases. *J Bone Joint Surg Am* 1982;64(5):700-712.

59. McKeon KE, McCormick JJ, Johnson JE, Klein SE: Intraosseous and extraosseous arterial anatomy of the adult navicular. *Foot Ankle Int* 2012;33(10):857-861.

60. Kitaoka HB, Luo ZP, An KN: Contact features of the talonavicular joint of the foot. *Clin Orthop Relat Res* 1996;325:290-295.

61. Lee S, Anderson RB: Stress fractures of the tarsal navicular. *Foot Ankle Clin* 2004;9(1):85-104.

62. Fitch KD, Blackwell JB, Gilmour WN: Operation for non-union of stress fracture of the tarsal navicular. *J Bone Joint Surg Br* 1989;71(1):105-110.

63. Pavlov H, Torg JS, Freiberger RH: Tarsal navicular stress fractures: Radiographic evaluation. *Radiology* 1983;148(3):641-645.

64. Ting A, King W, Yocum L, et al: Stress fractures of the tarsal navicular in long-distance runners. *Clin Sports Med* 1988;7(1):89-101.

65. Pinney SJ, Sangeorzan BJ: Fractures of the tarsal bones. *Orthop Clin North Am* 2001;32(1):21-33.

66. Saxena A, Fullem B, Hannaford D: Results of treatment of 22 navicular stress fractures and a new proposed radiographic classification system. *J Foot Ankle Surg* 2000;39(2):96-103.

67. Mallee WH, Weel H, van Dijk CN, van Tulder MW, Kerkhoffs GM, Lin CW: Surgical versus conservative treatment for high-risk stress fractures of the lower leg (anterior tibial cortex, navicular and fifth metatarsal base): A systematic review. *Br J Sports Med* 2015;49(6):370-376.

68. Smith JW, Arnoczky SP, Hersh A: The intraosseous blood supply of

the fifth metatarsal: Implications for proximal fracture healing. *Foot Ankle* 1992;13(3):143-152.

69. Shereff MJ, Yang QM, Kummer FJ, Frey CC, Greenidge N: Vascular anatomy of the fifth metatarsal. *Foot Ankle* 1991;11(6):350-353.

70. Jones R: Fracture of the base of the fifth metatarsal bone by indirect violence. *Ann Surg* 1902;35(6):697-700.2.

71. Den Hartog BD: Fracture of the proximal fifth metatarsal. *J Am Acad Orthop Surg* 2009;17(7):458-464.

72. Lawrence SJ, Botte MJ: Jones' fractures and related fractures of the proximal fifth metatarsal. *Foot Ankle* 1993;14(6):358-365.

73. Rettig AC, Shelbourne KD, Wilckens J: The surgical treatment of symptomatic nonunions of the proximal (metaphyseal) fifth metatarsal in athletes. *Am J Sports Med* 1992;20(1):50-54.

74. Rosenberg GA, Sferra JJ: Treatment strategies for acute fractures and nonunions of the proximal fifth metatarsal. *J Am Acad Orthop Surg* 2000;8(5):332-338.

75. Torg JS, Balduini FC, Zelko RR, Pavlov H, Peff TC, Das M: Fractures of the base of the fifth metatarsal distal to the tuberosity: Classification and guidelines for non-surgical and surgical management. *J Bone Joint Surg Am* 1984;66(2):209-214.

76. Porter DA, Duncan M, Meyer SJ: Fifth metatarsal Jones fracture fixation with a 4.5-mm cannulated stainless steel screw in the competitive and recreational athlete: A clinical and radiographic evaluation. *Am J Sports Med* 2005;33(5):726-733.

77. Murawski CD, Kennedy JG: Percutaneous internal fixation of proximal fifth metatarsal jones fractures (Zones II and III) with Charlotte Carolina screw and bone marrow aspirate concentrate: An outcome study in athletes. *Am J Sports Med* 2011;39(6):1295-1301.

78. Thevendran G, Deol RS, Calder JD: Fifth metatarsal fractures in the athlete: Evidence for management. *Foot Ankle Clin* 2013;18(2):237-254.

79. Mologne TS, Lundeen JM, Clapper MF, O'Brien TJ: Early screw fixation versus casting in the treatment of acute Jones fractures. *Am J Sports Med* 2005;33(7):970-975.

80. Low K, Noblin JD, Browne JE, Barnthouse CD, Scott AR: Jones fractures in the elite football player. *J Surg Orthop Adv* 2004;13(3):156-160.

81. Kerkhoffs GM, Versteegh VE, Sierevelt IN, Kloen P, van Dijk CN: Treatment of proximal metatarsal V fractures in athletes and non-athletes. *Br J Sports Med* 2012;46(9):644-648.

82. Lareau CR, Hsu AR, Anderson RB: Return to play in National Football League players after operative Jones fracture treatment. *Foot Ankle Int* 2016;37(1):8-16.

83. O'Malley M, DeSandis B, Allen A, Levitsky M, O'Malley Q, Williams R: Operative treatment of fifth metatarsal Jones fractures (zones II and III) in the NBA. *Foot Ankle Int* 2016;37(5):488-500.

84. DeLee JC, Evans JP, Julian J: Stress fracture of the fifth metatarsal. *Am J Sports Med* 1983;11(5):349-353.

85. Zelko RR, Torg JS, Rachun A: Proximal diaphyseal fractures of the fifth metatarsal—treatment of the fractures and their complications in athletes. *Am J Sports Med* 1979;7(2):95-101.

86. Chuckpaiwong B, Queen RM, Easley ME, Nunley JA: Distinguishing Jones and proximal diaphyseal fractures of the fifth metatarsal. *Clin Orthop Relat Res* 2008;466(8):1966-1970.

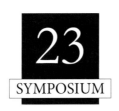

Management of Osteochondral Lesions of the Talus

Michael Isiah Sandlin, MD
Timothy P. Charlton, MD
Cyrus E. Taghavi, MD
Eric Giza, MD

Abstract

Management strategies for symptomatic osteochondral lesions of the talus are primarily surgical. Treatment options for symptomatic osteochondral lesions of the talus most commonly include bone marrow stimulation techniques, osteochondral autograft transplantation, osteochondral allograft transplantation, autologous chondrocyte implantation, matrix-induced autologous chondrocyte implantation, and particulated juvenile articular cartilage. The selection of the most appropriate treatment option should be based on the specifics of a talar lesion, in particular, lesion size.

Instr Course Lect 2017;66:293–299.

Osteochondral lesions of the talus (OLTs) are a common cause of chronic ankle pain and disability. Most OLTs are associated with prior trauma and may cause substantial long-term functional limitations.[1-3] The management of OLTs is complicated by the limited healing capacity and poor regenerative potential of articular cartilage.[4] Non-surgical treatment has been reported to be only moderately successful at mitigating symptoms and returning patients to their prior level of activity.[5,6] Tol et al[7] reported that patients who underwent surgical treatment of OLTs had substantially better outcomes compared with patients who underwent nonsurgical treatment of OLTs.

Nonsurgical Treatment

Often, nonsurgical management of OLTs is initially undertaken because many OLTs are discovered incidentally on imaging and are of an indeterminate age. Nonsurgical treatment may include cast or boot immobilization, activity modification, anti-inflammatory medications, and, possibly, corticosteroid injections. The success of nonsurgical treatment is limited. A large systematic review reported good to excellent overall outcomes in 45% of patients with OLTs who were treated nonsurgically.[7] In a study of 34 patients with OLTs who underwent nonsurgical treatment, Shearer et al[8] reported good or excellent outcomes in 54% of the patients at a mean follow-up of 38 months. Adjuvant nonsurgical treatment options include injections of hyaluronic acid formulations and platelet-rich plasma. Hyaluronic acid and platelet-rich plasma injections have been reported to improve pain and functional scores at 6-month follow-up; however, their long-term effectiveness is limited.[9,10]

Surgical Treatment

Surgical treatment is indicated for patients with symptomatic, focal OLTs

Dr. Charlton or an immediate family member has stock or stock options held in the Green Bay Packers Football Club and the Manchester United Football Club. Dr. Giza or an immediate family member is a member of a speakers' bureau or has made paid presentations on behalf of Amniox; serves as a paid consultant to Arthrex and Zimmer; and has received research or institutional support from Arthrex. Neither of the following authors nor any immediate family member has received anything of value from or has stock or stock options held in a commercial company or institution related directly or indirectly to the subject of this chapter: Dr. Sandlin and Dr. Taghavi.

in whom a trial of nonsurgical treatment fails. First-line surgical treatment options include reparative bone marrow stimulation (BMS) techniques, such as curettage, drilling, and microfracture. BMS techniques are typically performed arthroscopically and result in good to excellent outcomes in 72% to 85% of patients in whom they are performed.[7] Before arthroscopic BMS techniques were developed, BMS techniques typically were performed in an open manner with the use of tibial or fibular osteotomy. Open BMS techniques allowed for direct visualization of the lesion and potentially easier instrumentation but were complicated by a relatively high rate of degenerative ankle arthritis.[11] Care should be taken to evaluate patients with OLTs for ankle instability because cartilage treatment strategies are predicated on a stable joint. BMS techniques are unlikely to succeed in patients in whom ankle instability is present; therefore, ankle instability should be addressed either before or concurrent with the management of OLTs.

BMS Techniques

BMS techniques, which initially were developed to manage chondral injuries in the knee, have been successfully adopted to manage OLTs. Currently, microfracture is the most common initial BMS procedure used to manage OLTs because of its relative ease of use, ability to be performed arthroscopically, low cost, low morbidity, and quick recovery. BMS techniques rely on the penetration of subchondral bone, which allows stem cells to migrate from the marrow cavity into the prepared lesion site. Typically, stem cell proliferation results in fibrocartilaginous healing, which is biomechanically

inferior compared with hyaline cartilage.[12] Tol et al[7] reported good to excellent outcomes in 85% of patients with OLTs who underwent OLT excision and BMS. Excellent results, however, are not always retained over time. In a study of 50 patients with OLTs who underwent arthroscopic BMS, Ferkel et al[13] reported that the outcomes of 35% of the patients deteriorated 5 years postoperatively. Several studies have reported good outcomes in patients who undergo revision BMS procedures. In a study of 38 patients with OLTs who underwent arthroscopic curettage and drilling, Schuman et al[14] reported good to excellent results in 86% of the 22 patients in whom the procedure was a primary surgical treatment and 75% of the 16 patients in whom the procedure was a revision surgical treatment. In a study of 12 patients who underwent revision arthroscopy and débridement, Savva et al[15] reported improved mean American Orthopaedic Foot and Ankle Society ankle-hindfoot scores, with 11 patients reporting satisfaction with their clinical outcomes at a mean follow-up of 5.9 years.

Patient factors, including age, sex, body mass index, and duration of symptoms, have not consistently been reported to correlate with BMS outcomes;[13,16-18] however, lesion-specific factors appear to have a substantial influence on BMS outcomes. Patients with focal OLTs who undergo BMS have better outcomes compared with patients with degenerative, uncontained OLTs who undergo BMS.[16] Large OLTs (>1.29 to 1.50 cm²), delaminating OLTs, or cystic OLTs may not respond well to microfracture, and patients with these types of lesions have less reliable outcomes.[13,17-22] Chuckpaiwong et al[19] reported a strong correlation between the

size of an OLT and BMS outcomes, reporting excellent results in patients with OLTs smaller than 1.5 cm² who underwent BMS and inferior results in patients with larger OLTs who underwent BMS. Similar results were reported by Choi et al[18] and Cuttica et al,[17] with both studies reporting that OLTs larger than 1.5 cm² were associated with worse outcomes, and that the size of an OLT was the most important predictor of poor results. Some surgeons consider 100 mm² to 150 mm² as the consensus threshold limit for BMS procedures.

Other Treatment Options

A myriad of treatment options, including osteochondral autograft transplantation (OAT), osteochondral allograft transplantation, autologous chondrocyte implantation (ACI), matrix-induced ACI (MACI) with collagen or hyaluronic scaffolds, particulated juvenile articular cartilage implantation, and bone marrow aspirate concentrate (BMAC), have emerged in an attempt to improve the outcomes of patients with OLTs. The goal of these techniques is the replacement or regeneration of hyaline cartilage on the articular surface of the talus to provide the most durable and anatomically equivalent tissue possible.

Osteochondral Autograft Transplantation

OAT can be used as a primary or revision procedure after failed microfracture to manage OLTs larger than 1 cm². In OAT, the OLT is removed and replaced with one or more osteochondral plugs, which allow for bone-to-bone healing and hyaline articular cartilage replacement. Classically, autograft was harvested from a patient's knee; however, newer OAT techniques allow autograft harvest from the ipsilateral anterior talus.[23] Osteotomies are often required for OAT because perpendicular access to the OLT is necessary for optimal placement.

Several studies have reported positive results in patients who undergo OAT.[23-25] These positive results include good to excellent outcomes in 74% to 100% of patients who underwent OAT and histologic verification of the presence of hyaline cartilage at the site of an OLT.[6,17,23-25] In a study of 36 patients with OLTs (mean size, 1 cm^2) who underwent OAT mosaicplasty, Hangody et al[26] reported good to excellent outcomes in 94% of the patients at a mean follow-up of 4.7 years. In a larger study of 831 patients who underwent OAT mosaicplasty, Hangody and Füles[25] reported an overall donor site morbidity of 3% in patients in whom the osteochondral autograft was harvested from the superomedial or superolateral edges of the ipsilateral femoral condyle. In a recent systematic review of a subgroup of 212 patients with OLTs who underwent OAT, Zengerink et al[6] reported good to excellent outcomes in 87% of the patients; however, donor site morbidity was observed in 12% of the patients. Donor site morbidity in patients with OLTs who undergo OAT is an ongoing concern, which has led to increased interest in fresh osteochondral allograft transplantation. In addition to the concern for donor site morbidity, a recent prospective, randomized study reported no difference in the 2-year outcomes of patients with OLTs who underwent either microfracture, OAT, or simple chondroplasty.[20] These findings call into question the theoretical benefits of OAT compared with simpler, less expensive treatment options, such as microfracture or simple chondroplasty.

Osteochondral Allograft Transplantation

Fresh osteochondral allograft transplantation is a single-stage procedure that eliminates the potential for donor site morbidity because the graft is acquired from a fresh cadaver specimen. A preoperative CT scan should be obtained for patients in whom an osteochondral allograft is being considered to calculate the dimensions of the OLT for tissue bank analysis, which can take several months before a size-matched allograft becomes available. Typically, allograft acquisition requires 2 weeks to clear tissue cultures. After 3 weeks, an allograft may begin to show signs of deterioration.

Multiple recent studies have reported favorable results in patients with OLTs who undergo fresh talar osteochondral allograft transplantation, which can be performed in patients who have large, cystic shoulder OLTs that are not amenable to other treatment options.[27-31] In a retrospective study of eight patients with shoulder OLTs who underwent fresh osteochondral allograft transplantation, Adams et al[27] reported that all the patients had improved pain and functional scores at a mean follow-up of 48 months; however, radiographic lucencies at the graft site were observed in five of the eight patients (63%), and four of the eight patients (50%) required an additional surgical procedure. In a prospective study of 19 patients with substantial OLTs who underwent fresh osteochondral allograft transplantation, Berlet et al[28] reported improved pain and function scores in 12 patients at a mean follow-up of 3.3 years; however, radiographic lucencies at the graft site were observed in three patients, edema was observed at the graft site in four patients, an osteochondral allograft

failed to incorporate in one patient, and one patient underwent osteochondral allograft revision. In a study of 38 patients with OLTs who underwent fresh osteochondral allograft transplantation, El-Rashidy et al[29] reported good, very good, or excellent outcomes in 74% of the patients at mean follow-up of 37.7 months. The authors reported that allograft failure occurred in four of the patients (11%). In a prospective study of 15 patients with large cystic OLTs (>3,000 mm^3) who underwent fresh osteochondral allograft transplantation, Raikin et al[31] reported an 87% survival rate and good to excellent outcomes in 73% of the patients at a minimum follow-up of 2 years.

Disadvantages of fresh osteochondral allograft transplantation include the time interval for allograft availability, the potential for disease transmission, and the possible immunogenicity of an allograft, which can lead to rejection. Patients in whom fresh osteochondral allograft transplantation fails often require ankle arthrodesis.

Autologous Chondrocyte Implantation

ACI is a two-stage surgical procedure that attempts to fill an OLT with a patient's own transplanted chondrocytes. The first stage of ACI involves the harvest of chondrocytes from the edge of a patient's OLT or knee. These chondrocytes then undergo culture expansion in a laboratory for several weeks. In the second stage of ACI, the cultured chondrocytes are transplanted into the patient's OLT after the lesion has been débrided. A periosteal patch from the proximal tibia is sutured over the transplanted chondrocytes for containment. OLT margin cartilage has been used as a culture specimen to minimize donor site morbidity.[32] The indications for

ACI include well-contained, unipolar OLTs larger than 1 cm². Complications of ACI, including graft failure, delamination, and graft hypertrophy, are relatively low (3.8%).[33]

Multiple retrospective studies have reported good to excellent outcomes in patients who undergo ACI in the ankle joint.[34-37] In a study of 11 patients with OLTs who underwent ACI, Nam et al[38] reported good to excellent outcomes in 9 patients at a mean follow-up of 38 months. Complete OLT coverage was observed in 10 of the patients who underwent second-look arthroscopy; however; the authors reported a 20% rate of graft hypertrophy. Giannini et al[35] reported a histologic appearance of hyaline-like cartilage in eight patients who underwent second-look arthroscopy after ACI.

Matrix-Induced ACI

MACI, which is a second-generation ACI technique, is currently used in Europe for the management of OLTs. MACI eliminates the need for a periosteal patch by using a tissue-engineered bioabsorbable collagen membrane with implanted cultured autologous chondrocytes that is fixed to the site of an OLT with fibrin glue.[39] MACI does not require extensive joint exposure or osteotomy, which decreases surgical time and morbidity.[40,41] MACI also diminishes the risk of cell loss from an OLT, uneven cellular distribution, and periosteal hypertrophy.[42] Good to excellent outcomes have been reported in 70% to 92% of patients with OLTs who underwent mini-open or all-arthroscopic ACI or MACI as a primary or revision procedure.[37,38,43,44] In a study of 10 patients with full-thickness OLTs who underwent MACI, Giza et al[45] reported improved pain and functional scores

in 9 of the 10 patients at 1 year and 2 years postoperatively. Currently, MACI is not approved by the FDA for use in the United States.

Particulated Juvenile Articular Cartilage

Particulated juvenile articular cartilage is designed to form a hyaline-like cartilage mass within a prepared OLT.[46,47] Particulated juvenile articular cartilage has the ability to cover large OLTs without the requirements for preimplantation autologous chondrocyte harvest or a periosteal patch. Because a particulated juvenile articular cartilage graft is composed of juvenile cartilage cells, it has an increased cellular density compared with an adult articular cartilage graft and the potential for increased glycosaminoglycan production and type II collagen development, which are key to healthy articular cartilage.[48] Particulated juvenile articular cartilage implantation is a single-stage procedure that, typically, does not require osteotomy. Disadvantages of particulated juvenile articular cartilage include the possible immunogenicity of the particulated juvenile articular cartilage, disease transmission, and cost.

Current evidence for the use of particulated juvenile articular cartilage in patients with OLTs is based primarily on studies on its use for the management of patellar, femoral condyle, and trochlear osteochondral lesions of the knee. Patients with OLTs who underwent particulated juvenile articular cartilage implantation demonstrated improved pain and function 2 years postoperatively.[49,50] In a recent multicenter study of 23 patients with OLTs (24 ankles) who underwent particulated juvenile articular cartilage implantation, Coetzee et al[47] reported overall good to

excellent results in 78% of the patients at a mean follow-up of 16.2 months. Good to excellent outcomes were reported in 92% of patients who had OLTs that were 10 to 15 mm in size.

Bone Marrow Aspirate Concentrate

Biologic adjuncts, such as BMAC, are an increasingly common treatment strategy for patients who have soft-tissue, cartilage, and bony injuries. BMAC is obtained via aspiration of the bone marrow content, after which the cellular components are separated based on a centrifuge gradient that allows for the collection of both hematopoietic and mesenchymal stem cells. Pluripotent mesenchymal stem cells can be differentiated into both chondral and osseous progenitor cells, whereas hematopoietic cells as well as collected platelets and growth factors can help signal and propagate the cellular regenerative process. Wilke et al[51] reported that the introduction of BMAC into the full-thickness cartilage lesions of 12 horses improved cartilage repair, with several of the cartilage lesions having a propensity for type II hyaline-like cartilage. Improved cellular density, improved cellular orientation, and greater type II collagen content have been reported with the use of BMAC as an adjunct to microfracture and OAT in animal studies.[52,53]

Improved graft ingrowth, enhanced chondrocyte proliferation, and limited potential for articular fluid ingress around the graft plugs, which may lead to early failure, have been reported with the use of BMAC in human studies. In a study of 72 patients with large OLTs who underwent OAT with adjunct BMAC, Kennedy and Murawski[54] reported substantially improved mean Foot and Ankle Outcome Scores and

Medical Outcomes Study 12-Item Short Form scores at a minimum follow-up of 1 year; however, three patients had donor site knee pain postoperatively, and in one patient a perigraft cyst developed that required decompression at 28 months postoperatively. In a prospective study of 48 patients with OLTs who underwent microfracture with adjunct BMAC via a hyaluronic acid scaffold, Giannini et al[55] reported improved pain and functional scores as well as histologic verification of variable degrees of tissue remodeling at a minimum follow-up of 24 months.

 Video 23.1: Ankle and Cartilage Treatment in the Athlete. Eric Giza, MD (3 min)

Treatment Options

Good results have been reported in most patients with OLTs who undergo BMS; however, certain subsets of patients with OLTs who undergo BMS have poorer outcomes. Although several studies have reported that the size of an OLT is the primary factor in suboptimal microfracture outcomes, the size of an OLT that is most appropriate for each treatment option remains controversial.[22,56] The authors of this chapter used the best available evidence in the literature to create a treatment algorithm for OLTs based on lesion size (**Table 1**).

Summary

OLTs are a common source of ankle pain and functional disability. The management of OLTs with BMS techniques is reasonably effective in most patients; however, certain OLT characteristics, including size larger than 1.5 cm^2 and cystic changes, remain barriers to improved outcomes. Surgeons should

consider a treatment algorithm that is based on the best available evidence to aid in the selection of the most appropriate treatment option for patients with OLTs.

References

1. Berndt AL, Harty M: Transchondral fractures (osteochondritis dissecans) of the talus. *J Bone Joint Surg Am* 1959;41(7):988-1020.

2. Davidson AM, Steele HD, MacKenzie DA, Penny JA: A review of twenty-one cases of transchondral fracture of the talus. *J Trauma* 1967;7(3):378-415.

3. van Dijk CN: *On Diagnostic Strategies in Patients With Severe Ankle Sprain [Master's Thesis]*. Amsterdam, the Netherlands, University of Amsterdam, 1994.

4. Buckwalter JA, Rosenberg LC, Hunziker EB: Articular cartilage: Composition, structure, response to injury, and methods of facilitating repair, in Ewing JW, ed: *Articular Cartilage and Knee Joint Function: Basic Science and Arthroscopy*. New York, NY, Raven Press, 1990, pp 19-56.

5. Buckwalter JA, Mow VC, Ratcliffe A: Restoration of injured or degenerated articular cartilage. *J Am Acad Orthop Surg* 1994;2(4):192-201.

6. Zengerink M, Struijs PA, Tol JL, van Dijk CN: Treatment of osteochondral lesions of the talus: A systematic review. *Knee Surg Sports Traumatol Arthrosc* 2010;18(2):238-246.

7. Tol JL, Struijs PA, Bossuyt PM, Verhagen RA, van Dijk CN: Treatment strategies in osteochondral defects of the talar dome: A systematic review. *Foot Ankle Int* 2000;21(2):119-126.

8. Shearer C, Loomer R, Clement D: Nonoperatively managed stage 5 osteochondral talar lesions. *Foot Ankle Int* 2002;23(7):651-654.

9. Mei-Dan O, Maoz G, Swartzon M, et al: Treatment of osteochondritis dissecans of the ankle with hyaluronic acid injections: A prospective study. *Foot Ankle Int* 2008;29(12):1171-1178.

10. Mei-Dan O, Carmont MR, Laver L, Mann G, Maffulli N, Nyska M: Platelet-rich plasma or hyaluronate

Table 1	
Treatment Algorithm for Osteochondral Lesions of the Talus Based on Size	
OLT Size	**Treatment**
Small (<5 × 5 mm) with minimal cystic changes)	Microfracture, drilling, or curettage
Medium (5 × 5 mm to 10 × 10 mm) or smaller with cystic changes	Microfracture, drilling, or curettage
	MACI (not currently available for use in the United States), particulated juvenile articular cartilage, or bone marrow aspirate
Moderate (10 × 10 mm to 20 × 20 mm)	MACI (not currently available for use in the United States), particulated juvenile articular cartilage, or bone marrow aspirate
	ACI, OAT, or osteochondral allograft transplantation
Large (>20 × 20 mm)	OAT or osteochondral allograft transplantation
	Bulk allograft

ACI = autologous chondrocyte implantation, MACI = matrix-induced autologous chondrocyte implantation, OAT = osteochondral autograft transplantation, OLT = osteochondral lesion of the talus.

in the management of osteochondral lesions of the talus. *Am J Sports Med* 2012;40(3):534-541.

11. Gaulrapp H, Hagena FW, Wasmer G: Postoperative evaluation of osteochondrosis dissecans of the talus with special reference to medial malleolar osteotomy. *Z Orthop Ihre Grenzgeb* 1996;134(4):346-353.

12. Lynn AK, Brooks RA, Bonfield W, Rushton N: Repair of defects in articular joints: Prospects for material-based solutions in tissue engineering. *J Bone Joint Surg Br* 2004;86(8):1093-1099.

13. Ferkel RD, Zanotti RM, Komenda GA, et al: Arthroscopic treatment of chronic osteochondral lesions of the talus: Long-term results. *Am J Sports Med* 2008;36(9):1750-1762.

14. Schuman L, Struijs PA, van Dijk CN: Arthroscopic treatment for osteochondral defects of the talus: Results at follow-up at 2 to 11 years. *J Bone Joint Surg Br* 2002;84(3):364-368.

15. Savva N, Jabur M, Davies M, Saxby T: Osteochondral lesions of the talus: Results of repeat arthroscopic debridement. *Foot Ankle Int* 2007;28(6):669-673.

16. Becher C, Thermann H: Results of microfracture in the treatment of articular cartilage defects of the talus. *Foot Ankle Int* 2005;26(8):583-589.

17. Cuttica DJ, Smith WB, Hyer CF, Philbin TM, Berlet GC: Osteochondral lesions of the talus: Predictors of clinical outcome. *Foot Ankle Int* 2011;32(11):1045-1051.

18. Choi WJ, Park KK, Kim BS, Lee JW: Osteochondral lesion of the talus: Is there a critical defect size for poor outcome? *Am J Sports Med* 2009;37(10):1974-1980.

19. Chuckpaiwong B, Berkson EM, Theodore GH: Microfracture for osteochondral lesions of the ankle: Outcome analysis and outcome predictors of 105 cases. *Arthroscopy* 2008;24(1):106-112.

20. Gobbi A, Francisco RA, Lubowitz JH, Allegra F, Canata G: Osteochondral lesions of the talus: Randomized controlled trial comparing chondroplasty, microfracture, and osteochondral autograft transplantation. *Arthroscopy* 2006;22(10):1085-1092.

21. Scranton PE Jr, McDermott JE: Treatment of type V osteochondral lesions of the talus with ipsilateral knee osteochondral autografts. *Foot Ankle Int* 2001;22(5):380-384.

22. Robinson DE, Winson IG, Harries WJ, Kelly AJ: Arthroscopic treatment of osteochondral lesions of the talus. *J Bone Joint Surg Br* 2003;85(7):989-993.

23. Sammarco GJ, Makwana NK: Treatment of talar osteochondral lesions using local osteochondral graft. *Foot Ankle Int* 2002;23(8):693-698.

24. Al-Shaikh RA, Chou LB, Mann JA, Dreeben SM, Prieskorn D: Autologous osteochondral grafting for talar cartilage defects. *Foot Ankle Int* 2002;23(5):381-389.

25. Hangody L, Füles P: Autologous osteochondral mosaicplasty for the treatment of full-thickness defects of weight-bearing joints: Ten years of experimental and clinical experience. *J Bone Joint Surg Am* 2003;85(suppl 2):25-32.

26. Hangody L, Kish G, Módis L, et al: Mosaicplasty for the treatment of osteochondritis dissecans of the talus: Two to seven year results in 36 patients. *Foot Ankle Int* 2001;22(7):552-558.

27. Adams SB Jr, Viens NA, Easley ME, Stinnett SS, Nunley JA II: Midterm results of osteochondral lesions of the talar shoulder treated with fresh osteochondral allograft transplantation. *J Bone Joint Surg Am* 2011;93(7):648-654.

28. Berlet GC, Hyer CF, Philbin TM, Hartman JF, Wright ML: Does fresh osteochondral allograft transplantation of talar osteochondral defects improve function? *Clin Orthop Relat Res* 2011;469(8):2356-2366.

29. El-Rashidy H, Villacis D, Omar I, Kelikian AS: Fresh osteochondral allograft for the treatment of cartilage defects of the talus: A retrospective review. *J Bone Joint Surg Am* 2011;93(17):1634-1640.

30. Hahn DB, Aanstoos ME, Wilkins RM: Osteochondral lesions of the talus treated with fresh talar allografts. *Foot Ankle Int* 2010;31(4):277-282.

31. Raikin SM: Fresh osteochondral allografts for large-volume cystic osteochondral defects of the talus. *J Bone Joint Surg Am* 2009;91(12):2818-2826.

32. Giannini S, Buda R, Grigolo B, Vannini F, De Franceschi L, Facchini A: The detached osteochondral fragment as a source of cells for autologous chondrocyte implantation (ACI) in the ankle joint. *Osteoarthritis Cartilage* 2005;13(7):601-607.

33. Wood JJ, Malek MA, Frassica FJ, et al: Autologous cultured chondrocytes: Adverse events reported to the United States Food and Drug Administration. *J Bone Joint Surg Am* 2006;88(3):503-507.

34. Baums MH, Heidrich G, Schultz W, Steckel H, Kahl E, Klinger HM: Autologous chondrocyte transplantation for treating cartilage defects of the talus. *J Bone Joint Surg Am* 2006;88(2):303-308.

35. Giannini S, Buda R, Grigolo B, Vannini F: Autologous chondrocyte transplantation in osteochondral lesions of the ankle joint. *Foot Ankle Int* 2001;22(6):513-517.

36. Koulalis D, Schultz W, Psychogios B, Papagelopoulos PJ: Articular reconstruction of osteochondral defects of the talus through autologous chondrocyte transplantation. *Orthopedics* 2004;27(6):559-561.

37. Whittaker JP, Smith G, Makwana N, et al: Early results of autologous chondrocyte implantation in the talus. *J Bone Joint Surg Br* 2005;87(2):179-183.

38. Nam EK, Ferkel RD, Applegate GR: Autologous chondrocyte implantation of the ankle: A 2- to 5-year follow-up. *Am J Sports Med* 2009;37(2):274-284.

39. Vericel Corporation: Carticel package insert. Cambridge, MA, Vericel Corporation, November 2015. Available at: http://www.carticel.com. Accessed May 5, 2016.

40. Bartlett W, Skinner JA, Gooding CR, et al: Autologous chondrocyte implantation versus matrix-induced autologous chondrocyte implantation for osteochondral defects of the knee:

A prospective, randomised study. *J Bone Joint Surg Br* 2005;87(5):640-645.

41. Cherubino P, Grassi FA, Bulgheroni P, Ronga M: Autologous chondrocyte implantation using a bilayer collagen membrane: A preliminary report. *J Orthop Surg (Hong Kong)* 2003;11(1):10-15.

42. Brittberg M, Peterson L, Sjögren-Jansson E, Tallheden T, Lindahl A: Articular cartilage engineering with autologous chondrocyte transplantation: A review of recent developments. *J Bone Joint Surg Am* 2003;85(suppl 3):109-115.

43. Giannini S, Buda R, Ruffilli A, et al: Arthroscopic autologous chondrocyte implantation in the ankle joint. *Knee Surg Sports Traumatol Arthrosc* 2014;22(6):1311-1319.

44. Battaglia M, Vannini F, Buda R, et al: Arthroscopic autologous chondrocyte implantation in osteochondral lesions of the talus: Mid-term T2-mapping MRI evaluation. *Knee Surg Sports Traumatol Arthrosc* 2011;19(8):1376-1384.

45. Giza E, Sullivan M, Ocel D, et al: Matrix-induced autologous chondrocyte implantation of talus articular defects. *Foot Ankle Int* 2010;31(9):747-753.

46. McCormick F, Yanke A, Provencher MT, Cole BJ: Minced articular cartilage—basic science, surgical technique, and clinical application. *Sports Med Arthrosc* 2008;16(4):217-220.

47. Coetzee JC, Giza E, Schon LC, et al: Treatment of osteochondral lesions of the talus with particulated juvenile cartilage. *Foot Ankle Int* 2013;34(9):1205-1211.

48. Adkisson HD IV, Martin JA, Amendola RL, et al: The potential of human allogeneic juvenile chondrocytes for restoration of articular cartilage. *Am J Sports Med* 2010;38(7):1324-1333.

49. Bonner KF, Daner W, Yao JQ: 2-year postoperative evaluation of a patient with a symptomatic full-thickness patellar cartilage defect repaired with particulated juvenile cartilage tissue. *J Knee Surg* 2010;23(2):109-114.

50. Adams SB Jr, Yao JQ, Schon LC: Particulated juvenile articular cartilage allograft transplantation for osteochondral lesions of the talus. *Tech Foot Ankle Surg* 2011;10(2):92-98.

51. Wilke MM, Nydam DV, Nixon AJ: Enhanced early chondrogenesis in articular defects following arthroscopic mesenchymal stem cell implantation in an equine model. *J Orthop Res* 2007;25(7):913-925.

52. Fortier LA, Potter HG, Rickey EJ, et al: Concentrated bone marrow aspirate improves full-thickness cartilage repair compared with microfracture in the equine model. *J Bone Joint Surg Am* 2010;92(10):1927-1937.

53. Saw KY, Hussin P, Loke SC, et al: Articular cartilage regeneration with autologous marrow aspirate and hyaluronic acid: An experimental study in a goat model. *Arthroscopy* 2009;25(12):1391-1400.

54. Kennedy JG, Murawski CD: The treatment of osteochondral lesions of the talus with autologous osteochondral transplantation and bone marrow aspirate concentrate: Surgical technique. *Cartilage* 2011;2(4):327-336.

55. Giannini S, Buda R, Vannini F, Cavallo M, Grigolo B: One-step bone marrow-derived cell transplantation in talar osteochondral lesions. *Clin Orthop Relat Res* 2009;467(12):3307-3320.

56. Giannini S, Vannini F: Operative treatment of osteochondral lesions of the talar dome: Current concepts review. *Foot Ankle Int* 2004;25(3):168-175.

Video Reference

23.1: Giza E: Video. *Ankle and Cartilage Treatment in the Athlete*. Sacramento, CA, 2016.

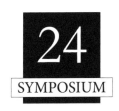

Lateral Ankle Instability and Peroneal Tendon Pathology

Michael Isiah Sandlin, MD
Cyrus E. Taghavi, MD
Timothy P. Charlton, MD
Richard D. Ferkel, MD

Abstract

Surgeons should understand the anatomic, vascular, biomechanical, and predisposing factors related to lateral ankle instability and peroneal tendon injuries, including peroneal tendinitis and tenosynovitis, peroneal tendon tears and ruptures, as well as peroneal tendon subluxation and dislocation. Surgeons should understand the treatment options and recommendations for patients who have lateral ankle instability and peroneal tendon injuries from the perspective of a sports medicine foot and ankle specialist. In addition, surgeons should be aware of arthroscopic approaches and an algorithm for the treatment of patients who have lateral ankle instability and peroneal tendon injuries.

Instr Course Lect 2017;66:301–312.

Lateral Ankle Instability

Ankle sprains are the most common sports-related injury that occur in athletes, contributing to approximately 20% of all athletic injuries.[1,2] The most common mechanism of injury involves forced ankle inversion with a plantar-flexed foot, which results in lateral ligamentous injury. The lateral ligament complex, which is the checkrein to pathologic range of motion, is easily overwhelmed. In patients who have a classic ankle sprain, the anterior talofibular ligament (ATFL) is injured first, after which varying degrees of injury to the calcaneofibular ligament (CFL) occur. The posterior talofibular ligament, which is the third structure of the lateral ankle ligament complex, typically is not involved in classic ankle sprains unless a higher-energy injury occurs, such as that which occurs in patients who sustain an ankle dislocation. Despite the successful outcomes achieved with nonsurgical treatment, 13% to 35% of patients who sustain an acute ankle sprain have residual symptoms, including pain, swelling, crepitance, functional limitations, and mechanical instability.[3,4] Unrecognized intra-articular injuries may contribute to these residual symptoms.[4,5] Factors that predispose patients to a persistently unstable and symptomatic ankle may include peroneal tendon weakness, proprioceptive dysfunction, tarsal coalition, gastrocnemius tightness, soleus tightness, genu varum, heel varus, or a posteriorly positioned fibula; some of these factors can be modified with nonsurgical management, and some of these factors cannot be modified with nonsurgical management.

Classification

Numerous systems have been developed to classify lateral ankle instability and ankle sprains. The American

Dr. Charlton or an immediate family member has stock or stock options held in the Green Bay Packers Football Club and the Manchester United Football Club. Dr. Ferkel or an immediate family member has received royalties from Smith & Nephew; serves as a paid consultant to Geistlich Pharma and Smith & Nephew; and serves as a board member, owner, officer, or committee member of the Arthroscopy Association of North America. Neither of the following authors nor any immediate family member has received anything of value from or has stock or stock options held in a commercial company or institution related directly or indirectly to the subject of this chapter: Dr. Sandlin and Dr. Taghavi.

Table 1

American Medical Association Standard Ankle Sprain Grading System

Grade	Characteristics
1	Microscopic tearing of the lateral ligaments
	Mild to moderate swelling
	Minimal to no ecchymosis
	Tenderness localized over ATFL
	No instability
	Patients able to bear weight
2	Partial ligament tearing
	Moderate to severe swelling
	Minimal to moderate ecchymosis
	Tenderness over ATFL and CFL
	Minimal instability
	Patients either partially or wholly unable to bear weight
3	Complete ligament rupture
	Severe swelling
	Severe ecchymosis
	Tenderness over ATFL, CFL, and PTFL
	Gross instability
	Patients unable to bear weight

ATFL = anterior talofibular ligament, CFL = calcaneofibular ligament, PTFL = posterior talofibular ligament.

Medical Association standard ankle sprain grading system[6] (**Table 1**), which has been adopted by the American Academy of Orthopaedic Surgeons, is the most commonly used ankle sprain classification system. Functional and/ or mechanical instability of the ankle may develop in patients who sustain an ankle sprain. Functional instability is defined as motion that is beyond voluntary control but does not exceed the normal physiologic limits of the joint. Mechanical instability is motion that is beyond voluntary control and exceeds the normal physiologic limits of the joint.[7]

Clinical Evaluation

History and Physical Examination

The clinical evaluation of an athlete with suspected lateral ankle instability should consist of a thorough history that includes the number and severity of ankle sprains, the position of the foot and ankle at the time of the injuries, and the activity and level of force required to elicit the injuries. The type of sport the athlete participates in also may help inform decision making on the appropriate treatment.

The physical examination begins with an observation of the position of the foot and ankle during standing and ambulation without shoes. An examination of the uninjured foot and ankle should be performed before the examination of the injured foot and ankle to give the surgeon a baseline from which to note differences. The assessment should include an evaluation of heel varus and cavus foot positioning, which may predispose patients to lateral ankle instability. An examination for peroneal tendon subluxation or dislocation with ankle circumduction and for peroneal tendon strength testing with resisted dorsiflexion and eversion may help with diagnosis. The ankle anterior drawer test in dorsiflexion and plantar flexion can help isolate CFL and ATFL laxity, respectively. Abnormal talar tilt or subtalar motion, both of which may suggest CFL or subtalar ligamentous injury, should be compared with that of the contralateral foot and ankle. Some studies advocate fluoroscopic stress testing of ATFL and CFL end points as well as assessment of subtalar joint opening and talar tilt.[8-12] A 10° talar tilt difference between neutral ankle position and varus stress suggests pathologic laxity.[10,13]

Imaging

On anterior drawer lateral fluoroscopic imaging, laxity is present if motion in the injured ankle is 10 mm greater compared with that in the contralateral ankle. MRI is the preferred imaging modality for evaluation of the lateral ligament complex. MRI also is useful to assess potential contributing pathology, including tears of the peroneal tendons or retinaculum, osteochondral lesions of the talus or tibial plafond, intra-articular loose bodies, and other abnormalities. In a study of 21 patients who had chronic lateral ankle instability, Ferkel and Chams[5] reported that 20 of the patients (95%) had associated intra-articular problems, most commonly synovitis (16 patients), adhesions (10 patients), chondromalacia (7 patients), ossicles (6 patients), loose bodies (5 patients), osteochondral lesions of the talus (4 patients), and osteophytes (4 patients). Komenda and Ferkel[14] reported a 93% rate of intra-articular pathology in patients who had unstable ankles. An evaluation of concurrent subtalar instability and CFL pathology is critical in the assessment of symptomatic patients who have undergone previous surgery. An examination under anesthesia and preligament reconstruction ankle arthroscopy also may aid in treatment.

Treatment

Nonsurgical Treatment

Treatment protocols for patients who have lateral ankle ligament ruptures have evolved. Currently, most patients who have an ankle sprain are treated nonsurgically, with surgery reserved for patients who have chronic, recurrent ankle sprains or patients with an ankle sprain who have persistent symptoms. The current best recommendations for the nonsurgical treatment of patients who have an ankle sprain include a comprehensive approach of functional treatment, brace support, and exercise therapy. Good evidence in the literature supports the use of the classic rest, ice (cryotherapy), compression, and elevation method.[15-19] The use of NSAIDs in the early phase of healing also is supported. Manual therapies to mobilize the injured ankle are not recommended.[20,21] Ultrasonography, laser stimulation therapy, and electrical stimulation therapy have not proven to be beneficial.[22-24] Despite historical precedence, the immobilization of a sprained ankle in a cast for more than 2 weeks is not recommended;[25] however, a short period of ankle immobilization in the acute phase of injury can help alleviate pain and may be a useful treatment adjunct.

For patients who have acute ankle sprains, functional treatment with the use of supportive bracing should begin as soon as tolerated. Supportive bracing may include lace-up or semirigid braces.

Elastic band wraps are less helpful because they may be associated with a delay in return to sport or work.[18,26] Taping may be an option for elite-level athletes who have ankle sprains; however, it may be associated with skin complications, and proper care is necessary.[26] Prophylactic ankle bracing and taping has been reported to reduce the incidence and severity of ankle sprains during the sporting season. Proprioceptive and functional exercise therapy, including home exercise programs, are essential components of the nonsurgical management of ankle sprains and may help improve outcomes.[15,27] Surgical treatment is rarely necessary for recreational athletes or nonathletic patients who have an acute ankle sprain because nonsurgical treatment with bracing, kinetic chain strengthening exercises, and proprioceptive training results in an approximately 90% success rate.[26] Surgical treatment should be considered for professional or elite-level athletes and those with instability recalcitrant to maximal nonsurgical treatment.[15]

Surgical Treatment

Surgical treatment for patients who have lateral ankle instability includes anatomic repair techniques, semianatomic repair techniques, and nonanatomic repair techniques. The modified Broström-Gould procedure, which is an anatomic repair technique, is the most commonly performed procedure for the management of lateral ankle instability. The modified Broström-Gould procedure involves direct repair of the ATFL and CFL, including ligament imbrication and fixation to bone. Augmentation with the inferior extensor retinaculum completes the modified Broström-Gould-procedure. The modified Broström-Gould procedure is

simple, is reliable, restores normal anatomy, maintains ankle range of motion, and provides excellent stability. Multiple studies have reported good to excellent results in 90% or more of patients with lateral ankle instability who underwent the modified Broström-Gould procedure.[28-31] Several studies have reported good outcomes with the use of arthroscopic Broström techniques.[32-34] Anatomic Broström procedures that use semitendinosus allograft or gracilis autograft have been recommended for patients who have greater levels of lateral ankle instability, patients who have long-standing lateral ankle instability and attenuated lateral ligaments, as well as patients undergoing revision procedures.[35-38] Additional indications for anatomic Broström procedures with the use of an allograft include high-demand vocations or athletic activities, elevated body mass index, and generalized ligament laxity.[35,37-39] Coughlin et al[9] described anatomic lateral ligament reconstruction of the ATFL and CFL with the use of a free gracilis tendon autograft. Clanton[11] performed anatomic reconstruction of the ATFL with the use of an allograft that had strength and stiffness similar to that of native ligaments. Dierckman and Ferkel[39] reported excellent results in patients with lateral ankle instability who underwent reconstruction with the use of scmitendinosus tendon allograft, which obviated the morbidity of autograft harvest.

Semianatomic repair techniques primarily include the modified Broström-Evans procedure, which involves repair of the ATFL and CFL with inferior extensor retinaculum augmentation and the use of a peroneus brevis tendon slip that serves as a static guard against inversion. In the modified Broström-Evans procedure, the anterior one-third of the peroneus brevis tendon slip is released proximally and left attached to the fifth metatarsal distally. The loose proximal slip is then tenodesed into the anterior distal fibula via a weave or interference screw technique to augment the lateral checkrein. In a study of 21 ankles that were managed with the Broström-Evans procedure, Girard et al[38] reported substantially improved stability, with no loss of eversion strength but substantial decreases in subtalar motion.

Nonanatomic repair techniques include the use of multiple different structural grafts and tenodeses, including allograft as well as peroneus brevis (Chrisman-Snook procedure) autograft, fascia lata autograft, Achilles tendon autograft, plantaris tendon autograft, palmaris longus tendon autograft, and semitendinosus autograft. Anatomic reconstruction has replaced many of these tenodesis procedures, which have been reported to limit subtalar motion and result in deteriorating long-term outcomes.[40-46]

Patients who have recurrent instability and patients in whom reconstructive procedures fail should be carefully assessed for unrecognized structural or mechanical abnormalities. In particular, patients should be evaluated for peroneal tendon pathology, osteochondral lesions of the talus, subtalar instability, and varus hindfoot positioning. In an athlete with varus hindfoot positioning, a Dwyer lateral calcaneal closing wedge osteotomy in combination with lateral ligament reconstruction (often with graft augmentation) is key. The Coleman block test can be used to assess hindfoot varus secondary to first ray plantar flexion, which can be managed with a dorsiflexion first metatarsal osteotomy at the time of lateral ligament reconstruction.

Postoperative Rehabilitation

Postoperative rehabilitation protocols may vary based on the demands of an athlete and his or her sport. The authors of this chapter consider the first 6 postoperative weeks the key to optimal soft-tissue healing and ligamentous stability. Postoperatively, the patient's leg is placed in a short-leg cast, which is bivalved in the recovery room. Initial follow-up is scheduled for 1 to 2 weeks postoperatively, at which time the wound is inspected, the sutures are removed, and the cast is changed. Weight bearing is initiated after the application of the second cast, with advancement to full weight bearing by the third postoperative week. Formal physical therapy is initiated at 6 weeks postoperatively, at which time the second cast is removed and the patient is transitioned to a compression stocking and controlled ankle motion boot. At 9 weeks postoperatively, the patient is transitioned to a normal shoe with the use of an ankle brace.

Patients are able to return to sports and/or active work duty without restrictions after they complete all four phases of postoperative rehabilitation.[39,47] The phases of postoperative rehabilitation are based on both time from surgery and patient progression. Typically, the first phase of postoperative rehabilitation, which focuses on edema and pain management, restoration of soft tissue and joint mobility, gait retraining, as well as proprioception, begins 4 to 6 weeks postoperatively. The second phase of postoperative rehabilitation, which focuses on returning gait and ankle range of motion to near-normal levels as well as increasing multidirectional

ankle strength, proprioceptive training, and edema control, takes place between 6 and 8 weeks postoperatively. Balance training, light-resistance band work, and pool therapy also are begun in the second phase of postoperative rehabilitation. The third phase of postoperative rehabilitation, which focuses on preparing the patient to return to sports and/or active work duty, takes place between 8 and 10 weeks postoperatively. Exercises in the third phase of postoperative rehabilitation include variable resistance and stability exercises as well as advancement to controlled single leg movements and activity-specific drills. The fourth and final phase of postoperative rehabilitation, which focuses on functional training for sports, including plyometrics as well as pivoting and cutting drills, and eventual return to sport, takes place between 11 and 18 weeks postoperatively. Reinjury is a concern in the fourth phase of postoperative rehabilitation, and the aid of a physical therapist to focus patients on the proper performance of drills is the key to avoid recurrent instability.

Some postoperative rehabilitation protocols include prolonged boot or brace immobilization at night to prevent passive plantar flexion and inversion. The authors of this chapter maintain the same postoperative rehabilitation protocol regardless of whether a patient underwent a Broström procedure or a repair with tendon augmentation. The authors of this chapter discuss with their patients the anticipated goal of return to game-level activity by 3 to 4 months postoperatively.

Peroneal Tendon Pathology

Peroneal tendon pathology includes a group of relatively uncommon but frequently underdiagnosed disorders that contribute to reports of posterolateral ankle pain and result in substantial functional limitations. Peroneal tendon injuries can be grouped into three primary categories of disorders: peroneal tendinitis and tenosynovitis; peroneal tendon tears and ruptures; and peroneal tendon subluxation and dislocation.[26] Peroneal tendinitis and tenosynovitis constitute most peroneal tendon injuries and more reliably respond to nonsurgical management compared with symptomatic peroneal tendon split tears and peroneal tendon subluxation and dislocation, all of which usually require surgical management. Factors that predispose patients to peroneal tendon pathology include structural conditions such as cavovarus foot positioning or varus hindfoot alignment that lead to increased stress on the peroneal tendons during activity. A posteriorly positioned fibula, a history of repetitive activities, acute ankle sprains, chronic ankle instability, and fractures also may predispose patients to peroneal tendon injury.

Clinical Evaluation
History and Physical Examination
The clinical evaluation of an athlete with a suspected peroneal tendon injury should consist of a thorough history and physical examination to confirm peroneal tendon injury, which is often misdiagnosed.[48] Patients with peroneal tendon injury most commonly complain of posterolateral ankle or hindfoot pain. Patients with peroneal tendon injury often are misdiagnosed with an ankle sprain, and a delay of up to 14 months in the diagnosis of a peroneal tendon injury is not uncommon.[48,49] The differential diagnosis for patients with peroneal tendon injury is broad, including lateral ankle instability,

osteochondral lesions of the talus, insertional Achilles tendinitis, sinus tarsi syndrome, fracture of the fifth metatarsal, calcaneocuboid joint arthritis, ankle or subtalar loose bodies, tarsal coalition, lumbosacral radiculopathy, sural nerve injury, peroneus quartus presence, malignant or benign tumor, and peroneal tubercle hypertrophy.[50] The history should include the duration of the complaint, a detailed location of the pain, and an assessment for the predisposing factors already mentioned. Alterations in type of footwear, inflammatory or neuromuscular conditions, diabetes mellitus, the use of fluoroquinolone antibiotics, and local steroid injections have been associated with peroneal tendon dysfunction.[51-53]

The physical examination begins with an observation of the standing alignment of the patient's ankle and hindfoot. Varus hindfoot or cavovarus foot positioning may be present. The Coleman block test can be used to determine if hindfoot varus is primary or secondary to a plantarflexed first ray or, alternatively, a result of forefoot valgus; this differentiation can aid in the selection of an appropriately molded orthotic device. The posterolateral ankle should be assessed for swelling, warmth, and tenderness, all of which Krause and Brodsky[54] reported to be the most reliable clinical findings associated with peroneal tendon pathology. Pain with passive or active hindfoot inversion/eversion or with resisted ankle dorsiflexion and foot eversion also indicates peroneal tendon pathology. Pain at the cuboid tunnel may indicate peroneus longus injury or os peroneum syndrome. Subtalar range of motion may be normal or limited by pain and tendon scarring. Anterior subluxation of the peroneal tendons over

the lateral malleolus may be obvious or subclinical. Palpation of the posterior fibular structures via active ankle circumduction and ankle dorsiflexion with the foot in eversion can help assess for peroneal tendon subluxation or gross dislocation.[55] An assessment of ankle joint stability and muscle strength testing also should be performed.

Imaging
Standard weight-bearing radiographs that include three views of the foot and ankle should be obtained in an athlete with a suspected peroneal tendon injury. Radiographs should be evaluated for osteochondral lesions of the talus; retromalleolar spurring; the presence and location of os peroneum syndrome; fracture or malunion of the calcaneus, fibula, or fifth metatarsal; joint arthrosis; and peroneal tubercle hypertrophy. Fracture of the fifth metatarsal tuberosity may indicate peroneus brevis injury or plantar fascia avulsion injury, and proximal migration of the os peroneum may suggest peroneus longus tendon rupture. In patients who have a peroneal tendon dislocation, ankle radiographs that demonstrate a cortical flake avulsion of the lateral malleolus may indicate superior retinacular rupture.[56] Hindfoot alignment radiographs or Harris heel radiographs can help identify varus hindfoot positioning as well as peroneal tubercle hypertrophy or retromalleolar groove spurs. CT, which allows for observation of the anatomic bony detail of the foot and ankle, can help identify the presence and size of tarsal coalitions. MRI is the preferred imaging modality for the evaluation of peroneal tendon pathology because it allows for excellent visualization of soft-tissue structures, peroneal tendon tears, tenosynovitis, retinacular tears,

retromalleolar groove depth and orientation, ankle ligament injury, and osteochondral lesions of the talus. Some surgeons recommend obtaining axial radiographs with the foot positioned in slight plantar flexion, which allows for a truer cross-sectional view of the tendons at the retromalleolar curve.

Steel and DeOrio[56] reported that the sensitivity of MRI for the diagnosis of peroneus brevis tears and peroneus longus tears was 80% and 100%, respectively; however, the sensitivity of MRI for the diagnosis of dual peroneal tendon injuries was only 60%. Other studies have reported less-than-ideal results with the use of MRI for the diagnosis of peroneus longus tears as well as a potential overestimation in the diagnosis of peroneal tendon disorders with the use of MRI.[57,58] Ultrasonography is increasingly being used to evaluate the peroneal tendons because of its low cost, lack of ionizing radiation, and high sensitivity for the diagnosis of peroneal tendon pathology. Ultrasonography is limited by technician proficiency but is able to demonstrate tendon thickening, fluid around the tendon, and partial or complete peroneal tendon ruptures. Peroneal tendon subluxation and dislocation can be observed on dynamic ultrasonography. Several studies have reported that the sensitivity and specificity of ultrasonography for the diagnosis of peroneal tendon subluxation and split peroneal tendon tears is more than 90%.[59,60]

Treatment

Peroneal Tendinitis and Tenosynovitis
Peroneal tendinitis and tenosynovitis are conditions that involve tendon or tendon sheath inflammation. Peroneal tendinitis and tenosynovitis are often related to overuse and repetitive activities; chronic ankle instability, direct trauma, gait abnormalities, and peroneal tubercle hypertrophy are contributing factors.[61-64] Chronic inflammation of the tendon or tendon sheath can lead to structural thickening, degeneration, and subsequent local scarring that limits tendon excursion and causes pain with motion.[65]

Typically, treatment is nonsurgical and consists of rest, possible short-term immobilization in a cast or a walking boot, activity modifications, NSAIDs, physical therapy, and orthotic use. Orthotic use should be informed by results of the Coleman block test. Lateral heel wedges are most effective in the management of hindfoot-driven pathology, and lateral forefoot wedges are most effective in the management of primary forefoot valgus. Recessed first ray positioning may be helpful for patients who have first ray plantar flexion. Steroid injections should be used judiciously to avoid iatrogenic tendon compromise. Open or arthroscopic peroneal tendon débridement and tenosynovectomy may be performed in patients with peroneal tendinitis or tenosynovitis in whom maximal nonsurgical treatment fails.[60,63,66] Care should be taken to address concomitant alignment deformities or associated pathologies, such as ankle instability, low-lying peroneus brevis muscle belly, or peroneus quartus presence, to increase successful patient outcomes.

Painful os peroneum syndrome is a related condition that involves pain at the cuboid tunnel in patients who have an intratendinous ossicle of the peroneus longus. Symptoms of painful os peroneum syndrome may be caused by ossicle fracture, tendon inflammation as a result of stenosis or compression, or partial or complete tendon tears around the ossicle. In patients who have a peroneus longus tendon tear, proximal migration of the os peroneum may be observed on radiographs, with concurrent loss of arch or first ray plantar flexion weakness noted on physical examination. Treatment for patients with painful os peroneum syndrome typically is symptomatic, and surgery rarely is indicated.[60]

Peroneal Tendon Tears
Peroneal tendon tears were first reported by the anatomist Arthur Meyers in 1924. An 11% to 37% incidence of peroneal tendon tears has been reported in cadaver model studies.[67] Peroneal tendon tears are believed to occur primarily as a result of repetitive movement and chronic attritional degeneration. Krause and Brodsky[54] hypothesized that chronic peroneal tendon subluxation at the level of the posterolateral corner of the distal fibula was the cause of most attritional split peroneal tendon tears. Split peroneal tendon tears also may result from stenosis within the retrofibular groove that is caused by crowding and increased tendon pressure secondary to a low-lying peroneus brevis muscle belly, tendon sheath inflammation, or peroneus quartus presence. Peroneal tendon tears also can result from acute direct trauma or ankle sprain. Peterson et al[68] described three critical avascular zones in the peroneal tendons that may contribute to tendinopathy. The peroneus brevis tendon has one avascular zone that is located at the turn of the distal fibula. The peroneus longus has two avascular zones: one zone at the same location as that in the peroneus brevis tendon and the other zone at the turn into the cuboid tunnel. These avascular zones correlate with the regions

of most frequent peroneal tendon injury; however, several recent studies have reported that the vascular supply to these tendon regions are adequate for healing.[69,70]

Nonsurgical treatment options for patients who have peroneal tendon tears include a short period of immobilization in a walking cast or boot, ankle bracing, orthotic use, NSAIDs, and physical therapy. Nonsurgical treatment can be effective for patients who have small peroneal tendon tears; however, surgery typically is required for patients who have large split peroneal tendon tears or complete peroneal tendon ruptures.[54,71]

Surgical treatment options for patients who have peroneal tendon tears vary depending on the severity of the injury and may include direct repair, tenodesis, flexor digitorum longus tendon transfer, or the use of an allograft. In a study of 20 patients with peroneus brevis tendon tears who underwent surgical treatment, Krause and Brodsky[54] proposed a new classification system that guided the surgical management of peroneal tendon tears. Grade 1 peroneal tendon tears that included damage to less than or equal to 50% of the cross-sectional area of the peroneal tendon were managed with débridement and tendon repair. Grade 2 peroneal tendon tears that included damage to more than 50% of the cross-sectional area of the peroneal tendon were managed with segmental resection and tenodesis. In addition, the authors recommended tendon stabilization for both grade 1 and grade 2 peroneal tendon tears to reduce overt or subclinical peroneal tendon subluxation, which the authors believed was the underlying cause of the peroneal tendon tears. The authors

reported that return to maximum function was prolonged, but that high levels of patient satisfaction were achieved.

Redfern and Myerson[71] proposed a treatment algorithm for patients who have peroneal tendon tears based on intraoperative findings. Type I peroneal tendon tears, in which both tendons are intact, were managed with excision of the torn segment and tubularization. Type II peroneal tendon tears, in which one tendon is irreparably torn and the other tendon is functional and has sufficient excursion, were managed with segment resection and proximal tenodesis. Type III peroneal tendon tears were classified as those in which both tendons were torn and nonfunctional. For type III peroneal tendon tears, if no proximal muscle excursion was present the authors recommended tendon transfer; if proximal muscle excursion was present and the tissue bed was free of scarring, the authors recommended one-stage tendon grafting; if proximal muscle excursion was present and the tissue bed had scarring, the authors recommended staged tendon grafting. The flexor digitorum longus is the most commonly transferred tendon in the acute setting because of its adequate excursion and because its strength profile is similar to that of the peroneal tendon. Multiple studies have reported satisfactory outcomes in patients with peroneal tendon tears who undergo flexor digitorum longus transfer.[72,73] In staged tendon transfer procedures, a partial tendon resection is performed and a Hunter rod is inserted in the first stage to allow for the formation of a pseudosynovial peroneal tendon sheath. In the second stage, which is performed 3 months after the first stage, the Hunter rod is removed, and either the flexor hallucis longus

tendon or the flexor digitorum longus tendon is transferred via the pseudosynovial tendon sheath to the base of the fifth metatarsal.[71] Any associated varus malalignment or ankle instability should be addressed simultaneously.

Good outcomes are achieved in most patients who undergo peroneal tendon tear repair. Sammarco[72] reported improved results in patients who had acute peroneal tendon tears compared with patients who had chronic peroneal tendon tears and in patients in whom one peroneal tendon was torn compared with patients in whom both peroneal tendons were torn. Krause and Brodsky[54] reported that most of their patients had satisfactory outcomes after peroneal tendon tears and underlying instability were addressed. In a study of seven patients with chronic rupture of both peroneal tendons who underwent staged reconstruction with the use of the Hunter rod technique, Wapner et al[74] reported that six of the patients had complete pain relief and returned to their preinjury level of function at a mean follow-up of 8.5 years. In a study of eight collegiate athletes who underwent primary peroneal tendon repair, Bassett and Speer[75] reported that all of the athletes returned to sport without recurrent symptoms. Steel and DeOrio[56] reported less successful outcomes in a study of 30 patients who underwent peroneal tendon tear repair, with only 46% of the patients able to return to sport at a mean follow-up of 31 months.

A consensus approach to the management of peroneal tendon tears conforms with the classification system for the management of peroneal tendon tears that was described by Krause and Brodsky.[54] A curved incision is centered over the fibular tip, and careful dissection is performed to avoid sural nerve injury. The common peroneal tendon sheath is opened just below the peroneal retinaculum; opening of the distinct tendon sheaths as they separate distally should be avoided, if possible. The tendons are then carefully inspected to determine the extent of the tear. If less than or equal to 50% of the cross-sectional area of the peroneal tendon is torn, the authors of this chapter excise the torn or degenerative tendon and tubularize the remaining limb. If more than 50% of the cross-sectional area of the peroneal tendon is torn, the authors of this chapter excise the torn or degenerative tendon and perform tenodesis. Fibular groove deepening also may be performed to reduce frictional attrition and the risk for recurrent tears or subluxation. Irreparable peroneal tendon tears and tears of both peroneal tendons are difficult and complex problems. Peroneal tendoscopy is an additional treatment consideration for patients with peroneal tendon pathology. For peroneal tendoscopy, portals are made approximately 2 cm proximal and 2 cm distal to the posterior edge of the malleolus. Small instrument, 2.7-mm and 1.9-mm 30° arthroscopes and a 2.9-mm shaver are used to débride the peroneal tendon and tenosynovium. Peroneal tendoscopy is a reasonable option for the evaluation of peroneal tendon integrity if a patient's MRI findings are inconclusive but his or her physical examination and history suggest peroneal tendon pathology.

Postoperative management may vary depending on the procedure that is performed. Typical postoperative management recommendations include immobilization in a splint or cast for 1 to 2 weeks postoperatively followed by transition to a walking cast or boot for an additional 2 to 3 weeks. Weight bearing is gradually increased after 2 weeks postoperatively, and physical therapy is initiated 4 to 6 weeks postoperatively.

Peroneal Tendon Subluxation and Dislocation

Peroneal tendon subluxation and dislocation are related conditions that were first described in a ballet dancer by Monteggia in 1803. Peroneal tendon subluxation and dislocation are frequently misdiagnosed as lateral ankle sprains in the acute setting. Most true peroneal tendon dislocations are of traumatic etiology as a result of sports such as snow skiing or football.[76] The superior peroneal retinaculum (SPR) is the primary restraint to peroneal tendon subluxation at the level of the ankle; injury to the SPR is required for pathologic tendon mobility to occur. Eckert and Davis[77] described the anatomy of the SPR, which includes the fibro-osseous retromalleolar groove through which the peroneal tendons travel, with the peroneus longus tendon positioned posterolaterally to the peroneus brevis tendon. The authors also described the contributions from the SPR, peroneal tendon sheath, CFL, posterior talofibular ligament, posteroinferior tibiofibular ligaments, and fibro-osseous retromalleolar groove. In addition, Eckert and Davis[77] described a classification system for SPR injuries. Grade I SPR injuries involve elevation of the SPR from the fibula and dislocation of the anterior peroneus longus tendon. Grade II SPR injuries involve rupture of the SPR with fibrocartilaginous rim avulsion from the posterior fibula. Grade III SPR injuries involve rupture of the SPR with cortical fragment avulsion from the fibula. Oden[78] added a grade IV SPR injury, which involves elevation of the SPR from the calcaneus.

The treatment of patients who have acute peroneal tendon dislocations may include an attempt at nonsurgical management. If the reduced peroneal tendon is stable, casting with the ankle positioned in neutral to slight plantar flexion and inversion may allow the retinaculum to heal to the posterolateral fibula.[50] Good results have been reported in approximately 50% of patients who undergo nonsurgical treatment, with athletes having a higher risk for recurrence.[77]

Recent studies advocate open or endoscopic repair of peroneal tendon subluxation or dislocation in high-demand patients or patients who have chronic pain that is associated with peroneal tendon subluxation.[50,76,79] McGarvey and Clanton[80] evaluated and grouped the various surgical techniques for the management of chronic peroneal tendon dislocation or subluxation into anatomic superior peroneal retinacular repair, retinacular reinforcement with tissue transfers, tendon rerouting procedures, bone block procedures, and fibular groove deepening procedures. In general, studies have reported good to excellent results in 90% of patients with peroneal tendon subluxation or dislocation who undergo surgical treatment.[81-84] In general, anatomic repair involves the creation of a posterolateral fibular osseous trough, the placement of three to four drill holes into the posterolateral fibular osseous trough, and repair of the retinaculum through the drill holes with the use of nonabsorbable suture.[81,82] Alternatively, the retinaculum can be fixed to the inferior edge of the fibular trough or augmented with a partial Achilles tendon slip, the goal of which includes diminishing the retromalleolar groove space and limiting excursion and the risk for dislocation. Both Maffulli et al[81] and Adachi et al[82] reported excellent results in patients who underwent retinacular repair techniques. Bone block procedures involve sagittal osteotomy of the fibula, with posterior displacement of the lateral segment to increase the required jump distance, and fixation of the bone block with screws. Higher rates of complications, including tendon irritation, nonunion, and tendon scarring, have been reported in patients who undergo bone block procedures.[50,83] Local tissue transfers from the plantaris tendon, peroneus brevis tendon, or posterior fibular periosteum as well as the use of an Achilles tendon slip also have been described.[50,81,82,84] Tendon rerouting procedures have been performed to reduce the recurrence of peroneal tendon subluxation. Typically, good results can be achieved in patients who undergo tendon re-routing procedures in which the peroneal tendons are transposed under the CFL.[85] Fibular groove-deepening procedures are performed under the assumption that a shallow retrofibular groove predisposes patients to peroneal tendon subluxation and dislocation. Fibular groove-deepening procedures involve deepening of the retrofibular groove via elevation of a posterior fibular cortical flap, removal of cancellous bone, and replacement of the posterior fibular cortical flap. Alternatively, vertical drilling of the posterior subcortical bone followed by tamping to collapse the posterior cortex into a deepened position can be performed. Excellent results with minimal recurrence have been reported in patients who undergo groove-deepening procedures.[50,79,81] General considerations for the surgical management of peroneal tendon dislocation or subluxation include avoiding isolated soft-tissue repairs in patients with chronic dislocations because of the high failure rate and addressing any associated pathology or malalignment at the time of surgery. The authors of this chapter prefer to perform fibular groove deepening combined with direct repair of the SPR in patients who have peroneal tendon subluxation or dislocation.

Summary

The approach of the authors of this chapter for a patient with suspected lateral ankle instability consists of a thorough patient history and a physical examination that includes a careful assessment for possible secondary diagnoses. Surgeons should be aware of combined injuries, including chronic lateral instability, osteochondral lesions of the talus, dislocating peroneal tendons, medial deltoid instability, syndesmotic injury, and subtalar instability. Surgeons should consider obtaining stress radiographs to help assess instability patterns. MRI is the preferred preoperative imaging modality for patients with suspected lateral ankle instability; however, many associated conditions will only be observed with the use of preligament reconstruction arthroscopy, which can aid in the assessment of associated injuries and may improve postoperative outcomes. The authors of this chapter recommend special caution in the treatment of patients who have generalized ligament laxity or larger athletes who participate in contact sports because they have a high risk for repair failure and may require semitendinosus hamstring augmentation in combination with the modified Broström-Gould procedure.

Peroneal tendon injuries are a relatively uncommon but clinically underdiagnosed cause of posterolateral ankle or hindfoot pain and functional disability. The clinical evaluation of a patient with a suspected peroneal tendon injury relies on a high level of suspicion for peroneal tendon injury and consists of a thorough patient history and a physical examination that includes an assessment of associated and contributing factors. MRI is the preferred preoperative imaging modality for the evaluation of peroneal tendon pathology. Nonsurgical treatment may be attempted but is less likely to be successful in patients who have chronic peroneal tendon injuries, peroneal tendon tears, and peroneal tendon subluxation or dislocation. Treatment options are based on addressing the specific peroneal tendon injury as well as any concomitant malalignment or instability patterns.

References

1. Gerber JP, Williams GN, Scoville CR, Arciero RA, Taylor DC: Persistent disability associated with ankle sprains: A prospective examination of an athletic population. *Foot Ankle Int* 1998;19(10):653-660.

2. Waterman BR, Owens BD, Davey S, Zacchilli MA, Belmont PJ Jr: The epidemiology of ankle sprains in the United States. *J Bone Joint Surg Am* 2010;92(13):2279-2284.

3. Korkala O, Tanskanen P, Mäkijärvi J, Sorvali T, Ylikoski M, Haapala J: Long-term results of the Evans procedure for lateral instability of the ankle. *J Bone Joint Surg Br* 1991;73(1):96-99.

4. Sammarco GJ, DiRaimondo CV: Surgical treatment of lateral ankle instability syndrome. *Am J Sports Med* 1988;16(5):501-511.

5. Ferkel RD, Chams RN: Chronic lateral instability: Arthroscopic findings and long-term results. *Foot Ankle Int* 2007;28(1):24-31.

6. American Medical Association, Committee on the Medical Aspects of Sports, Subcommittee on Classification of Sports Injuries: *Standard Nomenclature of Athletic Injuries.* Chicago, IL, American Medical Association, 1966.

7. Ferkel RD: *Arthroscopic Surgery: The Foot and Ankle.* Philadelphia, PA, Lippincott-Raven, 1996.

8. Coughlin MJ, Schenck RC Jr: Lateral ankle reconstruction. *Foot Ankle Int* 2001;22(3):256-258.

9. Coughlin MJ, Matt V, Schenck RC Jr: Augmented lateral ankle reconstruction using a free gracilis graft. *Orthopedics* 2002;25(1):31-35.

10. Coughlin MJ, Schenck RC Jr, Grebing BR, Treme G: Comprehensive reconstruction of the lateral ankle for chronic instability using a free gracilis graft. *Foot Ankle Int* 2004;25(4):231-241.

11. Clanton TO: Athletic injuries to the soft tissues of the foot and ankle, in Coughlin MJ, Mann RA, eds: *Surgery of the Foot and Ankle,* ed 7. St. Louis, MO, Mosby-Yearbook, 1999, pp 1090-1209.

12. Rubin G, Witten M: The talar-tilt angle and the fibular collateral ligaments: A method for the determination of talar tilt. *J Bone Joint Surg Am* 1960;42(2):311-326.

13. Schenck RC Jr, Coughlin MJ: Lateral ankle instability and revision surgery alternatives in the athlete. *Foot Ankle Clin* 2009;14(2):205-214.

14. Komenda GA, Ferkel RD: Arthroscopic findings associated with the unstable ankle. *Foot Ankle Int* 1999;20(11):708-713.

15. Kerkhoffs GM, van den Bekerom M, Elders LA, et al: Diagnosis, treatment and prevention of ankle sprains: An evidence-based clinical guideline. *Br J Sports Med* 2012;46(12):854-860.

16. Bleakley C, McDonough S, MacAuley D: The use of ice in the treatment of acute soft-tissue injury: A systematic review of randomized controlled trials. *Am J Sports Med* 2004;32(1):251-261.

17. Coté DJ, Prentice WE Jr, Hooker DN, Shields EW: Comparison of three treatment procedures for minimizing ankle sprain swelling. *Phys Ther* 1988;68(7):1072-1076.

18. Airaksinen O, Kolari PJ, Miettinen H: Elastic bandages and intermittent pneumatic compression for treatment of acute ankle sprains. *Arch Phys Med Rehabil* 1990;71(6):380-383.

19. Rucinkski TJ, Hooker DN, Prentice WE, Shields EW, Cote-Murray DJ: The effects of intermittent compression on edema in postacute ankle sprains. *J Orthop Sports Phys Ther* 1991;14(2):65-69.

20. Bleakley CM, McDonough SM, MacAuley DC: Some conservative strategies are effective when added to controlled mobilisation with external support after acute ankle sprain: A systematic review. *Aust J Physiother* 2008;54(1):7-20.

21. Brantingham JW, Globe G, Pollard H, Hicks M, Korporaal C, Hoskins W: Manipulative therapy for lower extremity conditions: Expansion of literature review. *J Manipulative Physiol Ther* 2009;32(1):53-71.

22. Barker AT, Barlow PS, Porter J, et al: A double-blind clinical trial of lower power pulsed shortwave therapy in the treatment of a soft tissue injury. *Physiotherapy* 1985;71(12):500-504.

23. Pennington GM, Danley DL, Sumko MH, Bucknell A, Nelson JH: Pulsed, non-thermal, high-frequency electromagnetic energy (DIAPULSE) in the treatment of grade I and grade II ankle sprains. *Mil Med* 1993;158(2):101-104.

24. Wilson DH: Treatment of soft-tissue injuries by pulsed electrical energy. *Br Med J* 1972;2(5808):269-270.

25. Kerkhoffs GM, Rowe BH, Assendelft WJ, Kelly KD, Struijs PA, van Dijk CN: Immobilisation for acute ankle sprain: A systematic review. *Arch Orthop Trauma Surg* 2001;121(8):462-471.

26. Kerkhoffs GM, Struijs PA, Marti RK, Blankevoort L, Assendelft WJ, van Dijk CN: Functional treatments for acute ruptures of the lateral ankle ligament: A systematic review. *Acta Orthop Scand* 2003;74(1):69-77.

27. van der Wees PJ, Lenssen AF, Hendriks EJ, Stomp DJ, Dekker J, de Bie RA: Effectiveness of exercise therapy and manual mobilisation in ankle sprain and functional instability: A systematic review. *Aust J Physiother* 2006;52(1):27-37.

28. Rechtin GR, McCarroll JR, Webster DA: Reconstruction for chronic lateral instability of the ankle: A review of twenty eight surgical patients. *Orthopedics* 1982;5(1):46-50.

29. Riegler HF: Reconstruction for lateral instability of the ankle. *J Bone Joint Surg Am* 1984;66(3):336-339.

30. Staples OS: Result study of ruptures of lateral ligaments of the ankle. *Clin Orthop Relat Res* 1972;85:50-58.

31. Ajis A, Younger AS, Maffulli N: Anatomic repair for chronic lateral ankle instability. *Foot Ankle Clin* 2006;11(3):539-545.

32. Corte-Real NM, Moreira RM: Arthroscopic repair of chronic lateral ankle instability. *Foot Ankle Int* 2009;30(3):213-217.

33. Drakos MC, Behrens SB, Paller D, Murphy C, DiGiovanni CW: Biomechanical comparison of an open vs arthroscopic approach for lateral ankle instability. *Foot Ankle Int* 2014;35(8):809-815.

34. Acevedo JI, Mangone P: Arthroscopic brostrom technique. *Foot Ankle Int* 2015;36(4):465-473.

35. Karlsson J, Bergsten T, Lansinger O, Peterson L: Reconstruction of the lateral ligaments of the ankle for chronic lateral instability. *J Bone Joint Surg Am* 1988;70(4):581-588.

36. Youn H, Kim YS, Lee J, Choi WJ, Lee JW: Percutaneous lateral ligament reconstruction with allograft for chronic lateral ankle instability. *Foot Ankle Int* 2012;33(2):99-104.

37. Karlsson J, Lansinger O: Chronic lateral instability of the ankle in athletes. *Sports Med* 1993;16(5):355-365.

38. Girard P, Anderson RB, Davis WH, Isear JA, Kiebzak GM: Clinical evaluation of the modified Brostrom-Evans procedure to restore ankle stability. *Foot Ankle Int* 1999;20(4):246-252.

39. Dierckman BD, Ferkel RD: Anatomic reconstruction with a semitendinosus allograft for chronic lateral ankle instability. *Am J Sports Med* 2015;43(8):1941-1950.

40. Colville MR, Marder RA, Zarins B: Reconstruction of the lateral ankle ligaments: A biomechanical analysis. *Am J Sports Med* 1992;20(5):594-600.

41. Colville MR: Reconstruction of the lateral ankle ligaments. *Instr Course Lect* 1995;44:341-348.

42. Bahr R, Pena F, Shine J, Lew WD, Tyrdal S, Engebretsen L: Biomechanics of ankle ligament reconstruction: An in vitro comparison of the Broström repair, Watson-Jones reconstruction, and a new anatomic reconstruction technique. *Am J Sports Med* 1997;25(4):424-432.

43. Savastano AA, Lowe EB Jr: Ankle sprains: Surgical treatment for recurrent sprains. Report of 10 patients treated with the Chrisman-Snook modification of the Elmslie procedure. *Am J Sports Med* 1980;8(3):208-211.

44. van der Rijt AJ, Evans GA: The long-term results of Watson-Jones tenodesis. *J Bone Joint Surg Br* 1984;66(3):371-375.

45. Snook GA, Chrisman OD, Wilson TC: Long-term results of the Chrisman-Snook operation for reconstruction of the lateral ligaments of the ankle. *J Bone Joint Surg Am* 1985;67(1):1-7.

46. Molloy R, Tisdel C: Failed treatment of peroneal tendon injuries. *Foot Ankle Clin* 2003;8(1):115-129, ix.

47. Donatelli R, Hall W, Prell BE, Linck G, Ferkel RD: Lateral ligament repair of the ankle, in Maxey L, Magnusson J, eds: *Rehabilitation for the Postsurgical Orthopedic Patient*, ed 3. St. Louis, MO, Elsevier-Mosby, 2013, pp 504-519.

48. Dombek MF, Lamm BM, Saltrick K, Mendicino RW, Catanzariti AR: Peroneal tendon tears: A retrospective review. *J Foot Ankle Surg* 2003;42(5):250-258.

49. Selmani E, Gjata V, Gjika E: Current concepts review: Peroneal tendon disorders. *Foot Ankle Int* 2006;27(3):221-228.

50. Rosenberg ZS, Feldman F, Singson RD, Price GJ: Peroneal tendon injury associated with calcaneal fractures: CT findings. *AJR Am J Roentgenol* 1987;149(1):125-129.

51. Vainio K: The rheumatoid foot; a clinical study with pathological and roentgenological comments. *Ann Chir Gynaecol Fenn Suppl* 1956;45(1):1-107.

52. Sharma P, Maffulli N: Tendon injury and tendinopathy: Healing and repair. *J Bone Joint Surg Am* 2005;87(1):187-202.

53. Niemi WJ, Savidakis J Jr, DeJesus JM: Peroneal subluxation: A comprehensive review of the literature with case presentations. *J Foot Ankle Surg* 1997;36(2):141-145.

54. Krause JO, Brodsky JW: Peroneus brevis tendon tears: Pathophysiology, surgical reconstruction, and clinical results. *Foot Ankle Int* 1998;19(5):271-279.

55. Church CC: Radiographic diagnosis of acute peroneal tendon dislocation. *AJR Am J Roentgenol* 1977;129(6):1065-1068.

56. Steel MW, DeOrio JK: Peroneal tendon tears: Return to sports after operative treatment. *Foot Ankle Int* 2007;28(1):49-54.

57. Brandes CB, Smith RW: Characterization of patients with primary peroneus longus tendinopathy: A review of twenty-two cases. *Foot Ankle Int* 2000;21(6):462-468.

58. Neustadter J, Raikin SM, Nazarian LN: Dynamic sonographic evaluation of peroneal tendon subluxation. *AJR Am J Roentgenol* 2004;183(4):985-988.

59. Magnano GM, Occhi M, Di Stadio M, Toma' P, Derchi LE: High-resolution US of non-traumatic recurrent dislocation of the peroneal tendons: A case report. *Pediatr Radiol* 1998;28(6):476-477.

60. Sobel M, Pavlov H, Geppert MJ, Thompson FM, DiCarlo EF, Davis WH: Painful os peroneum syndrome: A spectrum of conditions responsible for plantar lateral foot pain. *Foot Ankle Int* 1994;15(3):112-124.

61. Bonnin M, Tavernier T, Bouysset M: Split lesions of the peroneus brevis tendon in chronic ankle laxity. *Am J Sports Med* 1997;25(5):699-703.

62. Wind WM, Rohrbacher BJ: Peroneus longus and brevis rupture in a collegiate athlete. *Foot Ankle Int* 2001;22(2):140-143.

63. Bruce WD, Christofersen MR, Phillips DL: Stenosing tenosynovitis and impingement of the peroneal tendons associated with hypertrophy of the peroneal tubercle. *Foot Ankle Int* 1999;20(7):464-467.

64. Pierson JL, Inglis AE: Stenosing tenosynovitis of the peroneus longus tendon associated with hypertrophy of the peroneal tubercle and an os peroneum: A case report. *J Bone Joint Surg Am* 1992;74(3):440-442.

65. Gray JM, Alpar EK: Peroneal tenosynovitis following ankle sprains. *Injury* 2001;32(6):487-489.

66. Techner LM, DeCarlo RL: Peroneal tubercle osteochondroma. *J Foot Surg* 1992;31(3):234-237.

67. Sobel M, DiCarlo EF, Bohne WH, Collins L: Longitudinal splitting of the peroneus brevis tendon: An anatomic and histologic study of cadaveric material. *Foot Ankle* 1991;12(3):165-170.

68. Petersen W, Bobka T, Stein V, Tillmann B: Blood supply of the peroneal tendons: Injection and immunohistochemical studies of cadaver tendons. *Acta Orthop Scand* 2000;71(2):168-174.

69. Sobel M, Geppert MJ, Hannafin JA, Bohne WH, Arnoczky SP: Microvascular anatomy of the peroneal tendons. *Foot Ankle* 1992;13(8):469-472.

70. Sammarco GJ: Peroneal tendon injuries. *Orthop Clin North Am* 1994;25(1):135-145.

71. Redfern D, Myerson M: The management of concomitant tears of the peroneus longus and brevis tendons. *Foot Ankle Int* 2004;25(10):695-707.

72. Sammarco GJ: Peroneus longus tendon tears: Acute and chronic. *Foot Ankle Int* 1995;16(5):245-253.

73. Borton DC, Lucas P, Jomha NM, Cross MJ, Slater K: Operative reconstruction after transverse rupture of

the tendons of both peroneus longus and brevis: Surgical reconstruction by transfer of the flexor digitorum longus tendon. *J Bone Joint Surg Br* 1998;80(5):781-784.

74. Wapner KL, Taras JS, Lin SS, Chao W: Staged reconstruction for chronic rupture of both peroneal tendons using Hunter rod and flexor hallucis longus tendon transfer: A long-term followup study. *Foot Ankle Int* 2006;27(8):591-597.

75. Bassett FH III, Speer KP: Longitudinal rupture of the peroneal tendons. *Am J Sports Med* 1993;21(3):354-357.

76. Guillo S, Calder JD: Treatment of recurring peroneal tendon subluxation in athletes: Endoscopic repair of the retinaculum. *Foot Ankle Clin* 2013;18(2):293-300.

77. Eckert WR, Davis EA Jr: Acute rupture of the peroneal retinaculum. *J Bone Joint Surg Am* 1976;58(5):670-672.

78. Oden RR: Tendon injuries about the ankle resulting from skiing. *Clin Orthop Relat Res* 1987;216:63-69.

79. Porter D, McCarroll J, Knapp E, Torma J: Peroneal tendon subluxation in athletes: Fibular groove deepening and retinacular reconstruction. *Foot Ankle Int* 2005;26(6):436-441.

80. McGarvey WC, Clanton TO: Peroneal tendon dislocations. *Foot Ankle Clin* 1996;1(2):325-342.

81. Maffulli N, Ferran NA, Oliva F, Testa V: Recurrent subluxation of the peroneal tendons. *Am J Sports Med* 2006;34(6):986-992.

82. Adachi N, Fukuhara K, Tanaka H, Nakasa T, Ochi M: Superior retinaculoplasty for recurrent dislocation of peroneal tendons. *Foot Ankle Int* 2006;27(12):1074-1078.

83. Kelly RE: An operation for the chronic dislocation of the peroneal tendons. *Br J Surg* 1919;7(28):502-504.

84. Jones E: Operative treatment of chronic dislocation of the peroneal tendons. *J Bone Joint Surg Am* 1932;14(3):574-576.

85. Steinböck G, Pinsger M: Treatment of peroneal tendon dislocation by transposition under the calcaneofibular ligament. *Foot Ankle Int* 1994;15(3):107-111.

Spine

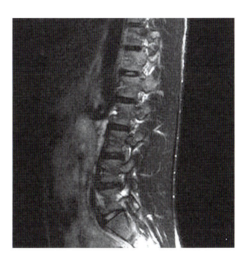

Differentiating Hip Pathology From Lumbar Spine Pathology: Key Points of Evaluation and Management

Aaron J. Buckland, MBBS, FRACS
Ryan Miyamoto, MD
Rakesh D. Patel, MD
James Slover, MS, MD
Afshin E. Razi, MD

Abstract

The diagnosis and treatment of patients who have both hip and lumbar spine pathologies may be a challenge because overlapping symptoms may delay a correct diagnosis and appropriate treatment. Common complaints of patients who have both hip and lumbar spine pathologies include low back pain with associated buttock, groin, thigh, and, possibly, knee pain. A thorough patient history should be obtained and a complete physical examination should be performed to identify the primary source of pain. Plain and advanced imaging studies and diagnostic injections can be used to further delineate the primary pathology and guide the appropriate sequence of treatment. Both the surgeon and the patient should understand that although one pathology is managed, management of the other pathology may be necessary because of persistent pain. The recognition of both entities may help reduce the likelihood of misdiagnosis, and the management of both entities in the appropriate sequence may help reduce the likelihood of persistent symptoms.

Instr Course Lect 2017;66:315–327.

Hip and lumbar spine pathologies often occur in combination, which may result in substantial disability.[1-3] Patients with both hip and lumbar spine pathology commonly have low back pain (LBP) with associated buttock, groin, thigh, and, possibly, knee pain. The diagnosis and treatment of these patients may be a challenge because overlapping symptoms may delay a correct diagnosis and, therefore, appropriate treatment.

Offierski and MacNab[4] originally described the term hip-spine syndrome in 1983. The authors classified hip-spine syndrome as simple, complex, secondary, or misdiagnosed. In patients with simple hip-spine syndrome, the primary source of symptoms is clear despite coexistent hip and lumbar spine pathologies. In patients with complex hip-spine syndrome, however, no clear source of symptoms is known despite a detailed physical examination. Patients with complex hip-spine syndrome require additional diagnostic tests, including diagnostic injections. In patients with secondary hip-spine syndrome, both pathologies are interdependent, and

Dr. Miyamoto or an immediate family member serves as a paid consultant to or is an employee of CONMED Linvatec and has stock or stock options held in Tornier. Dr. Patel or an immediate family member is a member of a speakers' bureau or has made paid presentations on behalf of Stryker Spine; and serves as a paid consultant to or is an employee of Globus Medical and Stryker. Dr. Slover or an immediate family member has received research or institutional support from Biomet and DJO Global. Dr. Razi or an immediate family member serves as a board member, owner, officer, or committee member of the American Academy of Orthopaedic Surgeons, the American Orthopaedic Association, and the Brooklyn Orthopaedic Society. Neither Dr. Buckland nor any immediate family member has received anything of value from or has stock or stock options held in a commercial company or institution related directly or indirectly to the subject of this chapter.

the symptoms of one region are secondary to the pathology of the other region. The authors reported that flexion contracture of the hip that results in compensatory hyperlordosis of the lumbar spine, which causes foraminal stenosis, especially at L3-4, is an example of secondary hip-spine syndrome. Similarly, scoliosis that causes pelvic obliquity and acetabular tilt may result in uncovering of the femoral head. In patients with misdiagnosed hip-spine syndrome, the primary source of pain is incorrectly diagnosed, which results in inappropriate, expensive treatment.

Hip and lumbar spine pathologies may mimic one another. Several studies have reported on the source of referred hip pain, which includes all lumbar nerve roots via the sciatic, obturator, and femoral nerves.[5,6] Surgeons should understand how to perform a comprehensive evaluation of and appropriately treat patients with potential hip and lumbar spine pathologies.

History

A thorough patient history is crucial to differentiate hip pathology from lumbar spine pathology. A thorough patient history begins with an assessment of the temporal onset, duration, severity, location, and character of the pain and the antecedent trauma. Surgeons must determine whether a patient has pain with activity, at rest, or both. Pain at night and the presence or absence of pain-free intervals may indicate a tumor or an infection. Traditionally, groin pain is associated with hip pathology, and buttock and back pain is associated with lumbar spine pathology; however, overlap exists between hip and lumbar spine pathologies. Pain from hip osteoarthritis (OA) can be localized to the groin (84%), buttock (76%), anterior

thigh (59%), posterior thigh (43%), anterior knee (69%), shin (47%), and calf (29%).[7,8] In general, difficulty with putting on shoes or getting in and out of a car are associated with hip pathology. A burning or electric character to pain may be suggestive of lumbar spine pathology, especially if accompanied by a nerve-root signature or associated numbness or weakness. The ability of a patient to ambulate with a forward posture, which is known as the shopping cart sign, or improvement in pain in a sitting position may indicate lumbar stenosis. The inability of a patient to lie on his or her side is likely caused by trochanteric bursitis rather than lumbar radiculopathy or intra-articular hip pathology. Clicking, snapping, or pain with movement of the hip likely indicates intra-articular hip pathology. Some patients may describe hip pain in which he or she grasps the lateral aspect of the hip with his or her thumb and index finger in the groin (C-sign). Changes in posture may highlight potential psoas pathology if pain is felt in the groin and thigh or spinal instability if pain is felt in the lower back. A history of startup groin pain (pain that usually improves after 5 to 10 steps and then gradually returns) may indicate a loose total hip arthroplasty (THA) component. Startup back or buttock pain may indicate spinal instability.

Physical Examination

The physical examination of a patient with potential hip and lumbar spine pathologies should include inspection and palpation of the affected areas, an observation of gait, and a comprehensive hip and spinal evaluation. Surgeons should observe a patient's posture, muscle atrophy, previous surgical scars, limb-length discrepancy, pelvic obliquity, and lower

limb and spinal alignment (coronal, sagittal, and rotational). If a limb-length discrepancy exists, blocks should be placed under the patient's short leg to correct pelvic obliquity before observing spinal alignment. The forward bend test should be performed to assess spinal rotational deformity; in a patient's attempt to achieve extension, pain may indicate lumbar stenosis or spinal instability. Palpation for areas of tenderness over the greater trochanter, sacroiliac joints, groin, buttock, and lumbar spine and evidence of step-off between spinous processes may be clues to the more likely pathology. An observation of a patient's gait may help surgeons assess for antalgic gait or the presence of an abductor lurch. Walking on the heels and toes may indicate subtle weakness as a result of L4 through S1 nerve involvement. The Trendelenburg test should be performed. Although a positive Trendelenburg test has been reported to indicate hip pathology, the test also may be positive in patients with L5 radiculopathy as a result of innervation of the gluteus medius and minimus muscles.

Hip range of motion testing should be performed, assessing for loss of internal rotation with pain at terminal range of motion, which indicates hip pathology.[9-12] Groin pain and thigh pain have been reported in 55% and 57% of patients with hip pathology, respectively; however, buttock pain and pain distal to the knee have been reported in 71% and 22% to 47% of patients with hip pathology, respectively.[5] The sensitivity and specificity of groin pain for hip dysfunction has been reported to be 84.3% and 70%, respectively. On physical examination, patients with pain caused by hip pathology are seven times more likely to have a limp and report

Table 1

Common Provocative Tests for Hip and Lumbar Spine Pathologies

Test	Description	Common Pathologies
Straight leg raise	With the patient positioned supine, the examined leg is raised with the knee extended.	Lumbar radiculopathy (lower lumbar nerves), with pain elicited from 30° to 60°
Contralateral straight leg raise	With the patient positioned supine, the contralateral leg is raised with the knee extended.	Lumbar radiculopathy (lower lumbar nerves), with pain elicited in the other leg from 30° to 60°
Femoral nerve stretch	With the patient positioned supine at the edge of the table or in the lateral position, the hip is extended and the knee is flexed.	Lumbar radiculopathy (upper lumbar nerves)
Thomas	In the supine position, the patient grasps one knee and flexes it to the chest. The test is positive if the examined leg does not extend fully.	Hip flexion contracture of the examined leg
Ober	With the patient lying on the unaffected side and the knee flexed to 90°, the symptomatic hip is brought from abduction to adduction.	Iliotibial band tightness
Anterior impingement (FADIR)	With the patient positioned supine, the hip is flexed to 90° and assessed under forced internal rotation and adduction	FAI, labral tear, or piriformis syndrome with groin pain
Posterior impingement (FABER)	With the patient positioned supine, the affected hip is placed in flexion, abduction, and external rotation	Sacroiliac joint dysfunction with buttock pain and intra-articular hip pathology (FAI) with anterior and lateral pain
Seated piriformis stretch	With the patient in a seated position, the hip is placed under flexion and adduction with the internal rotation test	A positive test, which re-creates posterior pain at the level of the piriformis or external rotators, indicates possible sciatic nerve entrapment.
Active piriformis contraction	The patient pushes the heel down into the table, abducting and externally rotating against resistance as the examiner monitors the piriformis.	Pain and weakness may indicate sciatic nerve entrapment.
Trendelenburg	With the patient standing on one leg, the opposite hemipelvis drops.	Weakness of gluteus medius on the standing leg

FABER = flexion, abduction, and external rotation; FADIR = flexion, adduction, and internal rotation; FAI = femoroacetabular impingement.

groin pain and are 14 times more likely to have limited internal rotation compared with patients with pain caused by lumbar spine pathology.[9]

A thorough neurologic examination of the upper and lower extremities for upper motor neuron signs is crucial. Several provocative tests can help clarify whether symptoms are caused by hip or lumbar spine pathology (**Table 1**). Positive provocative tests that likely indicate lumbar spine pathology include the straight leg raise, contralateral straight leg raise, and femoral nerve stretch tests. Surgeons should observe patients with hip flexion contracture, which may result in a false-positive femoral nerve stretch test. Positive provocative tests that likely indicate hip pathology include hip impingement tests, such as the flexion, adduction, and internal rotation test or the flexion, abduction, and external rotation (FABER) test; the snapping iliopsoas test; and instability tests. Compression at the sacroiliac joint and a positive FABER test may indicate sacroiliac joint arthritis.

Diagnostic Tests

Plain radiography is the first-line imaging modality that should be performed to determine the likely source of pathology. AP radiographs of the pelvis and cross-table lateral radiographs should be obtained in patients in whom hip OA is suspected. In addition to standing AP radiographs of the pelvis, 45° or 90° Dunn lateral or frog-lateral radiographs of the hip are useful to assess for femoral head asphericity, and false-profile radiographs are useful to assess for acetabular dysplasia. Radiographs of the spine should be obtained with the patient in a standing position, depending on pathology. If lumbar spine pathology is suspected, AP and lateral radiographs should be obtained; however, lateral flexion-extension radiographs can help identify instability or spondylolisthesis. If spinal malalignment is present, 36-inch AP and lateral standing radiographs should be obtained to assess alignment from the femoral heads to the lower cervical spine.

Although MRI and CT can help differentiate hip pathology from lumbar spine pathology, they are not first-line imaging modalities. MRIs of the spine can demonstrate nerve-root compression, epidural lesions, infection, and disk and soft-tissue pathology in the lumbar spine and the paraspinal muscles (including the psoas muscles). MRIs of the hip (with or without MRI arthrograms or delayed gadolinium-enhanced MRIs of cartilage) can demonstrate chondrolabral pathology, cartilage lesions, the ligamentum teres, and extra-articular soft-tissue pathology. CT scans of the lumbar spine aid in the evaluation of fusion, spondylolysis, stress fractures, or bony tumors and can be used in combination with CT myelograms for patients in whom MRI is contraindicated. Three-dimensional CT reconstructions of the hip allow surgeons to better assess for cam and pincer deformities, acetabular morphology, and suspected femoral neck stress fractures. CT scanograms can be used to assess for femoral rotational deformities. Care should be taken to correlate a patient's diagnostic tests with his or her history and physical examination because positive findings increase with patient age.

If the etiology of a patient's pain remains unclear or coexistent hip and lumbar spine pathologies are suspected, additional information may be required. Electrophysiologic studies can help differentiate radiculopathy from peripheral nerve disorders, such as neuropathy, if other diagnostic tests are equivocal. Normal electrophysiologic findings do not eliminate the possibility of radiculopathy.[13,14] Leriche syndrome, which is a form of internal iliac artery stenosis, can result in buttock and thigh pain. In patients with vascular claudication, symptoms typically are relieved with standing and may be located below the knees.[15] Patients with vascular claudication may have diminished pulses, skin discoloration, and loss of extremity hair. Vascular studies, including the ankle-brachial index, duplex ultrasonography, and magnetic resonance angiography, can help rule out peripheral vascular diseases. Selective nerve-root injections (transforaminal), epidural injections, and intra-articular hip injections can be used as a diagnostic or therapeutic modality. Hip injections have an 87% sensitivity and a 100% specificity for hip pathology and can help predict the success of surgical interventions such as THA.[16-18] The sensitivity of epidural steroid injections for lumbar spine pathology in the setting of hip-spine syndrome has been less well defined.[6]

Differential Diagnosis

The development of differential diagnoses for hip, spine, and other pathologies is based on the principles of probability and importance (**Table 2**). More common pathologies, such as hip OA or lumbar radiculopathy, are more probable in patients who have back and lower extremity pain; however, some pathologies, such as tumors, stress fractures, and infections, although they are less likely in patients who have back and lower extremity pain, cannot be missed because they may result in substantial consequences.

Hip Pathology
Arthritic Hip Pathology
Hip OA is diagnosed as either primary or secondary as a result of entities such as gout, chondrocalcinosis, or hemochromatosis. Often, hip OA occurs in combination with lumbar stenosis and back pain (**Figure 1**). Studies have reported that patients with persistent back pain after THA who undergo management of the lumbar spine have improved symptoms.[19-22] Other studies have reported the resolution of back pain after the management of hip disease in patients undergoing THA or arthroscopic hip surgery, such as that for the management of a labral tear.[23-25]

In a study of 25 patients with hip OA and LBP who underwent THA, Ben-Galim et al[23] reported improvement in both hip and back scores at a follow-up of 2 years. In a retrospective study of 3,206 patients with hip OA, 566 of whom also had LBP, who underwent THA, Prather et al[24] reported that, although all of the patients had improved pain and hip scores, the patients without LBP had greater improvement in function and pain relief, incurred fewer medical charges per episode of care, and spent fewer days in the hospital per episode of care compared with the patients who had LBP. In a study of 113 patients with pain extending into the back (21%), shin (7%), and calf (3%) who underwent THA, Hsieh et al[26] reported complete pain relief in 110 of the patients within 12 weeks postoperatively. In a study of 344 patients with hip OA, 170 of whom also had LBP, who underwent THA, Parvizi et al[25] reported the resolution of LBP in 66.4% of the 170 patients in whom it was noted preoperatively. Conversely, within 1 year postoperatively, LBP developed in 20% of the 174 patients in whom it was not noted preoperatively, which suggests that the management of hip pathology may exacerbate lumbar spine pathology. In a study of a cohort of patients who had exacerbated lumbar

Table 2
Differential Diagnoses for Hip, Spine, and Other Pathologies That May Mimic One Another

Intra-articular Hip Pathology	Extra-articular Hip Pathology	Spinal Pathology	Other Pathology
Hip osteoarthritis	Stress fracture	Lumbar stenosis with or without spondylolisthesis	Sacroiliac joint pathology
Septic arthritis	Greater trochanteric bursitis	Lumbar disk herniation	Sciatic nerve tumor
Stress fracture	Iliotibial band tendinitis	Foraminal stenosis	Intrapelvic tumors
Osteonecrosis	Gluteus medius or gluteus minimus tear	Facet cyst	Insufficiency fracture of the sacrum
Failed total hip arthroplasty	Iliopsoas tendinitis	Nerve-root sheath tumor	Peripheral vascular diseases (including Leriche syndrome)
Labral tear	Coxa saltans (internal or external snapping hip)	Spondylolysis and isthmic spondylolisthesis	Osteitis pubis
Femoroacetabular impingement	Piriformis syndrome	Iatrogenic cause (ie, misplaced pedicle screw)	Paget disease
Loose bodies (synovial chondromatosis, pigmented villonodular synovitis, osteochondritis dissecans)	Subgluteal space syndromes (deep gluteal, hamstring pathology, pudendal nerve, and ischiofemoral impingement)	Sagittal spinal malalignment	Peripheral neuropathy
Chondral damage	Adductor strain	Psoas pathology (abscess, hematoma, malpositioned hardware, transpsoas approach)	Shingles
Capsular laxity	None	None	Meralgia paresthetica
Ligamentum teres rupture	None	None	Sports hernia

spine symptoms after THA, McNamara et al[19] reported improved symptoms in the patients who underwent decompression. Pritchett[27] reported that 21 patients with lumbar stenosis who underwent THA had footdrop postoperatively. Therefore, decompression of symptomatic severe lumbar stenosis occasionally is recommended before THA.

Nonarthritic Hip Pathology
Femoroacetabular Impingement and Labral Tears
Femoroacetabular impingement (FAI) refers to altered geometry of the proximal femur and/or acetabulum, which leads to a conflict between the femoral neck and the acetabular rim. Long-standing symptomatic FAI may result in labral tears and, subsequently,

intra-articular chondral damage and early-onset OA. Cam impingement results from femoral head-neck junction abnormality, which affects the acetabulum. Pincer impingement results from acetabular overcoverage. Coexistent pathology is common in patients with FAI.

Clohisy et al[3] and Burnett et al[28] described the standard physical examination for patients in whom FAI is suspected, which includes hip range of motion, anterior impingement (flexion, adduction, and internal rotation), and posterior impingement (FABER) tests. Isometric strength testing and a gait analysis are the mainstays of a comprehensive physical examination. Groin pain has been reported in as many as 92% of patients with FAI, and a positive anterior impingement

test has been reported in as many as 88% of patients with FAI. Lateral hip pain, buttock pain, knee pain, and LBP have been reported in as many as 67%, 29%, 27%, and 23% of patients with FAI, respectively. Imaging studies that should be obtained in patients in whom FAI is suspected include plain radiographs and MRI arthrograms. Studies have reported that the intra-articular injection of bupivacaine during magnetic resonance arthrography is 92% sensitive, 97% specific, and 90% accurate for the diagnosis of FAI.[29-32] MRI can be used to assess asphericity (α angle) of the femoral head.

Greater Trochanteric Pain Syndrome
Greater trochanteric pain syndrome includes disorders that cause pain over the lateral hip, such as trochanteric

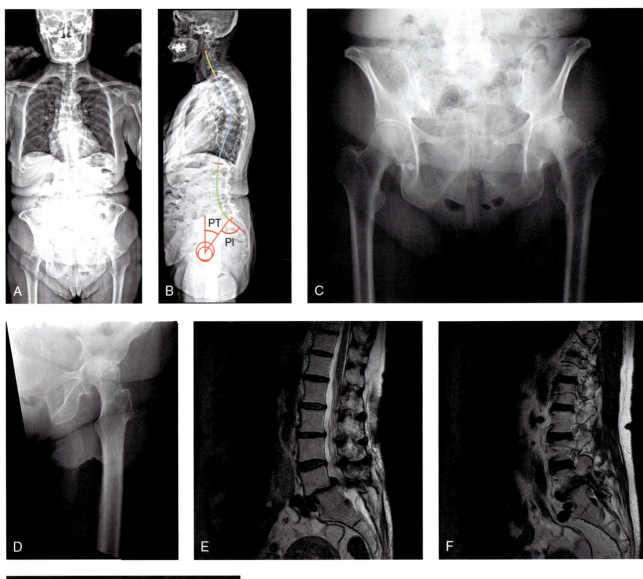

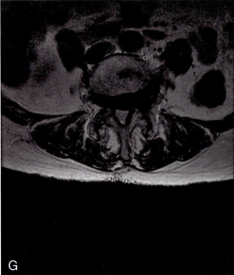

Figure 1 Images of a 75-year-old woman who had low back pain with associated left groin, lateral thigh, and knee pain. AP (**A**) and lateral (**B**) radiographs of the spine demonstrate pelvic tilt (PT) of 36°, pelvic incidence (PI) of 89°, lumbar lordosis of −59°, and PI-lumbar lordosis of 30°. In panel **B,** the yellow line indicates cervical spine alignment, the blue line indicates thoracic spine alignment, and the green line indicates lumbar spine alignment. AP radiograph of the pelvis (**C**) and lateral radiograph of the left hip (**D**) demonstrate avascular necrosis of the left femoral head with collapse and secondary arthritis of the left hip. Midline sagittal T2-weighted MRI of the lumbar spine (**E**), left of midline sagittal T2-weighted MRI of the lumbar spine (**F**), and axial T2-weighted MRI of the lumbar spine through L4-5 (**G**) show broad-based disk herniation with moderate to severe central and lateral recess lumbar stenosis. The patient was diagnosed with left hip osteoarthritis and L4-5 spondylolisthesis in combination with lateral recess and L4-5 foraminal stenosis left of midline. The patient underwent total hip arthroplasty of her left hip and had substantial pain relief in her back and lower extremity.

bursitis, external snapping hip, and gluteus minimus/medius dysfunction (tendinopathy/tears). Classic findings of greater trochanteric pain syndrome include pain with palpation over the lateral hip, a positive Ober test, the Trendelenburg sign, a Trendelenburg gait, and advanced abductor dysfunction. Hip abduction weakness and pain with resisted external rotation or pain with standing on one leg also are key physical examination findings of greater trochanteric pain syndrome. In a study of 24 patients with refractory greater trochanteric pain syndrome, Bird et al[33] reported that gluteus medius tears were observed on the MRIs of 45.8% of the patients.

Coxa Saltans (Snapping Hip Syndrome)
Internal snapping syndrome refers to the abrupt snapping of the iliopsoas tendon over the iliopectineal eminence as the hip moves from flexion into extension, which is accompanied by an audible snap, apprehension, and groin pain. External snapping syndrome refers to the snapping of the iliotibial band over the greater trochanter as the hip moves from extension into flexion. External rotation of the leg in extension followed by internal rotation of the hip as it moves into flexion can accentuate the snapping. Trochanteric bursitis is common in patients with snapping hip syndrome as a result of the thickened, tight iliotibial band.

Subgluteal Space Syndromes
Subgluteal space syndromes include deep gluteal syndrome, hamstring pathology, pudendal nerve impingement, and ischiofemoral impingement.[34,35] The subgluteal space is bordered by the posterior aspect of the femoral neck and is located anterior to the gluteus maximus,

lateral to the linea aspera, and medial to the sacrotuberous and falciform fascia below the sciatic notch. Deep gluteal syndrome involves sciatic nerve entrapment, which is most commonly caused by the piriformis, and results in diffuse buttock or posterior thigh pain and occasional radiating symptoms. A positive seated piriformis stretch test and a positive active piriformis contraction test are key physical examination findings of deep gluteal syndrome. Ischiofemoral impingement refers to the narrowing of the ischiofemoral space between the lesser trochanter and the ischial tuberosity. Patients with ischiofemoral impingement have atypical groin and/or posterior buttock pain. Pain in patients with ischiofemoral impingement is reproduced via a combination of hip extension, adduction, and external rotation. In patients with ischiofemoral impingement, MRI often demonstrates narrowing of the ischiofemoral space and an abnormal signal or edema in the quadratus femoris muscle.[36]

Stress Fractures
Stress fractures are classified as insufficiency fractures or fatigue fractures. The femoral neck is the most common site of stress fracture. A stress fracture should be suspected in long-distance runners; patients with metabolic bone diseases; patients being treated with long-term diphosphonate therapy; and patients who report groin, thigh, or knee pain. Pain in patients with a stress fracture is worse with weight bearing and improves with periods of rest. Technetium Tc-99m bone scanning and MRI are sensitive for the diagnosis of stress fracture.

Painful Total Hip Arthroplasty
Several unique factors must be considered in patients with pain after THA.

In most patients with pain after THA, a thorough history with regard to the surgery, the perioperative period, and the patient's recent health; a complete physical examination; and appropriate imaging studies will allow surgeons to correctly identify the source of pain. Early-onset pain may indicate an infection, implant instability, or heterotopic ossification. Late-onset pain may indicate an infection, synovitis, metallosis, osteolysis, instability or loosening of the implant, inadequate hip biomechanics (eg, inadequate offset, limb-length discrepancy), or soft-tissue (psoas, rectus femoris) inflammation or impingement. Acetabular loosening commonly results in groin pain and buttock pain. Thigh and/or knee pain may be caused by femoral loosening. Activity-related pain and startup pain are caused by component instability. Plain radiographs always are indicated in patients with pain after THA. Serial radiographs allow surgeons to assess changes in implant positioning, which may help isolate the source of pain. More advanced imaging studies, such as MRI, CT, and nuclear imaging, allow for a more detailed evaluation and should be obtained in patients in whom the source of pain is unclear. Laboratory studies (eg, complete blood count, erythrocyte sedimentation rate, C-reactive protein levels) and hip aspiration should be obtained in patients in whom they are warranted.

Lumbar Spine Pathology
Radiculopathy
Radicular pain may mimic referred hip pain in the groin, thigh, or buttock. Radiculopathy from the L1 through L3 nerve roots is more likely to mimic referred hip pain in these areas; however, L5 radiculopathy may result in referred pain in the buttock, the lateral aspect of

the hip, and the thigh. L5 radiculopathy may mimic meralgia paresthetica. Radiculopathy may occur as a result of several pathologies, including disk herniation, spondylolisthesis, foraminal stenosis, iatrogenic injury (ie, misplaced pedicle screw), facet cysts, or nerve sheath tumors. Typically, patients with radiculopathy report an electric character to lower extremity pain, which may be worse in a sitting position, in a standing position, or with a change in posture; however, the pain may not always have a nerve-root signature. Motor weakness, sensory deficits, and absent reflexes likely indicate radiculopathy rather than hip pathology. The straight leg raise test and the contralateral straight leg raise test are specific but less sensitive for the diagnosis of radiculopathy from the L4 through S1 nerve roots, and the femoral nerve stretch test is a provocative test for the diagnosis of L2 and L3 radiculopathy. Imaging studies that can be obtained to confirm radiculopathy include MRI, CT myelography, and/or electromyography. A diagnostic or therapeutic nerve-root block can be performed to further confirm radiculopathy; however, Saito et al[6] reported that nerve-root blocks mask hip pathology by interfering with sensory nerve pathways.

Neurogenic Claudication

Neurogenic claudication can manifest as buttock and posterior thigh pain with ambulation; however, patients with neurogenic claudication also may have thigh and leg aching or heaviness/weakness with ambulation, which are symptoms similar to those of patients with hip OA. Lumbar stenosis, with or without spondylolisthesis, is the underlying pathology in patients with neurogenic claudication. Vascular claudication must always be ruled out. Although patients with neurogenic claudication may have decreased ambulation tolerance as a result of leg pain, patients with lumbar stenosis can continue to ambulate by leaning forward with an ambulatory support, which is known as the shopping cart sign. Trochanteric bursitis is common in patients with lumbar stenosis and spondylolisthesis; therefore, it must be considered in the differential diagnosis.

Spondylolysis and Isthmic Spondylolisthesis

Typically, spondylolysis occurs in young athletes, especially those who participate in sports that require repeated hyperextension of the lumbar spine. Patients with spondylolysis have unilateral or bilateral LBP that may radiate to the buttock. The pain may improve with periods of rest, with bracing, or by avoiding hyperextension. Oblique lumbar radiographs may demonstrate a pars defect; however, CT often is required to confirm a diagnosis of spondylolysis. Pars defects can be active or inactive; therefore, technetium Tc-99 bone scans or single photon emission CT scans should be obtained. Selective injection of a pars defect can help surgeons determine if the lesion is substantial.

Isthmic spondylolisthesis refers to an anterior translation of the cephalad vertebra in patients with a pars defect. Patients with unstable isthmic spondylolisthesis may report startup pain when they first get out of bed or stand up from a chair that improves after a period of walking. Radiculopathy as a result of foraminal stenosis is common in patients with isthmic spondylolisthesis. Standing flexion-extension radiographs of the lumbar spine can aid in the evaluation of subtle instability.

Sacroiliac Joint Pathology

Patients with sacroiliac joint pathology may have unilateral or bilateral buttock pain. Typically, pain is worse with walking down a hill and when wearing a tight belt. Physical examination findings of sacroiliac joint pathology include tenderness to palpation, pain with compression over the sacroiliac joint, and a positive FABER test. The FABER test also may be positive in patients with posterior chondrolabral pathology of the hip. A sacroiliac joint injection can aid in differentiating posterior chondrolabral pathology of the hip from other hip pathology and lumbar spine pathology.

Psoas Pathology

Psoas pathology can manifest as groin and thigh pain and weakness on hip flexion. Causes of psoas pathology include psoas abscess, hematoma, malpositioned hardware (ie, pedicle screw), and the transpsoas approach for lumbar fusion. Patients with psoas pathology may report difficulty standing up from a chair or pain with full hip extension. Physical examination findings of psoas pathology include pain with resisted flexion and a positive psoas stretch test. MRI with contrast and laboratory tests (eg, erythrocyte sedimentation rate, C-reactive protein levels, complete blood count) are useful to assess for a suspected abscess, and CT is useful to assess for malpositioned hardware.

Sagittal Spinal Deformity

Adult degenerative scoliosis, which includes sagittal spine deformity (SSD), is a common pathology that affects 60% of individuals older than 65 years.[37] SSD may result in substantial pain and disability.[38,39] Hip OA is common in many patients with SSD. Although

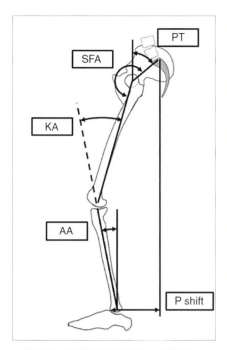

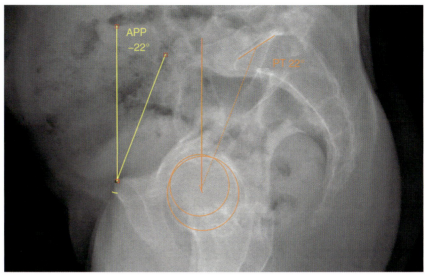

Figure 3   Lateral radiograph of a pelvis demonstrates that pelvic tilt (PT) can be determined by measuring the anterior pelvic plane (APP; denoted in yellow) or the position of the sacrum relative to the center of the hip (denoted in orange). (Reproduced with permission from Buckland AJ, Vigdorchik J, Schwab FJ, et al: Acetabular anteversion changes due to spinal deformity correction: Bridging the gap between hip and spine surgeons. *J Bone Joint Surg Am* 2015;97[23]:1913-1920.)

Figure 2   Illustration of a lower extremity shows the method for measuring lower limb compensatory mechanisms that are used by patients who have a sagittal spine deformity. Pelvic tilt (PT) is the angle between a line drawn from the center of the femoral head to the midpoint of the sacral plate and a vertical line to the floor. Posterior pelvic shift (P shift) is the offset between a vertical line from the posterosuperior corner of the sacral end plate to the floor and the anterior cortex of the distal tibia. The sacrofemoral angle (SFA), which measures hip extension, is the angle between a line drawn from the middle of the sacral end plate to the center axis of the hip and a line drawn from the center axis of the hip to the femoral axis. The knee flexion angle (KA) is the angle between the mechanical axis of the femur and the mechanical axis of the tibia. The ankle flexion angle (AA) is the angle between the mechanical axis of the tibia and a vertical line to the floor.

SSD is most commonly degenerative, it also may result from a fracture, Scheuermann kyphosis, spondylolisthesis, iatrogenic flatback, or neuromuscular disorders. Patients with SSD use several compensatory mechanisms, including lordosis of flexible spine segments, increased pelvic tilt (posterior tilt), posterior pelvic shift, and hip and knee flexion, in an attempt to stand in an upright position[40] (**Figure 2**). The abnormal mechanics of the gluteal muscles, paraspinal muscles, and quadriceps may result in back, buttock, and thigh pain. A fixed flexion deformity of the hip may prevent a patient from using hip extension to compensate for SSD. The pelvis is the common vital entity in SSD and hip OA.

Pelvic tilt can be measured using two different methods (**Figure 3**); however, the relationship between the two methods has yet to be defined. Pelvic tilt can be determined by measuring the angle between the anterior pelvic plane (from the anterior superior iliac spine to the pubic symphysis)[41] and a vertical line to the floor. Hip arthroplasty surgeons favor this method for the measurement of pelvic tilt because subcutaneous landmarks of the anterior pelvic plane aid in acetabular component orientation. However, the accuracy of the anterior pelvic plane has been called into question because of variable overlying soft tissues. Alternatively, pelvic tilt can be determined by measuring the angle between the plane from the bicoxofemoral axis to the center of the sacral plate and a vertical line to the floor. This method for the measurement of pelvic tilt has been reported to correlate with preoperative and postoperative health-related quality of life scores in patients with adult spine deformity. Spine surgeons attempt to achieve less than 20° of pelvic tilt in patients who undergo a spinal realignment procedure.

Acetabular anteversion is altered by the position of the pelvis. A reduction in pelvic tilt (anterior tilt) will functionally retrovert the acetabulum. Conversely, an increase in pelvic tilt

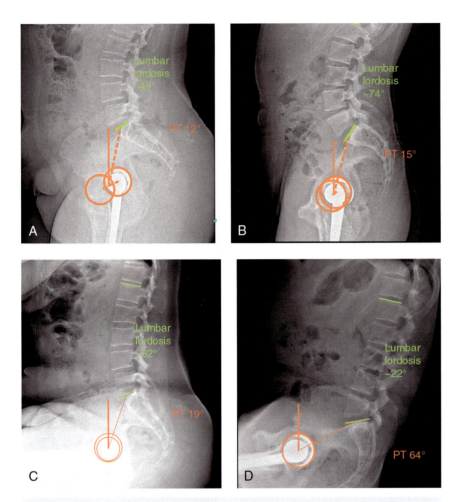

Figure 4 Lateral radiographs of the pelves of two different patients (patient 1: **A** and **C**; patient 2: **B** and **D**) demonstrate changes in pelvic tilt (PT) between standing (**A** and **B**) and sitting (**C** and **D**) positions. Note that, in both patients, PT increases in the sitting position as a result of decreasing lumbar lordosis; however, the increase in PT is different in each patient.

(posterior tilt) will functionally antevert the acetabulum. A 1° increase in pelvic tilt (posterior tilt) will result in a 0.7° increase in functional acetabular anteversion[42,43] and a nonlinear increase in functional inclination.

Pelvic tilt changes with posture. Several studies have suggested that pelvic tilt is similar in the supine and standing positions; however, this is not true in patients with SSD, and, therefore, supine radiographs of the pelvis in patients with SSD may not indicate the true functional position of the pelvis. In a sitting position, pelvic tilt increases approximately 22°[44] and acetabular anteversion increases approximately 15° (**Figure 4**). This increase in acetabular anteversion improves posterior coverage of the femoral head, which reduces the risk for dislocation and prevents anterior femoroacetabular implant impingement. Spinopelvic fusion eliminates the flexibility of the lumbar spine and a patient's ability to alter pelvic tilt during postural changes.[45] Similarly, a patient with increased pelvic tilt as a result of SSD will have less postural variation in pelvic tilt. Although a fixed flexion contracture may theoretically prevent a patient from increasing pelvic tilt to compensate for SSD and result in decompensation of a patient's SSD, pelvic tilt has not been reported to substantially change after THA.[46,47] The authors of this chapter cannot recommend THA as a surgical method to improve sagittal spine posture.

Pelvic tilt and acetabular anteversion increase as the severity of a patient's SSD increases. In a study of 33 patients (41 hips) with adult spine deformity who underwent spinal deformity correction, Buckland et al[48] reported that excessive acetabular prosthetic anteversion (>25°) was observed on the preoperative standing radiographs of 68% of the hips (**Figure 5**). Excessive acetabular prosthetic anteversion likely accounts for the increased risk for anterior dislocation in patients with ankylosing spondylitis[49] and may result in edge-loading, ceramic squeak, and increased bearing surface wear. The goal of spinal deformity correction is to increase lumbar lordosis and reduce pelvic tilt via instrumentation and fusion. Acetabular anteversion decreases as pelvic tilt decreases (**Figure 5**). Buckland et al[48] reported that the surgical realignment of SSD resulted in a mean decrease in acetabular anteversion of 5°; however, the authors reported that acetabular anteversion can decrease as much as 23°. The authors also reported that an iatrogenic increase in lumbar lordosis of 3.2° or a reduction in pelvic tilt of 1.1° resulted in 1° of acetabular retroversion.

The decision of whether to perform a spinal realignment procedure or THA as the initial intervention in patients in whom hip and lumbar spine pathologies occur in combination is a challenge. A thorough patient history should be obtained and a complete

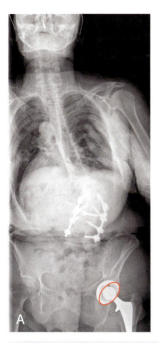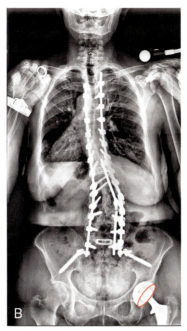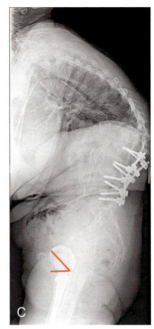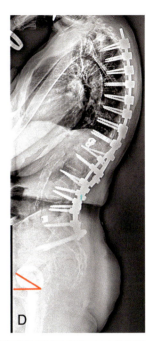

Figure 5 Preoperative (**A**) and postoperative (**B**) AP radiographs and preoperative (**C**) and postoperative (**D**) lateral radiographs of a spine demonstrate changes in acetabular anteversion after sagittal spine deformity correction. Note that the size of the acetabular ellipse (red oval) in panel **A** is decreased after deformity correction (**B**), which indicates decreased anteversion. The ante-inclination of the acetabulum (red angle) in panel **C** also is decreased after deformity correction (**D**). (Reproduced with permission from Buckland AJ, Vigdorchik J, Schwab FJ, et al: Acetabular anteversion changes due to spinal deformity correction: Bridging the gap between hip and spine surgeons. *J Bone Joint Surg Am* 2015;97[23]:1913-1920.)

physical examination of the spine and both of the hips should be performed to identify the primary source of a patient's pain. Patient preferences may guide whether the spine or the hip is managed first. If THA is being considered as the initial intervention in a patient with asymptomatic SSD, a pelvic tilt–adjusted acetabular orientation may help avoid excessive prosthetic anteversion.[50] If a spinal realignment procedure is likely to be performed after THA, the surgeon should consider the effect of the spinal surgery on the orientation of the acetabular component in the preoperative planning for THA. Spinal deformity correction should be performed before THA in patients in whom SSD is substantial and considerable spinal deformity correction is required.

Summary

In patients who have back and lower extremity pain, a systematic patient history and a comprehensive physical examination are necessary to identify the principal cause of pain. Diagnostic imaging studies and injections are used to further define the primary source of symptoms and guide the appropriate sequence of treatment. If symptoms persist after one pathology is managed, additional treatment may be necessary to address secondary causes of pain. The identification of both causes of pain may help reduce the likelihood of misdiagnosis and unnecessary treatment and, thus, reduce the likelihood of persistent symptoms.

References

1. Devin CJ, McCullough KA, Morris BJ, Yates AJ, Kang JD: Hip-spine syndrome. *J Am Acad Orthop Surg* 2012;20(7):434-442.

2. Byrd JW: Hip arthroscopy: Patient assessment and indications. *Instr Course Lect* 2003;52:711-719.

3. Clohisy JC, Knaus ER, Hunt DM, Lesher JM, Harris-Hayes M, Prather H: Clinical presentation of patients with symptomatic anterior hip impingement. *Clin Orthop Relat Res* 2009;467(3):638-644.

4. Offierski CM, MacNab I: Hip-spine syndrome. *Spine (Phila Pa 1976)* 1983;8(3):316-321.

5. Lesher JM, Dreyfuss P, Hager N, Kaplan M, Furman M: Hip joint pain referral patterns: A descriptive study. *Pain Med* 2008;9(1):22-25.

6. Saito J, Ohtori S, Kishida S, et al: Difficulty of diagnosing the origin of

lower leg pain in patients with both lumbar spinal stenosis and hip joint osteoarthritis. *Spine (Phila Pa 1976)* 2012;37(25):2089-2093.

7. Fogel GR, Esses SI: Hip spine syndrome: Management of coexisting radiculopathy and arthritis of the lower extremity. *Spine J* 2003;3(3):238-241.

8. Boden SD, Davis DO, Dina TS, Patronas NJ, Wiesel SW: Abnormal magnetic-resonance scans of the lumbar spine in asymptomatic subjects: A prospective investigation. *J Bone Joint Surg Am* 1990;72(3):403-408.

9. Brown MD, Gomez-Marin O, Brookfield KF, Li PS: Differential diagnosis of hip disease versus spine disease. *Clin Orthop Relat Res* 2004;419:280-284.

10. Almeida GP, de Souza VL, Sano SS, Saccol MF, Cohen M: Comparison of hip rotation range of motion in judo athletes with and without history of low back pain. *Man Ther* 2012;17(3):231-235.

11. Van Dillen LR, Bloom NJ, Gombatto SP, Susco TM: Hip rotation range of motion in people with and without low back pain who participate in rotation-related sports. *Phys Ther Sport* 2008;9(2):72-81.

12. Shum GL, Crosbie J, Lee RY: Symptomatic and asymptomatic movement coordination of the lumbar spine and hip during an everyday activity. *Spine (Phila Pa 1976)* 2005;30(23):E697-E702.

13. Cho SC, Ferrante MA, Levin KH, Harmon RL, So YT: Utility of electrodiagnostic testing in evaluating patients with lumbosacral radiculopathy: An evidence-based review. *Muscle Nerve* 2010;42(2):276-282.

14. Mondelli M, Aretini A, Arrigucci U, Ginanneschi F, Greco G, Sicurelli F: Clinical findings and electrodiagnostic testing in 108 consecutive cases of lumbosacral radiculopathy due to herniated disc. *Neurophysiol Clin* 2013;43(4):205-215.

15. Nadeau M, Rosas-Arellano MP, Gurr KR, et al: The reliability of differentiating neurogenic claudication from vascular claudication based on symptomatic presentation. *Can J Surg* 2013;56(6):372-377.

16. Crawford RW, Gie GA, Ling RS, Murray DW: Diagnostic value of intra-articular anaesthetic in primary osteoarthritis of the hip. *J Bone Joint Surg Br* 1998;80(2):279-281.

17. Yoong P, Guirguis R, Darrah R, Wijeratna M, Porteous MJ: Evaluation of ultrasound-guided diagnostic local anaesthetic hip joint injection for osteoarthritis. *Skeletal Radiol* 2012;41(8):981-985.

18. Kleiner JB, Thorne RP, Curd JG: The value of bupivicaine hip injection in the differentiation of coxarthrosis from lower extremity neuropathy. *J Rheumatol* 1991;18(3):422-427.

19. McNamara MJ, Barrett KG, Christie MJ, Spengler DM: Lumbar spinal stenosis and lower extremity arthroplasty. *J Arthroplasty* 1993;8(3):273-277.

20. Quintana JM, Escobar A, Aguirre U, Lafuente I, Arenaza JC: Predictors of health-related quality-of-life change after total hip arthroplasty. *Clin Orthop Relat Res* 2009;467(11):2886-2894.

21. Bischoff-Ferrari HA, Lingard EA, Losina E, et al: Psychosocial and geriatric correlates of functional status after total hip replacement. *Arthritis Rheum* 2004;51(5):829-835.

22. Bohl WR, Steffee AD: Lumbar spinal stenosis: A cause of continued pain and disability in patients after total hip arthroplasty. *Spine (Phila Pa 1976)* 1979;4(2):168-173.

23. Ben-Galim P, Ben-Galim T, Rand N, et al: Hip-spine syndrome: The effect of total hip replacement surgery on low back pain in severe osteoarthritis of the hip. *Spine (Phila Pa 1976)* 2007;32(19):2099-2102.

24. Prather H, Van Dillen LR, Kymes SM, Armbrecht MA, Stwalley D, Clohisy JC: Impact of coexistent lumbar spine disorders on clinical outcomes and physician charges associated with total hip arthroplasty. *Spine J* 2012;12(5):363-369.

25. Parvizi J, Pour AE, Hillibrand A, Goldberg G, Sharkey PF, Rothman RH: Back pain and total hip arthroplasty: A prospective natural history study. *Clin Orthop Relat Res* 2010;468(5):1325-1330.

26. Hsieh PH, Chang Y, Chen DW, Lee MS, Shih HN, Ueng SW: Pain distribution and response to total hip arthroplasty: A prospective observational study in 113 patients with end-stage hip disease. *J Orthop Sci* 2012;17(3):213-218.

27. Pritchett JW: Lumbar decompression to treat foot drop after hip arthroplasty. *Clin Orthop Relat Res* 1994;303:173-177.

28. Burnett RS, Della Rocca GJ, Prather H, Curry M, Maloney WJ, Clohisy JC: Clinical presentation of patients with tears of the acetabular labrum. *J Bone Joint Surg Am* 2006;88(7):1448-1457.

29. Toomayan GA, Holman WR, Major NM, Kozlowicz SM, Vail TP: Sensitivity of MR arthrography in the evaluation of acetabular labral tears. *AJR Am J Roentgenol* 2006;186(2):449-453.

30. Czerny C, Hofmann S, Neuhold A, et al: Lesions of the acetabular labrum: Accuracy of MR imaging and MR arthrography in detection and staging. *Radiology* 1996;200(1):225-230.

31. Byrd JW, Jones KS: Diagnostic accuracy of clinical assessment, magnetic resonance imaging, magnetic resonance arthrography, and intra-articular injection in hip arthroscopy patients. *Am J Sports Med* 2004;32(7):1668-1674.

32. Martin RL, Irrgang JJ, Sekiya JK: The diagnostic accuracy of a clinical examination in determining intra-articular hip pain for potential hip arthroscopy candidates. *Arthroscopy* 2008;24(9):1013-1018.

33. Bird PA, Oakley SP, Shnier R, Kirkham BW: Prospective evaluation of magnetic resonance imaging and physical examination findings in patients with greater trochanteric pain syndrome. *Arthritis Rheum* 2001;44(9):2138-2145.

34. Martin HD, Kivlan BR, Palmer IJ, Martin RL: Diagnostic accuracy of clinical tests for sciatic nerve entrapment in the gluteal region. *Knee Surg Sports Traumatol Arthrosc* 2014;22(4):882-888.

35. Martin HD, Shears SA, Johnson JC, Smathers AM, Palmer IJ: The endoscopic treatment of sciatic nerve

entrapment/deep gluteal syndrome. *Arthroscopy* 2011;27(2):172-181.

36. Stafford GH, Villar RN: Ischiofemoral impingement. *J Bone Joint Surg Br* 2011;93(10):1300-1302.

37. Schwab F, Dubey A, Gamez L, et al: Adult scoliosis: Prevalence, SF-36, and nutritional parameters in an elderly volunteer population. *Spine (Phila Pa 1976)* 2005;30(9):1082-1085.

38. Schwab FJ, Blondel B, Bess S, et al: Radiographical spinopelvic parameters and disability in the setting of adult spinal deformity: A prospective multicenter analysis. *Spine (Phila Pa 1976)* 2013;38(13):E803-E812.

39. Protopsaltis T, Schwab F, Bronsard N, et al: The T1 pelvic angle, a novel radiographic measure of global sagittal deformity, accounts for both spinal inclination and pelvic tilt and correlates with health-related quality of life. *J Bone Joint Surg Am* 2014;96(19):1631-1640.

40. Diebo BG, Ferrero E, Lafage R, et al: Recruitment of compensatory mechanisms in sagittal spinal malalignment is age and regional deformity dependent: A full-standing axis analysis of key radiographical parameters. *Spine (Phila Pa 1976)* 2015;40(9):642-649.

41. Lewinnek GE, Lewis JL, Tarr R, Compere CL, Zimmerman JR: Dislocations after total hip-replacement arthroplasties. *J Bone Joint Surg Am* 1978;60(2):217-220.

42. Lembeck B, Mueller O, Reize P, Wuelker N: Pelvic tilt makes acetabular cup navigation inaccurate. *Acta Orthop* 2005;76(4):517-523.

43. Maratt JD, Esposito CI, McLawhorn AS, Jerabek SA, Padgett DE, Mayman DJ: Pelvic tilt in patients undergoing total hip arthroplasty: When does it matter? *J Arthroplasty* 2015;30(3):387-391.

44. Philippot R, Wegrzyn J, Farizon F, Fessy MH: Pelvic balance in sagittal and Lewinnek reference planes in the standing, supine and sitting positions. *Orthop Traumatol Surg Res* 2009;95(1):70-76.

45. Lazennec JY, Brusson A, Rousseau MA: Lumbar-pelvic-femoral balance on sitting and standing lateral radiographs. *Orthop Traumatol Surg Res* 2013;99(1 suppl):S87-S103.

46. Blondel B, Parratte S, Tropiano P, Pauly V, Aubaniac JM, Argenson JN: Pelvic tilt measurement before and after total hip arthroplasty. *Orthop Traumatol Surg Res* 2009;95(8):568-572.

47. Murphy WS, Klingenstein G, Murphy SB, Zheng G: Pelvic tilt is minimally changed by total hip arthroplasty. *Clin Orthop Relat Res* 2013;471(2):417-421.

48. Buckland AJ, Vigdorchik J, Lafage R, et al: Paper No. 85. Acetabular anteversion changes in spinal deformity correction: Implications for hip and spine surgeons. *22nd International Meeting on Advanced Spine Techniques,* Kuala Lumpur, Malaysia, July 8-11, 2015.

49. Tang WM, Chiu KY: Primary total hip arthroplasty in patients with ankylosing spondylitis. *J Arthroplasty* 2000;15(1):52-58.

50. Babisch JW, Layher F, Amiot LP: The rationale for tilt-adjusted acetabular cup navigation. *J Bone Joint Surg Am* 2008;90(2):357-365.

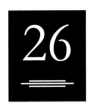

Surgical Management of Cervical Spondylotic Myelopathy

Chris A. Cornett, MD, MPT
James D. Kang, MD
Joon Yung Lee, MD
Clinton James Devin, MD
Emmett Gannon, MD
Elliott Kim, MD
Sean M. Esmende, MD

Abstract

Cervical spondylotic myelopathy (CSM) is a common cause of neurologic impairment in adults worldwide. Numerous studies have investigated the pathophysiology of CSM, which has provided surgeons with insight on the important factors that lead to the symptoms and deficits observed in patients who have CSM. However, further analysis of many unknown aspects of CSM is required to fully understand the disease and potential alternative treatment modalities. The diagnosis of CSM is based on a patient's history and physical examination and then confirmed with imaging studies. Progression, symptomatology, and imaging findings may vary by patient. Because of the variability of CSM, the disease course and a patient's response to treatment are difficult to predict. CSM can be managed either nonsurgically or it can be managed surgically via posterior or anterior cervical approaches, each of which has its own indications and possible complications.

Instr Course Lect 2017;66:329–351.

Cervical spondylotic myelopathy (CSM) is a degenerative disease that leads to compression of the cervical spinal cord. The neurologic deficits observed in patients who have CSM are caused by degenerative changes in the cervical vertebral column that lead to long-term narrowing of the cervical spinal canal.[1] CSM is the most common cause of cervical dysfunction in individuals older than 55 years, along with nontraumatic paraparesis and tetraparesis among all adults.[2,3] The disease progression of CSM is highly unpredictable, leading to deficits and compression that may vary in severity.[1,4] The etiology of CSM is believed to be multifactorial, being a combination of both environmental and heritable factors.[5] Static and dynamic mechanical factors substantially contribute to the pathophysiology of CSM.[6] Ischemia also plays a part in the progression of CSM; however, the importance of the role of ischemia in patients who have CSM is a topic of debate.[5,6]

The diagnosis of CSM is clinical, based on a patient's symptoms, history, physical examination findings, and imaging studies. Many conditions, some of which can lead to serious and/or permanent neurologic impairment if diagnosis is delayed, have characteristics similar to those of CSM. Therefore, surgeons must know the differential diagnosis for myelopathy and understand

Dr. Devin or an immediate family member serves as a paid consultant to or is an employee of DePuy and Exparel; has received research or institutional support from DePuy and Stryker; and serves as a board member, owner, officer, or committee member of the Cervical Spine Research Society and the North American Spine Society. None of the following authors nor any immediate family member has received anything of value from or has stock or stock options held in a commercial company or institution related directly or indirectly to the subject of this chapter: Dr. Cornett, Dr. Kang, Dr. Lee, Dr. Gannon, Dr. Kim, and Dr. Esmende.

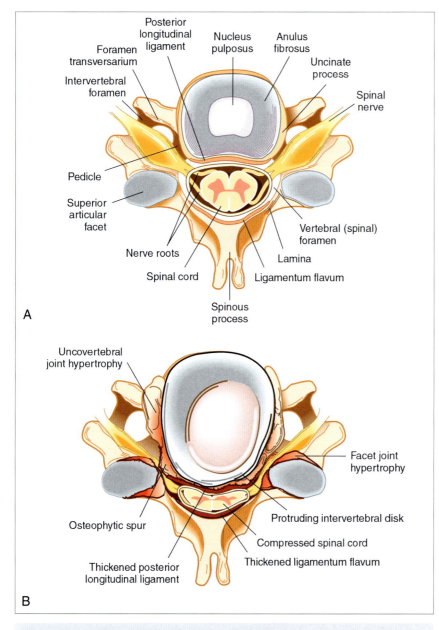

Figure 1 Axial view illustrations show a normal cervical spine (**A**) and a cervical spine with spondylosis and resultant spinal stenosis and spinal cord compression (**B**), which is consistent with the changes that are observed in patients who have cervical spondylotic myelopathy.

the role of the physical examination and imaging findings.[7] CSM can be managed nonsurgically or it can be managed surgically with decompression via either posterior or anterior approaches.[1] Fehlings et al[4] recommended a limited role for the nonsurgical management of CSM because of the highly unpredictable progression of CSM and the improved outcomes observed in patients with CSM who undergo surgical decompression.

Pathophysiology

Spondylosis of the cervical spine can eventually lead to myelopathy.

Anatomic knowledge of the cervical spine is important to understand how spondylotic changes can lead to the neurologic impairment observed in patients who have CSM. The structures of the spine that undergo the degenerative changes characteristic of CSM include the vertebrae, the intervertebral disks, the facet joints, the uncovertebral joints, the posterior longitudinal ligament, and the ligamentum flavum[8] (**Figure 1**). The pedicles and the lamina also play an important role because they are directly related to the size of the spinal canal. Degenerative changes, which can cause static compression, and dynamic factors can combine to cause myelopathy.

Static Factors

Static factors include the size of the spinal canal and the severity of the spondylotic changes. These two factors are tightly interwoven. The location and the amount of spondylosis, which itself leads to spinal stenosis, and the preexisting size of the spinal canal directly contribute to the amount of spinal cord compression observed. Therefore, the diameter of the central spinal canal plays an important role in patients who have CSM. The mean sagittal diameter of the central spinal canal between C3 and C7 is 17 to 18.5 mm (20 to 23 mm between C1 and C2), with the spinal cord itself being approximately 10 mm in diameter (range, 8.5 to 11.5 mm).[9,10] Edwards and LaRocca[11] reported that the size of the spinal canal is directly related to the development of myelopathy. The authors reported that individuals with a spinal canal diameter narrower than 10 mm had myelopathy, whereas individuals with a spinal canal diameter between 10 and 13 mm had premyelopathic findings. In addition, the authors reported that CSM symptoms were likely to develop in individuals with a spinal canal diameter between 13 and 17 mm, whereas CSM symptoms were less likely to develop in individuals with a wider spinal canal diameter (wider than 17 mm).[11,12] Similarly, studies have reported that a congenitally narrow spinal canal (narrower than 13 mm) is a substantial risk factor for the development of CSM.[11-14]

Dynamic Factors

Dynamic mechanical factors also contribute to the development of CSM. These dynamic factors are related to repetitive microtrauma of the spinal cord with flexion or extension, especially in individuals with an already compressed cervical spinal cord.[15] In extension, the spinal cord shortens, which leads to an increased cross-sectional area of the spinal cord.[16] In addition, the spinal canal diameter decreases secondary to inward buckling of the ligamentum flavum.[6,17] Therefore, extension places a substantial amount of strain on the spinal cord in patients who have underlying spondylosis because as the spinal cord itself widens, the spinal canal narrows. A pincer effect, in which the posteroinferior aspect of a cervical vertebral body compresses the spinal cord against the ligamentum flavum or the lamina of the next inferior level in extension, also has been described.[18,19] In flexion, the spinal cord lengthens and can compress against anterior osteophytic spurs.[2,18] These dynamic factors may further affect the spinal cord by causing ischemia because increased anterior and posterior compression can alter perfusion to the spinal cord.[20] Anterior compression affects the transverse arterioles, which are branches from the sulcal arteries, whereas posterior compression affects the intramedullary branches of the central gray matter.

Role of Ischemia

The importance of ischemia in the development of CSM is a subject of debate.[5] Numerous animal studies have used angiography or autoradiography to demonstrate evidence in support of ischemia as an important component in the etiology of CSM.[21-24] Breig et al[16] reported findings consistent with compromised perfusion to axonal pathways, namely the corticospinal tracts, secondary to stretching and curving of branches of the anterior spinal artery and the lateral plexus in cadaver models with CSM. The authors also demonstrated histopathologic ischemic changes to the white and gray matter of the spinal cord in cadaver models with CSM.[16] Moreover, ischemia may lead to a biochemical cascade that results in glutamate excitotoxicity, which can lead to cellular apoptosis.[25]

Demyelination, which is observed in patients who have chronic CSM, also is believed to be partially caused by the sensitivity of oligodendrocytes to ischemia.[26] In a recent animal study, Karadimas et al[27] reported that slow progressive compression of the cervical spinal cord disrupts the blood-spinal cord barrier, which may play a role with regard to the inflammation observed in patients who have CSM. However, other studies have questioned the importance of ischemia in patients who have CSM, which is supported by the finding of necrosis rather than apoptosis as the main pathway of cellular death after an ischemic injury.[28] This evidence is a key element in the argument against the importance of ischemia in patients who have CSM because apoptosis is the most likely pathway of oligodendrocyte and neuronal cell death in patients who have CSM.[28] Other studies, including a pathologic study in which

ischemia was reported to exist only in conjunction with severe spinal stenosis, also have supported a less important role of ischemia in patients who have CSM.[29,30] In addition, studies have reported no to mild evidence of ischemia in humans and animals with moderate CSM.[23,31,32] Ischemia most likely plays a role in patients who have CSM; however, further investigation with regard to the importance of its effect on the severity of CSM is required.

Other Factors

In addition to vascular disruption, other secondary mechanisms, including inflammation and apoptosis, play a role in the development of CSM.[6,15] The inflammation observed in patients who have CSM is believed to derive from both mechanical compression of the spinal cord and chronic ischemia.[28] On a cellular level, activated macrophages and microglia have been reported to be the predominant cell types observed in both the early and late phases of compression.[33] Similarly, apoptosis is believed to be a result of chronic ischemia and both local and systemic inflammatory conditions that are observed in patients who have CSM.[15] Evidence has supported the importance of apoptosis in oligodendrocytes and other neuronal cells with regard to the progression of CSM.[27] Moreover, studies have supported the notion that apoptosis most likely precedes axonal demyelination, which is a key event in the progression of CSM.[34,35] In an animal study on the relationship between mechanical compression and apoptosis, Karadimas et al[36] reported that decompression resulted in decreased cellular apoptosis. Overall, a very close relationship exists between the inflammation and apoptosis observed in patients who have CSM, and a Fas-mediated mechanism appears to play a predominant role with regard to both inflammation and apoptosis.[33] Yu et al[33] reported Fas-mediated apoptosis of neurons and oligodendrocytes and a Fas-mediated increase in inflammatory cells in humans and mice with compressed spinal cords. In addition, the authors reported that the use of an antibody to block Fas ligand reduced inflammation and promoted neurologic function in mice. Therefore, the authors hypothesized that targeting the Fas pathway may be helpful in humans who have CSM.[33]

Pathologic Findings

As a result of these molecular and mechanical factors, patients who have CSM undergo pathologic changes that most often correlate with the amount of spinal cord compression.[29] A clinicopathologic study reported lateral white-matter degeneration, which included the lateral corticospinal tracts, in patients who had mild spinal cord compression and gray-matter necrosis in patients who had more severe spinal cord compression.[30] Histologic changes observed in patients who have CSM include anterior and posterior horn atrophy, gliosis, vacuolations, axonal and neuronal loss, myelin pallor, demyelination of the descending axons, and degeneration of the ascending tracts.[1,16,30] The overall pathophysiology of CSM, which leads to these pathologic findings, is complex, and further investigation will aid in the development of advances for the diagnosis and management of CSM.

Clinical Evaluation

The diagnosis of CSM is based on a patient's history, physical examination, and imaging findings. The mean age of patients in whom a diagnosis of CSM is

Table 1

Japanese Orthopaedic Association Scale for Cervical Spondylotic Myelopathy

Factor		Finding	Points
Motor Function			
	Upper extremity	Unable to eat with a spoon or chopsticks	0
		Able to eat with a spoon but not chopsticks	1
		Possible to eat with chopsticks but not adequate	2
		Slightly clumsy in using chopsticks	3
		Normal	4
	Lower extremity	Impossible to walk	0
		Need a cane or other aid on flat ground	1
		Need a cane or other aid on stairs	2
		Possible to walk without a cane or other aid but slow	3
		Normal	4
Sensation			
	Upper extremity	Apparent sensory loss	0
		Minimal sensory loss	1
		Normal	2
	Lower extremity	Apparent sensory loss	0
		Minimal sensory loss	1
		Normal	2
	Trunk	Apparent sensory loss	0
		Minimal sensory loss	1
		Normal	2
Bladder Function		Complete retention	0
		Severe disturbance	1
		Mild disturbance	2
		Normal	3
Total for Normal Patients			17

Adapted with permission from Lebl DR, Bono CM: Update on the diagnosis and management of cervical spondylotic myelopathy. *J Am Acad Orthop Surg* 2015;23(11):648-660; and Hukuda S, Mochizuki T, Ogata M, Shichikawa K, Shimomura Y: Operations for cervical spondylotic myelopathy: A comparison of the results of anterior and posterior procedures. *J Bone Joint Surg Br* 1985;67(4):609-615.

made is 64 years. Patients in whom a diagnosis of CSM is made usually will not experience symptoms until at least age 40 years.[8,37] A diagnosis of CSM is more often made in males compared with females (2.7:1 ratio).[37] Frequently, patients who have CSM will report a subtle onset of symptoms; however, some patients who have CSM will experience an acute or subacute onset or worsening after a

fall or neck injury, such as a hyperextension or flexion injury.[8] Patients who have CSM may report symptoms such as neck pain, decreased dexterity, upper limb pain, upper and/or lower limb weakness, stiffness, impaired balance, and altered sensorium.[8] Patients who have CSM also may report autonomic dysfunction, such as increased urinary frequency, urgency, or incontinence.[1]

The Lhermitte sign, which is the feeling of shock-like sensations along the spine and into the arms and legs after neck extension or flexion, also has been reported in patients who have CSM.[8] Patients who have CSM may report the need to use a cane or walker or the necessity to use handrails when trying to navigate stairs, which may indicate acquired weakness or gait imbalance.[5] Patients who have CSM also may report difficulty with writing, using a telephone, buttoning a shirt, or performing other fine motor tasks.[5]

After an adequate history has been obtained, attention is centered on the physical examination. A basic neurologic and orthopaedic physical examination should include the testing of motor function, sensation, deep tendon reflexes, gait, balance, range of motion (ROM), and alignment. Upper motor neuron tests, such as the Hoffmann sign, the Babinski sign, and the inverted brachioradialis reflex test, and tests to assess for clonus should be performed if concern for CSM exists. Special tests for other peripheral nerve conditions, such as carpal and cubital tunnel syndromes, can help rule out other diagnoses. The physical examination findings that are suggestive of CSM include hyperreflexia of the upper or lower extremities, hyporeflexia, weakness, a positive Babinski sign, a positive Hoffmann sign, clonus, sensory loss, spasticity, and gait disturbance.[8] Positive upper motor neuron signs observed during the physical examination should raise concern for spinal cord compression, whereas positive lower motor neuron signs (ie, hyporeflexia) indicate nerve root compression.[5] Houten and Noce[38] reported that the Hoffmann sign is an invaluable test for patients who have

Table 2
Modified Japanese Orthopaedic Association Scale for Cervical Spondylotic Myelopathy

Factor		Finding	Points
Motor Function			
	Upper extremity	Inability to move hands	0
		Unable to use a spoon but able to move hands	1
		Unable to button a shirt but able to eat with a spoon	2
		Able to button a shirt with great difficulty	3
		Able to button a shirt with slight difficulty	4
		No dysfunction	5
	Lower extremity	Complete loss of motor and sensory function	0
		Sensory preservation without ability to move legs	1
		Ability to move legs but unable to walk	2
		Able to walk on a flat floor with a walking aid	3
		Able to walk up and/or down stairs with a handrail	4
		Moderate to substantial lack of stability but able to walk up and/or down stairs without a handrail	5
		Mild lack of stability but able to walk unaided with smooth reciprocation	6
		No dysfunction	7
Sensation		Complete loss of hand sensation	0
		Severe sensory loss or pain	1
		Mild sensory loss	2
		No sensory loss	3
Bladder Function		Inability to micturate voluntarily	0
		Marked difficulty with micturition	1
		Mild to moderate difficulty with micturition	2
		Normal micturition	3
Total for Normal Patients			18[a]

[a] If the total score is ≥15, the patient has mild cervical spondylotic myelopathy (CSM). If the total score ranges from 12 to 14, the patient has moderate CSM. If the total score is <12, the patient has severe CSM.

Adapted with permission from Lebl DR, Bono CM: Update on the diagnosis and management of cervical spondylotic myelopathy. *J Am Acad Orthop Surg* 2015;23(11):648-660; and Benzel EC, Lancon J, Kesterson L, Hadden T: Cervical laminectomy and dentate ligament section for cervical spondylotic myelopathy. *J Spinal Disord* 1991;4(3):286-295.

mild neurologic deficits because it is more likely to be positive compared with the Babinski sign. Moreover, the authors reported that the Hoffman sign also can be used for patients who have lumbar spine complaints because MRIs have revealed cervical spinal cord compression in 91% of patients who have a

positive Hoffmann sign bilaterally and 50% of patients who have a positive Hoffman sign unilaterally.[38] To assess the severity of CSM, surgeons can use one of several scales, including the Japanese Orthopaedic Association (JOA) scale (**Table 1**), the modified JOA scale (**Table 2**), and the Nurick classification system (**Table 3**); however, these scales are more often used for research than in the clinical setting.[8]

Differential Diagnosis

Many conditions have characteristics similar to those of CSM;[7] therefore, if surgeons are concerned with regard to a primary diagnosis of CSM, a broad differential diagnosis should be maintained. A differential diagnosis for myelopathy should include trauma; neoplasia; ossification of the posterior longitudinal ligament (OPLL); infection; inflammatory demyelinating conditions; noninfectious inflammatory states; and vascular, metabolic, hereditary, or toxic causes that explain a patient's history and physical examination findings[8] (**Table 4**). Patient symptoms or history that should raise immediate concern for urgent attention

Table 3
Nurick Classification System for Cervical Spondylotic Myelopathy

Grade	Root Signs	Cord Involvement	Gait	Employment
0	Yes	No	Normal	Possible
I	Yes	Yes	Normal	Possible
II	Yes	Yes	Mild abnormality	Possible
III	Yes	Yes	Severe abnormality	Impossible
IV	Yes	Yes	Only with assistance	Impossible

Reproduced from Lebl DR, Bono CM: Update on the diagnosis and management of cervical spondylotic myelopathy. *J Am Acad Orthop Surg* 2015;23(11):648-660.

Table 4
Differential Diagnosis for Cervical Spondylotic Myelopathy

Extrinsic to Spinal Cord

- Cervical spondylosis with stenosis
- Cervical disk herniation
- Congenital spinal stenosis
- Synovial cyst
- Extramedullary and extradural tumors
- Epidural abscess
- Osteomyelitis
- Diffuse idiopathic skeletal hyperostosis
- Rheumatoid arthritis or ankylosing spondylitis with upper cervical subluxation
- Trauma
  - Fracture
  - Central cord syndrome
- Ossification of the posterior longitudinal ligament
- Extramedullary hematopoiesis
- Paget disease
- Arachnoid cyst
- Fluorosis

Intrinsic to Spinal Cord

- Intramedullary spinal cord tumor
- Infection
  - Viral, including HIV, human T-lymphotropic virus, herpes zoster, West Nile, syphilis
  - Lyme disease
  - Intramedullary abscess (rarely)
- Inflammatory demyelination
  - Multiple sclerosis
  - Neuromyelitis optica
  - Acute transverse myelitis
  - Acute disseminated encephalomyelitis
- Noninfectious inflammatory
  - Systemic lupus erythematosus
  - Sjögren or Behçet syndrome
  - Sarcoidosis
  - Paraneoplastic
- Toxic, metabolic, hereditary
  - Vitamin B_{12}, vitamin E, copper, or folic acid deficiency
  - Nitrous oxide toxicity
  - Superficial siderosis
  - Radiation myelopathy
  - Hereditary spastic paraparesis
  - Adrenomyeloneuropathy

- Vascular
  - Spinal cord infarction
  - Arteriovenous malformation
  - Hematomyelia
  - Decompression sickness (Caisson disease)
- Other
  - Syringomyelia
  - Motor neuron disease
- Mimics
  - Parasagittal cerebral lesion, such as a tumor
  - Multiple strokes, brain stem stroke
  - Guillain-Barré syndrome
  - Conversion disorder

Adapted with permission from Bartleson JD, Deen HG: The cervical level, in *Spine Disorders: Medical and Surgical Management*. New York, NY, Cambridge University Press, 2009, pp 33-48.

include fever or chills, intravenous drug use, immunosuppressed states, a history of cancer, recent unexplained weight loss, recent trauma, or pain that has become severe or progressively worse.[8] HIV, human T-lymphotropic virus, herpes zoster, West Nile virus, Lyme disease, syphilis, osteomyelitis, and epidural abscess should all be considered with regard to an infectious origin of patient symptoms.[7,8] Multiple sclerosis and transverse myelitis are two inflammatory demyelinating conditions that should be included in the differential diagnosis. In addition, noninfectious inflammatory diseases, such as systemic lupus erythematosus, Sjögren syndrome, and sarcoidosis, should be considered. In patients who have rheumatoid arthritis or ankylosing spondylitis, surgeons must consider subluxation and/or malalignment as a potential cause of myelopathy. Potential metabolic causes of myelopathy include a deficiency of vitamin B_{12}, folic acid, copper, or vitamin E. The differential diagnosis for myelopathy is vast and can be overwhelming; therefore, appropriate referral to caregivers in other subspecialties (including neurology, infectious disease, or rheumatology) may be necessary if a surgeon is concerned that a patient's symptoms may be the result of another cause.

Diagnostic Studies

Diagnostic modalities that can be used in the diagnosis of CSM include plain radiography, MRI, CT myelography, nerve conduction velocity studies, electromyography, somatosensory-evoked potentials, and motor-evoked potentials. Plain radiographs of the cervical spine, including AP, lateral, and flexion/extension views, should be obtained in most patients in whom a diagnosis of

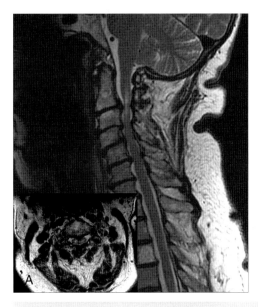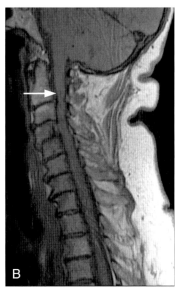

Figure 2   **A,** Sagittal T2-weighted MRI of a spine demonstrates a C2-C3 disk osteophyte complex with resultant impingement on the spinal cord and an associated hyperintense signal. Inset, Axial T2-weighted MRI of the spine at C2-C3 demonstrates deformation of the spinal cord and a hyperintense signal within the cord parenchyma. **B,** Sagittal T1-weighted MRI of a spine demonstrates a hypointense signal (arrow) just proximal to the C2-C3 disk level. (Reproduced from Lebl DR, Bono CM: Update on the diagnosis and management of cervical spondylotic myelopathy. *J Am Acad Orthop Surg* 2015;23[11]:648-660.)

CSM is suspected. Radiographs can help in the assessment of degenerative disk and joint disease, stenosis, alignment, and translational deformity or instability.[5,8] Lateral radiographs of the cervical spine are especially useful in determining spinal alignment, which can be classified as kyphotic, lordotic, neutral, or sigmoid shaped.[5] Plain radiographs also have been used to determine the amount of cervical stenosis via the Torg-Pavlov ratio, which is calculated by dividing the midsagittal diameter of the spinal canal by the AP diameter of the vertebral body at the same level.[5,8] A Torg-Pavlov ratio of less than 0.82 indicates concern for cervical stenosis; however, studies have reported that the Torg-Pavlov ratio is poorly correlated with the actual diameter of the spinal canal.[39,40]

The most helpful imaging modality in the evaluation of patients in whom a

diagnosis of CSM is suspected is MRI, which can be used to confirm a diagnosis of CSM and rule out many other diagnoses.[8] MRI is able to reveal the extent of spondylotic change, cervical stenosis, and spinal cord compression. In addition, signal changes observed on MRI have shown prognostic value because a hyperintense signal on a T2-weighted MRI combined with a hypointense signal on a T1-weighted MRI may correlate with a poorer postoperative prognosis[41-43] (**Figure 2**).

Diffusion tensor imaging has emerged as another potentially useful imaging modality for patients in whom a diagnosis of CSM is suspected. Diffusion tensor imaging is a promising tool that differentiates between symptomatic and asymptomatic myelopathy and assesses the neuronal status and grade of myelopathy in patients who

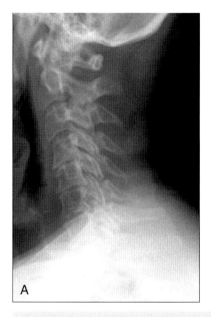
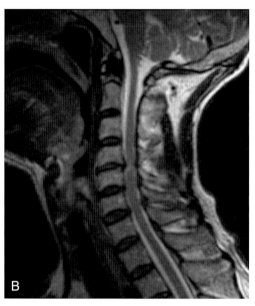
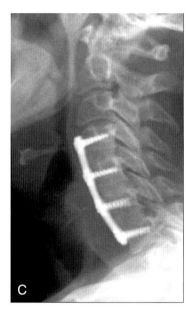

Figure 3 **A,** Preoperative lateral radiograph of a cervical spine demonstrates multilevel cervical spondylosis. **B,** Preoperative sagittal T2-weighted MRI of a cervical spine demonstrates myelomalacia of the spinal cord. **C,** Lateral radiograph of a cervical spine taken 1 year after three-level anterior cervical diskectomy and fusion demonstrates successful fusion and good alignment.

have CSM.[44,45] If MRI cannot be obtained, CT myelography is another imaging modality that can be used; however, CT myelography is more invasive than MRI and has associated risks because it requires an intrathecal injection.[5,8] Nerve conduction velocity studies and electromyography have been used to assist in the identification of impaired neural structures; however, these studies are best used to rule out other diagnoses. Somatosensory-evoked potentials and motor-evoked potentials have been suggested to have a high sensitivity for the detection of myelopathy; however,[46,47] they are most commonly used intraoperatively for monitoring purposes.[8]

Anterior Cervical Approaches
Anterior Cervical Diskectomy and Fusion

Anterior compression of the cervical spine or nerve roots is the most common indication for decompression via an anterior approach. Clinically, conditions such as cervical trauma, cervical disk herniation, OPLL, neoplasms, and infections can be successfully managed with decompression via an anterior cervical approach. Anterior cervical diskectomy and fusion (ACDF) is one of the most common procedures that spine surgeons perform. In treating patients who have one- or two-level disk CSM, most surgeons prefer to use an anterior cervical approach.[48] The clinical results of ACDF are gratifying. Overall, the complication rate in patients who undergo ACDF ranges from approximately 5% to 15%.[49,50]

In 1955, Robinson and Smith[51] described one of the two most common ACDF techniques; the second ACDF technique was described by Cloward[52] in 1958. Robinson and Smith[51] described an approach for cervical disk removal and replacement with an iliac crest autograft to promote fusion. Cloward[52] described a diskectomy with the use of

a cylindrical-shaped dowel for a graft. Numerous modifications have been made to these techniques; most spine surgeons use an iteration of the techniques initially described in the 1950s.[53]

ACDF allows for the removal of disk material and posterior osteophytes that impinge the spinal cord and nerve roots. The end plate is removed; the disk space is distracted, which leads to indirect decompression of the spinal canal and foramen; and a bone graft is inserted into the interspace (**Figure 3**). The height of the bone graft is typically 2 mm larger than the initial disk height to avoid loss of disk height after graft incorporation.[54] In general, ACDF alone is not recommended for the treatment of patients who have severe stenosis of the spinal canal because the overall AP diameter of the spinal canal is not increased by the procedure. Therefore, ACDF should be reserved for patients with myelopathy who have compression only at the level of the disk space.

Anterior Cervical Corpectomy and Fusion

Patients who have multilevel degenerative disk CSM in addition to kyphotic deformity of the cervical spine may require a corpectomy. Corpectomy is favored in certain clinical scenarios, such as OPLL, trauma, osteomyelitis, and neoplasms. Patients with neutral or kyphotic sagittal alignment of the cervical spine typically require corpectomy via an anterior approach. Correction of a fixed kyphotic cervical spine can be more reliably achieved with anterior cervical corpectomy and fusion (ACCF) compared with multilevel ACDF. Fusion rates after anterior decompression procedures that are performed across more than three disk levels may be higher in patients who undergo ACCF compared with patients who undergo ACDF, particularly in uninstrumented scenarios[55] (**Figure 4**).

After completing the soft-tissue exposure, the disk spaces above and below the vertebral body to be resected are exposed and incised. After the diskectomies are complete, a rongeur can be used to resect the ventral half of the vertebral body, and the remainder of the vertebral body can be removed with the use of a high-speed burr. ACCF allows for the expansion of a narrow osseous spinal canal and the simultaneous removal of large osteophytes from the vertebral end plates that impinge the spinal cord and nerve roots. Anatomic landmarks, such as the medial origin of the longus colli, the medial margin of the uncus, and the lateral curvature of the vertebral end plate, can be used to maintain midline orientation. The lateral extent of an ACCF is limited by the foramen transversarium, which contains the vertebral artery. Studies have reported that a total decompression

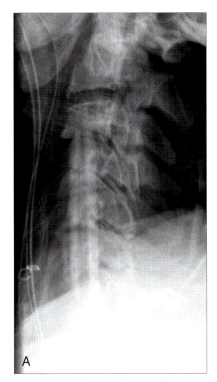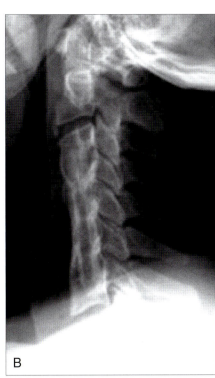

Figure 4   **A,** Lateral radiograph of a cervical spine demonstrates a fibular strut graft for a multilevel anterior cervical corpectomy and fusion (ACCF). **B,** Lateral radiograph of a cervical spine taken 1 year after ACCF demonstrates fibular strut graft consolidation.

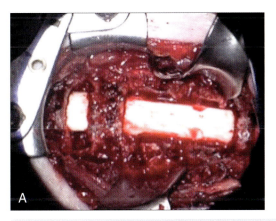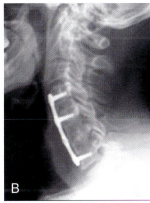

Figure 5   **A,** Intraoperative photograph of a cervical spine shows hybrid anterior decompression and graft placement. **B,** Lateral radiograph of a cervical spine taken after hybrid anterior diskectomy and corpectomy demonstrates successful fusion and good alignment.

of the central spinal canal of approximately 15 mm at C3 and 19 mm at C6 ensures a safety margin of 5 mm to the medial border of the foramen transversarium.[56]

Various modifications to ACCF have been described. A hybrid diskectomy-corpectomy technique is another option that can be used (**Figure 5**). Recent studies have reported that a hybrid diskectomy-corpectomy technique results in less blood loss and fewer complications compared with multilevel ACCF.[57] If retrovertebral disease is substantial, a hybrid diskectomy-corpectomy technique may be preferred. A hybrid diskectomy-corpectomy technique may avoid the biomechanical instability associated with multilevel ACCF.

Graft Choice

The material characteristics for the intervertebral graft include the iliac crest and the fibula as either an allograft or autograft. An autologous iliac crest graft tends to fuse rapidly, which is clearly advantageous; however, a fibular strut graft is a strong cortical circumferential graft that has a relatively high modulus of elasticity, and its length can be tailored as necessary. One distinct disadvantage of a fibular strut graft is the mismatch in bone mineral density from cancellous bone, which can cause pistoning of the fibular strut graft that penetrates the vertebral body. In patients who have osteoporosis, some level of graft subsidence is unavoidable but, typically, is not clinically important if the graft stabilizes.

Fibular strut allograft has been reported to incorporate slower compared with autologous iliac crest graft.[58] Typically, fibular strut autograft is not used because of the morbidity caused by graft harvest, which includes increased blood loss and increased surgical time.[59] Packing the fibular strut allograft with cancellous bone autograft taken from the iliac crest or the resected corpectomy bone itself has been reported to enhance fusion.[60] Despite the differences between iliac crest autograft and fibular strut allograft, a substantial difference with regard to pseudarthrosis

rates has not been consistently demonstrated.[61-63] Other options for anterior support include implants, such as polyetheretherketone and titanium cages; however, these implants still require bone grafting.

ACCF Versus ACDF

ACCF and ACDF are effective decompression techniques for the management of CSM; however, whether ACCF and ACDF offer equivalent outcomes for the management of multilevel CSM has yet to be determined. Hybrid diskectomy-corpectomy decompression is a plausible treatment option for patients with CSM who have substantial multilevel retrovertebral disease. For all anterior cervical approaches, stabilization is usually required and can be attained, depending on the patient, with the use of either anterior plating or posterior instrumentation. The location of compressive pathology, the size of the spinal canal, the alignment of the cervical spine, and the extent of retrovertebral osteophytes must all be considered in the selection of a specific procedure.

Posterior Cervical Approaches
Indications and Surgical Considerations

Anterior cervical approaches are very safe and straightforward and should be used for the treatment of patients who have direct anterior compressive pathology, focal stenosis, or cervical kyphosis; however, a posterior cervical approach may be more effective and a better treatment option for some patients. The use of an anterior approach alone in patients with multilevel congenital stenosis or instability in whom fusion of three or more levels is necessary has

proven to be insufficient. Sasso et al[64] reported that multilevel ACCF alone has a failure rate that increases from 6% in patients who undergo two-level fusion to 71% in patients who undergo three-level fusion. In a small, matched cohort analysis, Edwards et al[65] reported a higher rate of complications, including nonunion, adjacent segment problems, and dysphagia, as well as increased postoperative pain in patients with CSM who underwent multilevel ACCF compared with patients with CSM who underwent multilevel laminoplasty. In a meta-analysis that compared anterior cervical approaches with posterior cervical approaches for the treatment of patients with multilevel CSM, Zhu et al[66] reported that anterior cervical procedures alone were associated with significantly higher complication rates. A posterior cervical approach also can be used to augment ACCF in patients with multilevel CSM in whom preoperative kyphosis or a large anterior compressive lesion necessitates an anterior cervical approach. In a study of 40 patients with three- or four-level CSM who underwent combined anterior and posterior cervical approaches, Konya et al[67] reported improved neurologic function in all of the patients and fusion in all but one patient at 1-year follow-up.

Preoperative cervical sagittal alignment plays a substantial role in the selection of a surgical approach. In general, posterior cervical approaches allow for direct decompression of posterior lesions and provide an effective method for indirect decompression of anterior lesions by allowing posterior spinal cord drift. Sodeyama et al[68] reported that posterior spinal cord drift greater than 3 mm was associated with good clinical outcomes in patients who underwent laminoplasty; however, appropriate preoperative cervical sagittal alignment is required for posterior drift to occur. Yamazaki et al[69] reported that at least 10° of cervical lordosis is necessary to allow for adequate posterior drift and postoperative indirect decompression in patients with OPLL. Regardless of the location of pathology, appropriate cervical sagittal alignment is necessary to ensure favorable outcomes in patients who undergo posterior decompression. Suda et al[70] reported that a local kyphotic angle greater than 13° was the greatest risk factor for poor outcomes in patients who underwent laminoplasty alone. Therefore, in patients who have cervical kyphosis, surgeons should consider either performing an anterior decompression or addressing the kyphosis before performing a posterior decompression, such as laminoplasty.

If a high approach to the occipitocervical or axial cervical spine is necessary, a posterior cervical approach allows for better access from the occiput to C2. Isolated occipitoatlantal or atlantoaxial CSM is rare; however, unique causes, such as hypoplasia or dysplasia of the posterior arch of the atlas, ossification of the transverse ligament of the atlas, and hypertrophy of the dens, exist and must be addressed appropriately.[71-73] Good clinical outcomes were reported by Tsuruta et al[73] in a review of 13 case studies of atlas hypoplasia that were managed with posterior decompression. Furthermore, anterior cervical approaches may be associated with high morbidity, such as postoperative dysphagia, which is observed in patients who undergo odontoidectomies.[74] Not all patients who have anterior compressive lesions, even those in the subaxial spine, may benefit from anterior decompression. Patients with OPLL present a unique challenge for surgeons.

Although OPLL causes anterior compression, an anterior cervical approach can result in serious complications, including pseudarthrosis, graft failure, inadequate decompression, and a possible cerebrospinal fluid leak as a result of adherence to the dura.[75,76] However, Iwasaki et al[77] reported that the effectiveness of posterior decompression via laminoplasty was limited in patients with OPLL who had an occupying ratio greater than or equal to 60%; therefore, the authors recommended ACDF for patients with OPLL who have an occupying ratio greater than or equal to 60%.

Fujiyoshi et al[78] described the K-line, which is a radiographic marker that can be used to help determine the appropriate surgical approach for patients with OPLL. The K-line is a drawn line that connects the midpoints of the spinal canal at C2 and C7 on lateral radiographs of the cervical spine. Patients with OPLL that is posterior to the K-line have a substantially lower rate of neurologic recovery after posterior decompression. Taniyama et al[79] used a modified K-line, which is a drawn line that connects the midpoints of the spinal cord at C2 and C7 on a sagittal T1-weighted MRI, to predict the rate of residual anterior compression after laminoplasty. The authors reported that residual anterior compression was 26.6% more likely to occur in patients who had an anterior lesion that was within 4 mm of the modified K-line, and that the likelihood of residual anterior compression was substantially higher if an anterior lesion was closer to the modified K-line.

Altered anatomy may prevent the safe use of an anterior cervical approach. Patients who have undergone previous anterior neck surgery or radiation therapy may have a tissue bed that discourages an anterior cervical approach. In addition, anterior cervical approaches are associated with a much higher risk for dysphagia compared with posterior cervical approaches, which is a factor that may need to be considered if substantial concern for aspiration as a result of a history of dysphagia or an inability to protect the airway exists.[80] Furthermore, an appropriate preoperative evaluation of the anatomy and course of a patient's vertebral artery is warranted given that midline vertebral artery migration, which places the vertebral artery at risk in anterior cervical approaches, is reported in 7.6% of patients who have CSM.[81] Surgeons also should consider the need for surgical expediency in patients who have comorbidities or other risk factors that may place substantial time constraints on the surgical procedure. Studies have reported shorter surgical times for posterior cervical approaches compared with ACCF.[82,83] A careful assessment of the location of pathology, cervical sagittal alignment, the number of involved disk levels, and patient risk factors can help guide surgeons with regard to whether a posterior cervical approach is an effective treatment option.

Laminectomy

The primary indications for laminectomy include multilevel CSM in patients with lordosis and a spondylotic stiff spine in whom fusion may not be necessary. After an initial midline posterior cervical incision is made, care should be taken to avoid exposure of the facet joints. The technique for laminectomy involves thinning of the cortices at the junction of the laminae and lateral masses at the affected disk levels with the use of a high-speed burr. A Kerrison rongeur can be used to complete the final cut, or a Cobb elevator can be used to elevate the remaining bony segment; however, care must be taken to avoid violating the associated facet joint capsule to prevent iatrogenic instability.

Laminectomy should be avoided in patients in whom myeloradiculopathy exists and patients in whom resection of more than 50% of the facet joint is required to provide adequate decompression of the exiting nerve root. Biomechanical studies have reported that resection of more than 50% of the facet complex in combination with decompression results in substantial segmental hypermobility in the cervical spine, which necessitates fusion.[84] Although laminectomy without fusion was the traditional surgical treatment of choice for patients with CSM, it has been associated with a substantial rate of complications postoperatively (47%), including kyphosis and instability.[85-89] Furthermore, long-term follow-up studies have reported that the rate of neurologic improvement after laminectomy decreases with time; however, the rate of neurologic improvement after laminectomy has not necessarily been reported to correlate with the degree of kyphosis after laminectomy.[88,90] Although largely replaced by laminectomy with fusion, laminectomy without fusion is currently a viable option for the management of CSM in very specific patients, typically those with stable, severe spondylosis in whom appropriate preoperative cervical lordosis is present.[91]

Skip laminectomy is an alternative method of decompression that can be performed to reduce the morbidity that may be associated with traditional laminectomy or laminoplasty. Skip laminectomy attempts to decrease damage to the extensor mechanisms, decrease restriction on neck ROM, and prevent loss of cervical lordosis. Skip laminectomy involves standard laminectomies that are performed at select disk levels and partial laminectomies of the cephalad halves of the laminae that are performed at adjacent disk levels so that the muscular attachments of the respective spinous process can be left undisturbed.[92] In a study that compared the outcomes of 43 patients with CSM who underwent skip laminectomy with those of 51 control patients with CSM who underwent laminoplasty, Shiraishi et al[93] reported similar JOA scale scores at a mean follow-up of 2.6 years; however, the patients who underwent skip laminectomy had improved postoperative ROM, axial neck symptoms, and atrophy rates of the deep extensor muscles. In a prospective clinical trial of 41 patients with CSM who were randomized to either laminoplasty or skip laminectomy (21 and 20 patients, respectively), Yukawa et al[94] reported that the patients in both groups had similar JOA scale scores and comparable outcomes with regard to axial neck pain, ROM, and cervical alignment at a mean follow-up of 28.1 months. Skip laminectomy has limitations and is contraindicated in patients with extensive stenosis of the spinal canal who may require greater decompression than a skip laminectomy allows.[93]

Video 26.1: Surgical Management of Cervical Spondylotic Myelopathy. Chris A. Cornett, MD, MPT (3 min)

Laminectomy With Fusion

Laminectomy with fusion (**Figure 6**) is indicated for patients with multilevel CSM who have associated instability, patients who require an augment for multilevel anterior decompression, and patients who require decompression and an associated facetectomy. A detailed understanding of the cervical spine and its associated anatomy is necessary to attain successful outcomes and avoid complications. Occipital fixation may be necessary in patients who have CSM at a high cervical level. The mean thickness of the occipital skull at the external occipital protuberance is 13.8 mm, which decreases to a mean thickness of 8.3 mm at the inferior nuchal line.[95] Appropriate preoperative imaging, including CT, can be obtained to measure the thickness of the occiput for determining screw lengths. Imaging studies also can help guide decision making in patients who have abnormal anatomy. Surgeons attempting to provide fixation to the axial cervical spine should obtain a CT angiogram to better understand the anatomy of the vertebral artery. In a study of the magnetic resonance angiograms of 2,739 patients, Uchino et al[96] reported a 5% prevalence of vertebral artery variations, including persistent first intersegment artery, vertebral artery fenestration, and posteroinferior cerebellar artery originating at the C1-C2 level. CT angiography also is beneficial because it delineates the relationship of the internal carotid artery to the anterior aspect of the C1 vertebra. Currier et al[97] reported that the mean distance from the internal carotid artery to the C1 vertebra was 2.88 to 2.89 mm, which puts the internal carotid artery at risk during attempted C1 lateral mass screw placement, especially if bicortical fixation is attempted. Bony anatomy may vary at C1 in patients who have an arcuate foramen, which, if not appropriately identified preoperatively,

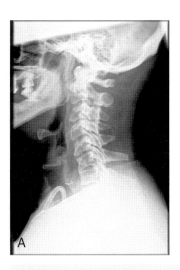 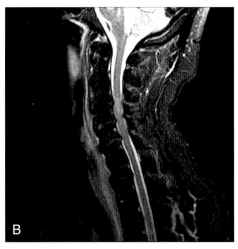 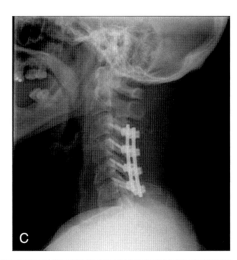

Figure 6   Images of the cervical spine of a patient with myelopathy and cervical stenosis from C3 through C6 who underwent laminectomy with fusion. **A,** Preoperative lateral radiograph demonstrates neutral to lordotic alignment, which is appropriate for a posterior cervical approach. **B,** Preoperative sagittal short tau inversion recovery MRI shows substantial cervical stenosis and myelomalacia. **C,** Lateral radiograph taken after laminectomy from C4 to C6, partial laminectomy at C3 and C7, and fusion from C3 to C6 demonstrates posterior instrumentation and good alignment.

can increase the risk for vertebral artery damage at C1 during the placement of lateral mass screws. Young et al[98] reported a 15.5% prevalence of arcuate foramen; therefore, appropriate identification of arcuate foramen on preoperative lateral radiographs of the cervical spine is warranted.

Traditionally, fusion of the axial cervical spine was accomplished with the use of wiring techniques. The Gallie method for fusion of the axial cervical spine involves sublaminar wire or cable that is passed under the posterior arch of the C1 vertebra and around the spinous process of the C2 vertebra to secure a bone graft and provide fusion of the posterior elements of C1-C2.[99] The Gallie method, however, provides little stability in rotation and allows for a substantial amount of motion.[100] Typically, the Gallie method requires additional postoperative immobilization, such as a halo vest, for reliable fusion.

The Brooks method, which is another technique for fusion of the axial cervical spine, has been reported to result in more reliable fixation and stability compared with the Gallie method.[100,101] The Brooks method for fusion of the axial cervical spine involves two sublaminar wires or cables that are passed under each side of the arch of the C1 vertebra and the C2 vertebra to secure two iliac crest bone grafts that are wedged between the posterior aspects of these disk levels. Typically, the Brooks method requires additional postoperative immobilization.

The advent of transarticular screw fixation of C1-C2, which was described by Jeanneret and Magerl,[102] eliminated the need for wiring and has been reported to result in the best biomechanical fixation of the axial cervical spine.[100] Substantial care must be taken, however, to ensure that appropriate reduction of C1-C2 has been performed and that potential vertebral artery anomalies have been identified to prevent any unwarranted complications, such as malreduction or vertebral artery injury.[103] The entry point for the transarticular screw is located along the inferomedial edge of the inferior articular process of C2. The transarticular screw is directed in a sagittal-cephalad orientation toward the posterior rim of the atlantoaxial joint through the lateral mass of C1.[102] Attaining the appropriate trajectory for transarticular screw placement without unnecessary exposure of the lower cervical spine may be difficult with the C1-C2 transarticular screw technique. To avoid this issue and attain the correct trajectory for transarticular screw placement, the transarticular screws and associated instruments can be tunneled percutaneously under the skin.

Segmental C1-C2 fixation with the use of C1 lateral mass screws is another method for fixation of the axial cervical spine that can result in high fusion rates.[104] Traditionally, segmental C1-C2 fixation with the use of C1 lateral mass screws was used to manipulate the C2 nerve root for appropriate placement of the C1 lateral mass screw; however, Squires and Molinari[105] reported no significant differences in Neck Disability

Index scores, analog pain, or satisfaction between patients who underwent C2 nerve root–sacrificing techniques compared with patients who underwent nerve root–sparing techniques. In a literature review of 20 studies that included 732 patients with C2 nerve root preservation and six studies that included 361 patients with C2 nerve root sacrifice, Elliott et al[106] reported that C2 nerve root sacrifice was associated with numbness in approximately 12% of patients. Few patients with C2 nerve root sacrifice had neuropathic pain, but approximately 5% of patients with C2 nerve root preservation had neuropathic pain. Furthermore, in a prospective study that compared C2 nerve root–sacrificing techniques with C2 nerve root–sparing techniques during segmental C1-C2 fixation with the use of C1 lateral mass screws, Dewan et al[107] reported that C2 nerve root sacrifice was associated with increased occipital numbness but had no effect on patient-reported outcomes. Sacrifice of the C2 nerve root may be necessary if a fixed dislocation exists between C1 and C2 or if a C1 or C2 laminectomy, in which the C1-C2 joint is the primary location of fusion, is required for decompression. Both pars screws and pedicle screws can be used to provide appropriate segmental fixation at the level of C2.[104,108]

C2 translaminar screw fixation, which is an alternative method of fixation at this level that was described by Wright,[109] can mitigate risk to an anomalous vertebral artery that prevents the safe placement of a pedicle or pars screw.[110] Furthermore, Ilgenfritz et al[111] described the use of laminar screws at C7, reporting no differences in pullout strength between C7 laminar screws compared with C7 pedicle screws.

Traditionally, wiring techniques, if combined with laminectomy, resulted in high fusion rates in the subaxial spine.[112,113] Wiring techniques involve passing wires through drill holes that are created in the articular processes after denudation, lateral to the area of the laminectomy, and securing bone graft to the posterior columns of the articular processes. Wiring techniques are a viable option for patients in whom lateral mass fixation may not be possible or patients in whom only a less invasive midline exposure is desired. Wiring techniques, however, have been replaced by lateral mass screw techniques because of the ease of the techniques and increased construct stiffness.[114] Lateral mass screw techniques for fixation of the cervical spine, which were first described by Roy-Camille et al,[115] use an entry point at the center of the posterior surface of the lateral mass that is perpendicular to the posterior surface of the lateral mass and angled 10° lateral to the sagittal plane. Montesano and Magerl[116] developed a technical variation to this technique, in which screws are placed 1 mm medial to the center of the lateral mass and parallel to the plane of the facet joint, with 25° of lateral angulation relative to the axial plane. The lateral mass screw technique described by Montesano and Magerl[116] has been reported to result in 40% greater pullout strength compared with the lateral mass screw technique described by Roy-Camille[115] but does not have any clear clinical advantage.[117,118] Bicortical screws increase the risk for injury to associated nerve roots and the vertebral artery and do not appear to have any clear biomechanical advantage.[119] Pedicle screw techniques for fixation of the cervical spine can result in greater pullout strength but increase the risk

for neurovascular injury that results from breaching of the pedicle walls, specifically in the region of C3 through C6 given the morphology and size of the pedicles in this region.[120-122] However, Park et al[123] reported the safe placement of pedicle screws in a cohort of 45 patients, achieving a 94.1% accuracy rate and only a 7.8% conversion rate to lateral mass screws.

Laminectomy with fusion can result in favorable clinical outcomes. In a study of 54 patients with CSM who underwent laminectomy with fusion, Gok et al[124] reported that 81% of the patients had improved Nurick grades at a mean follow-up of 17 months; however, 19% of the patients had stable but unimproved CSM. The authors reported that a higher preoperative Nurick grade was associated with more favorable postoperative outcomes and that an increased duration of preoperative CSM was associated with a decreased likelihood of CSM improvement.

Laminoplasty

Laminoplasty is a valuable option for posterior decompression in patients in whom fusion is not indicated (**Figure 7**). In an effort to maintain more motion, patients without spinal instability and no history of neck pain on clinical examination may achieve better results without fusion. In a small prospective randomized trial that compared cervical laminoplasty with cervical laminectomy and fusion, the patients who were randomized to laminoplasty had a 20% loss of ROM postoperatively, whereas the patients who were randomized to laminectomy with fusion had a 75% loss of ROM postoperatively.[125]

Hirabayashi et al[126] described a technique for open-door laminoplasty that

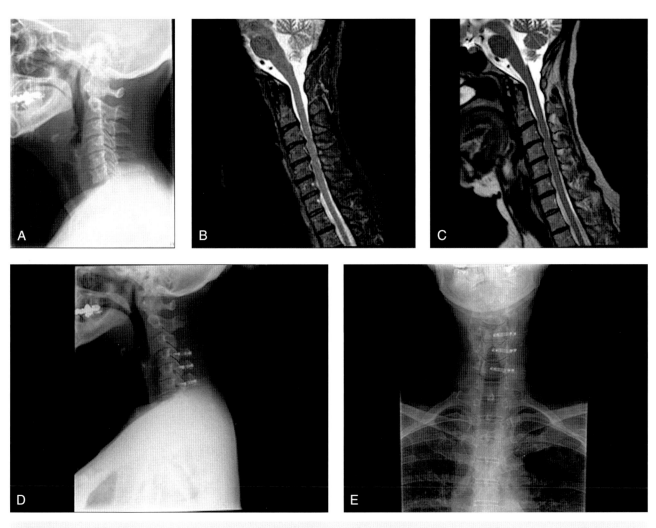

Figure 7 Images of the cervical spine of a patient with myelopathy and cervical stenosis from C3 through C7 who underwent laminoplasty from C4 to C6, complete laminectomy at C3, and partial laminectomy at C7. **A,** Preoperative lateral radiograph demonstrates degenerative changes and slight lordotic alignment. **B,** Preoperative sagittal short tau inversion recovery MRI shows substantial cervical stenosis and early myelomalacia. **C,** Preoperative sagittal T2-weighted MRI shows cervical stenosis. Postoperative lateral (**D**) and AP (**E**) radiographs demonstrate plate placement at C4, C5, and C6.

requires the creation of a bicortical trough at the junction of the lamina and the lateral mass with the use of a high-speed burr on the open door side, which typically is the side that is more symptomatic; a hinge is then made on the contralateral side by creating a unicortical trough in a similar fashion. The hinge increases the spinal canal diameter; keeping the hinge open usually requires some method of fixation, which can be achieved with the use of plates, simple bony suture techniques, suture anchors, spacers, or bone grafting.

Hoshi et al[127] subsequently described French-door laminoplasty, which uses a high-speed burr to create a sagittal split in the midline of the spinous process; a hinge is made by creating unicortical troughs in a manner similar to that used for open-door laminoplasty. The hinge is kept open with the use of plates, simple bony suture techniques, suture anchors, spacers, or bone grafting.

Although French-door laminoplasty is technically challenging and increases the risk for spinal cord injury, it is theoretically advantageous compared with open-door laminoplasty because it avoids the lateral epidural veins, which can increase bleeding, and because it allows for symmetric reconstruction of the posterior arch.

Midline T-saw laminoplasty, which was described by Tomita et al,[128] attempted to improve

French-door laminoplasty and avoid the associated technical challenges and safety concerns by using a T-saw instead of a high-speed burr to create the sagittal split in the spinous process. Furthermore, midline T-saw laminoplasty decreases the amount of bone loss that can occur with the use of a high-speed burr, which, theoretically, impairs reconstruction of the posterior arch. Regardless of the specific laminoplasty technique used, preservation of the C2 and C7 spinous process muscle attachments is important because it has been associated with a decrease in postoperative neck pain.[129,130]

The outcomes of laminoplasty are favorable in appropriately selected patients. Using the modified K-line, Taniyama et al[131] correlated the recovery rates of patients who underwent laminoplasty with preoperative nonlordotic alignment; however, recovery rates were not necessarily correlated with the amount of preoperative posterior spinal cord shift. Some studies reported that laminoplasty improved JOA scale scores by an average of as much as 55% and resulted in good long-term outcomes.[132,133] Compared with laminectomy and fusion, laminoplasty results in similar improvements in Nurick grades, modified JOA scale scores, and Odom outcomes.[134]

Although not a common procedure, laminoplasty with fusion results in distinct advantages, including reduction of perineural adhesions that can occur after laminectomy and a larger fusion bed along the hinge site.[135] In a study of 20 patients who underwent combined anterior cervical fusion with laminoplasty and posterior instrumented fusion, Yeh et al[135] reported significant improvements in JOA scale scores, Nurick grades, and Neck Disability

Index scores as well as no evidence of pseudarthrosis or hardware loosening at 24 months postoperatively.

Anterior Versus Posterior Approaches

The decision of which approach to use for the surgical management of CSM should be based primarily on the location and extent of the pathology. Lawrence et al[136] reported that both anterior and posterior cervical approaches are similarly effective with regard to outcomes. Fehlings et al[137] reported that patients with CSM attained considerable improvements after surgery via either anterior or posterior cervical approaches. The authors also reported that patients who underwent surgery via an anterior cervical approach were more likely to be younger (mean age, 53 years versus 63 years for patients who underwent surgery via an anterior cervical approach versus a posterior cervical approach, respectively), had more focal pathology, and had less severe CSM. Overall, Fehlings et al[137] reported that the efficacy of anterior and posterior cervical approaches for the management of CSM is equivalent.

Intraoperative Complications

The surgical management of CSM can lead to a variety of complications. To decrease the risk of complications, the surgeon should exercise efficiency during the procedure. Efficiency in the operating room decreases retractor time and swelling. Efficiency is gained through not only practice and repetition but also proper and thorough preoperative planning. Knowledge of cervical spine anatomy and possible anatomic variations is important to maintain appropriate retractor placement and attain

adequate exposure, which is easier with a careful and calculated dissection.

Recurrent Laryngeal Nerve Injury

A sore throat and mild hoarseness may occur after ventral cervical surgery; however, in most patients, these issues typically resolve within weeks or months of surgery without further intervention. Usually, the source of sore throat and mild hoarseness is edema caused by the endotracheal tube; however, laryngeal nerve injury also can occur and may result in permanent laryngeal dysfunction. Both the superior laryngeal nerve (SLN) and the recurrent laryngeal nerve (RLN) are at risk for injury during anterior exposure of the cervical spine, with vocal cord paralysis being the most common neurologic complication. The true incidence of RLN injury after anterior cervical spine surgery is approximately 1% to 2%.[138] With regard to specific cervical approaches, Beutler et al[138] reported that RLN injury occurs at a rate of 2.1% in patients who undergo ACDF, 3.5% in patients who undergo ACCF, and 9.5% in patients who undergo revision anterior spine surgery. Several proposed mechanisms for RLN injury include pressure- or stretch-induced neurapraxia, postoperative edema, and direct surgical trauma that results in inadvertent ligation of the nerve.

With a left-sided approach, the RLN loops under the arch of the aorta and resides within the tracheoesophageal groove. Conversely, the right RLN travels around the subclavian artery, passing dorsomedial to the side of the trachea and the esophagus. The right RLN is vulnerable because it travels from the subclavian artery to the tracheoesophageal groove. The inferior

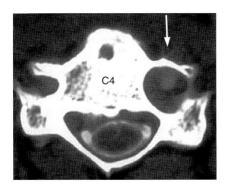

Figure 8 Axial CT demonstrates a left tortuous vertebral artery at C4 with an enlarged foramen (arrow).

thyroid artery on the right side is a key anatomic landmark for the identification of the right RLN. At the point at which the inferior thyroid artery enters the lower pole of the thyroid, the right RLN concomitantly enters the tracheoesophageal groove.

The external branch of the SLN is a branch of the vagus nerve and innervates the cricothyroid muscle. Above the level of C4, the superior thyroid artery is a key anatomic landmark for the identification of the SLN. Damage to either the SLN or the RLN may result in hoarseness, vocal fatigue, a weak cough, dysphagia, or aspiration.[139,140] Anatomic variations can occur on the right side, and a nonrecurrent RLN may be encountered. However, the frequency of a nonrecurrent RLN is quite low, occurring in substantially less than 1% of individuals.[141] Cannon[141] reported that a nonrecurrent RLN passes from the vagus nerve in the carotid sheath directly to the larynx. If a nonrecurrent RLN is encountered, it can be identified with the use of a nerve stimulator and via laryngoscopic examination of the vocal cords.

Endotracheal tube–related injury to the RLN also can occur. Monitoring of endotracheal cuff pressure and its release after the placement of retractors can decrease the rate of temporary vocal cord paralysis from 6.4% to 1.7%.[142] Endotracheal tube–related injury is believed to be caused by displacement of the larynx into the unyielding shaft of the endotracheal tube that is fixed distally by the balloon cuff and proximally by tape at the mouth. Deflation of the balloon cuff to allow the endotracheal tube to recenter in the larynx after placement of the cervical retractor system is believed to result in relief of pressure on the laryngeal wall.

Vertebral Artery Laceration

The reported incidence of vertebral arterial injury after cervical spine surgery is rare, occurring at a rate of 0.3% to 0.5%. Although rare, vertebral arterial injury is associated with morbidity. Axial and sagittal MRIs or CT scans should be reviewed to ensure that a normal vertebral artery path exists. In a study of 222 cadaver models, Curylo et al[143] reported a 2.7% incidence of a tortuous vertebral artery (**Figure 8**). Injury to the vertebral artery in patients who undergo anterior cervical surgery may result from excessive lateral placement of instruments, asymmetric dissection off midline, far lateral bone removal, or aggressive manipulation of the longus colli muscles.[144]

If vertebral artery injury occurs, primary repair of the artery is recommended. Often, bleeding can be controlled with gentle compression using hemostatic gelatin or oxidized cellulose, especially for smaller lacerations. If gentle compression is unsuccessful, direct proximal ligation should be performed. Visualization during repair of the artery is imperative and may require unroofing of the anterior aspect of the foramen transversarium to attain proximal control and perform direct microvascular repair. The surgeon should avoid blind placement of sutures in an attempt to control the hemorrhage because doing so can cause inadvertent damage to the cervical nerve roots. Returning the head to a neutral position from an extended position is recommended to ensure that the contralateral vertebral artery will not be mechanically occluded. An angiogram should be obtained to rule out an arteriovenous fistula or a pseudoaneurysm. Cerebellar infarction, isolated cranial nerve palsy, quadriparesis, and hemiplegia are rare but very morbid complications of vertebral artery laceration. To avoid vertebral artery injury, the surgeon should frequently reconfirm midline orientation. During diskectomy, the medial uncovertebral joint should be used as an anatomic guide for the lateral extent of dissection and drilling.

Esophageal Injury

In the upper cervical spine, injury to the esophagus or pharynx can occur, particularly in the region in which the hypopharynx is thin. If recognized intraoperatively, an esophageal perforation should be primarily repaired, and a nasogastric tube should be placed. A postoperative swallow study with water-soluble contrast should be subsequently obtained to assess the closure (**Figure 9**). Esophagoscopy or postesophagogram CT also may demonstrate a perforation. A growing mass in the neck or the presence of crepitus suggests a strong possibility of an esophageal perforation. In most patients, injury to the esophagus is typically not recognized during surgery and more often manifests clinically as a local infection, fistula, sepsis,

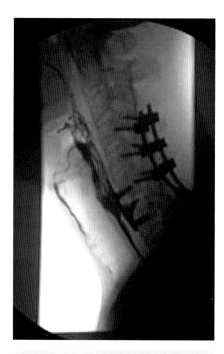

Figure 9 Lateral fluoroscopic image of a cervical spine from a swallow study shows inadequate closure of the esophagus, which is evidenced by a contrast leak.

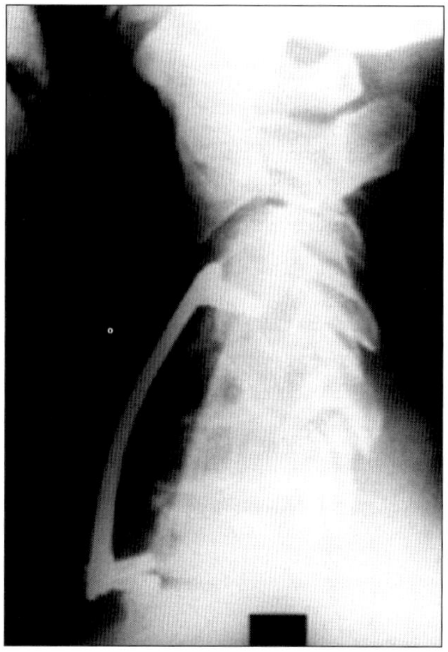

Figure 10 Lateral radiograph of a cervical spine demonstrates cavitation of a fibular strut graft in extension through the vertebral end plate.

or mediastinitis.[145] The muscles of the longus colli should be adequately freed laterally so that the teeth from self-retaining retractors can be placed safely underneath. The esophagus should be completely hidden by retractors to avoid injury from instrumentation.

Hardware- and Graft-Related Complications

Graft- and/or plate-related complications can occur in patients who undergo ACCF. The incidence of graft dislodgement increases as the number of corpectomy levels increases. For instance, the complication rate for patients who undergo one-level ACCF is 4.2%; however, the complication rate for patients who undergo four-level ACCF is 16.2%.[146]

In an attempt to reduce graft- and/or plate-related complications, long anterior cervical plating has been developed and used for graft stabilization. However, the use of a long anterior cervical plate is associated with a 9% to 50% rate of complications, depending on the number of corpectomy levels.[147] Foley et al[148] reported a 10.3% rate of graft/plate displacement in 39 patients who underwent multilevel anterior cervical corpectomy and plate fixation. Biomechanically, the plate acts as a distraction device that prevents settling of the graft onto the end plates. DiAngelo et al[149] reported that multilevel anterior plates increased stiffness and decreased local motion. However, the instantaneous axis of rotation is shifted anteriorly after an anterior plate is applied, which loads the graft in excessive extension and results in long-term graft cavitation through the end plate and subsequent kicking out of the lower vertebral body (**Figure 10**).

Posterior instrumentation moves the instantaneous axis of rotation posteriorly and essentially normalizes the axis.

Summary

CSM is a common cause of cervical spinal cord impairment, especially in adults. Surgeons must understand the differential diagnosis for myelopathy and recognize that patients may need immediate referral or treatment. The progression of CSM is unpredictable; therefore, a surgeon should discuss expectations and treatment options with a patient soon after a diagnosis is made. Although substantial knowledge on CSM is available, future research will help surgeons attain a better understanding of the disease process, which may lead to improved treatment options. If surgical intervention is warranted, surgeons must decide which approach is most appropriate for each patient and discuss with the patient the potential complications that may be encountered. Surgeons should be efficient in the operating room to decrease the risk for potential complications; this can be accomplished with careful and deliberate dissection as well as proper preoperative planning.

References

1. Kalsi-Ryan S, Karadimas SK, Fehlings MG: Cervical spondylotic myelopathy: The clinical phenomenon and the current pathobiology of an increasingly prevalent and devastating disorder. *Neuroscientist* 2013;19(4):409-421.

2. Young WF: Cervical spondylotic myelopathy: A common cause of spinal cord dysfunction in older persons. *Am Fam Physician* 2000;62(5):1064-1070, 1073.

3. Moore AP, Blumhardt LD: A prospective survey of the causes of non-traumatic spastic paraparesis and

tetraparesis in 585 patients. *Spinal Cord* 1997;35(6):361-367.

4. Fehlings MG, Wilson JR, Yoon ST, Rhee JM, Shamji MF, Lawrence BD: Symptomatic progression of cervical myelopathy and the role of non-surgical management: A consensus statement. *Spine (Phila Pa 1976)* 2013; 38(22 suppl 1):S19-S20.

5. Lebl DR, Bono CM: Update on the diagnosis and management of cervical spondylotic myelopathy. *J Am Acad Orthop Surg* 2015;23(11):648-660.

6. Fehlings MG, Skaf G: A review of the pathophysiology of cervical spondylotic myelopathy with insights for potential novel mechanisms drawn from traumatic spinal cord injury. *Spine (Phila Pa 1976)* 1998;23(24): 2730-2737.

7. Kim HJ, Tetreault LA, Massicotte EM, et al: Differential diagnosis for cervical spondylotic myelopathy: Literature review. *Spine (Phila Pa 1976)* 2013;38(22 suppl 1):S78-S88.

8. Tracy JA, Bartleson JD: Cervical spondylotic myelopathy. *Neurologist* 2010;16(3):176-187.

9. Burrows EH: The sagittal diameter of the spinal canal in cervical spondylosis. *Clin Radiol* 1963;14:77-86.

10. Payne EE, Spillane JD: The cervical spine; an anatomico-pathological study of 70 specimens (using a special technique) with particular reference to the problem of cervical spondylosis. *Brain* 1957;80(4):571-596.

11. Edwards WC, LaRocca H: The developmental segmental sagittal diameter of the cervical spinal canal in patients with cervical spondylosis. *Spine (Phila Pa 1976)* 1983;8(1):20-27.

12. Morishita Y, Naito M, Hymanson H, Miyazaki M, Wu G, Wang JC: The relationship between the cervical spinal canal diameter and the pathological changes in the cervical spine. *Eur Spine J* 2009;18(6):877-883.

13. Hayashi H, Okada K, Hamada M, Tada K, Ueno R: Etiologic factors of myelopathy: A radiographic evaluation of the aging changes in the cervical spine. *Clin Orthop Relat Res* 1987;214:200-209.

14. Gore DR: Roentgenographic findings in the cervical spine in asymptomatic persons: A ten-year follow-up. *Spine (Phila Pa 1976)* 2001;26(22):2463-2466.

15. Karadimas SK, Erwin WM, Ely CG, Dettori JR, Fehlings MG: Pathophysiology and natural history of cervical spondylotic myelopathy. *Spine (Phila Pa 1976)* 2013;38(22 suppl 1):S21-S36.

16. Breig A, Turnbull I, Hassler O: Effects of mechanical stresses on the spinal cord in cervical spondylosis: A study on fresh cadaver material. *J Neurosurg* 1966;25(1):45-56.

17. Parke WW: Correlative anatomy of cervical spondylotic myelopathy. *Spine (Phila Pa 1976)* 1988;13(7):831-837.

18. Penning L, van der Zwaag P: Biomechanical aspects of spondylotic myelopathy. *Acta Radiol Diagn (Stockh)* 1966;5:1090-1103.

19. White AA III, Panjabi MM: Biomechanical considerations in the surgical management of cervical spondylotic myelopathy. *Spine (Phila Pa 1976)* 1988;13(7):856-860.

20. Hashizume Y, Iijima S, Kishimoto H, Yanagi T: Pathology of spinal cord lesions caused by ossification of the posterior longitudinal ligament. *Acta Neuropathol* 1984;63(2):123-130.

21. Hukuda S, Wilson CB: Experimental cervical myelopathy: Effects of compression and ischemia on the canine cervical cord. *J Neurosurg* 1972;37(6):631-652.

22. Pathak M, Kim RC, Pribram H: Spinal cord infarction following vertebral angiography: Clinical and pathological findings. *J Spinal Cord Med* 2000;23(2):92-95.

23. Hoff J, Nishimura M, Pitts L, Vilnis V, Tuerk K, Lagger R: The role of ischemia in the pathogenesis of cervical spondylotic myelopathy: A review and new microangiopathic evidence. *Spine (Phila Pa 1976)* 1977;2(2):100-108.

24. Gooding MR, Wilson CB, Hoff JT: Experimental cervical myelopathy: Effects of ischemia and compression of the canine cervical spinal cord. *J Neurosurg* 1975;43(1):9-17.

25. Park E, Velumian AA, Fehlings MG: The role of excitotoxicity in secondary mechanisms of spinal cord injury: A

review with an emphasis on the implications for white matter degeneration. *J Neurotrauma* 2004;21(6):754-774.

26. Gledhill RF, Harrison BM, McDonald WI: Demyelination and remyelination after acute spinal cord compression. *Exp Neurol* 1973;38(3):472-487.

27. Karadimas SK, Moon ES, Yu WR, et al: A novel experimental model of cervical spondylotic myelopathy (CSM) to facilitate translational research. *Neurobiol Dis* 2013;54:43-58.

28. Karadimas SK, Gatzounis G, Fehlings MG: Pathobiology of cervical spondylotic myelopathy. *Eur Spine J* 2015;24(suppl 2):132-138.

29. Ogino H, Tada K, Okada K, et al: Canal diameter, anteroposterior compression ratio, and spondylotic myelopathy of the cervical spine. *Spine (Phila Pa 1976)* 1983;8(1):1-15.

30. Ono K, Ota H, Tada K, Yamamoto T: Cervical myelopathy secondary to multiple spondylotic protrusions: A clinicopathologic study. *Spine (Phila Pa 1976)* 1977;2(2):109-125.

31. Good DC, Couch JR, Wacaser L: "Numb, clumsy hands" and high cervical spondylosis. *Surg Neurol* 1984;22(3):285-291.

32. al-Mefty O, Harkey HL, Marawi I, et al: Experimental chronic compressive cervical myelopathy. *J Neurosurg* 1993;79(4):550-561.

33. Yu WR, Liu T, Kiehl TR, Fehlings MG: Human neuropathological and animal model evidence supporting a role for Fas-mediated apoptosis and inflammation in cervical spondylotic myelopathy. *Brain* 2011; 134(pt 5):1277-1292.

34. Baptiste DC, Fehlings MG: Pathophysiology of cervical myelopathy. *Spine J* 2006;6(6 suppl):190S-197S.

35. Bunge RP, Puckett WR, Becerra JL, Marcillo A, Quencer RM: Observations on the pathology of human spinal cord injury: A review and classification of 22 new cases with details from a case of chronic cord compression with extensive focal demyelination. *Adv Neurol* 1993;59:75-89.

36. Karadimas S, Moon ES, Fehlings MG: The sodium channel/glutamate blocker Riluzole is complementary to

decompression in a preclinical experimental model of cervical spondylotic myelopathy (CSM): Implications for translational clinical application. *Neurosurgery* 2012;71(2):543.

37. Northover JR, Wild JB, Braybrooke J, Blanco J: The epidemiology of cervical spondylotic myelopathy. *Skeletal Radiol* 2012;41(12):1543-1546.

38. Houten JK, Noce LA: Clinical correlations of cervical myelopathy and the Hoffmann sign. *J Neurosurg Spine* 2008;9(3):237-242.

39. Blackley HR, Plank LD, Robertson PA: Determining the sagittal dimensions of the canal of the cervical spine: The reliability of ratios of anatomical measurements. *J Bone Joint Surg Br* 1999;81(1):110-112.

40. Prasad SS, O'Malley M, Caplan M, Shackleford IM, Pydisetty RK: MRI measurements of the cervical spine and their correlation to Pavlov's ratio. *Spine (Phila Pa 1976)* 2003;28(12):1263-1268.

41. Suri A, Chabbra RP, Mehta VS, Gaikwad S, Pandey RM: Effect of intramedullary signal changes on the surgical outcome of patients with cervical spondylotic myelopathy. *Spine J* 2003;3(1):33-45.

42. Mastronardi L, Elsawaf A, Roperto R, et al: Prognostic relevance of the postoperative evolution of intramedullary spinal cord changes in signal intensity on magnetic resonance imaging after anterior decompression for cervical spondylotic myelopathy. *J Neurosurg Spine* 2007;7(6):615-622.

43. Tetreault LA, Dettori JR, Wilson JR, et al: Systematic review of magnetic resonance imaging characteristics that affect treatment decision making and predict clinical outcome in patients with cervical spondylotic myelopathy. *Spine (Phila Pa 1976)* 2013; 38(22 suppl 1):S89-S110.

44. Kerkovský M, Bednarík J, Dušek L, et al: Magnetic resonance diffusion tensor imaging in patients with cervical spondylotic spinal cord compression: Correlations between clinical and electrophysiological findings. *Spine (Phila Pa 1976)* 2012;37(1):48-56.

45. Rajasekaran S, Yerramshetty JS, Chittode VS, Kanna RM, Balamurali

G, Shetty AP: The assessment of neuronal status in normal and cervical spondylotic myelopathy using diffusion tensor imaging. *Spine (Phila Pa 1976)* 2014;39(15):1183-1189.

46. Nakai S, Sonoo M, Shimizu T: Somatosensory evoked potentials (SEPs) for the evaluation of cervical spondylotic myelopathy: Utility of the onset-latency parameters. *Clin Neurophysiol* 2008;119(10):2396-2404.

47. Simó M, Szirmai I, Arányi Z: Superior sensitivity of motor over somatosensory evoked potentials in the diagnosis of cervical spondylotic myelopathy. *Eur J Neurol* 2004;11(9):621-626.

48. Kawakami M, Tamaki T, Iwasaki H, Yoshida M, Ando M, Yamada H: A comparative study of surgical approaches for cervical compressive myelopathy. *Clin Orthop Relat Res* 2000;381:129-136.

49. Tew JM Jr, Mayfield FH: Complications of surgery of the anterior cervical spine. *Clin Neurosurg* 1976;23:424-434.

50. Dohn DF: Anterior interbody fusion for treatment of cervical-disk conditions. *JAMA* 1966;197(11):897-900.

51. Robinson RA, Smith GW: Anterolateral cervical disc removal and interbody fusion for cervical disc syndrome. *Bull Johns Hopkins Hosp* 1955;96:223-224.

52. Cloward RB: The anterior approach for removal of ruptured cervical disks. *J Neurosurg* 1958;15(6):602-617.

53. Brodke DS, Zdeblick TA: Modified Smith-Robinson procedure for anterior cervical discectomy and fusion. *Spine (Phila Pa 1976)* 1992; 17(10 suppl):S427-S430.

54. An HS, Evanich CJ, Nowicki BH, Haughton VM: Ideal thickness of Smith-Robinson graft for anterior cervical fusion: A cadaveric study with computed tomographic correlation. *Spine (Phila Pa 1976)* 1993;18(14):2043-2047.

55. Galler RM, Dogan S, Fifield MS, et al: Biomechanical comparison of instrumented and uninstrumented multilevel cervical discectomy versus corpectomy. *Spine (Phila Pa 1976)* 2007;32(11):1220-1226.

56. Vaccaro AR, Ring D, Scuderi G, Garfin SR: Vertebral artery location in relation to the vertebral body as determined by two-dimensional computed tomography evaluation. *Spine (Phila Pa 1976)* 1994;19(23):2637-2641.

57. Liu JM, Peng HW, Liu ZL, Long XH, Yu YQ, Huang SH: Hybrid decompression technique versus anterior cervical corpectomy and fusion for treating multilevel cervical spondylotic myelopathy: Which one is better? *World Neurosurg* 2015;84(6):2022-2029.

58. Eleraky MA, Llanos C, Sonntag VK: Cervical corpectomy: Report of 185 cases and review of the literature. *J Neurosurg* 1999;90(1 suppl):35-41.

59. Nassr A, Khan MH, Ali MH, et al: Donor-site complications of autogenous nonvascularized fibula strut graft harvest for anterior cervical corpectomy and fusion surgery: Experience with 163 consecutive cases. *Spine J* 2009;9(11):893-898.

60. Niu CC, Hai Y, Fredrickson BE, Yuan HA: Anterior cervical corpectomy and strut graft fusion using a different method. *Spine J* 2002;2(3):179-187.

61. Emery SE, Bohlman HH, Bolesta MJ, Jones PK: Anterior cervical decompression and arthrodesis for the treatment of cervical spondylotic myelopathy: Two to seventeen-year follow-up. *J Bone Joint Surg Am* 1998;80(7):941-951.

62. Fernyhough JC, White JI, LaRocca H: Fusion rates in multilevel cervical spondylosis comparing allograft fibula with autograft fibula in 126 patients. *Spine (Phila Pa 1976)* 1991; 16(10 suppl):S561-S564.

63. Ikenaga M, Shikata J, Tanaka C: Long-term results over 10 years of anterior corpectomy and fusion for multilevel cervical myelopathy. *Spine (Phila Pa 1976)* 2006;31(14):1568-1575.

64. Sasso RC, Ruggiero RA Jr, Reilly TM, Hall PV: Early reconstruction failures after multilevel cervical corpectomy. *Spine (Phila Pa 1976)* 2003;28(2):140-142.

65. Edwards CC II, Heller JG, Murakami H: Corpectomy versus laminoplasty for multilevel cervical myelopathy: An independent matched-cohort

analysis. *Spine (Phila Pa 1976)* 2002;27(11):1168-1175.

66. Zhu B, Xu Y, Liu X, Liu Z, Dang G: Anterior approach versus posterior approach for the treatment of multi-level cervical spondylotic myelopathy: A systemic review and meta-analysis. *Eur Spine J* 2013;22(7):1583-1593.

67. Konya D, Ozgen S, Gercek A, Pamir MN: Outcomes for combined anterior and posterior surgical approaches for patients with multisegmental cervical spondylotic myelopathy. *J Clin Neurosci* 2009;16(3):404-409.

68. Sodeyama T, Goto S, Mochizuki M, Takahashi J, Moriya H: Effect of decompression enlargement laminoplasty for posterior shifting of the spinal cord. *Spine (Phila Pa 1976)* 1999;24(15):1527-1532.

69. Yamazaki A, Homma T, Uchiyama S, Katsumi Y, Okumura H: Morphologic limitations of posterior decompression by midsagittal splitting method for myelopathy caused by ossification of the posterior longitudinal ligament in the cervical spine. *Spine (Phila Pa 1976)* 1999;24(1):32-34.

70. Suda K, Abumi K, Ito M, Shono Y, Kaneda K, Fujiya M: Local kyphosis reduces surgical outcomes of expansive open-door laminoplasty for cervical spondylotic myelopathy. *Spine (Phila Pa 1976)* 2003;28(12):1258-1262.

71. Tang JG, Hou SX, Shang WL, Wu WW: Cervical myelopathy caused by anomalies at the level of atlas. *Spine (Phila Pa 1976)* 2010;35(3):E77-E79.

72. Ma Z, Ma X, Yang H, Feng H, Chen C: Complex cervical spondylotic myelopathy: A report of two cases and literature review. *Eur Spine J* 2016;25(suppl 1):27-32.

73. Tsuruta W, Yanaka K, Okazaki M, Matsumura A, Nose T: Cervical myelopathy caused by hypoplasia of the atlas and ossification of the transverse ligament—case report. *Neurol Med Chir (Tokyo)* 2003;43(1):55-59.

74. Van Abel KM, Mallory GW, Kasperbauer JL, et al: Transnasal odontoid resection: Is there an anatomic explanation for differing swallowing outcomes? *Neurosurg Focus* 2014;37(4):E16.

75. Shinomiya K, Okamoto A, Kamikozuru M, Furuya K, Yamaura I: An analysis of failures in primary cervical anterior spinal cord decompression and fusion. *J Spinal Disord* 1993;6(4):277-288.

76. Epstein N: The surgical management of ossification of the posterior longitudinal ligament in 51 patients. *J Spinal Disord* 1993;6(5):432-455.

77. Iwasaki M, Okuda S, Miyauchi A, et al: Surgical strategy for cervical myelopathy due to ossification of the posterior longitudinal ligament: Part 2. Advantages of anterior decompression and fusion over laminoplasty. *Spine (Phila Pa 1976)* 2007;32(6):654-660.

78. Fujiyoshi T, Yamazaki M, Kawabe J, et al: A new concept for making decisions regarding the surgical approach for cervical ossification of the posterior longitudinal ligament: The K-line. *Spine (Phila Pa 1976)* 2008;33(26):E990-E993.

79. Taniyama T, Hirai T, Yamada T, et al: Modified K-line in magnetic resonance imaging predicts insufficient decompression of cervical laminoplasty. *Spine (Phila Pa 1976)* 2013;38(6):496-501.

80. Smith-Hammond CA, New KC, Pietrobon R, Curtis DJ, Scharver CH, Turner DA: Prospective analysis of incidence and risk factors of dysphagia in spine surgery patients: Comparison of anterior cervical, posterior cervical, and lumbar procedures. *Spine (Phila Pa 1976)* 2004;29(13):1441-1446.

81. Eskander MS, Drew JM, Aubin ME, et al: Vertebral artery anatomy: A review of two hundred fifty magnetic resonance imaging scans. *Spine (Phila Pa 1976)* 2010;35(23):2035-2040.

82. Shibuya S, Komatsubara S, Oka S, Kanda Y, Arima N, Yamamoto T: Differences between subtotal corpectomy and laminoplasty for cervical spondylotic myelopathy. *Spinal Cord* 2010;48(3):214-220.

83. Kristof RA, Kiefer T, Thudium M, et al: Comparison of ventral corpectomy and plate-screw-instrumented fusion with dorsal laminectomy and rod-screw-instrumented fusion for treatment of at least two vertebral-level spondylotic cervical myelopathy. *Eur Spine J* 2009;18(12):1951-1956.

84. Zdeblick TA, Zou D, Warden KE, McCabe R, Kunz D, Vanderby R: Cervical stability after foraminotomy: A biomechanical in vitro analysis. *J Bone Joint Surg Am* 1992;74(1):22-27.

85. Pal GP, Sherk HH: The vertical stability of the cervical spine. *Spine (Phila Pa 1976)* 1988;13(5):447-449.

86. Raynor RB, Moskovich R, Zidel P, Pugh J: Alterations in primary and coupled neck motions after facetectomy. *Neurosurgery* 1987;21(5):681-687.

87. Albert TJ, Vacarro A: Postlaminectomy kyphosis. *Spine (Phila Pa 1976)* 1998;23(24):2738-2745.

88. Kato Y, Iwasaki M, Fuji T, Yonenobu K, Ochi T: Long-term follow-up results of laminectomy for cervical myelopathy caused by ossification of the posterior longitudinal ligament. *J Neurosurg* 1998;89(2):217-223.

89. Kaptain GJ, Simmons NE, Replogle RE, Pobereskin L: Incidence and outcome of kyphotic deformity following laminectomy for cervical spondylotic myelopathy. *J Neurosurg* 2000; 93(2 suppl):199-204.

90. Arnold H, Feldmann U, Missler U: Chronic spondylogenic cervical myelopathy: A critical evaluation of surgical treatment after early and long-term follow-up. *Neurosurg Rev* 1993;16(2):105-109.

91. McAllister BD, Rebholz BJ, Wang JC: Is posterior fusion necessary with laminectomy in the cervical spine? *Surg Neurol Int* 2012;3(suppl 3):S225-S231.

92. Shiraishi T: Skip laminectomy—a new treatment for cervical spondylotic myelopathy, preserving bilateral muscular attachments to the spinous processes: A preliminary report. *Spine J* 2002;2(2):108-115.

93. Shiraishi T, Fukuda K, Yato Y, Nakamura M, Ikegami T: Results of skip laminectomy: Minimum 2-year follow-up study compared with open-door laminoplasty. *Spine (Phila Pa 1976)* 2003;28(24):2667-2672.

94. Yukawa Y, Kato F, Ito K, et al: Laminoplasty and skip laminectomy

for cervical compressive myelopathy: Range of motion, postoperative neck pain, and surgical outcomes in a randomized prospective study. *Spine (Phila Pa 1976)* 2007;32(18):1980-1985.

95. Roberts DA, Doherty BJ, Heggeness MH: Quantitative anatomy of the occiput and the biomechanics of occipital screw fixation. *Spine (Phila Pa 1976)* 1998;23(10):1100-1108.

96. Uchino A, Saito N, Watadani T, et al: Vertebral artery variations at the C1-2 level diagnosed by magnetic resonance angiography. *Neuroradiology* 2012;54(1):19-23.

97. Currier BL, Maus TP, Eck JC, Larson DR, Yaszemski MJ: Relationship of the internal carotid artery to the anterior aspect of the C1 vertebra: Implications for C1-C2 transarticular and C1 lateral mass fixation. *Spine (Phila Pa 1976)* 2008;33(6):635-639.

98. Young JP, Young PH, Ackermann MJ, Anderson PA, Riew KD: The ponticulus posticus: Implications for screw insertion into the first cervical lateral mass. *J Bone Joint Surg Am* 2005;87(11):2495-2498.

99. Gallie WE: Fractures and dislocations of the cervical spine. *Am J Surg* 1939;46(3):495-499.

100. Grob D, Crisco JJ III, Panjabi MM, Wang P, Dvorak J: Biomechanical evaluation of four different posterior atlantoaxial fixation techniques. *Spine (Phila Pa 1976)* 1992;17(5):480-490.

101. Brooks AL, Jenkins EB: Atlanto-axial arthrodesis by the wedge compression method. *J Bone Joint Surg Am* 1978;60(3):279-284.

102. Jeanneret B, Magerl F: Primary posterior fusion C1/2 in odontoid fractures: Indications, technique, and results of transarticular screw fixation. *J Spinal Disord* 1992;5(4):464-475.

103. Madawi AA, Casey AT, Solanki GA, Tuite G, Veres R, Crockard HA: Radiological and anatomical evaluation of the atlantoaxial transarticular screw fixation technique. *J Neurosurg* 1997;86(6):961-968.

104. Harms J, Melcher RP: Posterior C1-C2 fusion with polyaxial screw and rod fixation. *Spine (Phila Pa 1976)* 2001;26(22):2467-2471.

105. Squires J, Molinari RW: C1 lateral mass screw placement with intentional sacrifice of the C2 ganglion: Functional outcomes and morbidity in elderly patients. *Eur Spine J* 2010;19(8):1318-1324.

106. Elliott RE, Kang MM, Smith ML, Frempong-Boadu A: C2 nerve root sectioning in posterior atlantoaxial instrumented fusions: A structured review of literature. *World Neurosurg* 2012;78(6):697-708.

107. Dewan MC, Godil SS, Mendenhall SK, Devin CJ, McGirt MJ: C2 nerve root transection during C1 lateral mass screw fixation: Does it affect functionality and quality of life? *Neurosurgery* 2014;74(5):475-481.

108. Resnick DK, Benzel EC: C1-C2 pedicle screw fixation with rigid cantilever beam construct: Case report and technical note. *Neurosurgery* 2002;50(2):426-428.

109. Wright NM: Posterior C2 fixation using bilateral, crossing C2 laminar screws: Case series and technical note. *J Spinal Disord Tech* 2004;17(2):158-162.

110. Ebraheim N, Rollins JR Jr, Xu R, Jackson WT: Anatomic consideration of C2 pedicle screw placement. *Spine (Phila Pa 1976)* 1996;21(6):691-695.

111. Ilgenfritz RM, Gandhi AA, Fredericks DC, Grosland NM, Smucker JD: Considerations for the use of C7 crossing laminar screws in subaxial and cervicothoracic instrumentation. *Spine (Phila Pa 1976)* 2013;38(4):E199-E204.

112. Callahan RA, Johnson RM, Margolis RN, Keggi KJ, Albright JA, Southwick WO: Cervical facet fusion for control of instability following laminectomy. *J Bone Joint Surg Am* 1977;59(8):991-1002.

113. Epstein NE: Laminectomy with posterior wiring and fusion for cervical ossification of the posterior longitudinal ligament, spondylosis, ossification of the yellow ligament, stenosis, and instability: A study of 5 patients. *J Spinal Disord* 1999;12(6):461-466.

114. Gill K, Paschal S, Corin J, Ashman R, Bucholz RW: Posterior plating of the cervical spine: A biomechanical comparison of different posterior

fusion techniques. *Spine (Phila Pa 1976)* 1988;13(7):813-816.

115. Roy-Camille R, Saillant G, Mazel C: Internal fixation of the unstable cervical spine by a posterior osteosynthesis with plates and screws, in The Cervical Spine Research Society, Sherk HH, Dunn ES, Eismont FJ, et al, eds: *The Cervical Spine*. Philadelphia, PA, Lippincott, Williams & Wilkins, 1989, pp 390-403.

116. Montesano PX, Magerl F: Lateral mass plating, in The Cervical Spine Research Society, ed: *The Cervical Spine*. Philadelphia, PA, Lippincott-Raven, 1991, pp 509-514.

117. Montesano PX, Jauch E, Jonsson H Jr: Anatomic and biomechanical study of posterior cervical spine plate arthrodesis: An evaluation of two different techniques of screw placement. *J Spinal Disord* 1992;5(3):301-305.

118. Heller JG, Carlson GD, Abitbol JJ, Garfin SR: Anatomic comparison of the Roy-Camille and Magerl techniques for screw placement in the lower cervical spine. *Spine (Phila Pa 1976)* 1991;16(10 suppl):S552-S557.

119. Seybold EA, Baker JA, Criscitiello AA, Ordway NR, Park CK, Connolly PJ: Characteristics of unicortical and bicortical lateral mass screws in the cervical spine. *Spine (Phila Pa 1976)* 1999;24(22):2397-2403.

120. Jones EL, Heller JG, Silcox DH, Hutton WC: Cervical pedicle screws versus lateral mass screws: Anatomic feasibility and biomechanical comparison. *Spine (Phila Pa 1976)* 1997;22(9):977-982.

121. Karaikovic EE, Daubs MD, Madsen RW, Gaines RW Jr: Morphologic characteristics of human cervical pedicles. *Spine (Phila Pa 1976)* 1997;22(5):493-500.

122. Nakashima H, Yukawa Y, Imagama S, et al: Complications of cervical pedicle screw fixation for nontraumatic lesions: A multicenter study of 84 patients. *J Neurosurg Spine* 2012;16(3):238-247.

123. Park JH, Jeon SR, Roh SW, Kim JH, Rhim SC: The safety and accuracy of freehand pedicle screw placement in the subaxial cervical spine: A series of

45 consecutive patients. *Spine (Phila Pa 1976)* 2014;39(4):280-285.

124. Gok B, McLoughlin GS, Sciubba DM, et al: Surgical management of cervical spondylotic myelopathy with laminectomy and instrumented fusion. *Neurol Res* 2009;31(10):1097-1101.

125. Manzano GR, Casella G, Wang MY, Vanni S, Levi AD: A prospective, randomized trial comparing expansile cervical laminoplasty and cervical laminectomy and fusion for multilevel cervical myelopathy. *Neurosurgery* 2012;70(2):264-277.

126. Hirabayashi K, Watanabe K, Wakano K, Suzuki N, Satomi K, Ishii Y: Expansive open-door laminoplasty for cervical spinal stenotic myelopathy. *Spine (Phila Pa 1976)* 1983;8(7):693-699.

127. Hoshi K, Kurokawa T, Nakamura K, Hoshino Y, Saita K, Miyoshi K: Expansive cervical laminoplasties: Observations on comparative changes in spinous process lengths following longitudinal laminal divisions using autogenous bone or hydroxyapatite spacers. *Spinal Cord* 1996;34(12):725-728.

128. Tomita K, Kawahara N, Toribatake Y, Heller JG: Expansive midline T-saw laminoplasty (modified spinous process-splitting) for the management of cervical myelopathy. *Spine (Phila Pa 1976)* 1998;23(1):32-37.

129. Hosono N, Sakaura H, Mukai Y, Fujii R, Yoshikawa H: C3-6 laminoplasty takes over C3-7 laminoplasty with significantly lower incidence of axial neck pain. *Eur Spine J* 2006;15(9):1375-1379.

130. Sakaura H, Hosono N, Mukai Y, Fujimori T, Iwasaki M, Yoshikawa H: Preservation of muscles attached to the C2 and C7 spinous processes rather than subaxial deep extensors reduces adverse effects after cervical laminoplasty. *Spine (Phila Pa 1976)* 2010;35(16):E782-E786.

131. Taniyama T, Hirai T, Yoshii T, et al: Modified K-line in magnetic resonance imaging predicts clinical outcome in patients with nonlordotic alignment after laminoplasty for cervical spondylotic myelopathy. *Spine (Phila Pa 1976)* 2014;39(21):E1261-E1268.

132. Seichi A, Takeshita K, Ohishi I, et al: Long-term results of double-door laminoplasty for cervical stenotic myelopathy. *Spine (Phila Pa 1976)* 2001;26(5):479-487.

133. Kawaguchi Y, Kanamori M, Ishihara H, Ohmori K, Nakamura H, Kimura T: Minimum 10-year followup after en bloc cervical laminoplasty. *Clin Orthop Relat Res* 2003;411:129-139.

134. Highsmith JM, Dhall SS, Haid RW Jr, Rodts GE Jr, Mummaneni PV: Treatment of cervical stenotic myelopathy: A cost and outcome comparison of laminoplasty versus laminectomy and lateral mass fusion. *J Neurosurg Spine* 2011;14(5):619-625.

135. Yeh KT, Lee RP, Chen IH, et al: Laminoplasty instead of laminectomy as a decompression method in posterior instrumented fusion for degenerative cervical kyphosis with stenosis. *J Orthop Surg Res* 2015;10:138.

136. Lawrence BD, Jacobs WB, Norvell DC, Hermsmeyer JT, Chapman JR, Brodke DS: Anterior versus posterior approach for treatment of cervical spondylotic myelopathy: A systematic review. *Spine (Phila Pa 1976)* 2013; 38(22 suppl 1):S173-S182.

137. Fehlings MG, Barry S, Kopjar B, et al: Anterior versus posterior surgical approaches to treat cervical spondylotic myelopathy: Outcomes of the prospective multicenter AOSpine North America CSM study in 264 patients. *Spine (Phila Pa 1976)* 2013;38(26):2247-2252.

138. Beutler WJ, Sweeney CA, Connolly PJ: Recurrent laryngeal nerve injury with anterior cervical spine surgery risk with laterality of surgical approach. *Spine (Phila Pa 1976)* 2001;26(12):1337-1342.

139. Miscusi M, Bellitti A, Peschillo S, Polli FM, Missori P, Delfini R: Does recurrent laryngeal nerve anatomy condition the choice of the side for approaching the anterior cervical spine? *J Neurosurg Sci* 2007;51(2):61-64.

140. Melamed H, Harris MB, Awasthi D: Anatomic considerations of superior laryngeal nerve during anterior cervical spine procedures. *Spine (Phila Pa 1976)* 2002;27(4):E83-E86.

141. Cannon CR: The anomaly of nonrecurrent laryngeal nerve: Identification and management. *Otolaryngol Head Neck Surg* 1999;120(5):769-771.

142. Apfelbaum RI, Kriskovich MD, Haller JR: On the incidence, cause, and prevention of recurrent laryngeal nerve palsies during anterior cervical spine surgery. *Spine (Phila Pa 1976)* 2000;25(22):2906-2912.

143. Curylo LJ, Mason HC, Bohlman HH, Yoo JU: Tortuous course of the vertebral artery and anterior cervical decompression: A cadaveric and clinical case study. *Spine (Phila Pa 1976)* 2000;25(22):2860-2864.

144. Burke JP, Gerszten PC, Welch WC: Iatrogenic vertebral artery injury during anterior cervical spine surgery. *Spine J* 2005;5(5):508-514.

145. Dakwar E, Uribe JS, Padhya TA, Vale FL: Management of delayed esophageal perforations after anterior cervical spinal surgery. *J Neurosurg Spine* 2009;11(3):320-325.

146. Wang JC, Hart RA, Emery SE, Bohlman HH: Graft migration or displacement after multilevel cervical corpectomy and strut grafting. *Spine (Phila Pa 1976)* 2003;28(10):1016-1022.

147. Vaccaro AR, Falatyn SP, Scuderi GJ, et al: Early failure of long segment anterior cervical plate fixation. *J Spinal Disord* 1998;11(5):410-415.

148. Foley KT, DiAngelo DJ, Rampersaud YR, Vossel KA, Jansen TH: The in vitro effects of instrumentation on multilevel cervical strut-graft mechanics. *Spine (Phila Pa 1976)* 1999;24(22):2366-2376.

149. DiAngelo DJ, Foley KT, Vossel KA, Rampersaud YR, Jansen TH: Anterior cervical plating reverses load transfer through multilevel strut-grafts. *Spine (Phila Pa 1976)* 2000;25(7):783-795.

Video Reference

26.1: Cornett CA: Video. *Surgical Management of Cervical Spondylotic Myelopathy.* Omaha, NE, 2016.

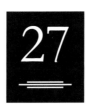

Adult Lumbar Scoliosis: Nonsurgical Versus Surgical Management

Jonathan Falakassa, MD

Serena S. Hu, MD

Abstract

Adult spinal deformity has become an increasingly recognized condition, with a 32% incidence in the adult population and a 68% incidence in the elderly population. Often, patients with adult spinal deformity are initially offered nonsurgical treatment for their symptoms despite the lack of data to support its efficacy because of the high complication rate associated with surgical treatment in this age group. Determining which patients would benefit the most from nonsurgical versus surgical treatment remains a challenge. Limited evidence exists to support guidelines on the most effective way to treat patients with adult spinal deformity. Treatment decisions for patients with adult spinal deformity often rely on individual surgeon experience and patient preferences.

Instr Course Lect 2017;66:353–360.

Adult spinal deformity (ASD) has become an increasingly recognized condition, with a 32% incidence in the adult population and a 68% incidence in the elderly population.[1] The number of patients with an ASD is expected to rise as the proportion of the population older than 65 years increases. Patients with ASD may have symptoms of pain, functional limitations, neurologic deficits, or progressive deformity.

Often, patients with ASD are initially offered nonsurgical treatment for their symptoms despite the lack of data to support its efficacy because of the high complication rate associated with surgical treatment in this age group. Complication and revision surgery rates associated with ASD surgery have been reported to be as high as 80% and 58%, respectively.[2,3] Determining which patients would benefit the most from

nonsurgical versus surgical treatment remains a challenge. Currently, limited level I evidence exists to help guide decision making.

Nonsurgical Management

In the absence of a progressive neurologic deficit, the initial treatment for patients with ASD should begin with nonsurgical treatment. A lack of consensus exists on the most successful nonsurgical clinical treatment option. Most patients are reluctant to consider major reconstructive surgery without an attempt at nonsurgical treatment. Many healthcare insurers require that surgeons document failure of nonsurgical treatment before proceeding with surgical treatment. Epidural steroid injections, physical therapy, bracing, and NSAIDs are currently the mainstays of nonsurgical treatment; however, a paucity of literature that supports the efficacy of nonsurgical management exists.

Epidural Steroid Injections

The use of epidural steroid injections for the management of ASD has grown

Dr. Hu or an immediate family member has received royalties from NuVasive; serves as a paid consultant to NuVasive; has stock or stock options held in NuVasive; and serves as a board member, owner, officer, or committee member of the American Orthopaedic Association. Neither Dr. Falakassa nor any immediate family member has received anything of value from or has stock or stock options held in a commercial company or institution related directly or indirectly to the subject of this chapter.

considerably. From 1999 to 2009, lumbar epidural steroid injections increased by nearly 900,000 injections per year.[4] Epidural steroid injections are often used to manage pain from spinal stenosis and radiculopathy that may be associated with adult lumbar scoliosis. Degenerative changes that lead to spinal stenosis can precede a spinal deformity, resulting in de novo scoliosis.[5] Lumbar stenosis that results from degenerative changes also can occur within a preexisting spinal deformity. Epidural steroid injections are widely used in patients who have lumbar spinal stenosis to manage leg pain caused by neurogenic claudication; however, rigorous data on the effectiveness and safety of these injections are lacking. In a double-blind, multisite study of 400 patients with spinal stenosis who were randomized to either epidural steroid injection with lidocaine or epidural injection of lidocaine alone, Friedly et al[6] failed to demonstrate any significant difference in Roland-Morris Disability Questionnaire scores or the intensity of leg pain between the patients in the two groups 6 weeks after injection. The authors concluded that the epidural injection of glucocorticoids in combination with lidocaine offered minimal or no short-term benefit compared with the epidural injection of lidocaine alone.

The use of epidural steroid injections for the management of radicular pain appears to be more promising. Lumbar radicular pain may be caused by foraminal stenosis and other lumbar spine conditions, such as lumbar disk herniation or facet cysts. Cooper et al[7] explored the effectiveness of transforaminal epidural steroid injections in a retrospective study of 61 patients who had degenerative scoliosis greater than 10° and complaints of

radicular pain. The authors defined a successful outcome as a patient who was both satisfied with his or her results and experienced at least a two-point improvement in Numeric Pain Rating Scale, Summary Pain, and Summary Function scores. The authors reported that 59.6% of the patients had a successful outcome 1 week after injection, 55.8% of the patients had a successful outcome 1 month after injection, 37.2% of the patients had a successful outcome 1 year after injection, and 27.3% of the patients had a successful outcome 2 years after injection ($P < 0.01$). However, the conclusions of the study are limited because the authors used historical recall. Ghahreman et al[8] conducted a prospective study of 150 patients with disk herniation and lumbar radicular pain who were randomized to either transforaminal steroid injection with local anesthetic, transforaminal injection of local anesthetic alone, transforaminal injection of normal saline, intramuscular steroid injection, or intramuscular injection of normal saline. Patients and outcome evaluators were blinded to the agent that was administered. The primary outcome measure was the proportion of patients who achieved at least 50% pain relief 1 month after injection. The authors reported that pain relief was achieved in a greater proportion of the patients who were treated with the transforaminal steroid injection in combination with local anesthetic (54%) compared with the patients who were treated with the transforaminal injection of local anesthetic alone (7%), the transforaminal injection of normal saline (19%), the intramuscular steroid injection (21%), or the intramuscular injection of normal saline (13%). The authors reported that pain relief was corroborated by significant

improvements in function and disability as well as reductions in the use of other healthcare resources. The patients with acute radicular pain and the patients with chronic radicular pain had equivalent outcomes; however, the number of patients who maintained pain relief diminished over time, with only 25% of patients reporting pain relief 12 months after injection. Overall, level III (weak) evidence exists for the use of transforaminal epidural steroid injections for the nonsurgical management of radiculopathy and/or spinal stenosis that is associated with adult lumbar scoliosis.

Physical Therapy

Physical therapy also is a commonly prescribed modality for the nonsurgical management of adult lumbar scoliosis. Between 1999 and 2009, physical therapy referrals for adults with degenerative spine disorders increased by 1.4 million visits per year.[4] Barrios et al[9] treated 30 patients who had adult degenerative scoliosis and Cobb angles that ranged from 25° to 65° for curve correction and pain control with the use of physiotherapy. The patients were initially treated with heat and lumbar traction, after which a traction device with pressure was applied to the apex of the deformity. Patients underwent 20 to 60 physical therapy sessions and were treated with the use of NSAIDs as necessary. The outcomes of the patients who underwent physiotherapy were compared with those of a control group of patients who had scoliosis that was not described in detail. The authors reported a statistically significant improvement in curve magnitude in the patients in the physiotherapy group (38.75%) compared with the patients in the control group (18.75%). The authors also reported a significant reduction in pain in the patients in the physiotherapy group, with 77% of the patients reported to be symptomatic before treatment compared with only 7% of the patients reported to be symptomatic after treatment. However, the method of pain assessment, therapy protocols, and independence of the radiographic reviewers were not well described, which makes the conclusions of the study difficult to extrapolate to specific patient populations. Mamyama et al[10] treated 69 skeletally mature patients who had scoliosis with the use of the side-shift exercise toward the concavity. The authors failed to demonstrate any substantial benefit of the side-shift exercise at a mean follow-up of 4.2 years, with the degree of curvature in most of the patients staying essentially the same or improving only slightly.

Bracing

Bracing is a well-accepted nonsurgical treatment modality that is used to prevent curve progression in skeletally immature patients who have adolescent idiopathic scoliosis with at-risk curves.[11] The use of bracing in skeletally mature patients who have adult lumbar scoliosis, however, has not been proven to be beneficial. In a case study of a woman with neurogenic claudication and adult scoliosis who underwent treatment with a custom lumbosacral orthosis, Weiss and Dallmayer[12] reported short-term improvement in the woman's ambulation distance but only a minimal decrease in her pain. In a study of 29 women (mean age, 41 years) with adult lumbar scoliosis and a mean Cobb angle of 37° who underwent treatment with a custom lumbosacral orthosis to restore sagittal balance, Weiss et al[13] reported that the patients reported immediate but only short-term pain relief with

the use of the brace, and 22 patients had stopped wearing the brace at a mean follow-up of 7.5 months. In an observational study of 67 patients with chronic low back pain (>24 months) and a diagnosis of scoliosis or hyperkyphosis who underwent treatment with a sagittal realignment brace, Weiss and Werkmann[14] reported that short-term pain reduction was achieved by increasing lumbar lordosis; however, no pain improvement was reported after 6 months of treatment. Similarly, in a retrospective analysis of studies on the treatment of patients who had degenerative scoliosis that was associated with stenosis, Ploumis et al[15] reported that the use of a lumbosacral orthosis or a thoracolumbosacral orthosis may provide temporary pain relief; however, the long-term use of a lumbosacral orthosis or a thoracolumbosacral orthosis was reported to be counterproductive because it may result in muscle wasting and has no effect on curve progression. Based on the limited number of studies and lack of support, level IV (very weak) evidence exists for the use of bracing for the nonsurgical management of adult scoliosis.

The potential risk for muscle deconditioning and spine off-loading with the use of bracing is a particularly important consideration in postmenopausal females who are at risk for osteoporosis. Proper nutrition and weight-bearing activities that increase loads on the spine in combination with adjunct pharmacologic treatment are preferred instead of bracing in this at-risk patient population.

Nonsteroidal Anti-inflammatory Drugs

NSAIDs, muscle relaxants, and narcotics are commonly prescribed to alleviate

the pain associated with adult lumbar scoliosis. Often, these oral medications are used intermittently to manage acute symptomatic and chronic musculoskeletal pain syndromes. Studies have reported that NSAIDs may be more effective compared with a placebo for the treatment of acute and chronic low back pain in patients who have degenerative spondylosis.[16] The use of muscle relaxants and narcotics, however, has not been reported to be as successful. In a recent double-blind study of 323 patients with acute, nontraumatic, nonradicular low back pain who were treated with naproxen and then randomized to either a placebo, cyclobenzaprine, or oxycodone/acetaminophen, Friedman et al[17] reported that the addition of cyclobenzaprine or oxycodone/acetaminophen to naproxen did not improve functional outcomes or pain at a follow-up of 1 week. Although a substantial decrease in postoperative pain medication has been reported in adults with degenerative scoliosis who were treated with narcotics preoperatively, no study has been performed that supports the use of narcotics for the nonsurgical treatment of adults with degenerative scoliosis.[18] In a recent, double-blind, placebo-controlled study of 24 patients with lumbar stenosis and neurogenic claudication who were randomized to either a placebo, oxymorphone hydrochloride, or propoxyphene/acetaminophen, Markman et al[19] failed to demonstrate a significant difference between the patients who were treated with oxymorphone hydrochloride or propoxyphene/acetaminophen and the patients who were treated with the placebo. Given the limited data that support their efficacy and the substantial risk associated with their chronic use, the authors of

Table 1

Indications for Surgical Management of Adult Spinal Deformity Based on Patient Age

Patient Age	Indications
<40 years	Thoracic curve greater than 50° with chronic pain that failed to resolve after nonsurgical treatment
	Severe deformity that is unacceptable to patient
>50 years	Documented curve progression in either the sagittal or coronal plane
	Back or radicular symptoms associated with lumbar stenosis
	Substantial loss of pulmonary function (not caused by pulmonary disease)

this chapter do not recommend the use of narcotics for the routine nonsurgical treatment of patients with adult lumbar scoliosis.

Unfortunately, the current literature has reported that the nonsurgical treatment of patients with adult lumbar scoliosis results in a substantial cost with no clear evidence of improved health status.[20] Glassman et al[20] followed 123 patients with adult scoliosis who underwent either nonsurgical treatment or did not undergo treatment for a minimum of 2 years. The authors collected data on the type and quantity of nonsurgical treatment used, including medication, physical therapy, exercise, injections/blocks, chiropractic care, pain management, bracing, and bed rest. The authors reported that the mean cost of nonsurgical management during the 2-year observation period was $10,815. Despite this expense, no improvement in health-related quality of life was observed in the patients who underwent nonsurgical treatment compared with the patients who did not undergo treatment; however, it should be noted that this study was not randomized, and whether nonsurgical treatment prevented the worsening of pain or the deterioration of function is unknown.

Surgical Decision Making

Sagittal balance has been accepted as a critical component of patient function. The importance of sagittal balance was first reported by Glassman et al.[21] Subsequently, Schwab et al[22] and Lafage et al[23] correlated sagittal balance with pelvic parameters and lumbar lordosis. An analysis of sagittal balance relies on full-length lateral radiographs that are obtained with the patient in a free-standing position and his or her fingers on the clavicles and the shoulders in 45° of forward elevation. In patients with positive sagittal balance, the sagittal vertical axis is greater than 50 mm anterior to the posterior aspect of the sacrum. Sagittal imbalance can occur as a result of loss of lumbar lordosis secondary to degenerative changes or prior surgeries in which patients underwent fusion in a hypolordotic position (flatback). As a compensatory mechanism to sagittal malalignment, a patient may rotate his or her pelvis into retroversion (increasing pelvic tilt) to maintain an upright posture. This compensatory mechanism may result in other compensatory changes, such as hip hyperextension and knee flexion, which can lead to contractures, increased difficulty in walking, and increased energy expenditure. Therefore,

an assessment of sagittal balance and spinopelvic alignment parameters, such as pelvic incidence and pelvic tilt, is critical for all patients who are candidates for fusion.

Pelvic incidence, which was first described by Duval-Beaupère,[24] is a fixed parameter in adults. A review of numerous radiographs from a database of the International Spine Study Group revealed a correlation between improved functional outcomes and a lumbar lordosis that is within 9° of a patient's pelvic incidence. In addition, improved sagittal balance parameters (ie, lumbar lordosis within 9° of pelvic incidence, sagittal vertical axis, and pelvic tilt) results in improved functional scores. Chen et al[25] reported that surgical treatment may be more appropriate for patients who have larger progressive deformities and sagittal plane imbalance. The authors also concluded that surgical treatment is generally inappropriate for patients who have mild symptoms, stable deformities, and no sagittal imbalance.

Determining which patients would benefit the most from nonsurgical versus surgical treatment remains a challenge. Limited evidence exists to support guidelines on the most effective way to treat patients with ASD. Treatment decisions for patients with ASD often rely on individual surgeon experience and patient preferences. Surgical decision making usually considers factors such as patient age, functional status, curve progression, bone quality, the extent of the deformity, and comorbidities.[26] Indications for the surgical management of ASD have been grouped into two categories based on patient age[27] (**Table 1**).

A critical component of patient counseling with regard to the surgical management of ASD includes understanding patient motivations and setting realistic expectations. Studies report that the surgical management of ASD in appropriately selected patients may result in an approximately 60% relief in back and leg pain and an approximately 40% improvement in disability at a follow-up of 2 years;[28,29] however, these data are based on averages of large patient populations with varying deformities, symptoms, and medical comorbidities. The identification of patients with ASD who are at both ends of the spectrum (ie, patients who will greatly benefit from surgery versus patients in whom the risks of surgery clearly outweigh the likely benefits) may aid in patient counseling and surgical decision making. In addition, understanding the factors that motivate patients to undergo surgical treatment for ASD may help surgeons better relate to their patients and aid in informed decision making.

In a retrospective review of a prospective, multicenter spinal deformity database, Smith et al[30] attempted to elucidate the predictors of marked improvement versus failure to improve in 276 patients with adult scoliosis who underwent surgical treatment. The authors identified the best and worst outcomes in younger (aged 18 to 45 years) and older (aged 46 to 85 years) patients who had adult scoliosis based on Oswestry Disability Index (ODI) and Scoliosis Research Society-22 (SRS-22) Questionnaire scores. In both younger and older patients who had adult scoliosis, predictors of best and worst outcomes included body mass index, depression/anxiety, narcotic use, tobacco use, and pain severity. Comorbidities, the severity of the deformity, surgical parameters, and complications did not appear

to be predictors of best and worst outcomes. The authors concluded that patient-related factors predominantly distinguished between patients with adult scoliosis in whom the best and worst outcomes were achieved. In a follow-up retrospective review of a prospective, multicenter database, Smith et al[31] attempted to elucidate the best and worst outcomes of 257 patients with ASD who underwent surgical treatment. The authors identified the best and worst outcomes based on 2-year follow-up ODI and SRS-22 Questionnaire scores. Smith et al[31] reinforced the findings of Smith et al,[30] reporting that several patient-specific factors, such as baseline depression, body mass index, comorbidities, and disability, were the strongest predictors of outcomes in patients with ASD who underwent surgical treatment. Smith et al[31] also reported that residual deformity in the sagittal vertical axis and complications correlated with worse outcomes in patients with ASD who underwent surgical treatment.

In a retrospective review of a prospective, multicenter database, Liu et al[32] attempted to clarify the factors associated with the successful nonsurgical treatment of patients with ASD. Using health-related quality of life measures, including the SRS-22 Questionnaire, the authors analyzed 215 patients with ASD at a minimum of 2 years after nonsurgical treatment. The authors concluded that patients with ASD who had lower SRS-22 Questionnaire pain scores (3.0 versus 3.6) and less coronal deformity in the thoracolumbar region (29.6° versus 36.5°) were most likely to benefit from nonsurgical treatment. Patients with ASD who had greater baseline SRS-22 Questionnaire pain scores and greater coronal deformities

in the thoracolumbar region that were associated with vertebral obliquity were less likely to benefit from nonsurgical treatment.

Understanding the motivations of patients with ASD who elect to undergo surgical treatment may aid in patient evaluation and counseling. In a retrospective-matched cohort study of patients with ASD, Pekmezci et al[26] reported that body mass index and comorbidities, as well as the incidence and severity of back and leg pain, were similar between the patients who underwent either surgical or nonsurgical treatment. The authors reported that the deterioration of functional status appeared to be the most important factor that led patients with ASD to seek surgical treatment. In a more recent prospective, randomized, observational study of 295 patients with adult symptomatic lumbar scoliosis, Neuman et al[33] reported that patients with ASD who sought surgical treatment had worse patient-related outcomes, worse back pain, worse back and leg pain during ambulation, and greater lumbar Cobb angles (56.5° versus 48.8°) compared with patients with ASD who sought nonsurgical treatment. Patients with ASD who sought surgical treatment had more symptomatic spinal stenosis (57% versus 39%) and worse patient-related outcome scores (Numeric Rating Scale back pain score [6.3 versus 5.5]; SRS-22 Questionnaire pain [2.8 versus 3.0], function [3.1 versus 3.4], and self-image [2.7 versus 3.1] scores; and ODI score [36.9 versus 31.8]) compared with patients with ASD who sought nonsurgical treatment. The authors also reported that older patients (aged 60 to 80 years) who had a lower educational level were more likely to seek nonsurgical treatment.

The surgical treatment of ASD often necessitates complex surgical procedures, including osteotomies, posterior long fusions to the pelvis, and combined anterior procedures to restore spinopelvic alignment and sagittal balance. Complication and revision surgery rates associated with ASD surgery have been reported to be as high as 80% and 58%, respectively.[2,3] Increased patient age is clearly associated with an increased rate of major short-term complications after the surgical treatment of ASD.[34] Perioperative complications (within 3 months of surgery) have been reported to occur in approximately 34% of patients who undergo surgical treatment for ASD.[35] Long-term complications (>3 months after surgery) have been reported to occur in 37% of patients who undergo surgical treatment for ASD. The rate of infection in patients with ASD who undergo surgical treatment has been reported to be higher compared with that of patients with adolescent deformity who undergo surgical treatment (3% to 5% versus 1% to 2%, respectively). Early complications that may require revision surgery include epidural hematoma resulting in neurologic compromise, early fixation failure, graft dislodgement, hardware malposition, and vena cava thrombosis. Late complications that may require revision surgery include pseudarthrosis (17%); junctional kyphosis (8%); and symptomatic hardware, including painful iliac screws that require removal (15%). Other complications include postsurgical vision loss (0.5% to 1%) and complications associated with prolonged anesthesia.[36]

A substantial cost is associated with the complex surgical procedures necessary for the surgical management of ASD. Given the current trends in healthcare reform, surgeons may soon be required to justify their surgical decisions both medically and economically. The current quality-adjusted life-year benchmark for a surgical procedure to be considered cost effective is less than $100,000. In a study of 541 patients with ASD who underwent surgical treatment, Terran et al[37] reported that the mean cost/quality-adjusted life-year at a follow-up of 5 years was $120,311. The authors reported that only 40.7% of the patients with ASD met the current quality-adjusted life-year benchmark. Factors associated with meeting the current quality-adjusted life-year benchmark included greater preoperative disability (based on ODI score), a diagnosis of idiopathic scoliosis, poor preoperative health-related quality-of-life scores, and fewer fusion levels. Further research is necessary to determine the overall economic value of surgical treatment for patients with ASD and help surgeons select patients who are most likely to meet the current quality-adjusted life-year benchmark.

Summary

The management of adult degenerative scoliosis continues to remain a challenge. Identification of the source of pain is crucial in the formulation of a treatment plan. The differentiation of pain associated with age-related degenerative changes from pain associated with scoliosis may be difficult. Nonsurgical treatment is recommended in patients with ASD who have mild or moderate pain and in elderly or systemically ill patients in whom surgery is not prudent. Surgical management of ASD may be associated with a high morbidity rate as a result of patient age, bone quality, and surgical complexity. Despite the lack of level I evidence on the efficacy of nonsurgical treatment in patients with ASD, it may be prudent to refrain from complex surgical deformity procedures in high-risk patients with ASD, particularly those with multiple medical comorbidities, advanced age, poor social and emotional state, and/or osteoporosis. Further studies are necessary to determine which patients with ASD benefit the most from nonsurgical treatment and which patients with ASD benefit the most from and have the fewest complications after surgical treatment. A determination of the optimal cost-benefit ratio for individual patients with ASD who are considering nonsurgical verus surgical treatment will help patients make better informed decisions.

References

1. Schwab F, Dubey A, Gamez L, et al: Adult scoliosis: Prevalence, SF-36, and nutritional parameters in an elderly volunteer population. *Spine (Phila Pa 1976)* 2005;30(9):1082-1085.

2. Carreon LY, Puno RM, Dimar JR II, Glassman SD, Johnson JR: Perioperative complications of posterior lumbar decompression and arthrodesis in older adults. *J Bone Joint Surg Am* 2003;85(11):2089-2092.

3. Edwards CC II, Bridwell KH, Patel A, Rinella AS, Berra A, Lenke LG: Long adult deformity fusions to L5 and the sacrum: A matched cohort analysis. *Spine (Phila Pa 1976)* 2004;29(18):1996-2005.

4. O'Lynnger TM, Zuckerman SL, Morone PJ, Dewan MC, Vasquez-Castellanos RA, Cheng JS: Trends for spine surgery for the elderly: Implications for access to healthcare in North America. *Neurosurgery* 2015;77(suppl 4):S136-S141

5. Crawford CH III, Glassman SD: Surgical treatment of lumbar spinal stenosis associated with adult scoliosis. *Instr Course Lect* 2009;58:669-676.

6. Friedly JL, Comstock BA, Turner JA, et al: A randomized trial of

epidural glucocorticoid injections for spinal stenosis. *N Engl J Med* 2014;371(1):11-21.

7. Cooper G, Lutz GE, Boachie-Adjei O, Lin J: Effectiveness of transforaminal epidural steroid injections in patients with degenerative lumbar scoliotic stenosis and radiculopathy. *Pain Physician* 2004;7(3):311-317.

8. Ghahreman A, Ferch R, Bogduk N: The efficacy of transforaminal injection of steroids for the treatment of lumbar radicular pain. *Pain Med* 2010;11(8):1149-1168.

9. Barrios C, Lapuente JP, Sastre S: Treatment of chronic pain in adult scoliosis. *Stud Health Technol Inform* 2002;88:290-303.

10. Mamyama T, Kitagawal T, Takeshita K, Nakainura K: Side shift exercise for idiopathic scoliosis after skeletal maturity. *Stud Health Technol Inform* 2002;91:361-364.

11. Weinstein SL, Dolan LA, Wright JG, Dobbs MB: Effects of bracing in adolescents with idiopathic scoliosis. *N Engl J Med* 2013;369(16):1512-1521.

12. Weiss HR, Dallmayer R: Brace treatment of spinal claudication in an adult with lumbar scoliosis—a case report. *Stud Health Technol Inform* 2006;123:586-589.

13. Weiss HR, Dallmayer R, Stephan C: First results of pain treatment in scoliosis patients using a sagittal realignment brace. *Stud Health Technol Inform* 2006;123:582-585.

14. Weiss HR, Werkmann M: Treatment of chronic low back pain in patients with spinal deformities using a sagittal re-alignment brace. *Scoliosis* 2009;4:7.

15. Ploumis A, Transfledt EE, Denis F: Degenerative lumbar scoliosis associated with spinal stenosis. *Spine J* 2007;7(4):428-436.

16. Roelofs PD, Deyo RA, Koes BW, Scholten RJ, van Tulder MW: Nonsteroidal anti-inflammatory drugs for low back pain: An updated Cochrane review. *Spine (Phila Pa 1976)* 2008;33(16):1766-1774.

17. Friedman BW, Dym AA, Davitt M, et al: Naproxen with cyclobenzaprine, oxycodone/acetaminophen, or placebo for treating acute low back pain:

A randomized clinical trial. *JAMA* 2015;314(15):1572-1580.

18. Mesfin A, Lenke LG, Bridwell KH, et al: Does preoperative narcotic use adversely affect outcomes and complications after spinal deformity surgery? A comparison of nonnarcotic- with narcotic-using groups. *Spine J* 2014;14(12):2819-2825.

19. Markman JD, Gewandter JS, Frazer ME, et al: A randomized, double-blind, placebo-controlled crossover trial of oxymorphone hydrochloride and propoxyphene/acetaminophen combination for the treatment of neurogenic claudication associated with lumbar spinal stenosis. *Spine (Phila Pa 1976)* 2015;40(10):684-691.

20. Glassman SD, Carreon LY, Shaffrey CI, et al: The costs and benefits of nonoperative management for adult scoliosis. *Spine (Phila Pa 1976)* 2010;35(5):578-582.

21. Glassman SD, Bridwell K, Dimar JR, Horton W, Berven S, Schwab F: The impact of positive sagittal balance in adult spinal deformity. *Spine (Phila Pa 1976)* 2005;30(18):2024-2029.

22. Schwab F, Patel A, Ungar B, Farcy JP, Lafage V: Adult spinal deformity-postoperative standing imbalance: How much can you tolerate? An overview of key parameters in assessing alignment and planning corrective surgery. *Spine (Phila Pa 1976)* 2010;35(25):2224-2231.

23. Lafage V, Schwab F, Patel A, Hawkinson N, Farcy JP: Pelvic tilt and truncal inclination: Two key radiographic parameters in the setting of adults with spinal deformity. *Spine (Phila Pa 1976)* 2009;34(17):E599-E606.

24. Duval-Beaupère G, Schmidt C, Cosson P: A Barycentremetric study of the sagittal shape of spine and pelvis: The conditions required for an economic standing position. *Ann Biomed Eng* 1992;20(4):451-462.

25. Chen PG, Daubs MD, Berven S, et al: Surgery for degenerative lumbar scoliosis: The development of appropriateness criteria. *Spine (Phila Pa 1976)* 2016;41(10):910-918.

26. Pekmezci M, Berven SH, Hu SS, Deviren V: The factors that play a

role in the decision-making process of adult deformity patients. *Spine (Phila Pa 1976)* 2009;34(8):813-817.

27. Bradford DS, Tay BK, Hu SS: Adult scoliosis: Surgical indications, operative management, complications, and outcomes. *Spine (Phila Pa 1976)* 1999;24(24):2617-2629.

28. Smith JS, Shaffrey CI, Berven S, et al: Improvement of back pain with operative and nonoperative treatment in adults with scoliosis. *Neurosurgery* 2009;65(1):86-94.

29. Smith JS, Shaffrey CI, Berven S, et al: Operative versus nonoperative treatment of leg pain in adults with scoliosis: A retrospective review of a prospective multicenter database with two-year follow-up. *Spine (Phila Pa 1976)* 2009;34(16):1693-1698.

30. Smith JS, Shaffrey CI, Glassman SD, et al: Clinical and radiographic parameters that distinguish between the best and worst outcomes of scoliosis surgery for adults. *Eur Spine J* 2013;22(2):402-410.

31. Smith JS, Shaffrey CI, Lafage V, et al: Comparison of best versus worst clinical outcomes for adult spinal deformity surgery: A retrospective review of a prospectively collected, multicenter database with 2-year follow-up. *J Neurosurg Spine* 2015;23(3):349-359.

32. Liu S, Diebo BG, Henry JK, et al: The benefit of nonoperative treatment for adult spinal deformity: Identifying predictors for reaching a minimal clinically important difference. *Spine J* 2016;16(2):210-218.

33. Neuman BJ, Baldus C, Zebala LP, et al: Patient factors that influence decision making: Randomization versus observational nonoperative versus observational operative treatment for adult symptomatic lumbar scoliosis. *Spine (Phila Pa 1976)* 2016;41(6):E349-E358.

34. Shaw R, Skovrlj B, Cho SK: Association between age and complications in adult scoliosis surgery: An analysis of the scoliosis research society morbidity and mortality database. *Spine (Phila Pa 1976)* 2016;41(6):508-514.

35. Emami A, Deviren V, Berven S, Smith JA, Hu SS, Bradford DS: Outcome and complications of long

fusions to the sacrum in adult spine deformity: Luque-galveston, combined iliac and sacral screws, and sacral fixation. *Spine (Phila Pa 1976)* 2002;27(7):776-786.

36. Goepfert CE, Ifune C, Tempelhoff R: Ischemic optic neuropathy: Are we any further? *Curr Opin Anaesthesiol* 2010;23(5):582-587.

37. Terran J, McHugh BJ, Fischer CR, et al: Surgical treatment for adult spinal deformity: Projected cost effectiveness at 5-year follow-up. *Ochsner J* 2014;14(1):14-22.

Realignment Planning in Adult Spinal Deformity: Formulas and Planning Tools

Themistocles Protopsaltis, MD
Dana L. Cruz, MD

Abstract

Adult spinal deformity is a complex pathologic process that has many etiologies and several mechanisms of compensation. A complete understanding of spinopelvic alignment is required to differentiate the origin of spinal deformity from its compensation and, ultimately, optimize surgical correction. Surgeons should understand the spinopelvic parameters involved in the evaluation of a patient who has an adult spinal deformity and their implications for treatment.

Instr Course Lect 2017;66:361–366.

Sagittal Alignment and Key Radiographic Parameters

Sagittal spine malalignment has been reported to correlate with disability.[1-5] The sagittal vertical axis (SVA) is a useful tool that is widely used to determine malalignment and its clinical effect in patients who have spinal deformity.[1] However, the SVA is limited because it alone does not sufficiently capture the complexities of standing alignment.[4-6] Several studies have reported that the pelvis is an important regulator of standing alignment.[4-6] For example, patients who have degenerative loss of lumbar lordosis (LL) compensate with pelvic retroversion to maintain an energetically economic position and horizontal gaze. Therefore, a sufficiently compensated patient may not demonstrate substantial deviation in the SVA. Accordingly, the SVA should always be considered in conjunction with pelvic tilt (PT), which is a measure of pelvic retroversion.

Another key parameter related to the pelvis is pelvic incidence (PI), which is a morphologic parameter that does not change after skeletal maturity.[6,7] Because PI is related to PT and sacral slope (SS; PI = PT + SS) and because SS is highly correlated with LL in asymptomatic patients, PI has recently emerged as a useful parameter to assess pathologic changes in patients who have LL.[7] Sagittal malalignment leads to alterations in pelvic version; however, because PI is a static parameter that is related to LL, surgeons can use the PI-LL relationship to determine optimal sagittal correction for each patient.[8]

Which Compensatory Mechanisms Should Be Assessed?

Patients who have sagittal spine deformity use a predictable compensatory response to optimize standing alignment.[4,9-12] A spinal deformity that is localized to one or more spinal regions will first lead to compensatory changes in the adjacent spinal regions, which are then followed by compensatory changes in the pelvis and, finally, compensatory changes in the lower extremities, as tolerated.[12] For example, some patients

Dr. Protopsaltis or an immediate family member is a member of a speakers' bureau or has made paid presentations on behalf of Medicrea; serves as a paid consultant to or is an employee of Medicrea; and has received research or institutional support from Zimmer. Neither Ms. Cruz nor any immediate family member has received anything of value from or has stock or stock options held in a commercial company or institution related directly or indirectly to the subject of this chapter.

who have lumbar flatback deformity will decrease their thoracic kyphosis (TK) to compensate for loss of LL.[11,12] This method of compensation requires good flexibility of the thoracic spine and the motor strength to maintain the hypokyphosis. In contrast, patients who have thoracic hyperkyphosis or thoracolumbar junctional kyphosis will often maintain hyperlordosis of their lumbar and cervical spine to optimize standing alignment.

As previously discussed, rotation of the pelvis is a key compensatory mechanism in the modulation of standing alignment.[4] In an unconscious effort to reposition the center of gravity over the feet, patients who have spinal deformity rotate the pelvis about the femoral heads, which thereby reduces standing energy expenditure. Pelvic retroversion has been reported to be one of the first compensatory mechanisms that is adopted by adult patients who have spinal deformity.[4,12] Patients who have severe degenerative hip arthritis and patients who have hip flexion contractures may be limited in their ability to effectively retrovert the pelvis and maintain economic posture in the setting of sagittal malalignment. Furthermore, patients who have poor motor strength, including frail and sarcopenic elderly patients, and patients who have neurodegenerative disorders may not be capable of effectively tilting the pelvis, even in the presence of severe malalignment.[13] Patients who have a small PT relative to their degree of spinal deformity will often demonstrate greater levels of disability.[4,5,13] These findings are counterintuitive given that increased PT is an early compensatory mechanism to sagittal deformity; however, in patients who have spinal deformity, the act of pelvic retroversion can contribute to fatigue,

pain, and even greater disability.[4] The most disabled class of patients with spinal deformity are those who have a combination of severe sagittal deformity and the inability to compensate with pelvic retroversion.[4,5,13]

Recognizing the relationship between PI, SS, and PT, it should be noted that the capacity to retrovert the pelvis is directly related to an individual's PI. Compared with a larger PI, a small PI decreases an individual's capacity to retrovert the pelvis. Therefore, patients who have a small PI rely on additional compensatory mechanisms or demonstrate greater disability secondary to a given deformity. Diebo et al[12] reported that larger magnitude spinal deformities lead to the activation of lower extremity compensatory mechanisms after pelvic and thoracic hypokyphosis compensatory mechanisms have been exhausted.

The use of several lower extremity compensatory mechanisms, including hip extension, knee flexion, and ankle flexion, have been reported in the literature.[8-10] Of these compensatory mechanisms, knee flexion is most important.[8-10] Hip extension is a component of the compensatory mechanism that facilitates pelvic retroversion and should not be considered separate from PT.[9,10] As compensation from pelvic retroversion is exhausted, knee flexion is activated to bring the body's center of gravity over the feet,[9,10] which has been reported to be a process that is quantified by pelvic shift.[6,10] In this manner, the compensatory mechanisms of knee flexion and pelvic shift quantify the same compensatory response in patients who have severe sagittal malalignment.[6,10] As knee flexion is activated, the pelvis shifts posteriorly and simultaneously allows for greater pelvic retroversion with less hip extension,

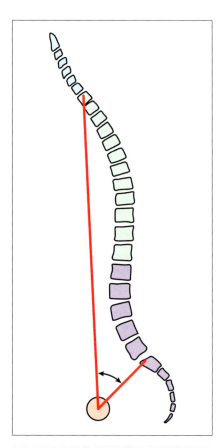

Figure 1   Illustration shows the T1 pelvic angle, which is the angle formed between a line that extends from the center of the femoral head to the centroid of the T1 vertebra and a line that extends from the center of the femoral head to the middle of the S1 end plate.

which affords decreased hip extension and improved energy expenditure.

Strategies to Account for Compensatory Mechanisms in Surgical Planning

Pelvic retroversion is the most important compensatory mechanism to account for in planning surgical correction for patients who have sagittal malalignment.[4] Failure to recognize increased PT in a patient who has a well-compensated lumbar flatback deformity or in a patient who has a large sagittal deformity with an increased SVA can lead to undercorrection, residual sagittal malalignment, persistent pain, and persistent disability postoperatively.[4,5]

The T1 pelvic angle (TPA) is a novel measure of sagittal alignment that simultaneously accounts for sagittal inclination and PT[5] (**Figure 1**). The TPA is useful in perioperative planning because it is a more direct measure of the geometry of a spinal deformity that is separate from pelvic and lower extremity compensation.[5] For the purposes of surgical planning, the TPA can be measured on full-length intraoperative radiographs (see case presentation 2, discussed later). Furthermore, the alignment goal for the TPA can be deduced intuitively. Because the TPA is the sum of T1 spinopelvic inclination and PT,[5] the correction used must bring spinal inclination back to a neutral or slightly negative position and restore PT to a normal range (15° to 25°, depending on a patient's age and PI). Therefore, the TPA of a well-aligned spine is less than 20° in most patients, and patients with a well-aligned spine do not have to recruit pelvic and lower extremity compensatory mechanisms to maintain standing alignment.

Other established radiographic parameters of sagittal alignment, such as the SVA and PT, can be modified by postural compensatory mechanisms, including pelvic retroversion and knee flexion. Further, because sagittal alignment measures such as the SVA and PT are described in free-standing individuals, they are inadequate in patients who require standing support. The TPA, however, is a sagittal alignment measure that is less dependent on postural factors; therefore, it can be measured with the patient placed in the prone, sitting,

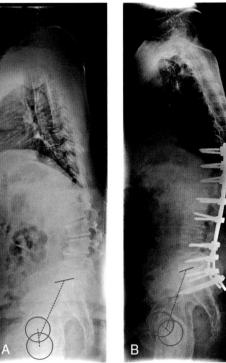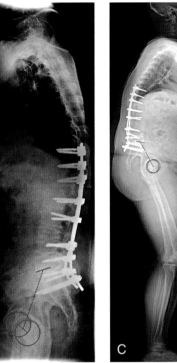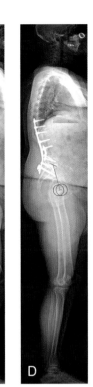

Figure 2   Radiographs of the spine of a 42-year-old man who had severe chronic low back pain with progressive weakness of the right lower extremity. **A,** Preoperative lateral standing radiograph demonstrates lumbar kyphosis with compensatory thoracic hypokyphosis and pelvic retroversion. **B,** Lateral standing radiograph taken after pedicle subtraction osteotomy was performed at the L3 vertebra demonstrates improved sagittal alignment; however, the T1 pelvic angle and pelvic tilt are elevated relative to age-specific ideals. **C,** Lateral standing radiograph taken 2 years postoperatively demonstrates hardware failure, which resulted in loss of sagittal alignment. **D,** Lateral standing radiograph taken after revision surgery demonstrates improved sagittal alignment without reliance on compensatory mechanisms that were used preoperatively. The blue lines and circles represent the bicoxofemoral axis from which the T1 pelvic angle and pelvic tilt are calculated.

or standing supported position, each of which provides the surgeon with different information. Similar to the SVA, the TPA has been reported to correlate with health-related quality-of-life measures.[5]

Surgeons can use the TPA to optimize postoperative correction of a patient's spine to fit his or her age. Protopsaltis et al[14] reported that a TPA target of 10° to 15° is optimal for middle-aged patients (40 to 65 years), and a TPA target of 15° to 25° is favorable for elderly patients (older than 65 years).

Although the TPA is valuable for assessment and corrective planning of global alignment, it is necessary to analyze thoracic and lumbar spinal alignment separately to assess optimal regional alignment. For example, it may be difficult to determine optimal regional alignment in patients who have pathologic loss of LL and pathologic or compensatory changes in the thoracic spine. Furthermore, identification of thoracic compensation via hypokyphosis is not well recognized in the literature. Fortunately, PI has been useful

Table 1
Radiographic Parameters for Primary Surgery in Case Presentation 1

Parameter	Preoperative	Postoperative
TPA	27°	21°
SVA	9 cm	5.2 cm
PT	34°	25°
PI-LL	48°	9°

PI-LL = pelvic incidence-lumbar lordosis relationship, PT = pelvic tilt, SVA = sagittal vertical axis, TPA = T1 pelvic angle.

Table 2
Radiographic Parameters for Revision Surgery in Case Presentation 1

Parameter	Preoperative	Postoperative
TPA	37°	14°
SVA	14 cm	2.3 cm
PT	29°	16°
PI-LL	38°	2°

PI-LL = pelvic incidence-lumbar lordosis relationship, PT = pelvic tilt, SVA = sagittal vertical axis, TPA = T1 pelvic angle.

in identifying the ideal LL for a given patient (LL = PI ± 10°).[4,6,8] However, because of the poor correlation between TK and PI, caution must be used in extrapolating an estimated TK for a given PI.[7]

In asymptomatic patients, TK correlates well with LL, and LL correlates well with PI.[7] Therefore, for patients who have pathologic loss of LL, the ideal LL can be calculated from the PI as previously discussed. Lafage et al[15] created an equation that determines the optimal LL for a given patient based on its closest correlates, which are PI and TK: LL = 1/2 × (PI + TK) + 10°. The equation can be solved for TK by substituting an ideal LL for a given PI, which leads to the following calculation for a patient who has uncompensated, expected TK: estimated TK = PI − 20°.[16] Compensation via thoracic hypokyphosis can be determined using this equation if actual TK is less than the estimated TK.

In a recent study of 219 adult patients with spinal deformity who underwent fusion from the pelvis to the lower thoracic spine, The International Spine Study Group[16] used the previously mentioned equation to calculate the presence of thoracic compensation, which predicted postoperative reciprocal thoracic hyperkyphosis. The authors reported that patients who exhibited preoperative thoracic compensation also were more likely to have postoperative proximal junctional kyphosis.[16] Therefore, identification of preoperative thoracic compensation via hypokyphosis aids in preoperative planning for deformity surgery because it allows the surgeon to anticipate and account for postoperative reciprocal kyphosis at the time that final target alignment is defined. Some surgeons have proposed the use of thoracic flexion/extension radiographs and other surgeons have proposed the use of sitting radiographs to help determine flexibility of the thoracic spine and anticipate reciprocal thoracic change relative to the pelvis after surgical correction.

Case Presentation 1

Case presentation 1 is a 42-year-old man who had severe, chronic low back pain with progressive weakness of the right lower extremity. Standing radiographs revealed kyphosis of the lumbar spine with compensatory thoracic hypokyphosis and pelvic retroversion (**Figure 2, A**). This case presentation demonstrates a patient who had extreme loss of LL; therefore, optimal correction of sagittal malalignment required restoration of LL. Given the patient's young age and low PI (43°), his LL should exceed his PI with a TPA less than 15°. Pedicle subtraction osteotomy was performed at the L3 vertebra; however, this procedure may not have been optimal for a patient his age (**Figure 2, B**). The patient had a TPA of 21° and a PI-LL relationship of 9° postoperatively (**Table 1**).

The patient suffered a rod breakage 2 years after the index procedure, which resulted in loss of sagittal alignment (**Figure 2, C**). He underwent pedicle subtraction osteotomy at the L4 vertebra as well as optimal regional and global correction. Compensatory mechanisms demonstrated by the patient preoperatively, including thoracic hypokyphosis and pelvic retroversion, resolved after revision surgery (**Figure 2, D**; **Table 2**).

Case Presentation 2

Case presentation 2 is a 65-year-old woman who had chronic low back pain 2 years after she underwent posterior fusion from the T5 vertebra to the sacrum. Full-length standing radiographs revealed instrumentation, mild proximal junction kyphosis, and global sagittal malalignment (**Figure 3, A**). Given the undercorrection of the patient's LL, which was evident from PI-LL relationship mismatch, and loss of thoracic flexibility secondary to fusion, the patient relied on pelvic retroversion and lower extremity compensatory mechanisms to maintain standing alignment. The goals of realignment included increasing the patient's LL to match her PI and correcting the patient's global malalignment to an age-appropriate target (TPA <24°). Pedicle subtraction osteotomy was performed at the L4 vertebra (**Figure 3, B**), after which the patient demonstrated improved sagittal alignment with decreased pelvic retroversion and relaxation of lower extremity compensatory mechanisms (**Figure 3, C; Table 3**).

Summary

Adult spinal deformity is a complex pathologic process that has many etiologies and several mechanisms of compensation. A complete understanding of spinopelvic alignment is required to differentiate the origin of spinal deformity from its compensation and, ultimately, optimize surgical correction. Compensatory mechanisms are activated in a predictable manner, beginning with adjacent spinal region compensatory changes and progressing to include pelvic and lower extremity compensatory changes, such as PT and knee flexion, as tolerated. Optimal sagittal correction can be determined preoperatively,

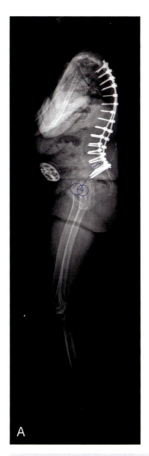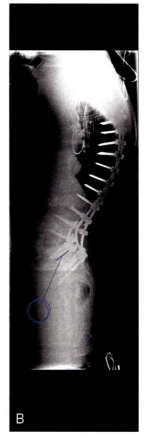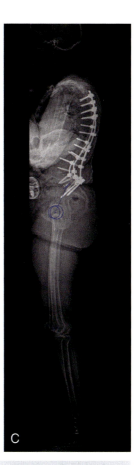

A   B   C

Figure 3   Radiographs of the spine of a 65-year-old woman who had chronic low back pain 2 years after she underwent posterior fusion from the T5 vertebra to the sacrum. **A,** Preoperative lateral standing radiograph demonstrates sagittal malalignment and the use of distal compensatory mechanisms, including pelvic retroversion and knee flexion. **B,** Intraoperative lateral radiograph demonstrates correction of the T1 pelvic angle and the pelvic incidence-lumbar lordosis relationship. **C,** Postoperative lateral standing radiograph demonstrates age-appropriate correction of the T1 pelvic angle and relaxation of lower extremity and pelvic compensatory mechanisms. The blue lines and circles represent the bicoxofemoral axis from which the T1 pelvic angle and pelvic tilt are calculated.

Table 3
Radiographic Parameters for Revision Surgery in Case Presentation 2

Parameter	Preoperative	Intraoperative	Postoperative
TPA	44°	17°	19°
SVA	55 mm	—	23 mm
PT	36°	—	23°
PI-LL	30°	2°	2°

PI-LL = pelvic incidence-lumbar lordosis relationship, PT = pelvic tilt, SVA = sagittal vertical axis, TPA = T1 pelvic angle.

executed intraoperatively, and verified postoperatively with the use of radiographic spinopelvic parameters such as the PI-LL relationship and the TPA.

References

1. Glassman SD, Bridwell K, Dimar JR, Horton W, Berven S, Schwab F: The impact of positive sagittal balance in adult spinal deformity. *Spine (Phila Pa 1976)* 2005;30(18):2024-2029.

2. Schwab F, Dubey A, Gamez L, et al: Adult scoliosis: Prevalence, SF-36, and nutritional parameters in an elderly volunteer population. *Spine (Phila Pa 1976)* 2005;30(9):1082-1085.

3. International Spine Study Group, Fu KMG, Bess RS, et al: Health impact comparison of different disease states and population norms to adult spinal deformity (ASD): A call for medical attention. *Spine J* 2012;12(9 suppl):S2.

4. Lafage V, Schwab F, Patel A, Hawkinson N, Farcy JP: Pelvic tilt and truncal inclination: Two key radiographic parameters in the setting of adults with spinal deformity. *Spine (Phila Pa 1976)* 2009;34(17):E599-E606.

5. Protopsaltis T, Schwab F, Bronsard N, et al: The T1 pelvic angle, a novel radiographic measure of global sagittal deformity, accounts for both spinal inclination and pelvic tilt and correlates with health-related quality of life. *J Bone Joint Surg Am* 2014;96(19):1631-1640.

6. Legaye J, Duval-Beaupère G, Hecquet J, Marty C: Pelvic incidence: A fundamental pelvic parameter for three-dimensional regulation of spinal sagittal curves. *Eur Spine J* 1998;7(2):99-103.

7. Vialle R, Levassor N, Rillardon L, Templier A, Skalli W, Guigui P: Radiographic analysis of the sagittal alignment and balance of the spine in asymptomatic subjects. *J Bone Joint Surg Am* 2005;87(2):260-267.

8. Schwab F, Ungar B, Blondel B, et al: Scoliosis Research Society-Schwab adult spinal deformity classification: A validation study. *Spine (Phila Pa 1976)* 2012;37(12):1077-1082.

9. Schwab F, Lafage V, Boyce R, Skalli W, Farcy JP: Gravity line analysis in adult volunteers: Age-related correlation with spinal parameters, pelvic parameters, and foot position. *Spine (Phila Pa 1976)* 2006;31(25):E959-E967.

10. Obeid I, Hauger O, Aunoble S, Bourghli A, Pellet N, Vital JM: Global analysis of sagittal spinal alignment in major deformities: Correlation between lack of lumbar lordosis and flexion of the knee. *Eur Spine J* 2011; 20(suppl 5):681-685.

11. Barrey C, Roussouly P, Perrin G, Le Huec JC: Sagittal balance disorders in severe degenerative spine: Can we identify the compensatory mechanisms? *Eur Spine J* 2011;20(suppl 5):626-633.

12. Diebo BG, Ferrero E, Lafage R, et al: Recruitment of compensatory mechanisms in sagittal spinal malalignment is age and regional deformity dependent: A full-standing axis analysis of key radiographical parameters. *Spine (Phila Pa 1976)* 2015;40(9):642-649.

13. Ferrero E, Vira S, Ames CP, et al: Analysis of an unexplored group of sagittal deformity patients: Low pelvic tilt despite positive sagittal malalignment. *Eur Spine J* 2015.

14. Protopsaltis TS, Maier SP, Smith JS, et al: Paper No. 2. Should our elderly spinal deformity patients have the same targets for correction and is there an optimal alignment target that results in less PJK? *21st International Meeting on Advanced Spine Techniques.* Valencia, Spain, July 16-19, 2014.

15. Lafage V, Schwab F, Vira S, Patel A, Ungar B, Farcy JP: Spino-pelvic parameters after surgery can be predicted: A preliminary formula and validation of standing alignment. *Spine (Phila Pa 1976)* 2011;36(13):1037-1045.

16. International Spine Study Group, Protopsaltis TS, Diebo BG, et al: Abstract No. 121. Identifying preoperative thoracic compensation and predicting postoperative reciprocal thoracic kyphosis and PJK. *30th North American Spine Society Annual Meeting*, Chicago, IL, October 14-17, 2015.

Minimally Invasive Lateral Approach for the Management of Adult Degenerative Scoliosis

Adam M. Wegner, MD, PhD
David M. Prior, MD
Eric O. Klineberg, MD

Abstract

Minimally invasive lateral releases for the correction of lumbar scoliosis are becoming an increasingly common treatment alternative to posterior osteotomies or surgery via an open anterior approach. Minimally invasive approaches minimize blood loss and morbidity, which may be important in older patients who often have substantial comorbidities. Anterior column realignment allows lumbar lordosis to be restored via a minimally invasive lateral approach, which restores sagittal balance and is correlated with improvements in health-related quality of life. Surgeons should understand the development of, the indications for, the surgical technique for, and the complications and early clinical outcomes of the minimally invasive lateral approach to the spine.

Instr Course Lect 2017;66:367–377.

Degenerative lumbar scoliosis can be a painful progressive condition that is associated with degenerative disk disease, facet hypertrophy, and loss of lumbar lordosis.[1] Nonsurgical management of symptomatic lumbar scoliosis includes physical therapy, medications, orthoses, and steroid injections. A recent multicenter trial reported that the surgical management of adult spinal deformity results in improved health-related quality of life compared with nonsurgical management.[2] Restoration of lumbar lordosis is the aspect of the surgical management of adult spinal deformity most important to achieve normalized sagittal plane balance, which has been associated with improved health-related quality of life.[3]

Traditionally, open decompression with segmental pedicle screw fixation, with or without posterior column or three-column osteotomies, depending on the rigidity of the deformity, has been the treatment of choice for patients with adult spinal deformity.[4] Interbody releases and fusion may offer patients who have amenable disk spaces some advantages compared with posterior-only approaches; these advantages include improved fusion and a lesser degree of lumbar lordosis without the substantial rate of rod fracture observed in patients who undergo posterior three-column osteotomies.[5]

Although posterior procedures are still the preferred treatment for patients who have rigid sagittal plane deformity, minimally invasive anterior releases offer substantial advantages with regard to the restoration of sagittal balance. Minimally invasive anterior releases are useful in patients who have minimal to

Dr. Klineberg or an immediate family member is a member of a speakers' bureau or has made paid presentations on behalf of AOSpine and K2M; serves as a paid consultant to or is an employee of DePuy and Stryker; and has received research or institutional support from AOSpine, the Orthopaedic Research and Education Foundation, and DePuy Synthes Spine. Neither of the following authors nor any immediate family member has received anything of value from or has stock or stock options held in a commercial company or institution related directly or indirectly to the subject of this chapter: Dr. Wegner and Dr. Prior.

moderate deformity and do not require invasive open anterior approaches, which are associated with substantial morbidity, including injury to vessels, hollow viscus injury, retrograde ejaculation, and injury to the sympathetic plexus.[6] Often, blood loss and surgical time can be diminished with the use of minimally invasive anterior releases.[7] However, several technical considerations that are unique to the minimally invasive lateral transpsoas approach must be considered. The lumbar plexus traverses the surgical field, the iliopsoas muscle can be injured, and hollow viscus organ and blood vessel injury can occur during the minimally invasive lateral transpsoas approach.

History

Traditional anterior releases for the management of lumber scoliosis were developed in the early 20th century for the management of spondylolisthesis and Pott disease and were performed via open anterior intra-abdominal transperitoneal or retroperitoneal approaches, which usually required exposure to be performed by a general surgeon.[8,9] The desired disk levels were exposed, and complete diskectomies were performed. Conflicting evidence exists on whether the addition of anterior lumbar interbody fusion (ALIF) compared with posterolateral lumbar or circumferential fusion improves fusion rates;[10] however, compared with ALIF alone, the addition of posterior instrumentation improves fusion rates.[11] Although the fusion rates of patients who undergo ALIF are similar compared with those of patients who undergo transforaminal interbody fusion, ALIF allows for disk height augmentation and more effectively restores lumbar lordosis and sagittal alignment.[12]

In addition to possible injury to vessels, nerves, or viscous structures, an anterior incision may be associated with substantial pain, bulging, and functional disturbance.[13] To avoid these complications, Obenchain[14] used a laparoscopic-assisted anterior spine approach for an L5-S1 diskectomy. Subsequently, McAfee et al[15] developed a minimally invasive endoscopic anterior retroperitoneal approach, which did not require carbon dioxide insufflation, avoided the peritoneum, and did not require dissection of the great vessels. The minimally invasive anterior retroperitoneal approach described by McAfee et al[15] requires substantial retraction of the psoas, which leads to psoas edema and hip flexion weakness postoperatively.

To avoid the complications of an anterior approach entirely, a minimally invasive lateral approach to the spine was developed. The first reported minimally invasive endoscopic lateral transpsoas approach was described in a study by Bergey et al.[16] The minimally invasive lateral transpsoas approach allows access up to L1 but is limited distally by the iliac crest. Often, L4-5 and L5-S1 are located below the bifurcation of the great vessels; therefore, an anterior approach allows for better access to those disk levels. Technically, lateral positioning allows the abdominal contents to fall away from the lumbar spine, which allows for better visualization; the anterior longitudinal ligament (ALL) and the posterior longitudinal ligament may be either left intact or, if desired, removed. In addition, a lateral approach allows for orthogonal access to the disk space and, compared with an anterior approach, minimizes the risk for instrument intrusion in the spinal canal.

A paradigm shift to minimally invasive lateral approaches to the lumbar spine occurred in conjunction with the development of the minimally invasive lateral transpsoas approach, which was first reported by Pimenta and Schaffa,[17] and a subsequent study on the technique for extreme lateral interbody fusion (XLIF).[18] XLIF allows access to the lateral aspect of the spine via the retroperitoneal fat and psoas muscle and avoids some of the pitfalls associated with open anterior approaches. XLIF eliminates the need to enter the peritoneum and avoids potential injury to the bowel or sympathetic plexus. XLIF also minimizes blood loss and results in quicker recovery times compared with traditional anterior approaches.[19] In addition, XLIF minimizes the need for assistance from general surgeons as well as the need to work around the great vessels and eliminates the restrictions and learning curve that are associated with minimally invasive endoscopic approaches. However, because the anatomy exposed via a lateral approach is not regularly encountered by most spine surgeons, XLIF is associated with a learning curve. In addition, the approach used for XLIF traverses the psoas muscle, which can result in pain or hip flexion weakness.[20,21]

XLIF may be superior compared with posterior interbody fusion techniques because it avoids direct entry in the spinal canal and manipulation of the dura and nerve roots; this minimizes the risk for postoperative epidural adhesions and allows for a larger graft to be safely placed, which may improve the graft footprint, provide greater contact area, and result in larger coronal and sagittal correction. XLIF allows for the restoration of disk height and the correction of sagittal plane deformity

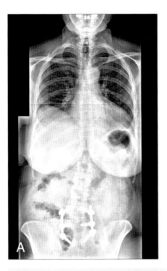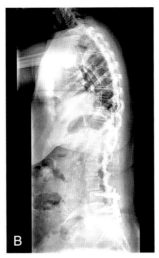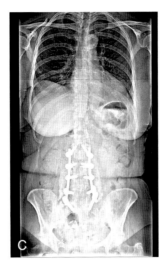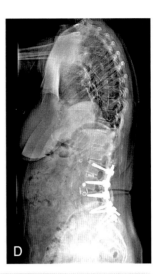

Figure 1   Preoperative AP (**A**) and lateral (**B**) standing radiographs of the spine of a woman with a flatback deformity and coronal imbalance. Postoperative AP (**C**) and lateral (**D**) standing radiographs of the spine of the woman shown in panels **A** and **B** taken after combined anterior release/extreme lateral interbody fusion with extension of posterior spinal fusion demonstrate improved lumbar lordosis and sagittal plane alignment.

(**Figure 1**), resulting in improved clinical outcomes.[22] Reasonable correction can be achieved in patients with correction goals of less than 5 cm in the sagittal plane and 10° in the coronal plane.[23] Correction is limited by the intact anterior and posterior longitudinal ligaments.

Anterior column realignment (ACR) is the most recent procedure that has emerged from the development of the minimally invasive lateral transpsoas approach to the lumbar spine.[24,25] A cadaver model study reported that the minimally invasive lateral transpsoas approach allows for ALL release, which may result in more correction, especially in the sagittal plane.[26] ACR consists of a minimally invasive lateral transpsoas approach to the spine, complete diskectomy, and direct release or resection of the ALL and anulus fibrosus; hyperlordotic interbody cages are then inserted to lengthen the anterior column, which may result in substantially increased lumbar lordosis. ACR allows for the correction of sagittal plane deformity and results in decreased surgical time and blood loss compared with posterior procedures, such as pedicle subtraction osteotomies;[6] this may be important in older patients who often have substantial comorbidities and are the individuals most affected by degenerative lumbar scoliosis.

Preoperative Evaluation

ACR via a minimally invasive direct lateral transpsoas approach may be considered in patients with fixed sagittal imbalance as a result of lumbar hypolordosis in whom previous instrumented fusion has been performed, degenerative spondylosis/spondylolisthesis, or other adult spinal deformities for which mobile disk spaces and an intact ALL are present. Appropriate patient selection is critical for this technique. Relative contraindications to ACR via a minimally invasive direct lateral transpsoas approach include solid arthrodesis, active infection, previous intra-abdominal surgical procedures that caused dense adherent scarring, and vascular injury.

ACR via a minimally invasive direct lateral transpsoas approach also may be contraindicated in patients with previous lumbosacral plexus injury or ankylosing conditions and patients in whom the ALL is no longer mobile.

The initial preoperative evaluation for patients who undergo minimally invasive surgical procedures is similar to that for patients who undergo open procedures and should include basic laboratory studies (complete blood count, basic metabolic panel, and, if appropriate, electrocardiography) and an overall preoperative health evaluation.[27] Appropriate clearance for surgery should be obtained from a patient's primary care provider. Nutrition and bone health should be optimized preoperatively because ACR achieves expansion against the bony integrity of the anterior column. In patients who have osteopenia/osteoporosis, vertebral bone quality and end plate strength should be maximized with the use of diphosphonates or recombinant parathyroid hormone.[27]

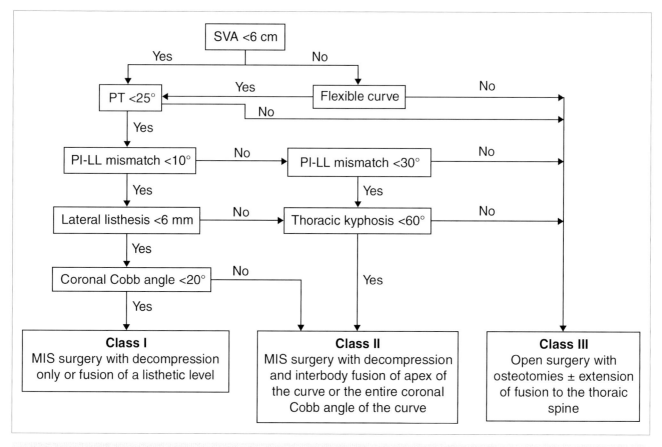

Figure 2 Algorithm proposed by Mummaneni et al[28] for the selection of appropriate patients for minimally invasive spinal (MIS) deformity surgery. PI-LL = pelvic incidence-lumbar lordosis, PT = pelvic tilt, SVA = sagittal vertical axis. (Reproduced with permission from Mummaneni PV, Shaffrey CI, Lenke LG, et al: The minimally invasive spinal deformity surgery algorithm: A reproducible rational framework for decision making in minimally invasive spinal deformity surgery. *Neurosurg Focus* 2014;36[5]:E6.)

Plain weight-bearing radiographs in either a standing or upright seated position should be obtained. For patients who have spondylolisthesis, dynamic flexion-extension radiographs also should be obtained. A careful consideration of overall sagittal alignment should guide the necessity of ACR. Positive sagittal imbalance is considered a C7 plumb line that is 5 cm or more anterior to the superoposterior end plate of the S1 vertebral segment and correlates with increased severity of symptoms.[3] Age-related changes exist in the normal patient population, with a propensity toward greater anterior sagittal alignment as patients age; therefore,

age-related realignment goals are appropriate. Parameters attained from weight-bearing radiographs should guide selection of the appropriate approach for the management of spinal deformity. Mummaneni et al[28] proposed an algorithm for the selection of appropriate patients for minimally invasive spinal deformity surgery, including those with a flexible deformity, a pelvic incidence-lumbar lordosis mismatch less than 30°, and thoracic kyphosis less than 60° (**Figure 2**).

Technique

After a patient has been appropriately selected for ACR, the surgeon must

consider the perioperative technical aspects of the minimally invasive direct lateral transpsoas approach. General anesthesia is necessary, and the patient should be placed in the lateral decubitus position on a flat-top radiolucent table with all of the bony prominences well padded. Traditional approaches to gain access to narrow disk spaces involved surgical table breaks, usually at the level of the greater trochanter, to create a flexion moment.[18] Greater emphasis on soft-tissue retraction and gentle manipulation of the iliac crest with the use of taping techniques in combination with flexion of the hips has obviated the need for more aggressive approaches that place the psoas and lumbar nerve roots on stretch. Access to the disk spaces from the thoracolumbar junction to L4-5 can be attained via the minimally invasive direct lateral transpsoas approach.

After the patient is appropriately positioned and anesthetized, preoperative fluoroscopic imaging should be obtained. Orthogonal fluoroscopic images that are referenced to the operating room floor are more reproducible compared with true AP and lateral fluoroscopic images that are obtained via manipulation of the fluoroscope. Flexion and extension of the surgical table as well as Trendelenburg or reverse Trendelenburg positioning can aid in achieving collinear vertebral end plates on lateral fluoroscopic images, and rotation of the surgical table can help center the spinous processes between the pedicles on AP fluoroscopic images (**Figure 3**). Surgeons must attain and maintain accurate fluoroscopic imaging at each disk level that will be instrumented to ensure accurate placement of retractors and instrumentation; surgical table adjustments may be necessary at each disk level. Maintenance of orientation of all retractors and instrumentation throughout the procedure aids in the accurate and safe placement of interbody grafts.

Skin incisions are either longitudinal or transverse, depending on the number of disk levels that will be instrumented. In general, one or two disk levels can be accessed via a single transverse incision; however, a longitudinal incision should be considered in patients in whom more than two disk levels will be instrumented. Separate fascial incisions may be created at each disk level. The anterior and posterior vertebral body margins are demarcated on the skin,

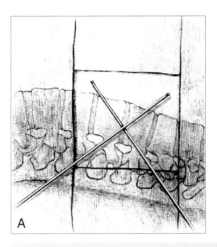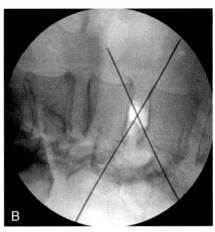

Figure 3   Rough sketch (**A**) and lateral fluoroscopic image (**B**) of a spine show perfect lateral imaging for the planning of Kirschner wire placement for minimally invasive spinal deformity surgery via the direct lateral transpsoas approach. (Panel B reproduced with permission from Ozgur BM, Aryan HE, Pimenta L, Taylor WR: Extreme lateral interbody fusion (XLIF): A novel surgical technique for anterior lumbar interbody fusion. *Spine J* 2006;6[4]: 435-443.)

and an appropriately centered skin incision is made. The subcutaneous tissue is dissected either sharply or bluntly, with hemostasis achieved via bipolar or Bovie electrocautery. The external oblique fascia, which is encountered just below the subcutaneous fat, is incised in line with the muscle fibers, and the external oblique muscle is bluntly dissected and retracted to reveal the internal oblique fascia. Between the layers of the abdominal wall musculature lie cutaneous branches of the ilioinguinal and iliohypogastric nerves[29] (**Figure 4**), which should be preserved if possible to avoid iatrogenic thigh and groin numbness. After all three layers of abdominal wall musculature have been dissected, the retroperitoneum can be entered.

The retroperitoneal fat is intimately associated with the ureter; therefore, blunt dissection should be undertaken to avoid injury to the ureter and to mobilize the peritoneal contents anterior to the surgical field. Blunt finger dissection and the use of endoscopic

Kittner dissectors aid in mobilization of the peritoneal contents. The psoas fascia is encountered next. The genitofemoral nerve is observed on the superficial aspect of the psoas fascia at the approximate level of the L3-4 disk space and further inferior, and the lumbar plexus is observed in the belly of the psoas muscle. At more rostral superior disk levels, the genitofemoral nerve lies in the belly of the psoas muscle. These neurovascular structures must be gently mobilized in a blunt fashion and must not be placed under unnecessary tension. The psoas fascia is incised longitudinally. The belly of the psoas muscle may then be either bluntly retracted or dilated through to allow for direct visualization of the disk space. A Kirschner wire may then be placed in the disk space and visualized under fluoroscopy to attain an ideal position for subsequent serial dilation and retractor placement (**Figure 5**).

A careful understanding of the anatomic location of nervous structures

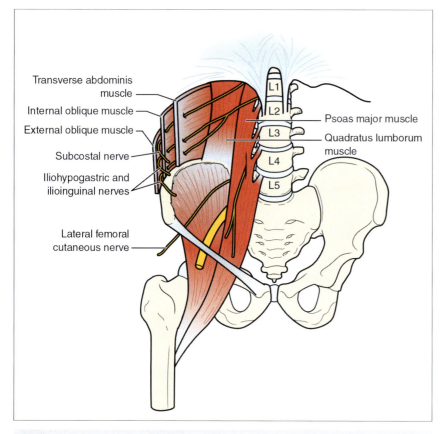

Figure 4 Illustration of a spine and pelvis shows the path of the four main nerves in the abdominal wall.

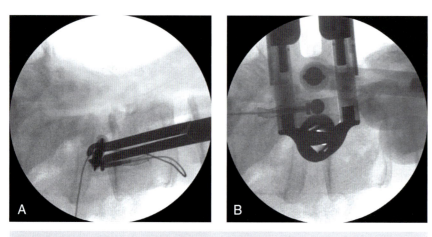

Figure 5 Lateral fluoroscopic images of a spine taken during minimally invasive spinal deformity surgery via the direct lateral transpsoas approach to L4-5 demonstrate initial dilator placement at the disk (**A**) and final retractor placement in the posterior aspect of the disk space (**B**). (Reproduced with permission from Benglis DM, Vanni S, Levi AD: An anatomical study of the lumbosacral plexus as related to the minimally invasive transpsoas approach to the lumbar spine. *J Neurosurg Spine* 2009;10[2]:139-144.)

guides the surgical approach. The lumbar root contributions to the lumbosacral plexus are oriented in a longitudinal fashion, with superior disk levels being posterior and each subsequent inferior contribution stemming from a more anterior position (**Figure 6**). The L1-2 contributions to the lumbosacral plexus are observed at the level of the posterior anulus of the L1-2 disk.[30] Neurophysiologic monitoring is required to allow for mapping of the neural structures and to avoid neural compression. Serial dilation and subsequent retractor placement may be performed with the use of triggered electromyography, with a minimum stimulation threshold of 10 mA indicating a safe work zone. Subsequent increases in the minimum amount of stimulation required for a response should indicate an increased risk of iatrogenic ischemic insult to the lumbar plexus, and the retractors should be appropriately adjusted.[31] Intraoperative neurophysiologic monitoring should be used as an adjunct measure of neurologic function.[32] Although direct stimulation of the retractors can help prevent iatrogenic neurapraxia as a result of stretch, it does not eliminate its occurrence.[31] The use of shallow docking techniques, in which retractors are placed superficial to the psoas fascia, decreases the likelihood of direct injury to the lumbar plexus and avoids aberrant retractor placement; however, shallow docking techniques should not supplant neurophysiologic monitoring and do not eliminate the risk for neurologic injury.[32] Accurate neurophysiologic monitoring requires cooperation with the anesthesiologist and the elimination of paralytic agents or certain inhalational anesthetics that may interfere with monitoring. The use of total intravenous anesthesia may be effective.

After the disk space is localized, a working corridor is created with the use

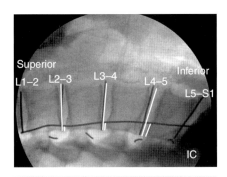

Figure 6   Lateral fluoroscopic image of a spine shows numbered disk spaces and marked white lines, which indicate the ratio of the location of the lumbar plexus from the posterior end plate to the total length of the end plate. IC = iliac crest. (Reproduced with permission from Benglis DM, Vanni S, Levi AD: An anatomical study of the lumbosacral plexus as related to the minimally invasive transpsoas approach to the lumbar spine. *J Neurosurg Spine* 2009;10[2]:139-144.)

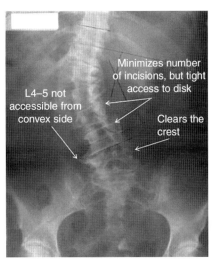

Figure 7   AP radiograph of a spine demonstrates planning for minimally invasive spinal deformity surgery via the direct lateral transpsoas approach. (Reproduced with permission from Pawar A, Hughes A, Girardi F, Sama A, Lebl D, Cammisa F: Lateral lumbar interbody fusion. *Asian Spine J* 2015;9[6]:978-983.)

of self-retaining retractor blades, which are secured to a table-mounted arm to provide stability. Sharp dissection of the posterior anulus fibrosus is performed, and the disk space is prepared in a standard fashion. Under direct and fluoroscopic visualization, Cobb elevators are advanced parallel to the end plate surface, with the sharp end toward the end plate, to detach the superior and inferior margins of a disk from its respective end plates. Care must be taken to not violate the subchondral bone of the end plates, which can lead to interbody graft subsidence.

After the disk space is freed of residual disk tissue, attention is turned to ALL release and subsequent ACR. The great vessels of patients who undergo ACR via the minimally invasive direct lateral transpsoas approach are located in close proximity to the anterior anulus fibrosus; therefore, extreme care must be taken to protect the great vessels during ALL release.[6] Under direct and

fluoroscopic visualization, blunt retractors should be gently placed anterior to the ALL and posterior to the great vessels before ALL release. The far side of the ALL is often difficult to directly visualize, and past-pointing of sharp instruments or inadvertent plunging of a knife blade poses a substantial risk to the aorta and vena cava. ALL release should be undertaken in a controlled manner and may be aided indirectly with the use of expandable cages or dilators, particularly for the last few fibers on the far side of the ALL. The knife blade should be passed such that the blade faces away from the great vessels and advanced under control and direct visualization. To release the remaining fibers, serial dilation with the use of trial grafts can be undertaken, with fluoroscopic imaging used to determine the extent of ALL release that has been achieved.[24]

If ALL release and ACR is required at multiple disk levels, each disk level should be fluoroscopically assessed independent of the previous disk level, with appropriate patient positioning adjustments made to obtain perfectly aligned orthogonal fluoroscopic images. For patients who have concomitant coronal plane imbalance, the surgeon should approach the spine from the concavity of the coronal deformity for instrumentation of multiple disk levels from a single incision. In general, the L4-5 disk level is the most inferior disk level for instrumentation via the minimally invasive direct lateral transpsoas approach. Surgeons should scrutinize preoperative images carefully to determine the feasibility of instrumentation at such an inferior disk level via the minimally invasive direct lateral transpsoas approach (**Figure 7**); if necessary, a more anteriorly oriented approach should be used.

Complications

The most commonly encountered postoperative sequelae of minimally invasive lateral lumbar fusion are transient hip flexion weakness, which results from manipulation and dissection through the psoas muscle, and proximal thigh sensory disturbances, which result from stretch injury to the ilioinguinal, iliohypogastric, genitofemoral, and lateral femoral cutaneous nerves during exposure and retraction.[29] Postoperative transient neurologic deficits are common, with more than 38% of patients reporting sensory disturbances, including groin pain, anterior thigh pain, and dysesthesias, and 24% of patients reporting motor deficits, most commonly thigh flexion weakness; however, most transient neurologic deficits resolve within the first

Table 1
Complications After Minimally Invasive Lateral Lumbar Fusion

Study (Year)[a]	Neurologic: Motor Weakness, Paresthesia			Psoas Weakness/ Dysfunction		Radiographic: Cage Subsidence, Implant Failure	
	No. Pts.	Total No. Pts. (%)	Deficit	No. Pts.	Total No. Pts. (%)	No. Pts.	Total No. Pts. (%)
Knight et al[20] (2009)	9	58 (15.5)	—	5	58 (8.6)	1	58 (1.7)
Isaacs et al[38] (2010)	8	107 (7.5)	—	5	107 (4.7)	—	—
Youssef et al[19] (2010)	—	84 (—)	—	1	85 (1.2)	4	84 (4.8)
Rodgers et al[34] (2011)	4	600 (0.7)	—	—	—	8	600 (1.3)
	—	—	MD[b]	25	324 (7.7)	54	840 (6.4)
	—	—	SD[c]	—	—	—	—
Cahill et al[37] (2012)	—	118 (1.7–4.8)	—	—	—	—	—
Aichmair et al[36] (2013)	—	293 (14.9–6.6)	SD	—	—	—	—
	—	293 (4.3–2.2)	MD	—	—	—	—
	—	293 (9.0–2.2)	TP	—	—	—	—
Le et al[39] (2013)	14	71 (19.7)	SD[d]	—	—	—	—
	—	71 (7.7)	SD[e]	—	—	—	—
Marchi et al[35] (2013)	14	74 (18.9)	—	14	74 (18.9)	41	98 (41.8)
Lykissas et al[33] (2014)	—	451 (9.3)	SD	—	—	—	(83)
	—	451 (3.2)	MD	—	—	—	—

MD = motor deficit, SD = sensory deficit, TP = thigh pain.

[a]All studies exhibited conflicts of interest.

[b]Motor (range, 0.7%–18.9%).

[c]Sensory (range, 2.2%–19.7%).

[d]Immediately postoperative.

[e]Three months postoperative.

Adapted from Kwon B, Kim DH: Lateral lumbar interbody fusion: Indications, outcomes, and complications. *J Am Acad Orthop Surg* 2016;24(2):96-105.

18 months postoperatively.[33] Postoperative transient neurologic deficits are associated with female sex, limited surgeon experience with minimally invasive lateral lumbar fusion, and more than two disk levels that are addressed during surgery. The incidence of the more common complications that occur after minimally invasive lateral lumbar fusion, including neurologic complications and psoas weakness, are summarized in **Table 1**.[19,20,33-39]

Surgeons should perform and document a sensory and motor examination as well as counsel the patient with regard to the potential complications of the surgical procedure before proceeding with minimally invasive lateral lumbar fusion. To help diminish potential complications, direct visualization of the lumbar plexus and other nerves encountered via the minimally invasive direct lateral transpsoas approach must be attained and shallow docking techniques can be used. Limiting the number of disk levels that are addressed, limiting retraction time, and neurophysiologic monitoring may help reduce the risk for iatrogenic nerve injury complications. Blunt dissection of the layers of abdominal musculature and direct visualization of each fascial layer can help reduce the risk for ilioinguinal and iliohypogastric nerve injury. In general, retraction time at each disk level should be less than

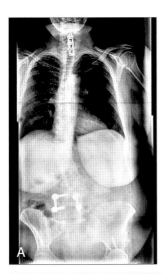 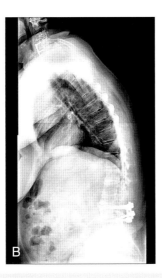 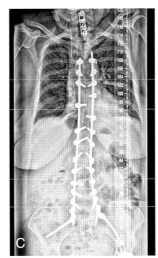 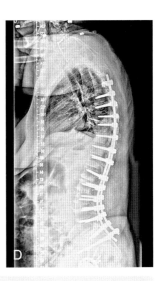

Figure 8   Images of the spine of a 66-year-old woman with back pain and bilateral radicular leg pain. Preoperative AP (**A**) and lateral (**B**) standing radiographs demonstrate lumbar hypolordosis and coronal imbalance, which resulted from a previous fusion. Postoperative AP (**C**) and lateral (**D**) standing radiographs taken after multilevel anterior column realignment and extreme lateral interbody fusion with extension of posterior spinal fusion demonstrate restoration of lumbar lordosis.

20 to 25 minutes.[31] Neurophysiologic monitoring often is unable to detect neurologic injury that occurs as a result of prolonged retraction and stretch. The perioperative intravenous administration of 10 mg of dexamethasone has been reported to reduce the risk for neurologic injury during the minimally invasive direct lateral transpsoas approach.[34] Mummaneni et al[28] avoid posterior retractor positioning in the disk space because it may result in lumbosacral plexus injury, especially at L4-5. The genitofemoral nerve courses in the psoas muscle belly proximally, piercing the psoas fascia and continuing on the anteromedial border of the psoas muscle more distally. The genitofemoral nerve can be directly visualized in line with the fibers of the psoas muscle and can be indirectly monitored via triggered electromyography.

Graft subsidence and subsequent loss of some lumbar lordosis that was gained after minimally invasive lateral lumbar fusion may occur via intraoperative end

plate violation in patients who have osteoporotic bone and is associated with a smaller cage footprint.[40] Management strategies for graft subsidence and subsequent loss of lumbar lordosis include revision posterior decompression and instrumentation as well as lateral plate instrumentation.

More serious complications of minimally invasive lateral lumbar fusion include distal lower extremity weakness, which results from lumbar plexus injury, as well as injury to hollow organs in the peritoneum, injury to the ureter, and injury to the great vessels. Although rare, peritoneal and vascular organ injuries can be avoided with the judicious use of direct visualization during approach and retractor placement as well as by not past-pointing sharp instruments beyond the margin of the retractors.

Outcomes

In general, the outcomes of ACR via the minimally invasive direct lateral transpsoas approach are favorable.

Restoration of lumbar lordosis may be substantial (**Figure 8**). Akbarnia et al[25] reported that mean lumbar lordosis improved from 16° preoperatively to 38° after ALL release, which then improved to 45° after supplemental posterior instrumentation. Saigal et al[24] reported 10° to 27° of improved segmental lumbar lordosis in patients who underwent anterior column release with the use of hyperlordotic cages. These improvements in lumbar lordosis are comparable with those achieved via three-column posterior osteotomies, which afford similar correction, but often result in a higher rate of complications including increased blood loss, neurologic injury, instrumentation failure, and pseudarthrosis.[41,42]

ACR via the minimally invasive direct lateral transpsoas approach is not performed in isolation. Posterior instrumentation and releases are the standard and may be performed at the time of the index surgery or in staged manner. A combined anterior/posterior approach results in considerable deformity correction in both the coronal and sagittal planes.[42,43] The minimally invasive direct lateral transpsoas approach is limited, and patients with large global sagittal imbalance may benefit from a combined approach that includes both anterior and posterior releases. Substantial lumbar lordosis, sagittal vertical axis, and Cobb angle improvements can be achieved in patients who undergo a combined approach that includes anterior release as well as open posterior instrumentation and release. Wang et al[43] reported a mean improvement in lumbar lordosis of 16.6°, a mean improvement in sagittal vertical axis of 34.1 mm, and a Cobb angle ceiling effect of 55° in the coronal plane in patients who underwent such an approach. Combined approaches that include anterior release as well as minimally invasive posterior instrumentation and release result in improved alignment but less substantial correction.[43] The use of a minimally invasive lateral approach for anterior release and interbody grafting in combination with posterior instrumentation and release allows for spinal deformity correction similar to that of open posterior deformity correction, with comparable complication rates and patient outcomes reported 5 years postoperatively.[44]

Summary

ACR via the minimally invasive direct lateral transpsoas approach is gaining popularity because it allows for the restoration of sagittal balance and results in less morbidity compared with open anterior or posterior-only approaches. Many approach-related complications can be avoided with knowledge of the unique anatomy exposed via a lateral approach and appropriate patient selection. The advantages of ACR via the minimally invasive direct lateral transpsoas approach include decreased blood loss and decreased surgical time. ACR via the minimally invasive direct lateral transpsoas approach is a powerful adjunct that is increasingly used for the surgical management of lumbar scoliosis.

References

1. Pritchett JW, Bortel DT: Degenerative symptomatic lumbar scoliosis. Spine (Phila Pa 1976) 1993;18(6):700-703.

2. Smith JS, Lafage V, Shaffrey CI, et al: Outcomes of operative and nonoperative treatment for adult spinal deformity: A prospective, multicenter, propensity-matched cohort assessment with minimum 2-year follow-up. Neurosurgery 2016;78(6):851-861.

3. Glassman SD, Bridwell K, Dimar JR, Horton W, Berven S, Schwab F: The impact of positive sagittal balance in adult spinal deformity. Spine (Phila Pa 1976) 2005;30(18):2024-2029.

4. Gill JB, Levin A, Burd T, Longley M: Corrective osteotomies in spine surgery. J Bone Joint Surg Am 2008;90(11):2509-2520.

5. Smith JS, Shaffrey E, Klineberg E, et al: Prospective multicenter assessment of risk factors for rod fracture following surgery for adult spinal deformity. J Neurosurg Spine 2014;21(6):994-1003.

6. Mobbs RJ, Phan K, Daly D, Rao PJ, Lennox A: Approach-related complications of anterior lumbar interbody fusion: Results of a combined spine and vascular surgical team. Global Spine J 2016;6(2):147-154.

7. Rodgers WB, Gerber EJ, Rodgers JA: Lumbar fusion in octogenarians: The promise of minimally invasive surgery. Spine (Phila Pa 1976) 2010;35(26 suppl):S355-S360.

8. Capener N: Spondylolisthesis. Br J Surg 1932;19(75):374-386.

9. Müller W: Transperitoneale freilegung der wirbelsäule bei tuberkulöser spondylitis. Dtsch Z Chirug 1906;85(1):128-135.

10. Lee CS, Hwang CJ, Lee DH, Kim YT, Lee HS: Fusion rates of instrumented lumbar spinal arthrodesis according to surgical approach: A systematic review of randomized trials. Clin Orthop Surg 2011;3(1):39-47.

11. McCarthy MJ, Ng L, Vermeersch G, Chan D: A radiological comparison of anterior fusion rates in anterior lumbar interbody fusion. Global Spine J 2012;2(4):195-206.

12. Jiang SD, Chen JW, Jiang LS: Which procedure is better for lumbar interbody fusion: Anterior lumbar interbody fusion or transforaminal lumbar interbody fusion? Arch Orthop Trauma Surg 2012;132(9):1259-1266.

13. Kim YB, Lenke LG, Kim YJ, et al: The morbidity of an anterior thoracolumbar approach: Adult spinal deformity patients with greater than five-year follow-up. Spine (Phila Pa 1976) 2009;34(8):822-826.

14. Obenchain TG: Laparoscopic lumbar discectomy: Case report. J Laparoendosc Surg 1991;1(3):145-149.

15. McAfee PC, Regan JJ, Geis WP, Fedder IL: Minimally invasive anterior retroperitoneal approach to the lumbar spine: Emphasis on the lateral BAK. Spine (Phila Pa 1976) 1998;23(13):1476-1484.

16. Bergey DL, Villavicencio AT, Goldstein T, Regan JJ: Endoscopic lateral transpsoas approach to the lumbar spine. Spine (Phila Pa 1976) 2004;29(15):1681-1688.

17. Pimenta L, Schaffa TL: Paper. Lateral endoscopic transpsoas retroperitoneal approach for lumbar spine surgery. Brazilian Spine Society Meeting. Belo Horizonte, Minas Gerais, Brazil, 2001.

18. Ozgur BM, Aryan HE, Pimenta L, Taylor WR: Extreme lateral interbody fusion (XLIF): A novel surgical technique for anterior lumbar interbody fusion. Spine J 2006;6(4):435-443.

19. Youssef JA, McAfee PC, Patty CA, et al: Minimally invasive surgery: Lateral approach interbody fusion: results and review. Spine (Phila Pa 1976) 2010;35(26 suppl):S302-S311.

20. Knight RQ, Schwaegler P, Hanscom D, Roh J: Direct lateral lumbar interbody fusion for degenerative

conditions: Early complication profile. *J Spinal Disord Tech* 2009;22(1):34-37.

21. Lee YP, Regev GJ, Chan J, et al: Evaluation of hip flexion strength following lateral lumbar interbody fusion. *Spine J* 2013;13(10):1259-1262.

22. Phillips FM, Isaacs RE, Rodgers WB, et al: Adult degenerative scoliosis treated with XLIF: Clinical and radiographical results of a prospective multicenter study with 24-month follow-up. *Spine (Phila Pa 1976)* 2013;38(21):1853-1861.

23. Costanzo G, Zoccali C, Maykowski P, Walter CM, Skoch J, Baaj AA: The role of minimally invasive lateral lumbar interbody fusion in sagittal balance correction and spinal deformity. *Eur Spine J* 2014;23(suppl 6):699-704.

24. Saigal R, Mundis GM Jr, Eastlack R, Uribe JS, Phillips FM, Akbarnia BA: Anterior column realignment (ACR) in adult sagittal deformity correction: Technique and review of the literature. *Spine (Phila Pa 1976)* 2016;41(suppl 8):S66-S73.

25. Akbarnia BA, Mundis GM Jr, Moazzaz P, et al: Anterior column realignment (ACR) for focal kyphotic spinal deformity using a lateral transpsoas approach and ALL release. *J Spinal Disord Tech* 2014;27(1):29-39.

26. Deukmedjian AR, Le TV, Baaj AA, Dakwar E, Smith DA, Uribe JS: Anterior longitudinal ligament release using the minimally invasive lateral retroperitoneal transpsoas approach: A cadaveric feasibility study and report of 4 clinical cases. *J Neurosurg Spine* 2012;17(6):530-539.

27. Halpin RJ, Sugrue PA, Gould RW, et al: Standardizing care for high-risk patients in spine surgery: The Northwestern high-risk spine protocol. *Spine (Phila Pa 1976)* 2010;35(25):2232-2238.

28. Mummaneni PV, Shaffrey CI, Lenke LG, et al: The minimally invasive spinal deformity surgery algorithm: A reproducible rational framework for decision making in minimally invasive spinal deformity surgery. *Neurosurg Focus* 2014;36(5):E6.

29. Dakwar E, Vale FL, Uribe JS: Trajectory of the main sensory and motor branches of the lumbar plexus outside the psoas muscle related to the lateral retroperitoneal transpsoas approach. *J Neurosurg Spine* 2011;14(2):290-295.

30. Benglis DM, Vanni S, Levi AD: An anatomical study of the lumbosacral plexus as related to the minimally invasive transpsoas approach to the lumbar spine. *J Neurosurg Spine* 2009;10(2):139-144.

31. Uribe JS: Neural anatomy, neuromonitoring and related complications in extreme lateral interbody fusion: Video lecture. *Eur Spine J* 2015;24(suppl 3):445-446.

32. Cheng I, Acosta F, Chang K, Pham M: Point-counterpoint: The use of neuromonitoring in lateral transpsoas surgery. *Spine (Phila Pa 1976)* 2016;41(suppl 8):S145-S151.

33. Lykissas MG, Aichmair A, Hughes AP, et al: Nerve injury after lateral lumbar interbody fusion: A review of 919 treated levels with identification of risk factors. *Spine J* 2014;14(5):749-758.

34. Rodgers WB, Gerber EJ, Patterson J: Intraoperative and early postoperative complications in extreme lateral interbody fusion: An analysis of 600 cases. *Spine (Phila Pa 1976)* 2011;36(1):26-32.

35. Marchi L, Abdala N, Oliveria L, Amaral R, Coutinho E, Pimenta L: Radiographic and clinical evaluation of cage subsidence after stand-alone lateral interbody fusion. *J Neurosurg Spine* 2013;19(1):110-118.

36. Aichmair A, Lykissas MG, Girardi FP, et al: An institutional six-year trend analysis of the neurological outcome after lateral lumbar interbody fusion: A 6-year trend analysis of a single institution. *Spine (Phila Pa 1976)* 2013;38(23):E1483-E1490.

37. Cahill KS, Martinez JL, Wang MY, Vanni S, Levi AD: Motor nerve injuries following the minimally invasive lateral transpsoas approach. *J Neurosurg Spine* 2012;17(3):227-231.

38. Isaacs RE, Hyde J, Goodrich JA, Rodgers WB, Phillips FM: A prospective, nonrandomized, multicenter evaluation of extreme lateral interbody fusion for the treatment of adult degenerative scoliosis: Perioperative outcomes and complications. *Spine (Phila Pa 1976)* 2010;35(26 suppl):S322-S330.

39. Le TV, Burkett CJ, Deukmedjian AR, Urible JS: Postoperative lumbar plexus injury after lumber retroperitoneal transpsoas minimally invasive lateral interbody fusion. *Spine (Phila Pa 1976)* 2013;38(1):E13-E20.

40. Kwon B, Kim DH: Lateral lumbar interbody fusion: Indications, outcomes, and complications. *J Am Acad Orthop Surg* 2016;24(2):96-105.

41. Hyun SJ, Rhim SC: Clinical outcomes and complications after pedicle subtraction osteotomy for fixed sagittal imbalance patients: A long-term follow-up data. *J Korean Neurosurg Soc* 2010;47(2):95-101.

42. Trobisch PD, Hwang SW, Drange S: PSO without neuromonitoring: Analysis of peri-op complication rate after lumbar pedicle subtraction osteotomy in adults. *Eur Spine J* 2016;25(8):2629-2632.

43. Wang MY, Mummaneni PV, Fu KM, et al: Less invasive surgery for treating adult spinal deformities: Ceiling effects for deformity correction with 3 different techniques. *Neurosurg Focus* 2014;36(5):E12.

44. Anand N, Baron EM, Khandehroo B, Kahwaty S: Long-term 2- to 5-year clinical and functional outcomes of minimally invasive surgery for adult scoliosis. *Spine (Phila Pa 1976)* 2013;38(18):1566-1575.

How to Decrease Complications in the Management of Adult Lumbar Scoliosis

Vijay Yanamadala, MD
Quinlan Buchlak, MPsych, MBIS
Jean-Christophe Leveque, MD
Rajiv Sethi, MD

Abstract

Complication rates that range from 25% to 80% have been reported for complex spine surgery. A comprehensive, standardized, and reproducible approach can substantially reduce the risk of complications in patients who undergo complex spine and deformity correction surgery. A systematic approach leverages multiple risk reduction strategies, including a multidisciplinary preoperative conference, two attending co-surgeons in the operating room, a dedicated complex spine anesthesia team, and the application of an intraoperative protocol to track coagulopathy and blood loss, to help reduce the likelihood of perioperative complications.

Instr Course Lect 2017;66:379–390.

Intraoperative adverse event rates of up to 10% have been reported in the literature for general spine surgery.[1-9] Overall complication rates that range from 25% to 80% have been reported for complex spine surgery, including deformity surgery.[10] A growing body of literature suggests that standardized protocols can help reduce complications in all surgical specialties.[11-18] Given the morbid nature of complex spine and deformity correction surgery,[4,7,15,18-24] a comprehensive, standardized, and reproducible approach can help maximize safety for patients who undergo these types of procedures.

Surgical complications can be categorized based on the time period in which they occur: intraoperative, postoperative short-term (first 90 days after surgery), and postoperative long-term (>90 days after surgery). Each of these time periods exposes the patient to unique risks. The surgical team must address the variable nature of these risks across each of these sequential time periods. Preventable intraoperative complications primarily include blood loss, coagulopathy, hypotensive sequelae, and surgeon error or misjudgment.[11] The literature on spine surgery contains both historical and recent reports of intraoperative blood loss that exceeds patients' baseline total estimated blood volumes, and it is clear that inadequate repletion during spine surgery can lead to critical hypotension and multiorgan system dysfunction.[25-32] In

Dr. Leveque or an immediate family member is a member of a speakers' bureau or has made paid presentations on behalf of NuVasive; serves as a paid consultant to or is an employee of K2M; and serves as a board member, owner, officer, or committee member of the Scoliosis Research Society. Dr. Sethi or an immediate family member serves as a paid consultant to or is an employee of K2M, NuVasive, and Orthofix; has received nonincome support (such as equipment or services), commercially derived honoraria, or other non-research–related funding (such as paid travel) from K2M; and serves as a board member, owner, officer, or committee member of the Scoliosis Research Society and the Washington State Orthopaedic Association. Neither of the following authors nor any immediate family member has received anything of value from or has stock or stock options held in a commercial company or institution related directly or indirectly to the subject of this chapter: Dr. Yanamadala and Mr. Buchlak.

the second time period, which stretches from the conclusion of the procedure through the first 90 days postoperatively, a patient is exposed to the risk of thromboembolism, local or systemic infection, hardware-related issues with neurologic sequelae or continued postoperative pain that requires revision surgery, poor wound healing, and complications that result from comorbid conditions. Long-term complications typically include hardware fatigue and failure, proximal and distal junctional failures, lack of fusion, and latent infection. Although many centers have developed individualized protocols to help address some of these complications individually,[30,33-38] the authors of this chapter firmly believe that a systematic and comprehensive approach to risk reduction is essential to achieve the best outcomes.

The comprehensive approach of the authors of this chapter is built on the concept that the entire team that cares for a patient from his or her preoperative state through his or her recovery plays a role in the overall outcome of the surgery. Therefore, the authors of this chapter have created a system that brings all relevant caregivers, including medical specialists, nursing staff, and physical therapists, to the table for a discussion on the specific factors that predispose a particular patient to the risk of complications and the ways in which a standardized approach can help prevent these complications. This framework, which is known as the Seattle Spine Team Protocol (SSTP), is structured on three key components: an in-person multidisciplinary preoperative complex spine conference, which helps assess the appropriateness of surgery and coordinates the entire spectrum of patient care from the preoperative state through discharge; a collaborative intraoperative surgical team that is focused on increasing efficiency and decreasing surgical time, which is accomplished with the use of two attending co-surgeons and a dedicated spine anesthesia team; and a rigorous intraoperative protocol that helps monitor and treat coagulopathy and blood loss.[11]

Figure 1 presents a conceptual diagram that shows how the risk mitigation strategies built into the SSTP are related to the most likely complex spine surgery complications. Multiple risk mitigation strategies address each likely intraoperative complication, which increases risk mitigation efficacy. This is important given that intraoperative complications may arise and progress rapidly as well as have severe postoperative consequences. The multidisciplinary preoperative conference helps mitigate many long- and short-term postoperative complications. A systematic approach to risk management comprehensively addresses all possible complication domains. The SSTP is a multidisciplinary protocol that helps decrease perioperative complications. The SSTP uses a system of constant process improvement in which iterative improvements are made to the system based on constant data tracking.

Initial Patient Evaluation

All patients with a diagnosis of scoliosis who are referred to the surgical spine clinic of the authors of this chapter undergo a thorough patient history and physical examination. The physical examination includes an assessment of a patient's functional status, including his or her mobility and ability to conduct activities of daily living, pain status, and current pain regimen. An Oswestry Low Back Pain Disability Questionnaire and a European Quality of Life-5 Dimensions Questionnaire are completed preoperatively by all patients. Smoking history, current smoking status, and current medications as well as any substantial comorbidities with respect to the cardiac, pulmonary, hemostatic, and neurologic systems are recorded.

For all patients, the authors of this chapter obtain standard preoperative imaging studies, including 36-inch standing AP and lateral spine radiographs as well as a dedicated lumbar spine radiograph with flexion-extension views. For patients who have symptoms of radiculopathy or neurogenic claudication, the authors of this chapter perform MRI of the lumbar spine. In conjunction with the thorough patient history and physical examination, the authors of this chapter carefully assess radiographs and MRI scans to determine if a patient would benefit from surgical intervention.

Radiographic evaluation includes measurement of sagittal and coronal balance, pelvic parameters, and Cobb angles of major and minor curves.[39] These measures, in conjunction with a patient's history, allow the authors of this chapter to tailor the surgical procedure so that it is most likely to alleviate a patient's symptoms and improve his or her functional status. A CT scan of the spine and a dual-energy x-ray absorptiometry scan are obtained in patients who are potential candidates for surgery.[33,40-42]

Preoperative Multidisciplinary Conference

After a patient is deemed a potential surgical candidate for the correction of a major lumbar kyphoscoliotic deformity, he or she enters the SSTP.

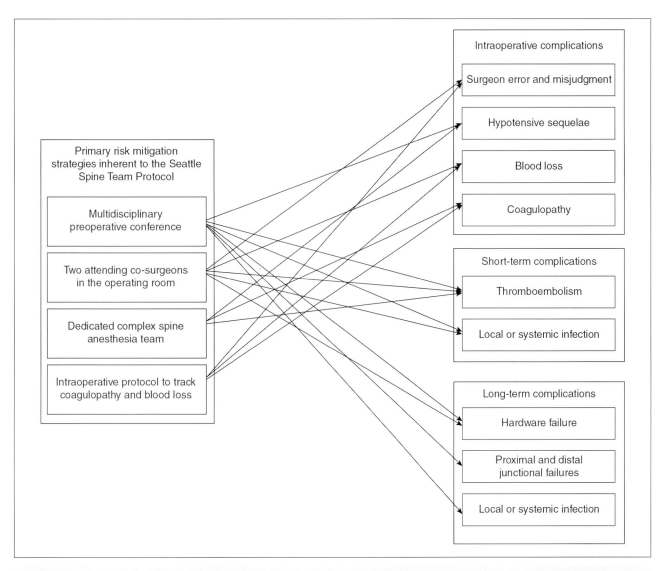

Figure 1   Conceptual diagram shows how perioperative complications are mitigated by the primary elements of the Seattle Spine Team Protocol.

All SSTP patients are presented at a monthly conference that is attended by an internist, a physical medicine and rehabilitation physician, at least two members of the dedicated complex spine anesthesia team, the nurses who coordinate the complex spine patient-education class, and the operating surgeons. The anesthesiologists and internist review each patient's history and medical issues before the conference. A written summary of each patient's medical history, relevant laboratory values, and screening tests (electrocardiogram, echocardiogram, etc) is then generated and sent to the conference participants.

Discussion on each patient focuses on both the proposed surgical correction as well as the relevant preoperative and postoperative medical issues. Conference discussions are predicated on the belief that both nonsurgeon (eg, internists and anesthesiologists) and surgeon members of the committee have equal power to decide if a patient is suitable for surgery. The authors of this chapter have discovered that, at most institutions, the surgeons wield the decision-making power for or against surgery, and the nonsurgeons who take care of patients postoperatively are often left wondering why a particular patient was ever selected for surgery. To prevent this type of scenario, the SSTP preoperative conference requires that each surgical patient have substantial, but not unanimous, support from all of the interested parties already mentioned. This means that patients who may appear to be surgically viable based on radiographic imaging, physical examination, and clinical history may be deemed unsafe for surgery because of factors or concerns raised by the nonsurgeon members. The primary surgeon then thoroughly discusses recommendations from the SSTP preoperative conference with the patient, and the patient is given the opportunity to ask questions and express his or her opinion on the recommendations.

The authors of this chapter firmly believe that the willingness to remove politics and economic incentives from the preoperative conference is important to ensure that an appropriate decision is made for each patient. In the past 5 years, the multidisciplinary medical team involved in the SSTP review process decided that approximately 25% of patients who initially presented at the conference had medical conditions that rendered them unsuitable for the extent of surgical treatment proposed. In many of these patients, the SSTP review process determined that risk of substantial harm from surgery outweighed the possibility of a good outcome, and a nonsurgical plan was proposed and pursued.[43] In some instances, patients may require medical optimization or further studies before a final decision can be made. These patients undergo a more in-depth evaluation or pretreatment based on the preoperative conference discussion and are then brought back for another review. The results of the preoperative conference are summarized and placed in a patient's medical record and also are discussed with the patient by the primary surgeon to aid in the shared decision-making process.

Patient Preparation and Preoperative Optimization

After a patient has been cleared at the preoperative conference, he or she enters the second phase of the SSTP. All patients attend a 2-hour patient-education class that is led by clinical nurses and one of the spinal deformity surgeons. This class focuses on the postoperative recovery period and includes printed materials as well as a question-and-answer session. All patients are then engaged in a lengthy consent process that involves a discussion of the potential complications that can occur during spine surgery, including bleeding, infection, proximal junctional kyphosis, hardware failure, postoperative neurologic injury, stroke, blindness, and death.[4,35,44-47]

After preliminary clearance by the preoperative conference, an internist performs a thorough preoperative patient evaluation. The need for further cardiac evaluation is based on American College of Cardiology/American Heart Association guidelines for perioperative risk stratification.[48] Pulmonary function tests are obtained preoperatively as indicated.[49] All patients with normal preoperative coagulation and hematologic panels have four units of packed red blood cells and four units of thawed plasma typed and crossed. If abnormalities in hematocrit levels or coagulation are discovered, additional workup that involves internal medicine and hematology is completed.

The Acute Pain Service, which is run by the Department of Anesthesiology, also evaluates all patients preoperatively to assess their baseline pain and current pain regimen. Based on this analysis, the Acute Pain Service creates a perioperative pain regimen for each patient. The attending anesthesiologists who direct the Acute Pain Service and supervise the resident and fellow team are closely involved with the complex spine surgery team; therefore, these anesthesiologists are cognizant of the unique issues with regard to patients who undergo complex spine surgery, the importance of early mobilization, and the importance of communication with members of the primary spine team who perform daily rounds. **Figure 2** presents the SSTP pain management pathway that is used in the treatment of complex spine patients.

Preoperative and Postoperative Multidisciplinary Coordination

On the morning of surgery, the primary surgeon contacts the intensivist or hospitalist who will care for the patient postoperatively. This discussion alerts the intensivist or hospitalist to the presence of a patient's preexisting comorbidities and the expected surgical course. Near the conclusion of the procedure, a member of the anesthesia team provides this same intensivist or hospitalist with an updated patient status. This update focuses on intraoperative events, total blood loss, and the physiologic state of the patient and facilitates the process of appropriate postoperative care team preparation. This operating room (OR)-to-floor discussion increases the efficiency and effectiveness of a patient's transition from the OR to intensive or floor care.

Extubation is routinely attempted in the OR, and, in the experience of the authors of this chapter, only a very small percentage of patients require transport to the intensive care unit (ICU) while intubated. On the first postoperative night, patients are

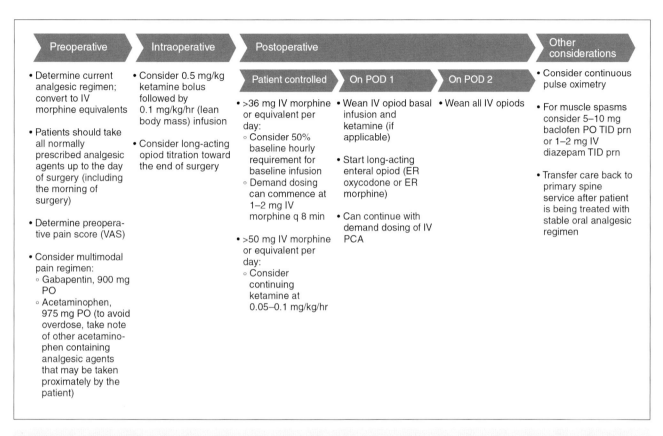

Figure 2 The Seattle Spine Team Protocol pain management pathway for the treatment of complex spine patients. ER = extended release, IV = intravenous, PCA = patient-controlled analgesia, PO = orally, POD = postoperative day, prn = when necessary, q = every, TID = three times a day, VAS = visual analog scale.

observed closely for any neurologic change, with strict control of hematocrit levels, coagulation factors, and platelet count. Initially, the authors of this chapter planned to transition all complex spine patients to the ICU for overnight observation before they were transferred to the general care floor on postoperative day 1. However, the involvement of the hospitalist team and floor nursing team in the SSTP pathway allowed the authors of this chapter to create a specialized step-down floor that is able to manage and monitor most complex spine patients, even on the first postoperative night, which decreases hospital stay costs and ICU burden. The floor nursing team helped create a standardized postoperative expectation for complex spine patients.

Complex spine patients are mobilized with physical therapy on postoperative days 1 through 3 and are typically discharged to home or to a skilled nursing facility between postoperative days 4 through 6.

Long-term follow-up is coordinated through the primary surgeon's office and generally involves follow-up appointments 2 weeks postoperatively for staple removal, 4 to 6 weeks postoperatively for surgeon follow-up, and every 3 to 6 months postoperatively thereafter for the first year followed by yearly follow-up visits. Full-length scoliosis radiographs are obtained at the first postoperative visit and every 6 months postoperatively for the first year and then yearly thereafter for a total of 5 years.

Intraoperative Process and Shared Decision Making

In addition to the standard OR team, the authors of this chapter have two attending surgeons perform surgery in tandem. The current practice of the authors of this chapter typically includes a neurosurgeon and an orthopaedic surgeon, both of whom have specialized spine training. Rather than having primary or secondary roles, both surgeons are viewed as equal members of the surgical team.[34] Multi-institutional studies have reported that this approach reduces OR time, blood loss, and overall complications.[34] The authors of this chapter also use a two-member anesthesia team, which consists of two dedicated anesthesiologists who have an interest in spinal deformity surgery, and an anesthesia technician. Orthopaedic or neurosurgical residents or fellows may scrub in on surgeries given that the protocol requirement of two attending surgeons is fulfilled.[34]

Figure 3 presents the optimal layout of the OR for a complex spine procedure. This layout provides the surgeons, scrub technicians, circulating registered nurse, anesthesia team, and neuromonitoring team with specific zones of operation. There are two large image screens on opposite walls. These screens are connected to the electronic medical record system and are used to display a range of radiologic imagery on demand. The OR team is able to view multiple radiographs, three-dimensional CT scans, and other imagery as necessary. A laboratory tracking board (**Figure 4**) and a blood tracking board (**Figure 5**) also are positioned on the wall. These boards provide the entire OR team with a clear visual summary of a patient's status and allow for efficient communication among all members of the OR team. These regularly updated informational display boards facilitate rapid decision making during critical moments and at structured hourly time points.

Adequate preparation for blood loss is ensured at the beginning of surgery. A rapid infuser, two cell saver units (one for each surgeon), a pulse oximeter with a plethysmographic variability index as well as real-time hemoglobin measures,[50] and a bispectral index monitor are used by the anesthesia team for continuous monitoring of the patient. After the anesthesia team induces the patient and places the central line, neuromonitoring leads are placed. It is the standard practice of the authors of this chapter to monitor somatosensory-evoked potentials, motor-evoked potentials, and lower extremity electromyography.[51-54] After the neuromonitoring leads are placed, the patient is placed in a Mayfield headrest (Ohio Medical Instrument) on a specialized spine surgical table.[35,55-57]

The authors of this chapter rigorously track important patient parameters throughout the surgery. Laboratory values, including arterial blood gas pressure, hemoglobin and hematocrit levels, platelet count, prothrombin time, international normalized ratio (INR), fibrinogen levels, D-dimer levels, ionized calcium levels, and lactate levels, are measured hourly. Working with the laboratory, the authors of this chapter established a rapid turnaround time (20 minutes) for these laboratory values. Laboratory values are called out in the OR as they are available and are then transcribed onto the laboratory tracking board in the OR (**Figure 4**). After all laboratory values for a particular hour have been returned, the surgical team and anesthesia team pause to review the patient's current physiologic state and progress in surgery as well as any challenges in either.

Tranexamic acid is currently part of the standardized treatment protocol at New York University–Langone Medical Center.[58] This protocol is different from that of most surgical centers, at which ongoing blood loss occurs and laboratory values are measured and replenished with the appropriate blood product. The authors of this chapter transfuse plasma after a patient receives one to two units of red blood cells or has an INR greater than 1.2. Although this coagulopathy has not been fully characterized, the authors of this chapter have observed that waiting until a patient's INR is greater than 1.5 or hematocrit level is less than 25% before beginning plasma transfusion is associated with increased amounts of subjective surgeon-observed bleeding and laboratory value derangements (eg, INR) that are difficult to correct. Although coagulopathy is ubiquitous in adult spinal deformity surgery, few protocols have been developed to track and manage it.[25,28,30-32,59] The etiology of coagulopathy during major spine surgery is unknown and likely represents both a dilution phenomenon and a consumptive element.[59]

Staged Surgery

Some surgeries for major spinal deformity should be performed in two stages. The primary stage is intended to place most or all of the required instrumentation, and the second stage is reserved for correction and final fixation in patients in whom the entire surgery cannot be safely completed in one sitting. The time between scheduled stages is typically 3 to 4 days. In patients who undergo staged surgery, a removable inferior vena cava filter is placed and is scheduled for removal 6 to 12 weeks after completion of the surgical procedure.[60,61] Inferior vena cava filters are placed only in patients who have surgery staged on different days. All patients are given 5,000 units of subcutaneous heparin three times a day on postoperative day 1. The authors of this chapter routinely have patients ambulate between the first and second stages of surgery.

Deformity correction hinges on several standard surgical strategies, including lumbar pedicle subtraction osteotomy and, more recently, multilevel minimally invasive lateral lumbar interbody fusion, which is often performed with hyperlordotic interbody grafts in patients who require correction of spinopelvic parameters. For surgical

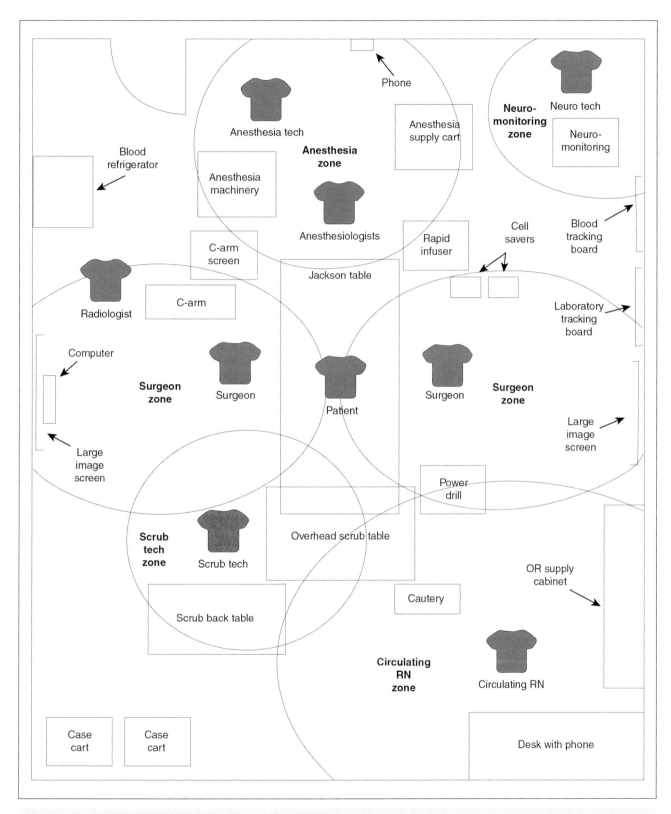

Figure 3   Illustration shows the optimal layout of the operating room (OR) for a complex spine procedure. This layout provides the surgeons, scrub technicians, circulating registered nurse (RN), anesthesia team, and neuromonitoring team with primary zones of operation. neuro = neurologic, tech = technician.

Time	Suction Canister	Cell Saver EBL	Field Irrigation	Total EBL	Hct	pH/BE	PT/INR	Platelet Count	Fibrinogen/D-dimer
9:00	N/A	N/A	N/A	N/A	33	7.38/-2.9	13.7/1.1	108	798/2.74
10:03	550	100	0	650	30	7.35/-4.5	14.2/1.1	100	647/2.65
11:00	650	550	0	1200	29	7.38/-3.6	15.3/1.2	95	497/2.94
12:00	800	1250	0	2050	31	7.34/-4.2	16.4/1.3	90	411/2.92
13:04	1300	1700	0	3000	21	7.31/-4.8	18.1/1.5	110	335/2.93
14:01	1500	2000	0	3500	31	7.30/-4.5	17.3/1.4	125	280/3.95
15:05	1600	2200	0	3800	29	7.33/-4.1	17.0/1.4	103	290/7.49

Figure 4 Example of a laboratory tracking board used to record and communicate laboratory values and estimated blood loss (EBL) during a complex spine procedure. This board displays hourly calculations of blood loss as well as key acid-base, red blood cell, and coagulation parameters. This board facilitates intrateam communication. Total EBL is calculated by adding suction canister and cell saver EBL and then subtracting field irrigation. BE = base excess, Hct = hematocrit, INR = international normalized ratio, N/A = not available, PT = prothrombin time.

plans that involve the lateral approach, the authors of this chapter generally perform the lateral surgery in the first stage to attain most of the release, correct lumbar lordosis, and relax lumbar coronal curvature. To complete the correction, the second stage involves pedicle screw instrumentation, iliac fixation, and smaller osteotomies. The decision for staged surgery is often made during the preoperative conference and is often affected by a patient's preoperative status and comorbidities that may increase the risk of a single-stage procedure. The guiding principle of the authors of this chapter in the decision to perform staged surgery involves minimizing a patient's total surgical time and blood loss; therefore, the authors of this chapter tailor their surgical plan with this primary objective in mind.

Postoperative Care

Near the conclusion of the surgery, the anesthesiologist contacts the intensivist or hospitalist to give a person-to-person report on the events of the surgery, blood loss, and the physiologic state of the patient. Extubation is routinely attempted in the OR. The authors of this chapter rarely keep patients intubated during transport to the ICU. Patients are observed overnight in the ICU, with strict control of hematocrit levels, coagulation factors, and platelet count. Most patients can be transferred to a general care floor on postoperative day 1. Patients are mobilized with physical therapy on postoperative days 1 through 3 and are discharged to home or to a skilled nursing facility between postoperative days 4 and 6.

At the institution of the authors of this chapter, a clinical care pathway has been developed to deliver optimal postoperative patient care. A clinical care pathway is an institution-specific tool that standardizes and optimizes care.[62] In general, clinical care pathways have been reported to reduce healthcare costs, increase efficiency, improve quality of care, reduce complications, and reduce hospital length of stay.[62-67] The authors of this chapter developed a lumbar spine fusion clinical care pathway that involves three key elements: (1) electronic order sets within a patient's electronic medical record; (2) review, clarification, and redesign of a patient's clinical care pathway, which is communicated to the patient, the patient's family, and staff; and (3) focused daily multidisciplinary communication channels. Initial data that have yet to be published suggest that this lumbar spine fusion clinical care pathway has reduced hospital length of stay and improved patient disposition.

Assessing Outcomes

Sethi et al[11] compared patients treated before and after the SSTP was implemented. Overall complication rates in the post-SSTP group were significantly lower compared with those in the pre-SSTP group (16% versus 52%, respectively; $P < 0.001$). Compared with the pre-SSTP group, the post-SSTP group had significantly lower return rates to the OR during the perioperative 90-day period (12.5% versus 0.8%, respectively; $P < 0.001$). In addition, compared with the pre-SSTP group, the post-SSTP group had lower rates of wound infection that required débridement (7.5% versus 1.6%, respectively), lower rates of deep vein thrombosis/pulmonary embolism (10% versus 3.2%, respectively), and lower rates of postoperative neurologic complications (2.5% versus 0.5%, respectively); however, these measures were not statistically significant. Compared with the pre-SSTP group, the post-SSTP group had dramatically lower rates of urinary tract infections that required antibiotics (32.5% versus 9.7%, respectively; $P < 0.001$).

Learning From Complications—Iterative Process Improvement

The SSTP is predicated on the principles of iterative continuous process improvement.[68] The hospital of the authors of this chapter uses a Lean process improvement system that is based on the Toyota production model.[69,70] Possible improvements to the SSTP that are identified by care team members are discussed and implemented if appropriate. To continue to improve the safety of patients who undergo complex spine surgery, all care team members are encouraged to provide input on the SSTP, which will be considered by the team. It is important to continually eliminate inefficiencies in the SSTP and arrange for the adequate provision of resources to ensure process timeliness (eg, the rapid provision of intraoperative laboratory test results). At regular points in time, a member of the complex spine surgery team conducts a review process that involves purposefully gathering information from all involved healthcare providers across the

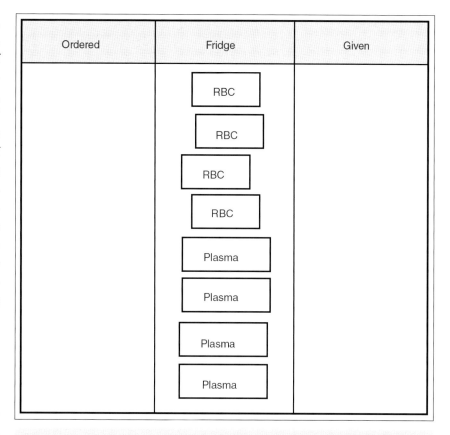

Figure 5   Example of a blood tracking board at the beginning of a complex spine procedure. According to the Seattle Spine Team Protocol, four units of packed red blood cells (RBCs) and four units of thawed plasma are kept in the refrigerator in the operating room. Thawed plasma is made available to avoid a delay if progressive consumptive coagulopathy occurs. As a unit is administered, the corresponding magnet is moved to the "Given" column. If additional blood products are ordered, additional magnets that represent the ordered units are added to the "Ordered" column. If the ordered product arrives in the operating room and is placed in the refrigerator, the corresponding magnet is moved to the "Fridge" column. This board provides the surgical team with visual control of the status of all blood products.

care process continuum. Perioperative data are constantly collected, tracked, and analyzed to generate insights into the efficiency and efficacy of the SSTP. A comprehensive constellation of variables is included in this tracking and analysis process. Results are regularly compared with and benchmarked against the most recent data published in the literature. Continuous improvement of the SSTP occurs by leveraging the ideas and insights of the broader hospital care team.

Summary

Current complication rates in adult spinal deformity surgery remain unacceptably high. Systems-based approaches can reduce complications and substantially mitigate risk. A clear multidisciplinary approach to complex spine surgery has been reported to reduce complications. A systematic multidisciplinary approach that integrates the entire patient-care experience is essential to ensure the highest quality and safety for patients who undergo complicated surgical procedures.

References

1. Rampersaud YR, Moro ER, Neary MA, et al: Intraoperative adverse events and related postoperative complications in spine surgery: Implications for enhancing patient safety founded on evidence-based protocols. *Spine (Phila Pa 1976)* 2006;31(13):1503-1510.

2. Bertram W, Harding I: Complications of spinal deformity and spinal stenosis surgery in adults greater than 50 years old. *J Bone Joint Surg Br* 2012; 94(supp X):105.

3. Booth KC, Bridwell KH, Lenke LG, Baldus CR, Blanke KM: Complications and predictive factors for the successful treatment of flatback deformity (fixed sagittal imbalance). *Spine (Phila Pa 1976)* 1999;24(16):1712-1720.

4. Cho SK, Bridwell KH, Lenke LG, et al: Major complications in revision adult deformity surgery: Risk factors and clinical outcomes with 2- to 7-year follow-up. *Spine (Phila Pa 1976)* 2012;37(6):489-500.

5. Daubs MD, Lenke LG, Cheh G, Stobbs G, Bridwell KH: Adult spinal deformity surgery: Complications and outcomes in patients over age 60. *Spine (Phila Pa 1976)* 2007;32(20):2238-2244.

6. Glassman SD, Hamill CL, Bridwell KH, Schwab FJ, Dimar JR, Lowe TG: The impact of perioperative complications on clinical outcome in adult deformity surgery. *Spine (Phila Pa 1976)* 2007;32(24):2764-2770.

7. Schwab FJ, Hawkinson N, Lafage V, et al: Risk factors for major perioperative complications in adult spinal deformity surgery: A multi-center review of 953 consecutive patients. *Eur Spine J* 2012;21(12):2603-2610.

8. Lenke LG, Fehlings MG, Schaffrey CI, Cheung KM, Carreon LY: Prospective, multicenter assessment of acute neurologic complications following complex adult spinal deformity surgery: The Scoli-Risk-1 Trial. *Spine J* 2013;13(9):S67.

9. Tormenti MJ, Maserati MB, Bonfield CM, et al: Perioperative surgical complications of transforaminal lumbar interbody fusion: A single-center experience. *J Neurosurg Spine* 2012;16(1):44-50.

10. Acosta FL Jr, McClendon J Jr, O'Shaughnessy BA, et al: Morbidity and mortality after spinal deformity surgery in patients 75 years and older: Complications and predictive factors. *J Neurosurg Spine* 2011;15(6):667-674.

11. Sethi RK, Pong RP, Leveque JC, Dean TC, Olivar SJ, Rupp SM: The Seattle Spine Team approach to adult deformity surgery: A systems-based approach to perioperative care and subsequent reduction in perioperative complication rates. *Spine Deform* 2014;2(2):95-103.

12. Haynes AB, Weiser TG, Berry WR, et al: A surgical safety checklist to reduce morbidity and mortality in a global population. *N Engl J Med* 2009;360(5):491-499.

13. Helmer KS, Robinson EK, Lally KP, et al: Standardized patient care guidelines reduce infectious morbidity in appendectomy patients. *Am J Surg* 2002;183(6):608-613.

14. Friedman SM, Mendelson DA, Kates SL, McCann RM: Geriatric co-management of proximal femur fractures: Total quality management and protocol-driven care result in better outcomes for a frail patient population. *J Am Geriatr Soc* 2008;56(7):1349-1356.

15. Halpin RJ, Sugrue PA, Gould RW, et al: Standardizing care for high-risk patients in spine surgery: The Northwestern high-risk spine protocol. *Spine (Phila Pa 1976)* 2010;35(25):2232-2238.

16. Fisher CG, Vaccaro AR, Whang PG, et al: Evidence-based recommendations for spine surgery. *Spine (Phila Pa 1976)* 2011;36(14):E897-E903.

17. Sugrue PA, Halpin RJ, Koski TR: Treatment algorithms and protocol practice in high-risk spine surgery. *Neurosurg Clin N Am* 2013;24(2):219-230.

18. Yadla S, Maltenfort MG, Ratliff JK, Harrop JS: Adult scoliosis surgery outcomes: A systematic review. *Neurosurg Focus* 2010;28(3):E3.

19. Akbarnia BA, Ogilvie JW, Hammerberg KW: Debate: Degenerative scoliosis. To operate or not to operate. *Spine (Phila Pa 1976)* 2006; 31(19, suppl):S195-S201.

20. Lee MJ, Hacquebord J, Varshney A, et al: Risk factors for medical complication after lumbar spine surgery: A multivariate analysis of 767 patients. *Spine (Phila Pa 1976)* 2011;36(21):1801-1806.

21. Kulkarni SS, Lowery GL, Ross RE, Ravi Sankar K, Lykomitros V: Arterial complications following anterior lumbar interbody fusion: Report of eight cases. *Eur Spine J* 2003;12(1):48-54.

22. Rajaraman V, Vingan R, Roth P, Heary RF, Conklin L, Jacobs GB: Visceral and vascular complications resulting from anterior lumbar interbody fusion. *J Neurosurg* 1999; 91(1, suppl):60-64.

23. Charosky S, Guigui P, Blamoutier A, Roussouly P, Chopin D; Study Group on Scoliosis: Complications and risk factors of primary adult scoliosis surgery: A multicenter study of 306 patients. *Spine (Phila Pa 1976)* 2012;37(8):693-700.

24. Sansur CA, Smith JS, Coe JD, et al: Scoliosis research society morbidity and mortality of adult scoliosis surgery. *Spine (Phila Pa 1976)* 2011;36(9):E593-E597.

25. Guay J, Haig M, Lortie L, Guertin MC, Poitras B: Predicting blood loss in surgery for idiopathic scoliosis. *Can J Anaesth* 1994;41(9):775-781.

26. Guay J, Reinberg C, Poitras B, et al: A trial of desmopressin to reduce blood loss in patients undergoing spinal fusion for idiopathic scoliosis. *Anesth Analg* 1992;75(3):405-410.

27. Phillips WA, Hensinger RN: Control of blood loss during scoliosis surgery. *Clin Orthop Relat Res* 1988;229:88-93.

28. Udén A, Nilsson IM, Willner S: Collagen-induced platelet aggregation and bleeding time in adolescent idiopathic scoliosis. *Acta Orthop Scand* 1980;51(5):773-777.

29. Yu X, Xiao H, Wang R, Huang Y: Prediction of massive blood loss in scoliosis surgery from preoperative variables. *Spine (Phila Pa 1976)* 2013;38(4):350-355.

30. Baldus CR, Bridwell KH, Lenke LG, Okubadejo GO: Can we safely reduce blood loss during lumbar pedicle subtraction osteotomy procedures

using tranexamic acid or aprotinin? A comparative study with controls. *Spine (Phila Pa 1976)* 2010;35(2):235-239.

31. Modi HN, Suh SW, Hong JY, Song SH, Yang JH: Intraoperative blood loss during different stages of scoliosis surgery: A prospective study. *Scoliosis* 2010;5:16.

32. Elgafy H, Bransford RJ, McGuire RA, Dettori JR, Fischer D: Blood loss in major spine surgery: Are there effective measures to decrease massive hemorrhage in major spine fusion surgery? *Spine (Phila Pa 1976)* 2010; 35(9, suppl):S47-S56.

33. Allen RT, Rihn JA, Glassman SD, Currier B, Albert TJ, Phillips FM: An evidence-based approach to spine surgery. *Am J Med Qual* 2009; 24(6, suppl):15S-24S.

34. Ames CP, Barry JJ, Keshavarzi S, Dede O, Weber MH, Deviren V: Perioperative outcomes and complications of pedicle subtraction osteotomy in cases with single versus two attending surgeons. *Spine Deform* 2013;1(1):51-58.

35. Baig MN, Lubow M, Immesoete P, Bergese SD, Hamdy EA, Mendel E: Vision loss after spine surgery: Review of the literature and recommendations. *Neurosurg Focus* 2007;23(5):E15.

36. Urban MK, Beckman J, Gordon M, Urquhart B, Boachie-Adjei O: The efficacy of antifibrinolytics in the reduction of blood loss during complex adult reconstructive spine surgery. *Spine (Phila Pa 1976)* 2001;26(10).1152-1156.

37. Beiner JM, Grauer J, Kwon BK, Vaccaro AR: Postoperative wound infections of the spine. *Neurosurg Focus* 2003;15(3):E14.

38. Fang A, Hu SS, Endres N, Bradford DS: Risk factors for infection after spinal surgery. *Spine (Phila Pa 1976)* 2005;30(12):1460-1465.

39. Schwab F, Ungar B, Blondel B, et al: Scoliosis Research Society-Schwab adult spinal deformity classification: A validation study. *Spine (Phila Pa 1976)* 2012;37(12):1077-1082.

40. Rabin R, de Charro F: EQ-5D: A measure of health status from the EuroQol Group. *Ann Med* 2001;33(5):337-343.

41. Jenkinson C, Coulter A, Wright L: Short form 36 (SF36) health survey questionnaire: Normative data for adults of working age. *BMJ* 1993;306(6890):1437-1440.

42. Rihn JA, Berven S, Allen T, et al: Defining value in spine care. *Am J Med Qual* 2009;24(6, suppl):4S-14S.

43. Sethi RK, Olivar SJ, Lavine S, et al: Poster No. 394. A multidisciplinary adult spinal deformity preoperative conference leads to a significant rejection rate. Presented at the 18th International Meeting on Advanced Spine Techniques (IMAST), Copenhagen, Denmark, July 13-16, 2011.

44. Drazin D, Shirzadi A, Rosner J, et al: Complications and outcomes after spinal deformity surgery in the elderly: Review of the existing literature and future directions. *Neurosurg Focus* 2011;31(4):E3.

45. Li G, Passias P, Kozanek M, et al: Adult scoliosis in patients over sixty-five years of age: Outcomes of operative versus nonoperative treatment at a minimum two-year follow-up. *Spine (Phila Pa 1976)* 2009;34(20):2165-2170.

46. Weiss HR, Goodall D: Rate of complications in scoliosis surgery - A systematic review of the Pub Med literature. *Scoliosis* 2008;3(9):9.

47. Sciubba DM, Yurter A, Smith JS, et al: A comprehensive review of complication rates after surgery for adult deformity: A reference for informed consent. *Spine Deform* 2015;3(6):575-594.

48. Eagle KA, Berger PB, Calkins H, et al: ACC/AHA guideline update for perioperative cardiovascular evaluation for noncardiac surgery— Executive summary: A report of the American College of Cardiology/ American Heart Association Task Force on Practice Guidelines (Committee to Update the 1996 Guidelines on Perioperative Cardiovascular Evaluation for Noncardiac Surgery). *J Am Coll Cardiol* 2002;39(3):542-553.

49. Jackson RP, Simmons EH, Stripinis D: Coronal and sagittal plane spinal deformities correlating with back pain and pulmonary function in adult idiopathic scoliosis. *Spine (Phila Pa 1976)* 1989;14(12):1391-1397.

50. Miller RD, Ward TA, Shiboski SC, Cohen NH: A comparison of three methods of hemoglobin monitoring in patients undergoing spine surgery. *Anesth Analg* 2011;112(4):858-863.

51. Fehlings MG, Brodke DS, Norvell DC, Dettori JR: The evidence for intraoperative neurophysiological monitoring in spine surgery: Does it make a difference? *Spine (Phila Pa 1976)* 2010;35(9, suppl):S37-S46.

52. Forbes HJ, Allen PW, Waller CS, et al: Spinal cord monitoring in scoliosis surgery: Experience with 1168 cases. *J Bone Joint Surg Br* 1991;73(3):487-491.

53. Langeloo DD, Lelivelt A, Louis Journée H, Slappendel R, de Kleuver M: Transcranial electrical motor-evoked potential monitoring during surgery for spinal deformity: A study of 145 patients. *Spine (Phila Pa 1976)* 2003;28(10):1043-1050.

54. Schwartz DM, Auerbach JD, Dormans JP, et al: Neurophysiological detection of impending spinal cord injury during scoliosis surgery. *J Bone Joint Surg Am* 2007;89(11):2440-2449.

55. Myers MA, Hamilton SR, Bogosian AJ, Smith CH, Wagner TA: Visual loss as a complication of spine surgery: A review of 37 cases. *Spine (Phila Pa 1976)* 1997;22(12):1325-1329.

56. Patil CG, Lad EM, Lad SP, Ho C, Boakye M: Visual loss after spine surgery: A population-based study. *Spine (Phila Pa 1976)* 2008;33(13):1491-1496.

57. Lee LA, Roth S, Posner KL, et al: The American Society of Anesthesiologists Postoperative Visual Loss Registry: Analysis of 93 spine surgery cases with postoperative visual loss. *Anesthesiology* 2006;105(4):652-659, quiz 867-868.

58. Verma K, Errico TJ, Vaz KM, Lonner BS: A prospective, randomized, double-blinded single-site control study comparing blood loss prevention of tranexamic acid (TXA) to epsilon aminocaproic acid (EACA) for corrective spinal surgery. *BMC Surg* 2010;10:13.

59. Raphael BG, Lackner H, Engler GL: Disseminated intravascular coagulation during surgery for scoliosis. *Clin Orthop Relat Res* 1982;162:41-46.

60. McClendon J Jr, O'shaughnessy BA, Smith TR, et al: Comprehensive assessment of prophylactic preoperative inferior vena cava filters for major spinal reconstruction in adults. *Spine (Phila Pa 1976)* 2012;37(13):1122-1129.

61. Dazley JM, Wain R, Vellinga RM, Cohen B, Agulnick MA: Prophylactic inferior vena cava filters prevent pulmonary embolisms in high-risk patients undergoing major spinal surgery. *J Spinal Disord Tech* 2012;25(4):190-195.

62. Campbell H, Hotchkiss R, Bradshaw N, Porteous M: Integrated care pathways. *BMJ* 1998;316(7125):133-137.

63. Stephen AE, Berger DL: Shortened length of stay and hospital cost reduction with implementation of an accelerated clinical care pathway after elective colon resection. *Surgery* 2003;133(3):277-282.

64. Archer SB, Burnett RJ, Flesch LV, et al: Implementation of a clinical pathway decreases length of stay and hospital charges for patients undergoing total colectomy and ileal pouch/anal anastomosis. *Surgery* 1997;122(4):699-705.

65. Pearson SD, Kleefield SF, Soukop JR, Cook EF, Lee TH: Critical pathways intervention to reduce length of hospital stay. *Am J Med* 2001;110(3):175-180.

66. Zehr KJ, Dawson PB, Yang SC, Heitmiller RF: Standardized clinical care pathways for major thoracic cases reduce hospital costs. *Ann Thorac Surg* 1998;66(3):914-919.

67. Rotter T, Kinsman L, James E, et al: Clinical pathways: Effects on professional practice, patient outcomes, length of stay and hospital costs. *Cochrane Database Syst Rev* 2010;3(3):CD006632.

68. Varkey P, Reller MK, Resar RK: Basics of quality improvement in health care. *Mayo Clin Proc* 2007;82(6):735-739.

69. Nelson-Peterson DL, Leppa CJ: Creating an environment for caring using lean principles of the Virginia Mason Production System. *J Nurs Adm* 2007;37(6):287-294.

70. Womack JP, Jones DT: *Lean Thinking: Banish Waste and Create Wealth in Your Corporation*, ed 2. New York, NY, Free Press, 2010.

Cervical Spine Injuries in the Athlete

Gregory D. Schroeder, MD

Alexander R. Vaccaro, MD, PhD, MBA

Abstract

Cervical spine injuries are common and range from relatively minor injuries, such as cervical muscle strains, to severe, life-threatening cervical fractures with spinal cord injuries. Although cervical spine injuries are most common in athletes who participate in contact and collision sports, such as rugby and American football, they also have been reported in athletes who participate in noncontact sports, such as baseball, gymnastics, and diving. Cervical spine injuries in athletes are not necessarily the result of substantial spine trauma; some athletes have chronic conditions, such as congenital stenosis, that increase their risk for a serious cervical spine injury after even minor trauma. Therefore, physicians who cover athletic events must have a thorough knowledge of cervical spine injures and the most appropriate methods for managing them. Although cervical spine injuries can be career-ending injuries, athletes often are able to return to play after appropriate treatment if the potential for substantial reinjury is minimized.

Instr Course Lect 2017;66:391–402.

Serious cervical spine injuries that result from athletic activity are rare; however, because cervical spine injuries can occur during almost any athletic event, including noncontact sports such as baseball, basketball, and gymnastics, physicians who cover any athletic event must have a thorough knowledge of the basic treatment principles for cervical spine injuries. Furthermore, although acute spinal cord injuries (SCIs) in athletes are rare, 2.4% of athletic-related hospitalizations are related to SCI,[1] and 9.2% of all SCIs in the United States are sustained during athletic activity.[2] Although muscle strains and soft-tissue contusions are the most common injuries observed in athletes,[1] all athletes in whom substantial cervical spine injury is suspected should be treated with spinal precautions and taken expeditiously to an SCI center for a complete evaluation given the possibility of a catastrophic injury if a cervical spine injury is missed.

Epidemiology

Cervical spine injuries that result from athletic activity most commonly occur in athletes younger than 30 years;[3,4] however, the exact mechanism of injury varies based on the regional popularity of different sports. In the United States, American football, wrestling, and gymnastics[3] are the most common sports in which cervical spine injuries are sustained. In Europe, rugby is the most common sport in which cervical

Dr. Schroeder or an immediate family member has received research or institutional support from Medtronic; and has received nonincome support (such as equipment or services), commercially derived honoraria, or other non-research–related funding (such as paid travel) from AOSpine and Medtronic. Dr. Vaccaro or an immediate family member has received royalties from Aesculap/B. Braun, Globus Medical, Medtronic, and Stryker; serves as a paid consultant to or is an employee of DePuy, Ellipse Technologies, Gerson Lehrman Group, Globus Medical, Guidepoint Global, Innovative Surgical Designs, MEDAcorp, Medtronic, Orthobullets, Stout Medical, and Stryker; has stock or stock options held in Advanced Spinal Intellectual Property, Avaz Surgical, Bonovo Orthopaedics, Computational Biodynamics, Cytonics, Dimension Prosthetics and Orthotics, ElectroCore Medical, Flagship Surgical, Flow Pharma, Gamma Spine, Globus Medical, InVivo Therapeutics, Innovative Surgical Designs, Location Based Intelligence, Paradigm Spine, Prime Surgeons, Progressive Spinal Technologies, Replication Medical, the Rothman Institute and related properties, Spine Medica, Spinology, Stout Medical, and VertiFlex; and serves as a board member, owner, officer, or committee member of AOSpine, the Association for Collaborative Spine Research, Flagship Surgical, Innovative Surgical Designs, and Prime Surgeons.

spine injuries are sustained, and in Canada, ice hockey is the most common sport in which cervical spine injuries are sustained.[4,5]

Cervical spine injuries are the most common injury to the axial skeleton in American football players; however, less than 1% of cervical spine injuries result in a cervical spine fracture or an SCI.[6] Although serious cervical spine injuries are relatively rare, 327 cervical SCIs (defined as any cervical spine fracture with concomitant neurologic symptoms) that resulted from American football were reported in the United States between 1977 and 2012. Of these 327 cervical SCIs, 8 occurred in athletes younger than high-school age, 266 occurred in high school athletes, 38 occurred in college athletes, and 15 occurred in professional athletes.[7]

The number of serious cervical spine injuries in American football players peaked in the 1960s, which correlates with the time at which players began tackling with the crown of their heads (spear tackling) and with the introduction of new helmet designs.[8] Recognizing the danger of spear tackling to both offensive and defensive players, spear tackling was banned in 1976; since then, the number of serious cervical spine injuries in American football players has markedly decreased.[8] Although the number of SCIs has decreased, cervical spine injuries are still common in American football players. In a study of the records of all 2,965 athletes who attended the National Football League (NFL) pre-draft Combine from 2003 to 2011, Schroeder et al[9] reported that a diagnosis of cervical spine disorder, pathology, or injury had been made in 4.8% of the athletes, with the three most common diagnoses being cervical spondylosis, cervical stenosis

(congenital, acquired, or a combination of both), and cervical herniated disk.

In Canada, 311 spinal column injuries and SCIs, 82.8% of which were cervical spine injuries, resulted from ice hockey between 1943 and 2005; these injuries were more common in males younger than 30 years.[4,10] These injuries most commonly occurred after skating into the boards (64.8%) and were most often the result of a player being pushed/checked from behind (35%).[4] Since 2001, the incidence of serious cervical spine injuries that result from ice hockey has dramatically decreased (69%). Tator et al[4] hypothesized that this decrease in the incidence of serious cervical spine injuries as a result of ice hockey is, in large part, the result of a rule change that prevents pushing/checking from behind as well as improved player and coach education.

Although cervical spine injuries that result from American football and ice hockey commonly occur during a structured athletic event, cervical spine injuries that result from other athletic activities often do not occur during organized practices and athletic events. Cervical spine injuries that result from diving more frequently occur during recreational diving than during competitive diving meets.[11,12] Similarly, cervical spine injuries that result from cycling are more common during recreational cycling than during competitive cycling.[13]

On-Field Management

Surgeons should exercise extreme caution in the initial evaluation of an athlete with a suspected cervical spine injury. Any athlete who sustains trauma to the cervical spine and reports cervical tenderness, pain, or decreased neck

range of motion should undergo a full neurologic examination. If a structural or neurologic injury other than a burner or stinger is suspected, the athlete's cervical spine should be immobilized with the use of a rigid cervical collar, and the athlete should be placed on a rigid backboard and transferred to the nearest SCI or trauma center. Although some studies have questioned the utility of a rigid backboard given its association with respiratory compromise, pain, and pressure sores in younger athletes,[14] the authors of this chapter believe that vigilant maintenance of spinal precautions supersedes these concerns. If an athlete is wearing a helmet, the facemask must be removed to gain access to the airway; however, to prevent unnecessary cervical spine movement, the rest of the helmet should remain in place until the athlete is in a controlled environment in which multiple individuals are available to aid in helmet removal.[8,15,16]

Cervical Spine Fractures and Dislocations
Upper Cervical Spine Fractures

Upper cervical spine fractures in athletes are rare. In a study of 196 high school and college American football players with cervical spine injuries, Boden et al[17] reported that only 9 (4.6%) of the cervical spine injuries occurred in the upper cervical spine. The sport most commonly associated with upper cervical spine injuries is mountain bicycling. In a study of 79 patients with cervical spine injuries that resulted from mountain bicycling, Dodwell et al[13] reported that approximately 17.7% of the cervical spine injuries were upper cervical spine fractures.

Because of the heterogeneity of upper cervical spine injuries, no single treatment algorithm is suitable for all athletes in whom these injuries occur. Highly unstable injuries, such as atlanto-occipital dissociations or injuries associated with C1-C2 instability, require surgical stabilization, whereas isolated C1 fractures without ligamentous disruption rarely require surgical management. Odontoid fractures are the most common upper cervical spine injury that occurs in athletes.[13] Because athletic injuries commonly occur in athletes younger than 30 years, most odontoid fractures can be managed with the use of a hard cervical collar or a halo vest.[18] However, odontoid screw fixation (**Figure 1**) or posterior C1-C2 arthrodesis should be considered in athletes with odontoid fractures that are associated with neurologic injury or odontoid fractures with more than 5 mm of displacement or 11° of angulation.[18] In addition, an increasing trend toward the management of type II odontoid fractures in younger athletes with the use of odontoid screw fixation rather than a hard cervical collar or a halo vest exists, even in the absence of substantial angulation or displacement.

Injuries to the Posterior Tension Band

Injuries to the posterior tension band are common athletic-related cervical spine injuries and often occur as a result of a substantial axial load across a slightly flexed neck.[16,17] In addition to disruption of the posterior tension band, injuries to the posterior tension band often are associated with a flexion-compression (teardrop) fragment, which is a small fracture of the antero-inferior vertebral body.[16,17,19] The most devastating injury to the posterior

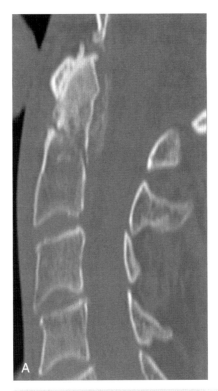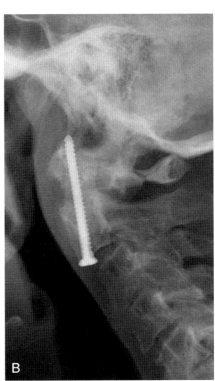

Figure 1 **A,** Sagittal CT scan of a spine with a type II odontoid fracture. **B,** Lateral radiograph of the spine shown in panel **A** taken after surgery with the use of an odontoid screw.

ligamentous complex is associated with bilateral facet dislocations. In a study of 36 rugby players with cervical spine fractures, MacLean and Hutchison[20] reported a substantial SCI in 90% of the rugby players who had a bilateral facet dislocation compared with only 58% of the rugby players who had other types of cervical spine injuries.

Surgical stabilization is necessary for almost all athletes in whom a posterior ligamentous complex injury is diagnosed (**Figure 2**). Facet fractures also can result in disruption of the posterior tension band; therefore, their management is controversial. The authors of this chapter recommend surgical stabilization for facet fractures that are displaced, greater than 1 cm in height, or involve more than 40% of the lateral mass.

Compression/Burst Fractures

Compression fractures, such as burst fractures, are another common cervical spine injury that occurs in athletes.[13,16,20] Compression fractures can occur if an athlete sustains an injury in which an axial force is transmitted across a neutrally aligned or slightly flexed cervical spine,[21] which results in an increase in intradiscal pressure and eventual failure of the vertebral body.[16] Compression fractures involve only the anterior column; therefore, compression fractures are never associated with neurologic injury. Burst fractures, however, involve the posterior vertebral wall; therefore, retropulsion of a burst fracture can lead to substantial neurologic sequelae. The incidence of neurologic injuries in athletes that result from a cervical burst fracture varies based on sport. MacLean

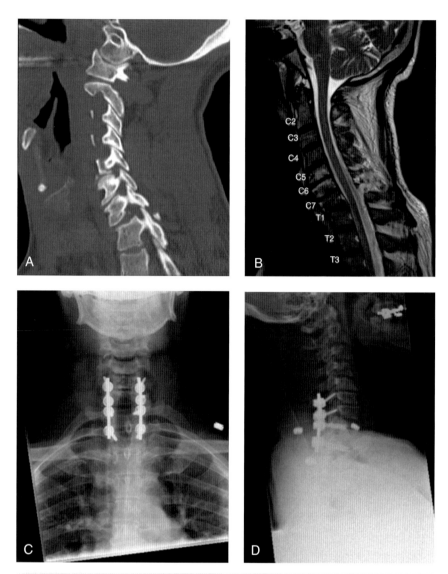

Figure 2 Images of the spine of a 25-year-old man who is a rugby player and who was neurologically intact after being thrown head first into the ground. Preoperative sagittal CT scan (**A**) and T2-weighted sagittal MRI (**B**) demonstrate a unilateral perched facet at C7-T1 with an associated facet fracture. AP (**C**) and lateral (**D**) radiographs taken after the patient underwent reduction and posterior cervical fusion from C6 through T2 demonstrate restoration of anatomic cervical spine alignment.

C7 burst fractures occur require close radiographic follow-up because early surgical intervention may be warranted. Similarly, cervical compression and burst fractures that result in substantial kyphosis or are associated with other fractures (such as facet fractures that are displaced, greater than 1 cm in height, or involve more than 40% of the lateral mass) also may require early surgical intervention.

Injuries to the Anterior Tension Band

Injuries to the anterior tension band/distraction-extension injuries in athletes are rare but often catastrophic.[23,24] These injuries occur after an accident in which an athlete's head is subjected to a large posteriorly directed force, which results in tensile failure of the anterior longitudinal ligament and the anterior anulus fibrosus.[21] In athletes with severe injuries to the anterior tension band/distraction-extension injuries, the superior vertebral body may translate posteriorly, which results in substantial SCI[25] (**Figure 4**).

Compared with injuries to the posterior tension band and compression fractures, substantially fewer athletes sustain injuries to the anterior tension band/distraction-extension injuries during athletic events. However, a cautious approach is warranted any time an athlete sustains a substantial hyperextension injury. Shelly et al[24] identified injuries to the anterior tension band/distraction-extension injuries in three rugby players, all of whom had an acute SCI. Because almost all injuries to the anterior tension band/distraction-extension injuries are unstable, the senior author of this chapter (A.R.V.) recommends that they be managed surgically.[25]

and Hutchison[13] reported no neurologic symptoms in rugby players who had a burst fracture; however, Dodwell et al[13] reported neurologic injury in 11 of 13 mountain bicyclists who had a cervical burst fracture.

Most isolated cervical compression and burst fractures that occur in athletes can be managed with the use of a hard cervical orthosis. Traditionally, surgical management is warranted only if neurologic injury or a concomitant injury to the posterior ligamentous complex exists[22] (**Figure 3**). The authors of this chapter have observed that younger athletes with C7 burst fractures have a high risk for substantial kyphotic deformity; therefore, athletes in whom

Return to Play After Cervical Spine Fracture

The decision to allow an athlete to return to play after a cervical spine fracture must be individualized based on the athlete and the sport. Currently, no high-level evidence is available to guide the return-to-play decision. All athletes who have persistent neurologic deficits should not return to athletic activity; however, many athletes with a united fracture or a solid fusion can return to athletic activity (**Table 1**). In addition to bony healing, athletes should have complete, painless cervical spine range of motion as well as full strength in the extremities and the neck muscles before returning to athletic activty.[26] Kepler and Vaccaro[26] proposed nine absolute contraindications to participation in intense athletic activity after cervical spine fracture: occipital-cervical arthrodesis, atlantoaxial instability, spear tackler's spine, residual subaxial spine instability, substantial sagittal malalignment, narrowing of the spinal canal as a result of retropulsed fragments, residual neurologic deficits, loss of cervical spine range of motion, and arthrodesis of three or more disk levels. Multiple other relative contraindications, such as upper cervical spine fracture that did not heal in the anatomic position; C1 ring fracture nonunion; two-level cervical arthrodesis; and congenital anomalies, such as os odontoideum, also have been proposed.[26]

Burners and Stingers

Burners and stingers are extremely common injuries in athletes, occurring in more than one-third of all rugby players during a single season and as many

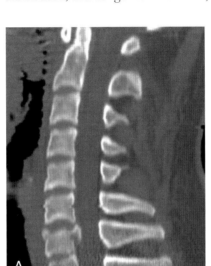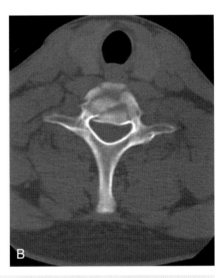

Figure 3 Sagittal (**A**) and axial (**B**) CT scans of the spine of a 30-year-old man who is a mountain bicyclist who was thrown from his bike and landed on the top of his head demonstrate a C7 burst fracture that was managed nonsurgically.

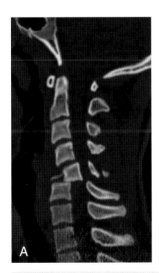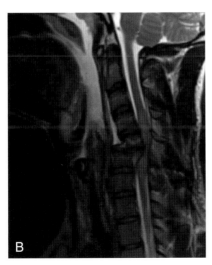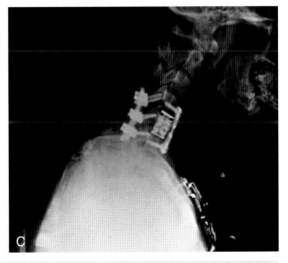

Figure 4 Images of the spine of a 19-year-old man who is a National Collegiate Athletic Association American football player who was injured during practice. Sagittal CT scan (**A**) and T2-weighted sagittal MRI (**B**) demonstrate a complete spinal cord injury. **C**, Lateral radiograph taken after the patient underwent an emergent C5 corpectomy and posterior fusion from C4 through C6 demonstrates decompression of the spinal canal and reconstruction of the vertebral column.

Table 1
Absolute and Relative Contraindications to Return to Play After Cervical Spine Fracture

Injury	Contraindication to Return to Play	Criteria for Return to Play
Any fracture associated with a residual neurologic deficit	Absolute	None
Any fracture in a patient with congenital stenosis	Absolute	None
Any fracture requiring occipital fusion	Absolute	None
Any fracture requiring C1-C2 fusion	Absolute	None
Any fracture requiring fusion of three or more levels	Absolute	None
Spear tackler's spine	Absolute	None
Minimally displaced C1 ring fracture	Relative	Solid union demonstrated on CT; no residual instability on flexion/extension radiographs; complete, painless range of motion of the cervical spine; and pre-injury muscle strength in the neck
C2 compression fracture	Relative	Solid union demonstrated on CT; no residual instability on flexion/extension radiographs; complete, painless range of motion of the cervical spine; and pre-injury muscle strength in the neck
All other upper cervical spine fractures managed nonsurgically	Relative	Solid union demonstrated on CT; no bony elements narrowing the spinal canal; no residual instability on flexion/extension radiographs; complete, painless range of motion of the cervical spine; and pre-injury muscle strength in the neck
Upper cervical spine fracture requiring surgical stabilization, excluding C1-C2 arthrodesis	Relative	Solid union or arthrodesis demonstrated on CT; no bony elements narrowing the spinal canal; no residual instability on flexion/extension radiographs; complete, painless range of motion of the cervical spine; and pre-injury muscle strength in the neck
Isolated compression fracture of the subaxial cervical spine	Relative	Solid union demonstrated on CT; no residual instability on flexion/extension radiographs; complete, painless range of motion of the cervical spine; and pre-injury muscle strength in the neck
Isolated stable burst fracture of the subaxial cervical spine	Relative	Solid union demonstrated on CT; no retropulsion of the fracture; no substantial sagittal malalignment (>11° compared with adjacent noninjured levels); no residual instability on flexion/extension radiographs; complete, painless range of motion of the cervical spine; and pre-injury muscle strength in the neck
Fracture disrupting the posterior bony (lateral mass or articular processes) or ligamentous tension band (excluding spinous or transverse process fractures) of the subaxial cervical spine	Relative	Solid union or arthrodesis demonstrated on CT; no bony fragments in the canal; no substantial sagittal malalignment (>11° compared with adjacent noninjured levels); surgical management involved fusion of less than three segments; no residual instability on flexion/extension radiographs; complete, painless range of motion of the cervical spine; and pre-injury muscle strength in the neck
Subaxial spinous process fracture	No	Complete, painless range of motion of the cervical spine and pre-injury muscle strength in the neck The presence of multiple contiguous spinous process fractures is not a further contraindication, but the presence of multiple fractures will likely necessitate a longer recovery until the patient has complete, painless range of motion
Transverse process fracture of the subaxial spine	No	Complete, painless range of motion of the cervical spine and pre-injury muscle strength in the neck

Reproduced from Schroeder G, Vaccaro A: Fractures of the cervical spine and spinal cord injuries, in Hecht A, ed: *Spine Injuries in Athletes*. Rosemont, IL, American Academy of Orthopaedic Surgeons, 2017, forthcoming.

as 65% of all college American football players during their 4-year college career.[27,28] Whether burners/stingers are the result of injury to the brachial plexus or the exiting cervical nerve root is a subject of debate in the literature.[29-32] Three major mechanisms of injury for athletes who sustain burners/stingers have been proposed: traction injury to the brachial plexus, which may occur after a lateral impact to the head causes contralateral lateral neck flexion and ipsilateral depression of the shoulder; direct compression of the brachial plexus at the Erb point; and compression of the exiting cervical nerve root in the neural foramen after the neck is forced into extension and lateral bending.[29-32]

The theory that burners/stingers are caused by compression of the exiting cervical nerve root in the neural foramen is largely based on a study by Meyer et al.[31] The authors reported that college American football players who had a Torg-Pavlov ratio[33] (**Figure 5**) less than 0.80 were three times more likely to sustain a burner/stinger compared with athletes who had a Torg-Pavlov ratio greater than 0.80.[31] Similarly, Kelly et al[29] reported that high school American football players with a history of burners/stingers had a significantly smaller Torg-Pavlov ratio compared with age-matched controls (0.88 versus 0.94, respectively; $P = 0.02$). Conversely, Clancy et al[34] reported brachial plexus axonotmesis on the electromyograms of 10 of 13 athletes who had burners/stingers, and Markey et al[30] consistently reported brachial plexus abnormalities in the nerve conduction velocity studies of 17 athletes with burners/stingers.

The reason for this discrepancy in the literature is likely because two different mechanisms of injury for burners/stingers exist: acute burners/stingers

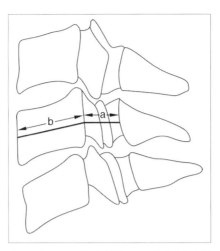

Figure 5 Illustration of part of a spine shows the Torg-Pavlov ratio, which is calculated by dividing the AP diameter of the spinal canal (a) by the AP diameter of the vertebral body (b) as measured on lateral extension radiographs. (Redrawn with permission from Torg JS, Pavlov H, Genuario SE, et al: Neurapraxia of the cervical spinal cord with transient quadriplegia. *J Bone Joint Surg Am* 1986;68[9]:1354-1370.)

result from injury to the brachial plexus, and chronic burner/stinger syndrome results from degenerative changes that narrow the neural foramen, which compresses the exiting cervical nerve root.[27] In a study of 55 athletes with burners/stingers, Levitz et al[27] reported that 93% of the athletes had advanced cervical spondylosis and neural foramen narrowing. Similarly, in a retrospective study of 103 athletes who attended the NFL pre-draft Combine, Presciutti et al[32] reported that the mean subaxial cervical space available for the cord (MSCSAC; **Figure 6**) was narrower in athletes who had chronic burners/stingers compared with athletes without chronic burners/stingers ($P < 0.01$). The authors reported that a MSCSAC of 5.0 mm or smaller had a sensitivity of 80% and a negative likelihood ratio of 0.23 for the prediction of chronic

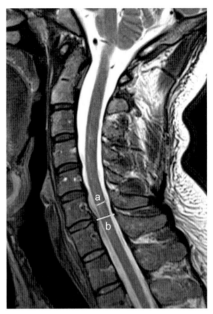

Figure 6 Sagittal T2-weighted MRI shows the mean subaxial cervical space available for the cord, which is calculated by subtracting the diameter of the spinal cord (a) from the diameter of the spinal canal (b) at the intervertebral disk level.

burners/stingers, and that a MSCSAC of 4.3 mm or smaller had a specificity of 96% and a positive likelihood ratio of 13.25 for prediction of recurrent burners/stingers.[32]

Regardless of the etiology, athletes with burners/stingers experience sudden pain and paresthesias in a single extremity that often is nondermatomal and may or may not be associated with weakness. Without intervention, symptoms should resolve in a short amount of time. Often, athletes will experience complete resolution of the symptoms caused by burners/stingers; these athletes may return to play if they have full strength and full range of motion.[35] However, many surgeons recommend a full neurologic workup for all athletes who sustain burners/stingers and do not allow athletes to return to play for the remainder of the season if they have sustained three or more burners/stingers within 1 year.[26,35] Surgeons must rule out transient cervical cord neurapraxia in athletes with a suspected burner/stinger. Any time an injury involves more than one extremity or symptoms do not rapidly and spontaneously resolve, the athlete should be transferred to the nearest SCI or trauma center for a thorough neurologic evaluation and workup.

Cervical Spine Stenosis

The safety of athletes with cervical spine stenosis who participate in athletic activity, particularly contact sports, is unclear. Schroeder et al[9] identified 10 athletes with absolute cervical spine stenosis (midsagittal diameter <10 mm) who attended the NFL pre-draft Combine and, despite such a diagnosis, were eventually drafted into the NFL. None of these athletes sustained an SCI in the NFL; however, cervical spine stenosis has repeatedly been reported to be associated with an increased risk for acute SCI.[33,36] Using multiple different imaging parameters, Aebli et al[36] compared the size of the spinal canals of 53 patients who had minor cervical spine injury and an associated SCI with those of 184 patients with minor cervical spine injury and no SCI. The authors reported that the patients with an SCI had a significantly smaller spinal canal compared with the patients without SCI. In addition, the authors reported that the midsagittal intervertebral disk space diameter was the most useful measurement for the prediction of SCI. A midsagittal intervertebral disk space diameter of 8 mm or smaller had a positive predictive value of 84% and a positive likelihood ratio of 15.6 for an SCI after minor cervical spine trauma.

Although some studies have proposed that asymptomatic athletes with an incidental diagnosis of cervical spine stenosis should be allowed to participate in contact sports,[9,26] these athletes have an increased risk for SCI and must be counseled on the risks of participation in athletic activity before returning to play. The authors of this chapter believe that any athlete with absolute cervical spine stenosis who has even a transient neurologic deficit or sensory disturbance should seriously consider not participating in contact sports.

In addition to permanent neurologic injury from SCI, athletes with cervical spine stenosis also have an increased risk for cervical cord neurapraxia (transient quadriparesis). Torg et al[37] identified 32 athletes who had an episode of transient quadriparesis and 17 athletes in whom congenital stenosis was observed on radiographs. The remaining 15 athletes all demonstrated evidence of congenital anomalies (such as Klippel-Feil syndrome), cervical disk herniation, or ligamentous instability. In a recent study of 10 athletes with transient quadriparesis, Bailes[38] reported that all of the athletes had cervical stenosis with a midsagittal diameter smaller than 12 mm at three or more disk levels. None of the athletes had evidence of myelomalacia, and none of the athletes underwent surgical decompression. Four of the athletes returned to professional American football, three of whom experienced no recurrent neurologic symptoms, and one of whom experienced three additional episodes of transient quadriparesis before he retired. Similarly, in a study of four professional athletes (three American football players and one basketball player) with transient quadriparesis, Brigham and Capo[39] reported that all of the athletes

underwent one-level anterior cervical diskectomy and fusion (ACDF) at the level of stenosis. Although all of the athletes initially returned to play, two of the athletes experienced a second episode of transient quadriparesis that occurred at an adjacent level within 2 years. The available literature on transient quadriparesis is limited; however, because of the high rate of recurrent symptoms (25% to 50%) observed in athletes who have transient quadriparesis, the authors of this chapter recommend against returning to athletic activity despite the opinion of many experts who consider recurrent symptoms a relative contraindication to return to play.

Cervical Disk Herniation

Cervical disk herniations in athletes, particularly those who participate in contact sports such as American football and rugby, are common[5,9,40-44] (**Table 2**). The symptoms of cervical disk herniation range from radicular pain to acute onset myelopathy to transient quadriparesis.[5,9,40-43] Using the NFL's Sports Injury Monitoring System, Gray et al[40] performed a retrospective analysis of 61 NFL players in whom a cervical disk herniation occurred between August 8, 2000, and January 5, 2012. The authors reported that linebackers (18%) and defensive backs (16%) were the NFL players in whom a cervical disk herniation most commonly occurred. Interestingly, C3-C4 (23%) and C5-C6 (23%) were the two most common disk levels that were affected in this patient population; comparatively, C6-C7 is the most common disk level that is affected in the general population. Unfortunately, the NFL's Sports Injury Monitoring System does not allow for the identification of individual

Table 2

Results of Treatment in Athletes With a Herniated Cervical Disk

Authors (Year)	Number of Patients	Sport	Procedure	Mean Patient Age in Years (Range)	Mean Follow-Up (Range)	Results
Andrews et al[5] (2008)	19	Professional rugby	One- or two-level ACDF for persistent cervical radiculopathy	28 (22–37)	17 mo (7 mo–5 yr)	14 patients returned to play 17 patients had partial or full resolution of symptoms
Hsu[41] (2011)	99	Professional American football	Surgical treatment (53); nonsurgical treatment (46)	Surgical, 28.4 (NR) Nonsurgical, 29.3 (NR)	10.4 yr (NR)	Patients who underwent surgical treatment were significantly more likely to return to play compared with patients who underwent nonsurgical treatment (72% versus 46%, P < 0.04); however, no difference in performance was reported based on treatment in the athletes who did return to play
Roberts et al[44] (2011)	11	Professional baseball	One-level ACDF (7); total disk arthroplasty (1); nonsurgical treatment (3)	30.7 (NR)	44 mo (NR)	7 of 8 patients who underwent surgical treatment returned to play; 1 of 3 patients who underwent nonsurgical treatment returned to play
Gray et al[40] (2013)	61	Professional American football	NR	NR	NR	Athletes missed a mean 93 days of play after injury
Maroon et al[42] (2013)	15	Professional American football (7); professional wrestling (8)	One-level ACDF	30.3 (22–40) Football, 31.3 (22–36) Wrestling, 29.0 (22–40)	NR	5 professional American football players returned to play; adjacent segment disease developed in 1 professional American football player who required a second ACDF All 8 professional wrestlers returned to play
Meredith et al[43] (2013)	16	Professional American football	One-level ACDF (3); nonsurgical treatment (13)	26.6 (20–31)	NR	1 of 3 patients who underwent surgical treatment returned to play; 8 of the 13 patients who underwent nonsurgical treatment returned to play
Schroeder et al[9] (2014)	27	Professional American football	Nonsurgical treatment (23); one-level ACDF (4)	NR	NR	Athletes with a previous herniated disk had no difference in career longevity or performance compared with matched control patients

ACDF = anterior cervical diskectomy and fusion, NR = not reported.

athletes; therefore, the authors were unable to determine the effect of cervical disk herniation on player performance.

Using public records, Hsu[41] identified 99 NFL players in whom a cervical disk herniation occurred during a 30-year period. Fifty-three players underwent surgical treatment, and 46 players underwent nonsurgical treatment. The authors reported that the players who underwent surgical treatment were significantly more likely to return to professional American football compared with the players who underwent nonsurgical treatment (72% versus 46%, respectively; P < 0.04). However, in the athletes who returned to professional American football, the authors reported no difference with regard to position-specific performance scores or the number of games started between

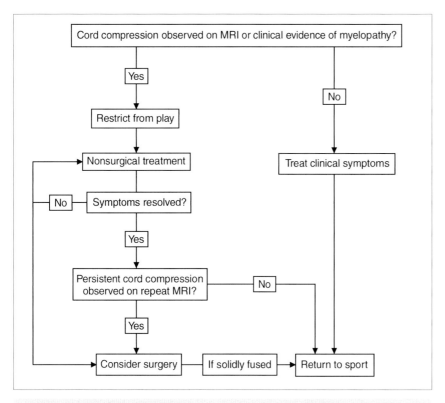

Figure 7 Return-to-play algorithm proposed by Meredith et al[43] for athletes with a herniated disk. Surgery is only considered for symptomatic patients. (Adapted with permission from Meredith DS, Jones KJ, Barnes R, Rodeo SA, Cammisa FP, Warren RF: Operative and nonoperative treatment of cervical disc herniation in National Football League athletes. *Am J Sports Med* 2013;41[9]:2054-2058.)

the athletes who underwent surgical treatment and the athletes who underwent nonsurgical treatment. Similarly, Schroeder et al[9] reported that asymptomatic athletes with a history of cervical disk herniation who attended the NFL pre-draft Combine demonstrated no difference with regard to the number of years played, number of games played, number of games started, or performance score ($P > 0.31$) in a comparison with matched controls without a history of a cervical disk herniation.

In a study of 16 NFL players with symptomatic cervical disk herniation who belonged to a single team, Meredith et al[43] reported that the most common symptom was isolated cervical radiculopathy, which occurred in 9 players;

however, 3 players had transient quadriparesis. Surgical treatment was recommended for all of the five players who had spinal cord compression; however, only three of the five players underwent ACDF. Two players decided to retire rather than undergo surgical treatment. Only one of the three players who underwent surgical treatment returned to play professional American football. Eight of the 13 players who underwent nonsurgical treatment returned to play professional American football.[43]

Because substantial disagreement exists in the literature with regard to whether surgical or nonsurgical treatment in American football players who have a cervical disk herniation leads to an increased return-to-play rate,[41,43] no

universally accepted treatment algorithm exists for athletes who have isolated radicular symptoms as a result of a cervical disk herniation. Few studies, however, would disagree that athletes who have persistent symptomatic spinal cord compression should undergo surgical treatment before returning to athletic activity (**Figure 7**). If an athlete requires surgical treatment, multiple studies have demonstrated the safety of returning to contact sports after one-level ACDF. In a study of 15 professional athletes (7 NFL players and 8 professional wrestlers) with cervical disk herniation who underwent one-level ACDF, Maroon et al[42] reported that 13 of the professional athletes were able to return to athletic activity. Before resuming athletic activity, all of the athletes had a solid fusion, full neck range of motion, and a normal neurologic examination. Similarly, in a study of 19 professional rugby players with persistent cervical radiculopathy who underwent ACDF, 17 of whom underwent one-level fusion and two of whom underwent two-level fusion, Andrews et al[5] reported that 13 of the players who underwent one-level fusion returned to rugby, and one of the players who underwent two-level fusion returned to rugby. The safety of athletes returning to contact sports after multilevel fusion is not well established in the literature. Commonly, three-level ACDF is considered an absolute contraindication to athletic activity, and two-level ACDF is considered a relative contraindication to athletic activity.[26]

Spear Tackler's Spine

Spear tackler's spine is a diagnosis that is unique to athletes who play American football. Spear tackler's spine occurs if an athlete repeatedly tackles with the crown of the head, which results in repetitive axial loads through a semiflexed spine.[19] The repeated force through the spine results in a loss of normal cervical lordosis, vertebral body abnormalities, and, eventually, cervical stenosis.[45] Although spear tackling is illegal in American football, physicians should be aware of the diagnosis because athletes with a diagnosis of spear tackler's spine have an increased risk for serious neurologic injuries and should not be permitted to participate in athletic activity.[45]

Summary

Cervical spine injuries are relatively common injuries in athletes and range from muscle sprains to complete SCIs. Physicians who cover athletic events should treat all athletes in whom a cervical spine injury is suspected with caution because a missed cervical spine injury can lead to a catastrophic neurologic outcome. Any athlete in whom a substantial cervical spine injury is suspected should be removed from athletic activity and taken expeditiously to an SCI or trauma center for a complete neurologic evaluation. Fortunately, most cervical spine injuries in athletes do not preclude participation in future athletic activity.

References

1. Nalliah RP, Anderson IM, Lee MK, Rampa S, Allareddy V, Allareddy V: Epidemiology of hospital-based emergency department visits due to sports injuries. *Pediatr Emerg Care* 2014;30(8):511-515.

2. UAB Spinal Cord Injury Model System Information Network: The UAB-SCIMS Information Network. University of Alabama School of Medicine, 2013. Available at: http://www.spinalcord.uab.edu. Accessed August 2014.

3. Bailes JE, Hadley MN, Quigley MR, Sonntag VK, Cerullo LJ: Management of athletic injuries of the cervical spine and spinal cord. *Neurosurgery* 1991;29(4):491-497.

4. Tator CH, Provvidenza C, Cassidy JD: Spinal injuries in Canadian ice hockey: An update to 2005. *Clin J Sport Med* 2009;19(6):451-456.

5. Andrews J, Jones A, Davies PR, Howes J, Ahuja S: Is return to professional rugby union likely after anterior cervical spinal surgery? *J Bone Joint Surg Br* 2008;90(5):619-621.

6. Mall NA, Buchowski J, Zebala L, Brophy RH, Wright RW, Matava MJ: Spine and axial skeleton injuries in the National Football League. *Am J Sports Med* 2012;40(8):1755-1761.

7. Mueller FO, Cantu RC: *Annual Survey of Catastrophic Football Injuries: 1977-2012,* 2015. Available at: http://nccsir.unc.edu/files/2014/05/FBAnnual2012.pdf. Accessed September 15, 2015.

8. Bailes JE, Petschauer M, Guskiewicz KM, Marano G: Management of cervical spine injuries in athletes. *J Athl Train* 2007;42(1):126-134.

9. Schroeder GD, Lynch TS, Gibbs DB, et al: The impact of a cervical spine diagnosis on the careers of National Football League athletes. *Spine (Phila Pa 1976)* 2014;39(12):947-952.

10. Tator CH, Provvidenza CF, Lapczak L, Carson J, Raymond D: Spinal injuries in Canadian ice hockey: Documentation of injuries sustained from 1943-1999. *Can J Neurol Sci* 2004;31(4):460-466.

11. Aito S, D'Andrea M, Werhagen L: Spinal cord injuries due to diving accidents. *Spinal Cord* 2005;43(2):109-116.

12. Tator CH, Edmonds VE, New ML: Diving: A frequent and potentially preventable cause of spinal cord injury. *Can Med Assoc J* 1981;124(10):1323-1324.

13. Dodwell ER, Kwon BK, Hughes B, et al: Spinal column and spinal cord injuries in mountain bikers: A 13-year review. *Am J Sports Med* 2010;38(8):1647-1652.

14. White CC IV, Domeier RM, Millin MG; Standards and Clinical Practice Committee, National Association of EMS Physicians: EMS spinal precautions and the use of the long backboard: Resource document to the position statement of the National Association of EMS Physicians and the American College of Surgeons Committee on Trauma. *Prehosp Emerg Care* 2014;18(2):306-314.

15. Anderson A, Tollefson B, Cohen R, Johnson J, Summers RL: A comparative study of American football helmet removal techniques using a cadaveric model of cervical spine injury. *J Miss State Med Assoc* 2011;52(4):103-105.

16. Banerjee R, Palumbo MA, Fadale PD: Catastrophic cervical spine injuries in the collision sport athlete, part 1: Epidemiology, functional anatomy, and diagnosis. *Am J Sports Med* 2004;32(4):1077-1087.

17. Boden BP, Tacchetti RL, Cantu RC, Knowles SB, Mueller FO: Catastrophic cervical spine injuries in high school and college football players. *Am J Sports Med* 2006;34(8):1223-1232.

18. Hsu WK, Anderson PA: Odontoid fractures: Update on management. *J Am Acad Orthop Surg* 2010;18(7):383-394.

19. Torg JS, Pavlov H, O'Neill MJ, Nichols CE Jr, Sennett B: The axial load teardrop fracture: A biomechanical, clinical and roentgenographic analysis. *Am J Sports Med* 1991;19(4):355-364.

20. MacLean JG, Hutchison JD: Serious neck injuries in U19 rugby union players: An audit of admissions to spinal injury units in Great Britain and Ireland. *Br J Sports Med* 2012;46(8):591-594.

21. Allen BL Jr, Ferguson RL, Lehmann TR, O'Brien RP: A mechanistic classification of closed, indirect fractures and dislocations of the lower cervical spine. *Spine (Phila Pa 1976)* 1982;7(1):1-27.

22. Vaccaro AR, Hulbert RJ, Patel AA, et al: The subaxial cervical spine injury classification system: A novel approach to recognize the importance of morphology, neurology, and integrity of the disco-ligamentous complex. *Spine (Phila Pa 1976)* 2007;32(21):2365-2374.

23. Rihn JA, Anderson DT, Lamb K, et al: Cervical spine injuries in American football. *Sports Med* 2009;39(9):697-708.

24. Shelly MJ, Butler JS, Timlin M, Walsh MG, Poynton AR, O'Byrne JM: Spinal injuries in Irish rugby: A ten-year review. *J Bone Joint Surg Br* 2006;88(6):771-775.

25. Vaccaro AR, Klein GR, Thaller JB, Rushton SA, Cotler JM, Albert TJ: Distraction extension injuries of the cervical spine. *J Spinal Disord* 2001;14(3):193-200.

26. Kepler CK, Vaccaro AR: Injuries and abnormalities of the cervical spine and return to play criteria. *Clin Sports Med* 2012;31(3):499-508.

27. Levitz CL, Reilly PJ, Torg JS: The pathomechanics of chronic, recurrent cervical nerve root neurapraxia: The chronic burner syndrome. *Am J Sports Med* 1997;25(1):73-76.

28. Kawasaki T, Ota C, Yoneda T, et al: Incidence of stingers in young rugby players. *Am J Sports Med* 2015;43(11):2809-2815.

29. Kelly JD IV, Aliquo D, Sitler MR, Odgers C, Moyer RA: Association of burners with cervical canal and foraminal stenosis. *Am J Sports Med* 2000;28(2):214-217.

30. Markey KL, Di Benedetto M, Curl WW: Upper trunk brachial plexopathy: The stinger syndrome. *Am J Sports Med* 1993;21(5):650-655.

31. Meyer SA, Schulte KR, Callaghan JJ, et al: Cervical spinal stenosis and stingers in collegiate football players. *Am J Sports Med* 1994;22(2):158-166.

32. Presciutti SM, DeLuca P, Marchetto P, Wilsey JT, Shaffrey C, Vaccaro AR: Mean subaxial space available for the cord index as a novel method of measuring cervical spine geometry to predict the chronic stinger syndrome in American football players. *J Neurosurg Spine* 2009;11(3):264-271.

33. Pavlov H, Torg JS, Robie B, Jahre C: Cervical spinal stenosis: Determination with vertebral body ratio method. *Radiology* 1987;164(3):771-775.

34. Clancy WG Jr, Brand RL, Bergfield JA: Upper trunk brachial plexus injuries in contact sports. *Am J Sports Med* 1977;5(5):209-216.

35. Weinberg J, Rokito S, Silber JS: Etiology, treatment, and prevention of athletic "stingers". *Clin Sports Med* 2003;22(3):493-500, viii.

36. Aebli N, Rüegg TB, Wicki AG, Petrou N, Krebs J: Predicting the risk and severity of acute spinal cord injury after a minor trauma to the cervical spine. *Spine J* 2013;13(6):597-604.

37. Torg JS, Pavlov H, Genuario SE, et al: Neurapraxia of the cervical spinal cord with transient quadriplegia. *J Bone Joint Surg Am* 1986;68(9):1354-1370.

38. Bailes JE: Experience with cervical stenosis and temporary paralysis in athletes. *J Neurosurg Spine* 2005;2(1):11-16.

39. Brigham CD, Capo J: Cervical spinal cord contusion in professional athletes: A case series with implications for return to play. *Spine (Phila Pa 1976)* 2013;38(4):315-323.

40. Gray BL, Buchowski JM, Bumpass DB, Lehman RA Jr, Mall NA, Matava MJ: Disc herniations in the National Football League. *Spine (Phila Pa 1976)* 2013;38(22):1934-1938.

41. Hsu WK: Outcomes following nonoperative and operative treatment for cervical disc herniations in National Football League athletes. *Spine (Phila Pa 1976)* 2011;36(10):800-805.

42. Maroon JC, Bost JW, Petraglia AL, et al: Outcomes after anterior cervical discectomy and fusion in professional athletes. *Neurosurgery* 2013;73(1):103-112.

43. Meredith DS, Jones KJ, Barnes R, Rodeo SA, Cammisa FP, Warren RF: Operative and nonoperative treatment of cervical disc herniation in National Football League athletes. *Am J Sports Med* 2013;41(9):2054-2058.

44. Roberts DW, Roc GJ, Hsu WK: Outcomes of cervical and lumbar disk herniations in Major League Baseball pitchers. *Orthopedics* 2011;34(8):602-609.

45. Torg JS, Sennett B, Pavlov H, Leventhal MR, Glasgow SG: Spear tackler's spine: An entity precluding participation in tackle football and collision activities that expose the cervical spine to axial energy inputs. *Am J Sports Med* 1993;21(5):640-649.

Lumbar Spine Injuries in the Athlete

Dustin H. Massel, BS

Kern Singh, MD

Abstract

Low back pain is the most common complaint expressed by adult patients in the primary care setting, and the incidence of low back pain in adolescents is rising. Adolescents who are involved in athletics most commonly suffer from spondylolysis, spondylolisthesis, mechanical low back pain, and herniated disks, whereas adult athletes most commonly suffer from lumbosacral strain and herniated or degenerative disks. Initial nonsurgical management aims to reduce inflammation and noninvasively strengthen damaged tissues. Although most patients who have low back pain will return to sports after nonsurgical treatment, surgery may be required in patients who have persistent or progressive neurologic symptoms.

Instr Course Lect 2017;66:403–408.

Approximately 60% to 80% of the general population will experience low back pain (LBP) at some point in their lives. Acute muscular or ligamentous strain of the lumbar spine will be diagnosed in approximately 70% of individuals who have LBP.[1-4] LBP is the most common type of pain reported by adult patients and, in general, is the result of acutely debilitating issues that resolve with nonsurgical treatment, such as rest, avoidance of the inciting activity, cold compression therapy, and over-the-counter anti-inflammatory drugs. In contrast to the general population, individuals who participate in sports suffer more severe injuries, most commonly to the cervical or lumbar spine, and require additional therapeutic measures.[5] Despite an overwhelming focus on full-contact sports (such as football, rugby, and hockey), low-contact and no-contact sports (such as soccer, basketball, volleyball, golf, figure skating, gymnastics,[6] and dance) also have led to substantial sports-related spine injuries that contribute to the increasing prevalence of LBP. Surgeons should have a thorough knowledge of the epidemiology, risk factors, and functional anatomy of lumbar spine injuries in athletes and understand how they can be managed, both surgically and nonsurgically.

Epidemiology and Risk Factors

Participation in sports is the fourth most common cause of spine injury (after motor vehicle accidents, falls, and violence), accounting for 9% to 15% of spine injuries annually.[2,6] Adolescents and young adults (most often those aged 13 to 14 years) often have nonspecific LBP that is incorrectly diagnosed as muscular or ligamentous strain.[7] Several studies have reported an increasing prevalence of LBP with age, with 11% to 71% of adolescents experiencing LBP by age 17 years.[3,7-10] These studies also reported that LBP will limit physical activity or interfere with schoolwork at any point in time in one-third of adolescents in whom LBP is experienced, and only one-fourth of adolescent patients who have LBP will seek medical treatment.[1,3,7-10]

Studies on the clinical presentation of adolescent patients with LBP have elucidated several kinetic and anatomic features that are associated with LBP. Fairbank et al[11] reported that LBP was associated with reduced lower extremity mobility, decreased hip and knee rotation, increased weight, and increased trunk length. The authors hypothesized that reduced lower extremity mobility leads to greater stress on the lumbar spine during physical activity, which results in LBP.[11,12] Mierau et al[12] reported that LBP was associated with a reduced straight leg raise and male sex; however, the authors were unable to determine whether a reduced straight leg raise was the result of nerve root irritation or reduced hamstring flexibility. Harreby et al[9] demonstrated similar findings and reported that LBP was associated with increased participation in competitive sports in boys and lifting or carrying heavy loads in a work environment.

Although it is known that numerous factors can cause or contribute to LBP in the general population, several studies have examined the etiology of LBP in athletes. Salminen et al[7] reported that approximately 50% of 14-year-old eighth grade students who experienced LBP could recall a specific incident from a sporting event that led to their symptoms. The authors hypothesized that the incidence of LBP in this population may have been a result of the timing of the study in conjunction with the adolescent growth spurt of the study's subjects and their involvement in activities that placed greater stress on the spine; however, this hypothesis was not examined further. Changstrom et al[13] reported

an increased risk for stress fractures in female athletes compared with male athletes, with the greatest risk for lumbar injury associated with participation in volleyball, football, and soccer. Although female athletes have a higher risk for stress fractures compared with male athletes, LBP is more frequently reported in boys than in girls.[3] In a study on spine injuries in dancers, Gottschlich and Young[14] reported that several common dance movements place the lumbar spine in hyperlordosis and predispose dancers to spondylolysis, spondylolisthesis, facet joint strain, piriformis syndrome, discogenic pain, and muscle spasms. Similarly, Kruse and Lemmen[6] examined LBP in gymnasts. Gymnastics requires flexibility, body holds that are physically demanding, and irregular body positioning that produces various amounts of hyperflexion, hyperextension, and traction or retraction forces, all of which increase a gymnast's risk for several pathologic processes. The authors reported that gymnasts have higher risk for bilateral pars defects and spondylolysis, spondylolisthesis, disk height reduction, thoracolumbar disk degeneration, bulging and herniated disks, and Schmorl nodes, all of which can result in LBP.[6]

Spinal health deteriorates with age. The replacement of muscle fibers with fat and fibrotic tissue reduces an individual's overall muscle mass at a rate of 1.25% per year after age 35 years, with more rapid muscle mass reduction after age 70 years.[4] Muscle mass reduction results in reduced vertebral stability and reduced maintenance of proper alignment, which causes progressive spinal deformity, scoliosis, and kyphosis. Facet osteoarthropathy and spinal stenosis in combination with degeneration of the intervertebral disks and a reduction in

bone mass (osteopenia or osteoporosis) results in LBP, radiculopathy, and neurogenic claudication.[4]

Differential Diagnosis

The most common causes of LBP in athletes are different for adolescents and adults. Micheli and Wood[15] performed a retrospective analysis of 100 adolescent athletes (age, ≤18 years) who had LBP and 100 adults who had acute LBP to determine whether any differences in the cause of pain existed. The authors reported that LBP was caused by spondylolysis, spondylolisthesis, hyperlordotic mechanical LBP, and herniated disks in more than two-thirds of the adolescent patients.[15] Conversely, LBP was caused by lumbosacral strain or had a herniated or degenerative discogenic origin in the adult patients. Despite the difference in the relative frequency of specific diagnoses for LBP, the differential diagnosis for lumbar spine pain and LBP in adolescent and adult athletes is quite extensive. Although spondylolysis, spondylolisthesis, discogenic LBP, and mechanical LBP are diagnosed more frequently in patients who have LBP, the less common causes of LBP that are listed in **Table 1** should not be overlooked or excluded in athletes who report LBP.

Spondylolysis and Spondylolisthesis

Spondylolysis and spondylolisthesis are common problems in both adolescents and adults. Spondylolysis refers to a pars interarticularis defect or stress fracture that leads to a reduction in vertebral stability. Pathologically, spondylolysis is the result of a traumatic microfracture and repetitive trauma that causes subsequent progression of the fracture or an initial stress fracture from repetitive loading of the lumbar spine in hyperlordotic extension. Participation in sports such as dance, gymnastics, football, volleyball, tennis, diving, and weight lifting has been associated with causative hyperlordosis.[2] Subsequent anterolisthetic progression of a bilateral spondylotic fracture demonstrates the complementary relationship between spondylolysis (L5) and spondylolisthesis (L5-S1).

Spondylolisthesis refers to the anterior subluxation of the cranial vertebra over the caudal vertebra. There are several types of spondylolisthesis; however, isthmic spondylolisthesis and degenerative spondylolisthesis are the most common types in adolescents and adults, respectively. Isthmic spondylolisthesis refers to an anterolisthetic progression that is caused by a bilateral pars defect. Degenerative spondylolisthesis refers to an anterolisthetic or retrolisthetic progression that is caused by degeneration of the intervertebral disks. The severity of spondylolisthesis is based on the classification system described by Meyerding: grade I, zero to 25% anterolisthetic progression; grade II, 25% to 50% anterolisthetic progression; grade III, 50% to 75% anterolisthetic progression; grade IV, 75% to 100% anterolisthetic progression; and grade V, complete anterolisthesis, which is known as spondyloptosis.

In general, patients with spondylolysis and spondylolisthesis will have nonspecific, localized, unilateral, or bilateral LBP that worsens with activity. Patients also may experience radiating buttock or leg pain, depending on the severity and progression of spondylolisthesis.[2,5] It is hypothesized that the stability and resilience of the intervertebral disks in adolescents halt the progression of the anterolisthesis; however, degeneration of the intervertebral disks

in the fourth and fifth decades of life results in progression to higher-grade spondylolisthesis and LBP and radicular leg pain. Adolescent patients who have nonspecific symptoms often are

misdiagnosed with muscular or ligamentous strains or spasms.

Surgeons may observe hyperlordosis of the lumbar spine and tightened hamstrings on physical examination

Table 1
Less Common Causes of Low Back Pain

Sacroiliac joint and lumbopelvic somatic dysfunction

Fractures

    Vertebral body

    Facet joint

    Spinous or transverse processes

    Pelvic

Tumors

    Benign

        Aneurysmal bone cyst

        Osteoid osteoma

        Osteoblastoma

    Malignant

        Primary

            Leukemia

            Lymphoma

            Ewing sarcoma (pelvis)

            Osteosarcoma (extremities)

        Metastatic

            Neurofibromatosis

Stenosis

    Congenital

    Acquired

Infections and inflammatory conditions

    Discitis (<10 years)

    Osteomyelitis

    Facet synovitis

    Osteitis pubis

    Sacroiliitis

    Tuberculosis

Seronegative spondyloarthropathies

    Psoriatic arthritis

    Enteropathic spondylitis (associated with Crohn disease and ulcerative colitis)

    Ankylosing spondylitis (HLA-B27)

    Reactive arthritis (Reiter syndrome)

Vascular

    Abdominal aortic aneurysm

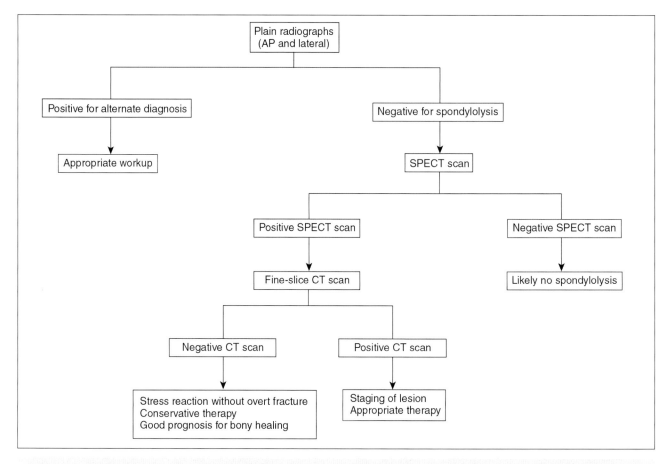

Figure 1   Algorithm shows the imaging workup for patients in whom a spondylolytic lesion is suspected. SPECT = single photon emission CT. (Adapted with permission from Kruse D, Lemmen B: Spine injuries in the sport of gymnastics. *Curr Sports Med Rep* 2009;8[1]:20-28.)

of patients who have spondylolysis and spondylolisthesis. Asking a patient to perform the stork test, in which one leg is hyperextended, will reproduce pain symptoms;[5] however, this test is nonspecific for spondylolysis and spondylolisthesis. Although spondylolysis often is not visible on plain radiographs, AP and lateral radiographs are obtained to assess for spondylolisthetic progression. Kruse and Lemmen[6] proposed an algorithmic approach for the imaging workup of patients in whom spondylolysis is suspected (**Figure 1**). If plain radiographs are negative for spondylolysis but a patient's history and physical examination indicate a possible fracture, a single photon emission CT

scan should be obtained to highlight metabolic activity at the fracture site.[6,14]

Management of spondylolysis and spondylolisthesis depends on the age and comorbidities of a patient as well as the severity and progression of the pathology. Acutely symptomatic spondylolysis and low-grade spondylolisthesis often are managed nonsurgically with rest, cold compression therapy, over-the-counter anti-inflammatory drugs, and activity modification.[2,5,14] In general, athletes are able to begin physical therapy, which includes range of motion and spine stabilization exercises, after 2 weeks of nonsurgical treatment if pain and symptoms have subsided. In addition, athletes may return to full-contact

sports after 4 to 6 weeks of nonsurgical treatment if adequate stability and strength have been attained and full range of motion and sport-specific movements can be achieved without pain. Prolonged activity modification is recommended for elderly patients who have concern for spondylolisthetic progression.

Symptoms caused by spondylolysis or spondylolisthesis often resolve after 2 to 6 weeks of nonsurgical management. Patients in whom spondylolysis is diagnosed before it progresses to fracture or anterolisthesis should rest and refrain from causative activities for 3 months postinjury;[16] however, 9% to 15% of patients who have symptomatic spondylolysis will require surgical treatment.[17] Although the timing from diagnosis to surgery is variable and dependent on several factors, surgical treatment with posterior spinal fusion is recommended for patients in whom more than 6 months of nonsurgical treatment fails or for patients with high-grade spondylolisthesis who have substantial neurologic compromise.[2,5,14]

Discogenic LBP

Intervertebral disks are gelatinous cushions, which are composed of a central nucleus pulposus surrounded by a collagen-based anulus fibrosus, that are designed to dissipate axial compressive force on the spine.[4,6] Acute disk injuries are common in athletes who perform activities that require a combination of flexion, rotation, and compression of the spine. This motion, and the subsequent disk herniation, is most commonly observed in athletes who participate in football, wrestling, hockey, dance, gymnastics, and golf.[4] Over time, several risk factors in combination with the aging process contribute to degeneration of the intervertebral disks. Chronic mechanical stress, obesity, tobacco use, and excessive axial loading put additional stress on the disks, which weakens the anulus fibrosus and causes microtears and subsequent bulging or herniation of the nucleus pulposus through the anulus fibrosus.

Patients with a herniated nucleus pulposus, whether focally or broadly herniated, can have symptoms that range from no symptoms to a combination of axial LBP and radicular leg pain. Patients often describe episodes of severe paraspinal axial pain and muscle spasms, with radiating pain in a dermatomal distribution that is exacerbated by activity, prolonged sitting, or standing and that recurs if lying supine. On physical examination, patients who have a herniated nucleus pulposus will exhibit a reduced ipsilateral and contralateral straight leg raise, reduced hamstring flexibility, and a positive slump test, which indicates dural irritation.[4,10] Radiographs are obtained to rule out vertebral abnormalities that affect normal anatomy; however, MRI is used to confirm diagnosis.[6]

Initially, patients are treated nonsurgically, with a specific emphasis on pain control with the use of over-the-counter anti-inflammatory drugs, opiates, or analgesic agents known to treat neuropathic pain, such as gabapentin. Physical therapy aims to relax the paraspinal muscles and break muscle spasms with the use of manual therapy, including massage and neuromuscular electrical stimulation, and strengthen abdominal and paraspinal musculature to improve core and spinal stability. Patients may discontinue physical therapy and return to sports after full, painless range of motion has been achieved and preinjury strength and conditioning has returned.[5] Epidural injections may be necessary in patients who continue to experience neuropathic and radicular symptoms; however, microdiskectomy should be considered in patients in whom neuropathic and radicular symptoms remain debilitating and in patients who have a progressive neurologic deficit.[4]

Mechanical LBP

Muscular or ligamentous lumbar strain is the most common cause of axial LBP in the general population and often is a preliminary diagnosis for acute LBP in the primary care setting.[2] Acute mechanical LBP, muscular hematomas, and contusions are frequently caused by acute traumatic, rotational, or flexional injuries or are the result of reduced hip and knee mobility, thoracic hyperkyphosis, lumbar hyperlordosis, overuse, or improper technique. A more thorough history, physical examination, and imaging workup are obtained in patients who have persistent pain or neurologic symptoms that do not resolve with nonsurgical treatment. Mechanical LBP is primarily managed with nonsurgical therapy that consists of rest, activity modification, stretching, ice, over-the-counter anti-inflammatory drugs, and muscle relaxant medications.[2,6,11] Physical therapy may be incorporated for patients who have more severe injuries and to help return elderly patients to normal function.

Summary

LBP is the most common complaint expressed by adult patients in the primary care setting, and the incidence of LBP in adolescents is rising. Adolescents who are involved in athletics most commonly suffer from spondylolysis, spondylolisthesis, mechanical LBP, and herniated disks, whereas adult athletes most commonly suffer from lumbosacral strain and herniated or degenerative disks. Initial nonsurgical management aims to reduce inflammation and noninvasively strengthen damaged tissues with the use of a combination of rest, activity modification, cold compression therapy, over-the-counter anti-inflammatory drugs, physical therapy, and epidural injections. Although most patients who have LBP will return to sports after nonsurgical treatment, surgery may be required in patients who have persistent or progressive neurologic symptoms.

References

1. Olsen TL, Anderson RL, Dearwater SR, et al: The epidemiology of low back pain in an adolescent population. *Am J Public Health* 1992;82(4):606-608.

2. Huang P, Anissipour A, McGee W, Lemak L: Return-to-play recommendations after cervical, thoracic, and lumbar spine injuries: A comprehensive review. *Sports Health* 2016;8(1):19-25.

3. Burton AK, Clarke RD, McClune TD, Tillotson KM: The natural history of low back pain in adolescents. *Spine (Phila Pa 1976)* 1996;21(20):2323-2328.

4. Borg-Stein J, Elson L, Brand E: The aging spine in sports. *Clin Sports Med* 2012;31(3):473-486.

5. Menzer H, Gill GK, Paterson A: Thoracic spine sports-related injuries. *Curr Sports Med Rep* 2015;14(1):34-40.

6. Kruse D, Lemmen B: Spine injuries in the sport of gymnastics. *Curr Sports Med Rep* 2009;8(1):20-28.

7. Salminen JJ, Pentti J, Terho P: Low back pain and disability in 14-year-old schoolchildren. *Acta Paediatr* 1992;81(12):1035-1039.

8. Skoffer B, Foldspang A: Physical activity and low-back pain in schoolchildren. *Eur Spine J* 2008;17(3):373-379.

9. Harreby M, Nygaard B, Jessen T, et al: Risk factors for low back pain in a cohort of 1389 Danish school children: An epidemiologic study. *Eur Spine J* 1999;8(6):444-450.

10. Balagué F, Nordin M: Back pain in children and teenagers. *Baillieres Clin Rheumatol* 1992;6(3):575-593.

11. Fairbank JC, Pynsent PB, Van Poortvliet JA, Phillips H: Influence of anthropometric factors and joint laxity in the incidence of adolescent back pain. *Spine (Phila Pa 1976)* 1984;9(5):461-464.

12. Mierau D, Cassidy JD, Yong-Hing K: Low-back pain and straight leg raising in children and adolescents. *Spine (Phila Pa 1976)* 1989;14(5):526-528.

13. Changstrom BG, Brou L, Khodaee M, Braund C, Comstock RD: Epidemiology of stress fracture injuries among US high school athletes, 2005-2006 through 2012-2013. *Am J Sports Med* 2015;43(1):26-33.

14. Gottschlich LM, Young CC: Spine injuries in dancers. *Curr Sports Med Rep* 2011;10(1):40-44.

15. Micheli LJ, Wood R: Back pain in young athletes: Significant differences from adults in causes and patterns. *Arch Pediatr Adolesc Med* 1995;149(1):15-18.

16. Standaert CJ, Herring SA: Expert opinion and controversies in sports and musculoskeletal medicine: The diagnosis and treatment of spondylolysis in adolescent athletes. *Arch Phys Med Rehabil* 2007;88(4):537-540.

17. Syrmou E, Tsitsopoulos PP, Marinopoulos D, Tsonidis C, Anagnostopoulos I, Tsitsopoulous PD: Spondylolysis: A review and reappraisal. *Hippokratia* 2010;14(1):17-21.

Adolescent Spondylolysis: Management and Return to Play

William C. Warner Jr, MD

Rodrigo Góes Medéa de Mendonça, MD

Abstract

The most common causes of low back pain in adolescents are spondylolysis and spondylolisthesis. Mechanical factors combined with rapid growth during adolescence place stress on the spine and can result in a stress fracture. Sports that require athletes to repeatedly place the spine in hyperextension may exacerbate both spondylolysis and spondylolisthesis. Many adolescent athletes with spondylolysis or low-grade spondylolisthesis have minimal symptoms and require no treatment or alteration in activity, including sports activity. For adolescents with spondylolysis or low-grade spondylolisthesis who have symptoms, nonsurgical treatment with activity restrictions and a structured rehabilitation program can help in return to most sports. Surgical treatment may be required for patients who have symptoms that are unresponsive to nonsurgical treatment and patients who have grade III or grade IV spondylolisthesis. Treatment and return to competitive sports must be individualized based on the severity and symptoms of the disease in each patient.

Instr Course Lect 2017;66:409–413.

Spondylolysis is a developmental or acquired defect of the pars interarticularis that can range from a stress reaction, to an incomplete or complete fracture, or even to a frank nonunion. Micheli and Wood[1] reported that the most common cause of back pain in young athletes is spondylolysis, which the authors diagnosed in 47% of patients who reported low back pain. The translation of one vertebral segment relative to the next caudal segment is referred to as spondylolisthesis. Progression of translation is uncommon but can occur during the adolescent growth spurt. Spondylolysis is bilateral in approximately 80% of patients and unilateral in approximately 20% of patients.[2] Spondylolysis most commonly affects the L5 vertebra (71% to 95% of patients), followed by the L4 vertebra (5% to 23% of patients) and the L3 vertebra (3% to 18% of patients).[3] Pars interarticularis fractures are found at more than one vertebra in 4% of patients and most commonly affect the L3-5 vertebrae.[4] The male-to-female ratio for spondylolysis is 2:1.[4] Several classification systems for spondylolysis and spondylolisthesis have been described based on etiologic and topographic criteria and whether the defect is developmental or traumatic;[5] however, most pars interarticularis defects in adolescent athletes are caused by acute or stress fractures.

Epidemiology

The incidence of spondylolysis and spondylolisthesis in the general population is 6% to 8%.[6] The high prevalence of spondylolysis and spondylolisthesis among athletes suggests that increased stresses placed on the lumbar spine may be an etiologic factor.[7] The incidence of spondylolysis and spondylolisthesis has been reported to be 15% to 50% in college football players[8] and 6% to 11% in gymnasts.[8,9] Wrestling, rowing, weightlifting, hockey, ballet, diving, swimming, running, golf, and baseball are other sports in which participants

Dr. Warner or an immediate family member serves as an unpaid consultant to Medtronic Sofamor Danek. Dr. Medéa de Mendonça has received research or institutional support from Medicrea.

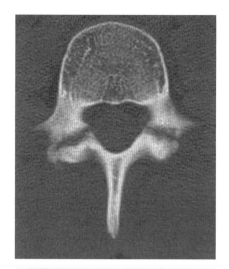

Figure 1 Axial CT scan of a spine demonstrates a bilateral pars interarticularis defect.

have a higher incidence of lumbar spine injuries.[10]

Pathophysiology

In adolescent athletes, spondylolysis and spondylolisthesis usually are caused by a combination of mechanical forces and anatomic factors that lead to the development of a pars interarticularis defect. In approximately 90% of patients, the pars interarticularis fails from inferior to superior,[11] which may be the result of a nutcracker effect.[12] Patients with increased thoracic kyphosis, such as those with Scheuermann disease, have a compensatory lumbar hyperlordosis that can cause increased stress on the pars interarticularis, which may result in an increased incidence of spondylolysis and spondylolisthesis.[13]

Adequate separation between adjacent articular facets allows the posterior elements of the spine to overlap one another during hyperextension. A recent anatomic study reported that individuals who lack sufficient distance between the facets in the cranial to caudal direction are likely to pinch the L5 lamina between the inferior facets of L4 and the superior facets of S1 during repetitive lumbar extension, which leads to the development of a pars interarticularis defect.[14] Another anatomic factor that can lead to spondylolysis is the orientation of the facet joint in the sagittal plane. The more the facet joint is rotated off the sagittal plane, the more force is transmitted to the pars interarticularis in hyperextension, which results in a pars interarticularis stress fracture.[15]

Vitamin D and calcium deficiencies also may play a role in the development of adult-onset spondylolysis.[16] Lappe et al[17] reported that, compared with a placebo group, female naval recruits who were being treated with a daily regimen of 2,000 mg of calcium and 800 IU of vitamin D had a 20% lower incidence of stress fractures.

Presentation

Often, adolescent athletes will have minimal symptoms, some of which consist of back or buttock pain. Symptoms often are aggravated by increased activity or participation in competitive sports. Pain may be acute or insidious in onset with activity for weeks or months, especially with hyperextension. Asking the patient to stand on one leg, which causes the spine to go into hyperextension, will reproduce the pain; this is known as a positive stork test. Pain may radiate into the buttock; however, true radicular symptoms are not common unless a substantial spondylolisthesis is present. Hamstring tightness or spasm may be found during an examination. Motor or sensory deficits are rare.

Diagnostic Tests

Initial imaging for patients with suspected spondylolysis or spondylolisthesis includes standing AP, lateral, and oblique radiographs of the lumbar spine. A recent study called into question whether routine oblique radiographs are useful and necessary in the workup for patients with suspected spondylolysis or spondylolisthesis.[18] Radiographic measurement of spondylolisthesis follows the method described by Meyerding,[19] which uses the percentage of displacement of the inferior aspect of the body of the L5 vertebra in relation to the superior border of the sacrum: grade 0, no displacement; grade I, zero to 25% displacement; grade II, 25% to 50% displacement; grade III, 50% to 75% displacement; grade IV, 75% to 100% displacement; and grade V, complete dissociation, which is known as spondyloptosis.

Isotope imaging with single photon emission CT is an extremely sensitive technique for the early diagnosis of acute spondylolysis.[20,21] Unfortunately, single photon emission CT is nonspecific, detects only 17% of chronic lesions,[22] and cannot distinguish between stress reactions and complete fractures.

CT is the preferred imaging modality for the detection of pars interarticularis fractures[21] (**Figure 1**). Some limitations of CT include low accuracy in distinguishing recent active fractures, stress reactions, and chronic nonunion. Another drawback of CT is increased radiation exposure.

MRI can help identify stress reactions and fractures in the pars interarticularis;[23,24] however, it is technique dependent, and T2-weighted fat-suppressed images in the oblique and sagittal planes are necessary to evaluate bone marrow edema in patients with acute lesions[25] (**Figure 2**). MRI is useful in the evaluation of disk pathology and any nerve root compression. The disadvantages of MRI are cost, availability, and the need for an experienced radiologist to read the image. Hollenberg et al[26] described an MRI classification system for spondylolysis: grade 0, normal; grade 1, bone marrow edema and intact cortices that are compatible with a stress reaction; grade 2, incomplete fracture with bone marrow edema; grade 3, complete active fracture with bone marrow edema; and grade 4, complete fracture without bone marrow edema.

Treatment
Nonsurgical Treatment
Nonsurgical treatment will allow most adolescent athletes who have spondylolysis or spondylolisthesis to return to sports. Nonsurgical treatment recommendations vary from rest and restriction of activities to bracing and a structured rehabilitation program. Treatment first begins with rest and the restriction of activities. El Rassi et al[27] reported a 42% compliance rate with restriction of activities, which highlights the need for patient, parent, and coach participation in the treatment plan. Brace treatment has been controversial because a standard thoracolumbosacral orthosis does not completely immobilize the lumbosacral junction. Bracing will restrict some motion of the lumbar spine but is most effective by forcing restriction of activities. Electrical stimulation has had varied results in attempts to heal acute pars interarticularis fractures.

A structured rehabilitation program is essential to allow patients to return to sports. A structured rehabilitation program consist of four phases: (1) acute, (2) subacute, (3) presport, and (4) sports conditioning. The acute phase focuses on improvement of pain and inflammation as well as rehabilitation of the lumbopelvic stabilizers. The subacute phase emphasizes core strengthening and restoration of trunk range of motion. Nonimpact cardio activities can begin during the subacute phase. The physical therapist will begin sports-simulated movements and increase a patient's strength and endurance during the presport phase. Sport-specific drills and impact cardio training are started in the sports conditioning phase, with the goal of returning patients to their desired sport.

The nonsurgical treatment and structured rehabilitation program usually takes 12 weeks to complete. Patients who have a stress reaction may progress faster, and some patients may require 4 to 5 months of rehabilitation before they are ready to return to sports. Patients who have early-stage pars interarticularis defects are the best candidates for nonsurgical treatment with a brace because they have a greater chance for bony healing.[28]

Surgical Treatment
Surgical management of spondylolysis is indicated in patients in whom a 6-month nonsurgical treatment program fails. The type of surgery performed is based on the location of the spondylolysis, any associated disk pathology, and any associated vertebral dysplasia. Either an intervertebral fusion or a repair of the pars interarticularis defect can be performed to surgically manage spondylolysis. Direct repair of a pars interarticularis defect and an L5-S1 fusion produce similar results in patients who have a pars interarticularis lesion at the L5 vertebra. Intervertebral fusion is preferred if there is associated disk pathology at L5-S1 or any associated dysplasia. Direct repair is recommended in patients

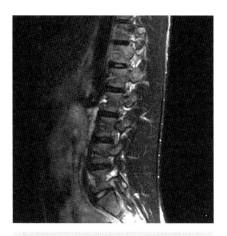

Figure 2 Sagittal T2-weighted MRI of a spine demonstrates increased signal in the pedicle and the pars interarticularis.

who have a pars interarticularis lesion at either the L4 or L3 vertebra.

Four repair techniques have been described for the management of spondylolysis: (1) the Scott wiring technique (**Figure 3, A**); (2) the Buck screw technique[29] (**Figure 3, B**); (3) the pedicle screw and hook technique (**Figure 3, C**); and (4) the U-rod technique (**Figure 3, D**). All four techniques have an 80% to 90% rate for return to sports. For the Scott wiring technique, wires are placed around the transverse process on each side and through the spinous process to compress the pars interarticularis defect. The Scott wiring technique is the least rigid of the four fixation methods yet still has a healing rate near 80%.[30,31] Direct intralaminar screw fixation of a pars defect, which was described by Buck,[29] is a minimally invasive, motion-preserving technique that has had good outcomes in 93% of patients. The use of pedicle screws and inflaminar hooks that are attached to a short rod allows for compression and stabilization of a pars interarticularis defect.[32,33] The pedicle screw and hook technique is the most rigid of the four

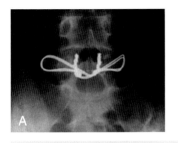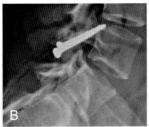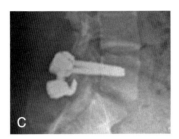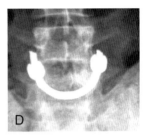

Figure 3   Radiographs of a spine demonstrate repair techniques for the management of spondylolysis. **A,** AP radiograph demonstrates the Scott wiring technique. **B,** Lateral radiograph demonstrates the Buck screw technique. **C,** Lateral radiograph demonstrates the pedicle screw and hook technique. **D,** AP radiograph demonstrates the U-rod technique. (Panel A reproduced with permission from Nozawa S, Shimizu K, Miyamoto K, Tanaka M: Repair of pars interarticularis defect by segmental wire fixation in young athletes with spondylolysis. *Am J Sports Med* 2003;31[3]: 359-364. Panel B reproduced with permission from Menga EN, Kebaish KM, Jain A, Carrino JA, Sponseller PD: Clinical results and functional outcomes after direct intralaminar screw repair of spondylolysis. *Spine (Phila Pa 1976)* 2014;39[1]:104-110. Panel C reproduced with permission from Drazin D, Shirzadi A, Jeswani S, et al: Direct surgical repair of spondylolysis in athletes: Indications, techniques, and outcomes. *Neurosurg Focus* 2011;31[5]:E9. Panel D reproduced with permission from Altaf F, Osei NA, Garrido E, et al: Repair of spondylolysis using compression with a modular link and screws. *J Bone Joint Surg Br* 2011;93[1]:73-77.)

fixation methods. A similar technique uses a U-shaped rod that is placed inferior to the spinous process to stabilize and compress the pars interarticularis defect.[34,35]

These four repair techniques for the management of spondylolysis have reported return-to-sports rates of 80% to 90%. Sairyo et al[36] reported that disk stresses at the cranial and caudal levels of the pars interarticularis defect were restored to normal after direct intralaminar screw fixation with the Buck screw technique. Several other studies have reported that the Buck screw technique is biomechanically superior to the other repair techniques for the management of spondylolysis.[37] In a biomechanical study that compared the four repair techniques for the management of spondylolysis, Fan et al[37] reported that all four techniques restored normal intervertebral rotation; however, the Scott wiring technique and the Buck screw technique provided less stability compared with the pedicle screw and hook technique and the U-rod technique. Mihara[38] reported

that the Buck screw technique restored more normal motion at both the involved and adjacent levels of pars interarticularis defects.

Return to sports after surgery varies from 6 to 9 months postoperatively. Return to sports for adolescent athletes who have spondylolisthesis is based on symptoms and the degree of listhesis. Patients who have grade I asymptomatic spondylolisthesis may return to play with no restriction. Patients who have grade II spondylolisthesis may return to play but should avoid high-risk activities that place a load on the lumbar spine in hyperextension. Patients who have grade III and grade IV spondylolisthesis often require fusion. Fusion may be considered in patients with grade I or grade II spondylolisthesis who have persistent symptoms despite 6 months of nonsurgical treatment.

Summary

Spondylolysis and spondylolisthesis are common causes of back pain in adolescent athletes. Nonsurgical treatment is successful in most adolescent athletes

who have symptomatic spondylolysis and spondylolisthesis. Athletes who undergo surgical treatment of spondylolysis, regardless of the repair technique used, may be able to return to sports, but their postoperative participation levels may vary. Ultimately, clearance of athletes for sports participation must be based on each patient's condition and chosen sport.

References

1. Micheli LJ, Wood R: Back pain in young athletes: Significant differences from adults in causes and patterns. *Arch Pediatr Adolesc Med* 1995;149(1):15-18.

2. Gurd DP: Back pain in the young athlete. *Sports Med Arthrosc* 2011;19(1):7-16.

3. Hirano K, Imagama S, Matsuyama Y, et al: Surgically treated cases of lumbar spondylolysis and isthmic spondylolisthesis: A multicenter study. *J Spinal Disord Tech* 2015;28(5):193-197.

4. Tallarico RA, Madom IA, Palumbo MA: Spondylolysis and spondylolisthesis in the athlete. *Sports Med Arthrosc* 2008;16(1):32-38.

5. Herman MJ, Pizzutillo PD: Spondylolysis and spondylolisthesis in the child and adolescent: A new

classification. *Clin Orthop Relat Res* 2005;434:46-54.

6. Fredrickson BE, Baker D, McHolick WJ, Yuan HA, Lubicky JP: The natural history of spondylolysis and spondylolisthesis. *J Bone Joint Surg Am* 1984;66(5):699-707.

7. Letts M, Smallman T, Afanasiev R, Gouw G: Fracture of the pars interarticularis in adolescent athletes: A clinical-biomechanical analysis. *J Pediatr Orthop* 1986;6(1):40-46.

8. McCarroll JR, Miller JM, Ritter MA: Lumbar spondylolysis and spondylolisthesis in college football players: A prospective study. *Am J Sports Med* 1986;14(5):404-406.

9. Dunn IF, Proctor MR, Day AL: Lumbar spine injuries in athletes. *Neurosurg Focus* 2006;21(4):E4.

10. Lawrence JP, Greene HS, Grauer JN: Back pain in athletes. *J Am Acad Orthop Surg* 2006;14(13):726-735.

11. Terai T, Sairyo K, Goel VK, et al: Spondylolysis originates in the ventral aspect of the pars interarticularis: A clinical and biomechanical study. *J Bone Joint Surg Br* 2010;92(8):1123-1127.

12. Dunn AJ, Campbell RS, Mayor PE, Rees D: Radiological findings and healing patterns of incomplete stress fractures of the pars interarticularis. *Skeletal Radiol* 2008;37(5):443-450.

13. Ogilvie JW, Sherman J: Spondylolysis in Scheuermann's disease. *Spine (Phila Pa 1976)* 1987;12(3):251-253.

14. Ward CV, Latimer B: Human evolution and the development of spondylolysis. *Spine (Phila Pa 1976)* 2005;30(16):1808-1814.

15. Don AS, Robertson PA: Facet joint orientation in spondylolysis and isthmic spondylolisthesis. *J Spinal Disord Tech* 2008;21(2):112-115.

16. Ravindra VM, Godzik J, Guan J, et al: Prevalence of vitamin D deficiency in patients undergoing elective spine surgery: A cross-sectional analysis. *World Neurosurg* 2015;83(6):1114-1119.

17. Lappe J, Cullen D, Haynatzki G, Recker R, Ahlf R, Thompson K: Calcium and vitamin d supplementation decreases incidence of stress fractures in female navy recruits. *J Bone Miner Res* 2008;23(5):741-749.

18. Beck NA, Miller R, Baldwin K, et al: Do oblique views add value in the diagnosis of spondylolysis in adolescents? *J Bone Joint Surg Am* 2013;95(10):e65.

19. Meyerding HW: Spondylolisthesis. *Surg Gynecol Obstet* 1932;54:371-377.

20. Bhatia NN, Chow G, Timon SJ, Watts HG: Diagnostic modalities for the evaluation of pediatric back pain: A prospective study. *J Pediatr Orthop* 2008;28(2):230-233.

21. Leone A, Cianfoni A, Cerase A, Magarelli N, Bonomo L: Lumbar spondylolysis: A review. *Skeletal Radiol* 2011;40(6):683-700.

22. Pennell RG, Maurer AH, Bonakdarpour A: Stress injuries of the pars interarticularis: Radiologic classification and indications for scintigraphy. *AJR Am J Roentgenol* 1985;145(4):763-766.

23. Sairyo K, Katoh S, Takata Y, et al: MRI signal changes of the pedicle as an indicator for early diagnosis of spondylolysis in children and adolescents: A clinical and biomechanical study. *Spine (Phila Pa 1976)* 2006;31(2):206-211.

24. Sakai T, Sairyo K, Mima S, Yasui N: Significance of magnetic resonance imaging signal change in the pedicle in the management of pediatric lumbar spondylolysis. *Spine (Phila Pa 1976)* 2010;35(14):E641-E645.

25. Rush JK, Astur N, Scott S, Kelly DM, Sawyer JR, Warner WC Jr: Use of magnetic resonance imaging in the evaluation of spondylolysis. *J Pediatr Orthop* 2015;35(3):271-275.

26. Hollenberg GM, Beattie PF, Meyers SP, Weinberg EP, Adams MJ: Stress reactions of the pars interarticularis: The development of a new MRI classification system. *Spine (Phila Pa 1976)* 2002;27(2):181-186.

27. El Rassi G, Takemitsu M, Glutting J, Shah SA: Effect of sports modification on clinical outcome in children and adolescent athletes with symptomatic lumbar spondylolysis. *Am J Phys Med Rehabil* 2013;92(12):1070-1074.

28. Cohen E, Stuecker RD: Magnetic resonance imaging in diagnosis and follow-up of impending spondylolysis in children and adolescents: Early treatment may prevent pars defects. *J Pediatr Orthop B* 2005;14(2):63-67.

29. Buck JE: Direct repair of the defect in spondylolisthesis: Preliminary report. *J Bone Joint Surg Br* 1970;52(3):432-437.

30. Johnson GV, Thompson AG: The Scott wiring technique for direct repair of lumbar spondylolysis. *J Bone Joint Surg Br* 1992;74(3):426-430.

31. Nozawa S, Shimizu K, Miyamoto K, Tanaka M: Repair of pars interarticularis defect by segmental wire fixation in young athletes with spondylolysis. *Am J Sports Med* 2003;31(3):359-364.

32. Kakiuchi M: Repair of the defect in spondylolysis: Durable fixation with pedicle screws and laminar hooks. *J Bone Joint Surg Am* 1997;79(6):818-825.

33. Roca J, Iborra M, Cavanilles-Walker JM, Albertí G: Direct repair of spondylolysis using a new pedicle screw hook fixation: Clinical and CT-assessed study. An analysis of 19 patients. *J Spinal Disord Tech* 2005;18(suppl):S82-S89.

34. Altaf F, Osei NA, Garrido E, et al: Repair of spondylolysis using compression with a modular link and screws. *J Bone Joint Surg Br* 2011;93(1):73-77.

35. Sumita T, Sairyo K, Shibuya I, et al: V-rod technique for direct repair surgery of pediatric lumbar spondylolysis combined with posterior apophyseal ring fracture. *Asian Spine J* 2013;7(2):115-118.

36. Sairyo K, Goel VK, Faizan A, Vadapalli S, Biyani S, Ebraheim N: Buck's direct repair of lumbar spondylolysis restores disc stresses at the involved and adjacent levels. *Clin Biomech (Bristol, Avon)* 2006;21(10):1020-1026.

37. Fan J, Yu GR, Liu F, Zhao J, Zhao WD: A biomechanical study on the direct repair of spondylolysis by different techniques of fixation. *Orthop Surg* 2010;2(1):46-51.

38. Mihara H, Onari K, Cheng BC, David SM, Zdeblick TA: The biomechanical effects of spondylolysis and its treatment. *Spine (Phila Pa 1976)* 2003;28(3):235-238.

Pediatrics

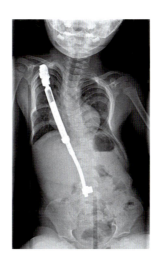

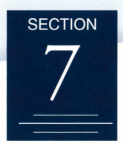

Pediatric Phalanx Fractures

Joshua M. Abzug, MD
Karan Dua, MD
Andrea Sesko Bauer, MD
Roger Cornwall, MD
Theresa O. Wyrick, MD

Abstract

Phalangeal fractures are the most common type of hand fracture that occurs in the pediatric population and account for the second highest number of emergency department visits in the United States for fractures. The incidence of phalangeal fractures is the highest in children aged 10 to 14 years, which coincides with the time that most children begin playing contact sports. Younger children are more likely to sustain a phalangeal fracture in the home setting as a result of crush and laceration injuries. Salter-Harris type II fractures of the proximal phalanx are the most common type of finger fracture. An unmineralized physis is biomechanically weaker compared with the surrounding ligamentous structures and mature bone, which make fractures about the physis likely. A thorough physical examination is necessary to assess the digital cascade for signs of rotational deformity and/or coronal malalignment. Plain radiographs of the hand and digits are sufficient to confirm a diagnosis of a phalangeal fracture. The management of phalangeal fractures is based on the initial severity of the injury and depends on the success of closed reduction techniques. Nondisplaced phalanx fractures are managed with splint immobilization. Stable, reduced phalanx fractures are immobilized but require close monitoring to ensure maintenance of fracture reduction. Unstable, displaced phalanx fractures require surgical management, preferably via closed reduction and percutaneous pinning.

Instr Course Lect 2017;66:417–427.

The hand is the most common location of injury in the pediatric and adolescent population.[1,2] In particular, the phalanges are the most frequently injured bones in the hand, with distal phalangeal and proximal phalangeal base fractures being the most diagnosed fractures.[3-5] Naranje et al[6] reported that the annual occurrence rate of phalangeal fractures was 27 per 1,000 patients aged 0 to 19 years, accounting for the second highest number of emergency departments visits in the United States for fractures. The fifth ray followed by the thumb are the most commonly injured phalanges.[7-9] The incidence of phalangeal fractures is the highest in children aged 10 to 14 years, which coincides with the time that most children begin playing contact sports.[6-9] A significant association exists between hand fractures that occur as a result of punching or fighting and psychiatric illness, such as depression and/or attention deficit hyperactivity disorder.[10] Toddlers and preschool-aged children are more likely to sustain a phalangeal

Dr. Abzug or an immediate family member is a member of a speakers' bureau or has made paid presentations on behalf of Checkpoint Surgical and serves as a paid consultant to or is an employee of AxoGen. Dr. Bauer or an immediate family member serves as a board member, owner, officer, or committee member of the American Society for Surgery of the Hand and the Pediatric Orthopaedic Society of North America. None of the following authors nor any immediate family member has received anything of value from or has stock or stock options held in a commercial company or institution related directly or indirectly to the subject of this chapter: Dr. Dua, Dr. Cornwall, and Dr. Wyrick.

fracture in the home setting as a result of crush and laceration injuries.[9] Two-thirds of all phalangeal fractures occur in males,[11] which likely is because of the number of adolescent males who participate in contact sports.[7]

Pathoanatomy

Surgeons must be familiar with the anatomy of the pediatric hand to understand how phalangeal fractures occur and can be optimally managed. Bone growth in children occurs through the physeal plate, which is located at the proximal end of the phalanges.[12] The phalangeal physes remain open until males and females are aged approximately 16.5 and 14.5 years, respectively.[2] Knowledge of these growth centers is important because iatrogenic physeal arrest may occur in patients with a physeal injury or patients who undergo multiple fracture reduction attempts.[12] An unmineralized physis is biomechanically weaker compared with the surrounding ligamentous structures and mature bone, which make fractures about the physis more likely than ligamentous injuries or diaphyseal fractures. In younger children, shear forces across the fingers stress the chondrocytes; this results in physeal injury, usually in the zone of hypertrophy, which is devoid of extracellular matrix as a result of ongoing cellular hypertrophy.[13]

The periosteum that surrounds pediatric bone is highly vascularized. The periosteum serves as a source for the differentiation of cells during fracture healing and, often, aids in the maintenance of fracture alignment after reduction. However, surgeons must understand that the periosteum may become entrapped at the fracture site, which may prevent adequate reduction.

Knowledge of tendon attachments in the pediatric hand is necessary to comprehensively manage phalangeal fractures and all associated injuries. The central slip of the extensor tendon attaches at the dorsal epiphysis of the middle phalanx, and the terminal extensor tendon attaches at the dorsal epiphysis of the distal phalanx. The flexor digitorum superficialis inserts on the volar shaft of the middle phalanx, and the flexor digitorum profundus as well as the flexor pollicis longus insert on the metadiaphyseal region of the distal phalanx.

Video 34.1: Pediatric Phalanx Fracture. Joshua M. Abzug, MD (19 sec)

Assessment of Injury

The clinical presentation of a child who has a pediatric phalanx fracture is based on the severity of the initial injury. The physical examination is an important aspect of the diagnostic workup of a child with a suspected phalangeal fracture. The skin should be inspected for abrasions, ecchymosis, and swelling. In patients who have a distal phalanx injury, the nail complex should be examined for a possible nail bed injury, Seymour fracture, or tuft fracture. Patients with a substantially displaced phalanx fracture and/or dislocation may have obvious deformity. The digital cascade must be assessed and compared with that of the uninjured hand to determine if any malrotation or deviation is present. An evaluation of active and passive range of motion via tenodesis grasp and release allows surgeons to assess the integrity of the tendons.

Typically, localized tenderness is present at the fracture site. The entire hand, wrist, and extremity should

be purposely palpated to rule out any concomitant injuries. A thorough neurovascular examination also should be performed. Digital sensation should be objectively measured with the use of the monofilament test and the static/moving two-point discrimination test, both of which are reliable tests in children aged at least 6 years.[14] In younger children who are not capable of performing such tests, digital sensation is assessed with the use of the sweat and/or wrinkle tests. The wrinkle test measures autonomic function of the peripheral nerves via placement of the hand in warm water for 10 minutes; wrinkles on the fingers indicate intact sensory function.[15] The wrinkle test, however, may be time consuming. The sweat test is easily performed by assessing the finger for the presence or absence of sweat.

PA and lateral radiographs of the injured finger should be obtained. Oblique radiographs are beneficial if an articular phalanx fracture is suspected. Three radiographic views of the hand are obtained in patients with injuries to multiple digits. In general, advanced imaging is not necessary.

Phalangeal Shaft and Base Fractures

In general, phalangeal shaft fractures are less common in the pediatric population compared with other phalangeal fracture patterns.[9,11] The principles of phalangeal shaft fracture management are based on initial fracture displacement and orientation. Very subtle signs of injury may be present; therefore, an assessment of the digital cascade for signs of rotational or angular deformity is necessary. Minimally or nondisplaced phalangeal shaft fractures are managed with the use of buddy taping and a splint for 3 to 4 weeks, after which early active range of motion is initiated.[12] Vertically oriented oblique and spiral phalangeal shaft fractures cannot be adequately immobilized with the use of buddy taping and a splint; therefore, a more rigid type of immobilization, such as a plaster or fiberglass cast, is necessary. Often, displaced phalangeal shaft fractures require closed reduction. Acceptable alignment may be difficult to maintain in patients who have an oblique, spiral, or comminuted phalangeal shaft fracture; therefore, fixation often is required.[16]

Typically, proximal phalangeal base fractures result from a finger being abducted beyond the acceptable limits of the metacarpophalangeal joint. The intrinsic and extrinsic muscles of the finger place an extension force on the distal aspect of the finger, which results in an apex volar deformity.[16] Salter-Harris type II fractures of the proximal phalanx are the most common type of finger fracture[17] and are referred to as extra-octave fractures if they occur in the little finger.[3] Phalangeal base fractures can extend through the physis or through the metaphysis only.[1,18] Salter-Harris type III epiphyseal fractures of the middle and proximal phalanx tend to occur in the adolescent population, with many studies reporting Salter-Harris type III epiphyseal fractures of the middle and proximal phalanx in climbing athletes.[19] Given the proximity of the fracture site to the physis in patients who have a proximal phalangeal base fracture, bone remodeling usually is substantial, even in patients who have a displaced phalangeal base fracture.[18] Rarely, open reduction and internal fixation is necessary in patients with phalangeal base fractures in whom the flexor tendon or soft

tissue becomes interposed at the fracture site, severe fracture comminution is present, and/or collateral ligament disruption occurs.[18]

Skier's/Gamekeeper's Thumb

The injury pattern associated with a skier's/gamekeeper's thumb that occurs in the pediatric population is different from that described in the adult population. Typically, a skier's/gamekeeper's thumb consists of a Salter-Harris type III fracture of the proximal phalangeal base of the thumb that avulses the insertion of the ulnar collateral ligament, which compromises the stability of the metacarpophalangeal joint.[3] The ulnar collateral ligament is the primary stabilizer of the first metacarpophalangeal joint and helps resist valgus stress. Therefore, in patients with substantial fracture displacement, closed reduction and percutaneous pinning (CRPP) or open reduction and internal fixation is necessary to restore ligament function. Depending on the size of the fracture fragment, open reduction and internal fixation can be performed with the use of Kirschner wires (K-wires), screws, the tension-band wire technique,[20] or suture anchors.[3]

Phalangeal Neck Fractures

Phalangeal neck fractures occur distal to the collateral ligament recess of the proximal or middle phalanx.[12] A number of terms are used to refer to phalangeal neck fractures (**Table 1**). Typically, patients with a phalangeal neck fracture have apex volar angulation with associated sagittal and subcondylar malalignment.[21] The adjacent interphalangeal joint hyperextends, and the proximal volar cortex fracture fragment creates a bony spike, which impedes flexion.[12]

Table 1
Terms Used to Refer to Pediatric Phalangeal Neck Fractures

Subcondylar fractures

Subcapital fractures

Cartilage cap fractures

Distal condylar phalangeal fractures

Supracondylar phalangeal fractures

Unicondylar phalangeal fractures

Bicondylar phalangeal fractures

Transcondylar phalangeal fractures

Avulsion phalangeal fractures

Phalangeal neck fractures are described based on the classification system that was proposed by Al-Qattan.[22] Type I phalangeal neck fractures are nondisplaced. Type II phalangeal neck fractures are displaced and have some remaining cortical contact. Type III phalangeal neck fractures are displaced and have rotational deformity.[22] Radiographs should be obtained with the hand in a position that allows for isolation of the affected digit from the other digits. Lateral radiographs warrant special attention because they are used to assess dorsal displacement. The subcondylar recess must be maintained to ensure full flexion of the digit.

The management of pediatric phalangeal neck fractures is based on the amount of fracture displacement. Nondisplaced phalangeal neck fractures are managed with immobilization for 3 to 4 weeks.[22,23] Displaced phalangeal neck fractures are inherently unstable in the sagittal plane, allowing for dorsal displacement of the distal fragment as a result of the lack of tendinous attachments to the cartilaginous cap;[24] this leads to disruption of the subcondylar fossa, which creates a mechanical block to finger flexion.[25] Therefore, displaced

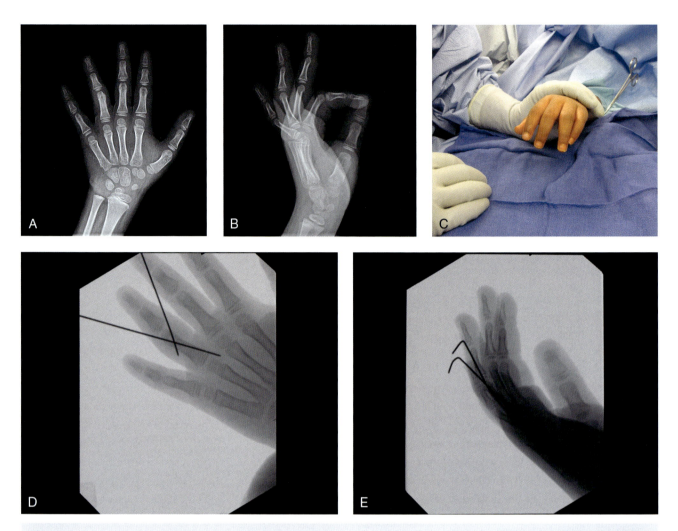

Figure 1 Images of the hand of a 5-year-old boy who caught his left ring finger in a door. PA (**A**) and lateral (**B**) radiographs demonstrate a proximal phalangeal neck/subchondral fracture of the left ring finger. Note the relatively benign appearance of the fracture. **C,** Intraoperative photograph shows the substantial angular deviation that was caused by the fracture. Intraoperative PA (**D**) and lateral (**E**) fluoroscopic images show closed reduction and percutaneous pinning of the fracture. (Copyright Joshua M. Abzug, MD, Timonium, MD.)

and angulated phalangeal neck fractures require surgical management, preferably via CRPP.[22,26-30] Matzon and Cornwall[31] proposed a stepwise algorithm for the surgical management of displaced phalangeal neck fractures, which begins with CRPP (**Figure 1**). For patients in whom CRPP is unsuccessful, percutaneous reduction and pinning is performed with the use of a temporary intrafocal K-wire as a joystick for reduction and osteoclasis as necessary. For patients in whom percutaneous reduction and pinning is unsuccessful, open reduction and percutaneous pinning is performed. Matzon and Cornwall[31] used this stepwise algorithm to guide the treatment of 61 children with a displaced phalangeal neck fracture, 80% of whom were treated with CRPP and 20% of whom were treated with percutaneous reduction and pinning. Percutaneous reduction and pinning was necessary in the patients who were treated more than 2 weeks postinjury. The authors reported that 92% of the patients had good to excellent outcomes, including fracture union, range of motion greater than 50° at the interphalangeal/distal interphalangeal (DIP) joint and greater than 90° at the proximal interphalangeal (PIP) joint, no residual deformity, and good to normal digit function.[31] Patients with a displaced phalangeal neck fracture who undergo percutaneous pinning have a decreased risk for malunion and nonunion compared with patients with a displaced phalangeal neck fracture who undergo only closed reduction; therefore, CRPP is the optimal treatment for patients who have a displaced phalangeal neck fracture.[21,22] However, in a recent study of 37 children with displaced phalangeal neck fractures, Park et al[24] reported that the outcomes of the patients in whom fracture reduction was achieved and maintained with the use of buddy taping and a short arm splint (PIP and DIP joints positioned in 40° to 50° and 10° to 20° of flexion, respectively) were similar compared with those of the patients who underwent CRPP.

The potential for bone remodeling decreases the further the fracture site is from the physis;[26,32,33] however, many studies have reported bone remodeling in pediatric patients with a phalangeal neck fracture, even in those with a displaced or angulated phalangeal neck fracture.[21,25,34-36] The patients in these studies could not be treated with closed reduction or osteoclasis techniques because of substantially delayed initial presentation. Successful bone remodeling is more likely to occur in patients who have a dorsally displaced phalangeal neck fracture with sagittal angulation compared with patients who have a phalangeal neck fracture with coronal malalignment.[34,36] Cortical contact at the fracture site is necessary in patients in whom treatment via observation and bone remodeling is considered. In addition, no coronal plane deformity should be present, the joint should be congruent, and the patient and his or her family must understand the prolonged process of bone remodeling, which may not be successful.[3,21] Salvage techniques are performed in patients in whom bone remodeling is unsuccessful.[37-39] Corrective osteotomy is associated with a high risk for osteonecrosis of the phalangeal condyles because of the limited collateral blood supply.[40] Therefore, the origin of the collateral ligaments should not be disturbed in patients in whom a corrective osteotomy is performed. Other techniques, including re-creation of the volar concavity of the subcondylar fossa, have been reported to decrease the risk for osteonecrosis in patients who require correction of a phalangeal neck malunion.[37]

Patients with a displaced proximal phalanx fracture, especially those with a phalangeal neck fracture, who undergo CRPP will have increased joint stiffness, more coronal plane deviation, and worse aesthetics compared with patients who have a nondisplaced proximal phalanx fracture.[41] Furthermore, patients with a phalangeal neck fracture who undergo either nonsurgical or surgical treatment are more likely to have decreased range of motion, malpositioning, and osteonecrosis compared with patients with other types of phalangeal fractures.[42]

Phalangeal Condyle Fractures

Phalangeal condyle fractures include lateral avulsion, unicondylar, bicondylar, and subcondylar shearing fractures with or without associated joint subluxation/dislocation.[3,27] Typically, phalangeal condyle fractures occur as a result of direct axial compression, avulsion forces, or subchondral shearing.[12] Often, phalangeal condyle fractures are very difficult to manage because of delayed initial presentation and variability in interpretation of the injury on radiographs. In addition, fracture comminution often is present in patients who have a phalangeal condyle fracture, which makes the management of the small articular fragments a technical challenge. Similar to patients with other types of phalangeal fractures, the injured finger of a patient with a suspected phalangeal condyle fracture may appear normal on PA radiographs. Therefore, lateral and oblique radiographs must be obtained to identify and understand the fracture pattern. A double-density sign, which indicates displaced offset of the phalangeal condyle, may be observed on true lateral radiographs.[3,12]

CRPP techniques are the preferred treatment for patients who have an acute phalangeal condyle fracture. Fracture reduction is achieved percutaneously with the assistance of a towel clip or the use of a K-wire as a joystick.[3] One or two 0.035-inch or 0.045-inch K-wires are then placed to stabilize the fracture. The patient's hand is immobilized for 4 weeks, after which the K-wires are removed, and range-of-motion exercises are initiated. Open reduction and internal fixation should be performed only if absolutely necessary because a high risk for osteonecrosis exists as a result of the blood supply of the condyles entering through the collateral ligament (**Figure 2**). Meticulous dissection must be performed to protect the soft-tissue envelope and minimize periosteal stripping.[39] If open reduction is performed, the subcondylar fossa should be débrided to prevent a mechanical block to finger flexion. Various fixation methods are available for patients who have a phalangeal condyle fracture. In a recent study of 13 cadaver models with intra-articular unicondylar fractures that underwent fixation with the use of either a single headless compression screw, a single lag screw, two K-wires, or one K-wire, Sirota et al[43] reported that all of the fixation methods were biomechanically equivalent and that no differences in

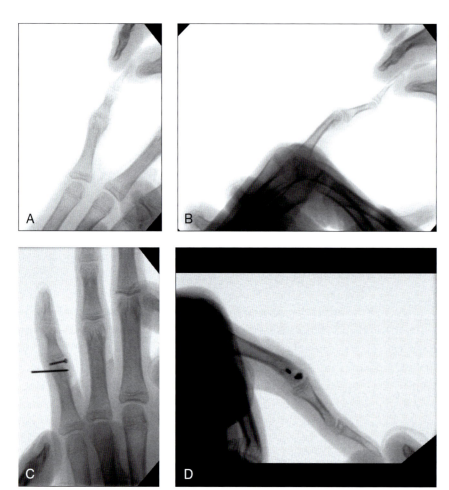

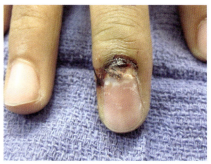

Figure 3   Clinical photograph of the long finger of a 12-year-old boy that was crushed in a car door shows a Seymour fracture. Note that the nail plate is superficial to the eponychial fold. (Copyright Joshua M. Abzug, MD, Timonium, MD.)

Figure 2   Images of the hand of a 13-year-old girl who injured her little finger while playing sports. PA (**A**) and lateral (**B**) fluoroscopic images show a phalangeal condyle fracture of the little finger. Note the lack of smooth contour about the phalangeal head in panel **B**. Postoperative PA (**C**) and lateral (**D**) radiographs demonstrate open reduction and internal fixation of the fracture. (Copyright Joshua M. Abzug, MD, Timonium, MD.)

fracture displacement existed between the fixation methods. Patients who require correction of a phalangeal condyle malunion should undergo a corrective osteotomy to restore as much articular congruity as possible.[3]

Seymour Fractures

Seymour fractures are juxtaepiphyseal injuries to the distal phalanx with concomitant nail bed lacerations.[44] Typically, Seymour fractures occur as a result of crush injuries to the distal phalanx. The associated nail bed laceration technically makes a Seymour fracture an open fracture. Often, the nail bed laceration is not visible; however, the nail plate typically is superficial to the eponychial fold, which makes the nail appear longer compared with the uninjured digits.[3,45] In some patients, the nail does not actually avulse through the eponychial fold; instead, the cuticle seal breaks when the nail bed is torn, which creates an open fracture.[3]

Because patients with a Seymour fracture often are not seen by a surgeon until a few days postinjury, eschar typically is present at the eponychial fold (**Figure 3**). Typically, the distal phalanx is in a flexed posture as a result of the imbalance between the terminal extensor tendon, which inserts on the epiphysis, and the flexor digitorum profundus tendon, which inserts on the metaphysis.[46] Because of this flexed posture of the distal phalanx, Seymour fractures often are misinterpreted as a bony mallet injury; however, displacement in Seymour fractures occurs at the site of the physis/fracture rather than the DIP joint. Concomitant tendon injuries are uncommon in patients who have a Seymour fracture because the physis is biomechanically weaker compared with the surrounding structures. Typically, Seymour fractures occur as a result of a volar force and the angulation of the diaphysis compared with the epiphysis.[44,46] PA radiographs of the injured finger of a patient with a suspected Seymour fracture may appear normal. Therefore, lateral radiographs, which will reflect the amount of fracture displacement and physeal widening, must be obtained to confirm a diagnosis of a Seymour fracture[46] (**Figure 4**).

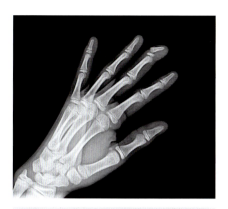

Figure 4 Oblique radiograph of a hand demonstrates a displaced physeal fracture of the distal phalanx of the long finger. Note the flexed posture of the long finger as a result of the relatively stronger force of the flexor digitorum profundus tendon. (Copyright Joshua M. Abzug, MD, Timonium, MD.)

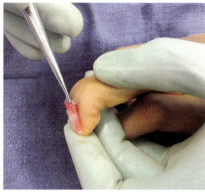

Figure 5 Clinical photograph of the long finger of the patient shown in Figure 3 shows hyperflexion of the digit to allow for extrusion of the germinal matrix, after which gentle débridement of the fracture site is performed. (Copyright Joshua M. Abzug, MD, Timonium, MD.)

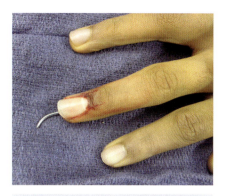

Figure 6 Clinical photograph of the long finger of the patient shown in Figures 3 and 5 taken after irrigation and débridement of the fracture site, nail bed repair, fixation of the Seymour fracture, and replacement of the nail plate. Note the proximal incisions, which were used to gain adequate exposure. (Copyright Joshua M. Abzug, MD, Timonium, MD.)

Closed Seymour fractures are managed with closed reduction and a splint, with weekly follow-up radiographs obtained to ensure maintenance of fracture reduction. Because children may not be compliant with splint wear, and follow-up radiographs may be difficult to interpret because of the adjacent digits, Seymour fractures often are managed surgically. The patient is prepared using sterile techniques, and a tourniquet is applied. The nail plate is removed with the use of blunt instruments, such as a Freer elevator and hemostat. Typically, the nail bed laceration in the germinal matrix allows for adequate exposure of the fracture site. Small oblique incisions that are directed proximally toward the DIP joint at the junction of paronychial and eponychial folds may be necessary to adequately visualize and expose the nail bed laceration. Hyperflexion of the digit also aids in visualization and allows for thorough irrigation and débridement of the fracture site (**Figure 5**). Surgeons must assess for soft tissue and nail matrix interposition at the fracture site; the

failure to remove interposed tissues may prevent anatomic reduction and lead to physeal arrest.[47] The distal fragment is extended to reduce the fracture, and a 0.035-inch or 0.045-inch K-wire is driven retrograde across the DIP joint to stabilize the fracture reduction. The nail bed laceration is then repaired with the use of 6-0 or 7-0 absorbable suture, after which the nail plate is appropriately cleansed, trimmed, and replaced beneath the eponychial fold (**Figure 6**). Patients who have an open injury are treated with parenteral antibiotics followed by a 5- to 7-day course of oral antibiotics.

Minimization of the time from injury to surgical treatment is important to decrease the risk for infection. In a recent study of 34 patients with 35 Seymour fractures, Reyes and Ho[48] reported no infections in the patients who were appropriately treated via irrigation and débridement, fracture reduction with or without K-wire stabilization, and antibiotics within 24 hours postinjury; however, a 15% infection rate was

reported in the patients who were partially treated within 24 hours postinjury, and a 45% infection rate was reported in the patients who were treated more than 24 hours postinjury. The failure to recognize and appropriately manage Seymour fractures may result in complications, including infection and/or osteomyelitis,[44] premature physeal closure,[45] nail bed deformity,[49] as well as dorsal rotation of the epiphysis that leads to articular deformity and extensor mechanism dysfunction.[50] Ganayem and Edelson[51] surgically managed six of seven Seymour fractures successfully and reported no evidence of deformity or infection at a mean follow-up of 18 months. Krushche-Mandl et al[52] surgically stabilized Seymour fractures in five patients successfully. The authors reported no evidence of infection at a mean follow-up of 10 years; however, a growth disturbance of the distal phalanx occurred in two of the patients, and nail dystrophy occurred in one of the patients.

Distal Tuft Fractures

Distal tuft fractures commonly occur in toddlers and preschool-aged children.[9] Typically, distal tuft fractures occur in the home setting as a result of a direct crush injury to the fingertip. A concomitant nail bed laceration and/or soft-tissue injury may be present in patients who have a distal tuft fracture. In patients who have an open distal tuft fracture, the injury should be irrigated as well as débrided, and antibiotics should be administered.

Most patients who have a closed distal tuft fracture are treated nonsurgically with the use of a mitten cast or with the use of a clam-shell splint that covers the injured area and restricts DIP joint motion but leaves the PIP joint free.[16] After 2 to 3 weeks of immobilization, active range of motion of the DIP joint is initiated, and a cap splint is used as necessary for fingertip sensitivity protection. Surgical treatment is reserved for patients with distal tuft fractures who have a near amputation or an unstable transverse fracture pattern. Complications of distal tuft fractures include cold intolerance, hyperesthesia, and numbness, all of which may last as long as 6 months postinjury.[16,53] Rarely, a fibrous nonunion may develop in patients with a distal tuft fracture but typically does not result in clinical consequences.[53]

Bony Mallet Injury

A bony mallet injury involves an injury to the extensor mechanism at the DIP joint as a result of an avulsion fracture at the attachment site of the extensor tendon on the epiphysis.[54] Typically, bony mallet injuries occur as a result of an axially directed load on an extended finger.[3] In a recent biomechanical study that simulated the mechanisms of hyperflexion and hyperextension injuries of the DIP joint in 103 cadaver models, Kreuder et al[55] reported that a hyperflexion injury of the DIP joint resulted in deformity of the extensor tendon aponeurosis, with or without a concomitant bony avulsion fragment, but did not affect the articular surface. Conversely, the authors reported that a hyperextension injury of the DIP joint resulted in a fracture of the dorsal lip of the distal phalanx but did not affect the extensor tendon aponeurosis.[55] Bony mallet injuries occur in patients in whom the extensor tendon avulses a fragment of the epiphysis, which results in an intra-articular fracture. This intra-articular fracture may extend to or through the metaphysis of the distal phalanx, resulting in a Salter-Harris type III or type IV fracture, respectively.[3]

Bony mallet injuries are described based on the Wehbé and Schneider[56] classification system, which divides bony mallet injuries into three types. Each type of bony mallet injury is divided into subtypes based on the amount of articular involvement[56] (**Table 2**). Patel et al[57] classified bony mallet injuries based on the time from injury to initial presentation. Patients with an acute bony mallet injury present less than 4 weeks postinjury, and patients

with a chronic bony mallet injury present more than 4 weeks postinjury.[57]

Limited information is available on the management of pediatric bony mallet injuries; however, surgeons typically treat pediatric patients who have a bony mallet injury based on the management principles used to treat adults who have a bony mallet injury. Ultimately, the goals of bony mallet injury management are to prevent an extensor lag deformity and a swan-neck deformity and to achieve adequate joint stability.[58] Nonsurgical treatment with splint or cast immobilization of the DIP joint in full extension is indicated in patients who have a bony mallet injury that involves less than one-third of the articular surface.[59] The PIP joint does not require splint immobilization because PIP joint extension does not contribute to tendon gapping.[60] Full-time immobilization of the DIP joint in extension for 6 to 8 weeks followed by 2 to 4 weeks of splinting at night is recommended for patients who have a bony mallet injury.[54,61] Care should be taken to avoid skin breakdown and ischemia.

Surgical treatment is indicated in patients who have a bony mallet injury that results in joint incongruence, that fails to maintain cortical bony contact after attempted reduction, with persistent volar subluxation of the

---

Table 2
Wehbé and Schneider Classification of Bony Mallet Injuries

Type	Subtype
I: No DIP joint subluxation	I: Less than one-third of articular surface involvement
II: DIP joint subluxation	II: Between one-third to two-thirds of articular surface involvement
III: Injury to epiphysis and physis	III: More than two-thirds of articular surface involvement

DIP = distal interphalangeal.

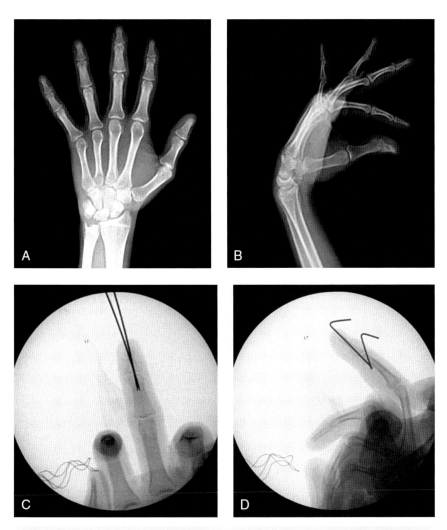

Figure 7   Images of the hand of a 15-year-old boy who jammed his long finger while playing basketball. PA (**A**) and lateral (**B**) radiographs demonstrate a bony mallet injury of the long finger. Note that the fracture fragment involves approximately 50% of the articular surface. Intraoperative PA (**C**) and lateral (**D**) fluoroscopic images show anatomic reduction via the extension-block pinning technique. (Copyright Joshua M. Abzug, MD, Timonium, MD.)

distal phalanx, or that involves more than one-third of the articular surface.[62,63] The percutaneous extension-block pinning technique, which was first described by Ishiguro,[64] is used to indirectly reduce a bony mallet injury (**Figure 7**). Other techniques for the surgical management of bony mallet injuries include tension band wiring, hook plating, internal suturing, pin fixation, and the use of bone anchors.[59,65-69] The outcomes of children with a bony mallet injury who undergo surgical treatment have not been studied. Ultimately, the amount of terminal extensor tendon shortening or lengthening determines a patient's final outcome. Terminal extensor tendon lengthening of 1 mm will result in 25° of extensor lag, and terminal extensor tendon shortening of 1 mm will result in severely restricted DIP joint flexion.[70] Surgeons should note that adults with a bony mallet injury who undergo surgical treatment have mild extensor lag (5° to 10°) and mild loss of range of motion postoperatively.[16]

Summary

Phalangeal fractures are one of the most common injuries that occur in the pediatric and adolescent population. The incidence of phalangeal fractures is the highest in children aged 10 to 14 years, which coincides with the time that most children begin playing contact sports. Younger children are more likely to sustain a phalangeal fracture in the home setting as a result of crush and laceration injuries. Knowledge of physeal anatomy and the secondary ossification centers is necessary to understand how phalangeal fractures occur. A thorough physical examination is necessary to assess the digital cascade for signs of rotational deformity and/or coronal malalignment. The management of phalangeal fractures is based on the amount of fracture displacement and depends on the success of closed reduction techniques. CRPP is the preferred treatment modality for the management of displaced phalanx fractures.

References

1. Barton NJ: Fractures of the phalanges of the hand in children. *Hand* 1979;11(2):134-143.

2. Hastings H II, Simmons BP: Hand fractures in children: A statistical analysis. *Clin Orthop Relat Res* 1984;188:120-130.

3. Cornwall R, Ricchetti ET: Pediatric phalanx fractures: Unique challenges and pitfalls. *Clin Orthop Relat Res* 2006;445:146-156.

4. Mahabir RC, Kazemi AR, Cannon WG, Courtemanche DJ: Pediatric hand fractures: A review. *Pediatr Emerg Care* 2001;17(3):153-156.

5. Rajesh A, Basu AK, Vaidhyanath R, Finlay D: Hand fractures: A study of their site and type in childhood. *Clin Radiol* 2001;56(8):667-669.

6. Naranje SM, Erali RA, Warner WC Jr, Sawyer JR, Kelly DM: Epidemiology of pediatric fractures presenting to emergency departments in the United States. *J Pediatr Orthop* 2016;36(4):e45-e48.

7. Chew EM, Chong AK: Hand fractures in children: Epidemiology and misdiagnosis in a tertiary referral hospital. *J Hand Surg Am* 2012;37(8):1684-1688.

8. Liu EH, Alqahtani S, Alsaaran RN, Ho ES, Zuker RM, Borschel GH: A prospective study of pediatric hand fractures and review of the literature. *Pediatr Emerg Care* 2014;30(5):299-304.

9. Vadivelu R, Dias JJ, Burke FD, Stanton J: Hand injuries in children: A prospective study. *J Pediatr Orthop* 2006;26(1):29-35.

10. Ozer K, Gillani S, Williams A, Hak DJ: Psychiatric risk factors in pediatric hand fractures. *J Pediatr Orthop* 2010;30(4):324-327.

11. Worlock PH, Stower MJ: The incidence and pattern of hand fractures in children. *J Hand Surg Br* 1986;11(2):198-200.

12. Nellans KW, Chung KC: Pediatric hand fractures. *Hand Clin* 2013;29(4):569-578.

13. Salter RB, Harris WR: Injuries involving the epiphyseal plate. *J Bone Joint Surg Am* 1963;45(3):587-622.

14. Cope EB, Antony JH: Normal values for the two-point discrimination test. *Pediatr Neurol* 1992;8(4):251-254.

15. Tindall A, Dawood R, Povlsen B: Case of the month: The skin wrinkle test. A simple nerve injury test for paediatric and uncooperative patients. *Emerg Med J* 2006;23(11):883-886.

16. Oetgen ME, Dodds SD: Nonoperative treatment of common finger injuries. *Curr Rev Musculoskelet Med* 2008;1(2):97-102.

17. Al-Qattan MM, Al-Zahrani K, Al-Boukai AA: The relative incidence of fractures at the base of the proximal phalanx of the fingers in children. *J Hand Surg Eur Vol* 2008;33(4):465-468.

18. Al-Qattan MM: Juxta-epiphyseal fractures of the base of the proximal phalanx of the fingers in children and adolescents. *J Hand Surg Br* 2002;27(1):24-30.

19. Desaldeleer AS, Le Nen D: Bilateral fracture of the base of the middle phalanx in a climber: Literature review and a case report. *Orthop Traumatol Surg Res* 2016;102(3):409-411.

20. Stahl S, Jupiter JB: Salter-Harris type III and IV epiphyseal fractures in the hand treated with tension-band wiring. *J Pediatr Orthop* 1999;19(2):233-235.

21. Cornwall R, Waters PM: Remodeling of phalangeal neck fracture malunions in children: Case report. *J Hand Surg Am* 2004;29(3):458-461.

22. Al-Qattan MM: Phalangeal neck fractures in children: Classification and outcome in 66 cases. *J Hand Surg Br* 2001;26(2):112-121.

23. Campbell RM Jr: Operative treatment of fractures and dislocations of the hand and wrist region in children. *Orthop Clin North Am* 1990;21(2):217-243.

24. Park KB, Lee KJ, Kwak YH: Comparison between buddy taping with a short-arm splint and operative treatment for phalangeal neck fractures in children. *J Pediatr Orthop* 2016;36(7):736-742.

25. Puckett BN, Gaston RG, Peljovich AE, Lourie GM, Floyd WE III: Remodeling potential of phalangeal distal condylar malunions in children. *J Hand Surg Am* 2012;37(1):34-41.

26. Graham TJ, Hastings HI: Fractures and dislocations in the child's hand, in Gupta A, Kay SPJ, Scheker LR, eds: *The Growing Hand: Diagnosis and Management of the Upper Extremity in Children*. London, United Kingdom, Harcourt, 2000, pp 591-607.

27. Graham TJ, Waters PM: Fractures and dislocations of the hand and carpus in children, in Beaty JH, Kasser JR, eds: *Rockwood and Wilkins' Fractures in Children,* ed 5. Philadelphia, PA, Lippincott, Williams & Wilkins, 2001, pp 269-379.

28. Stern PJ: Fractures of the metacarpals and phalanges, in Green DP, Hotchkiss RN, Pederson WC, eds: *Green's Operative Hand Surgery,* ed 4. New York, NY, Churchill Livingstone, 1999, pp 711-771.

29. Kang HJ, Sung SY, Ha JW, Yoon HK, Hahn SB: Operative treatment for proximal phalangeal neck fractures of the finger in children. *Yonsei Med J* 2005;46(4):491-495.

30. Janssen SJ, Molleman J, Guitton TG, Ring D; Science Of Variation Group: What middle phalanx base fracture characteristics are most reliable and useful for surgical decision-making? *Clin Orthop Relat Res* 2015;473(12):3943-3950.

31. Matzon JL, Cornwall R: A stepwise algorithm for surgical treatment of type II displaced pediatric phalangeal neck fractures. *J Hand Surg Am* 2014;39(3):467-473.

32. Green DP: Hand injuries in children. *Pediatr Clin North Am* 1977;24(4):903-918.

33. Armstrong PF, Joughin VE, Clarke HM: Pediatric fractures of the forearm, wrist, and hand, in Green NE, Swiontkowski MF, eds: *Skeletal Trauma in Children,* ed 2. Philadelphia, PA, Saunders, 1998, pp 161-257.

34. Hennrikus WL, Cohen MR: Complete remodelling of displaced fractures of the neck of the phalanx. *J Bone Joint Surg Br* 2003;85(2):273-274.

35. Crick JC, Franco RS, Conners JJ: Fractures about the interphalangeal joints in children. *J Orthop Trauma* 1987;1(4):318-325.

36. Tada K, Ikeda K, Tomita K: Malunion of fractures of the proximal phalangeal neck in children. *Scand J Plast Reconstr Surg Hand Surg* 2010;44(1):69-71.

37. Simmons BP, Peters TT: Subcondylar fossa reconstruction for malunion of fractures of the proximal phalanx in children. *J Hand Surg Am* 1987;12(6):1079-1082.

38. Waters PM, Taylor BA, Kuo AY: Percutaneous reduction of incipient malunion of phalangeal neck fractures in children. *J Hand Surg Am* 2004;29(4):707-711.

39. Topouchian V, Fitoussi F, Jehanno P, Frajman JM, Mazda K, Pennecot GF: Treatment of phalangeal neck fractures in children: Technical suggestion. *Chir Main* 2003;22(6):299-304.

40. Yousif NJ, Cunningham MW, Sanger JR, Gingrass RP, Matloub HS: The vascular supply to the proximal interphalangeal joint. *J Hand Surg Am* 1985;10(6 pt 1):852-861.

41. Boyer JS, London DA, Stepan JG, Goldfarb CA: Pediatric proximal phalanx fractures: Outcomes and complications after the surgical treatment of displaced fractures. *J Pediatr Orthop* 2015;35(3):219-223.

42. Huelsemann W, Singer G, Mann M, Winkler FJ, Habenicht R: Analysis of sequelae after pediatric phalangeal fractures. *Eur J Pediatr Surg* 2016;26(2):164-171.

43. Sirota MA, Parks BG, Higgins JP, Means KR Jr: Stability of fixation of proximal phalanx unicondylar fractures of the hand: A biomechanical cadaver study. *J Hand Surg Am* 2013;38(1):77-81.

44. Seymour N: Juxta-epiphysial fracture of the terminal phalanx of the finger. *J Bone Joint Surg Br* 1966;48(2):347-349.

45. Al-Qattan MM: Extra-articular transverse fractures of the base of the distal phalanx (Seymour's fracture) in children and adults. *J Hand Surg Br* 2001;26(3):201-206.

46. Abzug JM, Kozin SH: Seymour fractures. *J Hand Surg Am* 2013;38(11):2267 2270.

47. Banerjee A: Irreducible distal phalangeal epiphyseal injuries. *J Hand Surg Br* 1992;17(3):337-338.

48. Reyes BA, Ho CA: The high risk of infection with delayed treatment of open Seymour fractures: Salter-Harris I/II or juxta-epiphyseal fractures of the distal phalanx with associated nailbed laceration. *J Pediatr Orthop* 2015.

49. Egol K: Pediatric wrist and hand, in Egol KA, Koval KJ, Zuckerman JD, eds: *Handbook of Fractures,* ed 4. Philadelphia, PA, Lippincott, Williams & Wilkins, 2011, pp 660-680.

50. Waters PM, Benson LS: Dislocation of the distal phalanx epiphysis in toddlers. *J Hand Surg Am* 1993;18(4):581-585.

51. Ganayem M, Edelson G: Base of distal phalanx fracture in children: A mallet finger mimic. *J Pediatr Orthop* 2005;25(4):487-489.

52. Krusche-Mandl I, Köttstorfer J, Thalhammer G, Aldrian S, Erhart J, Platzer P: Seymour fractures: Retrospective analysis and therapeutic considerations. *J Hand Surg Am* 2013;38(2):258-264.

53. DaCruz DJ, Slade RJ, Malone W: Fractures of the distal phalanges. *J Hand Surg Br* 1988;13(3):350-352.

54. Alla SR, Deal ND, Dempsey IJ: Current concepts: Mallet finger. *Hand (N Y)* 2014;9(2):138-144.

55. Kreuder A, Pennig D, Boese CK, Eysel P, Oppermann J, Dargel J: Mallet finger: A simulation and analysis of hyperflexion versus hyperextension injuries. *Surg Radiol Anat* 2016;38(4):403-407.

56. Wehbé MA, Schneider LH: Mallet fractures. *J Bone Joint Surg Am* 1984;66(5):658-669.

57. Patel MR, Desai SS, Bassini-Lipson L: Conservative management of chronic mallet finger. *J Hand Surg Am* 1986;11(4):570-573.

58. Doyle JR: Extensor tendons: Acute injuries, in Green DP, Hotchkiss RN, Pederson WC, eds: *Green's Operative Hand Surgery,* ed 4. New York, NY, Churchill Livingstone, 1999, pp 1950-1987.

59. Miranda BH, Murugesan L, Grobbelaar AO, Jemec B: PBNR: Percutaneous blunt needle reduction of bony mallet injuries. *Tech Hand Up Extrem Surg* 2015;19(2):81-83.

60. Katzman BM, Klein DM, Mesa J, Geller J, Caligiuri DA: Immobilization of the mallet finger: Effects on the extensor tendon. *J Hand Surg Br* 1999;24(1):80-84.

61. Kalainov DM, Hoepfner PE, Hartigan BJ, Carroll C IV, Genuario J: Nonsurgical treatment of closed mallet finger fractures. *J Hand Surg Am* 2005;30(3):580-586.

62. Stark HH, Gainor BJ, Ashworth CR, Zemel NP, Rickard TA: Operative treatment of intra-articular fractures of the dorsal aspect of the distal phalanx of digits. *J Bone Joint Surg Am* 1987;69(6):892-896.

63. Pegoli L, Toh S, Arai K, Fukuda A, Nishikawa S, Vallejo IG: The Ishiguro extension block technique for the treatment of mallet finger fracture: Indications and clinical results. *J Hand Surg Br* 2003;28(1):15-17.

64. Ishiguro T: A new method of closed reduction for mallet fracture using extension-block Kirschner wire. *Cent Jpn J Orthop Trauma Surg* 1988;6:413-415.

65. Bischoff R, Buechler U, De Roche R, Jupiter J: Clinical results of tension band fixation of avulsion fractures of the hand. *J Hand Surg Am* 1994;19(6):1019-1026.

66. Damron TA, Engber WD: Surgical treatment of mallet finger fractures by tension band technique. *Clin Orthop Relat Res* 1994;300:133-140.

67. Bauze A, Bain GI: Internal suture for mallet finger fracture. *J Hand Surg Br* 1999;24(6):688-692.

68. Kakinoki R, Ohta S, Noguchi T, et al: A modified tension band wiring technique for treatment of the bony mallet finger. *Hand Surg* 2013;18(2):235-242.

69. Acar MA, Güzel Y, Güleç A, Uzer G, Elmadağ M: Clinical comparison of hook plate fixation versus extension block pinning for bony mallet finger: A retrospective comparison study. *J Hand Surg Eur Vol* 2015;40(8):832-839.

70. Schweitzer TP, Rayan GM: The terminal tendon of the digital extensor mechanism: Part II, kinematic study. *J Hand Surg Am* 2004;29(5):903-908.

Video Reference

34.1: Abzug JP: Video. *Pediatric Phalanx Fracture.* Timonium, MD, 2016.

Pediatric Scaphoid Fractures

Beverlie Ting, MD
Andrea Sesko Bauer, MD
Joshua M. Abzug, MD
Roger Cornwall, MD
Theresa O. Wyrick, MD
Donald S. Bae, MD

Abstract

Scaphoid fractures are the most common type of carpal injuries that occur in children and adolescents. The injury pattern seen in children and adolescents who have scaphoid fractures has recently shifted to resemble that of adults who have scaphoid fractures, with scaphoid waist fractures being the most common injury pattern. This shift has been attributed to increased body mass index in children and adolescents as well as more intense participation in extreme sports by both children and adolescents. The diagnosis of scaphoid fractures is based on both a clinical examination and radiographic findings. If a scaphoid fracture is clinically suspected but initial radiographs are negative, cast immobilization followed by repeat imaging can lead to accurate diagnosis of the injury. MRI can aid in the diagnosis of a scaphoid injury in pediatric patients with incomplete ossification of the scaphoid. Acute nondisplaced scaphoid fractures have a high rate of healing with cast immobilization; however, surgery should be considered in patients who have displaced scaphoid fractures with delayed presentation. In general, patients with scaphoid fractures who undergo appropriate treatment and achieve successful union have excellent long-term functional outcomes.

Instr Course Lect 2017;66:429–436.

Epidemiology

Scaphoid fractures are relatively uncommon in children and adolescents, representing only 0.39% of all pediatric fractures and 2.2% of all pediatric hand fractures.[1] The scaphoid is, however, the most commonly fractured carpal bone, and scaphoid fractures represent 87% of all pediatric carpal fractures.[2,3] Pediatric scaphoid fractures most commonly occur in patients aged 11 to 15 years, and 79% to 95% of pediatric scaphoid fractures occur in males.[4,5] Scaphoid fractures aer rare in children younger than 9 years.[6] The most frequent mechanism of injury for scaphoid fractures is a fall onto an extended wrist in ulnar deviation during sports participation.[3,4,7]

A recent retrospective analysis of 351 scaphoid fractures in patients aged 7 to 18 years who were treated between 1995 and 2010 suggested a shift in contemporary injury patterns in children and adolescents who have scaphoid fractures.[7] This shift in injury patterns was

Dr. Bauer or an immediate family member serves as a board member, owner, officer, or committee member of the American Society for Surgery of the Hand and the Pediatric Orthopaedic Society of North America. Dr. Abzug or an immediate family member is a member of a speakers' bureau or has made paid presentations on behalf of Checkpoint Surgical and serves as a paid consultant to or is an employee of AxoGen. Dr. Bae or an immediate family member has stock or stock options held in Cempra, Johnson & Johnson, Kythera Biopharmaceuticals, and Vivus and serves as a board member, owner, officer, or committee member of the American Academy of Orthopaedic Surgeons, the American Society for Surgery of the Hand, and the Pediatric Orthopaedic Society of North America. None of the following authors nor any immediate family member has received anything of value from or has stock or stock options held in a commercial company nor institution related directly or indirectly to the subject of this chapter: Dr. Ting, Dr. Cornwall, and Dr. Wyrick.

attributed to increased body mass index in children and adolescents as well as more intense participation in extreme sports, including football, basketball, snowboarding, and skateboarding, by both children and adolescents.[7] Historically, the distal pole of the scaphoid was the most frequently involved zone of injury in children and adolescents who sustained scaphoid fractures, accounting for 59% to 87% of all pediatric scaphoid fractures.[1,8,9] Currently, scaphoid waist fractures appear to be the most common injury pattern in children and adolescents who sustain scaphoid fractures, accounting for as many as 71% of all pediatric scaphoid fractures,[7] which is similar to the anatomic distribution of scaphoid fractures observed in adults. Although an increase in scaphoid waist fractures has been observed in children who have either closed or open physes, it is more pronounced in children who have closed physes (84% versus 68%, respectively).[7]

Although a scaphoid fracture is eventually diagnosed in only 6.7% of pediatric patients with wrist pain who arrive in an emergency department, surgeons should maintain a high level of suspicion for scaphoid injury to avoid the complications of a missed diagnosis.[6] It is estimated that as many as 37% of pediatric scaphoid fractures are not radiographically evident until follow-up radiographs are obtained.[1,2,10] Most clinically suspected scaphoid fractures that are not radiographically evident initially (45%) are identified at the first follow-up visit (mean, 2 weeks postinjury; range 8 to 31 days postinjury), and 84% of clinically suspected scaphoid fractures that are not radiographically evident initially are identified by the second follow-up visit (mean, 5 weeks postinjury; range, 2 to 9 weeks postinjury).

Anatomy

The scaphoid lies in the proximal carpal row and is adjacent to the lunate and the capitate. The scaphoid articulates proximally with the distal radius and distally with the trapezium and the trapezoid to form the scaphotrapeziotrapezoidal joint. The scaphoid's main blood supply is derived from two branches of the radial artery. The dorsal scaphoid branch of the radial artery runs along the dorsal ridge of the scaphoid in a retrograde fashion and supplies blood to the proximal 70% to 80% of the scaphoid, and the volar scaphoid branch of the radial artery supplies blood to the distal 20% to 30% of the scaphoid.[11] In males, the ossific nucleus of the scaphoid appears at 5 to 6 years of age, and enchondral ossification is complete by 15 years of age.[2] In females, the ossific nucleus appears earlier, at 4 to 5 years of age, and enchondral ossification is complete by 13 years of age. Bipartite scaphoids have been described; however, it remains unclear whether a bipartite scaphoid is a normal congenital variant or the result of asymptomatic nonunion.[12,13]

Classification

Scaphoid fractures are commonly classified based on the time from injury and the anatomic location of the fracture, both of which are factors with important treatment implications. In general, patients with scaphoid fractures that are less than 6 weeks postinjury have acute scaphoid injuries, and patients with scaphoid fractures that are more than 6 weeks postinjury have chronic scaphoid injuries.[7] Scaphoid fractures are typically divided into injuries of the proximal pole, the waist, or the distal pole, which include tuberosity fractures and avulsion fractures of the distal pole[2] (**Figure 1**). Historically, distal pole

fractures were the most common pediatric scaphoid fracture pattern; however, a notable rise in scaphoid waist injuries has occurred in the past decade.[7,8] This recent change in scaphoid fracture patterns is particularly important because patients with scaphoid waist fracture patterns have a higher risk for nonunion.[7]

Pediatric scaphoid fractures also can be classified based on the age of the patient and the degree of scaphoid ossification[9] (**Figure 2**). This classification system divides scaphoid fractures into three subcategories. Type I scaphoid fractures are pure chondral injuries and typically occur in patients younger than 8 years. Type I scaphoid fractures are rare and difficult to visualize on plain radiographs; therefore, MRI is typically required for diagnosis. Type II scaphoid fractures are osteochondral injuries and typically occur in patients aged 8 to 11 years. Type III scaphoid fractures are osseous injuries. Type III scaphoid injuries are the most common type of scaphoid fractures and typically occur in patients older than 11 years. This classification scheme emphasizes the difficulty in diagnosing scaphoid fractures that occur in patients with incomplete ossification of the scaphoid.

History and Physical Examination

The most frequent mechanism of injury for scaphoid fractures is a fall onto an extended wrist in ulnar deviation during sports participation.[3,4,7] Patients also may report history of a hyperflexion injury or a direct blow.[2] Snuffbox tenderness and tenderness to palpation over the distal pole of the scaphoid suggest a scaphoid fracture.[14] In a study of children in whom scaphoid fractures

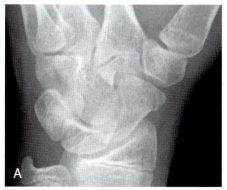 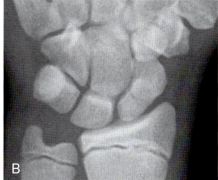 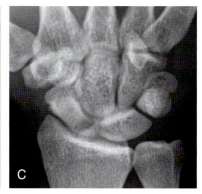

Figure 1 Wrist radiographs demonstrate various types of scaphoid fractures. **A,** Oblique radiograph demonstrates a scaphoid fracture of the distal pole. AP radiographs demonstrate scaphoid fractures of the waist (**B**) and the proximal pole (**C**). (Courtesy of Children's Orthopaedic Surgery Foundation, Boston, MA.)

were clinically suspected, Evenski et al[10] identified three statistically significant, independent predictors of a scaphoid fracture. The authors determined that patients who had volar tenderness over the scaphoid, pain with radial deviation, and pain with active wrist motion were 5.5, 9.8, and 5.5 times more likely, respectively, to have a true scaphoid fracture.[10]

Imaging

PA and lateral radiographs of the wrist as well as a PA radiograph of the wrist in ulnar deviation should be obtained if a scaphoid fracture is clinically suspected.[14] It is important to note that as many as 37% of pediatric scaphoid fractures are not radiographically evident until follow-up radiographs are obtained 4 to 12 days postinjury.[1,2,10] Therefore, immobilization followed by radiographs obtained 2 weeks postinjury is a common practice that often leads to timely scaphoid fracture identification. Although most scaphoid fractures are evident at the first follow-up visit, radiographic findings may not be observed in some patients until up to 9 weeks postinjury. Radiographic diagnosis of scaphoid fractures in children

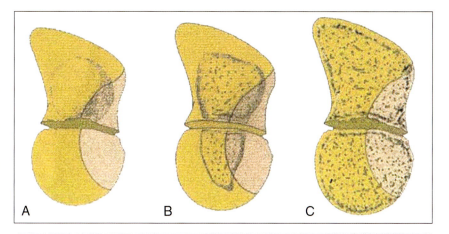

Figure 2 Illustration shows the classification system for pediatric scaphoid fractures. **A,** Type I fractures are pure chondral injuries. **B,** Type II fractures are osteochondral injuries. **C,** Type III fractures are osseous injuries. (Reproduced with permission from D'Arienzo M: Scaphoid fractures in children. *J Hand Surg Br* 2002;27[5]:424-426.)

and adolescents is further complicated by skeletal immaturity because the scaphoid is incompletely ossified.

The role of MRI within 48 to 72 hours of injury has been investigated to facilitate earlier diagnosis of scaphoid fracture and avoid unnecessary immobilization of children who have wrist pain.[15] In a study of 56 patients aged 6 to 15 years in whom scaphoid fractures were clinically suspected, Johnson et al[15] reported that 75% of patients in whom a scaphoid fracture was diagnosed with

MRI had initial radiographs that were negative. Furthermore, the authors reported that MRI aided in the correct diagnosis of adjacent carpal and radial injuries in patients who had no evidence of scaphoid fractures.[15] Proponents of MRI argue that the use of MRI can prevent unnecessary immobilization in as many as 58% of patients in whom scaphoid fractures are clinically suspected.[7,15] MRI has been reported to have a 100% negative predictive value for the diagnosis of acute scaphoid fractures.[16] Although early MRI may not be feasible or cost-effective in all patients who have a suspected scaphoid injury, it should be considered, especially for patients who have equivocal initial radiographs.[15]

CT also can be used to aid in the diagnosis and evaluation of patients who have scaphoid fractures; however, it is associated with a risk of radiation exposure. Furthermore, studies suggest that, compared with MRI, CT is not as sensitive in the diagnosis of acute scaphoid fractures.[17] In general, the authors of this chapter reserve CT for preoperative planning in patients who have scaphoid nonunion.

Associated Injuries

As many as 15% of patients with scaphoid fractures have associated injuries,[7] most of which occur as a result of high-energy mechanisms of injury.[2] A recent retrospective analysis of 351 pediatric patients who had scaphoid fractures reported that distal radius fractures (4.8%), transscaphoid perilunate dislocations (1.4%), ulnar styloid fractures (1.4%), and capitate fractures (1.1%) were the most common injuries associated with scaphoid fractures.[7] Other injuries associated with scaphoid fractures include trapezium fractures and radial head fractures.[2] Surgeons should maintain a high index of suspicion for concomitant scaphoid fracture in patients who sustain any of these fractures as a result of a high-energy mechanism of injury.

Management
Nonsurgical Treatment
Indications
Cast immobilization has been the mainstay of nonsurgical treatment for children and adolescents who have scaphoid

fractures.[1,9] Nonsurgical treatment for patients who have a clinically suspected scaphoid fracture involves immobilization followed by clinical and radiographic follow-up at 2 weeks postinjury. More than 90% of patients with acute nondisplaced scaphoid injuries who are treated with cast immobilization alone achieve successful union.[7] Bond et al[18] reported that percutaneous screw fixation of acute nondisplaced scaphoid fractures results in faster radiographic and clinical union compared with cast immobilization (7 weeks versus 12 weeks, respectively); however, because acute nondisplaced scaphoid fractures have a high rate of successful union, the authors of this chapter recommend a trial of cast immobilization. Conversely, fewer than one-fourth of patients with chronic scaphoid fractures (>6 weeks postinjury) who are treated with only cast immobilization achieve successful union.[6,7]

The duration of cast immobilization for patients who have scaphoid fractures varies widely. Several factors have been reported to influence the time to union in children who undergo cast immobilization and can help guide the duration of cast immobilization.[7,19] Union is defined as the absence of clinical signs of scaphoid fracture and more than 50% bridging trabeculae observed on radiographs.[7] Four factors that prolong time to healing in children who undergo cast immobilization are (1) the location of scaphoid waist or proximal pole fractures, (2) fracture displacement, (3) longer time to initial treatment, and (4) the presence of osteonecrosis.[7] In a study of pediatric patients who had scaphoid injuries, Gholson et al[7] reported that distal pole fractures, waist fractures, and proximal pole fractures healed after a median of 6 weeks, 9 weeks, and

15 weeks, respectively. The authors reported that displaced scaphoid fractures took 12 weeks longer to heal compared with nondisplaced scaphoid fractures (19 weeks versus 7 weeks, respectively), chronic scaphoid injuries took 9 weeks longer to heal compared with acute scaphoid injuries (16 weeks versus 7 weeks, respectively), and scaphoid fractures in patients who had osteonecrosis took 3 weeks longer to heal compared with scaphoid fractures in patients without evidence of osteonecrosis (13 weeks versus 10 weeks, respectively).[7] The authors recommended that the risk factors for nonunion after cast immobilization be discussed with patients and their families.[7]

The type of cast immobilization for patients who have scaphoid fractures also is a matter of debate. In a prospective study of 51 adults who had acute nondisplaced scaphoid injuries, Gellman et al[20] compared long arm-thumb spica cast immobilization with short arm-thumb spica cast immobilization. The authors reported that the patients who were initially treated with long arm-thumb spica cast immobilization for the first 6 weeks healed faster (mean time to healing, 9.5 weeks) compared with the patients who were initially treated with short arm-thumb spica cast immobilization (mean time to healing, 12.7 weeks).[20] Biomechanical studies have reported conflicting results with regard to scaphoid motion during forearm pronation and supination in cadaver models that were immobilized in short arm-thumb spica casts.[21,22] In a prospective, randomized trial of 62 adults who underwent immobilization of nondisplaced scaphoid fractures for 10 weeks in a short arm cast that either included or excluded the thumb, Buijze et al[23] reported greater evidence of union on the CT scans of the patients who were immobilized in a short arm cast that excluded the thumb. The authors reported that the overall union rate was 98%. More importantly, the authors reported no differences between the patients in the two groups with respect to wrist motion; grip strength; the Modified Mayo Wrist score; the Disabilities of the Arm, Shoulder and Hand score; or pain intensity.[23] Further investigation is necessary to determine the optimal mode of immobilization for patients who have nondisplaced scaphoid fractures.[5,7] The authors of this chapter immobilize nondisplaced scaphoid fractures in a short arm-thumb spica cast for the duration of healing.

Outcomes

In general, the functional outcomes of patients with acute scaphoid fractures who are treated with appropriate immobilization are favorable.[5,7] In a study of 56 patients younger than 14 years who underwent nonsurgical treatment for confirmed scaphoid fractures, Ahmed et al[6] reported that, at a mean follow-up of 70 months, 60% of the patients had no lasting functional limitations, and 25% of the patients had only mild or infrequent problems during participation in certain recreational sports. The authors reported that no patients had substantial limitations in their daily social or functional activities, and only one patient required surgical treatment as a result of delayed presentation at 5 months with evidence of nonunion. A more recent study investigated the long-term functional outcomes of 63 pediatric patients who underwent either surgical or nonsurgical treatment for scaphoid fractures.[24] The authors reported that, at a median follow-up of 6.3 years, all scaphoid fractures had

successfully healed, and 95% of the patients had excellent functional outcomes, with Modified Mayo Wrist and Disabilities of the Arm, Shoulder and Hand scores comparable with those of the general population. Although surgical treatment did not influence functional outcomes, the authors reported that chronic scaphoid fracture presentation and osteonecrosis were independent predictors of worse functional outcomes.[24]

Surgical Treatment
Indications

Surgical fixation is indicated in two types of patients: those who have acute displaced scaphoid fractures and those with scaphoid fractures in whom nonsurgical treatment with cast immobilization fails.[6] Surgical fixation also is indicated in patients who have chronic (>6 weeks postinjury) displaced scaphoid fractures, chronic nondisplaced waist fractures, and chronic nondisplaced proximal pole fractures; patients who have chronic scaphoid injuries deserve careful attention and must be advised that they have a high risk for nonunion with nonsurgical treatment.[7]

In patients who have nondisplaced scaphoid fractures, percutaneous screw fixation that is placed down the axis of the scaphoid can be performed via either the volar or dorsal approach with the use of cannulated compression screws.[25] Central screw placement has been reported to be biomechanically stronger compared with eccentric screw placement.[26]

In patients who have a substantial humpback deformity, open reduction and internal fixation is typically performed via the volar approach[27] (**Figure 3**). A radiolunate pin can be used to correct a dorsal intercalated segment

instability deformity and restore neutral lunate alignment before scaphoid fixation.[28] Scaphoid fixation can be achieved with the use of either Kirschner wires or headless variable-pitch compression screws and is often supplemented with the use of corticocancellous iliac crest bone graft.[27,29-32] Other techniques that have been described for the surgical treatment of scaphoid fractures include the Matti-Russe procedure with the use of autograft.[29,33]

Vascularized bone grafting for scaphoid nonunion is used far less frequently in children and adolescents compared with adults and is generally reserved for revision surgery in patients who have proximal pole nonunion with osteonecrosis. In these patients, vascularized radial bone grafting can lead to successful union.[19] In a case report on a pediatric patient who had osteonecrosis, Ben-Amotz et al[34] described scaphoid reconstruction with a vascularized medial femoral condyle graft, which is a procedure that is becoming increasingly popular in adults.

A high-energy perilunate injury that is known as a transscaphoid perilunate fracture-dislocation may occasionally be observed in conjunction with a scaphoid fracture. Although transscaphoid perilunate fracture-dislocations are less common in skeletally immature patients, they should generally be treated similar to transscaphoid perilunate fracture-dislocations in adults, with open reduction and internal fixation of the scaphoid and ligament repair/pin stabilization of the accompanying carpal dislocations.

Outcomes

Fracture location, fracture displacement, the presence of open physes, the use of bone graft, and the type of screw

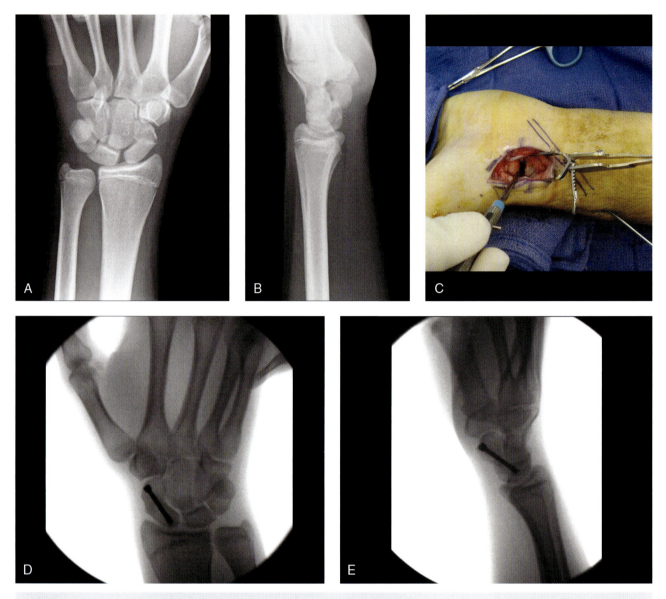

Figure 3   Images of the wrist of a skeletally immature boy show nonunion of a scaphoid waist fracture. Preoperative AP (**A**) and lateral (**B**) radiographs demonstrate a displaced waist fracture with dorsal intercalated segment instability deformity. **C,** Intraoperative photograph shows the volar approach for open reduction and internal fixation with the use of an iliac crest bone graft and a compression screw. Postoperative AP (**D**) and lateral (**E**) fluoroscopic images taken at final follow-up demonstrate restoration of scaphoid alignment with complete bony union. (Courtesy of Children's Orthopaedic Surgery Foundation, Boston, MA.)

used for fixation have been reported to influence the time to healing in patients who undergo surgical treatment for scaphoid fractures.[7] Children who undergo surgical fixation for the treatment of either acute scaphoid injuries or chronic scaphoid injuries will achieve high rates of union (98% and 96%, respectively).[7] Bae et al[24] investigated the functional outcomes of 63 pediatric patients aged 8 to 18 years with either acute or chronic scaphoid injuries who underwent either surgical or nonsurgical treatment. Although it is important to note that all of the patients in the study achieved bony union, the authors reported that, at a median follow-up of 6.3 years, 95% of the patients had a functional status equivalent to or better than that of the general population.[24] The authors also reported that chronic scaphoid injuries and osteonecrosis were independent predictors of worse functional outcomes.[24]

Postoperative Management

In general, patients who undergo surgical treatment for scaphoid fractures are immobilized in a short arm-thumb spica cast until union is achieved. Patients are monitored at regular intervals until radiographic union is achieved (usually between 6 and 12 weeks), after which elbow, forearm, and wrist exercises are started to restore range of motion. In general, patients are restricted from return to sports until 3 to 6 months postoperatively, depending on the rate of healing and rehabilitation.

Complications

Nonunion is a rare complication in patients who undergo appropriate treatment for an acute scaphoid injury;[1,29,35,36] however, as many as two-thirds of scaphoid fractures in children and adolescents are chronic injuries (>6 weeks postinjury).[4] Nonunion occurs in more than 65% of patients with chronic scaphoid injuries who undergo cast immobilization.[7] Fortunately, patients who undergo surgical fixation for the treatment of chronic scaphoid fractures have a healing rate of more than 90% to 95% and encouraging functional outcomes.[7,27,30] Complications reported after nonsurgical treatment with cast immobilization include refracture, malunion, collapse of the proximal pole, and persistent pain after radiographic healing.[7] Surgical fixation has been associated with limited wrist motion and painful hardware that requires removal.[7,18]

Summary

The diagnosis of pediatric scaphoid fractures is based on both a clinical examination and radiographic findings. Advanced imaging can aid in the diagnosis of a scaphoid injury in pediatric patients with incomplete ossification of the scaphoid. Although patients with acute nondisplaced scaphoid fractures have a high rate of healing with cast immobilization, surgery should be considered for patients who have displaced scaphoid fractures with delayed presentation. In general, patients with scaphoid fractures who undergo appropriate treatment and achieve successful union have excellent long-term functional outcomes.

References

1. Christodoulou AG, Colton CL: Scaphoid fractures in children. *J Pediatr Orthop* 1986;6(1):37-39.

2. Nafie SA: Fractures of the carpal bones in children. *Injury* 1987;18(2):117-119.

3. Brudvik C, Hove LM: Childhood fractures in Bergen, Norway: Identifying high-risk groups and activities. *J Pediatr Orthop* 2003;23(5):629-634.

4. Toh S, Miura H, Arai K, Yasumura M, Wada M, Tsubo K: Scaphoid fractures in children: Problems and treatment. *J Pediatr Orthop* 2003;23(2):216-221.

5. Gajdobranski D, Zivanović D, Mikov A, et al: Scaphoid fractures in children. *Srp Arh Celok Lek* 2014;142(7-8):444-449.

6. Ahmed I, Ashton F, Tay WK, Porter D: The pediatric fracture of the scaphoid in patients aged 13 years and under: An epidemiological study. *J Pediatr Orthop* 2014;34(2):150-154.

7. Gholson JJ, Bae DS, Zurakowski D, Waters PM: Scaphoid fractures in children and adolescents: Contemporary injury patterns and factors influencing time to union. *J Bone Joint Surg Am* 2011;93(13):1210-1219.

8. Vahvanen V, Westerlund M: Fracture of the carpal scaphoid in children: A clinical and roentgenological study of 108 cases. *Acta Orthop Scand* 1980;51(6):909-913.

9. D'Arienzo M: Scaphoid fractures in children. *J Hand Surg Br* 2002;27(5):424-426.

10. Evenski AJ, Adamczyk MJ, Steiner RP, Morscher MA, Riley PM: Clinically suspected scaphoid fractures in children. *J Pediatr Orthop* 2009;29(4):352-355.

11. Gelberman RH, Menon J: The vascularity of the scaphoid bone. *J Hand Surg Am* 1980;5(5):508-513.

12. Louis DS, Calhoun TP, Garn SM, Carroll RE, Burdi AR: Congenital bipartite scaphoid—fact or fiction? *J Bone Joint Surg Am* 1976;58(8):1108-1112.

13. Doman AN, Marcus NW: Congenital bipartite scaphoid. *J Hand Surg Am* 1990;15(6):869-873.

14. Cornwall R: The painful wrist in the pediatric athlete. *J Pediatr Orthop* 2010;30(2 suppl):S13-S16.

15. Johnson KJ, Haigh SF, Symonds KE: MRI in the management of scaphoid fractures in skeletally immature patients. *Pediatr Radiol* 2000;30(10):685-688.

16. Cook PA, Yu JS, Wiand W, Cook AJ II, Coleman CR, Cook AJ: Suspected scaphoid fractures in skeletally immature patients: Application of MRI. *J Comput Assist Tomogr* 1997;21(4):511-515.

17. Yin ZG, Zhang JB, Kan SL, Wang XG: Diagnostic accuracy of imaging modalities for suspected scaphoid fractures: Meta-analysis combined with latent class analysis. *J Bone Joint Surg Br* 2012;94(8):1077-1085.

18. Bond CD, Shin AY, McBride MT, Dao KD: Percutaneous screw fixation or cast immobilization for nondisplaced scaphoid fractures. *J Bone Joint Surg Am* 2001;83(4):483-488.

19. Waters PM, Stewart SL: Surgical treatment of nonunion and avascular necrosis of the proximal part of the scaphoid in adolescents. *J Bone Joint Surg Am* 2002;84(6):915-920.

20. Gellman H, Caputo RJ, Carter V, Aboulafia A, McKay M: Comparison of short and long thumb-spica casts for non-displaced fractures of the carpal scaphoid. *J Bone Joint Surg Am* 1989;71(3):354-357.

21. McAdams TR, Spisak S, Beaulieu CF, Ladd AL: The effect of pronation and supination on the minimally displaced

scaphoid fracture. *Clin Orthop Relat Res* 2003;411:255-259.

22. Kaneshiro SA, Failla JM, Tashman S: Scaphoid fracture displacement with forearm rotation in a short-arm thumb spica cast. *J Hand Surg Am* 1999;24(5):984-991.

23. Buijze GA, Goslings JC, Rhemrev SJ, et al: Cast immobilization with and without immobilization of the thumb for nondisplaced and minimally displaced scaphoid waist fractures: A multicenter, randomized, controlled trial. *J Hand Surg Am* 2014;39(4):621-627.

24. Bae DS, Gholson JJ, Zurakowski D, Waters PM: Functional outcomes after treatment of scaphoid fractures in children and adolescents. *J Pediatr Orthop* 2016;36(1):13-18.

25. Shin AY, Hofmeister EP: Percutaneous fixation of stable scaphoid fractures. *Tech Hand Up Extrem Surg* 2004;8(2):87-94.

26. McCallister WV, Knight J, Kaliappan R, Trumble TE: Central placement of the screw in simulated fractures of the scaphoid waist: A biomechanical study. *J Bone Joint Surg Am* 2003;85(1):72-77.

27. Chloros GD, Themistocleous GS, Wiesler ER, Benetos IS, Efstathopoulos DG, Soucacos PN: Pediatric scaphoid nonunion. *J Hand Surg Am* 2007;32(2):172-176.

28. Tomaino MM, King J, Pizillo M: Correction of lunate malalignment when bone grafting scaphoid nonunion with humpback deformity: Rationale and results of a technique revisited. *J Hand Surg Am* 2000;25(2):322-329.

29. Mintzer CM, Waters PM: Surgical treatment of pediatric scaphoid fracture nonunions. *J Pediatr Orthop* 1999;19(2):236-239.

30. Masquijo JJ, Willis BR: Scaphoid nonunions in children and adolescents: Surgical treatment with bone grafting and internal fixation. *J Pediatr Orthop* 2010;30(2):119-124.

31. Reigstad O, Thorkildsen R, Grimsgaard C, Reigstad A, Rokkum M: Excellent results after bone grafting and K-wire fixation for scaphoid nonunion surgery in skeletally immature patients: A midterm follow-up study of 11 adolescents after 6.9 years. *J Orthop Trauma* 2013;27(5):285-289.

32. Matsuki H, Ishikawa J, Iwasaki N, Uchiyama S, Minami A, Kato H: Non-vascularized bone graft with Herbert-type screw fixation for proximal pole scaphoid nonunion. *J Orthop Sci* 2011;16(6):749-755.

33. García-Mata S: Carpal scaphoid fracture nonunion in children. *J Pediatr Orthop* 2002;22(4):448-451.

34. Ben-Amotz O, Ho C, Sammer DM: Reconstruction of scaphoid non-union and total scaphoid avascular necrosis in a pediatric patient: A case report. *Hand (N Y)* 2015;10(3):477-481.

35. Düppe H, Johnell O, Lundborg G, Karlsson M, Redlund-Johnell I: Long-term results of fracture of the scaphoid: A follow-up study of more than thirty years. *J Bone Joint Surg Am* 1994;76(2):249-252.

36. Fabre O, De Boeck H, Haentjens P: Fractures and nonunions of the carpal scaphoid in children. *Acta Orthop Belg* 2001;67(2):121-125.

Pediatric Metacarpal Fractures

Jenna Godfrey, MD, MSPH
Roger Cornwall, MD

Abstract

Metacarpal fractures account for 10% to 35% of all pediatric hand fractures. Pediatric metacarpal fractures commonly occur in patients aged 13 to 16 years, with most injuries sustained during sports activities. Pseudoepiphyses can be confused with metacarpal fractures; however, a careful physical examination can help physicians distinguish the two. Thumb metacarpal base fractures that involve the physis warrant special attention. Thumb metacarpal base fractures with lateral metaphyseal fragments and pediatric Bennett fracture variants (Salter-Harris type III and type IV fractures) are unstable and require surgical management. Finger metacarpal base fractures, especially those in young children, are often the result of high-energy injuries and should increase a physician's concern for compartment syndrome. Metacarpal shaft fractures can result from a simple bending moment; however, they also can result from a rotational force, which may cause finger crossover that will not remodel and requires reduction. Metacarpal neck fractures account for three-fourths of all finger metacarpal fractures, and increasing acceptable alignment of the index finger through the little finger metacarpal necks (10°, 20°, 30°, and 40° across the digits, respectively) is commonly recommended. Metacarpal head fractures are rare intra-articular injuries that require anatomic fixation and may be underappreciated in children because of the complex geometry and largely cartilaginous nature of the metacarpal head.

Instr Course Lect 2017;66:437–445.

Epidemiology

Hand fractures are the most common type of fractures that occur in children.[1,2] Metacarpal fractures account for 10% to 35% of all pediatric hand fractures, with the little finger metacarpal being the most commonly injured metacarpal bone (54% to 80%).[2-5] Pediatric metacarpal fractures commonly occur in patients aged 13 to 16 years, with most injuries occurring in boys (68%).[2,3]

Sports related injury is the most common mechanism of injury, with most pediatric metacarpal fractures occurring at school (44%) and at the playground or sporting venues (32%).[2]

Anatomic Considerations in Children

Pediatric hand fractures differ from adult hand fractures in several respects. The soft-tissue structures tolerate a greater tensile load than the physis, which results in physeal fractures rather than ligamentous ruptures or tendon avulsions.[6] At the metacarpophalangeal (MCP) joint of the index, long, ring, and little fingers, the collateral ligaments attach to the epiphysis of both the metacarpal and phalanx, which most commonly results in a physeal injury to the proximal phalanx.[6] In the thumb, the radial and ulnar collateral ligaments attach to the epiphysis of the proximal phalanx and the metaphysis of the thumb metacarpal neck. Pediatric avulsion fractures of the base of

Neither of the following authors nor any immediate family member has received anything of value from or has stock or stock options held in a commercial company or institution related directly or indirectly to the subject of this chapter: Dr. Godfrey and Dr. Cornwall.

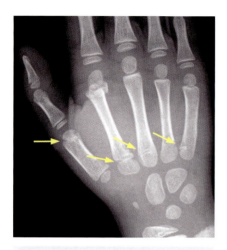

Figure 1 AP hand radiograph demonstrates physeal variation, with pseudoepiphyses (arrows) appreciated at the distal thumb metacarpal and the proximal index, long, and little finger metacarpals.

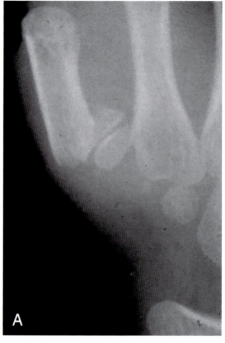

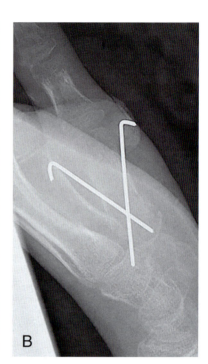

Figure 2 Radiographs of the hand of a patient who sustained a thumb metacarpal base fracture. **A,** AP view demonstrates an extraphyseal thumb metacarpal base fracture. **B,** Lateral view taken after reduction and pin fixation, which was performed to help maintain reduction during healing. (Reproduced with permission from Cornwall R: Pediatric hand fractures, in Budoff JE, ed: *Fractures of the Upper Extremity: A Master Skills Publication*. Chicago, IL, American Society for Surgery of the Hand, 2008.)

the proximal phalanx are equivalent to radial and ulnar collateral ligament avulsions in adults. The palmar plate originates from the metacarpal metaphyseal neck and inserts on the epiphysis of the proximal phalanx.[6]

Physeal injuries in the hand seldom result in growth arrest independently; however, late reduction (>7 to 10 days) or repeated reductions can result in physeal arrest.[6] The hypertrophic zone of the growth plate is most frequently fractured. Type I and type II Salter-Harris injuries typically heal with no sequelae; however, type III and type IV Salter-Harris injuries should be followed for 1 year postinjury to assess for growth arrest.[6] Angular deformity, especially in the plane of joint motion, reliably remodels in young children. Malrotation, however, does not reliably remodel and should be addressed with reduction and fixation as necessary.[6]

Physeal Variation

Normal metacarpal anatomy includes a proximal physis for the thumb metacarpal and distal physes for the index through little finger metacarpals. Pseudoepiphyses can occur and may easily be confused with a metacarpal fracture. Partial pseudoepiphyses, which appear as either notches or clefts at the nonepiphyseal end of the bone, most commonly occur in the metacarpals of the index (15%), little (7%), and long (0.49%) fingers[7] (**Figure 1**). Complete pseudoepiphyses, which appear as a complete cleft across the entire width of the metacarpal, most commonly occur in the metacarpals of the thumb (1.7%) and index finger (1.3%).[7] A careful physical examination specific for point tenderness that corresponds with a radiographic anomaly should help physicians reliably distinguish metacarpal fractures and anatomic variants.

Thumb Metacarpal Base Fractures

The three primary variants of pediatric thumb metacarpal base fractures are extraphyseal fractures through the metaphysis (**Figure 2**), type II Salter-Harris fractures that have either a medial or lateral metaphyseal fragment, and type III and type IV Salter-Harris fractures, which also are known as pediatric Bennett fractures[8,9] (**Figure 3**). The thumb metacarpal physis is located proximally, and the adjacent carpometacarpal (CMC) joint has six degrees of freedom, which supports good bone remodeling; however, bone remodeling depends on the direction and type of displacement as well as patient age.[8,10]

Maintenance of reduction in a thumb spica cast alone may be difficult

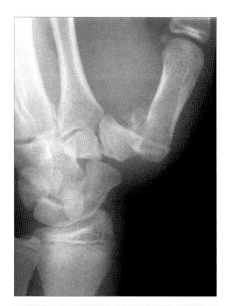

Figure 3 AP hand radiograph demonstrates an intra-articular thumb metacarpal base fracture with dislocation, which also is known as a pediatric Bennett fracture.

because the metacarpal base is located deep in the thenar eminence. Jehanno et al[8] reviewed 30 children who underwent closed reduction and spica cast application for thumb metacarpal base fractures to identify factors that convey instability. The study included children who had fracture displacement with angulation greater than 30° or had more than 1 mm of metaphyseal-epiphyseal displacement. One-half of the patients with metaphyseal thumb metacarpal base fractures and one-half of the patients with type II Salter-Harris thumb metacarpal base fractures with lateral metaphyseal fragments had displacement; however, no displacement occurred in the patients with type II Salter-Harris thumb metacarpal base fractures with a medial metaphyseal fragment.[8] The authors concluded that metaphyseal thumb metacarpal base fractures and type II Salter-Harris thumb metacarpal base fractures with

a lateral metaphyseal fragment that require reduction (>30° of angulation or >1 mm of metaphyseal-epiphyseal step-off) tend to be unstable and, therefore, benefit from pin fixation[8] (**Figure 2**). Type II Salter-Harris thumb metacarpal base fractures with medial metaphyseal fragments are stable and, therefore, can be managed with closed reduction and spica cast application alone.[8] Both metaphyseal thumb metacarpal base fractures and type II Salter-Harris thumb metacarpal base fractures with a lateral fragment lack stability in the medial cortex of the metacarpal and cannot counteract the pull of the adductor, which likely contributes to loss of reduction.

Pediatric Bennett fractures (type III and type IV Salter-Harris thumb metacarpal base fractures) are both inherently unstable and intra-articular injuries. Similar to adult injuries, the volar oblique ligament holds the volar lip of the epiphysis in place in children. Open reduction and surgical fixation is recommended in patients who have type III and type IV Salter-Harris thumb metacarpal base fractures to restore and help maintain joint alignment during healing.[9,11] Posttraumatic degenerative arthritis that results from poor articular alignment has been reported in patients who have type III and type IV Salter-Harris thumb metacarpal base fractures.[11]

Finger Metacarpal Base Fractures

Metacarpal base fractures account for 10% to 20% of all pediatric finger metacarpal fractures.[3,5,12] The metacarpal base of the little finger is most commonly injured, accounting for 72% to 80% of finger metacarpal base fractures.[3,5] Finger metacarpal base fractures are either

intra-articular or extra-articular. Extra-articular finger metacarpal fractures at the metaphyseal-diaphyseal junction, which are known as epibasal fractures, are the most common type of finger metacarpal base fractures in older children.[13] Dislocations of the CMC joint can occur simultaneously with finger metacarpal base fractures and are often observed in conjunction with little finger metacarpal base fractures as a result of the ligamentous laxity at this joint.[12] Multiple finger metacarpal base fractures that are caused by a crush injury should increase a physician's concern for severe soft-tissue injury and, more specifically, for compartment syndrome[12] (**Figure 4**).

Adequate imaging of finger metacarpal base fractures can be a challenge. Multiple pronated oblique radiographs may be necessary to assess the CMC joint of each metacarpal. High-frequency ultrasonography can help detect cortical irregularity and may be considered for patients in whom radiographs are equivocal.[14] CT of intra-articular finger metacarpal base fractures should be obtained to assess joint displacement (**Figure 5**). Minimally displaced extra-articular fractures will reliably heal and can be managed nonsurgically with cast immobilization.[12] However, intra-articular fractures and CMC joint dislocations are unstable and frequently require surgical fixation to maintain reduction (**Figure 5**).[12]

Metacarpal Shaft Fractures

Metacarpal shaft fractures are relatively uncommon in children, accounting for 8% to 11% of all pediatric metacarpal fractures.[3,5] The little finger metacarpal shaft is the most commonly injured metacarpal shaft, accounting for approximately one-half of reported metacarpal shaft fractures.[3,5] Metacarpal shaft fractures typically have either spiral or transverse fracture patterns. Spiral metacarpal shaft fracture patterns are the result of a rotational force, and reduction of a rotational deformity is often necessary[12,13] (**Figure 6**). Reduction is achieved by flexing the MCP joint and using the proximal phalanx as a lever to correct rotational alignment of the distal fragment.[12] Buddy taping helps maintain rotational control in a cast, which often is sufficient for stabilization during healing.

Transverse metacarpal shaft fracture patterns are the result of a bending moment, which can occur if a child's hand is stepped on during a sporting event.[12] In transverse metacarpal shaft fracture patterns, the fracture tends to angulate with the apex dorsally, with the metacarpal head flexed palmarly as a result of the pull of the interosseous muscles.[15] Transverse metacarpal shaft fractures can be easily reduced with the use of a gentle bending force and can be maintained in a well-molded cast with the MCP joints slightly flexed and the digits extended.[12,15] Translated transverse metacarpal shaft fractures are notoriously difficult to control in a cast after closed reduction; therefore, surgical fixation may be necessary. Several possible pin configurations can provide stability for translated transverse metacarpal shaft fractures: pinning to the adjacent stable metacarpals, intramedullary pins, and cross pins (**Figure 7**).

Definitive recommendations for acceptable angulation of metacarpal shaft fractures have not been established. In general, less angulation is

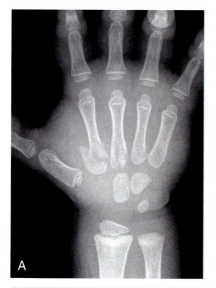
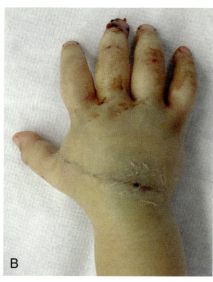

Figure 4 AP radiograph (**A**) and clinical photograph (**B**) of the hand of a young child who sustained a crush injury show multiple metacarpal base fractures. Note the substantial soft-tissue swelling. (Reproduced with permission from Cornwall R: Pediatric hand fractures, in Budoff JE, ed: *Fractures of the Upper Extremity: A Master Skills Publication*. Chicago, IL, American Society for Surgery of the Hand, 2008.)

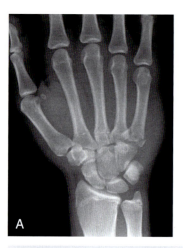
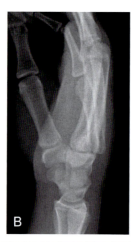
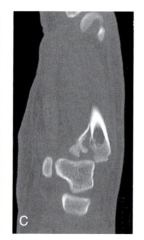
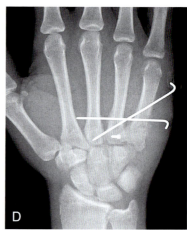

Figure 5 Images of the hand of a 16-year-old boy with an intra-articular metacarpal base fracture. AP (**A**) and lateral (**B**) radiographs demonstrate a fracture-dislocation at the carpometacarpal (CMC) joint of the ring finger. **C,** Sagittal CT scan of the ring finger demonstrates a CMC joint fracture-dislocation with a perched, dislocated joint. **D,** AP radiograph taken after open reduction and internal fixation of the CMC joint of the ring finger demonstrates pin stabilization from the little finger metacarpal fracture through to the stable long finger metacarpal.

tolerated in the index and long finger metacarpals (<10°), which have more stiff CMC joints, than in the ring and little finger metacarpals (20° and 30°, respectively), which have more mobile CMC joints.[15] Length-unstable long spiral or oblique metacarpal shaft fracture patterns and multiple metacarpal shaft fractures are indications for surgical fixation with the use of pins, plates, or flexible intramedullary nails.[12,16] Pin fixation allows for easy removal of the implant without the need for additional anesthesia but requires postoperative cast immobilization. Plate and screw constructs may be appropriate for unstable fractures; however, the surgical exposure required for their use may result in extensor tendon adhesions that require postoperative therapy, and children are not reliably amenable to immediate postoperative range of motion. Similarly, intramedullary devices can be used for the management of metacarpal shaft fractures; however, pins can provide a better fit in the narrow metacarpal canal of young children.

Metacarpal Neck Fractures

Metacarpal neck fractures account for three-fourths (70% to 79% in two studies) of all pediatric finger metacarpal fractures.[3,5] Most metacarpal neck fractures (60% to 67%) occur in the little finger metacarpal neck, which is referred to as a boxer's fracture[3,5] (**Figure 8**). The mechanism of injury for metacarpal neck fractures often involves a direct blow with a clenched fist on a hard surface.[13] The distal fragment flexes, causing an apex dorsal deformity, which results in loss of the normal contour of the knuckle and prominence of the metacarpal head in the palm. In children, metacarpal neck fractures may involve the physis.[12]

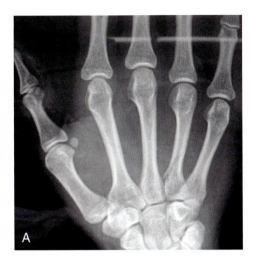
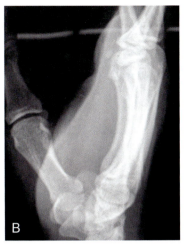
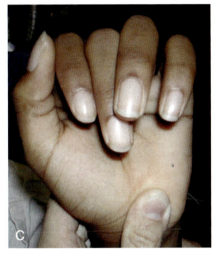
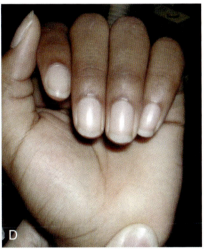

Figure 6   Images of the hand of a 17-year-old boy taken after he punched a wall. **A,** AP radiograph demonstrates a ring finger metacarpal fracture. **B,** Oblique radiograph demonstrates a ring finger metacarpal shaft fracture with no dorsal angulation. **C,** Clinical photograph shows that rotational deformity with ring finger crossover was appreciated during physical examination. **D,** Clinical photograph taken after reduction was performed in the clinic with the use of a local digital block shows resolution of the rotation deformity and ring finger crossover.

Careful physical examination of a patient who has a metacarpal neck fracture should include an assessment for rotational deformity. If the normal finger cascade that typically points toward the scaphoid tubercle is lost with the application of gentle flexion or if digit crossover is present, the distal fragment may be rotated. Swelling of the fourth webspace can result in a supination deformity of the MCP joint that mimics a rotational deformity of the fracture; however, passive adduction of the little finger during assessment of rotational alignment can control for this confounding effect. Lateral and oblique radiographs of the hand may be required to obtain a true lateral view of the affected metacarpal. Considerable debate exists with regard to acceptable alignment, with reports of up to 70° of angulation of the little

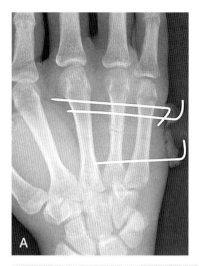
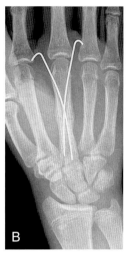
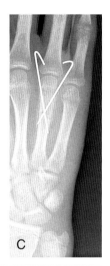

Figure 7 AP hand radiographs demonstrate percutaneous pin fixation options for the management of unstable transverse metacarpal shaft fractures. **A,** Pinning to the adjacent metacarpals, which maintains length. **B,** Using pins to create an intramedullary flexible nail construct. **C,** Cross pinning at the fracture site. (Reproduced with permission from Cornwall R: Pediatric hand fractures, in Budoff JE, ed: *Fractures of the Upper Extremity: A Master Skills Publication.* Chicago, IL, American Society for Surgery of the Hand, 2008.)

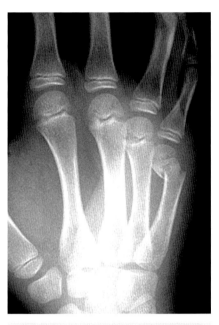

Figure 8 AP hand radiograph demonstrates a little finger metacarpal neck fracture with an apex dorsal deformity. (Reproduced with permission from Cornwall R: Finger metacarpal fractures and dislocations in children. *Hand Clin* 2006;22[1]:1-10.)

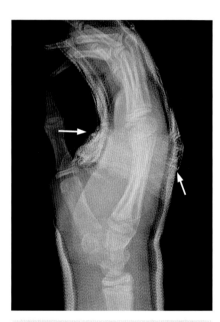

Figure 9 Lateral hand radiograph demonstrates that, in children, casting with the metacarpophalangeal joints in extension does not result in joint stiffness. Proper casting with the use of distal palmar and proximal dorsal molds (arrows) helps maintain reduction of metacarpal neck fractures during healing.

finger metacarpal in adults resulting in no functional deficits.[17] More conservative recommendations of 10°, 20°, 30°, and 40° for acceptable alignment of the index, long, ring, and little finger metacarpal necks, respectively, are more commonly used.[12]

Fracture reduction is easily accomplished with the use of the Jahss maneuver and a digital block. Flexion of the MCP and proximal interphalangeal joints to 90° relaxes the intrinsic muscles and tightens the collateral ligaments, which allows the proximal phalanx to be used to exert upward pressure on the metacarpal head, thus reducing the deformity.[18] Rotation of the phalanx in this position will help correct rotational malalignment. The reduced fracture can then be maintained in a cast with a palmar mold that exerts a similar upward force on the metacarpal head and a counter proximal dorsal mold (**Figure 9**). Casting with the MCP joints in flexion can be counterproductive to maintenance of the reduction and is not necessary because immobilization with the MCP joints in extension does not usually result in joint stiffness in children.[12] Typically, fracture healing is adequate 4 weeks after immobilization, at which point the cast is removed and range of motion is initiated. Patients can return to activity after they are pain free and full-digit range of motion has been achieved; however, physicians should warn patients and their parents/caretakers of the risk of refracture from a similar mechanism of injury, especially if the mechanism of injury was a punch. Whether the risk of refracture results from bone fragility or residual angulation secondary to the previous fracture or simply from a persistent pugilistic tendency is difficult to determine.

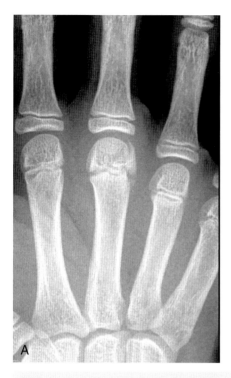
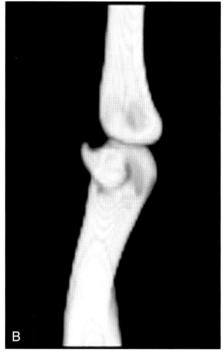
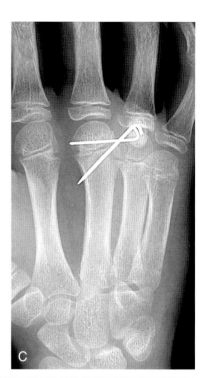

Figure 10 Images demonstrate the use of advanced imaging for better visualization of a pediatric metacarpal head fracture. **A,** AP hand radiograph demonstrates a long finger metacarpal head fracture, which may appear subtle on initial radiographs. A large intra-articular fragment of the long finger was better visualized on a three-dimensional sagittal CT reconstruction (**B**). **C,** AP hand radiograph demonstrates that open reduction and fixation was necessary to restore articular congruity. (Reproduced with permission from Cornwall R: Finger metacarpal fractures and dislocations in children. *Hand Clin* 2006;22[1]:1-10.)

Metacarpal Head Fractures

Pediatric epiphyseal fractures of the finger metacarpals are extremely rare. In a study of 284 pediatric finger metacarpal fractures, Fischer and McElfresh[19] reported only two type III Salter-Harris injuries (0.7%). In a study of 103 adult and pediatric metacarpal head fractures, McElfresh and Dobyns[20] reported only four type III Salter-Harris fractures (4%). A careful physical examination that reveals MCP joint effusion and limited motion in the absence of a more obvious metacarpal neck fracture should alert a physician to closely observe the metacarpal head. More advanced imaging studies, including CT, may be necessary to better visualize pediatric metacarpal head fractures (**Figure 10**).

Intra-articular incongruity inherently accompanies pediatric metacarpal head fractures; therefore, open reduction and fixation with the use of smooth pins, wires, or screws is recommended.[12] Osteonecrosis of the metacarpal head has been reported in patients who sustain metacarpal head fractures.[20] Osteonecrosis of the metacarpal head is thought to result from small vessel tamponade secondary to tense joint effusion.

Fight Bite Injuries at the MCP Joint

Trauma to the MCP joint and metacarpal head that is caused by penetration from an opponent's tooth is called a fight bite injury. Although less common in the pediatric population,

fight bite injuries, if missed, can result in devastating complications. Physicians should carefully assess for fight bite injuries, remembering that the skin wound in an open hand is proximal to the joint.[21] A high incidence of MCP joint penetration (64% to 95% in three studies) is present in patients who sustain fight bite injuries.[21-23] Fingers positioned in extension cause the capsule, the extensor tendon, and skin injuries to become staggered, which creates a closed environment that is susceptible to infection.[21] Because of these staggered injuries, a physician must examine patients for soft-tissue injuries with their metacarpal joints in flexion, which is the way they were positioned during injury. Inoculated (acute) injuries can be managed via immediate irrigation

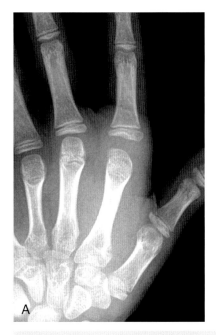
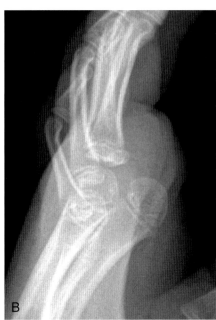

Figure 11   Radiographs of the hand of an 11-year-old girl who jammed her finger during physical education class. **A,** AP view demonstrates subtle widening of the metacarpophalangeal joint. The metacarpal and phalanx appear parallel on the lateral view (**B**), which indicates a complex complete metacarpophalangeal joint dislocation. (Reproduced with permission from Cornwall R: Finger metacarpal fractures and dislocations in children. *Hand Clin* 2006;22[1]:1-10.)

and prophylactic antibiotic drug coverage for oral flora; however, infected (subacute) injuries require surgical exploration and débridement of the joint. Metacarpal head fractures and osteochondral defects should be addressed after infection is controlled.

MCP Joint Dislocations

In children, MCP joint dislocations occur more frequently than proximal interphalangeal dislocations and often involve the thumb and index finger.[12] Finger MCP joint dislocations may appear subtle on radiographs, with MCP joint widening observed on AP views (the result of the interposed volar plate) and a hyperextended joint observed on lateral hand views.[13,24] Palpation of the metacarpal head in the palm can aid in the diagnosis of MCP joint dislocations.

MCP joint dislocations are classified as incomplete, simple complete, or complex complete.[25] In incomplete MCP joint dislocations, the collateral ligaments are intact. In simple complete MCP joint dislocations, the collateral ligaments and volar plate are torn but are not interposed. In complex complete MCP joint dislocations, the volar plate is interposed.[25] Radiographs of incomplete MCP joint dislocations and simple complete MCP joint dislocations reveal hyperextension of the joint, and radiographs of complex complete MCP joint dislocations reveal a parallel metacarpal and proximal phalanx[25] (**Figure 11**).

Closed reduction may be successful in patients who have incomplete MCP joint dislocations and patients who have simple complete MCP joint dislocations.

Simple complete MCP joint dislocations can be reduced in a closed manner by sliding the proximal phalanx over the metacarpal head. If, instead, traction and hyperextension maneuvers are used to reduce a simple complete MCP joint dislocation, the volar plate can become entrapped dorsally between the proximal phalanx and the metacarpal head, which transforms a simple complete MCP joint dislocation into a complex complete MCP joint dislocation. Therefore, longitudinal traction should never be used to reduce a simple complete MCP joint dislocation. Interposed structures of the thumb that can prevent reduction include the volar plate, flexor and adductor tendons, extensor expansion, joint capsule, and sesamoid bones.[25] In the fingers, the volar plate, flexor tendons, and lumbrical muscles can prevent reduction.

Open reduction is indicated for patients who have irreducible MCP joint dislocations. The dorsal approach is frequently used to avoid injury to the digital neurovascular bundle. In a study of four children who underwent surgical treatment for index finger MCP joint dislocations, Light and Ogden[24] reported an epiphyseal osteochondroma in one patient and osteonecrosis of the metacarpal head that led to subsequent deformity and growth arrest in another patient.

Summary

Pediatric metacarpal fractures are frequently encountered in the pediatric orthopaedic clinic. Pediatric metacarpal fractures occur most often in children aged 13 to 16 years as a result of an injury during a sporting event. A careful physical examination can help physicians distinguish between physeal variations and metacarpal fractures.

Metaphyseal thumb metacarpal base fractures, thumb metacarpal base fractures with lateral metaphyseal fragments, and pediatric Bennett fractures are unstable and require pin fixation. Physicians should be attentive to multiple metacarpal base fractures because they indicate a high-energy injury with substantial soft-tissue damage and a high risk for compartment syndrome. Metacarpal head fractures are rare but serious injuries that require open reduction to reduce intra-articular incongruity. Metacarpal neck fractures are the most common type of pediatric metacarpal injury and, typically, can be managed with closed reduction and a well-molded cast in which the finger MCP joints are only minimally flexed. Longitudinal traction should be avoided in the reduction of MCP joint dislocations.

References

1. Hastings H II, Simmons BP: Hand fractures in children: A statistical analysis. *Clin Orthop Relat Res* 1984;188:120-130.

2. Chew EM, Chong AK: Hand fractures in children: Epidemiology and misdiagnosis in a tertiary referral hospital. *J Hand Surg Am* 2012;37(8):1684-1688.

3. Rajesh A, Basu AK, Vaidhyanath R, Finlay D: Hand fractures: A study of their site and type in childhood. *Clin Radiol* 2001;56(8):667-669.

4. Valencia J, Leyva F, Gomez-Bajo GJ: Pediatric hand trauma. *Clin Orthop Relat Res* 2005;432:77-86.

5. Worlock PH, Stower MJ: The incidence and pattern of hand fractures in children. *J Hand Surg Br* 1986;11(2):198-200.

6. Smit A, Hooper G: Fractures in the child's hand. *Curr Orthop* 2006;20(6):461-466.

7. Limb D, Loughenbury PR: The prevalence of pseudoepiphyses in the metacarpals of the growing hand. *J Hand Surg Eur Vol* 2012;37(7):678-681.

8. Jehanno P, Iselin F, Frajman JM, Pennecot GF, Glicenstein J: Fractures of the base of the first metacarpal in children: Role of K-wire stabilisation. *Chir Main* 1999;18(3):184-190.

9. Yeh PC, Dodds SD: Pediatric hand fractures. *Tech Orthop* 2009;24(3):150-162.

10. Beatty E, Light TR, Belsole RJ, Ogden JA: Wrist and hand skeletal injuries in children. *Hand Clin* 1990;6(4):723-738.

11. Peljovich AE, Simmons BP: Traumatic arthritis of the hand and wrist in children. *Hand Clin* 2000;16(4):673-684.

12. Cornwall R: Finger metacarpal fractures and dislocations in children. *Hand Clin* 2006;22(1):1-10.

13. Sivit AP, Dupont EP, Sivit CJ: Pediatric hand injuries: Essentials you need to know. *Emerg Radiol* 2014;21(2):197-206.

14. Ruskis J, Kummer T: Diagnosis of metacarpal fracture with equivocal x-ray by point-of-care ultrasound: A case report. *Am J Emerg Med* 2014;32(7):821.e1-821.e3.

15. Dye TM: Metacarpal fractures. Medscape website. Updated August 24, 2015. Available at: http://emedicine.medscape.com/article/1239721-overview. Accessed January 11, 2016.

16. Lieber J, Härter B, Schmid E, Kirschner HJ, Schmittenbecher PP: Elastic stable intramedullary nailing (ESIN) of pediatric metacarpal fractures: Experiences with 66 cases. *Eur J Pediatr Surg* 2012;22(4):305-310.

17. Ford DJ, Ali MS, Steel WM: Fractures of the fifth metacarpal neck: Is reduction or immobilisation necessary? *J Hand Surg Br* 1989;14(2):165-167.

18. Jahss SA: Fractures of the metacarpals: A new method of reduction and immobilization. *J Bone Joint Surg Am* 1938;20(1):178-186.

19. Fischer MD, McElfresh EC: Physeal and periphyseal injuries of the hand: Patterns of injury and results of treatment. *Hand Clin* 1994;10(2):287-301.

20. McElfresh EC, Dobyns JH: Intra-articular metacarpal head fractures. *J Hand Surg Am* 1983;8(4):383-393.

21. Shewring DJ, Trickett RW, Subramanian KN, Hnyda R: The management of clenched fist 'fight bite' injuries of the hand. *J Hand Surg Eur Vol* 2015;40(8):819-824.

22. Patzakis MJ, Wilkins J, Bassett RL: Surgical findings in clenched-fist injuries. *Clin Orthop Relat Res* 1987;220:237-240.

23. Phair IC, Quinton DN: Clenched fist human bite injuries. *J Hand Surg Br* 1989;14(1):86-87.

24. Light TR, Ogden JA: Complex dislocation of the index metacarpophalangeal joint in children. *J Pediatr Orthop* 1988;8(3):300-305.

25. Maheshwari R, Sharma H, Duncan RD: Metacarpophalangeal joint dislocation of the thumb in children. *J Bone Joint Surg Br* 2007;89(2):227-229.

Pediatric Distal Radius Fractures

Karan Dua, MD

Joshua M. Abzug, MD

Andrea Sesko Bauer, MD

Roger Cornwall, MD

Theresa O. Wyrick, MD

Abstract

Distal radius fractures are the most common orthopaedic injury that occur in the pediatric population. The annual incidence of distal radius fractures has increased as a result of earlier participation in sporting activities, increased body mass index, and decreased bone mineral density. Most distal radius fractures are sustained after a fall onto an outstretched arm that results in axial compression on the extremity or from direct trauma to the extremity. Physeal fractures of the distal radius are described based on the Salter-Harris classification system. Extraphyseal fractures of the distal radius are described as incomplete or complete based on the amount of cortical involvement. A thorough physical examination of the upper extremity is necessary to rule out any associated injuries. PA and lateral radiographs of the wrist usually are sufficient to diagnose a distal radius fracture. The management of distal radius fractures is based on several factors, including patient age, fracture pattern, and the amount of growth remaining. Nonsurgical management is the most common treatment option for patients who have distal radius fractures because marked potential for remodeling exists. If substantial angulation or displacement is present, closed reduction maneuvers with or without percutaneous pinning should be performed. Patients with physeal fractures of the distal radius that may result in malunion who present more than 10 days postinjury should not undergo manipulation of any kind because of the increased risk for physeal arrest.

Instr Course Lect 2017;66:447–460.

Epidemiology

Distal radius fractures are the most common orthopaedic injury that occur in the pediatric population, accounting for as many as 20% to 31% of all fractures that occur during childhood.[1-6]

The annual incidence of distal radius fractures has increased in the past several decades as a result of increased participation in sporting activities, earlier participation in intense sporting activities, increased body mass index, and decreased bone mineral density.[7-9] Distal radius fractures are estimated to affect as many as 1 in 100 children in the United States.[5,10,11] A recent epidemiologic study reported that distal forearm fractures account for the highest number of emergency department visits in the United States for fractures, occurring at a rate of 32 per 1,000 patients aged 0 to 19 years.[12]

The incidence of distal radius fractures is the highest in females aged

Dr. Abzug or an immediate family member is a member of a speakers' bureau or has made paid presentations on behalf of Checkpoint Surgical and serves as a paid consultant to AxoGen. Dr. Bauer or an immediate family member serves as a board member, owner, officer, or committee member of the American Society for Surgery of the Hand and the Pediatric Orthopaedic Society of North America. None of the following authors nor any immediate family member has received anything of value from or has stock or stock options held in a commercial company or institution related directly or indirectly to the subject of this chapter: Dr. Dua, Dr. Cornwall, and Dr. Wyrick.

8 to 11 years and in males aged 11 to 14 years.[9] Traditionally, studies suggested that the highest incidence of distal radius fractures occurred at age 10 to 14 years in both sexes;[13,14] however, more recent studies confirm that children are most vulnerable to distal radius fractures at the onset of puberty,[1,11] with the rate of distal radius fractures substantially decreasing after puberty.[1,15] At the onset of puberty, children undergo rapid linear skeletal growth without an equal associated increase in bone mineralization, which leads to bone fragility and, subsequently, a higher risk for fractures.[1,16,17] In addition, adolescents tend to have increased bone porosity to allow for the increased calcium absorption that occurs during the rapid growth phase, which increases the risk for fracture.[1,18] A recent genomic study reported that sex-specific loci that influence bone mineral density and bone accretion, specifically of the distal radius, exist on the alleles of Caucasian children.[19] Conditions that lead to lower bone mineral density, including late menarche in females, theoretically increase the risk for distal radius fracture.[20] Childhood obesity may not adversely affect bone density and may, in fact, be a protective factor. A recent study reported that adolescents with obesity had a 0.45 higher radius cortical section modulus Z-score compared with nonobese patients ($P = 0.08$), most likely because of advanced skeletal maturity as well as greater muscle area and strength.[21] However, increased body mass index would be expected to increase the force transmitted through an outstretched arm during a fall. Therefore, the influence of the relationship between obesity and body mass index on distal radius fractures is still unclear.

Most distal radius fractures are sustained after a fall onto an outstretched arm that results in axial compression on the extremity or from direct trauma to the extremity. Males are twice as likely as females to sustain distal radius fractures.[22,23] In a recent epidemiologic study on emergency department visits for pediatric wrist fractures during a 16-year period, Shah et al[23] reported that children aged 0 to 36 months were more likely to sustain wrist fractures at home; children aged 3 to 10 years were more likely to sustain wrist fractures at a playground; and children aged 11 to 17 years were more likely to sustain wrist fractures during sport-related activities, especially football. The authors reported that the top five consumer product-related wrist fractures were associated with bicycles, football, playground activities, basketball, and soccer.[23] The incidence of distal radius fractures does not differ among races[1] or between urban and suburban populations.[9]

Pathoanatomy

A thorough knowledge of pediatric wrist anatomy is required to understand how distal radius fractures occur and can be optimally managed. The unmineralized physis is biomechanically weaker compared with the surrounding ligamentous structures and mature bone, which makes fractures through the physis extremely common. The epiphysis of the distal radius first appears in females aged 0.4 to 1.7 years and in males aged 0.5 and 2.3 years.[24] The distal ulnar epiphysis does not appear until age 7 years. The physis of the distal radius remains open until females and males are aged approximately 16.5 and 17.5 years, respectively.[24] Longitudinal bone growth in children occurs through the physis, with 75% of overall radius growth occurring through the distal physis.[25] Therefore, marked potential exists for distal radius remodeling, which is directly proportional to the amount of growth that remains before physeal closure. As much as 10° of volar-dorsal angulation remodeling can occur annually; therefore, as much as 20° of fracture angulation can be tolerated if more than 2 years of growth remain before physeal closure.[26] In patients who have distal radius fractures, remodeling potential is increased because of the elevated periosteum, which serves as a scaffold for cortical remodeling as callus and bone are deposited along the periosteal margin, and because of physeal growth.[27] Fung et al[28] reported that rapid remineralization and a transient elevation in bone mineral density occur in children who have a simple forearm fracture, which suggests that newly formed bone may be stronger around the fracture site.

The anatomy of the radius in relation to the ulna helps explain forearm biomechanics. The radius has a lateral bow, whereas the ulna is relatively straight; therefore, the axis of rotation of the forearm is directed obliquely from the center of the distal ulna to the proximal radial head.[27] The distal radioulnar joint is stabilized primarily by the triangular fibrocartilage complex and its association with the volar and dorsal radioulnar, radiocarpal, and ulnocarpal ligaments. The volar extrinsic ligaments tend to be stronger compared with the dorsal ligaments.[24] The triangular fibrocartilage complex extends from the radial sigmoid notch and inserts in the foveal region of the ulnar styloid. Distally, the triangular fibrocartilage complex inserts at the base of the fifth metacarpal and ulnar carpus via the ulnar collateral, ulnotriquetral, and ulnolunate ligaments.[24,29] In addition, the interosseous membrane at the diaphysis between the radius and ulna extends obliquely and distally to provide additional stability in the forearm.[27] Collectively, these articulations allow the radius to rotate around the immobile ulna, accounting for as much as 150° of forearm rotation, 50° of ulnar/radial deviation, and 120° of wrist flexion/extension.[29]

The noteworthy differences between pediatric and adult forearm anatomy include shorter shaft sizes, narrower medullary canals, more trabecular bone in the metaphysis, and thicker periosteum.[27] The thicker periosteum in pediatric patients helps maintain fracture reduction but can become entrapped at the fracture site, which can impede reduction.

Classification

Distal radius fractures can be described based on the location and pattern of the fracture; the amount of fracture displacement, angulation, and rotation; and the presence of associated injuries. Distal radius fractures are divided into two subgroups based on location: physeal fractures or extraphyseal fractures. Physeal fractures are described based on the Salter-Harris classification system.[30]

Typically, extraphyseal fractures of the distal radius involve the metaphysis of the distal radius. Extraphyseal fractures of the distal radius are described based on the amount of cortical involvement and the mechanism of injury. Torus/buckle fractures of the distal radius are incomplete fractures that result from a mechanical compressive axial load.[10] Torus/buckle fractures of the distal radius are inherently stable and have an intact cortex and periosteum on the opposite side (**Figure 1**). Greenstick fractures of the distal radius are

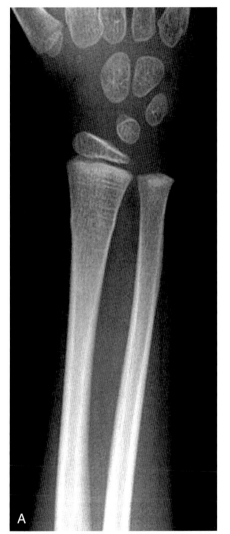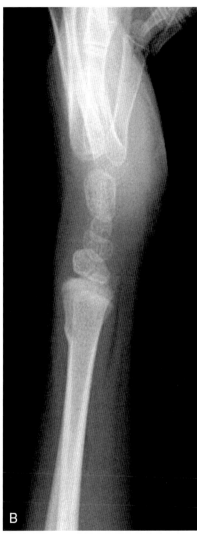

Figure 1 PA (**A**) and lateral (**B**) radiographs of a wrist demonstrate a torus/buckle fracture of the distal radius. (Courtesy of Theresa O. Wyrick, MD, Little Rock, AR.)

incomplete fractures that result from excessive rotational forces. Greenstick fractures of the distal radius involve complete disruption of only one cortex.[27] Complete distal radius fractures are inherently unstable because both cortices are disrupted. Typically, complete distal radius fractures result from excessive shear, bending, or rotational force and are dorsally angulated (apex of the fracture located volarly) with varying degrees of translation.

Assessment of Injury
Signs and Symptoms

The clinical presentation of distal radius fractures in children is predicated on the severity of the initial injury. Pain can be localized to the wrist in patients without visible deformity or an obvious joint effusion. If substantial fracture displacement or intra-articular fracture extension exists, a visible deformity and/or substantial swelling may be evident.

The physical examination is a vital part of the diagnostic workup of a child with a suspected distal radius fracture. The skin should be examined for any open wounds, swelling, lacerations, or abrasions. Spontaneous movement that is performed by a child during the physical examination may aid in obtaining information with regard to potential nerve injuries. Patients will have localized tenderness to palpation about the wrist. Surgeons must purposefully palpate various locations about the wrist to determine the location of maximal tenderness; such palpation can help diagnose a distal radius fracture, especially in patients with a physeal fracture of the distal radius in whom a fracture is not observed on radiographs. Associated wrist injuries, including fractures of the distal ulna, the ulnar styloid, and/or scaphoid, may be present.[31] Surgeons should clinically and radiographically assess for a Galeazzi fracture, which is a distal radius fracture with a concomitant distal radioulnar joint dislocation, by examining the distal radioulnar joint for dislocation or subluxation. A comparative examination of the uninjured extremity can help confirm or rule out a Galeazzi fracture.

Because the force of a fall onto an outstretched hand can be transmitted through the entire upper extremity, a systematic examination of the elbow, upper arm, and shoulder should be performed to rule out associated injuries. The most common concomitant injuries observed in patients who have distal radius fractures include radial head/neck fractures, supracondylar humerus fractures, and Monteggia fracture-dislocations.

A thorough neurovascular examination should always be performed in a child with a suspected distal radius fracture. Hand color and capillary refill should be noted to ensure that adequate perfusion is present. Nerve injury ranging in severity from neurapraxia to neurotmesis is associated with distal radius fractures and can involve the median, ulnar, and/or posterior interosseous nerves.[32] Sensation to light touch or two-point discrimination can be performed in the median, ulnar, and radial nerve distributions. Motor examination should include tests for posterior interosseous nerve function (thumb-interphalangeal joint hyperextension, finger-metacarpophalangeal joint extension with the wrist supported in neutral), median nerve function (thumb-interphalangeal joint flexion, distal interphalangeal joint flexion of the index finger), and ulnar nerve function (digital adduction/abduction, little finger distal interphalangeal joint flexion).

Surgeons should assess for nonaccidental trauma in all patients with fractures, especially in children younger than 3 years.[27] Patterns that are worrisome for abuse include physeal fractures of the distal radius in nonambulatory children.

Radiographic and Diagnostic Assessment

Plain radiography is the initial imaging modality used to assess patients in whom a distal radius fracture is suspected. Typically, PA and lateral radiographs of the wrist are sufficient to diagnose a distal radius fracture. Dedicated forearm radiographs may be necessary in patients in whom a more proximal fracture is suspected. Surgeons should obtain radiographs of any areas of tenderness to palpation that were noted during the physical examination of the upper extremity to rule out associated injuries.

Efforts have been made to standardize whether wrist radiographs should be obtained in patients who sustained wrist trauma. The Amsterdam Pediatric Wrist Rules is a clinical decision tool that was created to help surgeons decide if wrist radiographs are warranted.[33] Radiographs should be obtained if a patient has swelling of the distal radius, visible deformation, pain on palpation of the distal radius, pain on palpation of the anatomic snuffbox, or pain during supination. The sensitivity and specificity of the Amsterdam Pediatric Wrist Rules is 95.9% and 37.3%, respectively. Slaar et al[33] reported that the use of the Amsterdam Pediatric Wrist Rules led to a 22% reduction in ordered radiographs. A thorough knowledge of the radiographic anatomy of the distal radius is required to assess for a possible distal radius fracture on wrist radiographs. By skeletal maturity, approximately 11° of palmar tilt can be measured on lateral radiographs and 22° of radial inclination can be measured on PA radiographs. These are classic adult parameters. Because no parameters that are specific to age have been described, palmar tilt and radial inclination may be difficult to assess in young children with incomplete ossification (**Figure 2**).

To decrease radiation exposure that results from radiography, ultrasonography has become an increasingly popular imaging modality for patients in whom a distal radius fracture is suspected. A recent study reported that ultrasonography has a 99.5% sensitivity and specificity for the diagnosis of distal forearm fractures and allows for an examination of the surrounding soft tissue.[34] However, ultrasonography can be time consuming and requires specialized

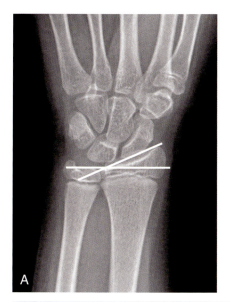 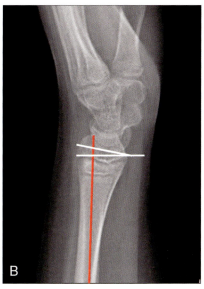 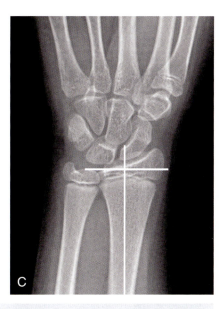

Figure 2   Radiographs of the wrist of a skeletally immature patient demonstrate measurements that are used to assess for a possible distal radius fracture. **A,** PA radiograph demonstrates measurement of radial inclination (white lines). **B,** Lateral radiograph demonstrates measurement of palmar tilt (white lines). The red line is parallel with the axis of the radial shaft. **C,** PA radiograph demonstrates measurement of ulnar variance (white lines). (Copyright Joshua M. Abzug, MD, Timonium, MD.)

training, whereas radiographs can be efficiently obtained in an inpatient or outpatient setting. Several studies have demonstrated the sensitivity and accuracy of ultrasonography for the diagnosis of distal radius fractures in adults and the value of ultrasonography to facilitate adequate reduction in adults with displaced fractures.[35,36]

Although MRI can be used to evaluate children in whom a distal radius injury is suspected, it usually is not necessary and requires sedation in younger children. Although CT can be used to evaluate children in whom a distal radius injury is suspected, it unnecessarily increases radiation exposure. These additional imaging modalities are rarely necessary in the evaluation of patients in whom a distal radius fracture is suspected. Preoperative planning for patients who have intraarticular distal radius fractures may be easier with CT.

Treatment and Outcomes
Nondisplaced or Minimally Displaced Fractures
Nondisplaced or minimally displaced distal radius fractures can be managed nonsurgically with the use of a splint or cast. Torus/buckle fractures of the distal radius are inherently stable injuries and do not require rigid immobilization because minimal risk for displacement or long-term sequelae exist.[10] A removable/prefabricated splint provides adequate stabilization for torus/buckle fractures of the distal radius, which should heal within 3 weeks of injury. Convenience and satisfaction is higher in patients with torus/buckle fractures of the distal radius who undergo nonsurgical treatment with the use of a prefabricated splint compared with those who undergo nonsurgical treatment with the use of a short arm cast.[37] Most patients prefer splints that can be removed at home by a family member.[10]

Extended clinical follow-up is not necessary for patients with torus/buckle fractures of the distal radius. Patients with torus/buckle fractures of the distal radius can follow up with their primary care provider, if necessary, and expect a full return to activity.[38] Although many studies have validated the use of splinting for pediatric torus/buckle fractures of the distal radius,[37,39-42] a consensus among surgeons on how to best manage torus/buckle fractures of the distal radius does not exist. Boutis et al[43] surveyed fellowship-trained pediatric orthopaedic surgeons and reported that only 29.1% (158 of 543) of the surgeons stated that they would use a removable splint to manage a torus/buckle fracture of the distal radius. The authors reported surgeon concerns for patient compliance, potential complications, and legal implications as the main barriers against the use of a removable splint.

Patients with greenstick fractures of the distal radius may have radial displacement and apex-ulnar angulation or rotational deformity, especially if a concomitant ulnar fracture is present. The risk for a greenstick fracture of the distal radius to progress to a complete distal radius fracture or extend into the compressed cortex always exists. Therefore, greenstick fractures of the distal radius require vigilance, and weekly follow-up radiographs should be obtained until adequate callus is observed. The type of immobilization used for patients with greenstick fractures of the distal radius is dictated by surgeon preference.[10] Most patients who have greenstick fractures of the distal radius can be treated effectively with the use of a short or long arm splint or cast for 4 to 6 weeks. Furthermore, debate exists regarding whether a pronated, neutral, or supinated resting position for an immobilized forearm best resists deforming forces. No obvious resting position for an immobilized forearm best prevents worsening angulation.[44] Long arm casts immobilize the elbow by limiting forearm rotation; however, children with greenstick fractures of the distal radius who are treated with a long arm cast will require more assistance with their daily activities. A short arm cast with an appropriate mold can provide the stability necessary for fracture healing. Attention to good casting techniques is critical, and methods for assessing cast quality are discussed later. Multiple studies have reported no differences in complication rates or loss of reduction among patients with greenstick fractures of the distal radius who underwent nonsurgical treatment with the use of prefabricated splints, short arm casts, or long arm casts.[45-47]

Typically, Salter-Harris type I and type II fractures of the distal radius displace dorsally and include apex-volar angulation. Patients with less than 50% displacement and acceptable angulation, as discussed later, can be treated with immobilization alone, without the need for reduction.[48] Typically, patients who have displaced Salter-Harris type II, type III, or type IV fractures of the distal radius require reduction maneuvers to achieve acceptable alignment.

Minimally displaced distal radius fractures or angulated metaphyseal fractures of the distal radius have remarkable remodeling potential because of the large amount of growth that occurs at the distal radial physis and the proximity of the fracture site to the physis. Parameters for coronal and sagittal alignment vary depending on the age of a patient.[24,49,50] In general, 20° to 30° of angulation in the sagittal plane will result in adequate remodeling, and as much as 50% displacement is tolerated in younger children. Bayonet apposition also may result in adequate remodeling in children younger than 10 years.[10,51] Most studies agree that rotational deformity will not result in adequate remodeling; however, Noonan and Price[27] reported that as much as 45° of malrotation in children younger than 9 years and as much as 30° of malrotation in children aged 9 years or older will not result in substantial functional deficits. Malrotation may be difficult to radiographically and clinically assess. Close inspection of the cortical diameters and bone alignment at the reduction site may indicate malrotation in patients in whom the cortical and medullary fracture lines do not exactly align radiographically. Rotation is assessed on AP radiographs of the

forearm. The radial tuberosity should be observed in profile and located 180° opposite of the radial styloid, which is observed in profile distally.

Although general acceptable alignment criteria for the nonsurgical management of distal radius fractures exist, indications for the surgical management of distal radius fractures vary. Bernthal et al[52] surveyed hand, pediatric, and general orthopaedic surgeons and reported that, based on initial radiographs, hand and general orthopaedic surgeons were 2.9 and 1.6 times more likely, respectively, to recommend surgical treatment for patients with distal radius fractures compared with pediatric surgeons. The authors also reported that hand and general orthopaedic surgeons were less likely to deem sagittal angulation less than 20°, coronal angulation less than 10°, and bayonet apposition less than 1 cm as acceptable alignment criteria compared with pediatric surgeons.

Displaced Fractures

The management of displaced distal radius fractures requires a more thorough consideration of treatment options that takes into account multiple factors to ensure optimal outcomes. Factors that should be considered in patients who have displaced distal radius fractures include the fracture pattern, the proximity of the fracture to the physis, concurrent injuries, patient age, and the amount of growth that remains before physeal closure. If substantial fracture displacement or rotational deformity exists or sagittal/coronal angulation is greater than the expected remodeling potential, a closed reduction should be performed. Patients with displaced distal radius fractures in whom initial closed

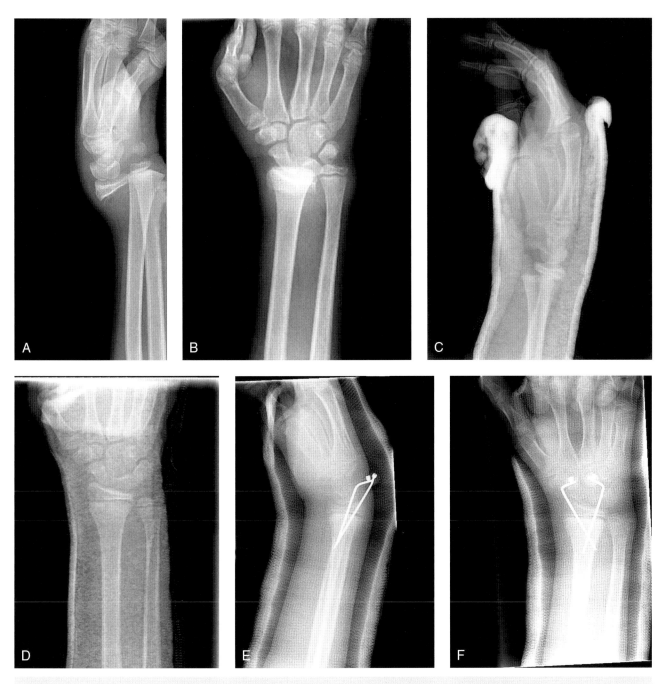

Figure 3   Radiographs of a wrist with a completely displaced fracture. Lateral (**A**) and PA (**B**) radiographs taken after initial injury demonstrate a completely displaced physeal fracture of the distal radius. Lateral (**C**) and PA (**D**) radiographs taken 3 days after anatomic closed reduction and immobilization demonstrate redisplacement. Lateral (**E**) and PA (**F**) radiographs taken after closed reduction and percutaneous pinning. (Courtesy of Theresa O. Wyrick, MD, Little Rock, AR.)

reduction is unsuccessful should undergo closed reduction and percutaneous pinning (CRPP) followed by open reduction and internal fixation (ORIF), if necessary (**Figure 3**).

Closed Reduction
Ideally, patients with a displaced distal radius fracture who undergo closed reduction should be either sedated or administered a local/regional anesthetic

agent. Various sedation and local/regional anesthetic agent protocols, including Bier block anesthesia, conscious sedation with ketamine, intranasal diamorphine with 50% oxygen and

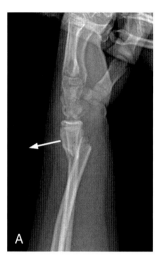 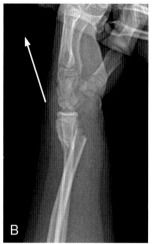 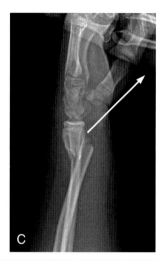 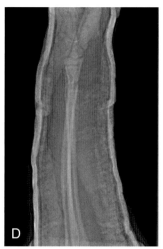

Figure 4   Lateral radiographs of the wrist of a skeletally immature patient with a completely displaced metaphyseal fracture of the distal radius demonstrate closed reduction. **A,** Dorsally directed pressure (arrow) is applied to the wrist to recreate the deformity that resulted in the fracture. **B,** Longitudinal traction (arrow) is applied to the distal fragment to unlock the fracture. **C,** Forced volar translation (arrow) is then applied to the distal fragment to achieve anatomic reduction (**D**). (Copyright Joshua M. Abzug, MD, Timonium, MD.)

nitrous oxide,[53] periosteal nerve block,[54] and local hematoma block, have been described for patients with displaced distal radius fractures who undergo a closed reduction.[55] Bear et al[55] reported no differences in pain control, patient satisfaction, and radiographic alignment between patients with distal radius fractures who underwent closed reduction with the use of a local hematoma block versus conscious sedation. However, the authors reported that closed reduction with the use of a local hematoma block significantly reduced the resources necessary to perform closed reduction and required a mean of 2.2 less hours in the emergency department.[55] In general, regional anesthesia is not well tolerated in children younger than 5 years; therefore, sedation may be required.

Typically, closed reduction of a displaced distal radius fracture is performed by applying traction to unlock the fracture fragments, after which the deformity is re-created. The fracture is then translated in the direction that will achieve anatomic reduction (**Figure 4**). In patients with more common extension-type injuries, the distal fragment is extended as traction is applied and then translated volarly to achieve reduction. After an acceptable reduction based on age, proximity to the physis, and remaining growth has been achieved, an assistant maintains the reduction as traction is applied, and the patient's arm is placed in a well-padded and molded splint or cast. A three-point mold or an interosseous mold should be used for patients with displaced distal radius fractures who undergo closed reduction. The use of a high-quality mold that has been verified by the three-point index and/or the cast index is imperative in the maintenance of fracture reduction. A three-point index value greater than 0.8 significantly increases the risk for redisplacement.[56] Both short and long arm immobilization, if applied properly, can be used to adequately manage displaced distal radius fractures and prevent redisplacement.[46,47] Plain radiographs or fluoroscopic images should be obtained after reduction and immobilization (**Figure 5**).

Many institutions have adopted the use of a mini C-arm in their emergency departments to assist surgeons in the closed reduction of fractures. Mini C-arm units have been reported to improve the quality of closed reduction of displaced distal radius fractures, decrease radiation exposure to surgeons, and decrease the need for repeat closed reduction attempts of displaced distal radius fractures.[57] Fluoroscopic imaging also has replaced the need for postreduction plain radiographs.[58] However, Sumko et al[59] contended the assertion that radiation exposure decreases with the use of a mini C-arm, and reported that the mean radiation exposure emitted during closed reduction of a distal radius fracture with the use of a mini C-arm was 63 millirems, which is significantly higher compared with the mean radiation exposure emitted by AP and lateral forearm radiographs (20 millirems). The authors also reported that less-experienced surgeons were exposed to more millirems per closed reduction compared with more advanced surgeons.

Patients are immobilized for 3 to 4 weeks after closed reduction, and parents should be properly educated on cast maintenance. Radiographs are recommended at scheduled follow-up intervals to ensure maintenance of reduction. Ideally, radiographs should be obtained every week for the first 2 to 3 weeks after closed reduction to monitor for redisplacement.[10] In a recent prospective study on the utility of outpatient follow-up radiographs after closed reduction of distal radius and forearm fractures, Luther et al[60] reported that 80% of patients who had radiographic loss of reduction demonstrated such loss of reduction within 2 weeks after closed reduction. The authors reported that radiographs obtained at a follow-up of 4 weeks after closed reduction did not change clinical decision making.[60]

Several risk factors, including casting technique, initial fracture displacement greater than 50%, the failure to achieve anatomic reduction,[61] dominant arm involvement, concomitant ulnar fracture,[60] and obesity,[62] are associated with loss of reduction. A recent retrospective study reported that children with obesity were more likely to require a closed reduction in an operating room after failed initial closed reduction in an emergency department and required more follow-up visits with radiographs compared with nonobese children.[62] Surgeons should be aware of the risk factors for redisplacement after closed reduction of distal radius fractures and inform patients accordingly.

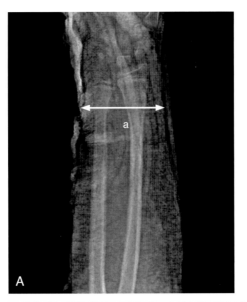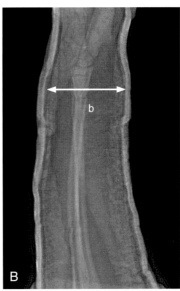

Figure 5 PA (**A**) and lateral (**B**) radiographs of the wrist of a skeletally immature patient with a metaphyseal fracture of the distal radius who underwent closed reduction and placement of the arm in a splint demonstrate the cast index. The cast index is calculated by dividing the distance between the inner edges of the cast or splint material at the fracture site on a lateral radiograph (line b) by the distance between the inner edges of the cast or splint material at the fracture site on a PA radiograph (line a). Ideally, the cast index should be equal to or less than 0.7 to prevent loss of reduction during immobilization. (Copyright Joshua M. Abzug, MD, Timonium, MD.)

Closed Reduction and Percutaneous Pinning

Irreducible fractures, displaced intra-articular fractures, open fractures, and floating elbow injuries (ipsilateral fractures of the humerus and forearm) are indications for surgical management. Patients with an ipsilateral supracondylar humerus fracture and a concomitant forearm fracture have a higher risk for compartment syndrome; surgical reduction and stabilization may help prevent compartment syndrome in these patients.[63] Closed reduction maneuvers should not be performed in patients with physeal fractures of the distal radius who present more than 10 days postinjury because of the increased risk for physeal arrest with delayed manipulation.[64] However, patients who have extraphyseal fractures of the

distal radius, even with early callous formation, can undergo late CRPP with osteoclasis as necessary if the deformity will not likely adequately remodel with growth.[65]

CRPP of a displaced distal radius fracture is achieved by administering a general anesthetic agent, after which a closed reduction maneuver is performed as previously described. A smooth 0.062-inch Kirschner wire (K-wire) is then placed either percutaneously or via a small incision over the radial styloid region. For extraphyseal fractures of the distal radius, the K-wire ideally should be placed just proximal to the physis. The reduction is maintained, and the K-wire is driven retrograde across the distal radius fracture to achieve bicortical fixation. A second K-wire can be inserted in either a crossing (dorsally via the fourth/fifth extensor compartment) or divergent (from radial styloid side) manner to provide additional stability. The K-wires are then bent and cut outside of the skin, and the patient's arm is placed in a short or long arm cast in neutral forearm rotation. Radiographs are obtained 5 to 7 days postoperatively to ensure maintenance of alignment. Radiographs are obtained 3 to 4 weeks postoperatively to confirm callous formation. After callous formation is confirmed, the cast and K-wires are removed in the office. Range of motion is assessed 6 to 8 weeks postoperatively to ensure that the patient has regained hand, wrist, and forearm motion. Follow-up visits should take place at 6-month intervals for 1 year or until growth is confirmed to ensure that physeal arrest did not occur.

In a prospective study of 68 children with displaced distal radius fractures who were randomized to either closed reduction or CRPP, McLauchlan et al[66] reported that 21% of the patients who were treated with closed reduction had a loss of reduction compared with zero of the patients who were treated with CRPP; however, 11% of the patients who were treated with CRPP had pin-site complications. The authors reported no functional differences between the patients in the two groups at a follow-up of 3 months.[66] Similarly, in a prospective study of 34 patients with displaced distal radius fractures who were randomized to either cast immobilization or CRPP, Miller et al[67] reported that 39% of the patients who were treated with cast immobilization required re-manipulation for loss of reduction, and 38% of the patients who were treated with CRPP had pin-related complications, including K-wire migration, pain, infection, tendon irritation,

and scarring, most of which resolved after K-wire removal.

Open Reduction and Internal Fixation

Pediatric patients seldom require ORIF for the management of distal radius fractures. However, ORIF should be performed in patients in whom satisfactory fracture reduction cannot be achieved via closed means, patients with displaced metadiaphyseal fractures of the distal radius that are unable to be stabilized via CRPP, patients who have open fractures, patients with suspected median neuropathy that does not improve after fracture reduction, patients with displaced intra-articular fractures, and patients with metadiaphyseal fractures of the distal radius that may result in a malunion that is unable to be reduced via osteoclasis. Children with late-presenting displaced physeal fractures of the distal radius who have less than 2 years of growth remaining should be observed closely until skeletal maturity to determine if remodeling in an acceptable position occurs. In patients who have more than 2 years of growth remaining, most deformities will adequately remodel; therefore, less close observation is warranted in these patients. A corrective osteotomy can be performed if the deformity or decreased motion persists. In most patients, distal radius fractures that require open reduction can be stabilized with the use of smooth pins. In the rare event that open reduction and plate fixation must be undertaken in a skeletally immature patient, surgeons should ensure that the plate does not cross the physis and that the screws are appropriately sized to prevent dorsal tendon irritation and, possibly, subsequent rupture. Plate fixation is indicated in patients with highly

oblique fracture patterns in whom pin fixation would not provide adequate biomechanical stabilization.

Complications

Physeal arrest occurs in 1% to 7% of patients who sustain physeal fractures of the distal radius[57,68] (**Figure 6**). Multiple and delayed attempts at reduction of a physeal fracture of the distal radius increase the risk for posttraumatic physeal arrest.[64] Ideally, manipulation should not be performed more than 10 days postinjury. If adequate remodeling does not occur, malunion can be corrected with an osteotomy that is performed at a later date.[69] In children who sustain a physeal fracture of the distal radius, repeat radiographs should be obtained every 3 months until normal growth resumes, which is observed as a lack of change in ulnar variance and/or parallel Park-Harris lines through the distal radius metaphysis on radiographs.[69] Surgical treatment should be considered in children with physeal arrest of the distal radius who have more than 2 mm of growth remaining because ulnar growth can lead to increased load transmission across the ulna, which, ultimately, can result in ulnar impaction and wrist pain. A completion epiphysiodesis of the distal radius and an epiphysiodesis of the distal ulna can be performed to prevent ulnar impaction and increased deformity.

Nonunion is a rare complication of forearm fractures in children. ORIF has been linked to a high rate of nonunion[70] as a result of iatrogenic surgical trauma that disrupts local blood circulation to the bone.[71] Delayed union (up to 3 months postinjury) and poor healing have been linked to inadequate immobilization and an insufficient duration of stabilization.[70,72,73] Patients who

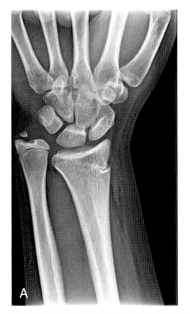 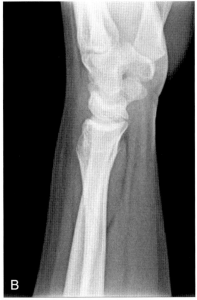 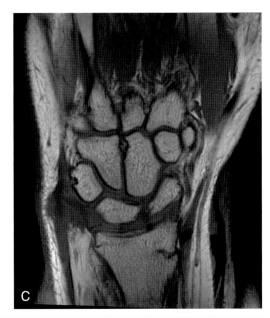

Figure 6   PA (**A**) and lateral (**B**) radiographs and coronal T1-weighted MRI (**C**) of a wrist taken 1.5 years after physeal fracture of the distal radius demonstrate physeal arrest of the distal radius with subsequent ulnar positive variance. (Courtesy of Theresa O. Wyrick, MD, Little Rock, AR.)

have a nonunion (lack of radiographic union at 3 to 6 months postinjury) that persists for more than 3 to 6 months will likely require surgical treatment to achieve fracture union.[2,74] Radioulnar synostosis is a rare complication that most commonly occurs in patients who sustained high-energy trauma or an associated head injury.[27] Radioulnar synostosis resection is not necessary in patients with a forearm that is in a neutral or pronated position; attempts at radioulnar synostosis resection often result in poor outcomes.[75]

Summary

Distal radius fractures are the most commonly managed fractures in the pediatric population. The highest incidence of distal radius fractures occurs at the onset of puberty, at which time linear skeletal growth is greater than bone mineralization. Physeal fractures of the distal radius are described based on the Salter-Harris classification system.

Extraphyseal fractures of the distal radius are incomplete if they involve one cortex or are complete if they involve both cortices. A thorough physical examination of the entire upper extremity should be performed in patients with a suspected distal radius fracture. PA and lateral radiographs of the wrist are sufficient to diagnose a distal radius fracture. Nondisplaced and minimally displaced distal radius fractures can be managed nonsurgically with the use of a splint or cast, depending on surgeon preference. Skeletally immature patients can tolerate as much as 20° to 30° of sagittal angulation and can expect sufficient remodeling without long-term sequelae. Patients who have distal radius fractures with substantial displacement or angulation require closed reduction maneuvers. Patients with physeal fractures of the distal radius with substantial angulation who present more than 10 days postinjury should not undergo manipulation because of the increased

risk for physeal arrest. CRPP should be performed in patients with displaced distal radius fractures in whom closed reduction and immobilization is inadequate. ORIF should be reserved as the last treatment option for patients with displaced distal radius fractures.

References

1. Nellans KW, Kowalski E, Chung KC: The epidemiology of distal radius fractures. *Hand Clin* 2012;28(2):113-125.

2. Randsborg PH, Gulbrandsen P, Saltytė Benth J, et al: Fractures in children: Epidemiology and activity-specific fracture rates. *J Bone Joint Surg Am* 2013;95(7):e42.

3. Ward WT, Rihn JA: The impact of trauma in an urban pediatric orthopaedic practice. *J Bone Joint Surg Am* 2006;88(12):2759-2764.

4. Landin LA: Fracture patterns in children: Analysis of 8,682 fractures with special reference to incidence, etiology and secular changes in a Swedish urban population 1950-1979. *Acta Orthop Scand Suppl* 1983;202:1-109.

5. Cheng JC, Shen WY: Limb fracture pattern in different pediatric age groups: A study of 3,350 children. *J Orthop Trauma* 1993;7(1):15-22.

6. Worlock P, Stower M: Fracture patterns in Nottingham children. *J Pediatr Orthop* 1986;6(6):656-660.

7. Skaggs DL, Loro ML, Pitukcheewanont P, Tolo V, Gilsanz V: Increased body weight and decreased radial cross-sectional dimensions in girls with forearm fractures. *J Bone Miner Res* 2001;16(7):1337-1342.

8. Goulding A, Jones IE, Taylor RW, Williams SM, Manning PJ: Bone mineral density and body composition in boys with distal forearm fractures: A dual-energy x-ray absorptiometry study. *J Pediatr* 2001;139(4):509-515.

9. Khosla S, Melton LJ III, Dekutoski MB, Achenbach SJ, Oberg AL, Riggs BL: Incidence of childhood distal forearm fractures over 30 years: A population-based study. *JAMA* 2003;290(11):1479-1485.

10. Bae DS, Howard AW: Distal radius fractures: What is the evidence? *J Pediatr Orthop* 2012;32(suppl 2):S128-S130.

11. Chung KC, Spilson SV: The frequency and epidemiology of hand and forearm fractures in the United States. *J Hand Surg Am* 2001;26(5):908-915.

12. Naranje SM, Erali RA, Warner WC Jr, Sawyer JR, Kelly DM: Epidemiology of pediatric fractures presenting to emergency departments in the united states. *J Pediatr Orthop* 2016;36(4):e45-e48.

13. Alffram PA, Bauer GC: Epidemiology of fractures of the forearm: A biomechanical investigation of bone strength. *J Bone Joint Surg Am* 1962;44(1):105-114.

14. Bailey DA, Wedge JH, McCulloch RG, Martin AD, Bernhardson SC: Epidemiology of fractures of the distal end of the radius in children as associated with growth. *J Bone Joint Surg Am* 1989;71(8):1225-1231.

15. Caspersen CJ, Pereira MA, Curran KM: Changes in physical activity patterns in the United States, by sex and cross-sectional age. *Med Sci Sports Exerc* 2000;32(9):1601-1609.

16. Krabbe S, Christiansen C, Rødbro P, Transbøl I: Effect of puberty on rates of bone growth and mineralisation: With observations in male delayed puberty. *Arch Dis Child* 1979;54(12):950-953.

17. Faulkner RA, Davison KS, Bailey DA, Mirwald RL, Baxter-Jones AD: Size-corrected BMD decreases during peak linear growth: Implications for fracture incidence during adolescence. *J Bone Miner Res* 2006;21(12):1864-1870.

18. Parfitt AM: The two faces of growth: Benefits and risks to bone integrity. *Osteoporos Int* 1994;4(6):382-398.

19. Chesi A, Mitchell JA, Kalkwarf HJ, et al: A trans-ethnic genome-wide association study identifies gender-specific loci influencing pediatric aBMD and BMC at the distal radius. *Hum Mol Genet* 2015;24(17):5053-5059.

20. Chevalley T, Bonjour JP, van Rietbergen B, Rizzoli R, Ferrari S: Fractures in healthy females followed from childhood to early adulthood are associated with later menarche age and with impaired bone microstructure at peak bone mass. *J Clin Endocrinol Metab* 2012;97(11):4174-4181.

21. Leonard MB, Zemel BS, Wrotniak BH, et al: Tibia and radius bone geometry and volumetric density in obese compared to non-obese adolescents. *Bone* 2015;73:69-76.

22. Ryan LM, Teach SJ, Searcy K, et al: Epidemiology of pediatric forearm fractures in Washington, DC. *J Trauma* 2010;69(4 suppl):S200-S205.

23. Shah NS, Buzas D, Zinberg EM: Epidemiologic dynamics contributing to pediatric wrist fractures in the United States. *Hand (N Y)* 2015;10(2):266-271.

24. Waters PM, Bae DS: Fractures of the distal radius and ulna, in Beaty JH, Kasser JR, eds: *Rockwood and Wilkins' Fractures in Children*, ed 7. Philadelphia, PA, Lippincott, Williams & Wilkins, 2010, pp 292-346.

25. Digby KH: The measurement of diaphysial growth in proximal and distal directions. *J Anat Physiol* 1916;50(pt 2):187-188.

26. Bae DS, Waters PM: Pediatric distal radius fractures and triangular fibrocartilage complex injuries. *Hand Clin* 2006;22(1):43-53.

27. Noonan KJ, Price CT: Forearm and distal radius fractures in children. *J Am Acad Orthop Surg* 1998;6(3):146-156.

28. Fung EB, Humphrey ML, Gildengorin G, Goldstein N, Hoffinger SA: Rapid remineralization of the distal radius after forearm fracture in children. *J Pediatr Orthop* 2011;31(2):138-143.

29. Fernandez DL, Palmer AK: Fractures of the distal radius, in Green D, Hotchkiss R, Pederson W, eds: *Green's Operative Hand Surgery,* ed 4. New York, NY, Churchill-Livingstone, 1999, pp 929-985.

30. Salter RB, Harris WR: Injuries involving the epiphyseal plate. *J Bone Joint Surg Am* 1963;45(3):587-622.

31. Pretell-Mazzini J, Carrigan RB: Simultaneous distal radial fractures and carpal bones injuries in children: A review article. *J Pediatr Orthop B* 2011;20(5):330-333.

32. Davis DR, Green DP: Forearm fractures in children: Pitfalls and complications. *Clin Orthop Relat Res* 1976;120:172-183.

33. Slaar A, Walenkamp MM, Bentohami A, et al: A clinical decision rule for the use of plain radiography in children after acute wrist injury: Development and external validation of the Amsterdam Pediatric Wrist Rules. *Pediatr Radiol* 2016;46(1):50-60.

34. Herren C, Sobottke R, Ringe MJ, et al: Ultrasound-guided diagnosis of fractures of the distal forearm in children. *Orthop Traumatol Surg Res* 2015;101(4):501-505.

35. Kozaci N, Ay MO, Akcimen M, et al: Evaluation of the effectiveness of bedside point-of-care ultrasound in the diagnosis and management of distal radius fractures. *Am J Emerg Med* 2015;33(1):67-71.

36. Chaar-Alvarez FM, Warkentine F, Cross K, Herr S, Paul RI: Bedside ultrasound diagnosis of nonangulated distal forearm fractures in the pediatric emergency department. *Pediatr Emerg Care* 2011;27(11):1027-1032.

37. Williams KG, Smith G, Luhmann SJ, Mao J, Gunn JD III, Luhmann JD: A randomized controlled trial of cast versus splint for distal radial buckle fracture: An evaluation of satisfaction, convenience, and preference. *Pediatr Emerg Care* 2013;29(5):555-559.

38. Koelink E, Schuh S, Howard A, Stimec J, Barra L, Boutis K: Primary care physician follow-up of distal radius buckle fractures. *Pediatrics* 2016;137(1):1-9.

39. Symons S, Rowsell M, Bhowal B, Dias JJ: Hospital versus home management of children with buckle fractures of the distal radius: A prospective, randomised trial. *J Bone Joint Surg Br* 2001;83(4):556-560.

40. Plint AC, Perry JJ, Correll R, Gaboury I, Lawton L: A randomized, controlled trial of removable splinting versus casting for wrist buckle fractures in children. *Pediatrics* 2006;117(3):691-697.

41. Davidson JS, Brown DJ, Barnes SN, Bruce CE: Simple treatment for torus fractures of the distal radius. *J Bone Joint Surg Br* 2001;83(8):1173-1175.

42. Khan KS, Grufferty A, Gallagher O, Moore DP, Fogarty E, Dowling F: A randomized trial of 'soft cast' for distal radius buckle fractures in children. *Acta Orthop Belg* 2007;73(5):594-597.

43. Boutis K, Howard A, Constantine E, Cuomo A, Somji Z, Narayanan UG: Evidence into practice: Pediatric orthopaedic surgeon use of removable splints for common pediatric fractures. *J Pediatr Orthop* 2015;35(1):18-23.

44. Boyer BA, Overton B, Schrader W, Riley P, Fleissner P: Position of immobilization for pediatric forearm fractures. *J Pediatr Orthop* 2002;22(2):185-187.

45. Boutis K, Willan A, Babyn P, Goeree R, Howard A: Cast versus splint in children with minimally angulated fractures of the distal radius: A randomized controlled trial. *CMAJ* 2010;182(14):1507-1512.

46. Bohm ER, Bubbar V, Yong Hing K, Dzus A: Above and below-the-elbow plaster casts for distal forearm fractures in children: A randomized controlled trial. *J Bone Joint Surg Am* 2006;88(1):1-8.

47. Webb GR, Galpin RD, Armstrong DG: Comparison of short and long arm plaster casts for displaced fractures in the distal third of the forearm in children. *J Bone Joint Surg Am* 2006;88(1):9-17.

48. Egol KA, Koval KJ, Zuckerman JD: *Handbook of Fractures,* ed 4. Philadelphia, PA, Lippincott, Williams & Wilkins, 2010.

49. Bae DS: Pediatric distal radius and forearm fractures. *J Hand Surg Am* 2008;33(10):1911-1923.

50. Skaggs DL, Frick S: Upper extremity fractures in children, in Weinstein SL, Flynn JM, eds: *Lovell and Winter's Pediatric Orthopaedics,* ed 7. Philadelphia, PA, Lippincott, Williams & Wilkins, 2013, pp 1694-1772.

51. Abzug JM, Kozin SH: Pediatric distal radius fractures, in Skaggs DL, Kocher MS, eds: *Master Techniques in Orthopaedic Surgery: Pediatrics,* ed 2. Philadelphia, PA, Wolters Kluwer, 2015, pp 67-81.

52. Bernthal NM, Mitchell S, Bales JG, Benhaim P, Silva M: Variation in practice habits in the treatment of pediatric distal radius fractures. *J Pediatr Orthop B* 2015;24(5):400-407.

53. Kurien T, Price KR, Pearson RG, Dieppe C, Hunter JB: Manipulation and reduction of paediatric fractures of the distal radius and forearm using intranasal diamorphine and 50% oxygen and nitrous oxide in the emergency department: A 2.5-year study. *Bone Joint J* 2016;98(1):131-136.

54. Tageldin ME, Alrashid M, Khoriati AA, Gadikoppula S, Atkinson HD: Periosteal nerve blocks for distal radius and ulna fracture manipulation– the technique and early results. *J Orthop Surg Res* 2015;10:134.

55. Bear DM, Friel NA, Lupo CL, Pitetti R, Ward WT: Hematoma block versus sedation for the reduction of distal radius fractures in children. *J Hand Surg Am* 2015;40(1):57-61.

56. Iltar S, Alemdaroğlu KB, Say F, Aydoğan NH: The value of the three-point index in predicting redisplacement of diaphyseal fractures of the forearm in children. *Bone Joint J* 2013;95(4):563-567.

57. Lee BS, Esterhai JL Jr, Das M: Fracture of the distal radial epiphysis: Characteristics and surgical treatment of premature, post-traumatic epiphyseal closure. *Clin Orthop Relat Res* 1984;185:90-96.

58. Shariett GQ, Kanegaye J, Wallace CD, McCaslin RI, Harley JR: Can portable bedside fluoroscopy replace standard, postreduction radiographs in the management of pediatric fractures? *Pediatr Emerg Care* 1999;15(4):249-251.

59. Sumko MJ, Hennrikus W, Slough J, et al: Measurement of radiation exposure when using the mini C-arm to reduce pediatric upper extremity fractures. *J Pediatr Orthop* 2016;36(2):122-125.

60. Luther G, Miller P, Waters PM, Bae DS: Radiographic evaluation during treatment of pediatric forearm fractures: Implications on clinical care and cost. *J Pediatr Orthop* 2016;36(5):465-471.

61. McQuinn AG, Jaarsma RL: Risk factors for redisplacement of pediatric distal forearm and distal radius fractures. *J Pediatr Orthop* 2012;32(7):687-692.

62. Auer RT, Mazzone P, Robinson L, Nyland J, Chan G: Childhood obesity increases the risk of failure in the treatment of distal forearm fractures. *J Pediatr Orthop* 2015.

63. Dhoju D, Shrestha D, Parajuli N, Dhakal G, Shrestha R: Ipsilateral supracondylar fracture and forearm bone injury in children: A retrospective review of thirty one cases. *Kathmandu Univ Med J (KUMJ)* 2011;9(34):11-16.

64. Valverde JA, Albiñana J, Certucha JA: Early posttraumatic physeal arrest in distal radius after a compression injury. *J Pediatr Orthop B* 1996;5(1):57-60.

65. Lefevre Y, Laville JM, Boullet F, Salmeron F: Early correction of paediatric malunited distal metaphyseal radius fractures using percutaneous callus osteoclasis ("Calloclasis"). *Orthop Traumatol Surg Res* 2012;98(4):450-454.

66. McLauchlan GJ, Cowan B, Annan IH, Robb JE: Management of completely displaced metaphyseal fractures of the distal radius in

children. A prospective, randomised controlled trial. *J Bone Joint Surg Br* 2002;84(3):413-417.

67. Miller BS, Taylor B, Widmann RF, Bae DS, Snyder BD, Waters PM: Cast immobilization versus percutaneous pin fixation of displaced distal radius fractures in children: A prospective, randomized study. *J Pediatr Orthop* 2005;25(4):490-494.

68. Buterbaugh GA, Palmer AK: Fractures and dislocations of the distal radioulnar joint. *Hand Clin* 1988;4(3):361-375.

69. Abzug JM, Little K, Kozin SH: Physeal arrest of the distal radius. *J Am Acad Orthop Surg* 2014;22(6):381-389.

70. Lewallen RP, Peterson HA: Nonunion of long bone fractures in children: A review of 30 cases. *J Pediatr Orthop* 1985;5(2):135-142.

71. Fernandez FF, Eberhardt O, Langendörfer M, Wirth T: Nonunion of forearm shaft fractures in children after intramedullary nailing. *J Pediatr Orthop B* 2009;18(6):289-295.

72. Song KS, Lee SW, Bae KC, Yeon CJ, Naik P: Primary nonunion of the distal radius fractures in healthy children. *J Pediatr Orthop B* 2016;25(2):165-169.

73. Prommersberger KJ, Fernandez DL: Nonunion of distal radius fractures. *Clin Orthop Relat Res* 2004;419:51-56.

74. De Raet J, Kemnitz S, Verhaven E: Nonunion of a pediatric distal radial metaphyseal fracture following open reduction and internal fixation: A case report and review of the literature. *Eur J Trauma Emerg Surg* 2008;34(2):173-176.

75. Vince KG, Miller JE: Cross-union complicating fracture of the forearm: Part II. Children. *J Bone Joint Surg Am* 1987;69(5):654-661.

Skeletally Immature Anterior Cruciate Ligament Injuries: Controversies and Management

Shital N. Parikh, MD, FACS
Bradley P. Jaquith, MD
Christopher M. Brusalis, BA
Lauren H. Redler, MD
Theodore J. Ganley, MD
Mininder S. Kocher, MD, MPH

Abstract

At one time, anterior cruciate ligament (ACL) tears in skeletally immature patients were considered rare. The recommended treatment option for skeletally immature patients with ACL tears was to modify activities until skeletal maturity, at which point definitive ACL reconstruction could be safely performed. The management of ACL tears in skeletally immature patients has evolved as a result of the increased frequency of ACL tears in younger patients and an increased awareness for the potential development or worsening of meniscal tears, chondral lesions, and degenerative changes that occur with the "wait-and-fix-later" approach. The surgical options for ACL reconstruction in skeletally immature patients include physeal-sparing, partial transphyseal, and complete transphyseal techniques. The timing and ideal technique for ACL reconstruction in skeletally immature patients are controversial. Accurate assessment of skeletal growth remaining and concerns for iatrogenic growth disturbances continually challenge treating physicians. Similar controversies with regard to the treatment of skeletally immature patients who have partial ACL tears or congenital absence of the ACL also exist.

Instr Course Lect 2017;66:461–474.

Dr. Parikh or an immediate family member serves as a board member, owner, officer, or committee member of the Pediatric Orthopaedic Society of North America. Dr. Kocher or an immediate family member serves as a paid consultant to or is an employee of OrthoPediatrics, Össur, and Smith & Nephew; has stock or stock options held in Fixes 4 Kids and Pivot Medical; has received research or institutional support from Össur; and serves as a board member, owner, officer, or committee member of the American Academy of Orthopaedic Surgeons, the ACL Study Group, the American Orthopaedic Society for Sports Medicine, Harvard Medical School, the Harvard T.H. Chan School of Public Health, the Herodicus Society, the Pediatric Orthopaedic Society of North America, the Pediatric Research in Sports Medicine Society, and the Steadman Philippon Research Institute. None of the following authors nor any immediate family member has received anything of value from or has stock or stock options held in a commercial company or institution related directly or indirectly to the subject of this chapter: Dr. Jaquith, Mr. Brusalis, Dr. Redler, and Dr. Ganley.

Anatomy

The anterior cruciate ligament (ACL) develops in utero. Before a gestational age of 24 weeks, the ACL appears as a confluence of ligament collagen fibers and periosteum of the distal femur and the proximal tibia on ultrasonography. At a gestational age of 24 weeks, vascular invasion into the epiphysis occurs. At a gestational age of 36 weeks, a secure epiphyseal attachment as well as interdigitation of collagen fibers with the surrounding bone, fibrocartilage, and mineralized fibrocartilage are observed.[1]

The ACL has two functional and anatomic bundles: the anteromedial bundle (AMB) and the posterolateral bundle (PLB), both of which are named based on their relative locations to their tibial insertions. The femoral ACL attachment is located on the posterior aspect of the medial surface of the lateral femoral condyle. The AMB originates at

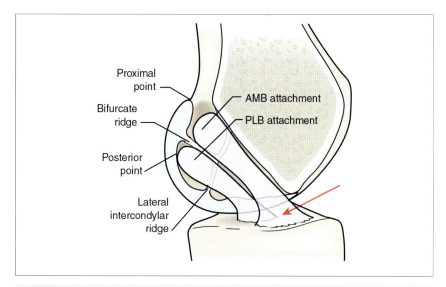

Figure 1   Illustration shows femoral anterior cruciate ligament (ACL) attachment terminology, which may be confusing because surgical anatomy is frequently described with the femur in a horizontal position. The anteromedial bundle (AMB) is attached more proximal and anterior compared with the posterolateral bundle (PLB), which is attached more distal and posterior. The bifurcate ridge separates the two bundles. The lateral intercondylar ridge, which also is known as the resident's ridge, forms the anterior border of the femoral ACL attachment. The AMB forms a comma-like crescent shape over the anterior aspect of the PLB (red arrow).

the most proximal portion of the femoral ACL footprint, which is between the intercondylar line and the cartilage margin, and inserts along the medial aspect of the intercondylar eminence. The PLB originates at the distal portion of the femoral ACL footprint and inserts just lateral to the central aspect of the intercondylar eminence[2,3] (**Figure 1**). At times, the terminology used to describe the femoral ACL attachment and the femoral tunnel position may be confusing because the femur is positioned horizontally during surgery; therefore, the commonly used nomenclature for the posterior position on the distal femur is actually the proximal position. The sizes of the bundles have been reported to vary with patient height, weight, and body mass index.[4]

The femoral intercondylar notch has been reported to steadily increase

in width until age 11 years, with less substantial growth occurring until skeletal maturity.[3] The lateral intercondylar ridge, which also is known as the resident's ridge, marks the anterior border of the femoral ACL footprint and can be used as a landmark for accurate femoral tunnel placement. The lateral intercondylar ridge is less commonly present and less clearly defined in younger patients. The lateral intercondylar ridge is present in 44% to 63% of patients aged 3 to 12 years compared with 88% of patients older than 12 years.[5]

Knowledge of distal femoral and proximal tibial physeal anatomy is critical if a surgeon is considering reconstruction techniques in a skeletally immature patient (**Figure 2**). The distal femoral physis contributes to 70% of total femoral length and 37% of total limb length, with a mean growth rate of

10 mm per year. The distance between the femoral physis and the femoral ACL origin has been reported to remain constant throughout development (mean, approximately 3 mm).[1] The proximal tibial physis contributes to approximately 55% of total tibial length and 25% of total limb length, with a mean growth rate of 6.4 mm per year. The distance between the tibial epiphysis and the tibial ACL footprint increases slightly, from 15.1 mm in preadolescents (aged 6 to 10 years) to 15.9 mm in adolescents (aged 11 to 15 years), as individuals reach skeletal maturity.[6] The maximum oblique tibial epiphyseal depth, which represents the length of the graft in the tibial tunnel for physeal-sparing reconstructions, has been reported to occur at a 50° angle from the plateau and does not change with age or sex. The mean maximum oblique depth in preadolescent and adolescent patients is approximately 30 mm.[6]

Epidemiology

The current literature suggests that the frequency of ACL tears in children and adolescents is increasing because of increased participation in competitive youth sports, earlier single-sport specialization, and an increased ability to detect ACL injuries as a result of increased physician awareness and easier access to advanced imaging.[7-10] Researchers at The Children's Hospital of Philadelphia reported a 400% increase in the incidence of ACL ruptures from 1999 to 2011.[11] A recent database study from New York State estimated that the incidence of ACL reconstructions per 100,000 people aged 3 to 20 years increased from 17.6 in 1990 to 50.9 in 2009.[12] With regard to high school sports in the United States, girls' soccer has the highest incidence of ACL injuries, with 14.08 injuries per 100,000 exposures. Football has the next highest incidence of ACL injuries, with 13.87 injuries per 100,000 exposures, but it has the highest total number of ACL injuries because of its greater number of participants.[9] Female athletes who play soccer and basketball have a higher incidence of ACL injuries than their male counterparts. In a study on acute traumatic knee hemarthrosis in adolescents, Abbasi et al[13] reported that 28% of males and 38% of females sustained ACL tears, which further confirms that female high school athletes appear to be more susceptible to ACL tears than their male counterparts.

Neuromuscular factors have been implicated as a reason for the higher incidence of ACL tears in female athletes. Landing, cutting, and pivoting maneuvers have been reported to be different in females and males.[14-16] Females perform these maneuvers with increased adduction and internal rotation of the femur, reduced hip and knee flexion angles, increased dynamic valgus, increased hip and knee flexion angles, increased quadriceps to hamstrings activation, and decreased muscle stiffness around the knee joint.[17] Prevention programs to address these neuromuscular factors have decreased ACL injuries in female soccer players.[18] Some studies have theorized that the ACL has receptors for estrogen and relaxin, and that the increased levels of these hormones in females leads to an increased risk for ACL injuries. Animal studies have suggested that higher levels of estrogen and relaxin change the elasticity of and weaken the ACL.[19-21] Mixed results have been reported on whether varying levels of sex hormones during the menstrual cycle lead to laxity; however, some studies have suggested that

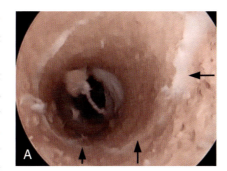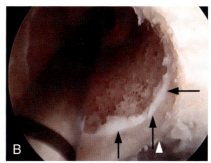

Figure 2   Arthroscopic images of transphyseal tunnels show the proximal tibial physis (black arrows; **A**) and the distal femoral physis (black arrows; **B**). The distance between the distal femoral physis and the posterior border of the lateral femoral condyle (arrowhead in panel **B**) is approximately 3 mm; therefore, care should be taken during notchplasty or femoral tunnel preparation to avoid physeal injury and potential growth disturbances.

females have a higher risk for ACL injury during the preovulatory phase because of higher estrogen levels.[22-25] In addition to female sex, other factors, such as decreased intercondylar notch width, increased posterior tibial slope, and a decreased intercondylar inclination angle, have been associated with an increased risk for ACL injury.[17,26]

Imaging and Skeletal Maturity Assessment
Magnetic Resonance Imaging
A normal ACL will appear on MRI as a straight structure that is parallel with the intercondylar notch, with fibers in continuity from the femur to the tibia. Because of adipose and synovial tissue, some increased signal intensity around the ACL is normal. In contrast, a torn ACL will have high signal intensity and edema within the ACL on a T2-weighted MRI, especially if the knee is imaged acutely. In addition, continuous fibers will not be identifiable from the femur to the tibia, and there will be a loss of the taut straight line of fibers. Detachment of the origin of the ACL from the lateral femoral condyle is best visualized on axial MRI. The stump of the ACL may be identifiable unless it is

scarred to the posterior cruciate ligament, in which case it may be obscured and not identifiable. In some patients who have ACL insufficiency, MRI also may show anterior subluxation of the tibia relative to the femur. Some bone bruising patterns, which are caused by the pivot-shift phenomenon, are pathognomonic for ACL injuries. The pivot-shift phenomenon is characterized by anterior subluxation of the tibia with valgus stress on the knee in 20° to 30° of flexion followed by reduction of the tibia with further flexion. The common locations of bone bruising after an acute ACL tear are the sulcus terminale of the lateral femoral condyle and the posterolateral tibial plateau. Concomitant injuries, including meniscal tears, chondral injuries, and other ligament injuries, often occur in patients who have ACL injuries; therefore, it is crucial that MRIs be carefully scrutinized to identify additional pathology.

Plain Radiographs
Imaging of a skeletally immature patient who has an ACL injury should include plain radiographs of the knee and, if the clinical evaluation suggests deformity (such as genu valgum or genu

Table 1
Criteria for Shorthand Bone Age Assessment

Radiographic Criteria	Bone Age (y)	
	Males	Females
Appearance of the hook of hamate ossific nucleus	12.5	10
Appearance of the thumb sesamoid ossific nucleus	13	11
Width of the proximal aspect of the distal radial epiphysis equals the width of the distal aspect of the distal radial metaphysis but has not yet begun to cap	13.5	—
Capping[a] of the distal radial epiphysis	14	12
Closure of the thumb distal phalanx physis	15	13
Closure of the index finger distal phalanx physis	15.5	13.5
Closure of the index finger proximal phalanx physis	16	14
Closure of the index finger distal metacarpal physis	—	15
Closure of the distal ulnar physis	—	16
Closure of the distal radial physis	—	17

[a]Presence of a rounded osseous peak that is oriented proximally (on the ulnar side).

varum), the entire limb. AP and lateral radiographs of the knee aid in the diagnosis of fractures or avulsions of the tibia and femur. Intercondylar notch and Merchant radiographs of the knee aid in the diagnosis of osteochondral fractures and osteochondritis dissecans lesions and in the assessment of the patellofemoral articulation. Standing radiographs of the entire limb obtained preoperatively can be compared with postoperative radiographs to evaluate for growth disturbances after ACL reconstruction.

An assessment of the status of skeletal maturity may be critical in the preoperative evaluation of younger patients. Surgeons should remember that chronologic age does not always match skeletal age. In many patients, skeletal age often lags behind chronologic age; therefore, an accurate assessment of bone age is critical to the selection of the appropriate surgical technique and graft for ACL reconstruction in skeletally immature patients.

Greulich and Pyle[27] introduced the *Radiographic Atlas of Skeletal Development of the Hand and Wrist* in 1959, and it is considered the preferred method for evaluation of bone age. Skeletal age is determined by comparing a patient's left hand and wrist radiograph with a corresponding image in the radiographic atlas. Alternatively, a knee radiograph can be used to determine skeletal age; however, this method is much less common.[28] Heyworth et al[29] developed a shorthand bone age system as a simple and more efficient alternative to the radiographic atlas. The shorthand bone age system uses a single, univariable criterion for each bone age rather than a multivariable subjective comparison with a radiographic atlas. The shorthand bone age system can be used to assess the skeletal maturity of males aged 12.5 to 16 years and females aged 10 to 16 years. The radiographic criteria and corresponding bone ages are listed in **Table 1**. A criterion can be used for bone age

assignments only if the criterion that follows is absent.

Sanders et al[30] developed a similar simplified staging system that involves the use of Tanner-Whitehouse III skeletal maturity assessment descriptors. The authors correlated this staging system with the timing of the curve acceleration phase in a cohort of 22 girls who had idiopathic scoliosis. The authors determined that the closure of the epiphysis of the distal phalanges can be used to divide patients between early and late adolescent stages.

Physiologic stage or biologic age, which can be established based on the Tanner and Whitehouse method, also plays an important part in determining a patient's skeletal maturity.[31] Physiologic stages include (1) prepubertal, (2) prepubertal–peak growth velocity, (3) pubertal–young adolescent, (4) pubertal–older adolescent, and (5) physiologic maturity. Several studies have shown the validity of reports from parents and families regarding a patient's physiologic Tanner stage.[32] A surgeon can confirm the reported physiologic stage of a patient at the time of surgery after general anesthesia is induced.

Natural History of ACL Tears
Historically, children and adolescents who suffered ACL tears were treated nonsurgically with a regimen of activity modification, bracing, and continued rehabilitation. Despite difficulty in ensuring pediatric patients adhered to activity modification, nonsurgical management was preferred because it avoided the risk of growth disturbance that was associated with the limited surgical treatment options that were previously available. ACL reconstruction performed after a patient reached

skeletal maturity circumvented the concern for iatrogenic physeal injury. The natural history of ACL tears, however, suggests that a delay in surgical intervention has inherent risks.[33-37] Without surgical reconstruction, many patients experience persistent instability, which results in secondary meniscal and chondral injuries that predispose patients to early degenerative knee arthritis and poor return to sport.

Several recent studies elucidated the consequences of the delayed surgical management of ACL injuries in skeletally immature patients. In a study of 56 pediatric patients who had ACL tears, Henry et al[38] compared the outcomes of a patient group who underwent surgical treatment at a mean time of 13.5 months postinjury with those of a patient group who underwent surgical treatment at a mean time of 30 months postinjury. The authors reported that the patients in the delayed treatment group had a significantly increased percentage of medial meniscal tears (41% versus 16%, $P = 0.01$) and a lower mean International Knee Documentation Committee Subjective Knee Evaluation Form score (83.4 versus 94.6, $P = 0.002$) compared with the patients in the early treatment group (**Figure 3**). In a logistic regression analysis of 70 patients, Lawrence et al[39] reported that patients who underwent ACL reconstruction more than 12 weeks postinjury had a fourfold greater risk of a medial meniscal tear compared with patients who underwent ACL reconstruction within the first 12 weeks of injury. The authors also reported that patients who delayed ACL reconstruction for more than 12 weeks postinjury had a significant increase in irreparable medial meniscal tears, an 11-fold increase in lateral chondral injury, and a threefold increase

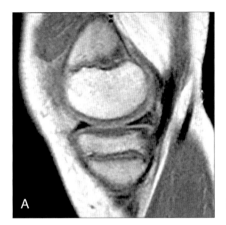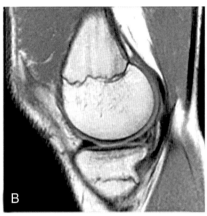

Figure 3   Sagittal T2-weighted MRIs of the knee of an 11.6-year old boy. **A,** Image taken 1 month after injury shows an anterior cruciate ligament tear with no meniscal injury. The patient was treated nonsurgically. **B,** Image taken 4 years after injury shows a grade III medial meniscal lesion. (Reproduced with permission from Henry J, Chotel F, Chouteau J, Fessy MH, Bérard J, Moyen B: Rupture of the anterior cruciate ligament in children: Early reconstruction with open physes or delayed reconstruction to skeletal maturity? *Knee Surg Sports Traumatol Arthrosc* 2009;17[7]:748-755.)

in patellotrochlear cartilage injury. The risk of meniscal and chondral injuries was increased if patients had a subjective sense of knee instability.

Anderson and Anderson[40] corroborated the association between delayed surgical treatment and increased incidence of medial meniscal and chondral injuries. The authors also associated delayed surgical intervention with increased incidence and severity of lateral meniscal tears. Moreover, the authors reported that the risk of secondary damage from ACL tears continues beyond the immediate postinjury time period.

Guenther et al[41] evaluated 112 Canadian adolescents, a population in whom healthcare delivery is often delayed, to assess the long-term prognosis of ACL injuries that were managed nonsurgically. The authors reported that medial meniscal tears and bucket-handle tears, in particular, increased in frequency more than 1 year after ACL injury. Despite a lack of studies with level I or level

II evidence, a growing body of literature has provided compelling evidence that complete ACL tears in skeletally immature patients result in poor clinical outcomes unless they are managed with early surgical intervention.[42]

Physeal Injury and Considerations

The risk of iatrogenic growth disturbance has contributed to controversy with regard to the management of complete ACL injuries in skeletally immature patients. Drill holes that are created during a transphyseal procedure can jeopardize the growth potential of the injured leg, which may result in a subsequent limb length discrepancy (LLD). In addition to limb shortening, other reported complications include limb overgrowth, femoral valgus deformity, and genu recurvatum.[30,43-46] Despite these concerns, several studies have reported that the risk of such injuries is minimal.[42,45,47-49] In a meta-analysis of 55 studies that encompassed 935

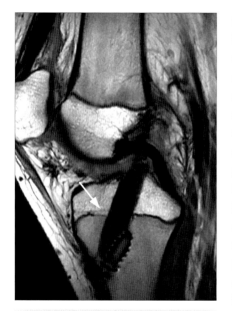

Figure 4 Sagittal MRI of the knee of a 14.6-year-old boy who underwent transphyseal anterior cruciate ligament reconstruction shows focal bone bridge formation (arrow) in the proximal tibial physis. (Reproduced with permission from Yoo WJ, Kocher MS, Micheli LJ: Growth plate disturbance after transphyseal reconstruction of the anterior cruciate ligament in skeletally immature adolescent patients: An MR imaging study. *J Pediatr Orthop* 2011;31[6]:691-696.)

patients who underwent various forms of ACL reconstruction, a 1.8% risk of LLD or angular deformity was calculated.[50] Another systematic review of 479 patients in 31 studies identified two patients who had LLD and three patients who had angular deformities.[42] Nonetheless, studies often focused on adolescent patients approaching skeletal maturity who had less risk of growth disturbance.[46]

Several factors that pertain to surgical technique predispose patients to physeal arrest. Studies of animal models have demonstrated that a large tunnel diameter relative to the cross-sectional area of the physis, graft fixation across the physis, and excessive graft tensioning are associated with an increased risk of growth disturbance.[51] A tunnel diameter that exceeds 12 mm, an overly oblique tunnel trajectory, dissection near the perichondrial ring of LaCroix, and extra-articular tenodesis also are associated with an increased risk of physeal growth disturbance.[45,46,52,53] Many angular deformities are secondary to either bony bars that form across the lateral distal femoral physis (54%) or fixation devices that traverse the tibial physis (27%).[45] Lawrence et al[54] suggested that all-epiphyseal techniques may not be immune to growth disturbance and postulated that thermal injury from nearby drilling, altered blood supply, and altered mechanical forces after graft placement may affect the adjacent physis.

Recent ongoing research has used MRI to better characterize physeal injuries. An injury threshold attempts to identify the maximum amount of physeal disruption permitted without causing clinical growth disturbance. In animal models, transphyseal tunnels that occupied less than 5% of the cross-sectional area of the physis did not result in growth disturbance; however, transphyseal tunnels that occupied more than 7% of the cross-sectional area of the physis did result in growth disturbance.[55,56] Kercher et al[57] used three-dimensional modeling to evaluate 31 adolescent patients after transphyseal ACL reconstruction. The use of 8-mm transphyseal tunnels corresponded with less than 3% of the cross-sectional area of the physis, which was less than the 7% injury threshold established in animal models. Using similar three-dimensional modeling, Shea et al[58] reported that the percentage of total physeal volume removed never exceeded 5.4% for a range of tibial tunnel sizes. In a review of 43 skeletally immature patients who had no clinically perceptible growth disturbance after transphyseal ACL reconstruction, Yoo et al[59] identified focal physeal disruption on the MRIs of 11.6% of the patients (**Figure 4**). Together, these studies explain the low rate of growth disturbance in adolescent patients who undergo transphyseal ACL reconstruction, but they also justify the need for physeal-sparing techniques in younger patients who have open physes. Because many growth disturbances occur without symptoms and at vastly different postoperative timeframes, patients should be monitored annually until they reach skeletal maturity.[46,54]

Surgical Techniques

Conventional surgical reconstruction techniques used in adults can cause iatrogenic growth disturbance as a result of damage to the distal femoral physis and/or the proximal tibial physis in skeletally immature patients. Surgical options to address ACL injuries in skeletally immature patients include primary ligament repair; extra-articular tenodesis; and reconstructions using physeal-sparing, partial transphyseal, and complete transphyseal techniques.

Primary Ligament Repair and Extra-Articular Tenodesis

Primary ACL repair and extra-articular tenodesis alone have poor results in children, adolescents, and adults.[33,60-62] In a study of 10 skeletally immature patients who underwent iliotibial band (ITB) tenodesis, McCarroll et al[62] reported that, based on KT-1000 arthrometer testing at a mean follow-up of 26 months, all patients had residual knee laxity, and five patients had instability. Despite these poor results, promising preliminary data exist on bridge-enhanced ACL reconstruction with a scaffold-assisted ACL repair model.[63]

Physeal-Sparing Reconstruction

Physeal-sparing reconstruction techniques include the all-epiphyseal technique and the combined extra- and intra-articular ITB technique. Anderson[64] first described the all-epiphyseal technique in 12 skeletally immature patients (**Figure 5, A**). At follow-up ranging from 2 to 8.2 years, the patients had a mean laxity of 1.5 mm, and no patients had residual instability. Laxity was determined via KT-1000 arthrometer testing, and instability was determined clinically.

Several modifications of Anderson's all-epiphyseal technique have been described. Lykissas et al[65] modified the all-epiphyseal technique to include split tibial tunnels, which decreases the diameter of a single tibial tunnel and avoids fixation in the tibial epiphysis (**Figure 5, B**). Lawrence et al[66] described a modification of the all-epiphyseal technique that uses inside-out retrograde tunnel preparation and retrograde interference screw fixation. McCarthy et al[67] modified the all-epiphyseal technique to include a retrograde-drilled all-epiphyseal tunnel and fixation with soft-tissue buttons on both the femur and tibia.

Nawabi et al[68] analyzed postoperative MRIs of the physes of 15 patients who underwent all-epiphyseal ACL reconstruction. The authors reported minimal tibial physeal violation in 10 patients. The mean area of total physeal disturbance was 2.1%. Minimal compromise (1.5%) of the femoral

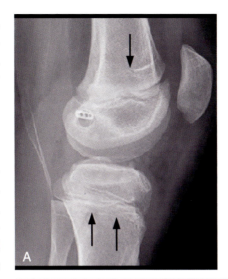 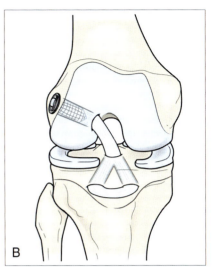

Figure 5   **A,** Lateral radiograph of a knee taken 1 year after reconstruction with the all-epiphyseal technique demonstrates continued growth (black arrows) with no growth disturbances. **B,** Illustration shows a modification of the all-epiphyseal technique, which uses split tibial tunnels. The graft is looped over a bone bridge to decrease the size of the tibial tunnel and avoid fixation on the tibial side.

physis was observed in one patient. The authors reported no growth arrest, articular surface violation, or osteonecrosis on MRI, and no postoperative angular deformities or substantial LLD were observed.

Cruz et al[69] reported on the safety of the all-epiphyseal technique in a review of 103 skeletally immature patients. At a mean follow-up of 21 months, the authors reported an overall complication rate of 16.5%, which included 11 reruptures (10.7%), one patient who had a clinical LLD of less than 1 cm (<1.0%), and two patients who had arthrofibrosis that required manipulation under anesthesia (1.9%). No associations were reported between the re-rupture rate and age, sex, graft type, graft thickness, body mass index, or associated injuries addressed during surgery.

Moderately encouraging results have been reported in a small series of patients who underwent surgery with physeal-sparing techniques in which a semitendinosus autograft was left attached to the Gerdy tubercle and an over-the-top position on the femur was used or in which a femoral epiphyseal-stapling technique was used.[55,70,71] Kocher et al[72] modified the combined extra- and intra-articular ITB technique, which was originally described by MacIntosh and Darby,[73] for skeletally immature patients. This modification uses arthroscopic assistance, altered graft fixation, and accelerated rehabilitation (**Figure 6**). Micheli et al[74] reported on the initial 17 patients (mean age, 11 years) who underwent combined intra-articular and extra-articular ACL reconstruction using the ITB technique. All of the knees were reported to be objectively stable via KT-1000 arthrometer testing, and the mean Lysholm Knee Scale score was 97.4. In a follow-up study on the series by Micheli et al,[74] Kocher et al[75] reported on 44 prepubescent patients (mean age, 10.3 years) who underwent combined

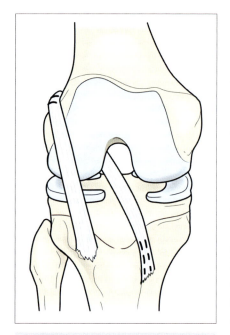

Figure 6 Illustration shows the iliotibial band technique, which uses extra-articular and intra-articular reconstruction to eliminate the need for femoral and tibial tunnels.

intra-articular and extra-articular ACL reconstruction using the ITB technique. At a follow-up ranging from 2 to 15.1 years, the authors reported a 4.5% revision surgery rate, a mean International Knee Documentation Committee Subjective Knee Evaluation Form score of 96.7 ± 6, a mean Lysholm Knee Scale score of 95.7 ± 6.7, a mean growth rate of 21.5 cm (range, 9.5 to 118.5 cm) after surgery, and no patients with growth disturbances. In a study of 21 skeletally immature patients who underwent combined intra-articular and extra-articular ACL reconstruction using the ITB technique, Willimon et al[76] reported excellent functional outcomes, a low revision surgery rate (14%), and no patients with growth disturbances at a minimum follow-up of 3 years.

Biomechanics data suggest that the ITB technique is better able to restore anteroposterior stability than the all-epiphyseal technique.[77] Currently, renewed interest in the extra-articular component of the ITB technique exists because it has been hypothesized that it simulates the anterolateral ligament.[78,79] The anterolateral ligament, which runs from the lateral femoral epicondyle to the anterolateral proximal tibia, is thought to be important for rotational stability of the knee. The addition of anterolateral ligament reconstruction has shown promising results in the adult sports medicine literature. In a study of 92 patients who underwent combined ACL and anterolateral ligament reconstruction, Sonnery-Cottett et al[80] reported a 1.1% revision surgery rate at a minimum follow-up of 2 years.

Partial Transphyseal Reconstruction

Partial transphyseal reconstructions violate only one physis, with a tunnel made through the proximal tibial physis and an over-the-top position or epiphyseal placement on the femur or with a tunnel made through the distal femoral physis and an epiphyseal tunnel in the tibia. Lipscomb and Anderson[43] performed combined intra-articular and extra-articular ACL reconstruction with the use of a transphyseal tibial tunnel and an epiphyseal femoral tunnel in 24 skeletally immature patients. The authors reported good results; however, an LLD developed in one patient. Andrews et al[81] used soft-tissue allografts with a transphyseal tibial tunnel and an over-the-top position on the femur in eight patients who had open physes. At a mean follow-up of 58 months, there were no growth disturbances; however, three patients had more than 3 mm of laxity, and one patient had a poor result. Lo et al[82] used soft-tissue autografts with a transtibial physeal

tunnel and an over-the-top position on the femur in five patients who had wide open physes. At a mean follow-up of 7.4 years, no patients had more than 3 mm of laxity, one patient had a poor result, and no patients had an LLD. Bisson et al[83] reported similar results in nine male patients with wide open physes who underwent reconstruction using hamstring autografts with a transtibial physeal technique and an over-the-top position on the femur. At a mean follow-up of 39 months (range, 24 to 72 months), the authors reported that seven patients had excellent results, with return to sport; a mean Lysholm Knee Scale score of 99; and, based on KT-1000 arthrometer testing, a mean laxity of 2.8 mm (range, 0 to 5.5 mm), and that reconstruction failed in two patients (one complete rupture at 10 months postoperatively and one partial rupture at 3 years postoperatively). The mean growth rate postoperatively was 10.7 cm (range, 4 to 22.9 cm), and no patients had LLD, angular deformity, or radiographic evidence of physeal injury.

Complete Transphyseal Reconstruction

Transphyseal reconstructions with tunnels that violate both the proximal tibial and distal femoral physes also have been advocated; however, these techniques are usually reserved for patients who have minimal skeletal growth remaining (**Figure 7**). Many studies have reported excellent results without LLD or angular deformities.[43,84-88]

Partial ACL Tears and Congenital Absence of the ACL

According to studies on pediatric knee injuries, partial ACL tears represent approximately one-quarter to one-half of all ACL injuries in the pediatric population.[87,89,90] In general, the management of partial ACL tears is controversial, and some pediatric studies and adult clinical series have yielded mixed results.[91-97] Treatment options for partial ACL tears include nonsurgical management with physical therapy and bracing, ACL augmentation, and ACL reconstruction. Kocher et al[98] nonsurgically treated 45 patients aged 17 years or younger who had arthroscopically documented partial ACL tears. Thirty-one percent of the patients underwent subsequent reconstruction. The factors that were associated with the need for subsequent reconstruction included tears that were greater than 50%, predominant PLB tears, a grade B pivot-shift test result on physical examination, and older age. In the patients who did not undergo subsequent reconstruction, functional outcomes were worse in those who had predominant PLB tears and tears that were greater than 50%. Based on these results, the authors recommended reconstruction in patients who have a partial ACL tear greater than 50%, an isolated PLB tear, and in whom the pivot-shift test is positive.

Congenital absence of the ACL is an extremely rare condition, with an incidence of 0.017 per 1,000 live births.[99] Congenital absence of the ACL has been reported as an isolated condition or associated with other abnormalities, such as femoral deficiency, fibular hemimelia, scoliosis, hip dysplasia, and dysplasia of the tibial intercondylar eminence.[100-104] Manner et al[105] classified dysplasia of the ACL based on tunnel view radiographs. In type I ACL dysplasia, partial closure of the femoral intercondylar notch and hypoplasia of the tibial eminence are observed, and

the ACL is hypoplastic or aplastic. In type II ACL dysplasia, additional hypoplasia of the posterior cruciate ligament is present, and hypoplasia of the intercondylar notch and tibial eminence are accentuated. In type III ACL dysplasia, the femoral intercondylar notch and tibial eminence are completely absent, with aplasia of both the ACL and posterior cruciate ligament (**Figure 8**). In general, treatment for congenital absence of the ACL is nonsurgical because most patients have low demands as a result of other associated anomalies and rarely report instability despite positive examination findings.[99] Some patients report medial compartment or patellofemoral knee pain that is caused by arthritis, which progresses slower than arthritis caused by an ACL rupture.[106] If symptomatic instability develops, it is likely the result of an event that altered knee homeostasis and caused the ACL deficiency to manifest.[107] In patients who undergo lower limb lengthening or deformity correction, ACL deficiency may manifest as progressive knee subluxation; therefore, routine monitoring of the knee joint is essential, and extension to a knee-spanning external fixator may be required. In patients who have symptomatic instability, ligamentous reconstruction may be warranted; however, ligamentous reconstruction can be technically difficult and may be associated with a higher failure rate.[99,108] Numerous case studies have reported reasonable results in patients who undergo reconstruction; however, no large series or long-term follow-up data are available.[99,109,110]

Summary

The incidence of ACL tears in skeletally immature patients is rising. The natural history of nonsurgically managed

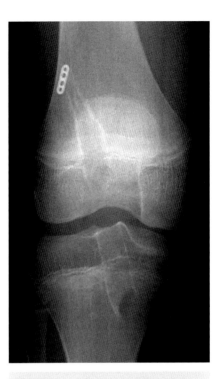

Figure 7   AP radiograph of the knee of a patient nearing skeletal maturity who underwent anterior cruciate ligament reconstruction with the transphyseal technique. The surgical principles for the transphyseal technique include the use of soft-tissue grafts, the placement of fixation away from the physis, and the avoidance of bone plugs or interference screws across the physis.

ACL injuries is largely unfavorable. Patients who have complete ACL tears should be considered for surgical reconstruction irrespective of their age. The authors of this chapter advocate an algorithm for the management of ACL injuries in skeletally immature patients that is based on the amount of skeletal growth remaining, which can be most accurately determined with an assessment of the physiologic Tanner stage and skeletal age. Chronologic age may be a poor guide for how much skeletal growth remains because of large variations in skeletal and physiologic maturity. In prepubescent patients

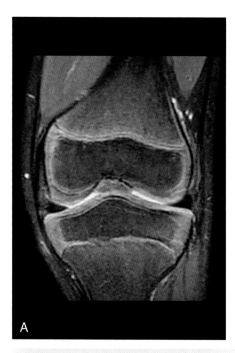
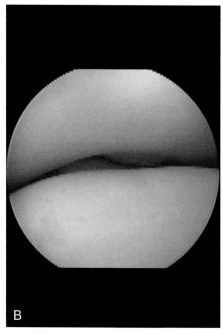
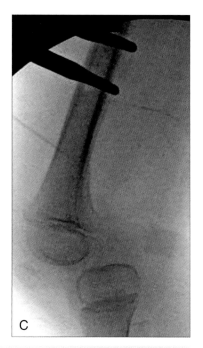

Figure 8 Images show congenital absence of the anterior cruciate ligament. **A,** Coronal T2-weighted MRI of a knee shows cartilage covering the tibial spine with complete aplasia of the cruciate ligaments. **B,** Arthroscopic image of the knee shown in panel **A** shows that the cartilage covers the entire convex tibial plateau. **C,** Lateral radiograph of a different knee taken during a femoral lengthening procedure for a congenital short femur demonstrates progressive subluxation of the knee joint as a result of congenital absence of the cruciate ligaments.

who have substantial skeletal growth remaining (Tanner stage 1 or stage 2, bone age ≤12 years in males, bone age ≤11 years in females), the authors of this chapter recommend physeal-sparing ACL reconstruction via either the all-epiphyseal technique or the combined intra- and extra-articular ITB technique. In pubescent adolescents who have moderate skeletal growth remaining (Tanner stage 3, bone age 13 to 16 years in males, bone age 12 to 14 years in females), the authors of this chapter recommend a transphyseal reconstruction with autogenous hamstring graft secured via metaphyseal fixation. For this group of patients, the authors of this chapter encourage physeal-respecting techniques by avoiding the placement of hardware or bone plugs across the distal femoral or proximal tibial physis, avoiding large-size tunnels, and minimizing over-the-top dissection and the extent of notchplasty. In older adolescents who are near skeletal maturity and, therefore, have minimal skeletal growth remaining (Tanner stage 4 or stage 5, bone age >15 years in males, bone age >14 years in females), adult-type ACL reconstructions with various graft choices and fixation techniques can be safely performed. ACL reconstruction is recommended for patients who have partial ACL tears greater than 50%, an isolated PLB tear, or in whom the pivot-shift test is positive. For patients who have congenital ACL deficiency, reconstruction is recommended only in select patients who have symptomatic instability or progressive knee subluxation during other reconstructive procedures.

References

1. Behr CT, Potter HG, Paletta GA Jr: The relationship of the femoral origin of the anterior cruciate ligament and the distal femoral physeal plate in the skeletally immature knee: An anatomic study. *Am J Sports Med* 2001;29(6):781-787.

2. LaPrade RF, Moulton SG, Nitri M, Mueller W, Engebretsen L: Clinically relevant anatomy and what anatomic reconstruction means. *Knee Surg Sports Traumatol Arthrosc* 2015;23(10):2950-2959.

3. Fabricant PD, Jones KJ, Delos D, et al: Reconstruction of the anterior cruciate ligament in the skeletally immature athlete: A review of current concepts. AAOS exhibit selection. *J Bone Joint Surg Am* 2013;95(5):e28.

4. Kopf S, Pombo MW, Szczodry M, Irrgang JJ, Fu FH: Size variability of the human anterior cruciate ligament insertion sites. *Am J Sports Med* 2011;39(1):108-113.

5. Liu RW, Farrow LD, Messerschmitt PJ, Gilmore A, Goodfellow DB, Cooperman DR: An anatomical study of the pediatric intercondylar notch. *J Pediatr Orthop* 2008;28(2):177-183.

6. Swami VG, Mabee M, Hui C, Jaremko JL: MRI anatomy of the tibial ACL attachment and proximal epiphysis in a large population of skeletally immature knees: Reference parameters for planning anatomic physeal-sparing ACL reconstruction. *Am J Sports Med* 2014;42(7):1644-1651.

7. DeLee JC, Curtis R: Anterior cruciate ligament insufficiency in children. *Clin Orthop Relat Res* 1983;172:112-118.

8. Bollen SR, Scott BW: Rupture of the anterior cruciate ligament—a quiet epidemic? *Injury* 1996;27(6):407-409.

9. Shea KG, Grimm NL, Ewing CK, Aoki SK: Youth sports anterior cruciate ligament and knee injury epidemiology: Who is getting injured? In what sports? When? *Clin Sports Med* 2011;30(4):691-706.

10. Johnston LD, Delva J, O'Malley PM: Sports participation and physical education in American secondary schools: Current levels and racial/ethnic and socioeconomic disparities. *Am J Prev Med* 2007;33(4, suppl):S195-S208.

11. Sampson NR, Beck NA: Knee injuries in children and adolescents: Has there been an increase in ACL and meniscus tears in recent years? Presented at the American Academy of Pediatrics 2011 National Conference and Exhibition. Boston, MA, October 15-18, 2011.

12. Dodwell ER, Lamont LE, Green DW, Pan TJ, Marx RG, Lyman S: 20 years of pediatric anterior cruciate ligament reconstruction in New York State. *Am J Sports Med* 2014;42(3):675-680.

13. Abbasi D, May MM, Wall EJ, Chan G, Parikh SN: MRI findings in adolescent patients with acute traumatic knee hemarthrosis. *J Pediatr Orthop* 2012;32(8):760-764.

14. Ford KR, Myer GD, Hewett TE: Valgus knee motion during landing in high school female and male basketball players. *Med Sci Sports Exerc* 2003;35(10):1745-1750.

15. Ford KR, Myer GD, Toms HE, Hewett TE: Gender differences in the kinematics of unanticipated cutting in young athletes. *Med Sci Sports Exerc* 2005;37(1):124-129.

16. McLean SG, Lipfert SW, van den Bogert AJ: Effect of gender and defensive opponent on the biomechanics of sidestep cutting. *Med Sci Sports Exerc* 2004;36(6):1008-1016.

17. Alentorn-Geli E, Myer GD, Silvers HJ, et al: Prevention of non-contact anterior cruciate ligament injuries in soccer players: Part 1. Mechanisms of injury and underlying risk factors. *Knee Surg Sports Traumatol Arthrosc* 2009;17(7):705-729.

18. Gilchrist J, Mandelbaum BR, Melancon H, et al: A randomized controlled trial to prevent noncontact anterior cruciate ligament injury in female collegiate soccer players. *Am J Sports Med* 2008;36(8):1476-1483.

19. Hattori K, Sano H, Komatsuda T, Saijo Y, Sugita T, Itoi E: Effect of estrogen on tissue elasticity of the ligament proper in rabbit anterior cruciate ligament: Measurements using scanning acoustic microscopy. *J Orthop Sci* 2010;15(4):584-588.

20. Komatsuda T, Sugita T, Sano H, et al: Does estrogen alter the mechanical properties of the anterior cruciate ligament? An experimental study in rabbits. *Acta Orthop* 2006;77(6):973-980.

21. Dragoo JL, Padrez K, Workman R, Lindsey DP: The effect of relaxin on the female anterior cruciate ligament: Analysis of mechanical properties in an animal model. *Knee* 2009;16(1):69-72.

22. Hewett TE, Zazulak BT, Myer GD: Effects of the menstrual cycle on anterior cruciate ligament injury risk: A systematic review. *Am J Sports Med* 2007;35(4):659-668.

23. Park SK, Stefanyshyn DJ, Loitz-Ramage B, Hart DA, Ronsky JL: Changing hormone levels during the menstrual cycle affect knee laxity and stiffness in healthy female subjects. *Am J Sports Med* 2009;37(3):588-598.

24. Abt JP, Sell TC, Laudner KG, et al: Neuromuscular and biomechanical characteristics do not vary across the menstrual cycle. *Knee Surg Sports Traumatol Arthrosc* 2007;15(7):901-907.

25. Hertel J, Williams NI, Olmsted-Kramer LC, Leidy HJ, Putukian M: Neuromuscular performance and knee laxity do not change across the menstrual cycle in female athletes. *Knee Surg Sports Traumatol Arthrosc* 2006;14(9):817-822.

26. Samora W, Beran MC, Parikh SN: Intercondylar roof inclination angle: Is it a risk factor for ACL tears or tibial spine fractures? *J Pediatr Orthop* 2016;36(6):e71-e74.

27. Greulich WW, Pyle SI: *Radiographic Atlas of Skeletal Development of the Hand and Wrist*, ed 2. Stanford, CA, Stanford University Press, 1959.

28. Pyle SI, Hoerr NL: *A Radiographic Standard of Reference for the Growing Knee*. Springfield, IL, C.C. Thomas, 1969.

29. Heyworth BE, Osei DA, Fabricant PD, et al: The shorthand bone age assessment: A simpler alternative to current methods. *J Pediatr Orthop* 2013;33(5):569-574.

30. Sanders JO, Khoury JG, Kishan S, et al: Predicting scoliosis progression from skeletal maturity: A simplified classification during adolescence. *J Bone Joint Surg Am* 2008;90(3):540-553.

31. Tanner JM, Whitehouse RH: *Atlas of Children's Growth: Normal Variation and Growth Disorders*. London, United Kingdom, Academic Press, 1982.

32. Coleman L, Coleman J: The measurement of puberty: A review. *J Adolesc* 2002;25(5):535-550.

33. Graf BK, Lange RH, Fujisaki CK, Landry GL, Saluja RK: Anterior cruciate ligament tears in skeletally immature patients: Meniscal pathology at presentation and after attempted conservative treatment. *Arthroscopy* 1992;8(2):229-233.

34. Mizuta H, Kubota K, Shiraishi M, Otsuka Y, Nagamoto N, Takagi K: The conservative treatment of complete tears of the anterior cruciate ligament in skeletally immature patients. *J Bone Joint Surg Br* 1995;77(6):890-894.

35. Millett PJ, Willis AA, Warren RF: Associated injuries in pediatric and adolescent anterior cruciate ligament tears: Does a delay in treatment

increase the risk of meniscal tear? *Arthroscopy* 2002;18(9):955-959.

36. Aichroth PM, Patel DV, Zorrilla P: The natural history and treatment of rupture of the anterior cruciate ligament in children and adolescents: A prospective review. *J Bone Joint Surg Br* 2002;84(1):38-41.

37. Dumont GD, Hogue GD, Padalecki JR, Okoro N, Wilson PL: Meniscal and chondral injuries associated with pediatric anterior cruciate ligament tears: Relationship of treatment time and patient-specific factors. *Am J Sports Med* 2012;40(9):2128-2133.

38. Henry J, Chotel F, Chouteau J, Fessy MH, Bérard J, Moyen B: Rupture of the anterior cruciate ligament in children: Early reconstruction with open physes or delayed reconstruction to skeletal maturity? *Knee Surg Sports Traumatol Arthrosc* 2009;17(7):748-755.

39. Lawrence JT, Argawal N, Ganley TJ: Degeneration of the knee joint in skeletally immature patients with a diagnosis of an anterior cruciate ligament tear: Is there harm in delay of treatment? *Am J Sports Med* 2011;39(12):2582-2587.

40. Anderson AF, Anderson CN: Correlation of meniscal and articular cartilage injuries in children and adolescents with timing of anterior cruciate ligament reconstruction. *Am J Sports Med* 2015;43(2):275-281.

41. Guenther ZD, Swami V, Dhillon SS, Jaremko JL: Meniscal injury after adolescent anterior cruciate ligament injury: How long are patients at risk? *Clin Orthop Relat Res* 2014;472(3):990-997.

42. Vavken P, Murray MM: Treating anterior cruciate ligament tears in skeletally immature patients. *Arthroscopy* 2011;27(5):704-716.

43. Lipscomb AB, Anderson AF: Tears of the anterior cruciate ligament in adolescents. *J Bone Joint Surg Am* 1986;68(1):19-28.

44. Robert HE, Casin C: Valgus and flexion deformity after reconstruction of the anterior cruciate ligament in a skeletally immature patient. *Knee Surg Sports Traumatol Arthrosc* 2010;18(10):1369-1373.

45. Kocher MS, Saxon HS, Hovis WD, Hawkins RJ: Management and complications of anterior cruciate ligament injuries in skeletally immature patients: Survey of the Herodicus Society and The ACL Study Group. *J Pediatr Orthop* 2002;22(4):452-457.

46. Shifflett GD, Green DW, Widmann RF, Marx RG: Growth arrest following ACL reconstruction with hamstring autograft in skeletally immature patients: A review of 4 cases. *J Pediatr Orthop* 2016;36(4):355-361.

47. Frank JS, Gambacorta PL: Anterior cruciate ligament injuries in the skeletally immature athlete: Diagnosis and management. *J Am Acad Orthop Surg* 2013;21(2):78-87.

48. Kaeding CC, Flanigan D, Donaldson C: Surgical techniques and outcomes after anterior cruciate ligament reconstruction in preadolescent patients. *Arthroscopy* 2010;26(11):1530-1538.

49. Barber FA: Anterior cruciate ligament reconstruction in the skeletally immature high-performance athlete: What to do and when to do it? *Arthroscopy* 2000;16(4):391-392.

50. Frosch KH, Stengel D, Brodhun T, et al: Outcomes and risks of operative treatment of rupture of the anterior cruciate ligament in children and adolescents. *Arthroscopy* 2010;26(11):1539-1550.

51. Edwards TB, Greene CC, Baratta RV, Zieske A, Willis RB: The effect of placing a tensioned graft across open growth plates: A gross and histologic analysis. *J Bone Joint Surg Am* 2001;83(5):725-734.

52. Chudik S, Beasley L, Potter H, Wickiewicz T, Warren R, Rodeo S: The influence of femoral technique for graft placement on anterior cruciate ligament reconstruction using a skeletally immature canine model with a rapidly growing physis. *Arthroscopy* 2007;23(12):1309-1319.e1.

53. Meller R, Kendoff D, Hankemeier S, et al: Hindlimb growth after a transphyseal reconstruction of the anterior cruciate ligament: A study in skeletally immature sheep with wide-open physes. *Am J Sports Med* 2008;36(12):2437-2443.

54. Lawrence JT, West RL, Garrett WE: Growth disturbance following ACL reconstruction with use of an epiphyseal femoral tunnel: A case report. *J Bone Joint Surg Am* 2011;93(8):e39.

55. Janarv PM, Nyström A, Werner S, Hirsch G: Anterior cruciate ligament injuries in skeletally immature patients. *J Pediatr Orthop* 1996;16(5):673-677.

56. Mäkelä EA, Vainionpää S, Vihtonen K, Mero M, Rokkanen P: The effect of trauma to the lower femoral epiphyseal plate: An experimental study in rabbits. *J Bone Joint Surg Br* 1988;70(2):187-191.

57. Kercher J, Xerogeanes J, Tannenbaum A, Al-Hakim R, Black JC, Zhao J: Anterior cruciate ligament reconstruction in the skeletally immature: An anatomical study utilizing 3-dimensional magnetic resonance imaging reconstructions. *J Pediatr Orthop* 2009;29(2):124-129.

58. Shea KG, Belzer J, Apel PJ, Nilsson K, Grimm NL, Pfeiffer RP: Volumetric injury of the physis during single-bundle anterior cruciate ligament reconstruction in children: A 3-dimensional study using magnetic resonance imaging. *Arthroscopy* 2009;25(12):1415-1422.

59. Yoo WJ, Kocher MS, Micheli LJ: Growth plate disturbance after transphyseal reconstruction of the anterior cruciate ligament in skeletally immature adolescent patients: An MR imaging study. *J Pediatr Orthop* 2011;31(6):691-696.

60. Clanton TO, DeLee JC, Sanders B, Neidre A: Knee ligament injuries in children. *J Bone Joint Surg Am* 1979;61(8):1195-1201.

61. Engebretsen L, Svenningsen S, Benum P: Poor results of anterior cruciate ligament repair in adolescence. *Acta Orthop Scand* 1988;59(6):684-686.

62. McCarroll JR, Rettig AC, Shelbourne KD: Anterior cruciate ligament injuries in the young athlete with open physes. *Am J Sports Med* 1988;16(1):44-47.

63. Proffen BL, Sieker JT, Murray MM: Bio-enhanced repair of the anterior cruciate ligament. *Arthroscopy* 2015;31(5):990-997.

64. Anderson AF: Transepiphyseal replacement of the anterior cruciate ligament using quadruple hamstring grafts in skeletally immature patients. *J Bone Joint Surg Am* 2004; 86(suppl 1, pt 2):201-209.

65. Lykissas MG, Nathan ST, Wall EJ: All-epiphyseal anterior cruciate ligament reconstruction in skeletally immature patients: A surgical technique using a split tibial tunnel. *Arthrosc Tech* 2012;1(1):e133-e139.

66. Lawrence JT, Bowers AL, Belding J, Cody SR, Ganley TJ: All-epiphyseal anterior cruciate ligament reconstruction in skeletally immature patients. *Clin Orthop Relat Res* 2010;468(7):1971-1977.

67. McCarthy MM, Graziano J, Green DW, Cordasco FA: All-epiphyseal, all-inside anterior cruciate ligament reconstruction technique for skeletally immature patients. *Arthrosc Tech* 2012;1(2):e231-e239.

68. Nawabi DH, Jones KJ, Lurie B, Potter HG, Green DW, Cordasco FA: All-inside, physeal-sparing anterior cruciate ligament reconstruction does not significantly compromise the physis in skeletally immature athletes: A postoperative physeal magnetic resonance imaging analysis. *Am J Sports Med* 2014;42(12):2933-2940.

69. Cruz AI Jr, Fabricant PD, McGraw M, Rozell JC, Ganley TJ, Wells L: All-epiphyseal ACL reconstruction in children: Review of safety and early complications. *J Pediatr Orthop* 2015.

70. Brief LP: Anterior cruciate ligament reconstruction without drill holes. *Arthroscopy* 1991;7(4):350-357.

71. Guzzanti V, Falciglia F, Stanitski CL: Physeal-sparing intraarticular anterior cruciate ligament reconstruction in preadolescents. *Am J Sports Med* 2003;31(6):949-953.

72. Kocher MS, Garg S, Micheli LJ: Physeal sparing reconstruction of the anterior cruciate ligament in skeletally immature prepubescent children and adolescents: Surgical technique. *J Bone Joint Surg Am* 2006;88(suppl 1, pt 2): 283-293.

73. MacIntosh DL, Darby TA: Lateral substitution reconstruction. *J Bone Joint Surg Br* 1976;58:142.

74. Micheli LJ, Rask B, Gerberg L: Anterior cruciate ligament reconstruction in patients who are prepubescent. *Clin Orthop Relat Res* 1999;364:40-47.

75. Kocher MS, Garg S, Micheli LJ: Physeal sparing reconstruction of the anterior cruciate ligament in skeletally immature prepubescent children and adolescents. *J Bone Joint Surg Am* 2005;87(11):2371-2379.

76. Willimon SC, Jones CR, Herzog MM, May KH, Leake MJ, Busch MT: Micheli anterior cruciate ligament reconstruction in skeletally immature youths: A retrospective case series with a mean 3-year follow-up. *Am J Sports Med* 2015;43(12):2974-2981.

77. Kennedy A, Coughlin DG, Metzger MF, et al: Biomechanical evaluation of pediatric anterior cruciate ligament reconstruction techniques. *Am J Sports Med* 2011;39(5):964-971.

78. Claes S, Vereecke E, Maes M, Victor J, Verdonk P, Bellemans J: Anatomy of the anterolateral ligament of the knee. *J Anat* 2013;223(4):321-328.

79. Kennedy MI, Claes S, Fuso FA, et al: The anterolateral ligament: An anatomic, radiographic, and biomechanical analysis. *Am J Sports Med* 2015;43(7):1606-1615.

80. Sonnery-Cottet B, Thaunat M, Freychet B, Pupim BH, Murphy CG, Claes S: Outcome of a combined anterior cruciate ligament and anterolateral ligament reconstruction technique with a minimum 2-year follow-up. *Am J Sports Med* 2015;43(7):1598-1605.

81. Andrews M, Noyes FR, Barber-Westin SD: Anterior cruciate ligament allograft reconstruction in the skeletally immature athlete. *Am J Sports Med* 1994;22(1):48-54.

82. Lo IK, Kirkley A, Fowler PJ, Miniaci A: The outcome of operatively treated anterior cruciate ligament disruptions in the skeletally immature child. *Arthroscopy* 1997;13(5):627-634.

83. Bisson LJ, Wickiewicz T, Levinson M, Warren R: ACL reconstruction in children with open physes. *Orthopedics* 1998;21(6):659-663.

84. McCarroll JR, Shelbourne KD, Porter DA, Rettig AC, Murray S: Patellar tendon graft reconstruction

for midsubstance anterior cruciate ligament rupture in junior high school athletes: An algorithm for management. *Am J Sports Med* 1994;22(4):478-484.

85. Matava MJ, Siegel MG: Arthroscopic reconstruction of the ACL with semitendinosus-gracilis autograft in skeletally immature adolescent patients. *Am J Knee Surg* 1997;10(2):60-69.

86. Aronowitz ER, Ganley TJ, Goode JR, Gregg JR, Meyer JS: Anterior cruciate ligament reconstruction in adolescents with open physes. *Am J Sports Med* 2000;28(2):168-175.

87. Kocher MS, DiCanzio J, Zurakowski D, Micheli LJ: Diagnostic performance of clinical examination and selective magnetic resonance imaging in the evaluation of intraarticular knee disorders in children and adolescents. *Am J Sports Med* 2001;29(3):292-296.

88. Redler LH, Brafman RT, Trentacosta N, Ahmad CS: Anterior cruciate ligament reconstruction in skeletally immature patients with transphyseal tunnels. *Arthroscopy* 2012;28(11):1710-1717.

89. Eiskjaer S, Larsen ST, Schmidt MB: The significance of hemarthrosis of the knee in children. *Arch Orthop Trauma Surg* 1988;107(2):96-98.

90. Kloeppel-Wirth S, Koltai JL, Dittmer H: Significance of arthroscopy in children with knee joint injuries. *Eur J Pediatr Surg* 1992;2(3):169-172.

91. Bak K, Scavenius M, Hansen S, Nørring K, Jensen KH, Jørgensen U: Isolated partial rupture of the anterior cruciate ligament: Long-term follow-up of 56 cases. *Knee Surg Sports Traumatol Arthrosc* 1997;5(2):66-71.

92. Barrack RL, Buckley SL, Bruckner JD, Kneisl JS, Alexander AH: Partial versus complete acute anterior cruciate ligament tears: The results of nonoperative treatment. *J Bone Joint Surg Br* 1990;72(4):622-624.

93. Buckley SL, Barrack RL, Alexander AH: The natural history of conservatively treated partial anterior cruciate ligament tears. *Am J Sports Med* 1989;17(2):221-225.

94. Fritschy D, Panoussopoulos A, Wallensten R, Peter R: Can we predict the

outcome of a partial rupture of the anterior cruciate ligament? A prospective study of 43 cases. *Knee Surg Sports Traumatol Arthrosc* 1997;5(1):2-5.

95. Kannus P, Järvinen M: Conservatively treated tears of the anterior cruciate ligament: Long-term results. *J Bone Joint Surg Am* 1987;69(7):1007-1012.

96. Lehnert M, Eisenschenk A, Zellner A: Results of conservative treatment of partial tears of the anterior cruciate ligament. *Int Orthop* 1993;17(4):219-223.

97. Messner K, Maletius W: Eighteen-to twenty-five-year follow-up after acute partial anterior cruciate ligament rupture. *Am J Sports Med* 1999;27(4):455-459.

98. Kocher MS, Micheli LJ, Zurakowski D, Luke A: Partial tears of the anterior cruciate ligament in children and adolescents. *Am J Sports Med* 2002;30(5):697-703.

99. Lee JJ, Oh WT, Shin KY, Ko MS, Choi CH: Ligament reconstruction in congenital absence of the anterior cruciate ligament: A case report. *Knee Surg Relat Res* 2011;23(4):240-243.

100. Barrett GR, Tomasin JD: Bilateral congenital absence of the anterior cruciate ligament. *Orthopedics* 1988;11(3):431-434.

101. Dejour H, Neyret P, Eberhard P, Walch G: Bilateral congenital absence of the anterior cruciate ligament and the internal menisci of the knee: A case report. *Rev Chir Orthop Reparatrice Appar Mot* 1990;76(5):329-332.

102. Noble J: Congenital absence of the anterior cruciate ligament associated with a ring meniscus. *J Bone Joint Surg Am* 1975;57(8):1165-1166.

103. Hu J, DU SX, Huang ZL, Xia X: Bilateral congenital absence of anterior cruciate ligaments associated with the scoliosis and hip dysplasia: A case report and review of the literature. *Chin Med J (Engl)* 2010;123(8):1099-1102.

104. Johansson E, Aparisi T: Missing cruciate ligament in congenital short femur. *J Bone Joint Surg Am* 1983;65(8):1109-1115.

105. Manner HM, Radler C, Ganger R, Grill F: Dysplasia of the cruciate ligaments: Radiographic assessment and classification. *J Bone Joint Surg Am* 2006;88(1):130-137.

106. Frikha R, Dahmene J, Ben Hamida R, Chaieb Z, Janhaoui N, Laziz Ben Ayeche M: Congenital absence of the anterior cruciate ligament: Eight cases in the same family. *Rev Chir Orthop Reparatrice Appar Mot* 2005;91(7):642-648.

107. Sonn KA, Caltoum CB: Congenital absence of the anterior cruciate ligament in monozygotic twins. *Int J Sports Med* 2014;35(13):1130-1133.

108. Carlioz H: Description and natural history of severe aplasia of the lower extremities. *Chir Pediatr* 1978;19(5-6):306-321.

109. Gabos PG, El Rassi G, Pahys J: Knee reconstruction in syndromes with congenital absence of the anterior cruciate ligament. *J Pediatr Orthop* 2005;25(2):210-214.

110. Chahla J, Pascual-Garrido C, Rodeo SA: Ligament reconstruction in congenital absence of the anterior cruciate ligament: A report of two cases. *HSS J* 2015;11(2):177-181.

Congenital Scoliosis: A Case-Based Approach

Frances A. Farley, MD

Laurel C. Blakemore, MD

Abstract

Congenital scoliosis is lateral curvature of the spine caused by vertebral anomalies. Congenital scoliosis is associated with congenital anomalies of other organ systems. Traditionally, treatment options for patients with congenital scoliosis focused on posterior spinal fusion. Current surgical treatment options for young children include growing rods, vertical expandable prosthetic titanium ribs, and, most recently, magnetic rods. Hemivertebrae resection is an important early treatment option for patients who have a hemivertebra. Intraoperative navigation may be an important tool that can be used to improve the accuracy of pedicle screw placement in patients who have abnormal pedicles.

Instr Course Lect 2017;66:475–480.

Congenital scoliosis is lateral curvature of the spine caused by vertebral anomalies that are misshapen.[1,2] Vertebral anomalies at birth result in scoliosis, which may be progressive. Congenital scoliosis is associated with congenital anomalies of other organ systems.[3] Traditionally, treatment options for patients with congenital scoliosis have focused on posterior spinal fusion.[4-7] Current surgical treatment options for young children include growing rods, vertical expandable prosthetic titanium ribs (VEPTRs),[8-10] and, most recently, magnetic rods. Surgeons should understand how to make a congenital scoliosis diagnosis, determine anomalies associated with congenital scoliosis, and manage congenital scoliosis.

Diagnosis and Associated Anomalies

A set of newborn twins were born with multiple congenital spine abnormalities, missing ribs, and rib fusions. Twin A had a tracheoesophageal fistula that was repaired at birth. Twin A also had a ventriculoseptal defect, a patent ductus arteriosus, as well as polydactyly and clubfoot of the left foot. Twin B had radioulnar synostosis, one kidney, and an atrioseptal defect.

VACTERL is an acronym for a developmental defect of the mesoderm.[11] The anomalies and their respective incidences that are present in a patient who has VACTERL include vertebral anomalies (60% to 80%), anal atresia (55% to 90%), cardiac defects (40% to 80%), tracheoesophageal fistula (50% to 80%), renal and radial anomalies (40% to 50%), and limb defects (40% to 50%).[11] Clubfoot and radioulnar synostosis are not usually associated with VACTERL; however, clubfoot and radioulnar synostosis are both limb abnormalities. VACTERL also is associated with maternal diabetes.[11] The mother of the newborn twins already mentioned had type 2 diabetes mellitus.

VACTERL was first described in 1972 by an emergency medicine physician and a physician who specialized

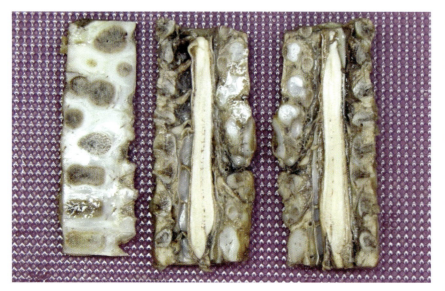

Figure 1 Photograph shows the pathologic spine specimen of an infant who was a twin. The vertebral bodies, cartilaginous end plates, and disk spaces are misshapen, disordered, and have ossification centers of different sizes. The spinal cord appears normal.

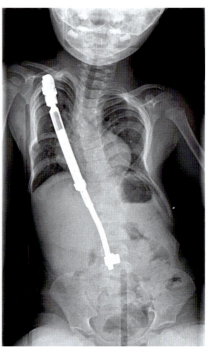

Figure 2 PA radiograph of the spine of the 2-year-old twin who underwent treatment with a VEPTR demonstrates stable kyphosis and mild scoliosis.

in dysmorphology. Most cases of VACTERL are sporadic, unlike that observed in the newborn twins already mentioned. Very few genetic anomalies (trisomy 21, deletion 22q11 syndrome) have been reported in patients who have VACTERL.[11] VACTERL is estimated to occur in 1 in 10,000 to 40,000 individuals.[11] VACTERL is believed to be the result of a developmental field defect that occurs during blastogenesis, which results in multiple mesodermal defects.[11] VACTERL is a polytypic defect that occurs in multiple organ systems.[11]

Twin A died in infancy. An autopsy of the spine of twin A revealed multiple abnormal ossification centers in the lower thoracic and upper lumbar spine, some of which had less ossification compared with adjacent normal vertebrae (**Figure 1**). Although cartilage surrounded the small round ossification centers of twin A, no identifiable adjacent disk material was present.

A VEPTR was placed to manage the multiple vertebral anomalies, congenital kyphosis, and multiple rib anomalies in twin B. The use of a VEPTR to manage congenital kyphosis is controversial because a VEPTR is a distraction device.[8] The authors of this chapter obtained a preoperative MRI of the spine of twin B, which revealed no evidence of spinal cord impingement. The authors planned to closely monitor the kyphosis of twin B. Radiographs of the spine of twin B that were obtained 2 years after the placement of the VEPTR revealed stable kyphosis and mild scoliosis (**Figure 2**).

Treatment
VEPTR and Magnetic Rods
A 2-year-old Caucasian boy with Jarcho-Levin syndrome had nephroblastomatosis and congenital heart disease with a thoracic aneurysm at infancy. The boy also had congenital scoliosis with multiple rib abnormalities and thoracic insufficiency

syndrome.[12,13] The boy underwent a thoracic aneurysm repair, chemotherapy, and a heminephrectomy. A left rib-to-rib VEPTR was placed, after which a right rib-to-spine VEPTR was placed.[13,14] At a later date, the left rib-to-rib VEPTR was removed, and the right rib-to-spine VEPTR was exchanged for a rib-to-spine magnetic rod (**Figure 3**). The scoliosis was stable by the time that the boy was aged 9 years.

Magnetic rods have been used in the past several years as an alternative to growing rods and VEPTRs because they can be lengthened in a clinic without the use of anesthesia.[15] The magnetic portion of a magnetic rod is coupled with an external remote control that is placed on a patient's skin and allows for lengthening of 5 mm, which usually occurs at 3-month intervals.[15]

Jarcho-Levin syndrome is a rare inherited growth disorder that is characterized by a short trunk and many vertebral and rib anomalies.[13,14] There are two types of Jarcho-Levin syndrome. The first type of Jarcho-Levin syndrome, present in the 2-year-old boy already mentioned, is spondylocostal dysostosis. Spondylocostal dysostosis, which can be autosomal dominant or recessive, is characterized by unilateral rib involvement and has an unknown natural history. The second type of Jarcho-Levin syndrome is spondylothoracic dysplasia. Spondylothoracic dysplasia is autosomal recessive, involves fusion of all of the ribs at the costovertebral junction (crablike chest), and has a high mortality rate.

Jarcho-Levin syndrome is believed to be caused by errors in the notch receptor pathway during somatogenesis.[16] Four genes have been associated with Jarcho-Levin syndrome.[16] The first gene associated with Jarcho-Levin syndrome is *DLL3* at 19q13.[16] The second gene associated with Jarcho-Levin syndrome is *MESP2* at 15q26.1. The *MESP2* gene is related to mesodermal development.[16] Both the *DLL3* gene and the *MESP2* gene are associated with notch pathway signaling, which is important in the development of the axial skeleton.[16] Other notch pathway genes have been implicated in families in whom Jarcho-Levin syndrome is present. The third gene associated with Jarcho-Levin syndrome is *LFNG* at 7p22. The fourth gene associated with Jarcho-Levin syndrome is *GDF6* at 8q22.1.[16] The genes associated with Jarcho-Levin syndrome may help elucidate the genetic mechanisms responsible for congenital scoliosis.

Hemivertebrae Resection

Surgical resection can be a sophisticated yet challenging treatment option for patients who have an isolated hemivertebra. First described in Australia in 1928, hemivertebrae resection was performed by Leatherman and Dickson[17] in 1975 via a staged anterior and posterior approach, which was associated with a substantial risk for neurologic injury. Bradford and Boachie-Adjei[18] and authors of subsequent studies[19-21] performed hemivertebrae resection via a single-stage simultaneous anterior and posterior approach. Currently, an all-posterior approach is most commonly used for hemivertebrae resection.

The ideal patient for hemivertebrae resection has progressive congenital scoliosis that is caused by a single hemivertebra in the thoracolumbar or lumbar region; however, hemivertebrae resection also can be accomplished at the lumbosacral or thoracic levels. Cervical hemivertebrae resection also has been performed but is associated with a higher risk for neurologic injury.[21] Most surgeons document curve progression before performing hemivertebrae resection; however, the identification of a hemivertebra at high risk for progression in a patient who already has a deformity may warrant immediate hemivertebrae resection.[22] The ideal age of a patient for hemivertebrae resection ranges from 18 months to 4 years; a reasonable chance of achieving fixation and restoring alignment with limited fusion exists for patients in this age range.

The preoperative evaluation for patients in whom a hemivertebrae resection is being considered should include plain radiographs with either bending or traction views as well as MRI to rule out intraspinal anomalies, which may be

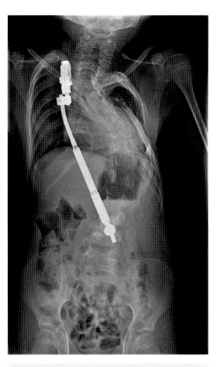

Figure 3 PA radiograph of the spine of a 2-year-old boy with Jarcho-Levin syndrome who underwent treatment with a rib-to-spine magnetic rod.

present in as many as 40% of patients with congenital scoliosis. Although concern for radiation exposure in young children exists, a three-dimensional CT reconstruction of the congenitally abnormal region can be invaluable in preoperative assessment and planning (**Figure 4, A**). The anterior hemivertebrae abnormality may not be at the same level as the posterior hemivertebrae abnormality; therefore, surgeons should examine three-dimensional CT reconstructions carefully before performing hemivertebrae resection to become familiar with the anatomic landmarks that will be encountered during surgery. Three-dimensional CT reconstructions also can aid in determining appropriate implant size and length.

Without in situ fixation and casting, implant options for fixation after

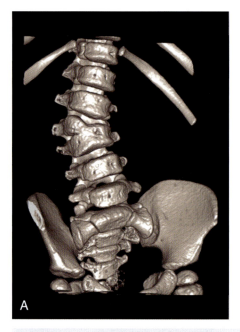

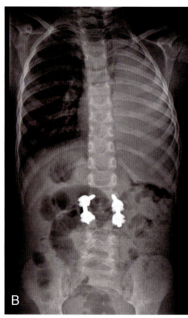

Figure 4 Images of the spine of a 3-year-old child. **A,** Three-dimensional coronal CT reconstruction demonstrates a L3 hemivertebrae. **B,** PA radiograph taken 2 years after hemivertebrae resection demonstrates correction of scoliosis.

hemivertebrae resection include hooks, wires, sublaminar tape, or pedicle screws. The most commonly used fixation constructs allow for compression on the convex side of the scoliosis and may include a rod on the concave side of the scoliosis. Postoperatively, the fixation typically is protected with immobilization in a cast, a thoracolumbosacral orthosis brace, or a cast followed by a transition to a thoracolumbosacral orthosis brace. The mean time for immobilization is 3 to 6 months postoperatively.

Correction achieved with hemivertebrae resection is good, with correction rates ranging from 50% to 70%[19,23] (**Figure 4, B**). However, complications after hemivertebrae resection are not uncommon and include implant failure as a result of pullout or pedicle fracture, rod fracture, infection, proximal junctional kyphosis, or subsequent

deformity that requires extension of fusion.[24-26] Hemivertebrae resection via an all-posterior approach appears to result in similar correction with fewer perioperative complications, such as ileus and pulmonary complications, compared with hemivertebrae resection via a simultaneous anterior and posterior approach.[27] Zhou et al[28] reported that resection of multiple hemivertebrae resulted in an 80% correction rate and complication rates comparable with those of patients who undergo hemivertebrae resection via a staged anterior and posterior approach. If curve progression and resultant spinal imbalance occur after hemivertebrae resection, bracing can be used to maintain alignment of the unfused segments. If necessary, guided growth techniques or definitive spinal fusion may be performed at a later date.

Intraoperative Navigation

Intraoperative navigation is advantageous in the management of any spinal deformity and, in particular, challenging congenital spinal deformities. Intraoperative navigation improves the accuracy of pedicle screw placement, decreases radiation exposure to the surgical team, and may decrease surgical time.[20,29,30] Currently, the potential risks of intraoperative navigation include increased radiation exposure to the patient, longer surgical time for surgeons in the early stages of their learning curve for intraoperative navigation, and, theoretically, a false sense of security/dependency that can result in serious errors if intraoperative navigation fails.

In the only study to date that specifically addressed the accuracy of intraoperative CT navigation, Larson et al[31] reported a very high rate of screw placement accuracy (99.3%) for the 142 screws that were placed in 14 consecutive patients who had congenital scoliosis. In a study that evaluated the accuracy of intraoperative CT navigation for pedicle screw placement in 21 consecutive patients with scoliosis based on the size of the pedicles that were instrumented, Jeswani et al[32] reported lateral screw placement in 3.4% of very small pedicles as well as in-out-in screw placement in 36.5% of small pedicles and 69.2% of very small pedicles. The authors did not identify any medial breaches. Both of these studies suggest that intraoperative navigation aids in the safe placement of pedicle screws in patients with small or difficult anatomy.

Summary

Patients with congenital scoliosis may have considerable comorbidities. The management of congenital scoliosis has evolved from spinal fusion to growth-sparing techniques and hemivertebrae resection, both of which have altered the natural history of congenital scoliosis. Congenital scoliosis is associated with congenital abnormalities of other organ systems, which may affect a child's morbidity. VACTERL is the most common abnormality associated with congenital scoliosis. Genetic identification of the rare Jarcho-Levin syndrome may help elucidate the genetic mechanisms responsible for congenital scoliosis.

References

1. McMaster MJ, Ohtsuka K: The natural history of congenital scoliosis: A study of two hundred and fifty-one patients. *J Bone Joint Surg Am* 1982;64(8):1128-1147.

2. McMaster MJ, Singh H: Natural history of congenital kyphosis and kyphoscoliosis: A study of one hundred and twelve patients. *J Bone Joint Surg Am* 1999;81(10):1367-1383.

3. Bowen RE, Scaduto AA, Banuelos S: Decreased body mass index and restrictive lung disease in congenital thoracic scoliosis. *J Pediatr Orthop* 2008;28(6):665-668.

4. Farley FA, Have KL, Hensinger RN, Streit J, Zhang L, Caird MS: Outcomes after spinal fusion for congenital scoliosis: Instrumented versus uninstrumented spinal fusion. *Spine (Phila Pa 1976)* 2011;36(2):E112-E122.

5. Nasca RJ, Stilling FH III, Stell HH: Progression of congenital scoliosis due to hemivertebrae and hemivertebrae with bars. *J Bone Joint Surg Am* 1975;57(4):456-466.

6. Vitale MG, Matsumoto H, Bye MR, et al: A retrospective cohort study of pulmonary function, radiographic measures, and quality of life in children with congenital scoliosis: An evaluation of patient outcomes after early spinal fusion. *Spine (Phila Pa 1976)* 2008;33(11):1242-1249.

7. Winter RB, Moe JH, Lonstein JE: Posterior spinal arthrodesis for congenital scoliosis: An analysis of the cases of two hundred and ninety patients, five to nineteen years old. *J Bone Joint Surg Am* 1984;66(8):1188-1197.

8. Campbell RM Jr, Adcox BM, Smith MD, et al: The effect of mid-thoracic VEPTR opening wedge thoracostomy on cervical tilt associated with congenital thoracic scoliosis in patients with thoracic insufficiency syndrome. *Spine (Phila Pa 1976)* 2007;32(20):2171-2177.

9. Campbell RM Jr, Hell-Vocke AK: Growth of the thoracic spine in congenital scoliosis after expansion thoracoplasty. *J Bone Joint Surg Am* 2003;85(3):409-420.

10. Farley FA, Li Y, Jong N, et al: Congenital scoliosis SRS-22 outcomes in children treated with observation, surgery, and VEPTR. *Spine (Phila Pa 1976)* 2014;39(22):1868-1874.

11. Bartels E, Schulz AC, Mora NW, et al: VATER/VACTERL association: Identification of seven new twin pairs, a systematic review of the literature, and a classical twin analysis. *Clin Dysmorphol* 2012;21(4):191-195.

12. Gadepalli SK, Hirschl RB, Tsai WC, et al: Vertical expandable prosthetic titanium rib device insertion: Does it improve pulmonary function? *J Pediatr Surg* 2011;46(1):77-80.

13. Ramirez N, Flynn JM, Emans JB, et al: Vertical expandable prosthetic titanium rib as treatment of thoracic insufficiency syndrome in spondylocostal dysplasia. *J Pediatr Orthop* 2010;30(6):521-526.

14. Karlin JG, Roth MK, Patil V, et al: Management of thoracic insufficiency syndrome in patients with Jarcho-Levin syndrome using VEPTRs (vertical expandable prosthetic titanium ribs). *J Bone Joint Surg Am* 2014;96(21):e181.

15. Hickey BA, Towriss C, Baxter G, et al: Early experience of MAGEC magnetic growing rods in the treatment of early onset scoliosis. *Eur Spine J* 2014;23(suppl 1):S61-S65.

16. Chapman G, Sparrow DB, Kremmer E, Dunwoodie SL: Notch inhibition by the ligand DELTA-LIKE 3 defines the mechanism of abnormal vertebral segmentation in spondylocostal dysostosis. *Hum Mol Genet* 2011;20(5):905-916.

17. Leatherman KD, Dickson RA: Two-stage corrective surgery for congenital deformities of the spine. *J Bone Joint Surg Br* 1979;61(3):324-328.

18. Bradford DS, Boachie-Adjei O: One-stage anterior and posterior hemivertebral resection and arthrodesis for congenital scoliosis. *J Bone Joint Surg Am* 1990;72(4):536-540.

19. Hedequist DJ, Hall JE, Emans JB: Hemivertebra excision in children via simultaneous anterior and posterior exposures. *J Pediatr Orthop* 2005;25(1):60-63.

20. Lange J, Karellas A, Street J, et al: Estimating the effective radiation dose imparted to patients by intraoperative cone-beam computed tomography in thoracolumbar spinal surgery. *Spine (Phila Pa 1976)* 2013;38(5):E306-E312.

21. Shono Y, Abumi K, Kaneda K: One-stage posterior hemivertebra resection and correction using segmental posterior instrumentation. *Spine (Phila Pa 1976)* 2001;26(7):752-757.

22. Marks DS, Qaimkhani SA: The natural history of congenital scoliosis and kyphosis. *Spine (Phila Pa 1976)* 2009;34(17):1751-1755.

23. Klemme WR, Polly DW Jr, Orchowski JR: Hemivertebral excision for congenital scoliosis in very young children. *J Pediatr Orthop* 2001;21(6):761-764.

24. Jalanko T, Rintala R, Puisto V, Helenius I: Hemivertebra resection for congenital scoliosis in young children: Comparison of clinical, radiographic, and health-related quality of life outcomes between the anteroposterior and posterolateral approaches. *Spine (Phila Pa 1976)* 2011;36(1):41-49.

25. Crostelli M, Mazza O, Mariani M: Posterior approach lumbar and thoracolumbar hemivertebra resection in congenital scoliosis in children under 10 years of age: Results with 3 years mean follow up. *Eur Spine J* 2014;23(1):209-215.

26. Ruf M, Jensen R, Letko L, Harms J: Hemivertebra resection and osteotomies in congenital spine deformity. *Spine (Phila Pa 1976)* 2009;34(17):1791-1799.

27. Mladenov K, Kunkel P, Stuecker R: Hemivertebra resection in children, results after single posterior approach and after combined anterior and posterior approach: A comparative study. *Eur Spine J* 2012;21(3):506-513.

28. Zhou C, Liu L, Song Y, et al: Hemivertebrae resection for unbalanced multiple hemivertebrae: Is it worth it? *Eur Spine J* 2014;23(3):536-542.

29. Tabaraee E, Gibson AG, Karahalios DG, Potts EA, Mobasser JP, Burch S: Intraoperative cone beam-computed tomography with navigation (O-ARM) versus conventional fluoroscopy (C-ARM): A cadaveric study comparing accuracy, efficiency, and safety for spinal instrumentation. *Spine (Phila Pa 1976)* 2013;38(22):1953-1958.

30. Van de Kelft E, Costa F, Van der Planken D, Schils F: A prospective multicenter registry on the accuracy of pedicle screw placement in the thoracic, lumbar, and sacral levels with the use of the O-arm imaging system and StealthStation Navigation. *Spine (Phila Pa 1976)* 2012;37(25):E1580-E1587.

31. Larson AN, Polly DW Jr, Guidera KJ, et al: The accuracy of navigation and 3D image-guided placement for the placement of pedicle screws in congenital spine deformity. *J Pediatr Orthop* 2012;32(6):e23-e29.

32. Jeswani S, Drazin D, Hsieh JC, et al: Instrumenting the small thoracic pedicle: The role of intraoperative computed tomography image-guided surgery. *Neurosurg Focus* 2014;36(3):E6.

Adolescent Idiopathic Scoliosis: Update on Bracing, Surgical Techniques, and Patient Safety

Venu M. Nemani, MD, PhD
Laurel C. Blakemore, MD
Lori A. Karol, MD
Daniel W. Green, MD, MS
Roger F. Widmann, MD

Abstract

The primary goal in the management of adolescent idiopathic scoliosis is to prevent the progression of spinal deformity either with the use of a brace or with surgery. The goals of surgery, if indicated, are to correct the spinal deformity safely and to preserve overall spinal balance and as many motion segments as possible, which maximizes the long-term health of a patient's spine. Recently, tremendous advances have been made in the surgical techniques that are used to correct adolescent idiopathic scoliosis, and improved tools have allowed surgeons to perform spinal deformity surgery as safely and with as few complications as possible. Surgeons should be aware of recent evidence that demonstrates the efficacy of bracing in patients who have adolescent idiopathic scoliosis. In addition, surgeons should understand recent advances in spinal deformity surgery with regard to fusion level selection, implant placement, three-dimensional deformity correction, and techniques that are used to minimize perioperative complications.

Instr Course Lect 2017;66:481–494.

Dr. Blakemore or an immediate family member is a member of a speakers' bureau or has made paid presentations on behalf of K2M; serves as a paid consultant to or is an employee of K2M; has received research or institutional support from K2M; and serves as a board member, owner, officer, or committee member of the International Congress on Early Onset Scoliosis, the Pediatric Orthopaedic Society of North America, and the Scoliosis Research Society. Dr. Karol or an immediate family member serves as a board member, owner, officer, or committee member of the Pediatric Orthopaedic Society of North America. Dr. Green or an immediate family member has received royalties from Arthrex and Pega Medical; and serves as a board member, owner, officer, or committee member of the American Academy of Orthopaedic Surgeons, the New York County Medical Society, the New York State Society of Orthopaedic Surgeons, and the Pediatric Orthopaedic Society of North America. Dr. Widmann or an immediate family member serves as a board member, owner, officer, or committee member of the Pediatric Orthopaedic Society of North America. Neither Dr. Nemani nor any immediate family member has received anything of value from or has stock or stock options held in a commercial company or institution related directly or indirectly to the subject of this chapter.

Adolescent idiopathic scoliosis (AIS) is the most common underlying diagnosis in pediatric patients who have spinal deformities. The primary goal in the surgical management of AIS is to prevent the progression of spinal deformity via arthrodesis of the spine in a balanced position with level shoulders centered over a level pelvis. Recent level I evidence conclusively demonstrated the efficacy of bracing in appropriately indicated patients with AIS who are compliant with brace wear. The goals of surgery, if indicated, are to correct the spinal deformity, improve cosmesis, and preserve as many motion segments as possible. In the past decade, advances in implants and surgical techniques and a better understanding of the three-dimensional nature of AIS have improved the ability of surgeons to achieve these goals. The safety of spinal fusion surgery also has improved, with new techniques that minimize transfusion requirements, improve intraoperative spinal cord monitoring, and provide better prophylaxis against infection. Surgeons should be aware of recent advances in the nonsurgical and surgical management of AIS.

Bracing

For decades, bracing has been used to manage AIS. Nachemson and Peterson[1] reported some of the earliest data on the effectiveness of bracing in patients with AIS; however, compliance with brace wear was not measured in early studies. Katz et al[2] were the first to prospectively examine the relationship between compliance with brace wear and the effectiveness of bracing in patients with AIS. In their study of 126 patients with AIS who underwent treatment with the use of a brace, Katz et al[2] reported a dose-response relationship between duration of brace wear and a successful outcome (defined as <6° of curve progression), reporting a successful outcome in 82% of the patients who wore the brace for more than 12 hours per day. This study demonstrated strong evidence that a patient's lack of compliance with brace wear was a confounding factor in earlier studies, which reported minimal to no effect of bracing on curve progression.

Weinstein et al[3] recently published the results of the Bracing in Adolescent Idiopathic Scoliosis Trial, which was a large multicenter study on the effect of bracing in 242 patients with AIS, 116 of whom were randomized to treatment with the use of a Boston-style brace or observation and 126 of whom chose to undergo treatment with the use of a Boston-style brace or observation. The authors reported that bracing significantly decreased the likelihood of curve progression to a threshold that required surgery (>50°) in the patients in both

the randomized and the self-chosen treatment groups.[3] In addition, the authors reported a strong dose-response relationship between duration of brace wear and a successful outcome, with 90% to 93% success rates reported in the patients who wore the brace for at least 12.9 hours per day. Karol et al[4] studied 222 patients with AIS to determine if compliance counseling influences compliance with brace wear and curve progression and reported that patients who undergo compliance counseling have decreased rates of curve progression and surgery.

Interestingly, in the studies by both Katz et al[2] and Weinstein et al,[3] many patients were poorly compliant with brace wear, and many patients who underwent observation alone had a curve that never reached a surgical threshold. This suggests that the current indications for bracing in patients who have AIS may be too broad and are an important avenue for further research. The indications for bracing in adolescents who have AIS must be further refined to avoid treatment with the use of a brace in those who have a curve that is not likely to progress and to encourage treatment with the use of a brace in those in whom it will be beneficial.

Computer-aided design/computer-aided manufacture (CAD/CAM) technology is the newest technology used to aid in the treatment of patients who have AIS. CAD/CAM technology digitally scans and captures the precise shape of a patient, which is then used to design and create a brace. The advantages are that a custom brace can be created more quickly compared with standard casting methods, can be created without having to fit a patient with a cast, and is more comfortable compared with a typical

Boston-style brace with an equivalent in-brace correction.[5] The use of CAD/CAM technology may provide surgeons with a better understanding of the three-dimensional nature of AIS specific to each patient, provide surgeons with a better understanding of curve flexibility, and allow for further improvements in brace adjustment to aid in optimal curve correction.[6]

Surgical Techniques

Tremendous advances have been made in the surgical techniques that are used to correct AIS. This chapter discusses several advances in the surgical techniques that are used to correct AIS, with an emphasis on those that occurred in the past 5 years, including fusion level selection, implant placement, and three-dimensional deformity correction.

Fusion Level Selection

The selection of appropriate fusion levels in patients who undergo surgical treatment for AIS is one of the most critical determinants of successful long-term clinical and radiographic outcomes. The Lenke classification of AIS was developed to address some of the limitations of the one-dimensional King-Moe classification of AIS.[7,8] The Lenke classification of AIS consists of three components: curve type (1 through 6), a lumbar spine modifier (A, B, or C), and a sagittal thoracic modifier (−, N, +). The six curve types are defined by specific radiographic characteristics that are observed on both AP radiographs (major curve and any minor curve with a Cobb angle ≥25° on side-bending radiographs) and lateral radiographs (kyphosis between T2 through T5 or T10 through L2 >20°). The Lenke classification

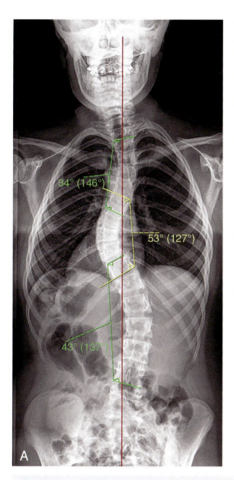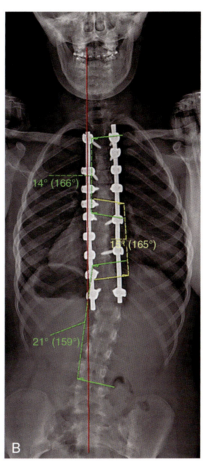

Table 1

Criteria for Consideration of Selective Thoracic Fusion in Patients With a Lenke Type 1C Curve

1. Lumbar curve smaller and more flexible compared with thoracic curve

2. Ratio of thoracic AVT to thoracolumbar/lumbar AVT >1.2 (thoracic curve more translated)[15]

3. Ratio of thoracic AVR to thoracolumbar/lumbar AVR >1.2 (thoracic curve more rotated)[15]

4. Clinical rotation of thoracolumbar/lumbar curve less compared with thoracic curve and clinically/cosmetically acceptable

5. Waist-crease asymmetry clinically acceptable

AVR = apical vertebral rotation, AVT = apical vertebral translation.

Figure 1   Preoperative (**A**) and postoperative (**B**) AP radiographs of the spine of a patient with a Lenke type 1C curve demonstrate adding on after selective thoracic fusion.

of AIS is an improvement compared with the King-Moe classification of AIS because it provides surgeons with objective criteria to classify curves as structural or nonstructural and proposes that only structural curves be fused at the time of surgery. The Lenke classification of AIS also is advantageous because it considers the sagittal plane in addition to the coronal plane, includes primary thoracolumbar and lumbar curves in addition to thoracic curves, and has improved interobserver and intraobserver reliability.[9]

The practice of the authors of this chapter for the selection of appropriate fusion levels in patients who undergo surgical treatment for AIS is largely guided by the Lenke classification of AIS and is well summarized in a recent study by Trobisch et al.[10] With the increasing popularity of correcting scoliosis with the use of constructs composed entirely of pedicle screws, the power/percent correction achieved has increased substantially.[11] In general, all structural curves should be included in the construct; however, decision making with regard to selective thoracic fusion (STF) continues to be a subject of debate.[12] STF in skeletally immature patients with AIS (especially those with an open triradiate cartilage) who have large, nonstructural thoracolumbar/

lumbar curves is associated with an increased risk for adding on and lumbar curve progression[13] (**Figure 1**). Criteria for consideration of STF in patients with a Lenke type 1C curve are listed in **Table 1**.[14,15]

In the selection of appropriate fusion levels in patients who undergo surgical treatment for AIS, surgeons must include the entire structural curve, with the lowest instrumented vertebra (LIV) being both neutral and stable. In skeletally mature or near skeletally mature patients with AIS, the King-Moe classification of AIS recommended fusion to the stable or neutral vertebra; however, currently, the authors of this chapter generally obey the last-touched rule, which involves LIV selection based on the most cephalad level that is just touched by the central sacral vertical line (CSVL; **Figure 2**). In a recent study of 104 patients who underwent surgical treatment for a Lenke type 1A (King-Moe type 2) curve, Qin et al[16] reported

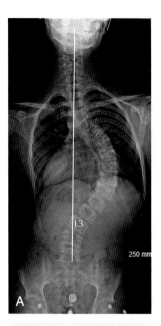 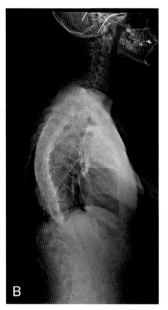 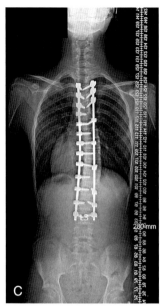 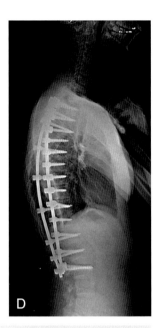

Figure 2 Preoperative AP (**A**) and lateral (**B**) radiographs and postoperative AP (**C**) and lateral (**D**) radiographs of the spine of a patient with severe adolescent idiopathic scoliosis demonstrate the use of the last-touched rule for lowest instrumented vertebra selection. (Courtesy of Michael P. Kelly, MD, Washington University, St. Louis, MO.)

that, at a minimum follow-up of 2 years, distal adding on was observed in 10% of the patients in whom a substantially touched vertebra (CSVL touching the pedicle or between the pedicles) was selected as the LIV and in 67% of the patients in whom a nonsubstantially touched vertebra (CSVL outside the pedicle) was selected as the LIV. In a study on the radiographic outcomes of patients who underwent surgical treatment using the last-touched rule for a Lenke type 1A curve, Lenke et al[17] reported that, at a minimum follow-up of 5 years, no distal adding-on was observed in the patients in whom a touched vertebra was selected as the LIV, whereas a significantly higher incidence of adding on was observed in the patients in whom a touched vertebra −1 was selected as the LIV.

In patients who have a Lenke type 1 curve with a nonstructural proximal thoracic curve and left shoulder elevation, the authors of this chapter

include the nonstructural proximal thoracic curve in the construct to prevent further elevation of the left shoulder. In the experience of the authors of this chapter, even nonstructural proximal thoracic curves are quite rigid, and not including the nonstructural proximal thoracic curve in the construct increases the risk for further elevation of an already elevated shoulder. The goal with regard to a patient's lumbar spine is to preserve as many motion segments as possible. In patients with AIS, the authors of this chapter almost never fuse to L5 and avoid fusion to L4 if possible. Stopping fusion at L3 is feasible if L3 is bisected by the CSVL, the disk wedging reverses below L3 on side-bending radiographs, and L3 is neutral or can be made neutral after deformity correction. If any of these criteria are not met, the surgeon should consider extending the fusion distally.

The Lenke classification of AIS is advantageous because it considers the

sagittal plane. Surgeons must include all structural curves determined by the T2 through T5 and T10 through L2 Cobb angles (**Figure 3**). The LIV should always be located in a neutral or lordotic region and should never be located in a kyphotic region, which increases the risk for distal junctional kyphosis.

Although the Lenke classification of AIS currently is the most advanced classification of AIS, it is a two-dimensional characterization of a complex three-dimensional deformity. In a recent study of the EOS images (EOS imaging) of 120 patients who underwent surgical treatment for AIS, Newton et al[18] reported that traditional two-dimensional radiographs significantly underestimate the amount of hypokyphosis in the thoracic spine of a typical patient with AIS because of concomitant axial plane deformity. EOS imaging, which allows surgeons to obtain both frontal and lateral whole-body, low-dose radiographs

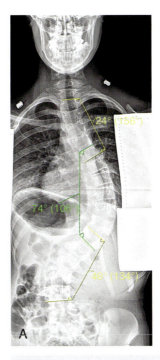
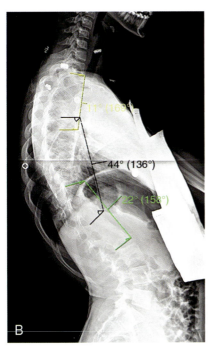
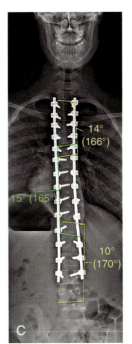
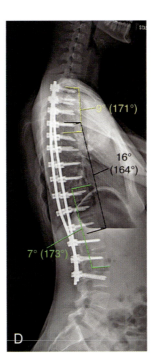

Figure 3   Preoperative AP (**A**) and lateral (**B**) radiographs and postoperative AP (**C**) and lateral (**D**) radiographs of the spine of a patient with a Lenke type 3 curve demonstrate marked thoracolumbar kyphosis. The thoracolumbar curve is considered structural based on the sagittal plane measurements and, therefore, was included in the construct; however, it would not be considered structural based on only the coronal plane measurements.

without any vertical distortion, has the potential to revolutionize surgeons' understanding of AIS because it also allows three-dimensional reconstructions of the spine to be obtained with the patient in a standing position.[19] In addition, patients who undergo EOS imaging are subjected to a much lower dose of ionizing radiation.[20] Another drawback of the current methods for classifying deformities is that they rely completely on radiographic measurements because a quantitative method to evaluate a clinical deformity is lacking. A patient with AIS who hides a deformity well may be treated differently (eg, STF versus fusion of both curves) compared with a patient with AIS who has an obvious clinical deformity even if the radiographic parameters of both of the patients are the same. New techniques that use surface topography to quantify a clinical deformity may help

characterize these patients and provide surgeons with better information to guide treatment.[21,22]

Thoracic Pedicle Screws

Thoracic pedicle screws have revolutionized the surgical management of AIS. Thoracic pedicle screws are advantageous compared with hooks and wires because they allow for superior fixation[23] and decreased spinal canal intrusion.[24] Although concerns exist with regard to the safety of thoracic pedicle screws given the many nearby vital structures in the scoliotic spine, the use of thoracic pedicle screws has been reported to be safe and accurate if the screws are placed by an experienced surgeon via a freehand technique using only anatomic landmarks.[25] However, many adjunctive techniques, including fluoroscopy, electronic conductivity-based gearshifts,[26] and intraoperative

computer navigation, continue to be used to aid in the accurate placement of thoracic pedicle screws.

Many studies have examined the breach rate of thoracic pedicle screws that are placed via various techniques. In a study of the postoperative CT scans of 60 patients (1,023 thoracic pedicle screws) with AIS who underwent thoracic pedicle screw placement via a freehand technique, Lehman et al[27] reported a 10.5% breach rate. Similar breach rates have been reported in other studies. In a meta-analysis that compared thoracic pedicle screw placement techniques, Kosmopoulos and Schizas[28] reported a placement accuracy rate of 95.2% in patients who underwent thoracic pedicle screw placement via in vivo-assisted navigation and a placement accuracy rate of 90.3% in patients who underwent thoracic pedicle screw placement without the use of navigation.[28] In a study of 45 pediatric patients who underwent surgery for AIS, Ughwanogho et al[29] compared screw placement via either a freehand technique or CT-guided navigation and reported increased accuracy in the patients in the CT-guided navigation group compared with the patients in the freehand technique group (97% versus 91%, respectively, with optimal or acceptable trajectory); however, the authors reported that CT-guided thoracic pedicle screw placement required more surgical time and was more expensive compared with freehand thoracic pedicle screw placement. Gelalis et al[30] reported similar results in a large systematic review of 1,105 patients (6,617 thoracic pedicle screws) with AIS who underwent thoracic pedicle screw placement. In all of the already mentioned studies, no neurologic, vascular, or other visceral complications and no other clinical sequelae from these breaches occurred.

Several factors must be considered in the decision of whether to use intraoperative navigation for the placement of thoracic pedicle screws in a patient with AIS. Surgical time may be substantially increased in patients who undergo thoracic pedicle screw placement via intraoperative navigation because of the registration (correlating intraoperative landmarks with preoperative or intraoperative imaging studies) that is required for intraoperative navigation. In particular, surgical time may be substantially increased in patients with a multilevel deformity in whom the best strategy is to separately register each spinal level; reduced navigational accuracy may occur if a single-registration strategy is used.[31,32] Additional surgical time may be substantial because point and surface matching for a single lumbar level

may require 6 to 8 minutes.[31] Increased surgical time may lead to increased blood loss and a higher rate of infection. However, for surgeons who are not familiar with thoracic pedicle screw placement via a freehand technique, the use of intraoperative navigation may reduce the surgical time necessary for thoracic pedicle screw placement. Surgeons also must consider radiation exposure to both the patient and the surgical team in the decision of whether to use intraoperative navigation for the placement of thoracic pedicle screws in a patient with AIS. Fluoroscopic-guided approaches are associated with substantial radiation exposure to both the patient and the surgical team, whereas CT-guided approaches typically are associated with radiation exposure to only the patient.[33-35] However, an increased risk for malignancy exists for both the patient and the surgeon as a result of the accumulation of radiation exposure from medical imaging, and although this has never been reported in children who undergo surgical treatment for AIS, it must be considered carefully.[36,37]

Although thoracic pedicle screws generally are considered safe if they are placed by an experienced surgeon, serious complications, such as neurologic deficit or vascular injury, may occur. Fortunately, these complications are rare. In a systematic review of 21 studies that included 1,666 patients (4,570 thoracic pedicle screws) who underwent thoracic pedicle screw placement, Hicks et al[38] reported an overall thoracic pedicle screw malposition rate of 4.2% (15.7% thoracic pedicle screw malposition rate in the studies in which postoperative CT scans were obtained) and a neurologic deficit rate of only 0.1%. Although descending aorta injuries that are caused by misplaced

thoracic pedicle screws have been reported in adult patients who undergo thoracic pedicle screw placement,[39] to the knowledge of the authors of this chapter, no major vascular injuries as a result of malpositioned thoracic pedicle screws have been reported in adolescent patients who undergo thoracic pedicle screw placement. Ultimately, surgeons should place thoracic pedicle screws via the technique with which they are the most comfortable and that will allow them to perform pedicle screw placement as safely and efficiently as possible.

Three-Dimensional Deformity Correction

In patients who undergo segmental spinal instrumentation with the use of thoracic pedicle screws, marked deformity correction in both the coronal and sagittal plane can be achieved by translating the spine to a precontoured rod via indirect correction of the axial plane rotational deformity. The concept of direct vertebral rotation (DVR), which uses towers that are attached to the thoracic pedicle screws to directly manipulate the vertebral bodies and correct the axial plane rotational deformity, was introduced by Lee et al.[40] DVR and increased correction of the axial plane rotational deformity are beneficial in patients with AIS because they allow for reduction of the rib hump deformity without a thoracoplasty. In their study of the CT scans of 38 patients with AIS who underwent segmental spinal instrumentation with the use of thoracic pedicle screws and either DVR or simple rod derotation, Lee et al[40] reported 42.5% deformity correction in the patients in the DVR group and only 2.4% deformity correction in the patients in the simple rod derotation group. The force that can be imparted to derotate a spine is increased if several thoracic pedicle screws are linked so that the force is distributed over multiple fixation points. Cheng et al[41] reported that a near-linear increase in relative torque could be applied to a derotation construct before failure as additional thoracic pedicle screws were linked, with quadrangularly linked thoracic pedicle screw constructs able to withstand 42.5 Nm of force before failure and single thoracic pedicle screws cut out of the pedicle, either laterally or into the spinal canal, able to withstand only 4 to 6 Nm of force. The linking of thoracic pedicle screws before DVR is essential because thoracic pedicle screw failure that occurs during a derotation maneuver may result in abutment of a thoracic pedicle screw on the spinal cord or the great vessels, which can have disastrous consequences.[42]

Most modern deformity correction techniques for patients who have AIS rely on differential rod contouring and materials, three-column fixation, and gradual reduction to multiple fixation points. The concave rod typically is bent into hyperkyphosis and often is stiffer compared with the underbent convex rod. Three-column fixation at multiple anchor points in combination with the ability to simultaneously achieve gradual reduction at those multiple levels of fixation allows for three-dimensional deformity correction. Most current instrumentation systems allow for gradual reduction of the spine to a precontoured rod across multiple fixation points, which distributes the corrective forces and reduces the risk for failure at the bone-screw interface.

Perioperative Safety

Ensuring the safety of patients who undergo surgical treatment for AIS is critical. In the past decade, many studies on the surgical treatment of patients with AIS have focused on achieving successful outcomes and minimizing complications. Several perioperative safety techniques for AIS surgery, including the management of intraoperative blood loss, intraoperative neuromonitoring, and perioperative antibiotic prophylaxis, are discussed.

Management of Intraoperative Blood Loss

Many factors affect intraoperative blood loss in patients who undergo a multilevel fusion procedure for the management of spinal deformity. Patient factors that affect intraoperative blood loss include the type of spinal deformity (idiopathic, neuromuscular, syndromic), the severity of the curve, and the size of the patient. Surgical factors that affect intraoperative blood loss include the duration of the surgery, prone positioning and maintenance of a free-hanging abdomen without compression, whether osteotomies are performed, intraoperative mean arterial pressure (MAP), whether blood salvage techniques are used (eg, cell saver), and whether antifibrinolytic agents are administered. The management of intraoperative blood loss is critical because allogeneic blood transfusions are not benign and may be associated with transfusion reactions, the transmission of blood-borne infections, and an increased rate of surgical site infection (SSI).[43-45] These complications of allogeneic blood transfusion may lead to increased costs, increased length of hospital stay, and, possibly, poor patient outcomes.

Although patient factors that affect intraoperative blood loss are difficult to alter, surgeons have the ability to control surgical factors that affect intraoperative blood loss. Several studies have reported that the maintenance of a patient's intraoperative MAP below 75 mm Hg may help reduce blood loss during spinal fusion surgery.[46,47] Maintenance of intraoperative MAP requires careful communication between the surgeon and the anesthesiologist. For spinal fusion surgery, a patient's intraoperative MAP should be maintained below 75 mm Hg during exposure and during anchor placement; however, a patient's intraoperative MAP should be raised to 80 to 90 mm Hg during any corrective maneuvers to maintain spinal cord perfusion pressure and decrease the risk for neurologic injury.[48]

The use of an intraoperative cell saver is another method that may help reduce the need for allogeneic blood transfusions. In a study of 54 patients with AIS who underwent spinal fusion surgery with or without the use of a cell saver, Bowen et al[49] reported that perioperative allogeneic blood transfusion rates were lower in the patients in whom an intraoperative cell saver was used (18%) compared with the patients in whom an intraoperative cell saver was not used (55%). However, other studies have questioned the efficacy of intraoperative cell savers with regard to reducing the need for allogeneic blood transfusions in patients who undergo AIS surgery.[50,51] In a recent randomized controlled trial of 110 patients with AIS in China who underwent spinal fusion surgery with or without the use of a cell saver, Liang et al[52] reported a decreased rate of perioperative allogeneic blood transfusions in the patients in whom an intraoperative cell saver was used. The added cost of a cell saver[53] and the potential negative physiologic effects of reinfusing washed blood[51,54,55] must be considered in the decision of whether to use a cell saver as part of a multimodal strategy to minimize intraoperative blood loss.

In the past several years, intriguing research has been performed with regard to the use of antifibrinolytic agents (epsilon-aminocaproic acid, aprotinin, tranexamic acid [TXA]) to help reduce intraoperative blood loss. Although aprotinin was highly effective with regard to the reduction of intraoperative blood loss, it no longer is used in the United States because it is associated with renal failure in patients who undergo cardiac surgery.[56] In a randomized controlled trial of 44 pediatric patients who underwent scoliosis surgery and were administered either TXA (100 mg/kg preoperatively followed by a 10 mg/kg/h infusion intraoperatively) or saline, Sethna et al[57] reported that intraoperative blood loss was reduced by 41% in the patients in the TXA group. In a Cochrane review of six studies that included 254 children who underwent scoliosis surgery and were administered either a placebo or an antifibrinolytic agent, Tzortzopoulou et al[58] reported that the use of TXA and epsilon-aminocaproic acid reduced the need for allogeneic blood transfusions. In a study of 106 adolescents with AIS who underwent spinal fusion surgery and were administered TXA (1 g preoperatively followed by a 100 mg/kg/h infusion intraoperatively), Yagi et al[59] reported a 43% reduction in intraoperative blood loss in the patients who were administered TXA compared with a group of patients in a historic cohort; however, these results may be confounded by overall improved surgical technique that occurred with time. In a recent prospective, randomized, double-blind study that compared the efficacy of TXA, epsilon-aminocaproic acid, and a placebo in 125 adolescents with AIS who underwent spinal fusion surgery, Verma et al[60] reported that TXA (10 mg/kg preoperatively followed by a 1 mg/kg/h infusion intraoperatively) and epsilon-aminocaproic acid (100 mg/kg preoperatively followed by a 10 mg/kg/h infusion intraoperatively) were equally effective at reducing intraoperative blood loss but not allogeneic blood transfusion rates. However, in a recent systematic review and meta-analysis of 18 studies that included 1,158 patients who underwent scoliosis surgery and were administered either an antifibrinolytic agent or a placebo, Wang et al[61] reported that TXA was likely more effective at reducing perioperative blood loss without increasing the risk for thromboembolic events compared with epsilon-aminocaproic acid. Several research studies are currently being conducted to determine the optimal antifibrinolytic dosing regimen, which will maximize the efficacy of antifibrinolytic agents and minimize the risk for toxicity, for patients who undergo scoliosis surgery.

Intraoperative Neuromonitoring

The use of intraoperative neuromonitoring (IONM) in patients who undergo spinal deformity surgery has been the standard of care since the publication of the landmark paper by Nash et al[62] in the mid 1970s. Although the incidence of new neurologic deficits in patients with AIS who undergo spinal deformity surgery is low,[63] a new neurologic deficit may be catastrophic and irreversible. The Stagnara wake-up test is the historic benchmark for the detection of neurologic deficits; however, the test is not time sensitive and is unable to quickly detect changes in neurologic function after an intraoperative maneuver (screw placement, deformity correction, completion of an osteotomy, etc.). The current benchmark for the detection of neurologic deficits is multimodal IONM, which involves the use of somatosensory-evoked potentials (SSEPs) in combination with some form of motor tract monitoring, such as descending neurogenic-evoked potentials or, more commonly, transcranial motor-evoked potentials (TcMEPs).

In a study of 1,121 patients with AIS who underwent scoliosis surgery, Schwartz et al[64] reported that both the sensitivity and specificity of TcMEPs for the detection of motor loss and the sensitivity and specificity of SSEPs for the detection of sensory loss were 100%. Importantly, the authors reported that changes in SSEPs lagged behind changes in TcMEPs by 5 to 10 minutes; therefore, the monitoring of TcMEPs in conjunction with SSEPs is critical to allow surgeons to quickly respond to IONM alerts. In a more recent study of 3,436 pediatric patients who underwent spine surgery, Thuet et al[65] reported potential neurologic deficits in 2.2% of the patients. The authors reported a 0.2% rate of false-negative results, and reported that the combined use of SSEPs; TcMEPs; descending neurogenic-evoked potentials; and nerve-root monitoring, such as electromyography, allowed for the detection of permanent neurologic status in 99.6% of the patients. In addition to monitoring SSEPs and TcMEPs, some surgeons use triggered electromyography in patients in whom thoracic pedicle screws are placed at or more caudad to T6 to assess for medial breaches that may not have been previously detected via manual palpation of the pedicle screw tract or via radiography.[66] The rate of postoperative neurologic deficits has decreased in pediatric patients who undergo spinal deformity surgery with the use of multimodal IONM.[67,68] The authors of this chapter recommend the use of multimodal IONM in the surgical treatment of patients with scoliosis, kyphosis, and spondylolisthesis (electromyography to monitor nerve-root function) as well as in patients who undergo any growing construct application or lengthening procedure. The use of IONM is absolutely mandatory in patients who undergo any three-column osteotomy, such as a vertebral column resection.

A surgical team must respond to IONM alerts, if they occur, quickly and in an organized manner to minimize the risk for permanent neurologic deficit. Vitale et al[69] recently published a best-practices guideline in the form of an intraoperative checklist to help surgeons respond to a situation that requires prompt action in a consistent, orderly, and thorough manner (**Table 2**). The field of pediatric spinal deformity lacks standardized methods for the surgical treatment of patients; therefore, more efforts to standardize the treatment of patients who have AIS, such as those similar to the already mentioned best-practices guideline, are necessary to improve outcomes and decrease complications.

Perioperative Antibiotic Prophylaxis

The rate of SSI in the adolescent spinal deformity population has been reported to range from 0.5% to 4.3%;[70-72] the rate of SSI in the neuromuscular population is much higher.[70,73,74] Patients in whom SSIs occur require repeated surgery for wound débridement,

Table 2	
Intraoperative Checklist for Response to Intraoperative Neuromonitoring Changes That Occur During Spinal Deformity Surgery	
Step	**Actions**
Surgical pause	Eliminate extraneous stimuli
	Gather experienced staff (anesthesiologist, neurophysiologist, nurse)
	Call for intraoperative imaging
Address anesthetic/ systemic issues	Optimize MAP, hematocrit level, pH level, and $PaCO_2$ level
	Ensure normothermia
	Discuss possible need for Stagnara wake-up test
Check technical/ neurophysiologic factors	Discuss status of anesthetic agents
	Check for degree of neuromuscular blockade and paralysis
	Check electrode and limb positioning
Check surgical factors	Review recent surgical events, such as implant placement, corrective maneuvers, traction, or osteotomy closure, and consider reversal
	Meticulous evaluation for spinal cord compression or spinal subluxation
	Intraoperative or perioperative imaging to evaluate implant placement

MAP = mean arterial pressure.

Adapted with permission from Vitale MG, Skaggs DL, Pace GI, et al: Best practices in intraoperative neuromonitoring in spine deformity surgery: Development of an intraoperative checklist to optimize response. *Spine Deform* 2014;2(5):333-339.

implant removal or exchange, and revision surgery, all of which are associated with considerable personal and societal costs.[75] Several recent studies have highlighted the substantial variability in the current practices of high-volume pediatric spine surgeons and the lack of high-quality evidence with regard to SSI prevention in patients who undergo pediatric spinal deformity surgery.[75,76] Vitale et al[77] recently published a best practice guideline for infection prophylaxis in high-risk pediatric patients who undergo spine surgery (**Table 3**). For the purposes of their study, the authors defined high risk as any fusion procedure other than a primary fusion in a patient who has AIS and no substantial comorbidities. This definition excludes

healthy adolescents with AIS who undergo spinal fusion surgery; however, the best practice guideline published by Vitale et al[77] is largely applicable, with a few exceptions, to any patient who undergoes scoliosis surgery. Unfortunately, the best practice guideline published by Vitale et al[77] was mostly based on expert opinion because very little high-quality evidence is available in the literature. Regardless, adherence to the criteria in the best practice guideline published by Vitale et al[77] will help surgeons standardize the surgical treatment of patients with AIS, which likely will result in fewer SSIs.

Intrawound vancomycin powder, which has become popular in the past 5 years, is an intriguing intervention

Table 3

Best Practice Guideline for the Prevention of Surgical Site Infection in High-Risk Pediatric Spine Surgery

1. Patients should undergo a chlorhexidine skin wash at home the night before surgery.
2. Preoperative urine cultures should be obtained, and patients should be treated if cultures are positive.[a]
3. Patients should receive a preoperative patient education sheet.
4. Patients should undergo a preoperative nutritional assessment.[a]
5. If hair is removed, clipping is preferable to shaving.
6. Patients should be administered perioperative intravenous cefazolin.
7. Patients should be administered perioperative intravenous prophylaxis for gram-negative bacilli.[a]
8. Adherence to perioperative microbial regimens should be monitored (ie, agent, timing, dosing, redosing, cessation).
9. Operating room access should be limited during scoliosis surgery if practical.
10. The use of ultraviolet lights in the operating room is not required.
11. Patients should undergo intraoperative wound irrigation.
12. Vancomycin powder should be used in the bone graft and/or the surgical site.
13. Impervious dressings are preferred postoperatively.
14. Postoperative dressing changes should be minimized as much as possible before discharge.

[a]These particular guidelines are not recommended for healthy patients with adolescent idiopathic scoliosis who undergo spine surgery but should be reserved for prophylaxis in high-risk pediatric patients who undergo spine surgery.

Adapted with permission from Vitale MG, Riedel MD, Glotzbecker MP, et al: Building consensus: Development of a best practice guideline (BPG) for surgical site infection (SSI) prevention in high-risk pediatric spine surgery. *J Pediatr Orthop* 2013;33(5):471-478.

that is used to reduce the rate of SSI in patients who undergo spine surgery. More than 60% of clinical isolates from wound infections of patients in the United States, including methicillin-resistant *Staphylococcus aureus* and coagulase-negative *Staphylococcus* species, are resistant to cephalosporins.[78,79] The use of intrawound vancomycin powder for infection prophylaxis in patients who undergo spine surgery was first reported by Sweet et al[80] in a retrospective cohort study of adult and pediatric patients who underwent thoracic and lumbar instrumented fusions. The authors reported that the rate of SSI decreased from 2.6% to 0.2% in the patients who were administered intrawound vancomycin powder compared with a group of patients in a historic cohort.[80]

The local application of vancomycin powder is beneficial because the drug can reach concentrations that are well above the minimum inhibitory concentration in the wound with essentially no risk for systemic absorption or systemic toxicity, even in children.[81-83] In a study of 20 rabbits that underwent spine surgery with the use of cefazolin and with or without the use of intrawound vancomycin powder, Zebala et al[84] reported that the use of intrawound vancomycin power in combination with intravenous cefazolin completely eliminated *S aureus* wound contamination, whereas the use of intravenous cefazolin alone

did not eliminate *S aureus* wound contamination. Several studies have reported that the use of intrawound vancomycin powder reduces the rate of SSI after spine surgery[85-88] and is a cost-effective intervention.[89,90] Because of the large number of patients that is necessary to perform a randomized controlled trial, high-quality evidence currently is lacking; however, the current collective evidence suggests that the use of intrawound vancomycin powder for infection prophylaxis in pediatric patients who undergo spine surgery is beneficial, is safe, and, in conjunction with other measures, reduces the rate of SSI with minimal to no increased risk for morbidity.

Summary

In the past several years, substantial advances have been made in the techniques that are used to manage AIS. Recent evidence has demonstrated the efficacy of bracing in appropriately indicated patients with AIS. More effective surgical techniques have been developed to maximize deformity correction in patients with AIS. Advances in perioperative safety techniques have minimized complications in patients who undergo surgical treatment for AIS. Surgeons must continue to search for opportunities to improve the safety of patients who undergo surgical treatment for AIS, which will further reduce complications and improve outcomes.

References

1. Nachemson AL, Peterson LE: Effectiveness of treatment with a brace in girls who have adolescent idiopathic scoliosis: A prospective, controlled study based on data from the Brace Study of the Scoliosis Research Society. *J Bone Joint Surg Am* 1995;77(6):815-822.

2. Katz DE, Herring JA, Browne RH, Kelly DM, Birch JG: Brace wear control of curve progression in adolescent idiopathic scoliosis. *J Bone Joint Surg Am* 2010;92(6):1343-1352.

3. Weinstein SL, Dolan LA, Wright JG, Dobbs MB: Effects of bracing in adolescents with idiopathic scoliosis. *N Engl J Med* 2013;369(16):1512-1521.

4. Karol LA, Virostek D, Felton K, Wheeler L: Effect of compliance counseling on brace use and success in patients with adolescent idiopathic scoliosis. *J Bone Joint Surg Am* 2016;98(1):9-14.

5. Sankar WN, Albrektson J, Lerman L, Tolo VT, Skaggs DL: Scoliosis in-brace curve correction and patient preference of CAD/CAM versus plaster molded TLSOs. *J Child Orthop* 2007;1(6):345-349.

6. Labelle H, Bellefleur C, Joncas J, Aubin CE, Cheriet F: Preliminary evaluation of a computer-assisted tool for the design and adjustment of braces in idiopathic scoliosis: A prospective and randomized study. *Spine (Phila Pa 1976)* 2007;32(8):835-843.

7. Lenke LG, Betz RR, Harms J, et al: Adolescent idiopathic scoliosis: A new classification to determine extent of spinal arthrodesis. *J Bone Joint Surg Am* 2001;83(8):1169-1181.

8. King HA, Moe JH, Bradford DS, Winter RB: The selection of fusion levels in thoracic idiopathic scoliosis. *J Bone Joint Surg Am* 1983;65(9):1302-1313.

9. Ogon M, Giesinger K, Behensky H, et al: Interobserver and intraobserver reliability of Lenke's new scoliosis classification system. *Spine (Phila Pa 1976)* 2002;27(8):858-862.

10. Trobisch PD, Ducoffe AR, Lonner BS, Errico TJ: Choosing fusion levels in adolescent idiopathic scoliosis. *J Am Acad Orthop Surg* 2013;21(9):519-528.

11. Kim YJ, Lenke LG, Cho SK, Bridwell KH, Sides B, Blanke K: Comparative analysis of pedicle screw versus hook instrumentation in posterior spinal fusion of adolescent idiopathic scoliosis. *Spine (Phila Pa 1976)* 2004;29(18):2040-2048.

12. Betz RR: Should all AIS 1C curves be fused selectively? *Spine (Phila Pa 1976)* 2016;41(suppl 7):S16-S17.

13. Sponseller PD, Betz R, Newton PO, et al: Differences in curve behavior after fusion in adolescent idiopathic scoliosis patients with open triradiate cartilages. *Spine (Phila Pa 1976)* 2009;34(8):827-831.

14. Fischer CR, Kim Y: Selective fusion for adolescent idiopathic scoliosis: A review of current operative strategy. *Eur Spine J* 2011;20(7):1048-1057.

15. Lenke LG, Bridwell KH, Baldus C, Blanke K: Preventing decompensation in King type II curves treated with Cotrel-Dubousset instrumentation: Strict guidelines for selective thoracic fusion. *Spine (Phila Pa 1976)* 1992; 17(8 suppl):S274-S281.

16. Qin X, Sun W, Xu L, Liu Z, Qiu Y, Zhu Z: Selecting the last "substantially" touching vertebra as lowest instrumented vertebra in Lenke type 1A Curve: Radiographic outcomes with a minimum of 2-year follow-up. *Spine (Phila Pa 1976)* 2016;41(12):E742-E750.

17. Lenke LG, Newton PO, Lehman RA, et al: Paper No. 5. Radiographic results of selecting the touched vertebra as the lowest instrumented vertebra in Lenke 1A AIS curves at a minimum five-year follow up. *49th Annual Meeting of the Scoliosis Research Society.* Anchorage, AK, September 10-13, 2014.

18. Newton PO, Fujimori T, Doan J, Reighard FG, Bastrom TP, Misaghi A: Defining the "three-dimensional sagittal plane" in thoracic adolescent idiopathic scoliosis. *J Bone Joint Surg Am* 2015;97(20):1694-1701.

19. Somoskeöy S, Tunyogi-Csapó M, Bogyó C, Illés T: Accuracy and reliability of coronal and sagittal spinal curvature data based on patient-specific three-dimensional models created by the EOS 2D/3D imaging system. *Spine J* 2012;12(11):1052-1059.

20. Deschênes S, Charron G, Beaudoin G, et al: Diagnostic imaging of spinal deformities: Reducing patients radiation dose with a new slot-scanning X-ray imager. *Spine (Phila Pa 1976)* 2010;35(9):989-994.

21. Komeili A, Westover L, Parent EC, El-Rich M, Adeeb S: Monitoring for idiopathic scoliosis curve progression using surface topography asymmetry analysis of the torso in adolescents. *Spine J* 2015;15(4):743-751.

22. Komeili A, Westover LM, Parent EC, Moreau M, El-Rich M, Adeeb S: Surface topography asymmetry maps categorizing external deformity in scoliosis. *Spine J* 2014;14(6): 973-83.e2.

23. Liljenqvist U, Hackenberg L, Link T, Halm H: Pullout strength of pedicle screws versus pedicle and laminar hooks in the thoracic spine. *Acta Orthop Belg* 2001;67(2):157-163.

24. Polly DW Jr, Potter BK, Kuklo T, Young S, Johnson C, Klemme WR: Volumetric spinal canal intrusion: A comparison between thoracic pedicle screws and thoracic hooks. *Spine (Phila Pa 1976)* 2004;29(1):63-69.

25. Kim YJ, Lenke LG, Bridwell KH, Cho YS, Riew KD: Free hand pedicle screw placement in the thoracic spine: Is it safe? *Spine (Phila Pa 1976)* 2004;29(3):333-342.

26. Ovadia D, Korn A, Fishkin M, Steinberg DM, Wientroub S, Ofiram E: The contribution of an electronic conductivity device to the safety of pedicle screw insertion in scoliosis surgery. *Spine (Phila Pa 1976)* 2011;36(20):E1314-E1321.

27. Lehman RA Jr, Lenke LG, Keeler KA, Kim YJ, Cheh G: Computed tomography evaluation of pedicle screws placed in the pediatric deformed spine over an 8-year period. *Spine (Phila Pa 1976)* 2007;32(24):2679-2684.

28. Kosmopoulos V, Schizas C: Pedicle screw placement accuracy: A meta-analysis. *Spine (Phila Pa 1976)* 2007;32(3):E111-E120.

29. Ughwanogho E, Patel NM, Baldwin KD, Sampson NR, Flynn JM: Computed tomography-guided navigation of thoracic pedicle screws for adolescent idiopathic scoliosis results in more accurate placement and less screw removal. *Spine (Phila Pa 1976)* 2012;37(8):E473-E478.

30. Gelalis ID, Paschos NK, Pakos EE, et al: Accuracy of pedicle screw placement: A systematic review of

prospective in vivo studies comparing free hand, fluoroscopy guidance and navigation techniques. *Eur Spine J* 2012;21(2):247-255.

31. Lee TC, Yang LC, Liliang PC, Su TM, Rau CS, Chen HJ: Single versus separate registration for computer-assisted lumbar pedicle screw placement. *Spine (Phila Pa 1976)* 2004;29(14):1585-1589.

32. Nottmeier EW, Crosby TL: Timing of paired points and surface matching registration in three-dimensional (3D) image-guided spinal surgery. *J Spinal Disord Tech* 2007;20(4):268-270.

33. Tabaraee E, Gibson AG, Karahalios DG, Potts EA, Mobasser JP, Burch S: Intraoperative cone beam-computed tomography with navigation (O-ARM) versus conventional fluoroscopy (C-ARM): A cadaveric study comparing accuracy, efficiency, and safety for spinal instrumentation. *Spine (Phila Pa 1976)* 2013;38(22):1953-1958.

34. Villard J, Ryang YM, Demetriades AK, et al: Radiation exposure to the surgeon and the patient during posterior lumbar spinal instrumentation: A prospective randomized comparison of navigated versus non-navigated freehand techniques. *Spine (Phila Pa 1976)* 2014;39(13):1004-1009.

35. Mendelsohn D, Strelzow J, Dea N, et al: Patient and surgeon radiation exposure during spinal instrumentation using intraoperative computed tomography-based navigation. *Spine J* 2016;16(3):343-354.

36. Brenner DJ, Hall EJ: Computed tomography—an increasing source of radiation exposure. *N Engl J Med* 2007;357(22):2277-2284.

37. Berrington de González A, Darby S: Risk of cancer from diagnostic X-rays: Estimates for the UK and 14 other countries. *Lancet* 2004;363(9406):345-351.

38. Hicks JM, Singla A, Shen FH, Arlet V: Complications of pedicle screw fixation in scoliosis surgery: A systematic review. *Spine (Phila Pa 1976)* 2010;35(11):E465-E470.

39. Kakkos SK, Shepard AD: Delayed presentation of aortic injury by pedicle screws: Report of two cases and review of the literature. *J Vasc Surg* 2008;47(5):1074-1082.

40. Lee SM, Suk SI, Chung ER: Direct vertebral rotation: A new technique of three-dimensional deformity correction with segmental pedicle screw fixation in adolescent idiopathic scoliosis. *Spine (Phila Pa 1976)* 2004;29(3):343-349.

41. Cheng I, Hay D, Iezza A, Lindsey D, Lenke LG: Biomechanical analysis of derotation of the thoracic spine using pedicle screws. *Spine (Phila Pa 1976)* 2010;35(10):1039-1043.

42. Wagner MR, Flores JB, Sanpera I, Herrera-Soto J: Aortic abutment after direct vertebral rotation: Plowing of pedicle screws. *Spine (Phila Pa 1976)* 2011;36(3):243-247.

43. Koutsoumbelis S, Hughes AP, Girardi FP, et al: Risk factors for postoperative infection following posterior lumbar instrumented arthrodesis. *J Bone Joint Surg Am* 2011;93(17):1627-1633.

44. Sharma S, Sharma P, Tyler LN: Transfusion of blood and blood products: Indications and complications. *Am Fam Physician* 2011;83(6):719-724.

45. Woods BI, Rosario BL, Chen A, et al: The association between perioperative allogeneic transfusion volume and postoperative infection in patients following lumbar spine surgery. *J Bone Joint Surg Am* 2013;95(23):2105-2110.

46. Malcolm-Smith NA, McMaster MJ: The use of induced hypotension to control bleeding during posterior fusion for scoliosis. *J Bone Joint Surg Br* 1983;65(3):255-258.

47. Pizov R, Segal E, Kaplan L, Floman Y, Perel A: The use of systolic pressure variation in hemodynamic monitoring during deliberate hypotension in spine surgery. *J Clin Anesth* 1990;2(2):96-100.

48. Yeoman PM, Gibson MJ, Hutchinson A, Crawshaw C, Bradshaw K, Beattie A: Influence of induced hypotension and spinal distraction on feline spinal somatosensory evoked potentials. *Br J Anaesth* 1989;63(3):315-320.

49. Bowen RE, Gardner S, Scaduto AA, Eagan M, Beckstead J: Efficacy of intraoperative cell salvage systems in pediatric idiopathic scoliosis patients undergoing posterior spinal fusion with segmental spinal instrumentation. *Spine (Phila Pa 1976)* 2010;35(2):246-251.

50. Siller TA, Dickson JH, Erwin WD: Efficacy and cost considerations of intraoperative autologous transfusion in spinal fusion for idiopathic scoliosis with predeposited blood. *Spine (Phila Pa 1976)* 1996;21(7):848-852.

51. Weiss JM, Skaggs D, Tanner J, Tolo V: Cell saver: Is it beneficial in scoliosis surgery? *J Child Orthop* 2007;1(4):221-227.

52. Liang J, Shen J, Chua S, et al: Does intraoperative cell salvage system effectively decrease the need for allogeneic transfusions in scoliotic patients undergoing posterior spinal fusion? A prospective randomized study. *Eur Spine J* 2015;24(2):270-275.

53. Miao YL, Ma HS, Guo WZ, et al: The efficacy and cost-effectiveness of cell saver use in instrumented posterior correction and fusion surgery for scoliosis in school-aged children and adolescents. *PLoS One* 2014;9(4):e92997.

54. Keverline JP, Sanders JO: Hematuria associated with low-volume cell saver in pediatric orthopaedics. *J Pediatr Orthop* 1998;18(5):594-597.

55. Murphy GJ, Rogers CS, Lansdowne WB, et al: Safety, efficacy, and cost of intraoperative cell salvage and autotransfusion after off-pump coronary artery bypass surgery: A randomized trial. *J Thorac Cardiovasc Surg* 2005;130(1):20-28.

56. Mangano DT, Tudor IC, Dietzel C; Multicenter Study of Perioperative Ischemia Research Group; Ischemia Research and Education Foundation: The risk associated with aprotinin in cardiac surgery. *N Engl J Med* 2006;354(4):353-365.

57. Sethna NF, Zurakowski D, Brustowicz RM, Bacsik J, Sullivan LJ, Shapiro F: Tranexamic acid reduces intraoperative blood loss in pediatric patients undergoing scoliosis surgery. *Anesthesiology* 2005;102(4):727-732.

58. Tzortzopoulou A, Cepeda MS, Schumann R, Carr DB: Antifibrinolytic agents for reducing blood loss in scoliosis surgery in children. *Cochrane Database Syst Rev* 2008;3:CD006883.

59. Yagi M, Hasegawa J, Nagoshi N, et al: Does the intraoperative tranexamic acid decrease operative blood loss during posterior spinal fusion for treatment of adolescent idiopathic scoliosis? *Spine (Phila Pa 1976)* 2012;37(21):E1336-E1342.

60. Verma K, Errico T, Diefenbach C, et al: The relative efficacy of antifibrinolytics in adolescent idiopathic scoliosis: A prospective randomized trial. *J Bone Joint Surg Am* 2014;96(10):e80.

61. Wang M, Zheng XF, Jiang LS: Efficacy and safety of antifibrinolytic agents in reducing perioperative blood loss and transfusion requirements in scoliosis surgery: A systematic review and meta-analysis. *PLoS One* 2015;10(9):e0137886.

62. Nash CL Jr, Lorig RA, Schatzinger LA, Brown RH: Spinal cord monitoring during operative treatment of the spine. *Clin Orthop Relat Res* 1977;126:100-105.

63. Hamilton DK, Smith JS, Sansur CA, et al: Rates of new neurological deficit associated with spine surgery based on 108,419 procedures: A report of the scoliosis research society morbidity and mortality committee. *Spine (Phila Pa 1976)* 2011;36(15):1218-1228.

64. Schwartz DM, Auerbach JD, Dormans JP, et al: Neurophysiological detection of impending spinal cord injury during scoliosis surgery. *J Bone Joint Surg Am* 2007;89(11):2440-2449.

65. Thuet ED, Winscher JC, Padberg AM, et al: Validity and reliability of intraoperative monitoring in pediatric spinal deformity surgery: A 23-year experience of 3436 surgical cases. *Spine (Phila Pa 1976)* 2010;35(20):1880-1886.

66. Raynor BL, Lenke LG, Kim Y, et al: Can triggered electromyograph thresholds predict safe thoracic pedicle screw placement? *Spine (Phila Pa 1976)* 2002;27(18):2030-2035.

67. Fehlings MG, Brodke DS, Norvell DC, Dettori JR: The evidence for intraoperative neurophysiological monitoring in spine surgery: Does it make a difference? *Spine (Phila Pa 1976)* 2010;35(9 suppl):S37-S46.

68. Winter RB: Neurologic safety in spinal deformity surgery. *Spine (Phila Pa 1976)* 1997;22(13):1527-1533.

69. Vitale MG, Skaggs DL, Pace GI, et al: Best practices in intraoperative neuromonitoring in spine deformity surgery: Development of an intraoperative checklist to optimize response. *Spine Deform* 2014;2(5):333-339.

70. Cahill PJ, Warnick DE, Lee MJ, et al: Infection after spinal fusion for pediatric spinal deformity: Thirty years of experience at a single institution. *Spine (Phila Pa 1976)* 2010;35(12):1211-1217.

71. Coe JD, Arlet V, Donaldson W, et al: Complications in spinal fusion for adolescent idiopathic scoliosis in the new millennium: A report of the Scoliosis Research Society Morbidity and Mortality Committee. *Spine (Phila Pa 1976)* 2006;31(3):345-349.

72. Rihn JA, Lee JY, Ward WT: Infection after the surgical treatment of adolescent idiopathic scoliosis: Evaluation of the diagnosis, treatment, and impact on clinical outcomes. *Spine (Phila Pa 1976)* 2008;33(3):289-294.

73. Benson ER, Thomson JD, Smith BG, Banta JV: Results and morbidity in a consecutive series of patients undergoing spinal fusion for neuromuscular scoliosis. *Spine (Phila Pa 1976)* 1998;23(21):2308-2318.

74. Sponseller PD, Shah SA, Abel MF, Newton PO, Letko L, Marks M: Infection rate after spine surgery in cerebral palsy is high and impairs results: Multicenter analysis of risk factors and treatment. *Clin Orthop Relat Res* 2010;468(3):711-716.

75. Glotzbecker MP, Vitale MG, Shea KG, Flynn JM; POSNA committee on the Quality, Safety, Value Initiative (QSVI): Surgeon practices regarding infection prevention for pediatric spinal surgery. *J Pediatr Orthop* 2013;33(7):694-699.

76. Glotzbecker MP, Riedel MD, Vitale MG, et al: What's the evidence? Systematic literature review of risk factors and preventive strategies for surgical site infection following pediatric spine surgery. *J Pediatr Orthop* 2013;33(5):479-487.

77. Vitale MG, Riedel MD, Glotzbecker MP, et al: Building consensus: Development of a best practice guideline (BPG) for surgical site infection (SSI) prevention in high-risk pediatric spine surgery. *J Pediatr Orthop* 2013;33(5):471-478.

78. Klevens RM, Edwards JR, Richards CL Jr, et al: Estimating health care-associated infections and deaths in U.S. hospitals, 2002. *Public Health Rep* 2007;122(2):160-166.

79. Klevens RM, Morrison MA, Nadle J, et al: Invasive methicillin-resistant Staphylococcus aureus infections in the United States. *JAMA* 2007;298(15):1763-1771.

80. Sweet FA, Roh M, Sliva C: Intrawound application of vancomycin for prophylaxis in instrumented thoracolumbar fusions: Efficacy, drug levels, and patient outcomes. *Spine (Phila Pa 1976)* 2011;36(24):2084-2088.

81. Armaghani SJ, Menge TJ, Lovejoy SA, Mencio GA, Martus JE: Safety of topical vancomycin for pediatric spinal deformity: Nontoxic serum levels with supratherapeutic drain levels. *Spine (Phila Pa 1976)* 2014;39(20):1683-1687.

82. Gans I, Dormans JP, Spiegel DA, et al: Adjunctive vancomycin powder in pediatric spine surgery is safe. *Spine (Phila Pa 1976)* 2013;38(19):1703-1707.

83. Ghobrial GM, Cadotte DW, Williams K Jr, Fehlings MG, Harrop JS: Complications from the use of intrawound vancomycin in lumbar spinal surgery: A systematic review. *Neurosurg Focus* 2015;39(4):E11.

84. Zebala LP, Chuntarapas T, Kelly MP, Talcott M, Greco S, Riew KD: Intrawound vancomycin powder eradicates surgical wound contamination: An in vivo rabbit study. *J Bone Joint Surg Am* 2014;96(1):46-51.

85. Chiang HY, Herwaldt LA, Blevins AE, Cho E, Schweizer ML: Effectiveness of local vancomycin powder to decrease surgical site infections: A meta-analysis. *Spine J* 2014;14(3):397-407.

86. Devin CJ, Chotai S, McGirt MJ, et al: Intrawound vancomycin decreases the risk of surgical site infection after

posterior spine surgery-A multicenter analysis. *Spine (Phila Pa 1976)* 2015.

87. Kang DG, Holekamp TF, Wagner SC, Lehman RA Jr: Intrasite vancomycin powder for the prevention of surgical site infection in spine surgery: A systematic literature review. *Spine J* 2015;15(4):762-770.

88. O'Neill KR, Smith JG, Abtahi AM, et al: Reduced surgical site infections in patients undergoing posterior spinal stabilization of traumatic injuries using vancomycin powder. *Spine J* 2011;11(7):641-646.

89. Theologis AA, Demirkiran G, Callahan M, Pekmezci M, Ames C, Deviren V: Local intrawound vancomycin powder decreases the risk of surgical site infections in complex adult deformity reconstruction: A cost analysis. *Spine (Phila Pa 1976)* 2014;39(22):1875-1880.

90. Emohare O, Ledonio CG, Hill BW, Davis RA, Polly DW Jr, Kang MM: Cost savings analysis of intrawound vancomycin powder in posterior spinal surgery. *Spine J* 2014;14(11):2710-2715.

Update in Pediatric Musculoskeletal Infections: When It Is, When It Isn't, and What to Do

Alexandre Arkader, MD

Christopher M. Brusalis, BA

William C. Warner Jr, MD

James H. Conway, MD

Kenneth Noonan, MD

Abstract

Musculoskeletal infections, including osteomyelitis, septic arthritis, and pyomyositis, are a substantial cause of morbidity in children and adolescents. The increased virulence of infectious agents and the increased prevalence of antimicrobial-resistant pathogens, particularly methicillin-resistant Staphylococcus aureus, *have resulted in a more complicated clinical course for diagnosis and management, which is evidenced by an increased length of hospital stays, incidence of complications, and number of surgical interventions. Musculoskeletal infections are a challenge for surgeons because they vary substantially in their presentation and in their required treatment, which is based on the causative organism, the location of the infection, and the age of the patient. The necessity for a prompt diagnosis is complicated by several diseases that may mimic musculoskeletal infection, including transient synovitis, autoimmune arthritis, and tumors. Recent innovations in diagnosis and management have provided surgeons with new options to differentiate musculoskeletal infections from these rapidly evolving disease pathologies. As diagnostic and treatment modalities improve, collaboration among surgeons from multiple disciplines is required to develop evidence-based clinical practice guidelines that minimize the effect of musculoskeletal infection and optimize clinical outcomes for patients.*

Instr Course Lect 2017;66:495–504.

Musculoskeletal infections are a substantial cause of morbidity and have potentially devastating consequences in children and adolescents.[1] Acute and subacute osteomyelitis have an estimated annual incidence of 13 per 100,000 children, which is twice the rate of septic arthritis, with an equal distribution between the sexes.[2,3] Musculoskeletal infections can extend length of hospital stays, with reports of mean hospital stays of 11 days for osteomyelitis, 8 days for pyomyositis, 6.4 days for septic arthritis, and 3.6 days for deep abscess.[1]

Although the early diagnosis of musculoskeletal infection is associated with improved patient outcomes, the myriad potential diagnoses that have

Dr. Arkader or an immediate family member serves as an unpaid consultant to OrthoPediatrics SAB. Dr. Warner or an immediate family member serves as an unpaid consultant to Medtronic Sofamor Danek. Dr. Conway or an immediate family member has received research or institutional support from Sanofi-Aventis and serves as a board member, owner, officer, or committee member of the Wisconsin Chapter of the American Academy of Pediatrics. Dr. Noonan or an immediate family member has received royalties from Biomet; serves as a paid consultant to or is an employee of Biomet; and has stock or stock options held in Fixx Orthopedics. Neither Mr. Brusalis nor any immediate family member has received anything of value from or has stock or stock options held in a commercial company or institution related directly or indirectly to the subject of this chapter.

shared characteristics with musculoskeletal infection is a challenge for surgeons.[4] In addition, the dynamic nature of infectious etiologies requires treatment regimens to evolve. The literature on musculoskeletal infections has expanded in recent years. Surgeons should understand the most recent advances in the field of musculoskeletal infection and be aware of evidence-based approaches to the identification and management of pediatric musculoskeletal infections.

Etiology

Primary septic arthritis is a result of hematogenous (most common) or direct inoculation. Secondary septic arthritis results from the spread of osteomyelitis in the joint and occurs at the point at which the metaphysis of the hip, shoulder, elbow, or ankle is intracapsular. Age plays a substantial role in the determination of the most likely causative organism. In children younger than 1 year, staphylococcal species cause most of the common nosocomial-acquired infections, and group B streptococci cause many neonatal community-acquired infections. In children younger than 5 years, *Staphylococcus aureus*, *Kingella kingae*, and *Streptococcus pneumoniae* are the predominant pathogens. The incidence of *Haemophilus influenzae* type b has decreased substantially with immunization.[1] *S aureus* is the primary source of musculoskeletal infection in children older than 5 years. *Neisseria gonorrhoeae* is a source of musculoskeletal infection in sexually active adolescents and should be considered in younger patients if sexual abuse is suspected or identified.

Despite this age-based variation in causative organism, *S aureus* is the dominant causative agent of infection. A distinction must be made between methicillin-susceptible *S aureus* (MSSA), community-acquired methicillin-resistant *S aureus* (CA-MRSA), and hospital-acquired MRSA. Bacteria gain resistance to β-lactam antibiotics via four types of staphylococcal cassette chromosomes, which are mobile forms of genetic material that can transfer specific genes from one genome to another. These four mobile elements allow transfer of the mecA gene to *S aureus*, with type I through type III staphylococcal cassette chromosomes conferring β-lactam resistance to hospital-acquired MRSA and type IV staphylococcal cassette chromosomes conferring β-lactam resistance to CA-MRSA. In turn, the mecA gene encodes for a form of penicillin-binding protein that has a low affinity for β-lactam antibiotics, which renders *S aureus* resistant to β-lactam antibiotics.[5-7]

The Panton–Valentine leukocidin (PVL) locus is another important genetic mutation that confers enhanced virulence to certain staphylococcal species.[5] Approximately 2% of patients with hospital-acquired MRSA possess the PVL gene, and most patients with CA-MRSA possess the PVL gene. The PVL gene encodes for the production of cytotoxin, which causes hospital-acquired MRSA and CA-MRSA to create lesions via lysis of neutrophils and cell necrosis.[7] PVL-positive strains of MSSA also have been reported to cause infection that is characterized by extensive cell necrosis.[8]

The prevalence of MRSA is rising, with reports of a threefold to tenfold increase in septic arthritis and acute osteomyelitis in the past decade.[9-11] In general, patients with MRSA have more extensive local soft-tissue destruction, a more rapid spread of infection, and higher overall mortality rates.[9] Studies have reported that MRSA leads to an increased length of hospital stay, a greater need for surgical intervention, and admission to an intensive care unit.[10,12-14] In addition, patients with MRSA have an increased risk for complications, including persistent bacteremia, deep vein thrombosis, septic pulmonary emboli, and pathologic fracture.[15,16]

In parallel with the emergence of MRSA as a substantial cause of musculoskeletal infection, other organisms also have been increasingly recognized as causative agents of infection.[17] *K kingae*, a gram-negative coccobacillus, is a substantial cause of osteoarthritis infection in children younger than 4 years[18-20] and may account for as many as 50% of septic arthritis cases in children younger than 2 years.[19,20] *K kingae* is able to be identified as a result of improved culture techniques and the use of molecular diagnostic methods, such as *K kingae*-specific real-time polymerase chain reaction (PCR).[21] *K kingae* is common in the oropharyngeal flora of young children.[22] *K kingae* produces a repeats-in-toxin cytotoxin, which allows it to colonize the respiratory tract, invade the bloodstream, and, ultimately, infect bone and joint tissue.[23] A recently developed oropharyngeal swab PCR assay that was conducted in 40 children demonstrated a 100% sensitivity and a 90.5% specificity for the diagnosis of *K kingae*.[24]

Although *K kingae* more often presents as a subacute infection, the musculoskeletal system is the most common site of infection for invasive *K kingae* strains.[25] Patients appear only mildly ill and have normal or modest elevations in erythrocyte sedimentation rate (ESR) and C-reactive protein (CRP) levels.[25] *Pseudomonas*, enteric gram-negative bacteria, fungal osteomyelitis, and anaerobic osteomyelitis are rare in healthy patients but can be substantial pathogens or co-pathogens that lead to a poor treatment response.[26,27]

Evaluation

The adoption of a multidisciplinary team facilitates an efficient approach to the diagnostic workup of a patient with musculoskeletal infection. In addition to obtaining a complete history of illness, a physical examination must be performed with the understanding that findings vary based on the stage of infection; early infection may reveal few abnormal findings.[28] A systematic review of more than 12,000 patients identified pain (81%), localized signs and symptoms (70%), reduced range of motion (50%), and reduced weight bearing (50%) as the most frequent clinical findings.[17]

Children with septic arthritis often are younger than 2 years. The hip is the most common location of septic arthritis. The physical examination of a patient with septic arthritis will reveal an irritable joint with the hip in flexion, external rotation, and abduction. Infants may only have malaise and/or listlessness. In a retrospective analysis of 27 children with MRSA, Vander Have et al[13] reported that 17 of the children had a temperature higher than 101.3°F (38.5°C). Given the risk of complications associated with delayed diagnosis, it is important to recognize atypical presentations of infection.

Laboratory Studies

Patients who have a suspected musculoskeletal infection warrant routine laboratory studies, including a complete blood count with differential, blood chemistries, ESR, CRP levels, and blood cultures.[5,29] Pääkkönen et al[30] demonstrated the value of measuring ESR and CRP levels at the time a patient is admitted to the hospital in a review of 265 children who had a culture-positive osteoarticular infection. The authors reported that 94% of the patients had an ESR that exceeded 20 mm/h, and 95% of the patients had a CRP level greater than 200 mg/L. The continued measurement of CRP levels to monitor a patient's response to antibiotic therapy has been reported to shorten the length of hospital stay.[31] Although the early initiation of antibiotics is important, it is critical to obtain blood cultures before beginning antibiotic therapy because it may be a surgeon's only opportunity to obtain a positive culture that helps guide subsequent treatment.[5,29]

If concern for a septic joint exists, a synovial fluid analysis via joint aspiration is essential. Synovial fluid analysis findings that strongly favor the diagnosis of infection include a cloudy or purulent synovial fluid appearance; a white blood cell count greater than 100,000 cells/μL with more than 90% polymorphonuclear neutrophils; and a glucose level 50 mg/dL less than serum glucose levels. Gram stain and cultures with susceptibility testing should be ordered and include aerobic and anaerobic cultures because some aerobic pathogens grow better in microaerophilic conditions. Immunocompromised patients, patients who fail to respond to treatment, and children from particular endemic regions should have specimens sent for fungal as well as mycobacterial stains and cultures.[32] A Lyme titer (usually an enzyme-linked immunosorbent assay with Western blotting) and a Lyme PCR from joint fluid should be considered in patients from other endemic regions. Lyme disease can often present as monoarticular arthritis of the knee, and patients who have Lyme disease typically appear to have less toxicity compared with patients who have pyogenic septic arthritis.

The use of PCR and 16-second ribosomal RNA gene sequencing is an emerging and rapid method that is used to identify bacteria, particularly MRSA. Although not widely available, the routine use of PCR and 16-second ribosomal RNA gene sequencing is advantageous for the identification of an infectious etiology in patients with low inoculum, in patients with difficult-to-culture organisms, and in patients in whom antibiotics have been started.

The creation of diagnostic algorithms that are based on clinical and laboratory data to help establish the likelihood of infection in patients with various clinical presentations and distinguish between MSSA and MRSA is a particular area of active research. Patients who have MSSA and MRSA appear to have no differences in symptom duration before hospital admission, and the presence of MSSA and MRSA cannot be accurately predicted based on antibiotic use before hospital admission.[33,34] MRSA is associated with higher ESR, CRP levels, and white blood cell (WBC) count.[12,33,34] Ju et al[11] designed a clinical prediction algorithm to differentiate between MRSA and MSSA based on four predictor parameters: a temperature higher than 100.4°F (38°C), a WBC count greater than 12,000 cells/μL, a hematocrit level less than 34%, and a CRP level greater than 13 mg/L. The authors applied the clinical prediction algorithm in a retrospective analysis of 129 children, and reported that the probability of MRSA osteomyelitis increased with the addition of each predictor: zero for no predictors, 1% for one predictor, 10% for two predictors, 45% for three predictors, and 92% for all four predictors. However, Wade Schrader et al[35] reported that the presence of all four predictors from the clinical prediction algorithm described by Ju et al[11] resulted in a probability of MRSA infection of approximately 50%. The poor performance of the clinical prediction algorithm described by Ju et al[11] suggests that regional differences in bacterial strains and/or patient populations are critical to the interpretation of laboratory data.[36]

Recent investigations have focused on the early diagnosis and management of musculoskeletal infections.[37] Serum procalcitonin has emerged as a new marker for infection. The normally low level of serum procalcitonin (<0.1 ng/mL) in humans is increased drastically if bacterial endotoxin is present.[38] A prospective study of 82 patients reported that a serum procalcitonin level greater than 0.4 ng/mL was 85.2% sensitive and 87.3% specific for the diagnosis of septic arthritis and acute osteomyelitis.[39] Further studies are necessary to evaluate the clinical utility of serum procalcitonin as a marker for infection.

Real-time PCR may help guide antibiotic therapy until culture results become available. In a study of tissue specimens from 20 children, the sensitivity of real-time PCR for the diagnosis of septic arthritis was higher compared with that of traditional microbiological culture (0.79 versus 0.47, respectively); however, both methods had a specificity for the diagnosis of septic arthritis of 1.00.[40]

Imaging Studies

Radiographs should always be obtained in patients with a suspected musculoskeletal infection. Although radiographs are often normal in the initial phases of infection, periosteal reaction, osteolysis, joint space widening, and soft-tissue changes may develop. Ultrasonography may help identify soft-tissue swelling, subperiosteal abscess, and joint effusion as well as aid in joint aspiration (**Figure 1**).

MRI is beneficial if the diagnosis of acute hematogenous osteomyelitis remains unclear after clinical evaluation and radiographic imaging. MRI can reveal fluid collections, effusion, or other potential bone involvement and can help rule out concomitant pathology.[41] In addition, MRI more readily identifies the full extent of infection and can increase suspicion for septic arthritis, osteomyelitis, pyomyositis, subperiosteal abscess, or a combination of these entities[41-44] (**Figure 2**). To increase the availability of MRI, one pediatric institution successfully implemented a daily imaging timeframe dedicated for patients with suspected musculoskeletal infection.[29]

Although gadolinium-enhanced MRI has been reported to detect the presence of abscess, there is conflicting evidence on whether the routine use of gadolinium-enhanced MRI is warranted. Kan et al[45] reported no statistically significant improvement in the sensitivity of pregadolinium MRI (89%) and postgadolinium MRI (91%) for the diagnosis of osteomyelitis. Conversely, Browne et al[46] reported that contrast-enhanced MRI was useful in the diagnosis of infection in patients younger than 18 months, identifying 7 of 9 infections of unossified growth cartilage that appeared normal on noncontrast MRI.

A posttreatment protocol that incorporated positron emission tomography

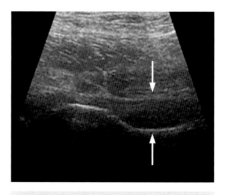

Figure 1 Point-of-care ultrasonogram of a left hip shows joint effusion (arrows).

and CT was reported to be superior in the differentiation of infection and reparative activity in pediatric patients who were recovering from acute osteomyelitis compared with MRI.[47] Ongoing efforts are being made to evaluate and standardize posttreatment protocols; however, a diagnostic algorithm that reliably translates between all geographic regions has yet to be successfully developed and implemented.[37]

Differential Diagnosis

Many of the signs and symptoms of musculoskeletal infection are nonspecific, and the differential diagnosis for a child with a limp and/or pain, with or without a fever, is broad. Three differential diagnoses that should be considered are transient synovitis, juvenile idiopathic arthritis, and neoplastic conditions.

Transient Synovitis

Transient synovitis, which is an inflammation of the synovium, can occur in any large joint but is most common in the hip. The incidence of transient synovitis is 0.2%, with a 2:1 male-to-female ratio and a mean age of presentation of 6 years.[48] Often, patients with transient synovitis have a history of upper

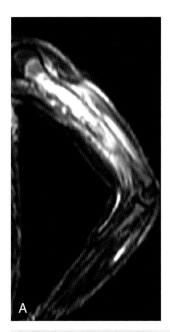
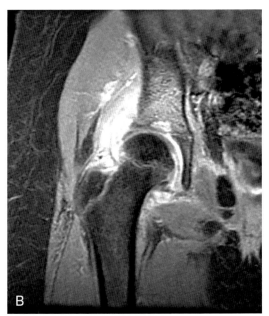

Figure 2   A, Sagittal T2-weighted MRI of a humerus shows a hyperintense signal within the humeral shaft, which is evidence of acute osteomyelitis. Note that the amount of bony involvement may be overestimated because areas of inflammation return a similar pattern. **B,** Coronal T1-weighted MRI of a right hip shows features of acute osteomyelitis, including soft-tissue edema, mild effusion, and an area of hyperintensity in the acetabulum.

respiratory infection. Transient synovitis presents acutely as an irritable hip in a limping child who has decreased internal rotation on physical examination. Patients with transient synovitis often have a less severe clinical presentation (less pain and lower fever) compared with patients who have septic arthritis. Transient synovitis usually is self-limited and only requires symptomatic treatment for 1 to 2 weeks. Patients with transient synovitis have a recurrence rate as high as 20%.[49]

The Kocher criteria were developed as a set of clinical prediction rules to help surgeons differentiate between septic arthritis and transient synovitis of the hip and have been successfully applied in other anatomic locations.[50,51] Four predictors (a history of fever, non–weight-bearing status, an ESR greater than 40 mm/h, and a serum WBC count greater than 12,000 cells/μL) correlate with an increased probability of septic arthritis. Caird et al[52] reported that a CRP level greater than 20 mg/L was a strong independent predictor for septic arthritis, whereas a normal CRP level indicated a decreased likelihood of infection. Such clinical prediction rules are not intended for strict use and should not be a substitute for clinical judgment.

Juvenile Idiopathic Arthritis

Juvenile idiopathic arthritis is an autoimmune-mediated disorder that is characterized by chronic joint inflammation. The estimated incidence of juvenile idiopathic arthritis is 6 per 10,000 children, most commonly occurring in children aged 7 to 12 years.[53] Patients with juvenile idiopathic arthritis often have a fever, a rash, and joint involvement. The pattern of joint involvement is often migratory and polyarticular; however, it can be monoarticular or pauciarticular. Diagnostic criteria for juvenile idiopathic arthritis include a fever for at least 2 weeks and joint effusion for at least 6 weeks.[54] Juvenile idiopathic arthritis most commonly occurs in the knee (two-thirds of patients), followed by the ankle. Synovial fluid analysis findings that indicate juvenile idiopathic arthritis include a WBC count between 25,000 to 100,000 cells/μL with fewer than 75% polymorphonuclear neutrophils and an intermediate glucose level.

Neoplastic Conditions

Surgeons who evaluate children with joint involvement and/or limb pain must always consider the possibility of malignancy.[55] **Table 1** lists examples of neoplasms that resemble infection. Patients who have musculoskeletal manifestations of acute leukemia are sometimes misdiagnosed with osteomyelitis or septic arthritis.[56-58] Because of their small bone marrow reserve, 50% to 75% of children with acute leukemia have skeletal lesions, and 30% of children with acute leukemia have musculoskeletal symptoms. Occasionally, neoplastic conditions may be associated with normal peripheral hematologic counts.[58]

Treatment

Treatment of musculoskeletal infection is time-sensitive. The release of proteolytic enzymes in the joint leads to articular damage within 8 hours of onset, which increases intracapsular pressure and, ultimately, causes venous stasis and osteonecrosis. Early empiric antibiotic therapy and drainage with irrigation are the primary treatment methods for

Table 1

Neoplastic Conditions That Resemble Infection

Neoplasm	Infection	Common Features	Distinguishing Features of Neoplasm
Leukemia	Acute osteomyelitis	Fatigue, fever, pallor, bone and joint pain Increased ESR, increased CRP	Leukopenia, peripheral blood smear often has immature leukocytes Anemia, neutropenia, or thrombocytopenia in 80% of patients
Osteosarcoma	Acute osteomyelitis	Pain associated with a mass Location: metaphysis, knee, shoulder	Normal laboratory results (elevated alkaline phosphatase level)
Ewing sarcoma	Acute osteomyelitis	Pain associated with a palpable mass Fever, weight loss, night pain, sweats, or chills	Imaging: moth-eaten pattern of bone destruction in diaphyseal/metadiaphyseal region
Chondroblastoma	Subacute osteomyelitis	Insidious onset with localized tenderness in the involved bone and adjacent joint Joint effusion, limp, muscle wasting	Histopathology: compact areas of chondroblasts with well-defined cytoplasmic borders that are surrounded by scattered multinucleated giant cells Chicken-wire appearance
Primary lymphoma of bone	Chronic osteomyelitis	Insidious pain associated with a bone lesion Imaging: poorly defined sclerotic lesion, more often in long bone metaphysis	Histopathology: tumor stains positive for CD20, Ki-67, CD45, CD19
Metastatic neuroblastoma	Chronic osteomyelitis	Pain, limp, fever, and metastatic lesion in long bone metaphysis	Elevated VMA or HVA urinary or serum levels

CD = cluster of differentiation, CRP = C-reactive protein level, ESR = erythrocyte sedimentation rate, HVA = homovanillic acid, VMA = vanillylmandelic acid.

septic arthritis. Surgical intervention may be required in some patients who have osteomyelitis.

Septic Arthritis

Empiric intravenous antibiotic therapy is a mainstay of treatment for MSSA. Although a recent report suggested that the administration of antibiotics before culture samples are obtained may not interfere with aerobic culture results,[59] most surgeons strongly recommend withholding antibiotics until blood cultures and, if appropriate, joint fluid cultures have been obtained. In children younger than 5 years, either a semisynthetic penicillin derivative with activity against staphylococci (eg, oxacillin or nafcillin) or a first-generation cephalosporin is used for treatment; however, a second- or third- generation cephalosporin may instead be used for treatment to provide additional coverage for respiratory pathogens (eg, streptococci, *Kingella*) and Lyme disease.[22] In children aged 5 to 12 years, a first-generation cephalosporin is most commonly used for treatment. For sexually active adolescents, a more advanced-generation cephalosporin is often used for treatment to provide coverage for gonococcus. Surgeons must be aware of a child's immunization status because children that have not been immunized against *H influenzae* type b are at risk for septic arthritis and have an increased risk for meningitis.

Adjustments to this antibiotic regimen is recommended in regions in which CA-MRSA accounts for at least 10% of *S aureus* isolates. Vancomycin or clindamycin is used in combination with MSSA-specific antibiotics as first-line agents, depending on local susceptibility patterns.[59] Higher doses of vancomycin are recommended for many patients with musculoskeletal infections to optimize antibiotic penetration. If clindamycin is used to treat MRSA, the hospital laboratory should perform an erythromycin-clindamycin D-zone test to detect inducible clindamycin resistance.

Empiric antibiotic regimens for patients who have septic arthritis are adjusted for regional susceptibility patterns and modified as culture results become available. In general, the total duration of antibiotic therapy for patients who have septic arthritis ranges from 2 to 4 weeks, depending on the pathogen and clinical response.[60] Conversion from parenteral antibiotic therapy to enteral antibiotic therapy varies widely based on a large number of factors but generally occurs after a patient has substantial clinical improvement, a substantial decrease in inflammatory markers, and a resolution of systemic symptoms.

CRP levels can be used to monitor a patient's early response to antibiotic therapy, and ESR is more effective for monitoring a patient's response to antibiotic therapy over a longer period of time. Equivalent outcomes were reported in select uncomplicated patients with acute osteomyelitis who were transitioned to an oral antibiotic agent after a short course of intravenous antibiotic therapy and patients with acute osteomyelitis those who underwent prolonged intravenous antibiotic therapy alone.[61] The transition to an oral antibiotic agent that is guided by a combination of clinical findings and CRP levels also reduces the risk of complications associated with a peripherally placed central intravenous catheter.[62] Antibiotic resistance is a pervasive issue, with increasing reports of drug-resistant organisms that cause infections.

Joint decompression (arthrotomy or arthroscopy) is always necessary for patients who have septic arthritis. All areas of devitalized tissue, including soft-tissue collections, joint effusions, and subperiosteal abscesses, must be débrided.[29] Although arthrotomy has been the preferred surgical technique, arthroscopy has been reported to result in equivalent outcomes.[63,64] Drains are used on a patient-by-patient basis for up to 2 to 3 days postoperatively to allow for continued efflux of blood and fluids that may serve as a nidus for infection; however, evidence to support the use of drains is sparse. If drainage persists beyond 2 to 3 days postoperatively, the patient should undergo repeat surgical decompression. Revision surgery also is warranted if patients do not show clinical and laboratory improvement. Serial aspirations may be a useful alternative for patients in whom surgical intervention is contraindicated. In a study of 34 children who had septic arthritis of the hip joint, Givon et al[65] reported that repeat joint aspiration with the guidance of ultrasonography was a safe and effective alternative to surgical intervention, allowing 24 of the patients to avoid surgery.

Acute Osteomyelitis

Similar to patients with septic arthritis, antibiotic selection for patients who have acute osteomyelitis is based on empiric antibiotic regimens that are adjusted as culture results become available. Traditionally, the suggested duration of antibiotic therapy for patients who have acute osteomyelitis ranges from 4 to 6 weeks;[60] however, recent evidence suggests that a shorter duration of antibiotic therapy may be sufficient for uncomplicated patients. In a randomized controlled trial of 131 children who had acute osteomyelitis, Peltola et al[61] reported that a 20-day course of oral antibiotic therapy after 2 to 4 days of intravenous antibiotic therapy was equivalent to a 30-day course of oral antibiotic therapy after 2 to 4 days of intravenous antibiotic therapy. Irrigation and débridement are not necessarily required in patients who have acute osteomyelitis because antibiotics may be sufficient to clear infection. Surgery may be delayed or avoided in patients who are clinically stable and have positive blood cultures and in patients who are not clinically stable for surgery. Radiographic imaging features that favor surgical intervention include the presence of subperiosteal abscess, evidence of bone necrosis, or direct invasion of the growth plate. Because acute osteomyelitis more directly involves metaphyseal bone, surgical intervention, if performed, often incorporates a cortical window that is created under fluoroscopic guidance to help decompress devitalized tissue without damaging the adjacent physis.[5,29]

Patients who have acute osteomyelitis must be monitored for several known complications, including persistent bacteremia, deep vein thrombosis, and pathologic fractures.[16,66] Hollmig et al[15] reported that children older than 8 years with MRSA and a CRP level greater than 60 mg/L had a 40% increased risk for deep vein thrombosis. Some studies recommend the use of ultrasonography in all patients who have a bone or joint MRSA infection to evaluate for deep vein thrombosis.[5] After discharge from the hospital, the frequency of clinical and laboratory monitoring for medication toxicities and response to antibiotic therapy is on a patient-by-patient basis. Because of the long-term effects of some complications of acute osteomyelitis, such as growth arrest leading to limb-length discrepancy and/or angular deformity, continued follow-up care is essential.[5] Other long-term complications of acute osteomyelitis include osteonecrosis, chronic osteomyelitis, gait abnormalities, and premature arthritis.

Improvement in the ability to treat pediatric musculoskeletal infections ultimately requires multidisciplinary coordination.[67] Copley et al[68] organized a team that consisted of individuals from several hospital services, including orthopaedics, general pediatrics, infectious disease, nursing, and social work, to implement treatment guidelines for patients who had osteomyelitis. The treatment guidelines for patients who had osteomyelitis included MRI that was performed within 24 hours of admission, antibiotics that were withheld until culture results were available, ESR and CRP levels that were measured every 48 hours during a patient's hospital stay, and intravenous antibiotics that were continued until CRP levels were less than 20 mg/L with a benign clinical course. Patients were not discharged until they were afebrile, were pain free, were cleared by a physical therapist, had a CRP level less than 20 mg/L, and had home antibiotics arranged. The authors reported that, compared with patients with osteomyelitis who were treated before the implementation of the treatment guidelines, patients with osteomyelitis who were treated after the implementation of the treatment guidelines trended toward a shorter length of hospital stay and a lower hospital readmission rate.

Summary

Although MRSA has become a substantial cause of musculoskeletal infections in children, new diagnostic tools have allowed for better recognition of other infectious agents, including *K kingae*, streptococcal species, fungi, mycobacteria, *Pseudomonas*, and anaerobic species. In addition to traditional clinical evaluation and laboratory markers, the early, judicious use of MRI may help differentiate infectious causes from noninfectious diagnoses, including neoplastic conditions. Antibiotic selection should be made with a consideration of regional antibiotic susceptibilities, and response to antibiotic treatment should be confirmed via careful serial physical examinations and monitoring of ESR and CRP levels. Close follow-up care

after initial diagnosis and treatment of infection is critical given that complications of infection include deep vein thrombosis, pathologic fracture, chronic osteomyelitis, and growth arrest.

Technologic advances may provide surgeons with a greater ability to identify specific causative organisms; however, current diagnostic algorithms that differentiate between multiple overlapping disease presentations have failed to translate between different geographic regions. Ultimately, collaboration between orthopaedic surgeons and other clinical and administrative personnel is necessary to optimize the management of pediatric musculoskeletal infections.

References

1. Gafur OA, Copley LA, Hollmig ST, Browne RH, Thornton LA, Crawford SE: The impact of the current epidemiology of pediatric musculoskeletal infection on evaluation and treatment guidelines. *J Pediatr Orthop* 2008;28(7):777-785.

2. Riise OR, Kirkhus E, Handeland KS, et al: Childhood osteomyelitis-incidence and differentiation from other acute onset musculoskeletal features in a population-based study. *BMC Pediatr* 2008;8:45.

3. Dodwell ER: Osteomyelitis and septic arthritis in children: Current concepts. *Curr Opin Pediatr* 2013;25(1):58-63.

4. Blyth MJ, Kincaid R, Craigen MA, Bennet GC: The changing epidemiology of acute and subacute haematogenous osteomyelitis in children. *J Bone Joint Surg Br* 2001;83(1):99-102.

5. Pendleton A, Kocher MS: Methicillin-resistant staphylococcus aureus bone and joint infections in children. *J Am Acad Orthop Surg* 2015;23(1):29-37.

6. Hiramatsu K, Cui L, Kuroda M, Ito T: The emergence and evolution of methicillin-resistant Staphylococcus aureus. *Trends Microbiol* 2001;9(10):486-493.

7. Chambers HF, Deleo FR: Waves of resistance: Staphylococcus aureus in the antibiotic era. *Nat Rev Microbiol* 2009;7(9):629-641.

8. Boan P, Tan HL, Pearson J, Coombs G, Heath CH, Robinson JO: Epidemiological, clinical, outcome and antibiotic susceptibility differences between PVL positive and PVL negative Staphylococcus aureus infections in Western Australia: A case control study. *BMC Infect Dis* 2015;15:10.

9. Arnold SR, Elias D, Buckingham SC, et al: Changing patterns of acute hematogenous osteomyelitis and septic arthritis: Emergence of community-associated methicillin-resistant Staphylococcus aureus. *J Pediatr Orthop* 2006;26(6):703-708.

10. Sarkissian EJ, Gans I, Gunderson MA, Myers SH, Spiegel DA, Flynn JM: Community-acquired methicillin-resistant staphylococcus aureus musculoskeletal infections: Emerging trends over the past decade. *J Pediatr Orthop* 2016;36(3):323-327.

11. Ju KL, Zurakowski D, Kocher MS: Differentiating between methicillin-resistant and methicillin-sensitive Staphylococcus aureus osteomyelitis in children: An evidence-based clinical prediction algorithm. *J Bone Joint Surg Am* 2011;93(18):1693-1701.

12. Hawkshead JJ III, Patel NB, Steele RW, Heinrich SD: Comparative severity of pediatric osteomyelitis attributable to methicillin-resistant versus methicillin-sensitive Staphylococcus aureus. *J Pediatr Orthop* 2009;29(1):85-90.

13. Vander Have KL, Karmazyn B, Verma M, et al: Community-associated methicillin-resistant Staphylococcus aureus in acute musculoskeletal infection in children: A game changer. *J Pediatr Orthop* 2009;29(8):927-931.

14. Goergens ED, McEvoy A, Watson M, Barrett IR: Acute osteomyelitis and septic arthritis in children. *J Paediatr Child Health* 2005;41(1-2):59-62.

15. Hollmig ST, Copley LA, Browne RH, Grande LM, Wilson PL: Deep venous thrombosis associated with osteomyelitis in children. *J Bone Joint Surg Am* 2007;89(7):1517-1523.

16. Belthur MV, Birchansky SB, Verdugo AA, et al: Pathologic fractures in children with acute Staphylococcus aureus osteomyelitis. *J Bone Joint Surg Am* 2012;94(1):34-42.

17. Dartnell J, Ramachandran M, Katchburian M: Haematogenous acute and subacute paediatric osteomyelitis: A systematic review of the literature. *J Bone Joint Surg Br* 2012;94(5):584-595.

18. Chometon S, Benito Y, Chaker M, et al: Specific real-time polymerase chain reaction places Kingella kingae as the most common cause of osteoarticular infections in young children. *Pediatr Infect Dis J* 2007;26(5):377-381.

19. Ceroni D, Cherkaoui A, Ferey S, Kaelin A, Schrenzel J: Kingella kingae osteoarticular infections in young children: Clinical features and contribution of a new specific real-time PCR assay to the diagnosis. *J Pediatr Orthop* 2010;30(3):301-304.

20. Ilharreborde B, Bidet P, Lorrot M, et al: New real-time PCR-based method for Kingella kingae DNA detection: Application to samples collected from 89 children with acute arthritis. *J Clin Microbiol* 2009;47(6):1837-1841.

21. Yagupsky P: Kingella kingae: From medical rarity to an emerging paediatric pathogen. *Lancet Infect Dis* 2004;4(6):358-367.

22. Yagupsky P, Weiss-Salz I, Fluss R, et al: Dissemination of Kingella kingae in the community and long-term persistence of invasive clones. *Pediatr Infect Dis J* 2009,28(8):707-710.

23. Kehl-Fie TE, St Geme JW III: Identification and characterization of an RTX toxin in the emerging pathogen Kingella kingae. *J Bacteriol* 2007;189(2):430-436.

24. Ceroni D, Dubois-Ferriere V, Cherkaoui A, et al: Detection of Kingella kingae osteoarticular infections in children by oropharyngeal swab PCR. *Pediatrics* 2013;131(1):e230-e235.

25. Dubnov-Raz G, Ephros M, Garty BZ, et al: Invasive pediatric Kingella kingae infections: A nationwide collaborative study. *Pediatr Infect Dis J* 2010;29(7):639-643.

26. Gamaletsou MN, Kontoyiannis DP, Sipsas NV, et al: Candida osteomyelitis: Analysis of 207 pediatric and adult cases (1970-2011). *Clin Infect Dis* 2012;55(10):1338-1351.

27. Espinosa CM, Davis MM, Gilsdorf JR: Anaerobic osteomyelitis in children. *Pediatr Infect Dis J* 2011; 30(5):422-423.

28. Copley LA, Barton T, Garcia C, et al: A proposed scoring system for assessment of severity of illness in pediatric acute hematogenous osteomyelitis using objective clinical and laboratory findings. *Pediatr Infect Dis J* 2014; 33(1):35-41.

29. Copley LA: Pediatric musculoskeletal infection: Trends and antibiotic recommendations. *J Am Acad Orthop Surg* 2009;17(10):618-626.

30. Pääkkönen M, Kallio MJ, Kallio PE, Peltola H: Sensitivity of erythrocyte sedimentation rate and C-reactive protein in childhood bone and joint infections. *Clin Orthop Relat Res* 2010;468(3):861-866.

31. Pääkkönen M, Kallio MJ, Kallio PE, Peltola H: Shortened hospital stay for childhood bone and joint infections: Analysis of 265 prospectively collected culture-positive cases in 1983-2005. *Scand J Infect Dis* 2012;44(9):683-688.

32. Section J, Gibbons SD, Barton T, Greenberg DE, Jo CH, Copley LA: Microbiological culture methods for pediatric musculoskeletal infection: A guideline for optimal use. *J Bone Joint Surg Am* 2015;97(6):441-449.

33. Saavedra-Lozano J, Mejías A, Ahmad N, et al: Changing trends in acute osteomyelitis in children: Impact of methicillin-resistant Staphylococcus aureus infections. *J Pediatr Orthop* 2008;28(5):569-575.

34. Erdem G, Salazar R, Kimata C, et al: Staphylococcus aureus osteomyelitis in Hawaii. *Clin Pediatr (Phila)* 2010;49(5):477-484.

35. Wade Shrader M, Nowlin M, Segal LS: Independent analysis of a clinical predictive algorithm to identify methicillin-resistant Staphylococcus aureus osteomyelitis in children. *J Pediatr Orthop* 2013;33(7):759-762.

36. Luhmann SJ, Jones A, Schootman M, Gordon JE, Schoenecker PL, Luhmann JD: Differentiation between septic arthritis and transient synovitis of the hip in children with clinical prediction algorithms. *J Bone Joint Surg Am* 2004;86(5):956-962.

37. Montgomery NI, Rosenfeld S: Pediatric osteoarticular infection update. *J Pediatr Orthop* 2015;35(1):74-81.

38. Barassi A, Pallotti F, Melzi d'Eril G: Biological variation of procalcitonin in healthy individuals. *Clin Chem* 2004;50(10):1878.

39. Maharajan K, Patro DK, Menon J, et al: Serum Procalcitonin is a sensitive and specific marker in the diagnosis of septic arthritis and acute osteomyelitis. *J Orthop Surg Res* 2013;8:19.

40. Choe H, Inaba Y, Kobayashi N, et al: Use of real-time polymerase chain reaction for the diagnosis of infection and differentiation between gram-positive and gram-negative septic arthritis in children. *J Pediatr Orthop* 2013;33(3):e28-e33.

41. Monsalve J, Kan JH, Schallert EK, Bisset GS, Zhang W, Rosenfeld SB: Septic arthritis in children: Frequency of coexisting unsuspected osteomyelitis and implications on imaging work-up and management. *AJR Am J Roentgenol* 2015;204(6):1289-1295.

42. Mignemi ME, Menge TJ, Cole HA, et al: Epidemiology, diagnosis, and treatment of pericapsular pyomyositis of the hip in children. *J Pediatr Orthop* 2014;34(3):316-325.

43. Courtney PM, Flynn JM, Jaramillo D, Horn BD, Calabro K, Spiegel DA: Clinical indications for repeat MRI in children with acute hematogenous osteomyelitis. *J Pediatr Orthop* 2010;30(8):883-887.

44. Jaramillo D, Treves ST, Kasser JR, Harper M, Sundel R, Laor T: Osteomyelitis and septic arthritis in children: Appropriate use of imaging to guide treatment. *AJR Am J Roentgenol* 1995;165(2):399-403.

45. Kan JH, Young RS, Yu C, Hernanz-Schulman M: Clinical impact of gadolinium in the MRI diagnosis of musculoskeletal infection in children. *Pediatr Radiol* 2010;40(7):1197-1205.

46. Browne LP, Guillerman RP, Orth RC, Patel J, Mason EO, Kaplan SL: Community-acquired staphylococcal musculoskeletal infection in infants and young children: Necessity of contrast-enhanced MRI for the diagnosis of growth cartilage involvement. *AJR Am J Roentgenol* 2012;198(1):194-199.

47. Warmann SW, Dittmann H, Seitz G, Bares R, Fuchs J, Schäfer JF: Follow-up of acute osteomyelitis in children: The possible role of PET/CT in selected cases. *J Pediatr Surg* 2011;46(8):1550-1556.

48. Landin LA, Danielsson LG, Wattsgård C: Transient synovitis of the hip: Its incidence, epidemiology and relation to Perthes' disease. *J Bone Joint Surg Br* 1987;69(2):238-242.

49. Asche SS, van Rijn RM, Bessems JH, Krul M, Bierma-Zeinstra SM: What is the clinical course of transient synovitis in children: A systematic review of the literature. *Chiropr Man Therap* 2013;21(1):39.

50. Kocher MS, Zurakowski D, Kasser JR: Differentiating between septic arthritis and transient synovitis of the hip in children: An evidence-based clinical prediction algorithm. *J Bone Joint Surg Am* 1999;81(12):1662-1670.

51. Kocher MS, Mandiga R, Zurakowski D, Barnewolt C, Kasser JR: Validation of a clinical prediction rule for the differentiation between septic arthritis and transient synovitis of the hip in children. *J Bone Joint Surg Am* 2004;86(8):1629-1635.

52. Caird MS, Flynn JM, Leung YL, Millman JE, D'Italia JG, Dormans JP: Factors distinguishing septic arthritis from transient synovitis of the hip in children: A prospective study. *J Bone Joint Surg Am* 2006;88(6):1251-1257.

53. Behrens EM, Beukelman T, Gallo L, et al: Evaluation of the presentation of systemic onset juvenile rheumatoid arthritis: Data from the Pennsylvania Systemic Onset Juvenile Arthritis Registry (PASOJAR). *J Rheumatol* 2008;35(2):343-348.

54. Petty RE, Southwood TR, Manners P, et al: International League of Associations for Rheumatology classification of juvenile idiopathic arthritis: Second revision, Edmonton, 2001. *J Rheumatol* 2004;31(2):390-392.

55. Brix N, Rosthøj S, Herlin T, Hasle H: Arthritis as presenting manifestation of acute lymphoblastic leukaemia in children. *Arch Dis Child* 2015;100(9):821-825.

56. Sinigaglia R, Gigante C, Bisinella G, Varotto S, Zanesco L, Turra S: Musculoskeletal manifestations in pediatric acute leukemia. *J Pediatr Orthop* 2008;28(1):20-28.

57. Riccio I, Marcarelli M, Del Regno N, et al: Musculoskeletal problems in pediatric acute leukemia. *J Pediatr Orthop B* 2013;22(3):264-269.

58. Cabral DA, Tucker LB: Malignancies in children who initially present with rheumatic complaints. *J Pediatr* 1999;134(1):53-57.

59. Kaplan SL: Recent lessons for the management of bone and joint infections. *J Infect* 2014;68(suppl 1):S51-S56.

60. Vinod MB, Matussek J, Curtis N, Graham HK, Carapetis JR: Duration of antibiotics in children with osteomyelitis and septic arthritis. *J Paediatr Child Health* 2002;38(4):363-367.

61. Peltola H, Pääkkönen M, Kallio P, Kallio MJ; Osteomyelitis-Septic Arthritis Study Group: Short- versus long-term antimicrobial treatment for acute hematogenous osteomyelitis of childhood: Prospective, randomized trial on 131 culture-positive cases. *Pediatr Infect Dis J* 2010;29(12):1123-1128.

62. Arnold JC, Cannavino CR, Ross MK, et al: Acute bacterial osteoarticular infections: Eight-year analysis of C-reactive protein for oral step-down therapy. *Pediatrics* 2012;130(4):e821-e828.

63. El-Sayed AM: Treatment of early septic arthritis of the hip in children: Comparison of results of open arthrotomy versus arthroscopic drainage. *J Child Orthop* 2008;2(3):229-237.

64. Nusem I, Jabur MK, Playford EG: Arthroscopic treatment of septic arthritis of the hip. *Arthroscopy* 2006;22(8):902.e1-902.e3.

65. Givon U, Liberman B, Schindler A, Blankstein A, Ganel A: Treatment of septic arthritis of the hip joint by repeated ultrasound-guided aspirations. *J Pediatr Orthop* 2004;24(3):266-270.

66. Lee CY, Lee YS, Tsao PC, Jeng MJ, Soong WJ: Musculoskeletal sepsis associated with deep vein thrombosis in a child. *Pediatr Neonatol* 2016;57(3):244-247.

67. Kocher MS, Mandiga R, Murphy JM, et al: A clinical practice guideline for treatment of septic arthritis in children: Efficacy in improving process of care and effect on outcome of septic arthritis of the hip. *J Bone Joint Surg Am* 2003;85(6):994-999.

68. Copley LA, Kinsler MA, Gheen T, Shar A, Sun D, Browne R: The impact of evidence-based clinical practice guidelines applied by a multidisciplinary team for the care of children with osteomyelitis. *J Bone Joint Surg Am* 2013;95(8):686-693.

Sports Medicine

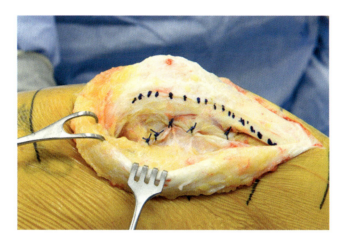

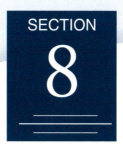

The Four Most Common Types of Knee Cartilage Damage Encountered in Practice: How and Why Orthopaedic Surgeons Manage Them

Brian J. Chilelli, MD
Brian J. Cole, MD, MBA
Jack Farr, MD
Christian Lattermann, MD
Andreas H. Gomoll, MD

Abstract

Cartilage damage of the knee is common and may present in patients as a variety of symptoms. These conditions can be classified based on location, etiology, and/or pathophysiology. A systematic approach to the evaluation and classification of chondral injuries helps improve definitive management. The four most common types of knee cartilage damage are osteochondritis dissecans, incidental chondral defects, patellofemoral defects, and defects encountered after meniscectomy.

Instr Course Lect 2017;66:507–530.

The field of cartilage repair continues to evolve rapidly, with new products regularly introduced in clinical practice. Concurrently, established procedures for cartilage repair, such as autologous chondrocyte implantation (ACI) and osteochondral allograft transplantation, have undergone improvements in techniques and availability. Collectively, these changes help make cartilage repair accessible to a wide range of patients and surgeons for a variety of indications. Education on cartilage repair also has evolved to incorporate a more case-based approach. Surgeons should understand the epidemiology of as well as how to diagnose and manage the four most common types of knee cartilage damage encountered in clinical practice: incidental chondral defects, osteochondritis dissecans (OCD), patellofemoral defects, and defects encountered after meniscectomy.

Incidental Chondral Defects

Chondral or osteochondral lesions have been reported in as many as 61% to 66% of patients who undergo knee arthroscopy.[1-3] Chondral and osteochondral lesions may be traumatic, idiopathic, or associated with repetitive microtrauma. Cartilage damage often is associated with injuries to other anatomic knee structures and may be observed in conjunction with malalignment. Meniscal derangement and acute anterior cruciate ligament (ACL) tears are highly correlated with chondral lesions.[4,5] Compressive and shear forces at the time of injury can lead to disruption of the osteochondral unit. In addition, chronic ligamentous instability or meniscal derangement can alter knee biomechanics and increase joint contact forces, which may result in damage to chondral surfaces and the underlying subchondral bone.

In a recent systematic review, Brophy et al[4] reported a 16% to 46% incidence of severe articular cartilage injury in patients who had acute ACL tears. Studies have reported a higher incidence of chondral and osteochondral injury with increasing time from ACL injury.[4,6-12] Sometimes the treating surgeon may be aware of a chondral defect based on preoperative imaging; at other times, a chondral defect may be unexpectedly discovered during arthroscopy that is performed to manage other ligamentous or meniscal injuries. The natural history of articular cartilage defects is not completely understood; however, full-thickness chondral defects are known to lack the ability to spontaneously heal.[13-15] If left untreated, chondral defects can lead to progressive joint degeneration and eventual osteoarthritis.[16,17] Because of poor understanding of the independent variables associated with defect progression, close monitoring of asymptomatic defects, rather than surgery, often is selected as a management strategy. Patients who have a suspected genetic predisposition to chondral or osteochondral lesions (parent who underwent arthroplasty in their 40s or 50s) as well as patients

with marked malalignment or meniscal deficiency warrant closer monitoring.

Clinical Evaluation

Patients with symptomatic chondral defects typically have nonspecific knee pain and swelling. Mechanical symptoms, such as catching and locking, as well as instability may be present. Traumatic etiologies often are associated with a specific event, such as a fall or a twisting injury while playing sports. Conversely, idiopathic lesions and lesions associated with repetitive microtrauma may have more of an insidious onset, without a specific event that the patient can recall. After a detailed history with regard to the onset of symptoms is obtained, a comprehensive physical examination should be performed. The physical examination begins with a gait analysis followed by an assessment for effusion, deformity, contracture, malalignment, and patellar maltracking, paying close attention for possible mechanical blockage or

crepitus. Unfortunately, neither a patient's history nor physical examination are sensitive or specific for cartilage defects versus other intra-articular derangements.

Imaging

Radiographic studies include standing AP, lateral, Merchant, and 45° flexion PA views. Full limb-length radiographs may help determine mechanical alignment in select patients or in patients with known chondral defects. MRI can help effectively evaluate for articular cartilage and subchondral edema. Although determining the size of a lesion on imaging is helpful for prognostic purposes and can help guide surgical management, MRI frequently underestimates lesion size by as much as 60%.[18] Ligamentous and meniscal structures should be assessed for any evidence of injury.

Treatment

Nonsurgical Treatment

Initial management for most articular cartilage lesions consists of activity modification, anti-inflammatory medications, injections, bracing, and physical therapy. Patients who continue to be symptomatic despite nonsurgical treatment should be evaluated for possible surgical treatment. Age, activity level, patient expectations, defect size, and associated injuries are important factors in the determination of whether a patient is a surgical candidate. Patients who are considered surgical candidates must understand that most cartilage-restoring procedures require extensive rehabilitation and that they will be unable to return to activities for an extended period of time. In addition, patients should understand that high-impact activities, such as running

Dr. Cole or an immediate family member has received royalties from Arthrex, DJ Orthopaedics, and Elsevier; serves as a paid consultant to Arthrex, Regentis Biomaterials, and Zimmer; has stock or stock options held in Carticept and Regentis Biomaterials; has received research or institutional support from Aesculap/B. Braun, Arthrex, Cytori Therapeutics, Medipost, the National Institutes of Health (NIAMS & NICHD), and Zimmer; has received nonincome support (such as equipment or services), commercially derived honoraria, or other non-research–related funding (such as paid travel) from Athletico Physical Therapy, Össur, Smith & Nephew, and Tornier; and serves as a board member, owner, officer, or committee member of the American Orthopaedic Society for Sports Medicine, the American Shoulder and Elbow Surgeons, the Arthroscopy Association of North America, and the International Cartilage Repair Society. Dr. Farr or an immediate family member has received royalties from DePuy and Arthrex; is a member of a speakers' bureau or has made paid presentations on behalf of Arthrex, ArthroCare, MedShape, Moximed, and Osiris Therapeutics; serves as a paid consultant to Ceterix Orthopaedics, Genzyme, Arthrex, DePuy, Mitek, RTI Biologics, Zimmer, Stryker, Advanced Bio-Surfaces, NuOrtho Surgical, Schwartz Biomedical, Knee Creations, Science for BioMaterials, BioRegeneration Technologies, NuTech Medical, Moximed, MedShape, and ArthroCare; has stock or stock options held in MedShape; has received research or institutional support from Genzyme, DePuy, Mitek, RTI Biologics, Zimmer, Knee Creations, NuTech Medical, Moximed, ArthroCare, and Histogenics; and serves as a board member, owner, officer, or committee member of the Cartilage Research Foundation, the Patellofemoral Foundation, the International Patellofemoral Study Group, and the International Cartilage Repair Society. Dr. Lattermann or an immediate family member serves as a paid consultant to CartiHeal and Vericel; has received research or institutional support from Smith & Nephew; and serves as a board member, owner, officer, or committee member of the International Cartilage Repair Society and the German Speaking Arthroscopy Society. Dr. Gomoll or an immediate family member has received royalties from NuTech; serves as a paid consultant to Aesculap/B. Braun, CartiHeal, Geistlich Pharma, Novartis, NuTech, Regentis Biomaterials, and Vericel; has received research or institutional support from JRF Ortho and Science for BioMaterials; and serves as a board member, owner, officer, or committee member of the International Cartilage Repair Society. Neither Dr. Chilelli nor any immediate family member has received anything of value from or has stock or stock options held in a commercial company or institution related directly or indirectly to the subject of this chapter.

and basketball, are discouraged, but not necessarily contraindicated, postoperatively depending on the surgical procedure selected and the outcome desired.

Surgical Treatment

The goal of surgical treatment for patients who have symptomatic chondral defects is to restore the osteochondral unit in an anatomic fashion with maintenance of the supporting subchondral bone and repair tissue that closely resembles native articular cartilage. However, if a chondral lesion is incidentally found at the time of ACL reconstruction or meniscal surgery, the symptomatology is less clear. In general, the lesion should be documented and possibly managed with chondroplasty based on its appearance. National Football League players who underwent microfracture for the management of articular cartilage lesions were 4.4 times less likely to return to professional football compared with National Football League players who underwent chondroplasty alone.[19] Acute cartilage repair is discouraged because it is unknown whether a particular lesion is or will be symptomatic. Furthermore, most cartilage repair rehabilitation protocols differ from those of the primary procedure, especially a simple meniscectomy. A patient who is faced with drastically and unexpectedly different postoperative weight-bearing restrictions will, most likely, be unhappy. Postoperatively, the patient and the family should be counseled on the surgical findings and instructed on when to seek a reevaluation (eg, if persistent pain and swelling occur). A scheduled follow-up, with or without repeat MRI, is advised in certain high-risk patients, such as younger patients with a lateral meniscal deficiency or a large lateral femoral condyle OCD lesion.

Arthroscopic Débridement and Chondroplasty

Arthroscopy can be used for both diagnostic and therapeutic purposes. Direct visualization via arthroscopy can help a surgeon determine the exact size and location of a defect, which provides the surgeon with a guide for definitive cartilage repair treatment options if they are necessary in the future. Arthroscopy is particularly helpful because MRI frequently underestimates lesion size.[18] During arthroscopy, a surgeon may be tempted to débride lesions in the patellofemoral joint despite a patient being clinically asymptomatic. In these patients, the surgeon is advised to document the damage but refrain from débridement because it can convert an asymptomatic lesion into a clinically symptomatic lesion. Although arthroscopic débridement and chondroplasty can help improve a patient's clinical symptoms, it is not curative.

Arthroscopic débridement and chondroplasty also can be a useful procedure for patients who may not be good candidates for cartilage restoration (based on age, advanced degenerative changes, body mass index, and participation in athletics) or patients who are unwilling to adhere to a strict postoperative rehabilitation protocol; however, data on the long-term efficacy of arthroscopic débridement and chondroplasty are lacking.

Marrow Stimulation (Microfracture)

Marrow stimulation in the form of drilling or microfracture can be used to treat patients who have small chondral defects (<2 cm^2) of the knee. The ideal patient for marrow stimulation is younger than 40 years and has a focal chondral defect of the medial or lateral femoral condyle. In a study of 72 patients with chondral defects of the

knee who underwent microfracture, Steadman et al[20] reported significant improvements in mean Tegner activity and Lysholm Knee Scale scores as well as good to excellent Medical Outcomes Study 36-Item Short Form (SF-36) and Western Ontario and McMaster Universities Osteoarthritis Index scores at a mean follow-up of 11 years. In a study of 109 patients with chondral defects of the knee who underwent microfracture, Gobbi et al[21] reported that, at a mean follow-up of 6 years, mean Lysholm Knee Scale scores improved and International Knee Documentation Committee (IKDC) Subjective Knee Evaluation Form scores were normal or near normal in 70% of the patients who had a mean defect size of 4 cm^2. After further analysis, the authors reported that a lesion size less than 2 cm^2 and an age younger than 40 years were associated with a better rate of return to high-impact sports.

Many other studies have reported good short-term results after microfracture; however, the recent literature suggests that outcomes after microfracture may deteriorate with time. Goyal et al[22] reported that microfracture resulted in good short-term outcomes in low-demand patients who had small lesions; however, the authors reported that failure could be expected 5 years after microfracture regardless of lesion size. Gobbi et al[23] reported good short- and long-term clinical results in patients with small lesions who underwent microfracture but acknowledged that deterioration of clinical outcomes should be expected 2 to 5 years postoperatively. A systematic review of 3,000 patients reported improved knee function 24 months after microfracture; however, data on outcomes more than 24 months after microfracture were

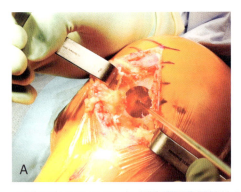
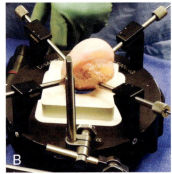
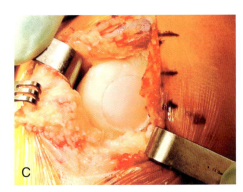

Figure 1   Photographs of a knee with an osteochondral defect that was treated with osteochondral allograft transplantation. **A,** Intraoperative photograph taken after preparation of the osteochondral defect shows removal of unhealthy cartilage and the underlying subchondral bone. **B,** Clinical photograph shows a fresh femoral hemicondyle that was used to obtain an osteochondral allograft cylinder. **C,** Intraoperative photograph taken after osteochondral allograft transplantation that was performed with the use of the press-fit technique. (Reproduced from Gomoll AH, Chilelli BJ: Articular cartilage of the knee, in Miller MD, ed: *Orthopaedic Knowledge Update: Sports Medicine*, ed 5. Rosemont, IL, American Academy of Orthopaedic Surgeons, 2016, 221-236.)

insufficient.[24] Modifications to the microfracture technique, such as the creation of smaller holes via nanofracture or the augmentation of microfracture with a dehydrated micronized articular cartilage allograft scaffold combined with platelet rich plasma, are currently being investigated.[25,26]

Osteochondral Autograft Transfer/Mosaicplasty

Osteochondral autograft transfer (OAT) is best suited for patients who have small chondral or osteochondral lesions (<2 to 3 cm²) of the femoral condyles. OAT addresses abnormal or deficient subchondral bone and restores mature hyaline cartilage. Multiple osteochondral cylinders are transferred via mosaicplasty for patients who have lesions larger than 1 cm².

In a study of athletes who underwent OAT, Hangody et al[27] reported good to excellent outcomes at a mean follow-up of 9.6 years in 91% of patients who were treated for femoral condyle lesions, 86% of patients who were treated for tibial lesions, and 74% of patients who were treated for patellofemoral lesions. In

a study of 73 patients who underwent OAT, Solheim et al[28] reported that, at a mean follow-up of 7 years, 88% of the patients said that they would undergo the procedure again; however, the authors reported a deterioration of results from 1 year postoperatively to 5 to 9 years postoperatively. In a long-term outcomes study of 73 patients who underwent OAT, Solheim et al[29] reported poor outcomes in 40% of the patients at a long-term follow-up that ranged from 10 to 14 years. A further analysis revealed that the poor outcomes were associated with patients who were older than 40 years (59%), were women (61%), and had defects larger than 3 cm² (57%). Conversely, patients who were younger than 40 years and had a defect smaller than 3 cm² had a failure rate of only 12.5% and a mean Lysholm Knee Scale score of 82. Long-term donor site morbidity after graft harvest has been reported to be approximately 3%.[30]

Osteochondral Allograft Transplantation

Osteochondral allograft transplantation is ideal for patients who have large chondral or osteochondral lesions

(>2 to 4 cm²; **Figure 1**). Osteochondral allograft transplantation can be performed to treat patients who have uncontained defects and used as a salvage option in patients in whom other cartilage repair procedures fail. Similar to OAT, osteochondral allograft transplantation addresses subchondral bone abnormalities and restores mature articular cartilage.

In a recent long-term outcomes study of 58 patients who underwent fresh osteochondral allograft transplantation, Raz et al[31] reported that graft survival was 91%, 84%, 69%, and 59% at 10, 15, 20, and 25 years postoperatively, respectively. The mean modified Hospital for Special Surgery score was 86 for patients who had a surviving graft 15 years postoperatively. In a systematic review of 19 studies, which included 644 knees that were managed with osteochondral allograft transplantation, Chahal et al[32] reported an overall satisfaction rate of 86% at a mean follow-up of 58 months, with little to no arthritis reported in 65% of the patients at final follow-up. The mean age of the patients across all of the studies

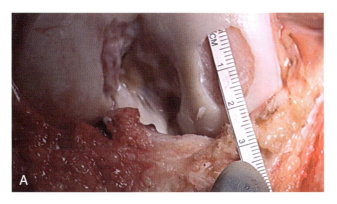
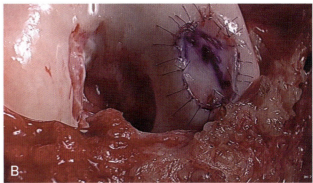
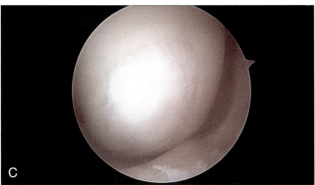

Figure 2   Images of a knee with a chondral defect that was treated with autologous chondrocyte implantation (ACI). **A,** Intraoperative photograph shows a chondral defect of the medial femoral condyle that has been prepared for ACI. **B,** Intraoperative photograph shows that autologous chondrocytes have been injected beneath a type I/III collagen membrane and sealed with 6-0 absorbable braided suture and fibrin glue. **C,** Arthroscopic image shows the medial femoral condyle 10 months after ACI.

that were included was 37 years, and the mean defect size across all of the studies that were included was 6.3 cm².

Video 42.1: Autologous Chondrocyte Implantation. Jack Farr, MD (3 min)

Autologous Chondrocyte Implantation

ACI is an articular cartilage-restoring procedure that is used to treat patients who have medium to large full-thickness chondral defects (>2 to 4 cm²) of the knee (**Figure 2**). The size of a defect being managed with ACI is not limited; however, contained defects rather than uncontained defects are preferred. Since ACI was originally described in 1994, newer second- and third-generation ACI techniques have been routinely used in the United States and Europe.[33-36]

Saris et al[37] conducted a randomized controlled trial of 144 patients with a mean lesion size of 4.8 cm² who underwent either matrix-applied ACI or microfracture. The authors reported that the patients who underwent matrix-applied ACI had significant improvements in mean Knee Injury and Osteoarthritis Outcome Scores (KOOS) and knee-related quality of life scores 2 years postoperatively. The authors reported that management with matrix-applied ACI for cartilage defects larger than 3 cm² was both statistically and clinically better and had similar structural repair tissue and safety compared with microfracture. Several other studies have reported favorable midterm results after ACI.[38-40] In a long-term study of 224 patients who underwent ACI, Peterson et al[41] reported that, at a mean follow-up of 12.8 years, 74% of the patients described their postoperative status as better or the same as that in previous years, and 92% of the patients stated that they were satisfied

and would undergo ACI again. In a study of 210 patients with a mean defect size of 8.4 cm² who underwent ACI, Minas et al[42] reported that, at 10 years postoperatively, survivorship was 71%, and 75% of the patients had improved function.

Particulated Juvenile Articular Cartilage

Particulated juvenile articular cartilage (PJAC) for the management of chondral defects of the knee has recently gained popularity and consists of small, minced pieces of juvenile articular cartilage allograft that were obtained from donors aged 13 years or younger. PJAC is applied to a prepared defect in a monolayer and attached with a fibrin sealant.[43] Although outcome studies on the use of PJAC are limited, short-term results are encouraging.

In the largest outcomes study to date, Farr et al[44] followed 29 defects (11 trochlear defects and 18 femoral condyle defects; mean defect size, 2.7 cm²) in 25 patients who underwent treatment with PJAC. The authors reported statistically significant increases in mean IKDC Subjective Knee Evaluation Form scores as well as KOOS pain, symptoms, activities of daily living, and sports and recreation subscale scores at 24 months postoperatively. Postoperative biopsy samples obtained from eight patients revealed a mixture of hyaline and fibrocartilage; however, immunohistologic results confirmed a higher percentage of hyaline cartilage with excellent integration of the PJAC in the surrounding native cartilage. The advantages of PJAC include the lack of donor site morbidity, the ability to perform a one-stage procedure, and the likely increased chondrocytic differentiation potential of the juvenile tissue.[45,46] Further studies are necessary to determine the long-term efficacy and durability of PJAC. Additional treatment options that use a cryopreserved three-dimensional sheet of meshed allograft cartilage are currently being investigated as an alternative to PJAC.

Osteochondritis Dissecans

OCD is an idiopathic condition that primarily affects subchondral bone and has the potential to disrupt overlying articular cartilage. Pain and dysfunction can result from OCD. OCD most often occurs in the skeletally immature population and the young adult population. The exact prevalence of OCD is unknown; however, estimates between 15 and 29 per 100,000 individuals have been reported.[47,48] The incidence of OCD is higher in males compared with females, with male-to-female ratios ranging from 2:1 to 4:1.[49-52] The most common site of OCD in the knee is the

medial femoral condyle (60% to 80%), followed by the lateral femoral condyle (15% to 32.5%) and the patella (5% to 10%).[48,52,53]

OCD is divided into juvenile (open physes) and adult (closed physes) forms; this distinction is important because patients with juvenile OCD have a higher likelihood to spontaneously heal with nonsurgical treatment, whereas patients with adult OCD often follow a progressive disease course that results in fragment detachment.[54] Despite several theories on the etiology of OCD, the exact cause of OCD is unknown. The term "osteochondritis" was initially selected to describe an inflammatory condition, but this has since been deemed unlikely. Various theories on the pathophysiology of OCD include endocrine disorders, abnormal ossification, vascular insufficiency, repetitive microtrauma, and genetic predisposition.[48,55-57] Several studies have attempted to relate sports activity to OCD, which would suggest repetitive microtrauma as a potential cause;[48,58,59] however, inconsistent histologic analyses have resulted in a lack of consensus on the exact etiology of OCD.[60]

Clinical Evaluation

Typically, patients with OCD have an insidious onset of nonspecific pain that often is exacerbated by activity and may be accompanied by effusions. Mechanical symptoms, such as catching and locking, may occur, especially in patients who have unstable OCD lesions. Some patients may have an antalgic gait or an obligate external rotation gait, both of which are used to avoid tibial spine impingement on the medial femoral condyle defect.[61] The physical examination should focus on an assessment

of the knee for effusion, mechanical blockage, associated ligamentous laxity, and tenderness to palpation.

Imaging

Initial imaging studies include weight-bearing AP, lateral, and Merchant radiographs. In addition, 45° flexion PA radiographs are particularly helpful to evaluate OCD lesions along the posterior femoral condyles.[62] Contralateral knee radiographs can be considered given the high incidence of bilateral involvement.[59] The radiographs should be scrutinized for radiolucencies, subchondral cysts, sclerosis, fragmentation, loose bodies, joint space narrowing, and physeal status. If an OCD lesion is suspected, MRI can help in diagnosis and characterization of the defect.[63-65] The size, location, and depth of the OCD lesion can be determined with MRI. The articular surface overlying abnormal subchondral bone is analyzed for any evidence of disruption. MRI classification systems have been proposed to help predict the stability of OCD lesions;[66,67] however, the appearance of OCD lesions on MRI is often inconsistent with clinical symptoms and arthroscopic findings.[65,68,69] Anatomic detail of the subchondral bone can be difficult to assess on MRI in patients who have diffuse subchondral edema; therefore, CT or CT arthrography can be used to assess the fine anatomy of subchondral bone. In patients in whom nonsurgical treatment fails, full limb-length radiographs can help determine mechanical alignment and aid in surgical decision making.

Treatment
Nonsurgical Treatment
The goal of nonsurgical treatment for patients who have an OCD lesion is

to attain healing, which is most often observed in patients who have juvenile OCD.[53,70,71] Nonsurgical treatment consists of activity modification, limited weight bearing, immobilization, physical therapy, and anti-inflammatory medications. Running, jumping, sports, and physical education class activities should be restricted. No studies have reported that one form of nonsurgical treatment is better than another, and no data support a specific duration of nonsurgical treatment.[72] The authors of this chapter restrict activity and consider limited weight bearing with crutches but without immobilization. Crutches should not be used longer than 12 to 16 weeks because of the potential for atrophy and weakness. Physical therapy is initiated to maintain motion and facilitate quadriceps and hamstring strengthening. Radiographs should be obtained at 3 and 6 months to assess for lesion healing. If healing is observed, patients are allowed to gradually return to activities.

In a study of 42 skeletally immature patients with stable OCD lesions who underwent 6 months of nonsurgical treatment, Wall et al[70] reported progressive healing in two-thirds of the patients. The authors reported that large OCD lesions, swelling, and/or mechanical symptoms were poor prognostic factors for healing. Similarly, Hefti et al[59] reported a better prognosis, no effusion, and a classic lesion location (lateral aspect of the medial femoral condyle) in younger patients with small OCD lesions (<2 cm²) who underwent nonsurgical treatment; however, the authors reported that unstable OCD lesions were best managed with surgery. Sales de Gauzy et al[71] reported complete radiographic healing in 30 of 31 OCD lesions in 24 children

(mean age, 11 years 4 months) who underwent a nonsurgical treatment regimen of activity restriction alone. Other studies have reported successful healing in only 50% of patients who were treated nonsurgically.[53,73,74] Surgical treatment should be considered in patients who remain symptomatic despite 6 months of nonsurgical treatment and in patients who have unstable OCD lesions that are unlikely to heal. However, patients who have mechanical symptoms as a result of displaced or grossly unstable OCD lesions often are indicated for immediate surgical treatment.

Surgical Treatment

Surgical treatment should be considered in patients in whom nonsurgical treatment fails and in patients who have unstable OCD lesions, especially in the setting of mechanical symptoms. Surgical options for the management of OCD lesions include arthroscopic fragment excision and débridement, drilling, arthroscopic/open reduction and internal fixation, microfracture, OAT, osteochondral allograft transplantation, and ACI; however, no consensus on the preferred surgical option exists. Factors such as patient age, mechanical alignment, and lesion characteristics (size, location, depth, and stability) should be considered in the development of the surgical plan. In addition, the treating surgeon should approach abnormal subchondral bone and the overlying articular surface as an intimately related osteochondral unit. The goal of reparative and restorative procedures is to reestablish the osteochondral unit in an anatomic fashion and, thus, restore joint congruity and normal kinematics of the knee.

Arthroscopic Fragment Excision and Débridement

Arthroscopy can be used for diagnostic, palliative, and reparative purposes. For patients who have unstable OCD lesions with evidence of a loose fragment that has little capacity to heal with osteosynthesis or drilling, arthroscopic fragment excision and débridement can provide short-term relief of pain and mechanical symptoms. However, some long-term studies have reported a high rate of progressive radiographic degeneration in patients with large OCD lesions (>2 cm²) who underwent arthroscopic fragment excision and débridement.[75-77] Based on the available literature, débridement alone in younger patients is not considered an ideal long-term treatment. Close postoperative observation with the potential for early cartilage restoration may be considered, especially in younger patients who have lateral femoral condyle lesions.

Drilling

Arthroscopic or arthroscopic-aided drilling can be effective for the management of OCD lesions, especially in children with OCD lesions who have open growth plates and an intact chondral surface.[78-81] Drilling can be performed via an anterograde (transarticular) approach with penetration of intact articular cartilage or via a retrograde (extra-articular) approach with preservation of intact articular cartilage. The goal of drilling is to promote subchondral healing by creating vascular channels from the underlying marrow. No current evidence supports one drilling approach over another. Anterograde drilling is less technically challenging but disrupts an intact chondral surface. Retrograde drilling is more technically challenging but avoids articular

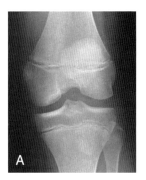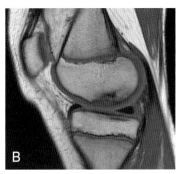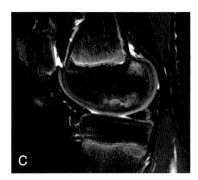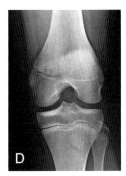

Figure 3 Images of the knee of a skeletally immature patient with an osteochondritis dissecans (OCD) lesion who underwent arthroscopic drilling. **A,** AP radiograph demonstrates an OCD lesion on the lateral aspect of the medial femoral condyle. Sagittal T1-weighted proton-density (**B**) and sagittal T2-weighted fat-saturated (**C**) MRIs confirm abnormal subchondral bone with an intact chondral surface. **D,** AP radiograph taken 3 months after retrograde drilling demonstrates complete healing of the OCD lesion.

cartilage penetration. The authors of this chapter prefer to perform retrograde drilling in skeletally immature patients who have an intact articular surface with no arthroscopic evidence of fragment instability (**Figure 3**). The use of fluoroscopy is encouraged because of the risk for physeal injury with a retrograde approach.

Arthroscopic/Open Reduction and Internal Fixation

Partially detached or hinged fragments can be reduced and fixed to intact underlying subchondral bone via an arthroscopic or open approach.[82] The fixation of loose osteochondral fragments also can be considered based on the intraoperative appearance of the fragment. Partially detached chondral or osteochondral flaps are hinged open, after which débridement, curettage, and microfracture or drilling of the subchondral bone is performed. Substantial subchondral bone deficiency or cysts should be addressed with local autograft bone that is harvested from the intercondylar notch or the ipsilateral proximal tibia, being mindful of potentially open physes. Fixation devices include cannulated metal

headless compression screws and bioabsorbable screws or pins. Headless, cannulated, titanium, variably pitched implants allow for excellent compression and placement below the articular surface, which helps avoid prominent hardware and potential third-body wear (**Figure 4**). Screws should be removed after healing of the defect at 6 to 12 weeks postoperatively. Bioabsorbable implants have shown promise; however, questions remain with regard to their compression strength and enzymatic breakdown, which can lead to large subchondral cysts in some patients.[83-87] In addition, complete resorption may take years, during which time the implant can become prominent if the OCD lesion fails to heal and disintegrates around the implant, risking injury to the opposing articular surface. Therefore, the authors of this chapter prefer to use headless metal compression screws for fixation, which are then removed at 6 to 12 weeks postoperatively.

Implant removal is performed to assess lesion healing and remove unstable fragments. After implant removal, 8 additional weeks of postoperative full weight bearing are recommended to prepare the patient for return to

higher level activities and avoid concern for damage that could be caused by a prominent screw that may be associated with fragment settling. In a study on the outcomes of patients with OCD lesions who underwent various surgical treatments, Pascual-Garrido et al[88] reported that patients who underwent arthroscopic internal fixation had a greater improvement in outcome scores compared with those who underwent osteochondral allograft transplantation.

Marrow Stimulation (Microfracture)

Marrow stimulation can be performed in patients who have an unstable OCD lesion if the osteochondral fragment is considered unsalvageable. Marrow stimulation involves penetration of the subchondral bone to liberate mesenchymal stem cells from the trabecular bone. These mesenchymal stem cells flow into the OCD lesion and biologically induce the formation of fibrocartilage repair tissue.

Although several studies have reported good outcomes after marrow stimulation, the long-term durability of the procedure has been questioned. Gudas et al[89] randomized 50 children (aged 18 years or younger) with OCD lesions to either a microfracture group or an OAT group. After 1 year, both groups had significant clinical improvement, with good to excellent results reported in 23 of 25 patients (92%) in the OAT group and 19 of 22 patients (86%) in the microfracture group. Although outcomes were stable in the OAT group at a follow-up of 4.2 years (19 of 23 patients [83%] had good to excellent results), only 12 of 19 patients (63%) in the microfracture group had similar results. In addition, microfracture failed in 9 patients (41%). Patients with OCD lesions that were larger than 3 cm^2 who underwent microfracture had worse outcomes compared with patients with OCD lesions that were less than 3 cm^2 who underwent microfracture. Microfracture is a viable option for patients who have small defects (<2 to 3 cm^2) without substantial subchondral bone deficiency (<6 mm). Postoperative rehabilitation that includes protected weight bearing and immediate range of motion is critical to enhance surgical outcomes.

OAT/Mosaicplasty

OAT may be considered in patients who have subchondral bone deficiency and a disrupted articular surface. OAT is most effective for patients who have small OCD lesions (<2 to 3 cm^2). OAT involves preparation of the osteochondral defect and transfer of an osteochondral cylinder from a low–weight-bearing region of the knee (such as the intercondylar notch or the periphery of the trochlea) to the OCD lesion. OCD lesions larger than 1 cm^2 require the use of multiple plugs, which is referred to as mosaicplasty. Because of the potential donor site morbidity that is associated with the use of multiple plugs, the authors of this chapter

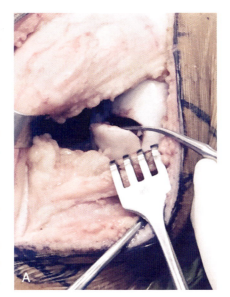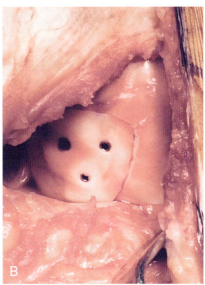

Figure 4   Intraoperative photographs of a knee with an osteochondritis dissecans (OCD) lesion that was treated with open reduction and internal fixation. **A,** Photograph shows a hinged OCD lesion on the lateral femoral condyle. **B,** Photograph shows open reduction and internal fixation of the OCD lesion with the use of headless, cannulated, titanium, variably pitched screws.

prefer to perform mosaicplasty only in patients who have small OCD lesions.

OAT also can be used as an alternate form of fixation in lieu of screws. Miniaci and Tytherleigh-Strong[90] performed OAT mosaicplasty in 20 patients to secure OCD fragments. The harvested osteochondral cylinders were placed through the central aspect of the OCD fragment and, occasionally, along the periphery of the OCD fragment to create a biologic splint. At a follow-up of 18 months, all of the patients had normal IKDC Subjective Knee Evaluation Form scores. In addition, MRI demonstrated bone healing and cartilage healing at 6 months and 9 months postoperatively, respectively.

Osteochondral Allograft Transplantation

Patients who have large OCD lesions (>2 to 4 cm^2) may be treated with osteochondral allograft transplantation. Osteochondral allograft transplantation

is ideal for patients who have OCD defects with subchondral bone deficiency (>8 to 10 mm) because it restores the entire osteochondral unit. Osteochondral allograft transplantation also can be used as a salvage procedure in patients in whom other cartilage repair procedures fail.

In a study of 64 patients with OCD lesions who underwent fresh osteochondral allograft transplantation, Emmerson et al[91] reported good to excellent results in 72% of the patients at a mean follow-up of 7.7 years. All of the patients underwent previous surgical procedures before osteochondral allograft transplantation. In a more recent study of 39 patients (43 knees) who underwent fresh osteochondral allograft transplantation, Murphy et al[92] reported that, at a follow-up of 10 years, graft survivorship was 90%, and 88% of the knees in which the grafts were in situ were rated good to excellent. The cohort consisted of 26 pediatric and adolescent knees in which an OCD lesion was the underlying cause of the defect.

Autologous Chondrocyte Implantation
Similar to osteochondral allograft transplantation, ACI can be performed in patients who have large OCD lesions (>2 to 4 cm²) and used as a salvage option in patients in whom other cartilage repair procedures fail. Modifications to ACI have been described for patients with more than 8 to 10 mm of subchondral bone loss. This modified ACI technique, which has been referred to as the sandwich technique, involves autologous bone grafting of the subchondral defect followed by the application of a collagen membrane on which ACI is performed.[93,94]

In a study of 58 patients with OCD lesions who underwent ACI, Peterson et al[93] reported successful clinical results in more than 90% of the patients at a mean follow-up of 5.6 years. Mean Wallgren-Tegner activity scale, Lysholm Knee Scale, and visual analog scale scores improved, and 93% of the patients reported improvement on a patient self-assessment questionnaire. Forty-eight of the patients underwent a mean of 2.1 surgical procedures before ACI, and the mean duration of symptoms was 7.8 years. The sandwich technique was performed in seven patients who had a defect depth greater than 10 mm. In a study of 32 patients with OCD lesions who underwent ACI for the management of at least one failed non-ACI procedure, Cole et al[95] reported successful results in 85% of the patients at a follow-up of 48 months. The authors performed ACI with the use of a traditional single-layer technique rather than the sandwich technique.

Patellofemoral Defects

Patellofemoral pain is one of the most common musculoskeletal conditions, with etiologies including acute trauma, overuse, chronic patellar maltracking, and patellar instability. Patellofemoral chondral defects can result from these etiologies or may be idiopathic. In a systematic review of 11 studies that included 931 athletes, Flanigan et al[96] reported patellofemoral chondral defects in 37% of the athletes. Retrospective studies that were based on a large number of consecutive knee arthroscopies have reported that, after the medial femoral condyle, the patella is the second most common site for chondral defects.[1,97] Numerous studies have reported that chondral and osteochondral lesions are observed in as many as 95% of patients who sustain a patellar dislocation.[98-101] The inferior aspect of the medial patellar facet is the most common defect site after patellar dislocation.[98] Although a large percentage of patients who have patellofemoral chondral lesions respond favorably to nonsurgical treatment, surgical treatment should be considered in the subset of patients who remain symptomatic despite nonsurgical treatment. Successful management of patellofemoral chondral lesions can be challenging because of the complex biomechanical environment of the patellofemoral joint. Therefore, a careful evaluation of the underlying pathomechanics of the patellofemoral joint is necessary to ensure a successful surgical outcome.

Clinical Evaluation

Typically, patients with patellofemoral cartilage injuries have anterior knee pain that is worse with activity. Activities that involve loaded knee flexion, such as squatting, kneeling, and the use of stairs, often elicit pain. Intermittent swelling is common, and catching or locking can result from an unstable chondral flap. Some patients may have patellar instability (acute or chronic) and recall a specific event associated with their dislocation or subluxation. The physical examination should focus on an assessment of the knee for effusion, patellar mobility, and tracking with range of motion. Generalized ligamentous laxity, lower extremity alignment and rotation (femoral neck anteversion and tibial torsion), hip strength, and core strength should be evaluated.

Imaging

Routine radiographs, including standing AP, lateral, Merchant, and 45° flexion PA views, should be obtained. The radiographs are evaluated for fractures, loose bodies, joint space narrowing, osteophytes, patella alta, patellar tilt, and patellar subluxation. MRI is particularly useful to help diagnose and characterize chondral and osteochondral defects of the patellofemoral joint. In addition, MRI helps evaluate the integrity of the medial patellofemoral ligament (MPFL) and the tibial tubercle-trochlear groove (TT-TG) as well as assess the TT-TG distance, the TT-posterior cruciate ligament (PCL) distance, patellar height, and the presence of trochlear dysplasia. The TT-TG distance is a measure of tibial tubercle lateralization, which is calculated by measuring the medial to lateral distance between the center of the trochlear groove and the center of the tibial tubercle. The TT-PCL distance is measured from the medial aspect of the PCL, close to its tibial insertion, to the center of the tibial tubercle. Both MRI and CT can help calculate the TT-TG distance in patients who have patellar instability; however, recent data suggest that MRI may underestimate this distance.[102-104] The TT-TG distance often is misleading for a variety of reasons and should not be used in isolation. Measurement of the TT-PCL distance helps resolve underestimated TT-TG.[105] Given the high incidence of chondral and osteochondral injuries after patellar dislocation, many surgeons routinely obtain MRI after patellar dislocation, even after a primary dislocation, because, often, substantial chondral or osteochondral avulsions may be missed on radiographs. The medial patella and the lateral femoral condyle are the most commonly injured sites after patellar dislocation. The lateral femoral condyle can be particularly difficult to evaluate. Edema is commonly observed; however, because of the convexity of the mostly peripherally located defect zone, actual cartilage damage can easily be missed.

Treatment

Nonsurgical Treatment

Initial management for most patellofemoral chondral defects should consist of nonsurgical measures, with attention to the core-to-floor approach. The exception to nonsurgical management includes patients who have mechanical symptoms resulting from a displaced chondral flap or an osteochondral fragment. A detailed discussion on the management of acute patellar dislocations is beyond the scope of this chapter. Nonsurgical treatment focuses on activity modification, anti-inflammatory medications, physical therapy, bracing, and intra-articular injections (cortisone or viscosupplementation). Physical therapy focuses on patellar stabilization; functional pelvic, valgus, and rotational control; and core,

hip, and lower extremity strengthening. Physical therapy effectively alleviates patellofemoral pain by reducing mechanical stress in the joint and improving patellar tracking.[106,107] Nonsurgical treatment should be attempted for 6 weeks to 6 months, depending on a patient's progress.

Surgical Treatment

Patients in whom nonsurgical treatment fails or patients who have displaced chondral or osteochondral injuries should be considered for surgical treatment. Surgical treatment is individualized based on defect characteristics (size, location, stability, and status of the subchondral bone) and associated conditions, such as malalignment and instability. Other factors that should be considered in the development of the surgical plan include patient age, activity level, goals, and expectations, as well as a willingness to participate in postoperative rehabilitation. Surgical options for the management of patellofemoral defects include open reduction and internal fixation of the chondral/osteochondral fragment, microfracture with or without augments, OAT, osteochondral allograft transplantation, ACI, PJAC, realignment procedures (tibial tubercle osteotomy [TTO], lateral release/lengthening, and MPFL reconstruction), tibial and femoral rotational osteotomies, and patellofemoral arthroplasty.

Loose Body Repair, Removal, and/or Chondroplasty

Small chondral or osteochondral loose bodies that result from patellar dislocation can be removed arthroscopically. The removal of these fragments helps eliminate mechanical symptoms and prevents third-body wear. Associated

patellofemoral defects can be further evaluated and addressed with open reduction and internal fixation if the fragment is amenable and in an age-appropriate patient. Alternatively, stabilization chondroplasty can be performed to address loose chondral flaps. If large osteochondral fragments are suspected preoperatively or encountered during arthroscopy, primary in situ fixation with metal screws or bioabsorbable implants should be considered. Small partial- or full-thickness chondral lesions (<1 cm^2) may require only chondroplasty, especially if they are located at the inferior aspect of the medial patellar facet, which experiences limited loading.

The anterior lateral femoral condyle is the second most common defect site after patellar dislocation; however, it is difficult to visualize through the standard lateral arthroscopic viewing portal. Frequently, the defect bed is covered with early repair tissue that is similar to that observed after marrow stimulation, particularly in patients who have an osteochondral defect. Large acute defects observed within 6 weeks of injury can be managed with a marrow-stimulation rehabilitation protocol to maximize the healing potential of this regenerative tissue.

Marrow Stimulation (Microfracture)

Microfracture can be used to treat patients who have small full-thickness chondral defects (<2 cm^2) of the patella or trochlea. Performing patellar microfracture via an arthroscopic approach is technically challenging because it is difficult to position the instruments perpendicular to the defect. Unfortunately, few outcome studies have evaluated patellofemoral defects in isolation; most studies combine data on femoral condyle defects with that of patello-femoral defects.

Kreuz et al[108] followed 70 patients who underwent microfracture for the management of full-thickness chondral defects that involved various compartments of the knee. Thirty-two patients had femoral condyle defects, 11 patients had tibial defects, 16 patients had trochlear defects, and 11 patients had patellar defects. The authors reported good results in all of the patients at 6 months and 18 months postoperatively but reported deteriorating outcome scores and MRI defect filling at 36 months postoperatively. In addition, greater deterioration was reported in the patients who had trochlear and patellar defects compared with the patients who had femoral condyle defects; this is a concern given the known long-term deterioration that occurs after microfracture in other areas of the knee. Therefore, microfracture should be reserved only for patients who have small lesions, most of which are located in the inferior pole or the lateral patellar facet.

OAT/Mosaicplasty
OAT may be considered in patients who have small full-thickness chondral or osteochondral defects (<2 cm^2) of the patella or the trochlea. OAT restores the osteochondral unit with hyaline cartilage and native bone. OAT is a viable option for patients who have patellofemoral defects; however, the procedure is more complicated in these patients because it requires the complex contour of the patella and trochlea to be matched with donor cylinders that commonly lack the same thickness of native patellofemoral cartilage.[109]

In a study of 10 consecutive patients with patellar defects (mean defect size, 1.2 cm^2) who underwent OAT, Figueroa et al[110] reported improved mean Lysholm Knee Scale scores (73.8 to 95) and no complications at a mean follow-up of 37.3 months. Follow-up MRI obtained at 8 months postoperatively were favorable, with all of the grafts being flush to the adjacent cartilage and, in most patients, no fissures in the graft-receptor interface. In a study of 22 patients with patellar defects (mean defect size, 1.65 cm^2) who underwent OAT, Nho et al[111] reported improved mean IKDC Subjective Knee Evaluation Form (47.2 to 74.4), Activities of Daily Living Scale of the Knee Outcome Survey (60.1 to 84.7), and SF-36 (64.0 to 79.4) scores at a mean follow-up of 28.7 months. Similarly, in a study of 33 patients with symptomatic patellar defects (1 to 2.5 cm^2) who underwent OAT, Astur et al[112] reported statistically significant improvements in mean Lysholm Knee Scale, Kujala Anterior Knee Pain Scale, Fulkerson Knee Instability Scale, and SF-36 scores 2 years postoperatively. The authors reported that MRI obtained 2 years postoperatively revealed full graft integration in all patients.

Conversely, Bentley et al[113] reported a high failure rate in patients with patellar chondral lesions who underwent mosaicplasty. The authors conducted a prospective randomized study of 100 patients with osteochondral defects who underwent either ACI or mosaicplasty. Of the 100 patients, 5 underwent mosaicplasty for the management of patellar defects. All of the patellar mosaicplasty procedures had failed at a mean follow-up of 1.7 years. Therefore, OAT may be considered in patients who have small lesions (<2 cm^2); however, higher failure rates should be expected in patients with larger defects that require more donor cylinders.

Patellar cartilage is approximately twice as thick as medial or lateral trochlear cartilage (the usual donor site). This difference in cartilage thickness will lead to subchondral bone mismatch and may be a stress riser. In addition, many patients with patellar lesions have patellar instability or malalignment, in which the lateral trochlea, in particular, is overloaded. The selection of the donor site in these patients is difficult and may be impossible without causing further damage to the patellofemoral joint.

Osteochondral Allograft Transplantation
Osteochondral allograft transplantation restores the entire osteochondral unit and is ideal for patients who have large defects (>2 to 4 cm^2). Similar to OAT, osteochondral allograft transplantation is a technically demanding procedure because of the concave and convex contour of the patella and trochlea. In a retrospective study of 14 fresh patellofemoral allografts that were implanted in the knees of 11 patients, Torga Spak and Teitge[114] reported that eight grafts were in place at final follow-up (mean, 10 years; range, 2.6 to 17.5 years), four of which were in place for more than 10 years and two of which were in place for more than 5 years. Of the nonsurviving allografts, three were in place for more than 10 years. Ten of the 11 patients in the study said that they would undergo the procedure again.

In a study of 20 fresh osteochondral allografts that were used to manage patellofemoral lesions in the knees of 18 patients, Jamali et al[115] reported a failure rate of 25% and a revision surgery rate of 53%. In a recent prospective study of 27 patients (28 knees) with isolated full-thickness patellar injuries who underwent osteochondral allograft transplantation, Gracitelli

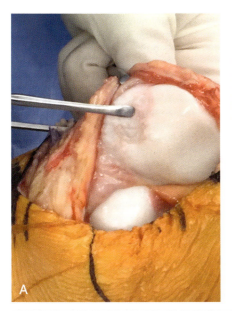 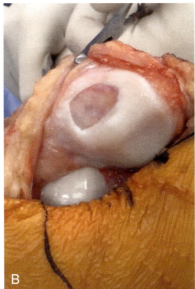 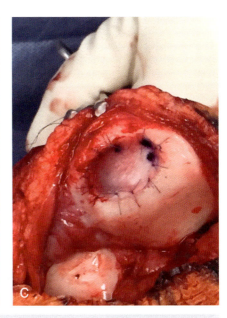

Figure 5   Intraoperative photographs of a knee with a patellofemoral defect that was treated with autologous chondrocyte implantation (ACI). **A,** Photograph shows a large chondral defect of the medial patellar facet. **B,** Photograph shows the removal of unhealthy articular cartilage from the medial patellar facet before ACI. **C,** Photograph shows the medial patellar facet after ACI.

et al[116] reported that survivorship was 78.1% at 5 and 10 years postoperatively and 55.8% at 15 years postoperatively. Seventeen of the 28 knees (60.7%) underwent additional surgery after osteochondral allograft transplantation, and osteochondral allograft transplantation failed in 8 of the 28 knees (28.6%). Despite the high revision surgery rate, 89% of the patients in whom osteochondral allograft transplantation was successful said that they were extremely satisfied or satisfied with the results of the procedure. The authors reported that the outcomes of their study were inferior compared with the published outcomes of osteochondral allograft transplantation for the management of femoral condyle injuries. Chahal et al[32] discovered a similar trend in a systematic review of 19 studies of 644 knees that were managed with osteochondral allograft transplantation and reported that osteochondral allograft transplantation results in inferior outcomes in patients

who have patellofemoral defects compared with patients who have tibial and femoral condyle lesions.

Autologous Chondrocyte Implantation
ACI is a surgical option for patients who have medium to large chondral defects (>2 to 4 cm²) of the patellofemoral joint (**Figure 5**). Compared with OAT and osteochondral allograft transplantation, matching the contour of the native morphology of the patellofemoral chondral surfaces is technically easier with ACI (**Figure 6**). In a large multicenter study of 110 patients with patellar cartilage defects who underwent ACI, Gomoll et al[117] reported statistically significant and clinically important improvements in all physical outcome scale scores at a minimum follow-up of 4 years. The authors reported that mean IKDC Subjective Knee Evaluation Form scores improved from 40.2 to 69.4, mean modified Cincinnati Knee Rating Scale scores improved

from 3.2 to 6.2, and mean Western Ontario and McMaster Universities Osteoarthritis Index scores improved from 50.4 to 28.6. The authors noted that 92% of the patients said that they would undergo the procedure again, and 86% of the patients rated their knees as good or excellent at final follow-up.

Particulated Juvenile Articular Cartilage
PJAC is a surgical option for the treatment of patients who have patellofemoral defects of any size. Similar to ACI, matching the contour of the native patellofemoral surface is technically easier with PJAC compared with OAT or osteochondral allograft transplantation. PJAC is particularly useful for the management of patellofemoral lesions in patients in whom concomitant osteochondral allograft transplantation is necessary to manage femoral condyle defects because PJAC can be ordered on short notice after an osteochondral allograft has been matched (**Figure 7**). In

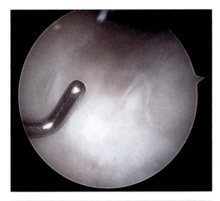

Figure 6 Arthroscopic image of a knee taken 10 months after autologous chondrocyte implantation for the management of a chondral lesion of the femoral trochlea shows that the anatomic contour of the trochlea was restored.

a study of 13 patients (15 knees) with patellar chondral defects who underwent treatment with PJAC, Tompkins et al[118] reported that, at a mean follow-up of 28.8 months, mean IKDC Subjective Knee Evaluation Form, visual analog scale, and KOOS scores were favorable, and the mean fill of the defect based on MRI was 89%. The authors reported that two patients required knee manipulation under anesthesia for arthrofibrosis, and three patients required revision surgery for symptomatic grafts.

Video 42.2: Anteromedialization. Jack Farr, MD (2 min)

Video 42.3: Lateral Lengthening. Jack Farr, MD (2 min)

Video 42.4: Medial Patellofemoral Ligament Reconstruction. Jack Farr, MD (4 min)

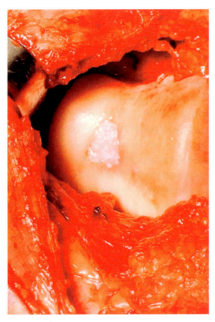

Figure 7 Intraoperative photograph of the knee of a patient shows a femoral trochlear defect that was managed with particulated juvenile articular cartilage at the same time that a lateral femoral condyle osteochondral defect was managed with osteochondral allograft transplantation.

Osteotomy

TTO for the treatment of patients who have patellar instability or patellofemoral disease has been extensively studied. TTO typically involves anteromedialization of the tibial tubercle.[119,120] Decreased lateral patellofemoral contact pressures have been demonstrated in biomechanical models after TTO.[121,122] Therefore, patients who have defects of the lateral patella or the trochlea are ideal candidates for and have the greatest potential to benefit from TTO.

Studies on the use of TTO in conjunction with cartilage repair have been recently published in the literature. Peterson et al[39] reported disappointing early results in patients with patellar defects who underwent ACI, with good to excellent results reported in only two of

seven patients (29%). The authors performed realignment procedures, if they were necessary, in the latter 14 patients in the study, which resulted in good to excellent results in 11 of the 14 patients (79%). In a study that compared the outcomes of patients who underwent patellar ACI with or without concomitant extensor realignment, Henderson et al[123] reported superior mean modified Cincinnati Knee Rating Scale scores, function, mean SF-36 scores, and IKDC Subjective Knee Evaluation Form scores in the patients who underwent ACI in conjunction with extensor realignment compared with those who underwent ACI without extensor realignment. The authors reported that an unloading osteotomy may improve the outcomes of select patients who have normal patellofemoral biomechanics; however, both of the groups in the study included a substantial number of patients who had lateral patellar facet defects, which would be expected to respond positively to an unloading osteotomy, thus amplifying the differences the authors reported between the groups.

Pascual-Garrido et al[88] reported that ACI in conjunction with anteromedialization resulted in improved outcomes compared with ACI alone. Gillogly et al[124] reported good to excellent results at a mean follow-up of 7.6 years in 83% of patients who underwent ACI in conjunction with TTO. The authors reported that ACI in conjunction with TTO failed in only one patient, who subsequently underwent patellofemoral arthroplasty 5.9 years after the index procedure. A recent systematic review reported significantly greater improvements in multiple clinical outcomes in patients with patellofemoral chondral defects who underwent ACI in combination with osteotomy compared with those with patellofemoral chondral defects who underwent ACI alone.[125]

Conversely, a recent, large, multicenter study reported no significant difference between patients who underwent patellofemoral ACI with or without concomitant TTO.[117] However, the authors noted that most of the patients in the study (70%) had panpatellar defects, which would be expected to improve less after ACI with concomitant TTO, and, overall, the rate of ACI in conjunction with TTO was quite high (68%). The authors stressed that TTO is indicated in patients who have an abnormal biomechanical environment, and reported that the outcomes of patients who underwent patellar ACI in conjunction with TTO were similar compared with those of patients who underwent femoral condyle ACI.

Patellar instability must be addressed in patients with patellofemoral chondral defects who undergo cartilage restoration. Therefore, TTO should be considered in patients who have an elevated TT-TG distance (>15 mm) and patellar instability. Lateral retinacular lengthening typically is performed in combination with TTO. MPFL reconstruction can be performed in combination with TTO in select patients, most of whom typically have an acute or chronically disrupted MPFL and intraoperative evidence of continued lateral maltracking or instability despite distal realignment and lateral retinacular lengthening.

Video 42.5: Patellofemoral Arthroplasty. Jack Farr, MD (9 min)

Patellofemoral Arthroplasty

Patellofemoral arthroplasty is a primary surgical option for the treatment of patients who have advanced diffuse patellofemoral degeneration and is a salvage option in patients in whom cartilage procedures fail. Historically, a high failure rate and mediocre results were associated with patellofemoral arthroplasty; however, newer implant designs and techniques have substantially improved patient outcomes and implant survivorship.[126]

The Meniscectomized Knee

Meniscus tears are one of the most common knee injuries and frequently require surgical management. The meniscus is a critically important structure that minimizes joint contact stresses by providing maximum contact area. The meniscus also has a crucial role in proprioception and knee stability. In a loaded knee, the medial meniscus transmits 50% of the medial compartment load, and the lateral meniscus transmits 70% of the lateral compartment load.[127] Medial meniscus tears are twice as likely to occur compared with lateral meniscus tears. Meniscal surgery is performed in approximately 35 to 61 per 100,000 individuals.[128-130]

Biomechanical studies have reported that meniscectomy results in higher contact forces and lower contact areas compared with meniscal repair;[131] however, because of patient factors and tear characteristics, meniscal tears are not always amenable to repair. Contact forces have been reported to increase by as much as 65% after partial meniscectomy and 235% after total meniscectomy.[131] A change in contact forces may cause medial and/or lateral knee pain secondary to compartment overload, which may lead to progressive articular cartilage degeneration. In a prospective 40-year follow-up study of 53 patients who underwent total meniscectomy as adolescents, Pengas et al[132] reported that meniscectomy led to symptomatic knee osteoarthritis later in all of the patients, with a 132-fold increase in the rate of total knee replacement compared with that of age-matched control patients. Roos et al[133] reported that patients who underwent meniscectomy had a 14.0 relative risk for advanced osteoarthritis compared with age- and sex-matched control patients. Many other studies have reported a strong association between meniscectomy and radiographic and symptomatic osteoarthritis.[134-136]

Clinical Evaluation

Patients who are symptomatic and have undergone meniscectomy may have a wide variety of complaints; however, localized joint line pain or focal pain in the medial or lateral compartment are common. The surgeon should obtain a thorough history, including the time from previous surgery, the duration of current symptoms, and the activities or factors that precipitate pain. Some patients experience pain only with high-impact activities; other patients may experience pain with normal weight-bearing activities. The physical examination begins with a gait analysis followed by an assessment for effusion, deformity, contracture, ligamentous instability, malalignment, and patellar maltracking.

Imaging

Routine radiographs, including standing AP, lateral, Merchant, and 45° flexion PA views, should be obtained. The radiographs are evaluated for fractures, loose bodies, osteophytes, and joint space narrowing. Full limb-length

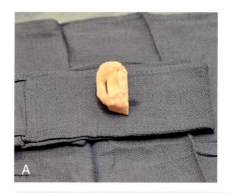
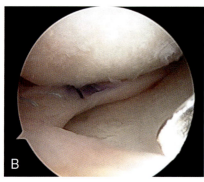

Figure 8 Images show meniscal allograft transplantation. **A,** Clinical photograph shows a meniscal allograft before transplantation. **B,** Arthroscopic image of a knee taken after suture fixation of the meniscal allograft.

radiographs may help determine mechanical alignment. MRI is used to evaluate for meniscal insufficiency and associated relevant chondral or osteochondral defects.

Treatment

Nonsurgical Treatment

Initial management should consist of nonsurgical treatment, including anti-inflammatory medications, activity modification, physical therapy, and injections (cortisone or viscosupplementation). An unloader brace can be effective in patients who have unilateral compartment overload as a result of malalignment or meniscal deficiency. Nonsurgical treatment may help alleviate symptoms; however, in many patients, nonsurgical treatment is only palliative in nature. Younger patients, especially those younger than 30 years, who have meniscal deficiency should be monitored closely because joint degeneration can occur quickly, especially after lateral meniscectomy.[136] A short period of time in which surgical intervention can be attempted to provide pain relief and potentially alter the progression of degenerative disease may exist.

Surgical Treatment

Surgical treatment should be considered in patients who are symptomatic and in patients in whom nonsurgical treatment fails, especially younger patients who have a high risk for rapid joint deterioration. Surgical options include meniscal allograft transplantation (MAT), osteotomy, cartilage repair, unicompartmental knee arthroplasty (UKA), and total knee arthroplasty (TKA). Factors such as patient age, goals, and activity level as well as the extent of the disease process should be considered in the development of the surgical plan.

Meniscal Allograft Transplantation

MAT may be considered in younger patients who have meniscal deficiency (**Figure 8**). The first human MAT was performed in 1984; since then, physicians' understanding of MAT has evolved.[137] Biomechanical studies report improved intra-articular contact area and pressures in patients who undergo MAT.[138,139] The primary indication for MAT is a symptomatic knee compartment in a patient with a history of total or subtotal meniscectomy.[140] No consensus on the upper age limit for MAT exists; however, 50 to 55 years is

typically used as a cutoff. Controversy on the amount of acceptable chondral loss for MAT exists; however, ideally, articular cartilage defects that are greater than International Cartilage Repair Society grade III should be focal and small so that they can be addressed in conjunction with cartilage repair.[141] Contraindications to MAT include obesity, ligamentous instability (unless it is addressed before or in conjunction with MAT), previous joint infection, and squaring of the femoral condyles.[142,143] Patients who have more than 3° of varus or valgus malalignment should be considered for a concurrent osteotomy (high tibial osteotomy or distal femoral osteotomy).

Isolated MAT is an appropriate treatment option for younger patients who have meniscal deficiency, neutral alignment, and no chondral damage. Conversely, younger patients who have medial meniscal deficiency, varus malalignment, and a medial chondral defect may benefit from medial MAT, high tibial osteotomy, and cartilage repair. In a study of 18 patients who underwent MAT, osteotomy, and cartilage repair, Harris et al[144] reported statistically significant improvements in mean IKDC Subjective Knee Evaluation Form scores; mean Lysholm Knee Scale scores; and KOOS pain, activities of daily living, sports and recreation, and quality of life subscale scores at a mean follow-up of 6.5 years. Thirteen revision surgeries were performed in 10 patients (55.5% reoperation rate); however, only one patient (5.6%) was converted to TKA.

Overall, survival rates and patient satisfaction have been positive after MAT. In a study of 172 patients who underwent MAT, McCormick et al[145] reported a 95% survival rate at a mean follow-up of 5 years. In a study of 30 patients who underwent MAT, Vundelinckx et al[146] reported that, at a mean follow-up of 12 years 8 months, 90% of the patients said that they were very satisfied or satisfied with the procedure and would undergo MAT again. In a systematic review of 55 studies on MAT, Rosso et al[147] reported that MAT provides good clinical results at short-term and midterm follow-up, with improvement in knee function and acceptable failure and complication rates. Although MAT has been associated with favorable outcomes, treating surgeons must carefully identify proper candidates for MAT. Younger patients who have realistic expectations and are willing to comply with a rigorous postoperative rehabilitation are ideal. If multiple procedures are indicated, a staged procedure in which extra-articular and intra-articular procedures are grouped together based on surgeon comfort level may be considered.

Video 42.6: High Tibial Valgus Osteotomy. Jack Farr, MD (7 min)

Osteotomy

An osteotomy (distal femoral or proximal tibial) is a joint-preserving procedure that can be used to treat patients younger than 50 years who have early compartment osteoarthritis. A varus-producing distal femoral osteotomy is indicated in patients who have lateral compartment disease, and a valgus-producing proximal tibial osteotomy is indicated in patients who have medial compartment disease (**Figure 9**). Osteotomy is advantageous for younger patients because long-term activities are not restricted, and the need for

joint arthroplasty may be delayed or prevented.

Opening and closing wedge osteotomies have been described in the literature; however, a paucity of studies support one technique over another.[148,149] As a result of improved plating technology and various bone graft substitutes, opening wedge osteotomy has become the preferred technique.[150,151] In a study of 47 consecutive adults (younger than 55 years) who underwent proximal tibial opening wedge osteotomy for the management of medial compartment osteoarthritis and genu varus alignment, LaPrade et al[152] reported that, at a mean follow-up of 3.6 years, mean modified Cincinnati Knee Rating Scale scores improved from 42.9 to 65.1, and only three patients (6%) required revision osteotomy or conversion to TKA. In a recent systematic review of 21 studies, which included 1,065 patients who were treated for unicompartmental knee osteoarthritis, Brouwer et al[153] reported that valgus high tibial osteotomy reduced pain and improved knee function in patients who had medial compartment knee osteoarthritis.

Although less commonly used, varus-producing distal femoral osteotomy has resulted in encouraging outcomes in patients who have lateral compartment disease and genu valgus alignment.[154-156] The authors of this chapter prefer to perform osteotomy in patients with malalignment and isolated medial or lateral compartment disease who are younger than 55 years because they tend to be more active and may not be willing to comply with the postoperative activity restrictions associated with UKA. Conversely, UKA is a good option for less active patients aged 55 to 70 years who have isolated unicompartmental disease.

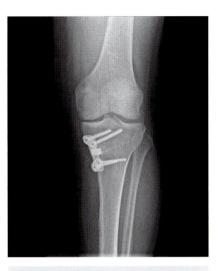

Figure 9 AP radiograph of the knee of a patient who was treated with a medial high tibial opening wedge osteotomy.

Cartilage Repair

Younger patients who have focal chondral defects as well as meniscal deficiency and/or malalignment may benefit from cartilage repair surgery in conjunction with other procedures, such as osteotomy or MAT. Cartilage repair options include microfracture, OAT, PJAC, ACI, and osteochondral allograft transplantation. The decision on which repair technique to use depends on both patient factors and the characteristics of the chondral lesion. Small lesions (<2 to 3 cm²) are best managed with microfracture, OAT, or PJAC. Large lesions (>2 to 3 cm²) are best managed with ACI or osteochondral allograft transplantation. If abnormal or deficient subchondral bone is present, OAT or osteochondral allograft transplantation should be considered to restore the entire osteochondral unit. The authors of this chapter recommend that additional patellofemoral or tibial defects be managed with ACI or PJAC (the use of ACI is off-label in the patella and tibia).

In a study of 30 patients who underwent 31 combined MAT and cartilage restoration procedures, Rue et al[157] reported statistically significant improvements in mean Lysholm Knee Scale and IKDC Subjective Knee Evaluation Form scores at a mean follow-up of 3.1 years. The cartilage restoration procedures in the study included ACI and osteochondral allograft transplantation. In a case series of 36 patients who underwent MAT in combination with ACI, Farr et al[158] reported statistically significant improvement in standardized outcome survey, visual analog pain scale, and satisfaction scores at a minimum follow-up of 2 years. The authors reported that, before the 2-year follow-up, the procedure failed in four patients, all of whom required revision surgery. In a study of 48 patients who underwent MAT in combination with osteochondral allograft transplantation, Getgood et al[159] reported that, at a mean follow-up of 6.8 years, revision surgery was required in 26 of the 48 patients (54.2%), but the procedure failed in only 11 patients (22.9%). The authors reported statistically significant improvements in all outcome scores of the patients who had grafts that were still in place at the last follow-up. In addition, 90% of the patients said that they would undergo the procedure again, and 78% of the patients were extremely satisfied or satisfied with their outcomes.

Arthroplasty

UKA and TKA are treatment options for patients who have advanced degeneration of the knee. Because of the more limited life span of implants in younger patients, arthroplasty, especially TKA, should be reserved for patients older than 55 years who have lower physical demands. UKA and TKA also can be used as a salvage option for patients in whom cartilage surgery fails. Patients who have isolated unicompartmental disease can be successfully treated with UKA, whereas patients who have more diffuse disease that involves more than one compartment are better treated with TKA. In a study of 54 consecutive patients who underwent lateral UKA, Lustig et al[160] reported that implant survival was 94.4% at 10 years postoperatively and 91.4% at 15 years postoperatively. The authors reported that the most common reason for revision surgery to TKA was progression of medial compartment osteoarthritis. Similarly, implant survival rates as high as 94% to 100% have been reported 10 years after medial compartment arthroplasty.[161-163]

Summary

The evaluation and treatment decision-making process for patients who have articular cartilage injuries will continue to evolve in conjunction with advances made in cartilage repair surgery. A systematic approach to the evaluation and classification of chondral lesions is of the utmost importance in the development of treatment algorithms. Treatment algorithms should be tailored based on patient factors, lesion characteristics, and associated injuries. Patients with an asymptomatic chondral or osteochondral defect should be observed rather than considered for surgical treatment.

Nonsurgical management is the mainstay of initial treatment for most patients who have symptomatic articular cartilage injuries. Nonsurgical treatment has proved successful, especially in patients who have juvenile OCD, incidental chondral defects, and certain patellofemoral defects that are associated with patellar instability or maltracking. Surgical treatment is reserved for patients in whom nonsurgical treatment fails, patients who have mechanical symptoms, and patients who have a high risk of rapid joint degeneration. Incidental chondral defects that are found at the time of arthroscopy should be documented and, possibly, managed with chondroplasty; more advanced cartilage repair techniques should not be attempted acutely for many reasons.

Cartilage repair surgery may be considered in patients who have symptomatic chondral defects and meet surgical indications. A preoperative discussion is important to establish realistic postoperative expectations and discuss possible postoperative complications. First-line surgical treatment options include arthroscopic débridement and chondroplasty, marrow stimulation (microfracture), drilling, arthroscopic/open reduction and internal fixation, OAT, osteochondral allograft transplantation, ACI, and PJAC. Careful attention should be paid to articular cartilage and underlying subchondral bone in the decision of which surgical technique should be used to reestablish the osteochondral unit. Cartilage repair surgery can be combined with other procedures, such as osteotomy and MAT, in select patients. Multiple procedures can be performed concomitantly or in a staged fashion based on a surgeon's comfort level. Salvage options for patients in whom cartilage surgery fails include osteochondral allograft transplantation, ACI, sandwich bone graft techniques, partial joint arthroplasty, and total joint arthroplasty.

References

1. Curl WW, Krome J, Gordon ES, Rushing J, Smith BP, Poehling GG: Cartilage injuries: A review of 31,516

knee arthroscopies. *Arthroscopy* 1997;13(4):456-460.

2. Arøen A, Løken S, Heir S, et al: Articular cartilage lesions in 993 consecutive knee arthroscopies. *Am J Sports Med* 2004;32(1):211-215.

3. Hjelle K, Solheim E, Strand T, Muri R, Brittberg M: Articular cartilage defects in 1,000 knee arthroscopies. *Arthroscopy* 2002;18(7):730-734.

4. Brophy RH, Zeltser D, Wright RW, Flanigan D: Anterior cruciate ligament reconstruction and concomitant articular cartilage injury: Incidence and treatment. *Arthroscopy* 2010;26(1):112-120.

5. Lewandrowski KU, Müller J, Schollmeier G: Concomitant meniscal and articular cartilage lesions in the femorotibial joint. *Am J Sports Med* 1997;25(4):486-494.

6. Church S, Keating JF: Reconstruction of the anterior cruciate ligament: Timing of surgery and the incidence of meniscal tears and degenerative change. *J Bone Joint Surg Br* 2005;87(12):1639-1642.

7. Joseph C, Pathak SS, Aravinda M, Rajan D: Is ACL reconstruction only for athletes? A study of the incidence of meniscal and cartilage injuries in an ACL-deficient athlete and non-athlete population: An Indian experience. *Int Orthop* 2008;32(1):57-61.

8. Maffulli N, Binfield PM, King JB: Articular cartilage lesions in the symptomatic anterior cruciate ligament-deficient knee. *Arthroscopy* 2003;19(7):685-690.

9. Takeda T, Matsumoto H, Fujikawa K: Influence of secondary damage to menisci and articular cartilage on return to sports after anterior cruciate ligament reconstruction. *J Orthop Sci* 1997;2(4):215-221.

10. Vasara AI, Jurvelin JS, Peterson L, Kiviranta I: Arthroscopic cartilage indentation and cartilage lesions of anterior cruciate ligament-deficient knees. *Am J Sports Med* 2005;33(3):408-414.

11. Slauterbeck JR, Kousa P, Clifton BC, et al: Geographic mapping of meniscus and cartilage lesions associated with anterior cruciate ligament injuries. *J Bone Joint Surg Am* 2009;91(9):2094-2103.

12. Murrell GA, Maddali S, Horovitz L, Oakley SP, Warren RF: The effects of time course after anterior cruciate ligament injury in correlation with meniscal and cartilage loss. *Am J Sports Med* 2001;29(1):9-14.

13. Newman AP: Articular cartilage repair. *Am J Sports Med* 1998;26(2):309-324.

14. O'Driscoll SW: The healing and regeneration of articular cartilage. *J Bone Joint Surg Am* 1998;80(12):1795-1812.

15. Shapiro F, Koide S, Glimcher MJ: Cell origin and differentiation in the repair of full-thickness defects of articular cartilage. *J Bone Joint Surg Am* 1993;75(4):532-553.

16. Lefkoe TP, Trafton PG, Ehrlich MG, et al: An experimental model of femoral condylar defect leading to osteoarthrosis. *J Orthop Trauma* 1993;7(5):458-467.

17. Messner K, Maletius W: The long-term prognosis for severe damage to weight-bearing cartilage in the knee: A 14-year clinical and radiographic follow-up in 28 young athletes. *Acta Orthop Scand* 1996;67(2):165-168.

18. Gomoll AH, Yoshioka H, Watanabe A, Dunn JC, Minas T: Preoperative measurement of cartilage defects by MRI underestimates lesion size. *Cartilage* 2011;2(4):389-393.

19. Scillia AJ, Aune KT, Andrachuk JS, et al: Return to play after chondroplasty of the knee in National Football League athletes. *Am J Sports Med* 2015;43(3):663-668.

20. Steadman JR, Briggs KK, Rodrigo JJ, Kocher MS, Gill TJ, Rodkey WG: Outcomes of microfracture for traumatic chondral defects of the knee: Average 11-year follow-up. *Arthroscopy* 2003;19(5):477-484.

21. Gobbi A, Nunag P, Malinowski K: Treatment of full thickness chondral lesions of the knee with microfracture in a group of athletes. *Knee Surg Sports Traumatol Arthrosc* 2005;13(3):213-221.

22. Goyal D, Keyhani S, Lee EH, Hui JH: Evidence-based status of microfracture technique: A systematic review of level I and II studies. *Arthroscopy* 2013;29(9):1579-1588.

23. Gobbi A, Karnatzikos G, Kumar A: Long-term results after microfracture treatment for full-thickness knee chondral lesions in athletes. *Knee Surg Sports Traumatol Arthrosc* 2014;22(9):1986-1996.

24. Mithoefer K, McAdams T, Williams RJ, Kreuz PC, Mandelbaum BR: Clinical efficacy of the microfracture technique for articular cartilage repair in the knee: An evidence-based systematic analysis. *Am J Sports Med* 2009;37(10):2053-2063.

25. Abrams GD, Mall NA, Fortier LA, Roller BL, Cole BJ: Biocartilage: Background and operative technique. *Oper Tech Sports Med* 2013;21(2):116-124.

26. Benthien JP, Behrens P: Nanofractured autologous matrix induced chondrogenesis (NAMIC©)—Further development of collagen membrane aided chondrogenesis combined with subchondral needling: A technical note. *Knee* 2015;22(5):411-415.

27. Hangody L, Dobos J, Baló E, Pánics G, Hangody LR, Berkes I: Clinical experiences with autologous osteochondral mosaicplasty in an athletic population: A 17-year prospective multicenter study. *Am J Sports Med* 2010;38(6):1125-1133.

28. Solheim E, Hegna J, Øyen J, Austgulen OK, Harlem T, Strand T: Osteochondral autografting (mosaicplasty) in articular cartilage defects in the knee: Results at 5 to 9 years. *Knee* 2010;17(1):84-87.

29. Solheim E, Hegna J, Øyen J, Harlem T, Strand T: Results at 10 to 14 years after osteochondral autografting (mosaicplasty) in articular cartilage defects in the knee. *Knee* 2013;20(4):287-290.

30. Hangody L, Ráthonyi GK, Duska Z, Vásárhelyi G, Füles P, Módis L: Autologous osteochondral mosaicplasty: Surgical technique. *J Bone Joint Surg Am* 2004;86(suppl 1):65-72.

31. Raz G, Safir OA, Backstein DJ, Lee PT, Gross AE: Distal femoral fresh osteochondral allografts: Follow-up at a mean of twenty-two years. *J Bone Joint Surg Am* 2014;96(13):1101-1107.

32. Chahal J, Gross AE, Gross C, et al: Outcomes of osteochondral allograft transplantation in the knee. *Arthroscopy* 2013;29(3):575-588.

33. Brittberg M, Lindahl A, Nilsson A, Ohlsson C, Isaksson O, Peterson L: Treatment of deep cartilage defects in the knee with autologous chondrocyte transplantation. *N Engl J Med* 1994;331(14):889-895.

34. Gooding CR, Bartlett W, Bentley G, Skinner JA, Carrington R, Flanagan A: A prospective, randomised study comparing two techniques of autologous chondrocyte implantation for osteochondral defects in the knee: Periosteum covered versus type I/III collagen covered. *Knee* 2006;13(3):203-210.

35. Steinwachs MR, Kreuz PC: Clinical results of autologous chondrocyte transplantation (ACT) using a collagen membrane, in Hendrich C, Nöth U, Eulert J, eds: *Cartilage Surgery and Future Perspectives*. Berlin, Germany, Springer-Verlag, 2003, pp 37-47.

36. Gomoll AH, Probst C, Farr J, Cole BJ, Minas T: Use of a type I/III bilayer collagen membrane decreases reoperation rates for symptomatic hypertrophy after autologous chondrocyte implantation. *Am J Sports Med* 2009;37(suppl 1):20S-23S.

37. Saris D, Price A, Widuchowski W, et al: Matrix-applied characterized autologous chondrocytes versus microfracture: Two-year follow-up of a prospective randomized trial. *Am J Sports Med* 2014;42(6):1384-1394.

38. McNickle AG, L'Heureux DR, Yanke AB, Cole BJ: Outcomes of autologous chondrocyte implantation in a diverse patient population. *Am J Sports Med* 2009;37(7):1344-1350.

39. Peterson L, Minas T, Brittberg M, Nilsson A, Sjögren-Jansson E, Lindahl A: Two- to 9-year outcome after autologous chondrocyte transplantation of the knee. *Clin Orthop Relat Res* 2000;374:212-234.

40. Minas T: Autologous chondrocyte implantation for focal chondral defects of the knee. *Clin Orthop Relat Res* 2001;(391 suppl):S349-S361.

41. Peterson L, Vasiliadis HS, Brittberg M, Lindahl A: Autologous chondrocyte implantation: A long-term follow-up. *Am J Sports Med* 2010;38(6):1117-1124.

42. Minas T, Von Keudell A, Bryant T, Gomoll AH: The John Insall Award: A minimum 10-year outcome study of autologous chondrocyte implantation. *Clin Orthop Relat Res* 2014;472(1):41-51.

43. Farr J, Yao JQ: Chondral defect repair with particulated juvenile cartilage allograft. *Cartilage* 2011;2(4):346-353.

44. Farr J, Tabet SK, Margerrison E, Cole BJ: Clinical, radiographic, and histological outcomes after cartilage repair with particulated juvenile articular cartilage: A 2-year prospective study. *Am J Sports Med* 2014;42(6):1417-1425.

45. Liu H, Zhao Z, Clarke RB, Gao J, Garrett IR, Margerrison EE: Enhanced tissue regeneration potential of juvenile articular cartilage. *Am J Sports Med* 2013;41(11):2658-2667.

46. Adkisson HD IV, Martin JA, Amendola RL, et al: The potential of human allogeneic juvenile chondrocytes for restoration of articular cartilage. *Am J Sports Med* 2010;38(7):1324-1333.

47. Hughston JC, Hergenroeder PT, Courtenay BG: Osteochondritis dissecans of the femoral condyles. *J Bone Joint Surg Am* 1984;66(9):1340-1348.

48. Lindén B: The incidence of osteochondritis dissecans in the condyles of the femur. *Acta Orthop Scand* 1976;47(6):664-667.

49. Kocher MS, Tucker R, Ganley TJ, Flynn JM: Management of osteochondritis dissecans of the knee: Current concepts review. *Am J Sports Med* 2006;34(7):1181-1191.

50. Crawford DC, Safran MR: Osteochondritis dissecans of the knee. *J Am Acad Orthop Surg* 2006;14(2):90-100.

51. Grimm NL, Weiss JM, Kessler JI, Aoki SK: Osteochondritis dissecans of the knee: Pathoanatomy, epidemiology, and diagnosis. *Clin Sports Med* 2014;33(2):181-188.

52. Kessler JI, Nikizad H, Shea KG, Jacobs JC Jr, Bebchuk JD, Weiss JM: The demographics and epidemiology of osteochondritis dissecans of the knee in children and adolescents. *Am J Sports Med* 2014;42(2):320-326.

53. Cahill BR, Phillips MR, Navarro R: The results of conservative management of juvenile osteochondritis dissecans using joint scintigraphy: A prospective study. *Am J Sports Med* 1989;17(5):601-606.

54. Cahill BR: Osteochondritis dissecans of the knee: Treatment of juvenile and adult forms. *J Am Acad Orthop Surg* 1995;3(4):237-247.

55. Tóth F, Nissi MJ, Ellermann JM, et al: Novel application of magnetic resonance imaging demonstrates characteristic differences in vasculature at predilection sites of osteochondritis dissecans. *Am J Sports Med* 2015;43(10):2522-2527.

56. Andrew TA, Spivey J, Lindebaum RH: Familial osteochondritis dissecans and dwarfism. *Acta Orthop Scand* 1981;52(5):519-523.

57. Kozlowski K, Middleton R: Familial osteochondritis dissecans: A dysplasia of articular cartilage? *Skeletal Radiol* 1985;13(3):207-210.

58. Koch S, Kampen WU, Laprell H: Cartilage and bone morphology in osteochondritis dissecans. *Knee Surg Sports Traumatol Arthrosc* 1997;5(1):42-45.

59. Hefti F, Beguiristain J, Krauspe R, et al: Osteochondritis dissecans: A multicenter study of the European Pediatric Orthopedic Society. *J Pediatr Orthop B* 1999;8(4):231-245.

60. Shea KG, Jacobs JC Jr, Carey JL, Anderson AF, Oxford JT: Osteochondritis dissecans knee histology studies have variable findings and theories of etiology. *Clin Orthop Relat Res* 2013;471(4):1127-1136.

61. Wilson JN: A diagnostic sign in osteochondritis dissecans of the knee. *J Bone Joint Surg Am* 1967;49(3):477-480.

62. Harding WG III: Diagnosis of ostechondritis dissecans of the femoral condyles: The value of the lateral x-ray view. *Clin Orthop Relat Res* 1977;123:25-26.

63. De Smet AA, Fisher DR, Graf BK, Lange RH: Osteochondritis dissecans of the knee: Value of MR imaging in determining lesion stability and the presence of articular

cartilage defects. *AJR Am J Roentgenol* 1990;155(3):549-553.

64. Nelson DW, DiPaola J, Colville M, Schmidgall J: Osteochondritis dissecans of the talus and knee: Prospective comparison of MR and arthroscopic classifications. *J Comput Assist Tomogr* 1990;14(5):804-808.

65. O'Connor MA, Palaniappan M, Khan N, Bruce CE: Osteochondritis dissecans of the knee in children: A comparison of MRI and arthroscopic findings. *J Bone Joint Surg Br* 2002;84(2):258-262.

66. De Smet AA, Ilahi OA, Graf BK: Reassessment of the MR criteria for stability of osteochondritis dissecans in the knee and ankle. *Skeletal Radiol* 1996;25(2):159-163.

67. Dipaola JD, Nelson DW, Colville MR: Characterizing osteochondral lesions by magnetic resonance imaging. *Arthroscopy* 1991;7(1):101-104.

68. Heywood CS, Benke MT, Brindle K, Fine KM: Correlation of magnetic resonance imaging to arthroscopic findings of stability in juvenile osteochondritis dissecans. *Arthroscopy* 2011;27(2):194-199.

69. Samora WP, Chevillet J, Adler B, Young GS, Klingele KE: Juvenile osteochondritis dissecans of the knee: Predictors of lesion stability. *J Pediatr Orthop* 2012;32(1):1-4.

70. Wall EJ, Vourazeris J, Myer GD, et al: The healing potential of stable juvenile osteochondritis dissecans knee lesions. *J Bone Joint Surg Am* 2008;90(12):2655-2664.

71. Sales de Gauzy J, Mansat C, Darodes PH, Cahuzac JP: Natural course of osteochondritis dissecans in children. *J Pediatr Orthop B* 1999;8(1):26-28.

72. Chambers HG, Shea KG, Anderson AF, et al: Diagnosis and treatment of osteochondritis dissecans. *J Am Acad Orthop Surg* 2011;19(5):297-306.

73. Pill SG, Ganley TJ, Milam RA, Lou JE, Meyer JS, Flynn JM: Role of magnetic resonance imaging and clinical criteria in predicting successful nonoperative treatment of osteochondritis dissecans in children. *J Pediatr Orthop* 2003;23(1):102-108.

74. Cepero S, Ullot R, Sastre S: Osteochondritis of the femoral condyles in children and adolescents: Our experience over the last 28 years. *J Pediatr Orthop B* 2005;14(1):24-29.

75. Wright RW, McLean M, Matava MJ, Shively RA: Osteochondritis dissecans of the knee: Long-term results of excision of the fragment. *Clin Orthop Relat Res* 2004;424:239-243.

76. Anderson AF, Richards DB, Pagnani MJ, Hovis WD: Antegrade drilling for osteochondritis dissecans of the knee. *Arthroscopy* 1997;13(3):319-324.

77. Murray JR, Chitnavis J, Dixon P, et al: Osteochondritis dissecans of the knee; long-term clinical outcome following arthroscopic debridement. *Knee* 2007;14(2):94-98.

78. Lebolt JR, Wall EJ: Retroarticular drilling and bone grafting of juvenile osteochondritis dissecans of the knee. *Arthroscopy* 2007;23(7):794.e1-794.e4.

79. Boughanem J, Riaz R, Patel RM, Sarwark JF: Functional and radiographic outcomes of juvenile osteochondritis dissecans of the knee treated with extra-articular retrograde drilling. *Am J Sports Med* 2011;39(10):2212-2217.

80. Aglietti P, Buzzi R, Bassi PB, Fioriti M: Arthroscopic drilling in juvenile osteochondritis dissecans of the medial femoral condyle. *Arthroscopy* 1994;10(3):286-291.

81. Anderson AF, Pagnani MJ: Osteochondritis dissecans of the femoral condyles: Long-term results of excision of the fragment. *Am J Sports Med* 1997;25(6):830-834.

82. Gomoll AH, Flik KR, Hayden JK, Cole BJ, Bush-Joseph CA, Bach BR Jr: Internal fixation of unstable Cahill Type-2C osteochondritis dissecans lesions of the knee in adolescent patients. *Orthopedics* 2007;30(6):487-490.

83. Tegnander A, Engebretsen L, Bergh K, Eide E, Holen KJ, Iversen OJ: Activation of the complement system and adverse effects of biodegradable pins of polylactic acid (Biofix) in osteochondritis dissecans. *Acta Orthop Scand* 1994;65(4):472-475.

84. Tabaddor RR, Banffy MB, Andersen JS, et al: Fixation of juvenile osteochondritis dissecans lesions of the knee using poly 96L/4D-lactide copolymer bioabsorbable implants. *J Pediatr Orthop* 2010;30(1):14-20.

85. Camathias C, Festring JD, Gaston MS: Bioabsorbable lag screw fixation of knee osteochondritis dissecans in the skeletally immature. *J Pediatr Orthop B* 2011;20(2):74-80.

86. Millington KL, Shah JP, Dahm DL, Levy BA, Stuart MJ: Bioabsorbable fixation of unstable osteochondritis dissecans lesions. *Am J Sports Med* 2010;38(10):2065-2070.

87. Nuzzo MS, Posner M, Warme WJ, Medina F, Wicker R, Owens BD: Compression force and pullout strength comparison of bioabsorbable implants for osteochondral lesion fixation. *Am J Orthop (Belle Mead NJ)* 2011;40(4):E61-E63.

88. Pascual-Garrido C, Slabaugh MA, L'Heureux DR, Friel NA, Cole BJ: Recommendations and treatment outcomes for patellofemoral articular cartilage defects with autologous chondrocyte implantation: Prospective evaluation at average 4-year follow-up. *Am J Sports Med* 2009;37(suppl 1):33S-41S.

89. Gudas R, Simonaityte R, Cekanauskas E, Tamosiūnas R: A prospective, randomized clinical study of osteochondral autologous transplantation versus microfracture for the treatment of osteochondritis dissecans in the knee joint in children. *J Pediatr Orthop* 2009;29(7):741-748.

90. Miniaci A, Tytherleigh-Strong G: Fixation of unstable osteochondritis dissecans lesions of the knee using arthroscopic autogenous osteochondral grafting (mosaicplasty). *Arthroscopy* 2007;23(8):845-851.

91. Emmerson BC, Görtz S, Jamali AA, Chung C, Amiel D, Bugbee WD: Fresh osteochondral allografting in the treatment of osteochondritis dissecans of the femoral condyle. *Am J Sports Med* 2007;35(6):907-914.

92. Murphy RT, Pennock AT, Bugbee WD: Osteochondral allograft transplantation of the knee in the pediatric and adolescent population. *Am J Sports Med* 2014;42(3):635-640.

93. Peterson L, Minas T, Brittberg M, Lindahl A: Treatment of

osteochondritis dissecans of the knee with autologous chondrocyte transplantation: Results at two to ten years. *J Bone Joint Surg Am* 2003;85(suppl 2):17-24.

94. Bartlett W, Skinner JA, Gooding CR, et al: Autologous chondrocyte implantation versus matrix-induced autologous chondrocyte implantation for osteochondral defects of the knee: A prospective, randomised study. *J Bone Joint Surg Br* 2005;87(5):640-645.

95. Cole BJ, DeBerardino T, Brewster R, et al: Outcomes of autologous chondrocyte implantation in study of the treatment of articular repair (STAR) patients with osteochondritis dissecans. *Am J Sports Med* 2012;40(9):2015-2022.

96. Flanigan DC, Harris JD, Trinh TQ, Siston RA, Brophy RH: Prevalence of chondral defects in athletes' knees: A systematic review. *Med Sci Sports Exerc* 2010;42(10):1795-1801.

97. Widuchowski W, Lukasik P, Kwiatkowski G, et al: Isolated full thickness chondral injuries: Prevalance and outcome of treatment. A retrospective study of 5233 knee arthroscopies. *Acta Chir Orthop Traumatol Cech* 2008;75(5):382-386.

98. Nomura E, Inoue M, Kurimura M: Chondral and osteochondral injuries associated with acute patellar dislocation. *Arthroscopy* 2003;19(7):717-721.

99. Stanitski CL, Paletta GA Jr: Articular cartilage injury with acute patellar dislocation in adolescents: Arthroscopic and radiographic correlation. *Am J Sports Med* 1998;26(1):52-55.

100. Vähäsarja V, Kinnuen P, Serlo W: Arthroscopy of the acute traumatic knee in children: Prospective study of 138 cases. *Acta Orthop Scand* 1993;64(5):580-582.

101. Hawkins RJ, Bell RH, Anisette G: Acute patellar dislocations: The natural history. *Am J Sports Med* 1986;14(2):117-120.

102. Schoettle PB, Zanetti M, Seifert B, Pfirrmann CW, Fucentese SF, Romero J: The tibial tuberosity-trochlear groove distance; a comparative study between CT and MRI scanning. *Knee* 2006;13(1):26-31.

103. Ho CP, James EW, Surowiec RK, et al: Systematic technique-dependent differences in CT versus MRI measurement of the tibial tubercle-trochlear groove distance. *Am J Sports Med* 2015;43(3):675-682.

104. Camp CL, Stuart MJ, Krych AJ, et al: CT and MRI measurements of tibial tubercle-trochlear groove distances are not equivalent in patients with patellar instability. *Am J Sports Med* 2013;41(8):1835-1840.

105. Seitlinger G, Scheurecker G, Högler R, Labey L, Innocenti B, Hofmann S: Tibial tubercle-posterior cruciate ligament distance: A new measurement to define the position of the tibial tubercle in patients with patellar dislocation. *Am J Sports Med* 2012;40(5):1119-1125.

106. Wong YM, Chan ST, Tang KW, Ng GY: Two modes of weight training programs and patellar stabilization. *J Athl Train* 2009;44(3):264-271.

107. Chiu JK, Wong YM, Yung PS, Ng GY: The effects of quadriceps strengthening on pain, function, and patellofemoral joint contact area in persons with patellofemoral pain. *Am J Phys Med Rehabil* 2012;91(2):98-106.

108. Kreuz PC, Steinwachs MR, Erggelet C, et al: Results after microfracture of full-thickness chondral defects in different compartments in the knee. *Osteoarthritis Cartilage* 2006;14(11):1119-1125.

109. Gomoll AH, Minas T, Farr J, Cole BJ: Treatment of chondral defects in the patellofemoral joint. *J Knee Surg* 2006;19(4):285-295.

110. Figueroa D, Meleán P, Calvo R, Gili F, Zilleruelo N, Vaisman A: Osteochondral autografts in full thickness patella cartilage lesions. *Knee* 2011;18(4):220-223.

111. Nho SJ, Foo LF, Green DM, et al: Magnetic resonance imaging and clinical evaluation of patellar resurfacing with press-fit osteochondral autograft plugs. *Am J Sports Med* 2008;36(6):1101-1109.

112. Astur DC, Arliani GG, Binz M, et al: Autologous osteochondral transplantation for treating patellar chondral injuries: Evaluation, treatment, and outcomes of a two-year

follow-up study. *J Bone Joint Surg Am* 2014;96(10):816-823.

113. Bentley G, Biant LC, Carrington RW, et al: A prospective, randomised comparison of autologous chondrocyte implantation versus mosaicplasty for osteochondral defects in the knee. *J Bone Joint Surg Br* 2003;85(2):223-230.

114. Torga Spak R, Teitge RA: Fresh osteochondral allografts for patellofemoral arthritis: Long-term followup. *Clin Orthop Relat Res* 2006;444:193-200.

115. Jamali AA, Emmerson BC, Chung C, Convery FR, Bugbee WD: Fresh osteochondral allografts: Results in the patellofemoral joint. *Clin Orthop Relat Res* 2005;437:176-185.

116. Gracitelli GC, Meric G, Pulido PA, Görtz S, De Young AJ, Bugbee WD: Fresh osteochondral allograft transplantation for isolated patellar cartilage injury. *Am J Sports Med* 2015;43(4):879-884.

117. Gomoll AH, Gillogly SD, Cole BJ, et al: Autologous chondrocyte implantation in the patella: A multicenter experience. *Am J Sports Med* 2014;42(5):1074-1081.

118. Tompkins M, Hamann JC, Diduch DR, et al: Preliminary results of a novel single-stage cartilage restoration technique: Particulated juvenile articular cartilage allograft for chondral defects of the patella. *Arthroscopy* 2013;29(10):1661-1670.

119. Fulkerson JP, Becker GJ, Meaney JA, Miranda M, Folcik MA: Anteromedial tibial tubercle transfer without bone graft. *Am J Sports Med* 1990;18(5):490-497.

120. Preston CF, Fulkerson EW, Meislin R, Di Cesare PE: Osteotomy about the knee: Applications, techniques, and results. *J Knee Surg* 2005;18(4):258-272.

121. Stephen JM, Lumpaopong P, Dodds AL, Williams A, Amis AA: The effect of tibial tuberosity medialization and lateralization on patellofemoral joint kinematics, contact mechanics, and stability. *Am J Sports Med* 2015;43(1):186-194.

122. Beck PR, Thomas AL, Farr J, Lewis PB, Cole BJ: Trochlear contact pressures after anteromedialization

of the tibial tubercle. *Am J Sports Med* 2005;33(11):1710-1715.

123. Henderson IJ, Lavigne P: Periosteal autologous chondrocyte implantation for patellar chondral defect in patients with normal and abnormal patellar tracking. *Knee* 2006;13(4):274-279.

124. Gillogly SD, Arnold RM: Autologous chondrocyte implantation and anteromedialization for isolated patellar articular cartilage lesions: 5- to 11-year follow-up. *Am J Sports Med* 2014;42(4):912-920.

125. Trinh TQ, Harris JD, Siston RA, Flanigan DC: Improved outcomes with combined autologous chondrocyte implantation and patellofemoral osteotomy versus isolated autologous chondrocyte implantation. *Arthroscopy* 2013;29(3):566-574.

126. Lustig S: Patellofemoral arthroplasty. *Orthop Traumatol Surg Res* 2014; 100(1 suppl):S35-S43.

127. Seedholm BB, Dowson D, Wright V: Proceedings: Functions of the menisci. A preliminary study. *Ann Rheum Dis* 1974;33(1):111.

128. Campbell SE, Sanders TG, Morrison WB: MR imaging of meniscal cysts: Incidence, location, and clinical significance. *AJR Am J Roentgenol* 2001;177(2):409-413.

129. Baker BE, Peckham AC, Pupparo F, Sanborn JC: Review of meniscal injury and associated sports. *Am J Sports Med* 1985;13(1):1-4.

130. Jameson SS, Dowen D, James P, Serrano-Pedraza I, Reed MR, Deehan DJ: The burden of arthroscopy of the knee: A contemporary analysis of data from the English NHS. *J Bone Joint Surg Br* 2011;93(10):1327-1333.

131. Baratz ME, Fu FH, Mengato R: Meniscal tears: The effect of meniscectomy and of repair on intraarticular contact areas and stress in the human knee. A preliminary report. *Am J Sports Med* 1986;14(4):270-275.

132. Pengas IP, Assiotis A, Nash W, Hatcher J, Banks J, McNicholas MJ: Total meniscectomy in adolescents: A 40-year follow-up. *J Bone Joint Surg Br* 2012;94(12):1649-1654.

133. Roos EM, Ostenberg A, Roos H, Ekdahl C, Lohmander LS: Long-term outcome of meniscectomy: Symptoms, function, and performance tests in patients with or without radiographic osteoarthritis compared to matched controls. *Osteoarthritis Cartilage* 2001;9(4):316-324.

134. Englund M, Roos EM, Lohmander LS: Impact of type of meniscal tear on radiographic and symptomatic knee osteoarthritis: A sixteen-year followup of meniscectomy with matched controls. *Arthritis Rheum* 2003;48(8):2178-2187.

135. McNicholas MJ, Rowley DI, McGurty D, et al: Total meniscectomy in adolescence: A thirty-year follow-up. *J Bone Joint Surg Br* 2000;82(2):217-221.

136. Alford JW, Cole BJ: Cartilage restoration, part 2: Techniques, outcomes, and future directions. *Am J Sports Med* 2005;33(3):443-460.

137. Milachowski KA, Weismeier K, Wirth CJ: Homologous meniscus transplantation: Experimental and clinical results. *Int Orthop* 1989;13(1):1-11.

138. Paletta GA Jr, Manning T, Snell E, Parker R, Bergfeld J: The effect of allograft meniscal replacement on intraarticular contact area and pressures in the human knee: A biomechanical study. *Am J Sports Med* 1997;25(5):692-698.

139. Alhalki MM, Hull ML, Howell SM: Contact mechanics of the medial tibial plateau after implantation of a medial meniscal allograft: A human cadaveric study. *Am J Sports Med* 2000;28(3):370-376.

140. Smith NA, Costa ML, Spalding T: Meniscal allograft transplantation: Rationale for treatment. *Bone Joint J* 2015;97(5):590-594.

141. Gomoll AH, Filardo G, Almqvist FK, et al: Surgical treatment for early osteoarthritis: Part II. Allografts and concurrent procedures. *Knee Surg Sports Traumatol Arthrosc* 2012;20(3):468-486.

142. Verdonk P, Van Laer M, ElAttar M, Almqvist KF, Verdonk R: Results and indications, in Beaufils P, Verdonk R, eds: *The Meniscus*. Berlin, Germany, Springer, 2010, pp 349-363.

143. Cole BJ, Carter TR, Rodeo SA: Allograft meniscal transplantation: Background, techniques, and results. *Instr Course Lect* 2003;52:383-396.

144. Harris JD, Hussey K, Wilson H, et al: Biological knee reconstruction for combined malalignment, meniscal deficiency, and articular cartilage disease. *Arthroscopy* 2015;31(2):275-282.

145. McCormick F, Harris JD, Abrams GD, et al: Survival and reoperation rates after meniscal allograft transplantation: Analysis of failures for 172 consecutive transplants at a minimum 2-year follow-up. *Am J Sports Med* 2014;42(4):892-897.

146. Vundelinckx B, Vanlauwe J, Bellemans J: Long-term subjective, clinical, and radiographic outcome evaluation of meniscal allograft transplantation in the knee. *Am J Sports Med* 2014;42(7):1592-1599.

147. Rosso F, Bisicchia S, Bonasia DE, Amendola A: Meniscal allograft transplantation: A systematic review. *Am J Sports Med* 2015;43(4):998-1007.

148. Smith TO, Sexton D, Mitchell P, Hing CB: Opening- or closing-wedged high tibial osteotomy: A meta-analysis of clinical and radiological outcomes. *Knee* 2011;18(6):361-368.

149. Brouwer RW, Bierma-Zeinstra SM, van Raaij TM, Verhaar J: Osteotomy for medial compartment arthritis of the knee using a closing wedge or an opening wedge controlled by a Puddu plate: A one-year randomised, controlled study. *J Bone Joint Surg Br* 2006;88(11):1454-1459.

150. Lobenhoffer P, De Simoni C, Staubli AE: Open-wedge high-tibial osteotomy with rigid plate fixation. *Tech Knee Surg* 2002;1(2):93-105.

151. Stoffel K, Stachowiak G, Kuster M: Open wedge high tibial osteotomy: Biomechanical investigation of the modified Arthrex Osteotomy Plate (Puddu Plate) and the TomoFix Plate. *Clin Biomech (Bristol, Avon)* 2004;19(9):944-950.

152. Laprade RF, Spiridonov SI, Nystrom LM, Jansson KS: Prospective outcomes of young and middle-aged adults with medial compartment osteoarthritis treated with a proximal

tibial opening wedge osteotomy. *Arthroscopy* 2012;28(3):354-364.

153. Brouwer RW, Huizinga MR, Duivenvoorden T, et al: Osteotomy for treating knee arthritis. *Cochrane Database Syst Rev* 2014;12:CD004019.

154. Wang JW, Hsu CC: Distal femoral varus osteotomy for osteoarthritis of the knee. *J Bone Joint Surg Am* 2005;87(1):127-133.

155. Saithna A, Kundra R, Getgood A, Spalding T: Opening wedge distal femoral varus osteotomy for lateral compartment osteoarthritis in the valgus knee. *Knee* 2014;21(1):172-175.

156. Cameron JI, McCauley JC, Kermanshahi AY, Bugbee WD: Lateral opening-wedge distal femoral osteotomy: Pain relief, functional improvement, and survivorship at 5 years. *Clin Orthop Relat Res* 2015;473(6):2009-2015.

157. Rue JP, Yanke AB, Busam ML, McNickle AG, Cole BJ: Meniscus transplantation and cartilage repair: Minimum 2-year follow-up. *Am J Sports Med* 2008;36(9):1770-1778.

158. Farr J, Rawal A, Marberry KM: Concomitant meniscal allograft transplantation and autologous chondrocyte implantation: Minimum 2-year follow-up. *Am J Sports Med* 2007;35(9):1459-1466.

159. Getgood A, Gelber J, Gortz S, De Young A, Bugbee W: Combined osteochondral allograft and meniscal allograft transplantation: A survivorship analysis. *Knee Surg Sports Traumatol Arthrosc* 2015;23(4):946-953.

160. Lustig S, Lording T, Frank F, Debette C, Servien E, Neyret P: Progression of medial osteoarthritis and long term results of lateral unicompartmental arthroplasty: 10 to 18 year follow-up of 54 consecutive implants. *Knee* 2014;21(suppl 1):S26-S32.

161. Murray DW, Goodfellow JW, O'Connor JJ: The Oxford medial unicompartmental arthroplasty: A ten-year survival study. *J Bone Joint Surg Br* 1998;80(6):983-989.

162. Keys GW, Ul-Abiddin Z, Toh EM: Analysis of first forty Oxford medial unicompartmental knee replacement from a small district hospital in UK. *Knee* 2004;11(5):375-377.

163. Rajasekhar C, Das S, Smith A: Unicompartmental knee arthroplasty: 2- to 12-year results in a community hospital. *J Bone Joint Surg Br* 2004;86(7):983-985.

Video References

42.1: Farr J: Video. *Autologous Chondrocyte Implantation*. Indianapolis, IN, 2016.

42.2: Farr J: Video. *Anteromedialization*. Indianapolis, IN, 2016.

42.3: Farr J: Video. *Lateral Lengthening*. Indianapolis, IN, 2016.

42.4: Farr J: Video. *Medial Patellofemoral Ligament Reconstruction*. Indianapolis, IN, 2016.

42.5: Farr J: Video. *Patellofemoral Arthroplasty*. Indianapolis, IN, 2016.

42.6: Farr J: Video. *High Tibial Valgus Osteotomy*. Indianapolis, IN, 2016.

Management of Patellofemoral Arthritis: From Cartilage Restoration to Arthroplasty

Brian A. Mosier, MD
Elizabeth A. Arendt, MD
Diane L. Dahm, MD
David Dejour, MD
Andreas H. Gomoll, MD

Abstract

The management of patellofemoral cartilage lesions is controversial and should begin with a comprehensive nonsurgical treatment plan. Patients with patellofemoral cartilage lesions in whom nonsurgical treatment fails may be candidates for surgical treatment. Surgical treatment strategies for the management of patellofemoral cartilage lesions are guided by the size, quality, and location of the defect. Recent advancements in cartilage restoration and arthroplasty techniques as well as appropriate patient selection and meticulous surgical technique have resulted in promising outcomes for patients with patellofemoral cartilage lesions who undergo surgical treatment.

Instr Course Lect 2017;66:531–542.

Patients who have anterior knee pain may be a diagnostic challenge because anterior knee pain can have multifactorial etiologies and vast differential diagnoses. This chapter focuses on patients who have patellofemoral pain that is caused by chondral lesions. Asymptomatic full-thickness fissures and defects of the patellar articular cartilage are the most common findings in patients who undergo knee arthroscopy.[1] An accurate patient history and physical examination as well as thorough imaging studies must be obtained to definitively attribute the source of a patient's pain to patellofemoral cartilage lesions. The key to achieving successful outcomes in the treatment of patients who have patellofemoral cartilage lesions is to decipher which structural defects need to be managed and identify other associated pathomechanical factors that need to be addressed. A clear treatment plan must be presented to patients who have patellofemoral cartilage lesions to gain their confidence and motivate them to take an active role in their recovery.

Dr. Arendt or an immediate family member serves as a paid consultant to or is an employee of Smith & Nephew and Tornier; and serves as a board member, owner, officer, or committee member of the American Orthopaedic Society for Sports Medicine and the International Society of Arthroscopy, Knee Surgery and Orthopaedic Sports Medicine. Dr. Dahm or an immediate family member has received royalties from Tenex Health; has stock or stock options held in Tenex Health; and serves as a board member, owner, officer, or committee member of the American Academy of Orthopaedic Surgeons and the Arthroscopy Association of North America. Dr. Dejour or an immediate family member has received royalties from Arthrex and SBM; serves as a paid consultant to or is an employee of Smith & Nephew; and serves as a board member, owner, officer, or committee member of the European Society of Sports Traumatology, Knee Surgery & Arthroscopy and the Société Française de Chirurgie Orthopédique et Traumatologique. Dr. Gomoll or an immediate family member has received royalties from Nutech; serves as a paid consultant to or is an employee of Aesculap/B. Braun, CartiHeal, Geistlich, Norvartis, Nutech, Regentis Biomaterials, and Vericel; has received research or institutional support from JRF Ortho and SBM; and serves as a board member, owner, officer, or committee member of the International Cartilage Repair Society. Neither Dr. Mosier nor any immediate family member has received anything of value from or has stock or stock options held in a commercial company or institution related directly or indirectly to the subject of this chapter.

History

Surgeons must obtain a thorough patient history to achieve an accurate diagnosis. The initial patient assessment may be difficult because articular cartilage is aneural; therefore, any pain that is perceived by a patient is caused by patellar or trochlear chondrosis of other tissues. Patients who have larger chondral or osteochondral defects may report mechanical symptoms or recurrent effusions. Patients who have an acute injury, such as a fracture or dislocation sustained as a result of direct trauma, may have recurrent dislocations or symptomatic loose bodies. Risk factors for instability must be assessed in patients who have a more insidious onset of symptoms or low-energy mechanisms of dislocation/subluxation. Pain that is exacerbated by activities that increase patellofemoral joint loading, including traversing stairs and squatting, is common in almost all patients who have symptomatic patellofemoral chondral lesions. Patellofemoral joint loading occurs as the knee is brought into increasing degrees of flexion as the patient traverses stairs. The patella acts as a lever arm for the extensor mechanism and enters the trochlear groove with the knee in 20° of flexion, with maximum contact occurring with the knee in 90° of flexion.[2,3]

Physical Examination

The physical examination should include an extensive evaluation of the patellofemoral compartment as well as the entire knee and lower extremity. A gait analysis and a single leg stance test should be performed to assess for signs of an antalgic gait, dynamic internal rotation of the femur, or valgus alignment. The proximal core musculature, hip abductors, quadriceps, hamstrings, gastrocnemius, soleus, and iliotibial band should be tested for strength and flexibility. Active and passive motion should be assessed, and patellar tracking should be observed for any signs of lateral deviation (J sign) that suggest trochlear dysplasia or an incompetent medial patellofemoral ligament. Patients with painful palpable crepitus with the knee in low angles of flexion may have a supratrochlear spur or trochlear dysplasia. Medial/lateral displacement of the patella should be measured with the knee in 0° and 20° of flexion, noting the direction of movement that causes apprehension. Typically, the direction of movement is assessed by dividing the trochlea into four quadrants. Patellar translation of three quadrants or more indicates pathologic laxity. Patients with tight lateral structures may have medial translation in less than one quadrant.[4] Palpation of the retinaculum may elicit medial pain in patients who sustained a recent dislocation and an injury to the medial patellofemoral ligament and may elicit lateral pain in patients who have chronic lateral maltracking and lateral chondrosis. Patients also should be evaluated for excessive femoral anteversion, genu valgum, and generalized ligamentous laxity, which should be classified based on the criteria described by Beighton and Horan.[5]

Imaging

The initial assessment should include standard AP weight-bearing radiographs, PA weight-bearing radiographs with the knee in 45° of flexion, bilateral Merchant radiographs, and true lateral radiographs with the knee in 30° of flexion. Standard AP and flexed PA radiographs help rule out arthritic changes at the tibiofemoral articulation. Bilateral Merchant radiographs allow surgeons to assess patellofemoral morphology, such as patellar tilt and subluxation; however, the bony relationship observed on plain radiographs does not always correlate with the chondral surface of the patellofemoral articulation,[6] especially because dysplasia usually affects the more proximal aspect of the trochlea, which typically is not able to be visualized on bilateral Merchant radiographs. True lateral radiographs that are obtained with the knee in 30° of flexion allow surgeons to assess trochlear morphology and patellar height, which can be determined with the use of the Insall-Salvati, Caton-Deschamps, or Blackburne-Peel patellar height ratios. The authors of this chapter prefer to use the Caton-Deschamps patellar height ratio, which is calculated by dividing the distance from the distal-most aspect of the patellar articular surface to the anterosuperior aspect of the tibia by the length of the patellar articular surface (**Figure 1**), because it can be used to describe positional change after distalization (in contrast with the Insall-Salvati ratio, which remains unchanged after distalization). Normal patellar height ratios are between 0.8 and 1.2. Lateral radiographs also can be used to assess trochlear morphology for evidence of dysplasia, which is indicated by the presence of the crossing sign or a supratrochlear spur (**Figure 2**). The crossing sign is observed on lateral radiographs if the radiographic line that represents the deepest part of the trochlear grooves extends beyond the anterior margin of the medial and lateral condyles. The crossing sign indicates that the trochlear groove is essentially flat or convex.[7] The presence of a supratrochlear spur on lateral radiographs represents a bony prominence at the proximal-most aspect of the trochlear groove.[7] Full-length alignment radio-graphs can be used to measure the mechanical axis of patients who have coronal plane malalignment; surgeons should rule out marked valgus alignment in these patients because it may contribute to patellofemoral instability.

CT can be used to accurately assess patellar tilt, subluxation, patellar height, and the tibial tuberosity-trochlear groove distance (TT-TG).[8] The TT-TG distance is calculated by measuring the distance between two parallel lines (one drawn through the anterior-most portion of the tibial tubercle and another drawn through the deepest portion of the trochlear groove), both of which are drawn perpendicular to the posterior femoral condylar axis.[9] DeJour et al[10] reported that most asymptomatic patients have a TT-TG distance of 13 mm. A TT-TG distance greater than 15 mm is associated with lateral patellar instability, and most symptomatic patients have a TT-TG distance greater than 20 mm.[9] CT also can be used to assess for rotational abnormalities such as femoral anteversion or tibial torsion.

MRI can be used to accurately assess the TT-TG distance (**Figure 3**), the tibial tuberosity-posterior cruciate ligament (TT-PCL) distance (**Figure 4**), the Caton-Deschamps patellar height ratio, articular cartilage, and subchondral bone.[11] The TT-PCL distance is assessed in patients who have severe trochlear dysplasia. The TT-PCL distance is independent of the shape of the trochlea, and a TT-PCL distance greater than 24 mm is considered abnormal.[12] MRI is advantageous because ionizing radiation is not used and it offers cartilage-specific imaging sequences (eg, proton density fat suppressed), which allow for better characterization of the location, size, and

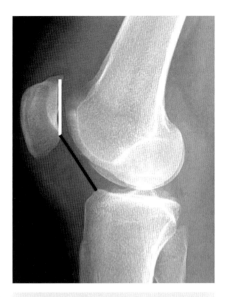

Figure 1 Lateral radiograph of a knee demonstrates the Caton-Deschamps patellar height ratio, which is calculated by dividing the distance from the inferior-most aspect of the patellar articular surface to the anterosuperior aspect of the tibia (black line) by the length of the patellar articular surface (white line).

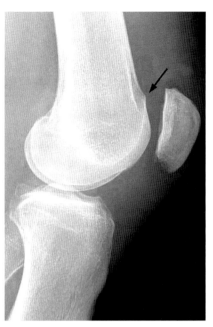

Figure 2 Lateral radiograph of a knee demonstrates a supratrochlear spur (arrow).

depth of a defect compared with older imaging sequences (T1-weighted, T2-weighted, short tau inversion recovery). Subchondral edema and cystic changes also can be observed on MRIs.

Treatment
Nonsurgical Treatment
Most patients with patellofemoral pain who undergo nonsurgical treatment with the assistance of a well-trained physical therapist will experience pain relief. Often, patients with full-thickness cartilage defects in whom nonsurgical treatment fails will require surgical treatment. The goal of nonsurgical treatment is to reduce pain/swelling, improve patellar tracking, improve flexibility, and restore normal gait patterns. The importance of soft-tissue balance with regard to the

restoration of normal knee kinematics via capsular stretching and vastus medialis strengthening has been a mainstay of nonsurgical treatment. Improved hip and trunk muscular control with regard to dynamic function of the lower extremity has recently been reported to result in good outcomes.[13] Improved strength and endurance of the hip and core musculature has been reported to result in positive changes in the frontal plane kinematics of the lower extremity.[14] Most patients with patellofemoral pain who undergo nonsurgical treatment with the assistance of a well-trained physical therapist will experience pain relief and not require surgical treatment.

Surgical Treatment
Cartilage Restoration
Patellofemoral cartilage lesions are difficult to manage because of the inherent complexity of the patellofemoral joint.

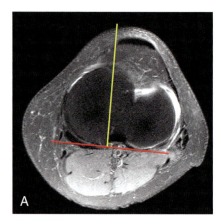 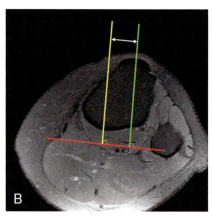

Figure 3   Axial T2-weighted MRIs of a knee demonstrate the method for measuring tibial tuberosity-trochlear groove (TT-TG) distance. **A,** A baseline (red line) is drawn tangent to the posterior femoral condyles at the level of the Roman arch. A line (yellow line) that is perpendicular to the baseline is drawn through the deepest point of the TG. **B,** A line (green line) that is perpendicular to the baseline is drawn at the midpoint of the TT at the level of the patellar tendon attachment. The distance between the yellow line and the green line (double arrow line) is the TT-TG distance.

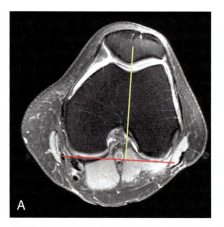 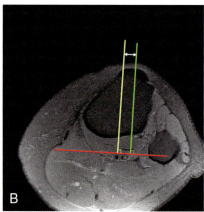

Figure 4   Axial T2-weighted MRIs of a knee demonstrate the method for measuring tibial tuberosity-posterior cruciate ligament (TT-PCL) distance. **A,** A baseline (red line) is drawn tangent to the medial and lateral posterotibial plateaus 1 cm distal to the tibial plateau. A line (yellow line) that is perpendicular to the baseline is drawn through the medial margin of the PCL. **B,** A line (green line) that is perpendicular to the baseline is drawn at the midpoint of the TT at the level of the patellar tendon attachment. The distance between the yellow line and the green line (double arrow line) is the TT-PCL distance.

The differential cartilage thickness, articular contour, and high shear stress encountered in the patellofemoral joint limit the available cartilage restoration options and require meticulous surgical technique to achieve successful outcomes. Patients must be assessed for contraindications to cartilage restoration techniques that may increase the risk for a poor outcome (**Table 1**).

The use of concomitant procedures with the cartilage restoration techniques discussed later is beyond the scope of this chapter; however, a brief mention of tibial tubercle osteotomy (TTO) is warranted. Techniques for the correction of malalignment have evolved; however, an anteromedialization osteotomy helps correct alignment and unloads the patellofemoral joint. The authors of this chapter perform an anteromedialization osteotomy in patients who have patellar chondrosis and a TT-TG distance greater than 20 mm. An anteromedialization osteotomy is especially useful for patients in whom most of the pathology is located on the inferior pole of the patella or the lateral facet.

Débridement/Chondroplasty

The role of débridement in the management of patellar and trochlear cartilage lesions has not been well described in the literature. Mechanical and thermal débridement techniques have been described for all compartments in the knee; however, controversy exists with regard to the extent and magnitude of chondrocyte death associated with these techniques.[15-18] In general, chondroplasty is limited to incidental findings that are encountered during arthroscopy, such as the removal of an irregular chondral flap that is less than 1 to 2 cm^2 in size, which may or may not be related to a patient's mechanical symptoms. One of the most important technical goals of débridement is the creation of stable vertical walls, which may be difficult given the unique anatomy of the patella. Surgeons must avoid deepening partial-thickness defects and exposing subchondral bone during the débridement of patellar defects because doing so can lead to subchondral cyst formation and poor functional outcomes.[19]

The results of chondroplasty for the management of patellofemoral

Table 1

Cartilage Restoration Techniques for Patients With High-Grade Patellofemoral Chondrosis

Technique	Indications	Contraindications	Technical Pearls
Chondroplasty/débridement	Unstable chondral flaps with mechanical symptoms Incidental finding	Large areas of chondrosis Bipolar lesions	Creation of stable walls if practical
Microfracture	Trochlear lesions <2 cm^2 Lower demand patients	Larger lesions Uncontained lesions Bipolar lesions Patellar lesions BMI >35	Creation of stable vertical walls Removal of calcified layer Preservation of bone bridge at least 2-3 mm between holes
Osteochondral autograft transfer	Trochlear or patellar lesions <2 cm^2	Larger lesions Uncontained lesions	Perpendicular placement of plugs Avoid excessive force when seating plugs Avoid harvesting plugs from ipsilateral side of trochlea
Autologous chondrocyte implantation	Trochlear or patellar lesions >3-4 cm^2 Off-label in United States for patellar lesions	Uncontained lesions BMI >35	Avoid damage to subchondral plate
Fresh osteochondral allograft transplantation	Salvage procedure for younger patients who have arthritis and/or in whom restoration procedures fail Trochlear or patellar lesions Technically challenging	Inadequate patellar thickness Advanced arthritis	Morphologic- and size-matched fresh allograft Minimize graft thickness The larger the bony portion, the more likely the patient will become antibody positive

BMI = body mass index.

cartilage lesions are limited. Federico et al[20] reviewed the records of 36 patients who underwent arthroscopic débridement for the management of isolated patellar lesions that caused patellofemoral pain, which was refractory to a minimum of 4 months of nonsurgical treatment. All of the patients had isolated International Cartilage Repair Society grade 2 or grade 3 lesions and no history of patellar instability or malalignment. The authors reported that the mean Fulkerson-Shea Patellofemoral Joint Evaluation score improved from 51.9 to 78.8. Good to excellent results were reported in 58% of the patients who had traumatic lesions and 41% of the patients who had atraumatic lesions.

Marrow Stimulation

The management of patellar and trochlear cartilage lesions with the use of marrow stimulation techniques, such as microfracture, requires the strict adherence to specific principles to achieve successful outcomes. These principles include the thorough débridement of soft tissue from the base, removal of the calcified layer, creation of perpendicular vertical walls, and creation of microfracture holes that are placed 2 to 4 mm apart. The management of patellofemoral cartilage lesions with the use of microfracture may be a challenge. The trochlea is easily accessed, and microfracture can be performed without much technical difficulty; however, the patella may present a

substantial challenge based on lesion location, and a mini-arthrotomy may be required to ensure proper technique. The mobility of the patella may make arthroscopic microfracture techniques difficult. Mechanical devices, such as drills, Kirschner wires, or other proprietary attachments, may be used as an alternative to traditional awl techniques. Penetration of the calcified layer allows mesenchymal cells from the marrow to populate the defect, which results in a fibrocartilaginous scar that fills the lesion. The tissue that is formed is mainly type I collagen, which lends itself to poor durability given the high shear stresses that are encountered in the patellofemoral joint. Kreuz et al[21] supported the poor durability of

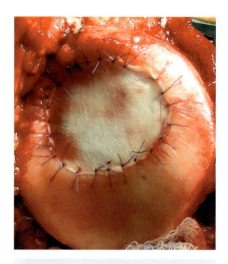

Figure 5 Intraoperative photograph of a knee with a patellar lesion that was managed with autologous chondrocyte implantation. Note that the collagen membrane is secured with the use of 6-0 absorbable sutures, after which fibrin glue is used to create a watertight seal.

fibrocartilage in a study of 85 patients with full-thickness cartilage lesions who underwent microfracture. The authors reported short-term improvement followed by a precipitous decline in function 2 years after microfracture. The decline in function in patients who undergo microfracture is likely caused by the limited peripheral integration and poor histologic quality of the repair tissue because it is mainly type I collagen.[22]

Little high-quality evidence exists for the use of microfracture for the management of patellofemoral cartilage lesions.[22] Currently, microfracture should be limited to and used cautiously in patients who have patellofemoral cartilage lesions smaller than 2 cm². If microfracture is undertaken, execution of proper surgical technique via the creation of properly spaced holes that are perpendicular to the subchondral plate is extremely important to prevent damage to the subchondral plate and avoid

intralesional osteophyte formation, which may have a detrimental effect on subsequent revision procedures, such as autologous chondrocyte implantation (ACI).[23,24]

ACI and Cell-Based Techniques

In 1997, the FDA approved the use of ACI for the management of large defects of the femoral condyles and trochlea. Good long-term outcomes have been reported in patients who have undergone ACI for the management of patellar and bipolar defects; however, the use of ACI for the management of such defects is considered off-label in the United States.[25] Indications for ACI include large (>3 to 4 cm²) full-thickness defects of the femoral condyles or trochlea. Surgeons should carefully assess a patient's subchondral plate on preoperative imaging because patients with substantial abnormality of the subchondral plate, including cystic changes, may require concurrent bone grafting or a cartilage restoration technique other than ACI. Contraindications for ACI include obesity, smoking history, and inflammatory or global osteoarthritis.

ACI is a two-stage cartilage restoration technique. In the first stage of ACI, arthroscopy is performed to harvest a small piece of articular cartilage and assess the global health of the knee, including the chondral surfaces, the menisci, and the cruciate ligaments. The harvested biopsy specimen should be a 200- to 300-mg piece of full-thickness articular cartilage that is taken from the superior and lateral portions of the intercondylar notch. Chondrocytes from the harvested biopsy specimen are enzymatically released and expanded in a cell culture for 2 weeks, after which they are cryopreserved.

After the physician and patient decide to proceed with ACI, the chondrocytes are grown for several more weeks, after which they are shipped to the surgical center.

In the second stage of ACI, the defect is débrided of any poor-quality tissue, and stable vertical shoulders are created. The calcified cartilage layer is removed with the use of meticulous surgical technique to avoid damage to the subchondral plate and to maintain hemostasis. Occasionally, débridement of degenerated tissue in the patella may result in an uncontained defect. Ideally, surgeons should leave a small rim of tissue to which sutures can be sewn rather than use suture anchors. With first-generation ACI techniques, a periosteal patch was used; however, because of overgrowth problems, a collagen membrane currently is routinely used. The collagen membrane is secured with the use of 6-0 absorbable sutures, after which fibrin glue is used to create a watertight seal (**Figure 5**). A small superior opening allows for injection of the chondrocytes. Because the cartilage of the trochlea and patella is thick, a 0.4-mL vial of chondrocytes may not adequately fill the defect. Saline or a second vial of chondrocytes may be added to completely fill the defect. The authors of this chapter routinely order at least two vials of chondrocytes to ensure appropriate cell concentration.

The initial outcomes of ACI for the management of patellofemoral cartilage lesions were disappointing. Brittberg et al[26] reported that only two of seven patients with patellar facet defects who underwent ACI had good or excellent outcomes, whereas 14 of 16 patients with femoral condyle defects who underwent ACI had good or excellent outcomes. Increased understanding of patellofemoral anatomy, kinematics, and ACI implantation techniques as well as the use of concurrent procedures to correct alignment have substantially improved outcomes. In a study of 34 patients with full-thickness patellofemoral cartilage lesions who underwent ACI, Gobbi et al[27] reported statistically significant improvement in all outcome scores at a follow-up of 2 years and 5 years, with the mean International Knee Documentation Committee score improving from 46.09 preoperatively to 77.06 at a follow-up of 5 years. In a multicenter case series of 40 patients with isolated full-thickness trochlear lesions who underwent ACI, Mandelbaum et al[28] reported improved functional outcomes at a mean follow-up of 59 months. In a recent multicenter series of 110 patients with cartilage lesions of the patella, including bipolar defects, who underwent ACI, Gomoll et al[25] reported that, at a minimum follow-up of 4 years, 84% of the patients had good to excellent outcomes, and 92% of the patients stated that they would undergo ACI again. Consistently good outcomes have been reported in patients with lesions of the inferior pole or lateral facet who undergo TTO in combination with ACI.[29] Currently, the use of TTO in combination with ACI for the management of medial facet defects is controversial, whereas improved outcomes have been reported in patients with lateral or panpatellar lesions who undergo TTO in combination with ACI.

Particulated or minced cartilage techniques are quickly gaining use in the United States because they are easy to perform and are less expensive compared with ACI. The indications for particulated cartilage implantation are the same as those for ACI. Particulated cartilage allograft is implanted after a defect is prepared and adequate hemostasis is attained. The particulated cartilage allograft is placed in the defect and secured with fibrin glue. Improvements in symptom relief and function that are maintained 2 years postoperatively have been reported in patients with patellofemoral cartilage defects who undergo particulated cartilage techniques.[30]

Osteochondral Autograft Transfer

The use of osteochondral autograft transfer (OAT) for the management of femoral condyle defects has resulted in successful outcomes.[31] The use of OAT for the management of patellofemoral cartilage defects has not resulted in good outcomes, which likely is because OAT uses grafts from the periphery of the trochlea or the intercondylar notch. The mismatch in contour that occurs as a result of the unique anatomy of the patella and trochlea leads to increased contact pressures if the OAT plug is left proud or to rim loading if the OAT plug is recessed. The cartilage in the patella and central trochlea is substantially thicker compared with that of the sites from which OAT plugs are typically harvested. The step-off that is created by the bony portion of the OAT plug that extends beyond the native subchondral plate is believed to create a stress riser, which may result in cyst formation and graft failure.[32]

The use of OAT for the management of patellofemoral cartilage defects is limited to patients who have small (<2 to 4 cm²) lesions of the patella and trochlea; however, meticulous surgical technique is required (**Figure 6**). The results of OAT for the management of patellofemoral cartilage defects have been inconsistent. Hangody and Füles[31] reported good to excellent outcomes in 79% of patients who underwent OAT for the management of patellar and/or trochlear defects. In a study of 22 patients with patellar defects who underwent OAT, Nho et al[33] reported that the mean International Knee Documentation Committee score increased from 47.2 preoperatively to 74.4 at a mean follow-up of 28.7 months. Miniaci et al[34] reported good to excellent outcomes in eight patients who underwent OAT for the management of full-thickness patellar defects. In a controlled trial of 100 patients with osteochondral defects of the knee who were randomized to either ACI or mosaicplasty, Bentley et al[35] reported that OAT failed in 100% of the patients who had patellar defects. Meticulous surgical technique is extremely important in patients with patellofemoral cartilage lesions who undergo OAT. Proud OAT plugs may result in increased contact stresses, which, given the high shear stress environment of the patellofemoral joint, can lead to poor outcomes. Mismatch of the subchondral bone and cartilage junction between the OAT plug and the implant site may result in mechanical instability with fibrous union and, subsequently, cyst formation.[32,36] In many patients, a mini-arthrotomy is required to improve visualization and ensure that the OAT plug fits properly, particularly in the patella, which is not accessible arthroscopically.

Osteochondral Allograft Transplantation

The use of osteochondral allografts increased after the FDA imposed stricter guidelines for the procurement and storage of allograft tissues, which decreased the risk for disease transmission.[37] Osteochondral allograft transplantation is

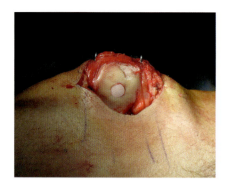

Figure 6 Intraoperative photograph of a knee with an osteochondral allograft transfer plug, which was used to manage a small, well-contained chondral lesion of the lateral patellar facet.

a considerable challenge in patients who have patellofemoral cartilage lesions because it may be difficult to morphologically match patella to patella. Osteochondral allograft transplantation is the most challenging cartilage restoration technique for the management of patellofemoral cartilage defects because only one attempt at the procedure is realistically feasible. In general, osteochondral allograft transplantation is indicated for patients who have full-thickness defects with abnormal subchondral bone. Usually, larger osteochondral shell allografts can be used in patients younger than 40 years who have larger, uncontained lesions or bipolar lesions that are not amenable to other cartilage restoration techniques.

Osteochondral allograft transplantation is performed via an arthrotomy. Defects that are amenable to a large osteochondral allograft are prepared, and a size- and shape-matched osteochondral allograft plug is press fit in the prepared defect. Osteochondral shell allograft transplantation can be used as a salvage procedure for patients who have large and irregular patellofemoral cartilage defects. In osteochondral shell allograft transplantation, the patella is prepared in the same manner as that for patellar arthroplasty, conserving a minimum of 12 to 15 mm of bone, which is required to prevent fracture. The trochlea is prepared with a cut that is made in a single plane just proximal to the roof of the intercondylar notch; the cut is then carried just cephalad to the proximal aspect of the trochlea without notching the anterior femoral cortex. The osteochondral allografts are cut and then secured outside of the articulating surface with the use of biocompression or metal screws. Thorough irrigation of the bony portion of the osteochondral allograft is important to decrease the number of marrow elements in the tissue, which are believed to be the only source of immunogenic reaction.[37] The incidence of immunogenic reactions in patients who undergo osteochondral allograft transplantation is rare as a result of thorough irrigation practices and because chondrocytes are believed to be immune privileged.

The outcomes of patients with patellofemoral cartilage lesions who undergo osteochondral allograft transplantation are less promising compared with those of patients with condylar lesions who undergo osteochondral allograft transplantation. In a retrospective review of 18 patients (20 knees) who underwent osteochondral allograft transplantation, Jamali et al[38] reported good to excellent outcomes in 60% of the patients at a mean follow-up of 94 months. In a series of 11 patients (14 knees) with patellofemoral arthritis who underwent fresh osteochondral allograft transplantation, Torga Spak and Teitge[39] reported graft survival in 57% of the patients at a follow-up of 10 years, which is less favorable compared with osteochondral allograft survival in other knee compartments.[40] The failure rates observed in these already mentioned studies also are higher compared with those observed in patients who undergo ACI or patellofemoral arthroplasty; therefore, narrow indications exist for use of osteochondral allografts given the potential for failure. However, patients younger than 40 years with diffuse degenerative patellofemoral joint changes in whom nonsurgical treatment fails are candidates for osteochondral allograft transplantation because of the lack of surgical alternatives.

Partial Lateral Facetectomy and Lateral Retinacular Lengthening

Partial lateral facetectomy and lateral retinacular lengthening is a relatively simple resection arthroplasty technique that is used to treat patients with isolated lateral patellar arthrosis or bipolar lesions of the lateral patellofemoral joint in whom nonsurgical treatment fails. In general, isolated patellofemoral arthritis is a slow disease process that is well tolerated.[41,42] Patients with isolated patellofemoral arthritis most often report pain during knee flexion as they traverse stairs and while rising from a chair. On physical examination, patients with isolated patellofemoral arthritis often have lateral patellar tenderness and a decreased ability to translate the patella medially.[43] Frequently, imaging studies of patients with isolated patellofemoral arthritis reveal substantial lateral patellofemoral joint space narrowing, with pseudolateral patellar tilt and a large trailing osteophyte observed on axial radiographs or MRIs.

The indications for partial lateral facetectomy and lateral retinacular lengthening include isolated lateral facet arthrosis and patellar tilt in patients who do not have substantial subluxation or a current history of patellofemoral instability. Axial MRIs should reveal a large trailing osteophyte and minimal evidence of tibiofemoral arthritis. Patients should have had a positive response to McConnell taping as well as strength gains during physical therapy without improvements in pain relief. The authors of this chapter prefer to perform partial lateral facetectomy and lateral retinacular lengthening via an open technique. The authors of this chapter prefer to perform partial lateral facetectomy in combination with lateral retinacular lengthening because it allows surgeons to better balance patellofemoral forces and reduces the risk for excessive medial translation. For partial lateral retinacular lengthening, a longitudinal incision is made adjacent to the lateral border of the patella, after which the patellar contribution of the iliotibial band is divided. The lateral patellofemoral ligament and capsule are incised in a more lateral location and are dissected medially from the underlying osteophyte, which is then removed with the use of an oscillating saw. The iliotibial band contribution that was transected at the lateral border of the patella is then sewn to the edge of the lateral patellofemoral ligament and capsule, which effectively lengthens the lateral soft tissues approximately 10 to 15 mm (**Figure 7**).

Satisfactory mid- to long-term outcomes have been reported in patients with isolated patellofemoral arthritis who undergo partial lateral facetectomy and lateral retinacular lengthening. In a study of 11 patients with isolated lateral patellofemoral osteoarthritis who underwent partial lateral facetectomy, Yercan et al[44] reported a statistically significant improvement in the mean Knee Society score, which improved

from 150 preoperatively to 176 at a final follow-up of 14 years. In a study of 63 patients (66 knees) with patellofemoral arthritis who underwent partial lateral facetectomy and lateral retinacular lengthening, Paulos et al[45] reported that, at a mean follow-up of 5 years, 80% of the patients had symptomatic relief, and 88% of the patients stated that they were very satisfied or satisfied and willing to undergo the procedure again. The longest follow-up study of patients with isolated patellofemoral arthritis who underwent partial lateral facetectomy was reported in a study by Wetzels et al.[46] The authors reported that 50% of 155 patients with isolated patellofemoral arthritis who underwent partial lateral facetectomy were satisfied at a mean follow-up of 10.9 years. The outcomes of partial lateral facetectomy and lateral retinacular lengthening in patients with end-stage, isolated, lateral patellar arthrosis who are not yet candidates for total knee arthroplasty or patellofemoral arthroplasty are satisfactory; however, surgeons should ensure that the expectations of patients in whom partial lateral facetectomy and lateral retinacular lengthening is being considered match expected surgical outcomes.

Patellofemoral Arthroplasty

The management of diffuse, symptomatic patellofemoral arthritis may be a challenge for orthopaedic surgeons. Patellofemoral arthroplasty is emerging as a viable option for patients who have isolated patellofemoral arthritis with pain that is refractory to nonsurgical treatment and patients in whom cartilage restoration techniques fail. In active patients younger than 40 years, diffuse, isolated patellofemoral arthritis is either posttraumatic in origin or, more commonly, the result of trochlear

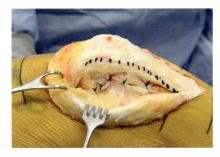

Figure 7   Intraoperative photograph of a knee that underwent partial lateral retinacular lengthening as part of a cartilage transplant procedure. The patellofemoral joint was accessed via a lateral parapatellar approach. The superficial layer (iliotibial band contribution to the patella) was divided at the lateral edge of the patella (dotted line). The deep layer (patellofemoral ligament and capsule) was divided approximately 2 cm away from the lateral edge of the patella. On closure, the edge of the superficial and deep layers were sutured to each other with the use of interrupted stitches, which effectively lengthened the lateral soft tissues by 2 cm.

dysplasia with or without recurrent episodes of patellar dislocation. Patellofemoral arthroplasty that was performed with the use of first-generation implants resulted in revision surgery rates as high as 63%.[47] Patellofemoral arthroplasty that is performed with the use of second-generation implants has resulted in improved outcomes, with studies reporting good and excellent outcomes in 80% to 90% of patients at a midterm follow up of 6 to 7 years.[48]

Second-generation patellofemoral arthroplasty implants are designed to better match the radius of curvature of the trochlear groove and have wider anterior flanges, which allows for extension more proximally, compared with first-generation patellofemoral arthroplasty implants. The wider mediolateral dimension and greater proximal extension of second-generation

Table 2

Results of Patellofemoral Arthroplasty With Second-Generation Implants

Authors (Year)	No. of Patients (Knees)	Mean Patient Age in Years (Range)	Mean Follow-up (Range)	Outcomes	Survival
Ackroyd et al[53] (2007)	85 (109)	68 (46–86)	5.2 yr (5–8 yr)	Median BPS: Pre, 15; Post, 35 Median Melbourne score: Pre, 10; Post, 25 Median OKS: Pre, 18; Post, 39	No knees revised during the study period 1 patient required distal soft-tissue realignment for patellar maltracking
Mont et al[51] (2012)	47 (53)	49 (27–67)	7 yr (4–8 yr)	Mean objective KSS: Pre, 64; Post, 87 Mean functional KSS: Pre, 48; Post, 82	5 patients underwent revision to TKR by mean follow-up of 7 years Kaplan Meier Survivorship: 95% at mean follow-up of 5 years; 82% at mean follow-up of 7 years
Morris et al[50] (2013)	30 (37)	55 (32–80)	31 mo (12–80 mo)	Mean pain KSS: Pre, 10.6; Post, 33.8 Mean clinical KSS: Pre, 59.4; Post, 82.4 Mean functional KSS: Pre, 56; Post, 62.8	No revisions 2 secondary surgeries (1 for arthrofibrosis, 1 for adhesions and painful crepitus)
Dahm et al[52] (2014)	59 (NR)	56 (± 10.4)	4 yr (2–6 yr)	Post KSS: 89 Post UCLA: 6.6	No reported failures or complications
Akhbari et al[54] (2015)	57 (61)	66.1 (± 10.1)	5.09 yr (12–124 mo)	Median HKS: Pre, 40; Post, 80 Mean OKS: Pre, 20.8; Post, 31.8	96.3% survivorship at mean follow-up of 5 years 2 patients underwent revision to TKR

BPS = Bristol pain score, HKS = Hungerford and Kenna score, KSS = Knee Society score, Melbourne = Melbourne patellar score, NR = not reported, OKS = Oxford knee score, Post = postoperative, Pre = preoperative, TKR = total knee replacement, UCLA = University of California–Los Angeles Activity score.

patellofemoral arthroplasty implants is less constraining compared with first-generation patellofemoral arthroplasty implants, which allows for enhanced patellar tracking. The most common cause of failure in patients who undergo patellofemoral arthroplasty with the use of second-generation implants is the progression of tibiofemoral arthritis.[49] Importantly, patients with radiographic evidence of trochlear dysplasia preoperatively have less progression of tibiofemoral arthritis postoperatively. Although long-term follow-up of patients who undergo patellofemoral arthroplasty with the use of second-generation implants is lacking, studies have reported that, with appropriate patient selection and meticulous surgical technique, patellofemoral arthroplasty with the use of second-generation implants is a reliable alternative to total knee arthroplasty in active patients younger than 40 years who have isolated, diffuse patellofemoral arthritis[50-54] (**Table 2**).

Summary

Patients who have anterior knee pain may be a diagnostic and therapeutic challenge. A full assessment of the knee and the lower extremity alignment of patients who have anterior knee pain must be performed to address any additional pathologic conditions that may compromise the integrity and durability of proposed cartilage restoration techniques. Multiple cartilage restoration techniques have been reported to result in acceptable outcomes; however, given the complex structure of the patellofemoral joint, meticulous surgical technique is required to ensure the durability of the repair or reconstruction.

References

1. Curl WW, Krome J, Gordon ES, et al: Cartilage injuries: A review of 31,516 knee arthroscopies. *Arthroscopy* 1997;13(4):456-460.

2. Beynnon BD, Johnson RJ, Coughlin KM: Relevant biomechanics of the knee, in DeLee JC, Drez D Jr, Miller MD, eds: *Orthopaedic Sports Medicine: Principles and Practice,* ed 2. Philadelphia, PA, Saunders, 2003, pp 1577-1595.

3. Fu FH, Seel MJ, Berger RA: Patellofemoral biomechanics, in Fox JM, Del Pizzo W, eds: *The Patellofemoral Joint.* New York, NY, McGraw-Hill, 1993, pp 49-62.

4. Post WR: Clinical evaluation of patients with patellofemoral disorders. *Arthroscopy* 1999;15(8):841-851.

5. Beighton P, Horan F: Orthopaedic aspects of the Ehlers-Danlos syndrome. *J Bone Joint Surg Br* 1969;51(3):444-453.

6. Stäubli HU, Dürrenmatt U, Porcellini B, Rauschning W: Anatomy and surface geometry of the patellofemoral joint in the axial plane. *J Bone Joint Surg Br* 1999;81(3):452-458.

7. Dejour D, Le Coultre B: Osteotomies in patello-femoral instabilities. *Sports Med Arthrosc* 2007;15(1):39-46.

8. Tavernier T, Dejour D: Knee imaging: What is the best modality. *J Radiol* 2001;82(3 pt 2):387-405, 407-408.

9. Schoettle PB, Zanetti M, Seifert B, Pfirrmann CW, Fucentese SF, Romero J: The tibial tuberosity-trochlear groove distance; a comparative study between CT and MRI scanning. *Knee* 2006;13(1):26-31.

10. Dejour H, Walch G, Nove-Josserand L, Guier C: Factors of patellar instability: An anatomic radiographic study. *Knee Surg Sports Traumatol Arthrosc* 1994;2(1):19-26.

11. Camp CL, Stuart MJ, Krych AJ, et al: CT and MRI measurements of tibial tubercle-trochlear groove distances are not equivalent in patients with patellar instability. *Am J Sports Med* 2013;41(8):1835-1840.

12. Seitlinger G, Scheurecker G, Högler R, Labey L, Innocenti B, Hofmann S: Tibial tubercle-posterior cruciate ligament distance: A new measurement to define the position of the tibial tubercle in patients with patellar dislocation. *Am J Sports Med* 2012;40(5):1119-1125.

13. Werner S: Anterior knee pain: An update of physical therapy. *Knee Surg Sports Traumatol Arthrosc* 2014;22(10):2286-2294.

14. Baldon Rde M, Piva SR, Scattone Silva R, Serrão FV: Evaluating eccentric hip torque and trunk endurance as mediators of changes in lower limb and trunk kinematics in response to functional stabilization training in women with patellofemoral pain. *Am J Sports Med* 2015;43(6):1485-1493.

15. Kosy JD, Schranz PJ, Toms AD, Eyres KS, Mandalia VI: The use of radiofrequency energy for arthroscopic chondroplasty in the knee. *Arthroscopy* 2011;27(5):695-703.

16. Lotto ML, Wright EJ, Appleby D, Zelicof SB, Lemos MJ, Lubowitz JH: Ex vivo comparison of mechanical versus thermal chondroplasty: Assessment of tissue effect at the surgical endpoint. *Arthroscopy* 2008;24(4):410-415.

17. Kaplan LD, Chu CR, Bradley JP, Fu FH, Studer RK: Recovery of chondrocyte metabolic activity after thermal exposure. *Am J Sports Med* 2003;31(3):392-398.

18. Kaplan LD, Ionescu D, Ernsthausen JM, Bradley JP, Fu FH, Farkas DL: Temperature requirements for altering the morphology of osteoarthritic and nonarthritic articular cartilage: In vitro thermal alteration of articular cartilage. *Am J Sports Med* 2004;32(3):688-692.

19. Galloway MT, Noyes FR: Cystic degeneration of the patella after arthroscopic chondroplasty and subchondral bone perforation. *Arthroscopy* 1992;8(3):366-369.

20. Federico DJ, Reider B: Results of isolated patellar debridement for patellofemoral pain in patients with normal patellar alignment. *Am J Sports Med* 1997;25(5):663-669.

21. Kreuz PC, Steinwachs MR, Erggelet C, et al: Results after microfracture of full-thickness chondral defects in different compartments in the knee. *Osteoarthritis Cartilage* 2006;14(11):1119-1125.

22. Mithoefer K, McAdams T, Williams RJ, Kreuz PC, Mandelbaum BR: Clinical efficacy of the microfracture technique for articular cartilage repair in the knee: An evidence-based systematic analysis. *Am J Sports Med* 2009;37(10):2053-2063.

23. Minas T, Gomoll AH, Rosenberger R, Royce RO, Bryant T: Increased failure rate of autologous chondrocyte implantation after previous treatment with marrow stimulation techniques. *Am J Sports Med* 2009;37(5):902-908.

24. Jungmann PM, Salzmann GM, Schmal H, Pestka JM, Südkamp NP, Niemeyer P: Autologous chondrocyte implantation for treatment of cartilage defects of the knee: What predicts the need for reintervention? *Am J Sports Med* 2012;40(1):58-67.

25. Gomoll AH, Gillogly SD, Cole BJ, et al: Autologous chondrocyte implantation in the patella: A multicenter experience. *Am J Sports Med* 2014;42(5):1074-1081

26. Brittberg M, Lindahl A, Nilsson A, Ohlsson C, Isaksson O, Peterson L: Treatment of deep cartilage defects in the knee with autologous chondrocyte transplantation. *N Engl J Med* 1994;331(14):889-895.

27. Gobbi A, Kon E, Berruto M, et al: Patellofemoral full-thickness chondral defects treated with second-generation autologous chondrocyte implantation: Results at 5 years' follow-up. *Am J Sports Med* 2009;37(6):1083-1092.

28. Mandelbaum B, Browne JE, Fu F, et al: Treatment outcomes of autologous chondrocyte implantation for full-thickness articular cartilage defects of the trochlea. *Am J Sports Med* 2007;35(6):915-921.

29. Henderson IJ, Lavigne P: Periosteal autologous chondrocyte implantation for patellar chondral defect in patients with normal and abnormal patellar tracking. *Knee* 2006;13(4):274-279.

30. Bonner KF, Daner W, Yao JQ: 2-year postoperative evaluation of a patient with a symptomatic full-thickness patellar cartilage defect repaired with particulated juvenile cartilage tissue. *J Knee Surg* 2010;23(2):109-114.

31. Hangody L, Füles P: Autologous osteochondral mosaicplasty for the treatment of full-thickness defects of weight-bearing joints: Ten years of experimental and clinical experience. *J Bone Joint Surg Am* 2003;85(suppl 2):25-32.

32. von Rechenberg B, Akens MK, Nadler D, et al: Changes in subchondral bone in cartilage resurfacing—an experimental study in sheep using different types of osteochondral grafts. *Osteoarthritis Cartilage* 2003;11(4):265-277.

33. Nho SJ, Foo LF, Green DM, et al: Magnetic resonance imaging and clinical evaluation of patellar resurfacing with press-fit osteochondral autograft plugs. *Am J Sports Med* 2008;36(6):1101-1109.

34. Miniaci A, Jambor C, Petrigliano FA: Autologous osteochondral transplantation, in Williams RJ, ed: *Cartilage Repair Strategies*. Totowa, NJ, Humana Press, 2007.

35. Bentley G, Biant LC, Carrington RW, et al: A prospective, randomised comparison of autologous chondrocyte implantation versus mosaicplasty for osteochondral defects in the knee. *J Bone Joint Surg Br* 2003;85(2):223-230.

36. Koh JL, Kowalski A, Lautenschlager E: The effect of angled osteochondral grafting on contact pressure: A biomechanical study. *Am J Sports Med* 2006;34(1):116-119.

37. Torrie AM, Kesler WW, Elkin J, Gallo RA: Osteochondral allograft. *Curr Rev Musculoskelet Med* 2015;8(4):413-422.

38. Jamali AA, Emmerson BC, Chung C, Convery FR, Bugbee WD: Fresh osteochondral allografts: Results in the patellofemoral joint. *Clin Orthop Relat Res* 2005;437:176-185.

39. Torga Spak R, Teitge RA: Fresh osteochondral allografts for patellofemoral arthritis: Long-term followup. *Clin Orthop Relat Res* 2006;443:193-200.

40. Demange M, Gomoll AH: The use of osteochondral allografts in the management of cartilage defects. *Curr Rev Musculoskelet Med* 2012;5(3):229-235.

41. Dejour D, Allain J: Isolated patellofemoral osteoarthritis. *Rev Chir Orthop* 2004;90(suppl 5):S69-129.

42. Grelsamer RP, Dejour D, Gould J: The pathophysiology of patellofemoral arthritis. *Orthop Clin North Am* 2008;39(3):269-274, v.

43. Kolowich PA, Paulos LE, Rosenberg TD, Farnsworth S: Lateral release of the patella: Indications and contraindications. *Am J Sports Med* 1990;18(4):359-365.

44. Yercan HS, Ait Si Selmi T, Neyret P: The treatment of patellofemoral osteoarthritis with partial lateral facetectomy. *Clin Orthop Relat Res* 2005;436:14-19.

45. Paulos LE, O'Connor DL, Karistinos A: Partial lateral patellar facetectomy for treatment of arthritis due to lateral patellar compression syndrome. *Arthroscopy* 2008;24(5):547-553.

46. Wetzels T, Bellemans J: Patellofemoral osteoarthritis treated by partial lateral facetectomy: Results at long-term follow up. *Knee* 2012;19(4):411-415.

47. Tauro B, Ackroyd CE, Newman JH, Shah NA: The Lubinus patellofemoral arthroplasty: A five- to ten-year prospective study. *J Bone Joint Surg Br* 2001;83(5):696-701.

48. Sisto DJ, Sarin VK: Custom patellofemoral arthroplasty of the knee. *J Bone Joint Surg Am* 2006;88(7):1475-1480.

49. Lustig S, Magnussen RA, Dahm DL, Parker D: Patellofemoral arthroplasty, where are we today? *Knee Surg Sports Traumatol Arthrosc* 2012;20(7):1216-1226.

50. Morris MJ, Lombardi AV Jr, Berend KR, Hurst JM, Adams JB: Clinical results of patellofemoral arthroplasty. *J Arthroplasty* 2013;28(9 suppl):199-201.

51. Mont MA, Johnson AJ, Naziri Q, Kolisek FR, Leadbetter WB: Patellofemoral arthroplasty: 7-year mean follow-up. *J Arthroplasty* 2012;27(3):358-361.

52. Dahm DL, Kalisvaart MM, Stuart MJ, Slettedahl SW: Patellofemoral arthroplasty: Outcomes and factors associated with early progression of tibiofemoral arthritis. *Knee Surg Sports Traumatol Arthrosc* 2014;22(10):2554-2559.

53. Ackroyd CE, Newman JH, Evans R, Eldridge JD, Joslin CC: The Avon patellofemoral arthroplasty: Five-year survivorship and functional results. *J Bone Joint Surg Br* 2007;89(3):310-315.

54. Akhbari P, Malak T, Dawson-Bowling S, East D, Miles K, Butler-Manuel PA: The Avon patellofemoral joint replacement: Mid-term prospective results from an independent centre. *Clin Orthop Surg* 2015;7(2):171-176.

International Perspective on Revision Anterior Cruciate Ligament Reconstruction: What Have We Been Missing?

Mohammad Humza Ansari, BS
Steven Claes, MD, PhD
Daniel C. Wascher, MD
Philippe Neyret, MD
Michael J. Stuart, MD
Aaron J. Krych, MD

Abstract

Primary anterior cruciate ligament (ACL) reconstruction is a common orthopaedic procedure. A graft failure rate of 5% to 10% after primary ACL reconstruction has resulted in an increased need for revision ACL reconstruction. ACL reconstruction failure etiologies include trauma, technical errors, and biologic factors. Based on the current literature, the outcomes of revision ACL reconstruction are clearly inferior compared with those of primary reconstruction. A thorough patient evaluation, including surgical history, a physical examination, and imaging studies, is crucial in the assessment of a failed ACL reconstruction. Tunnel malposition, which is a technical error, is the most common reason for ACL reconstruction failure. Tunnel positioning and widening are important factors to consider in the decision to perform either one-stage or two-stage revision ACL reconstruction. Other concomitant factors such as malalignment, pathologic posterior tibial slope, and meniscal or ligamentous deficiency (in particular, deficiency of the anterolateral ligament) must be considered and addressed to achieve an optimal outcome. Patients who have a positive pivot shift test and rotational instability may require extra-articular anterolateral ligament reconstruction. In addition, patients who have severe pathologic tibial slope and anterior tibial translation may require a tibial deflexion osteotomy.

Instr Course Lect 2017;66:543–556.

Anterior cruciate ligament (ACL) reconstruction is one of the most common procedures in orthopaedic surgery and is generally successful in reducing symptomatic instability. Given that more than 200,000 primary ACL reconstructions are performed each year, the current graft rupture rate of 5% has led to numerous revision ACL reconstructions.[1,2] Graft rupture is not the only cause of failure that may require revision ACL reconstruction. Unsatisfactory outcomes after ACL reconstruction may result from intraoperative or postoperative complications, concomitant cartilage or meniscal injuries, or persistent instability with an intact graft[3] (**Figure 1**). Successful revision ACL reconstruction requires identification of the most likely reason for primary ACL reconstruction failure.

ACL Reconstruction Failure Etiology

In a large systematic review of revision ACL reconstruction, primary ACL reconstruction failure etiologies were categorized as traumatic reinjuries (49%), technical errors (46%), and biologic

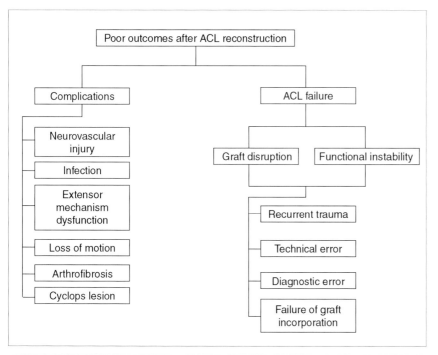

Figure 1 Flowchart shows various etiologies of poor outcomes after anterior cruciate ligament (ACL) reconstruction.

ACL reconstruction, which reflects the technical demands of ACL reconstruction.[7] Wasserstein et al[8] reported that academic center status was a risk factor for ACL reconstruction failure, which may confirm that surgeon trainees negatively influence ACL reconstruction outcomes.

Untreated secondary instability at the time of the index surgery also is a key reason for ACL reconstruction failure. Ligamentous instability can result from injuries to the posterolateral corner, the posterior cruciate ligament, the medial collateral ligament (MCL), or the anterolateral ligament (ALL). In addition, there may be meniscal root detachment, an unrecognized hidden tear of the medial meniscus (the so-called "ramp lesion"), or a lack of the posterior horn of the medial meniscus.[9,10] A thorough workup for revision ACL reconstruction must include an evaluation of the secondary restraints of the knee and the integrity of the posterior horn of the medial meniscus.

Another cause of ACL reconstruction failure is a lack of biologic graft healing; this may be more common in younger patients who undergo allograft ACL reconstruction. van Eck et al[11] reported that patients younger than 25 years had a higher risk for graft failure after allograft ACL reconstruction. Several possible reasons for allograft biologic failure exist. Early ACL reconstruction allograft failure may result from a possible immune response and subsequent lack of graft incorporation or ligamentization. A second reason for early ACL reconstruction allograft biologic failure is premature return to high-level activities before complete graft healing and remodeling. A meta-analysis by Krych et al[12] reported that irradiation, which

factors (5%).[4] A study of 148 patients in whom ACL reconstruction failed reported that 64% of the failures were caused by tunnel malposition (a technical error). Other reasons for failure included traumatic reinjury (24%), synthetic graft (6%), posterolateral instability (3%), graft elongation (2%), and tunnel dilation (2%).[5] Femoral socket

malposition is the most common technical error that causes recurrent instability after ACL reconstruction. Most of the ACL reconstructions performed in the United States are done by surgeons who perform fewer than 10 ACL reconstructions per year.[6] Thus, there appears to be a correlation between surgeon volume and outcomes after

Dr. Claes or an immediate family member is a member of a speakers' bureau or has made paid presentations on behalf of Arthrex and Smith & Nephew, and serves as a paid consultant to or is an employee of Arthrex. Dr. Wascher or an immediate family member has received research or institutional support from Arthrex and Smith & Nephew, and serves as a board member, owner, officer, or committee member of the American Orthopaedic Society for Sports Medicine. Dr. Neyret or an immediate family member has received royalties from Tornier; is a member of a speakers' bureau or has made paid presentations on behalf of Tornier; serves as a paid consultant to or is an employee of Blue Belt Technologies, Smith & Nephew, and Tornier; has received research or institutional support from Tornier, Resoimplant, and the Tissue Bank of France; has received nonincome support (such as equipment or services), commercially derived honoraria, or other non-research–related funding (such as paid travel) from Tornier, the Tissue Bank of France, and Resoimplant; and serves as a board member, owner, officer, or committee member of the Anterior Cruciate Ligament Study Group, the Knee Society, the International Society of Arthroscopy, Knee Surgery and Orthopaedic Sports Medicine, and the European Federation of National Associations of Orthopedics and Traumatology. Dr. Stuart has received royalties from Arthrex; serves as a paid consultant to or is an employee of Arthrex; and has received research or institutional support from Stryker. Dr. Krych or an immediate family member serves as a paid consultant to or is an employee of Arthrex, and has received research or institutional support from the Arthritis Foundation and Histogenics. Neither Mr. Ansari nor any immediate family member has received anything of value from or has stock or stock options held in a commercial company or institution related directly or indirectly to the subject of this chapter.

is used to sterilize grafts, may increase the risk for graft failure by possibly delaying graft remodeling. Finally, higher tension loads on an ACL graft may contribute to delayed healing and subsequent failure. A recent study of a large number of primary ACL reconstructions from the Danish Knee Ligament Reconstruction Register suggested that an anatomic graft position may result in increased biomechanical loads, leading to poor biologic healing and subsequent graft failure. The study reported that the relative risk of graft rupture was two times greater in patients who underwent anteromedial drilling of the femoral tunnel compared with patients who underwent transtibial drilling. This increased risk for graft rupture may be caused by increased tension on an anatomic ACL graft that is positioned with anteromedial drilling versus a vertically oriented nonanatomic graft that is positioned with transtibial drilling.[13] Currently, ACL graft healing mechanisms are poorly understood, and even ACL reconstruction with an allograft can result in incomplete incorporation.

An often overlooked reason for graft failure is poor lower extremity biodynamics. Insufficient muscle control can contribute to graft rupture and will not improve after surgery. The correction of a patient's lower extremity biodynamics is crucial to prevent secondary ACL injury after ACL reconstruction. Lower extremity biodynamics can be assessed with the four measures of neuromuscular asymmetry: excessive frontal plane knee mechanics, hip rotational control deficits, knee flexor deficits, and postural control deficits.[14] If pathologic lower extremity biodynamics are not corrected before ACL reconstruction,

then any graft, no matter how strong or anatomic, will fail. Fortunately, lower extremity biodynamics can be addressed before ACL reconstruction and during postoperative rehabilitation.[14]

Current Results of Revision ACL Reconstruction

Because of an increased number of concomitant injuries at the time of revision ACL reconstruction, it is important to note the treatment results of these concomitant injuries.[15] Wright et al[4] reported that 56% of patients underwent a partial meniscectomy and 14% of patients underwent a meniscal repair at the time of revision ACL reconstruction. With respect to articular cartilage, the authors reported that 79% of patients had grade I or grade II lesions, and 21% of patients had grade III or grade IV lesions, with an almost even distribution between medial, lateral, and patellofemoral locations. Concomitant chondral lesions correlate with worse Lysholm Knee Scale and International Knee Documentation Committee (IKDC) Subjective Knee Evaluation Form scores.[5] The Lysholm Knee Scale allows for the evaluation of instability symptoms after ligament surgery. In addition, even at short-term to midterm follow-up, radiographic osteoarthritic changes occur in 37% to 80% of patients.[16]

In a systematic review of 863 patients from 21 studies who underwent revision ACL reconstruction, Wright et al[4] reported that, at a follow-up of 2 years, objective graft failure occurred in 14% of the patients, and the mean Lysholm Knee Scale score and mean IKDC Subjective Knee Evaluation Form score were 82 and 75, respectively. The IKDC Subjective Knee Evaluation Form score reported by the authors was

a concern because severely abnormal knee function is defined by an IKDC Subjective Knee Evaluation Form score less than 75.4.[17] Therefore, the authors concluded that the outcomes of revision ACL reconstruction are worse compared with those of primary ACL reconstruction.[4] The return-to-sport results after revision ACL reconstruction are highly variable. Kamath et al[16] reported that as many as 40% of athletes who undergo revision ACL reconstruction are unable to return to the same level of competition.

Unfortunately, the current results of revision ACL reconstruction are much less positive compared with patients' expectations after revision ACL reconstruction. Feucht et al[18] reported that unrealistic patient expectations negatively influence patient-reported outcomes after revision ACL reconstruction. The authors reported that, after revision ACL reconstruction, 84% of patients expected the same level of activity, 92% of patients expected no pain or only minor pain with high-demand activities, 94% of patients expected no instability or only minor instability during sport activities, and 96% of patients expected no or only a slightly increased risk of future osteoarthritis. Surgeons must set realistic goals that reflect the current outcomes of revision ACL reconstruction for patients who undergo revision ACL reconstruction.

Revision ACL reconstruction may fail in some patients. Griffith et al[19] reported that repeat revision ACL reconstruction may improve functional outcomes for patients in whom revision ACL reconstruction fails. The presence of grade III or grade IV chondral lesions and a body mass index greater than 28 kg/m² are associated with

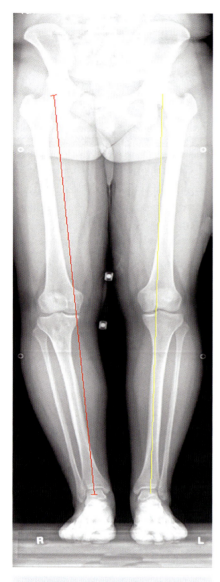

Figure 2 AP long leg alignment radiograph of the lower limbs of an 18-year-old woman in whom right knee anterior cruciate ligament reconstruction failed demonstrates asymmetric varus alignment. Varus thrust was observed on physical examination. The red and yellow lines indicate the mechanical axis of each limb.

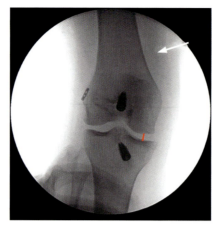

Figure 3 AP valgus stress radiograph of the knee of a patient in whom anterior cruciate ligament reconstruction failed twice demonstrates increased valgus laxity (arrow) and opening of the medial compartment (red line).

Approach and Preoperative Patient Evaluation

A thorough patient evaluation must include a careful review of previous clinical notes, surgical reports, and arthroscopic images. Medical records should be examined, with careful attention given to the surgical report of the time since the index surgery, the type of graft that was used, and the type of fixation that was used. In addition, a patient's history helps establish whether the failed ACL reconstruction was a true reinjury or a minor reinjury with failure to return to full activity. This distinction is important because early ACL reconstruction failure or a minor reinjury may suggest that the knee never regained stability. Early ACL reconstruction failure, which is defined as that occurring less than 5 months postoperatively, is likely caused by poor surgical technique, incomplete graft incorporation, a loss of graft fixation, overly aggressive rehabilitation, or a premature return to

worse outcomes after repeat revision ACL reconstruction.[19] Importantly, most patients do not return to the same activity levels after repeat revision ACL reconstruction.[19]

high-demand activities.[16] Later ACL reconstruction failure suggests that stability was restored after primary ACL reconstruction, but a traumatic reinjury occurred.

A careful physical examination is important during the preoperative patient evaluation phase. A gait analysis provides the surgeon with information about overall mechanics and alignment. An examination of the contralateral knee helps create a baseline for range of motion and ligament laxity. The surgeon should carefully observe for any concurrent ligamentous deficiencies in the knee. Well-performed Lachman and pivot shift tests can help distinguish between a completely torn graft and an intact graft with persistent rotational laxity.

Imaging is useful to determine the cause for graft failure. A long leg alignment radiograph helps assess alignment asymmetries (**Figure 2**). If a fibular collateral ligament, MCL, or posterolateral corner injury is suspected, varus and valgus stress radiographs can help quantify the severity of the injury (**Figure 3**). A single-leg-stance radiograph may be obtained if increased posterior tibial slope or anterior tibial translation is suspected (**Figure 4**). A Rosenberg radiograph can help assess joint space narrowing (**Figure 5**). Advanced imaging, such as MRI or CT, can aid in mapping the location, size, and position of previous tunnels as well as locating the bioabsorbable screw. MRI can reveal the status of the meniscus and the articular cartilage of the affected joint. An axial MRI that is obtained in the operating room may be preferred to assess the position of the femoral tunnel because it is obtained with the knee in 90° of flexion (**Figure 6**).

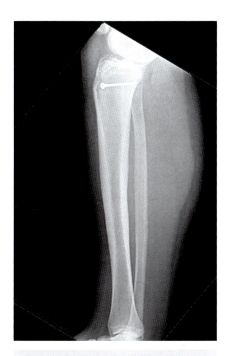

Figure 4   Lateral single-leg-stance radiograph of the leg of an 18-year old man who failed anterior cruciate ligament reconstruction three times demonstrates increased posterior tibial slope and static anterior tibial translation.

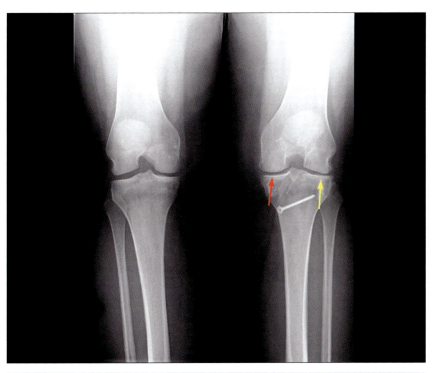

Figure 5   AP Rosenberg radiograph of both knees of a patient demonstrates medial (red arrow) and lateral (yellow arrow) joint space narrowing in the left knee in comparison with the contralateral knee.

Tunnel Position Assessment

Morgan et al[20] reported that technical error is the most common reason for primary ACL reconstruction failure, with the most common error being femoral tunnel malposition. In their study of 117 patients who had femoral tunnel malposition after revision ACL reconstruction, the authors reported that malposition was too vertical in 36% of the patients, too anterior in 30% of the patients, both too vertical and too anterior in 27% of the patients, and compromised because of the position and size in 8% of the patients. In an analysis of the techniques that were used for revision ACL reconstruction, the authors reported the use of an entirely new femoral tunnel in 79.8% of the patients, a blended femoral tunnel in 14% of the patients, an added second

femoral tunnel in 4.4% of the patients, and the same compromised femoral tunnel aperture in 1.8% of the patients.

The tibial socket and tunnel position are assessed by noting the point posterior to the intersection of the Blumensaat line (the roof of the intercondylar notch) and the tibial plateau as well as the point anterior to the midpoint of the tibial plateau. The femoral socket is noted at the point posterior to the intersection of the Blumensaat line and the posterior femoral cortex (**Figure 7**). Three-dimensional CT reconstruction can assist in measuring dimensions, determining geometric shape, and identifying sclerotic bone. Compared with CT, MRI is inferior in assessment of tunnel positioning.[21] Attention should be given to whether hardware needs to be removed. If reaming is required

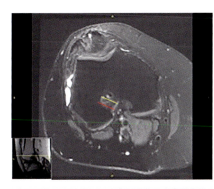

Figure 6   Axial T2-weighted MRI of a knee demonstrates the position of the femoral tunnel and hardware in a more anterior position. The red and yellow lines indicate the position of the femoral tunnel. Inset, Sagittal MRI of the knee taken at the same level as the axial MRI.

through previous hardware, appropriate removal instruments should be available.

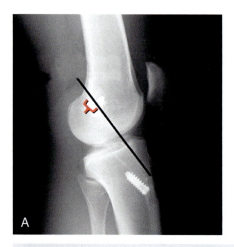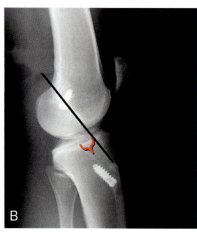

Figure 7 Lateral knee radiographs demonstrate assessment of the tibial tunnel (**A**) and the femoral socket (**B**), both of which are indicated by red brackets. The black line indicates the Blumensaat line.

One-Stage ACL Reconstruction

If tunnel widening is less than 16 mm in all the imaging planes or if severe tunnel malposition is present, one-stage ACL reconstruction should be considered. Multiple approaches can be used, depending on the assessment of tunnel positions. In patients who have a poorly placed, nonanatomic tunnel, a new tunnel is reamed with a new aperture and trajectory. In patients who have a well-placed tunnel with mild widening, the previous tunnel is used with the same aperture and a new trajectory, which has been described as a divergent cone approach.[22] An outside-in technique with an antegrade screw or an inside-out technique with a retrograde screw can be used, with backup fixation added if necessary. A third option involves a blended tunnel with an aperture and trajectory that communicates with the previous tunnel. In this technique, a large allograft bone block, stacked interference screws, a biocomposite screw and reaming, or allograft dowel bone grafting can be used.

Optimal graft choice also is an important factor to consider. Recent data support that the use of allografts should be avoided in athletes younger than 25 years. In a study that compared the use of autograft versus allograft in 1,205 patients who underwent revision ACL reconstruction, the MARS Group[23] reported that the use of autograft predicted an improved Knee Injury and Osteoarthritis Outcome Score, IKDC Subjective Knee Evaluation Form score, and Marx Activity Rating Scale score and resulted in patients being 2.8 times less likely to sustain a graft rupture.

Two-Stage ACL Reconstruction

Whereas one-stage ACL reconstruction combines concomitant meniscus and cartilage treatment, hardware removal, tunnel débridement, and ACL reconstruction, two-stage ACL reconstruction requires bone grafting of widened tunnels and delays definitive ACL reconstruction 6 months after the first stage of surgery. If tunnel widening is more than 16 mm in any imaging plane or if slight tunnel malposition is present, a two-stage ACL reconstruction is recommended. The first stage requires meniscus and cartilage treatment, hardware removal, tunnel débridement, and bone grafting. Bone grafting requires meticulous débridement of graft material, fibrous tissue, and sclerotic bone from the previous tunnel. The tunnel is then densely packed with cancellous allograft (with or without platelet-rich plasma), cancellous autograft, an allograft dowel, or bone substitute. Radiographs are evaluated 4 to 6 months postoperatively to assess for signs of bone healing, which include blurring of the margins and reactive sclerosis. If the bone is incorporating well, revision ACL reconstruction can be considered 6 months postoperatively.

Unnecessary delayed revision ACL reconstruction may result in worse outcomes. In a study that separated patients in whom primary ACL reconstruction has failed into those who underwent early revision ACL reconstruction (<6 months) versus delayed revision ACL reconstruction, Ohly et al[24] reported a higher incidence of cartilage injury in the patients who underwent delayed revision ACL reconstruction (24% for patients who underwent early revision ACL reconstruction versus 52% for patients who underwent delayed revision ACL reconstruction). The authors also reported a correlation between radiographic osteoarthritic changes and the duration of symptoms before revision ACL reconstruction.[24] These findings have implications for the selection of one-stage versus two-stage revision ACL reconstruction. In two-stage revision ACL reconstruction, knee instability will be prolonged, which increases the potential for chondrosis and meniscal injury. Typically, the surgeon can consider the use of an ACL derotational brace and require the patient to avoid cutting, pivoting, jumping, and impact activities while the bone graft is healing to avoid further injury to the knee. Consequently, one-stage revision ACL reconstruction should be performed in all patients in whom it is feasible. Conversely, if the risk for repeat ACL reconstruction failure is high with one-stage revision ACL reconstruction, two-stage revision ACL reconstruction should be considered.

The Role of the ALL
Rotational Knee Laxity

An important goal of ACL reconstruction is to eliminate the pivot shift phenomenon. The results of the pivot shift test directly correlate with functional outcomes after ACL reconstruction.[25] A positive pivot shift test indicates persistent rotational laxity, which is an important issue after both single-bundle and double-bundle ACL reconstruction.[26,27] Although recurrent instability after ACL reconstruction is not uncommon, 50% to 70% of patients with recurrent instability had no obvious traumatic reinjury.[4,28] Persistent rotational laxity, among other causes, may explain why only 45% to 65% of athletes return to their preinjury activity level after ACL reconstruction.[29]

Biomechanical principles indicate that a centrally located structure, such as the ACL, is limited in completely controlling internal tibial rotation. An eccentrically located ligament, however, is more effective at restraining rotational forces. The ALL is a distinct ligamentous structure on the lateral aspect of the knee that courses obliquely from the lateral aspect of the lateral

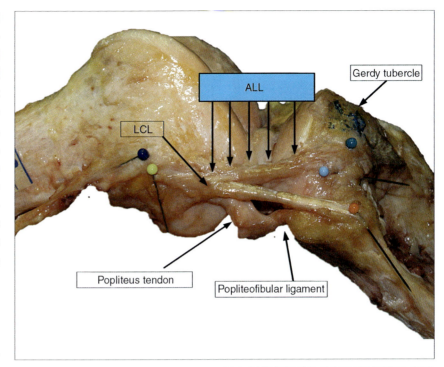

Figure 8   Lateral clinical photograph of a knee specimen shows the relationship of the anterolateral ligament (ALL) to its surrounding structures. The black pin indicates the lateral femoral condyle. The light blue pin indicates the fibular head. The yellow and green pins indicate the proximal and distal ends of the ALL, respectively. The orange pin indicates the fibular head attachment of the lateral collateral ligament (LCL). (Reproduced with permission from Claes S, Vereecke E, Maes M, Victor J, Verdonk P, Bellemans J: Anatomy of the anterolateral ligament of the knee. *J Anat* 2013;223[4]:321-328.)

femoral condyle toward the anterolateral tibia and inserts between the Gerdy tubercle and the anterior margin of the fibular head[30-33] (**Figure 8**). The ALL controls internal rotation of the tibia, and, therefore, affects the pivot shift phenomenon. Thus, the ALL is a subject of great interest with regard to persistent rotational laxity after ACL reconstruction.[33-35]

Extra-articular ACL Reconstruction

In the 1970s, extra-articular ACL reconstruction techniques began using a type of iliotibial band (ITB) tenodesis to overcome anterolateral knee instability.[36,37] Because of inconsistent results, however, extra-articular

ACL reconstruction was largely abandoned, especially in the United States. Given the current knowledge of the anatomy and function of the ALL, extra-articular ACL reconstruction is currently regarded as nonanatomic ALL reconstruction.

Several studies have recently reported excellent results after extra-articular ACL reconstruction to augment traditional ACL reconstruction. Clinical studies have reported that lateral augmentation has been especially useful for controlling rotational laxity in ACL-reconstructed knees.[38-40] A laboratory study by Monaco et al[40] reported that anatomic ACL reconstruction and lateral ITB tenodesis were synergic in restraining the pivot shift phenomenon.

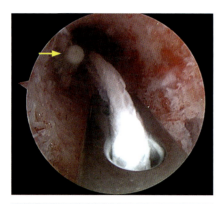

Figure 9 Arthroscopic image of a knee shows the anterior cruciate ligament (ACL) femoral socket from the anteromedial portal. The tip of the anchor from the femoral anterolateral ligament (ALL; arrow) is inside the ACL femoral socket. This can be avoided by placing an ALL guide pin and checking for coalescence before the ALL socket is reamed.

Although the intuitive benefits of an extra-articular ACL reconstruction in the setting of revision ACL reconstruction may be important, literature on the topic is relatively sparse. In a multicenter study of 163 patients who underwent revision ACL reconstruction during a 10-year period, Trojani et al[41] reported that the addition of a lateral extra-articular ITB tenodesis resulted in a significantly lower residual pivot shift rate. Although ITB tenodesis techniques have been useful in select patients, emerging knowledge on the precise anatomy and function of the ALL continues to drive the development of minimally invasive anatomic ALL reconstruction techniques and further decreases persistent rotational laxity and graft re-rupture rates after revision ACL reconstruction.

Anatomic ALL Reconstruction

ALL reconstruction initially requires an examination under anesthesia to confirm the presence of substantial rotational instability, which is confirmed by a high-grade pivot shift. ALL reconstruction fixes an autograft or allograft hamstring tendon (gracilis or semitendinosus) on the anatomic attachment sites of the native ALL in both the femur and the tibia. Both single- and V-strand techniques have been proposed to mimic the native footprint of the ALL.[42]

An incision is planned over the main landmark for the femoral socket, which is the lateral epicondyle, in a proximal direction. The tibial incision is marked at a point that is equidistant between the fibular head and the Gerdy tubercle, just distal to the tibial joint line. The placement of two guide pins, one on the femur and one on the tibia, is recommended before socket creation. The femoral incision is made first, the ITB is split in line with its fibers, and the fibular collateral ligament is identified and protected. A 2.4-mm guidewire is advanced anteriorly and distally (to avoid the ACL femoral socket, which is located posterior and proximal on the lateral femoral condyle) at a point 4.7 mm proximal and posterior to the fibular collateral ligament attachment.[31] The surgeon should avoid the ACL femoral socket, and the femoral ALL socket should be drilled before ACL graft insertion to prevent injury. After the guide pin for the femoral ALL has been placed, an arthroscope can be used in the anteromedial portal to ensure that no coalescence exists in the previously created ACL femoral socket (**Figure 9**).

A second tibial longitudinal skin incision is made, and soft-tissue dissection is then performed at the site of the tibial fixation socket. The 2.4-mm guidewire is then placed on the anatomic insertion of the ALL, approximately 9 mm distal to the tibial joint line and halfway between the Gerdy tubercle and the fibular head. Fluoroscopy can help ensure accurate placement on the tibia, avoid subchondral bone and joint penetration, as well as avoid coalescence of the ACL tibial tunnel.[43] Similar to the femur, after the tibial ALL guide pin has been placed, an arthroscope can be used in the tibial tunnel to ensure that no coalescence exists before the tibial ALL socket is reamed. At this point, a suture can be passed deep to the ITB and around the femoral and tibial guide pins to check for ALL isometry. Typically, the ALL will loosen in flexion and slightly tighten between 0° and 30° of extension; if this is satisfactory, two 4.5-mm sockets with a depth of 20 mm are drilled.[42]

After ACL reconstruction, the ALL graft is secured into the femoral and tibial bone sockets with an appropriate tap and 4.75-mm diameter, bioabsorbable, fully threaded, knotless anchors. The whipstitched end of the ALL graft is secured into the femoral socket, and the graft is tensioned from the tibial end after the shuttling suture is used to pass the graft deep to the ITB and through the distal skin incision (**Figure 10**). An anchor is then used to secure the graft distally on the tibia while the graft is tensioned. Different techniques for graft fixation using the principles discussed earlier have been successful; however, optimal knee flexion for ALL graft tensioning is currently controversial. Currently, an ALL graft typically is tensioned between full extension and 30° of knee flexion.[42,44]

Outcomes

Limited data on the outcomes of combined ACL and ALL reconstruction are available. Sonnery-Cottet et al[44] conducted a promising study of 92 patients who underwent combined ACL and ALL reconstruction, 83 of whom were available at a minimum follow-up of 2 years. The authors reported significant improvement ($P < 0.0001$) in Lysholm Knee Scale as well as IKDC Subjective and Objective Knee Evaluation Form scores. A slightly lower Tegner Activity Scale score ($P < 0.01$) was reported at final follow-up. Postoperatively, 76 patients (91.6%) had a negative (grade 0) pivot shift, and 7 patients (8.4%) had a grade 1 pivot shift. In addition, 59 patients (71.1%) returned to the same activity level postoperatively, and 24 patients (28.9%) returned to a lower level of activity postoperatively, 14 of whom returned to a lower level of activity for reasons unrelated to the knee injury. More data are necessary to determine the outcomes and comparative efficacy of combined ACL and ALL reconstruction.

Tibial Deflexion Osteotomy

Other structures, in addition to the ACL, help prevent abnormal anterior tibial translation. Osseous anatomy affects tibial translation and applied loads to the ACL. Theoretically, an increase in posterior tibial slope will cause the femoral condyles to slide posteriorly with weight bearing, which results in a relative anterior tibial translation and increases loads on a native or graft ACL. A computer model predicted increased loads on the ACL during walking in patients who had a higher degree of posterior tibial slope.[45] Multiple cadaver model studies reported that a 5° to 10° increase in tibial slope resulted in increased anterior tibial translation, with one study reporting increased ACL strain.[46-48] Clinically,

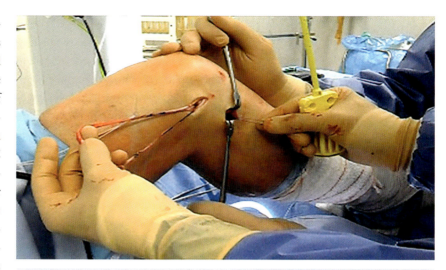

Figure 10   Intraoperative photograph of a knee shows anterolateral ligament graft passage under the iliotibial band after femoral fixation.

this same phenomenon was demonstrated with the use of lateral single-leg-stance radiographs.[49] Increased posterior tibial slope that results in increased anterior tibial translation occurs in patients who have an intact ACL as well as patients who have chronic ACL deficiency. An iatrogenic increase in posterior tibial slope also has an effect on anterior tibial translation. An iatrogenic increase in posterior tibial slope is most commonly caused by a valgus-producing opening wedge high tibial osteotomy for the management of medial compartment degenerative change in a varus knee. Increased anterior tibial translation results from an osteotomy that alters the tibial slope.[50] Several studies have observed the relationship between tibial slope and ACL injuries. Most studies have reported increased posterior tibial slope in ACL-injured populations compared with control groups.[51-55] A recent study reported an increased lateral posterior tibial slope in patients in whom early ACL reconstruction graft failure occured.[56]

Indications

Although posterior tibial slope has an effect on anterior tibial translation and ACL graft loads, it rarely is the only cause of ACL reconstruction graft failure. A tibial deflexion osteotomy is a technically difficult procedure and entails a long rehabilitation period; therefore, it is indicated only in select patients. A careful physical examination and radiographic evaluation are required to identify patients who are ideal candidates for tibial deflexion osteotomy, most of whom will be undergoing revision ACL reconstruction rather than primary ACL reconstruction.

Clinically, most patients will have marked symptoms of instability with activity. Markedly positive Lachman and pivot shift tests will be evident on physical examination despite a patient having undergone ACL reconstruction. Posterior tibial slope is determined with a lateral radiograph by measuring the angle between a line drawn perpendicular to the long axis of the tibia and a line drawn tangent to the tibial plateau. Normally, this angle

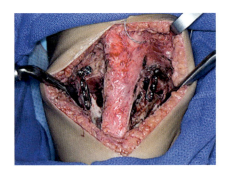

Figure 11 Intraoperative photograph of a knee shows exposure for a tibial deflexion osteotomy. Note the subperiosteal elevation of the medial and lateral structures with bent retractors in place. The plates are fixed to the proximal bone segment before closing the osteotomy and securing the distal segment with compression plates. The low-profile L-shaped plates allow for placement of the tibial tunnel and fixation for revision anterior cruciate ligament reconstruction if both procedures are performed in a single stage.

is between 9° and 11° medially and 6° and 8° laterally.[57] In addition, anterior tibial translation is measured with the use of comparative monopodal single-leg-stance radiographs.[49] Tibial deflexion osteotomy is indicated only in patients who have both a posterior tibial slope greater than 13° and anterior tibial translation greater than or equal to 10 mm compared with the contralateral knee[58] (**Figure 4**). The posterior soft-tissue slope is relatively reduced if the posterior horns of the menisci are intact because the posterior horns of the menisci are higher compared with the anterior horns of the menisci.[59] In the experience of the authors of this chapter, the greatest effects of posterior tibial slope on anterior tibial translation are observed in patients who have early degenerative changes and patients who have undergone prior meniscectomy. These

patients may have an increased posterior soft-tissue slope that is not easily correctable. Similar to treatment of all patients who undergo revision ACL reconstruction, the authors of this chapter recommend preoperative three-dimensional CT to accurately identify the location of previous tunnels and preoperative MRI to evaluate for meniscal and chondral pathology.

Technique

A longitudinal anterior incision is made; however, modifications may be required depending on previous incisions. The incision extends from the distal third of the patella to a point just distal to the tibial tuberosity. If available, the authors of this chapter prefer to harvest a bone-patellar tendon-bone graft from the ipsilateral knee. If that site has been harvested previously, a bone-patellar tendon-bone graft from the contralateral knee or a bone-patellar tendon-bone allograft can be used. The ACL femoral and tibial tunnels are created. The authors of this chapter prefer to drill a complete tibial tunnel rather than a blind socket to ensure appropriate graft placement after the osteotomy.

After the tunnels are created, a tibial deflexion osteotomy is performed. The knee is flexed to 90° to minimize risk to the posterior neurovascular structures. The osteotomy is performed just proximal to the attachment of the patellar tendon on the tibial tubercle. The medial and lateral borders of the patellar tendon are identified, and dissection is performed posterior to the patellar tendon to expose the proximal tibia. On the medial side, the superficial MCL is elevated off the tibia at the anticipated level of the osteotomy, and a Hohmann retractor is inserted for protection. On the lateral side, the superior aspect of

the tibialis anterior muscle is elevated off the tibia to expose the bone at the level of the cut (**Figure 11**). Using fluoroscopic guidance, a guide pin is drilled medial to the patellar tendon. The guide pin enters the tibia a few millimeters proximal to the tibial tubercle, approximately 3 cm below the joint line. The guide pin is angled proximally toward the posterior cruciate ligament insertion and advanced into the posterior tibial cortex. The surgeon must ensure that the guide pin and the oscillating saw do not excessively penetrate the posterior cortex to avoid neurovascular injury.

After the successful placement of the first guide pin, a second guide pin is placed parallel to the first guide pin just lateral to the patellar tendon. The guide pins must enter the posterior cortex proximal to the tibial insertion of the posterior capsule to ensure the integrity of the posterior hinge during closure of the osteotomy. A second set of guide pins is placed at the superior aspect of the planned osteotomy. In general, 1 mm of anterior cortex closure will result in an approximately 2° decrease in posterior tibial slope.[58] Therefore, if 10° of posterior tibial slope correction is desired, the second set of guide pins should be placed anteriorly 5 mm above the first set of guide pins and converge at the posterior cortex. An oscillating saw is used to make osteotomy cuts along the inferior surface of the guide pins, taking care to protect the patellar tendon and the MCL. The oscillating saw must cut the medial and lateral cortices completely; however, the posterior cortex should be kept intact. The anterior bone wedge is removed, and a 3.5-mm drill bit osteotome is used to perforate the posterior tibial cortex in multiple locations (**Figure 12**). If the posterior hinge is adequately weakened

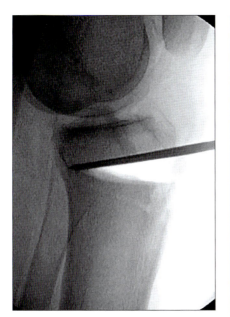

Figure 12   Lateral intraoperative fluoroscopic image of a knee shows a tibial deflexion osteotomy. An osteotome is carefully used to penetrate the posterior cortex without causing destabilization.

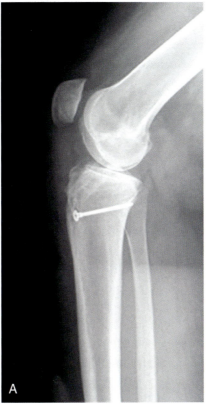

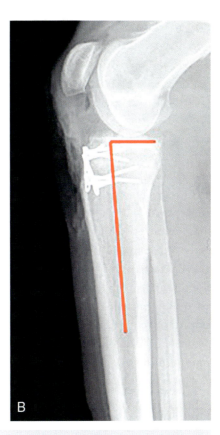

Figure 13   Lateral radiographs of a knee with an increased posterior tibial slope taken before (**A**) and after (**B**) tibial deflexion osteotomy. Note the 5° of posterior tibial slope correction, which is indicated by the red line in panel **B**.

by the drill holes, the osteotomy site will close slightly.

The knee is gently extended to close the osteotomy. Because of the tendency to create a varus angulation of the tibia, care should be taken to ensure symmetric closure of the osteotomy. Fixation is achieved with the use of two large staples or small locking plates that are placed on both sides of the patellar tendon. Care must be taken to ensure that the medial staple does not enter the tibial tunnel. After fixation of the osteotomy is achieved, an appropriate size reamer is passed through the tibial tunnel to smooth out any irregularities caused by the osteotomy. The bone-patellar tendon-bone graft is passed and secured according to the preference of the surgeon.

Although tibial deflexion osteotomy has little effect on patellar height, and the authors of this chapter have not noted any adverse effects after the procedure, the change in posterior tibial slope frequently leads to excessive genu recurvatum. Because genu recurvatum can lead to stretching of the graft and early failure, the authors of this chapter perform a posteromedial capsular advancement to normalize extension in patients in whom genu recurvatum occurs. Dissection is extended to the posteromedial aspect of the knee, and the posterior capsule is sharply released from its origin on the posterior femur. Two suture anchors are placed along the capsular attachment, and sutures are brought through the capsule 5 to 10 mm distally to advance the capsule. The sutures are tied in 10° of flexion to re-tension the capsule and eliminate hyperextension. Alternatively, if a flexion contracture is present, tibial deflexion osteotomy often will help reestablish full terminal extension.

Rehabilitation

The rehabilitation program after tibial deflexion osteotomy prevents hyperextension and avoids the placement of excessive stress on the ACL graft. The knee is placed in a hinged brace, and passive motion from 10° to 90° is allowed. A continuous passive motion machine helps minimize stiffness. Full extension is avoided for the first 6 weeks postoperatively to allow for healing of the posteromedial capsular advancement. Patients should not bear weight for 8 weeks postoperatively. Anticoagulation therapy should be continued until the patient is able to fully bear weight.

Patients may progress to a normal revision ACL reconstruction protocol after 8 weeks postoperatively.

Complications

Potential complications of tibial deflexion osteotomy include infection, stiffness, venous thromboembolism, and osteotomy-specific complications. Neurovascular injury may occur if the guide pins or saw blade extend beyond the posterior tibial cortex. Nonunion of the osteotomy and overcorrection or undercorrection of the posterior tibial slope may occur. Care must be taken to avoid iatrogenic varus deformity during closure of the osteotomy. Thorough preoperative planning and meticulous surgical technique will minimize the risk for complications.

Outcomes

The authors of this chapter are aware of only one study that analyzed outcomes after tibial deflexion osteotomy. In a study of 22 patients who underwent tibial deflexion osteotomy, 18 of whom underwent concomitant ACL reconstruction, Dejour et al[60] reported better results in the patients who underwent combined tibial deflexion osteotomy and ACL reconstruction and recommended the combined procedure. Good outcomes also were reported in a case study of a patient with bilateral congenital absence of the ACL who underwent combined ACL reconstruction and tibial deflexion osteotomy.[61] Unfortunately, no studies comparing the outcomes of patients who underwent revision ACL reconstruction with or without an associated tibial deflexion osteotomy for the management of chronic anterior instability and increased posterior tibial slope are available in the literature. The authors

of this chapter have observed that tibial deflexion osteotomy reliably corrects posterior tibial slope (**Figure 13**). Further studies are necessary to clearly identify the role and efficacy of tibial deflexion osteotomy.

Summary

Revision ACL reconstruction can be a challenging procedure. In general, the outcomes of revision ACL reconstruction are less favorable compared with those of primary ACL reconstruction. Meticulous technique, with careful attention given to tunnel and socket placement, is critical. In many patients in whom ACL reconstruction fails, the ALL is insufficient, and ALL reconstruction should be considered in the setting of revision ACL reconstruction. Although uncommon, excessive posterior tibial slope can contribute to ACL reconstruction graft failure and should be evaluated and, occasionally, corrected. In addition, safe postoperative rehabilitation and adequate graft healing must be complete before any sports activities are initiated. A comprehensive approach to revision ACL reconstruction will help improve clinical outcomes.

References

1. Gifstad T, Foss OA, Engebretsen L, et al: Lower risk of revision with patellar tendon autografts compared with hamstring autografts: A registry study based on 45,998 primary ACL reconstructions in Scandinavia. *Am J Sports Med* 2014;42(10):2319-2328.

2. Leathers MP, Merz A, Wong J, Scott T, Wang JC, Hame SL: Trends and demographics in anterior cruciate ligament reconstruction in the United States. *J Knee Surg* 2015;28(5):390-394.

3. George MS, Dunn WR, Spindler KP: Current concepts review: Revision anterior cruciate ligament reconstruction. *Am J Sports Med* 2006;34(12):2026-2037.

4. Wright RW, Gill CS, Chen L, et al: Outcome of revision anterior cruciate ligament reconstruction: A systematic review. *J Bone Joint Surg Am* 2012;94(6):531-536.

5. Diamantopoulos AP, Lorbach O, Paessler HH: Anterior cruciate ligament revision reconstruction: Results in 107 patients. *Am J Sports Med* 2008;36(5):851-860.

6. Jain N, Pietrobon R, Guller U, Shankar A, Ahluwalia AS, Higgins LD: Effect of provider volume on resource utilization for surgical procedures of the knee. *Knee Surg Sports Traumatol Arthrosc* 2005;13(4):302-312.

7. Leroux T, Wasserstein D, Dwyer T, et al: The epidemiology of revision anterior cruciate ligament reconstruction in Ontario, Canada. *Am J Sports Med* 2014;42(11):2666-2672.

8. Wasserstein D, Khoshbin A, Dwyer T, et al: Risk factors for recurrent anterior cruciate ligament reconstruction: A population study in Ontario, Canada, with 5-year follow-up. *Am J Sports Med* 2013;41(9):2099-2107.

9. Peltier A, Lording T, Maubisson L, Ballis R, Neyret P, Lustig S: The role of the meniscotibial ligament in posteromedial rotational knee stability. *Knee Surg Sports Traumatol Arthrosc* 2015;23(10):2967-2973.

10. Sonnery-Cottet B, Conteduca J, Thaunat M, Gunepin FX, Seil R: Hidden lesions of the posterior horn of the medial meniscus: A systematic arthroscopic exploration of the concealed portion of the knee. *Am J Sports Med* 2014;42(4):921-926.

11. van Eck CF, Schkrohowsky JG, Working ZM, Irrgang JJ, Fu FH: Prospective analysis of failure rate and predictors of failure after anatomic anterior cruciate ligament reconstruction with allograft. *Am J Sports Med* 2012;40(4):800-807.

12. Krych AJ, Jackson JD, Hoskin TL, Dahm DL: A meta-analysis of patellar tendon autograft versus patellar tendon allograft in anterior cruciate ligament reconstruction. *Arthroscopy* 2008;24(3):292-298.

13. Rahr-Wagner L, Thillemann TM, Pedersen AB, Lind MC: Increased risk of revision after anteromedial

compared with transtibial drilling of the femoral tunnel during primary anterior cruciate ligament reconstruction: Results from the Danish Knee Ligament Reconstruction Register. *Arthroscopy* 2013;29(1):98-105.

14. Hewett TE, Di Stasi SL, Myer GD: Current concepts for injury prevention in athletes after anterior cruciate ligament reconstruction. *Am J Sports Med* 2013;41(1):216-224.

15. Thomas NP, Kankate R, Wandless F, Pandit H: Revision anterior cruciate ligament reconstruction using a 2-stage technique with bone grafting of the tibial tunnel. *Am J Sports Med* 2005;33(11):1701-1709.

16. Kamath GV, Redfern JC, Greis PE, Burks RT: Revision anterior cruciate ligament reconstruction. *Am J Sports Med* 2011;39(1):199-217.

17. Irrgang JJ, Ho H, Harner CD, Fu FH: Use of the International Knee Documentation Committee guidelines to assess outcome following anterior cruciate ligament reconstruction. *Knee Surg Sports Traumatol Arthrosc* 1998;6(2):107-114.

18. Feucht MJ, Cotic M, Saier T, et al: Patient expectations of primary and revision anterior cruciate ligament reconstruction. *Knee Surg Sports Traumatol Arthrosc* 2016;24(1):201-207.

19. Griffith TB, Allen BJ, Levy BA, Stuart MJ, Dahm DL: Outcomes of repeat revision anterior cruciate ligament reconstruction. *Am J Sports Med* 2013;41(6):1296-1301.

20. Morgan JA, Dahm D, Levy B, Stuart MJ; MARS Study Group: Femoral tunnel malposition in ACL revision reconstruction. *J Knee Surg* 2012;25(5):361-368.

21. Marchant MH Jr, Willimon SC, Vinson E, Pietrobon R, Garrett WE, Higgins LD: Comparison of plain radiography, computed tomography, and magnetic resonance imaging in the evaluation of bone tunnel widening after anterior cruciate ligament reconstruction. *Knee Surg Sports Traumatol Arthrosc* 2010;18(8):1059-1064.

22. Bach Jr BR, Mazzocca AD, Fox JA, Rue JPH: Revision ACL reconstruction. *Orthopaedic Knowledge Online Journal*. Rosemont, IL,

American Academy of Orthopaedic Surgeons. Available at: http://www.aaos.org/OKOJ/vol5/issue4/SPO002/?ssopc=1.

23. MARS Group: Effect of graft choice on the outcome of revision anterior cruciate ligament reconstruction in the Multicenter ACL Revision Study (MARS) Cohort. *Am J Sports Med* 2014;42(10):2301-2310.

24. Ohly NE, Murray IR, Keating JF: Revision anterior cruciate ligament reconstruction: Timing of surgery and the incidence of meniscal tears and degenerative change. *J Bone Joint Surg Br* 2007;89(8):1051-1054.

25. Ayeni OR, Chahal M, Tran MN, Sprague S: Pivot shift as an outcome measure for ACL reconstruction: A systematic review. *Knee Surg Sports Traumatol Arthrosc* 2012;20(4):767-777.

26. Suomalainen P, Järvelä T, Paakkala A, Kannus P, Järvinen M: Double-bundle versus single-bundle anterior cruciate ligament reconstruction: A prospective randomized study with 5-year results. *Am J Sports Med* 2012;40(7):1511-1518.

27. Meredick RB, Vance KJ, Appleby D, Lubowitz JH: Outcome of single-bundle versus double-bundle reconstruction of the anterior cruciate ligament: A meta-analysis. *Am J Sports Med* 2008;36(7):1414-1421.

28. Mayr R, Rosenberger R, Agraharam D, Smekal V, El Attal R: Revision anterior cruciate ligament reconstruction: An update. *Arch Orthop Trauma Surg* 2012;132(9):1299-1313.

29. Ardern CL, Taylor NF, Feller JA, Webster KE: Fifty-five per cent return to competitive sport following anterior cruciate ligament reconstruction surgery: An updated systematic review and meta-analysis including aspects of physical functioning and contextual factors. *Br J Sports Med* 2014;48(21):1543-1552.

30. Claes S, Vereecke E, Maes M, Victor J, Verdonk P, Bellemans J: Anatomy of the anterolateral ligament of the knee. *J Anat* 2013;223(4):321-328.

31. Kennedy MI, Claes S, Fuso FA, et al: The anterolateral ligament: An anatomic, radiographic, and biomechanical analysis. *Am J Sports Med* 2015;43(7):1606-1615.

32. Dodds AL, Halewood C, Gupte CM, Williams A, Amis AA: The anterolateral ligament: Anatomy, length changes and association with the Segond fracture. *Bone Joint J* 2014;96(3):325-331.

33. Cavaignac E, Wytrykowski K, Reina N, et al: Ultrasonographic identification of the anterolateral ligament of the knee. *Arthroscopy* 2016;32(1):120-126.

34. Parsons EM, Gee AO, Spiekerman C, Cavanagh PR: The biomechanical function of the anterolateral ligament of the knee. *Am J Sports Med* 2015;43(3):669-674.

35. Lutz C, Sonnery-Cottet B, Niglis L, Freychet B, Clavert P, Imbert P: Behavior of the anterolateral structures of the knee during internal rotation. *Orthop Traumatol Surg Res* 2015;101(5):523-528.

36. Duthon VB, Magnussen RA, Servien E, Neyret P: ACL reconstruction and extra-articular tenodesis. *Clin Sports Med* 2013;32(1):141-153.

37. Dodds AL, Gupte CM, Neyret P, Williams AM, Amis AA: Extra-articular techniques in anterior cruciate ligament reconstruction: A literature review. *J Bone Joint Surg Br* 2011;93(11):1440-1448.

38. Marcacci M, Zaffagnini S, Giordano G, Iacono F, Presti ML: Anterior cruciate ligament reconstruction associated with extra-articular tenodesis: A prospective clinical and radiographic evaluation with 10- to 13-year follow-up. *Am J Sports Med* 2009;37(4):707-714.

39. Pernin J, Verdonk P, Si Selmi TA, Massin P, Neyret P: Long-term follow-up of 24.5 years after intra-articular anterior cruciate ligament reconstruction with lateral extra-articular augmentation. *Am J Sports Med* 2010;38(6):1094-1102.

40. Monaco E, Maestri B, Conteduca F, Mazza D, Iorio C, Ferretti A: Extra-articular ACL reconstruction and pivot shift: In vivo dynamic evaluation with navigation. *Am J Sports Med* 2014;42(7):1669-1674.

41. Trojani C, Beaufils P, Burdin G, et al: Revision ACL reconstruction: Influence of a lateral tenodesis.

Knee Surg Sports Traumatol Arthrosc 2012;20(8):1565-1570.

42. Smith JO, Yasen SK, Lord B, Wilson AJ: Combined anterolateral ligament and anatomic anterior cruciate ligament reconstruction of the knee. *Knee Surg Sports Traumatol Arthrosc* 2015;23(11):3151-3156.

43. Rezansoff AJ, Caterine S, Spencer L, Tran MN, Litchfield RB, Getgood AM: Radiographic landmarks for surgical reconstruction of the anterolateral ligament of the knee. *Knee Surg Sports Traumatol Arthrosc* 2015;23(11):3196-3201.

44. Sonnery-Cottet B, Thaunat M, Freychet B, Pupim BH, Murphy CG, Claes S: Outcome of a combined anterior cruciate ligament and anterolateral ligament reconstruction technique with a minimum 2-year follow-up. *Am J Sports Med* 2015;43(7):1598-1605.

45. Shelburne KB, Kim HJ, Sterett WI, Pandy MG: Effect of posterior tibial slope on knee biomechanics during functional activity. *J Orthop Res* 2011;29(2):223-231.

46. Fening SD, Kovacic J, Kambic H, McLean S, Scott J, Miniaci A: The effects of modified posterior tibial slope on anterior cruciate ligament strain and knee kinematics: A human cadaveric study. *J Knee Surg* 2008;21(3):205-211.

47. Giffin JR, Vogrin TM, Zantop T, Woo SL, Harner CD: Effects of increasing tibial slope on the biomechanics of the knee. *Am J Sports Med* 2004;32(2):376-382.

48. McLean SG, Oh YK, Palmer ML, et al: The relationship between anterior tibial acceleration, tibial slope, and ACL strain during a simulated jump landing task. *J Bone Joint Surg Am* 2011;93(14):1310-1317.

49. Dejour H, Bonnin M: Tibial translation after anterior cruciate ligament rupture: Two radiological tests compared. *J Bone Joint Surg Br* 1994;76(5):745-749.

50. Dejour H, Neyret P, Boileau P, Donell ST: Anterior cruciate reconstruction combined with valgus tibial osteotomy. *Clin Orthop Relat Res* 1994;299:220-228.

51. Bisson LJ, Gurske-DePerio J: Axial and sagittal knee geometry as a risk factor for noncontact anterior cruciate ligament tear: A case-control study. *Arthroscopy* 2010;26(7):901-906.

52. Brandon ML, Haynes PT, Bonamo JR, Flynn MI, Barrett GR, Sherman MF: The association between posterior-inferior tibial slope and anterior cruciate ligament insufficiency. *Arthroscopy* 2006;22(8):894-899.

53. Hohmann E, Bryant A, Reaburn P, Tetsworth K: Is there a correlation between posterior tibial slope and non-contact anterior cruciate ligament injuries? *Knee Surg Sports Traumatol Arthrosc* 2011;19(suppl 1):S109-S114.

54. Stijak L, Herzog RF, Schai P: Is there an influence of the tibial slope of the lateral condyle on the ACL lesion? A case-control study. *Knee Surg Sports Traumatol Arthrosc* 2008;16(2):112-117.

55. Todd MS, Lalliss S, Garcia E, DeBerardino TM, Cameron KL: The relationship between posterior tibial slope and anterior cruciate ligament injuries. *Am J Sports Med* 2010;38(1):63-67.

56. Christensen JJ, Krych AJ, Engasser WM, Vanhees MK, Collins MS, Dahm DL: Lateral tibial posterior slope is increased in patients with early graft failure after anterior cruciate ligament reconstruction. *Am J Sports Med* 2015;43(10):2510-2514.

57. Giffin JR, Shannon FJ: The role of the high tibial osteotomy in the unstable knee. *Sports Med Arthrosc* 2007;15(1):23-31.

58. Neyret P, Zuppi G, Aït Si Selmi T: Tibial deflexion osteotomy. *Oper Tech Sports Med* 2000;8:61-66.

59. Agneskirchner JD, Hurschler C, Stukenborg-Colsman C, Imhoff AB, Lobenhoffer P: Effect of high tibial flexion osteotomy on cartilage pressure and joint kinematics: A biomechanical study in human cadaveric knees. Winner of the AGA-DonJoy Award 2004. *Arch Orthop Trauma Surg* 2004;124(9):575-584.

60. Dejour D, Kuhn A, Dejour H: Tibial deflexion osteotomy and chronic anterior laxity: A series of 22 cases. *Rev Chir Orthop Repar Appar Mot* 1998;84(2):28-29.

61. Dejour H, Neyret P, Eberhard P, Walch G: Bilateral congenital absence of the anterior cruciate ligament and the internal menisci of the knee: A case report. *Rev Chir Orthop Reparatrice Appar Mot* 1990;76(5):329-332.

Concussion in Sports: What Do Orthopaedic Surgeons Need to Know?

Patrick J. Cahill, MD
Christian Refakis, BA
Eileen Storey, BA
William C. Warner Jr, MD

Abstract

A concussion is a relatively common sports-related injury that affects athletes of all ages. Although not expected to replace sports medicine physicians and neurologists with regard to the management of concussions, orthopaedic surgeons, particularly those who are fellowship-trained in sports medicine, must have a current knowledge base of what a concussion is, how a concussion is diagnosed, and how a concussion should be managed. Orthopaedic surgeons should understand the pathophysiology, assessment, and management of concussion so that they have a basic comprehension of this injury that is at the forefront of the academic literature and North American media. This understanding will prepare orthopaedic surgeons to work in concert with and assist sports medicine physicians, athletic trainers, and physical therapists in providing comprehensive care for athletes with a concussion.

Instr Course Lect 2017;66:557–566.

Although concussion has been a topic of investigation for many years, media scrutiny of concussion has increased in the past decade as a result of several high-profile athletes who sustained a concussion, which has highlighted the potential long-term sequelae associated with repeated head trauma.[1] This media attention has triggered a concomitant increase in medical and academic attention that is dedicated to understanding concussion. Although the scientific community has not yet discovered sufficient evidence that directly links recurrent head trauma to the development of severe medical conditions such as chronic traumatic encephalopathy (CTE), substantial advances in how to better identify and manage concussions have been made. Emerging concussion awareness and subsequent policy changes have made concussion a national public health issue by demonstrating that concussion affects not only professional athletes but also youth- and collegiate-level athletes.

In the past decade, the increase in reported concussions across all ages and all sports has led to the development of several concussion management guidelines, including those published by the Concussion in Sport Group in the 2012 Zurich Consensus statement[2] and those published by the

Dr. Cahill or an immediate family member is a member of a speakers' bureau or has made paid presentations on behalf of DePuy, Ellipse Technologies, Globus Medical, and Medtronic; serves as a paid consultant to or is an employee of DePuy, Ellipse Technologies, and Medtronic; has received nonincome support (such as equipment or services), commercially derived honoraria, or other non-research–related funding (such as paid travel) from DePuy Synthes Spine and Medtronic; and serves as a board member, owner, officer, or committee member of the American Academy of Orthopaedic Surgeons, the Pediatric Orthopaedic Society of North America, and the Scoliosis Research Society. Dr. Warner or an immediate family member serves as an unpaid consultant to Medtronic Sofamor Danek. Neither of the following authors nor any immediate family member has received anything of value from or has stock or stock options held in a commercial company or institution related directly or indirectly to the subject of this chapter: Mr. Refakis and Ms. Storey.

Table 1
Multisport Concussion Incidence in High School and College Athletes[a]

Sport	High School[b]	NCAA[c]
Male baseball	0.05	0.07; CI, 0.06–0.08
Male basketball	0.16	0.16; CI, 0.14–0.17
Female basketball	0.21	0.22; CI, 0.20–0.24
Female field hockey	0.22	0.18; CI, 0.15–0.21
Male football	0.64	0.37; CI, 0.36–0.38
Female gymnastics	0.07	0.16; CI, 0.12–0.20
Male ice hockey	0.54	0.41; CI, 0.37–0.44
Female ice hockey	NA	0.91; CI, 0.71–1.11
Male lacrosse	0.40	0.26; CI, 0.23–0.29
Female lacrosse	0.35	0.25; CI, 0.22–0.28
Male soccer	0.19	0.28; CI, 0.25–0.30
Female soccer	0.34	0.41; CI, 0.38–0.44
Female softball	0.16	0.14; CI, 0.12–0.16
Female volleyball	0.06	0.09; CI, 0.07–0.10
Male wrestling	0.22	0.25; CI, 0.22–0.27
Male spring football	NA	0.54; CI, 0.50–0.58
Cheerleading	0.14	NA
Male track	0.02	NA
Female track	0.02	NA
Male swimming/diving	0.01	NA
Female swimming/diving	0.02	NA
Total concussions	**0.25**	**0.28; CI, 0.27–0.28**

CI = confidence interval (95%, unless otherwise stated), NA = not applicable, NCAA = National Collegiate Athletic Association.

[a]Rates are reported as concussions per 1,000 athletic exposures.

[b]Data from Marar M, McIlvain NM, Fields SK, Comstock RD: Epidemiology of concussions among United States high school athletes in 20 sports. *Am J Sports Med* 2012;40(4):747-755.

[c]Data from Hootman JM, Dick R, Agel J: Epidemology of collegiate injuries for 15 sports: Summary and recommendations for injury prevention initiatives. *J Athl Train* 2007;42(2):311-319.

Adapted with permission from Clay MB, Glober KL, Lowe DT: Epidemiology of concussion in sport: A literature review. *J Chiropr Med* 2013;12(4):230-251.

American Academy of Neurology in 2013.[3] Despite these standardized concussion management guidelines, the heterogeneity of concussion and the lack of objective measures to identify a concussion have led to variation and confusion with regard to proper diagnosis and management, which has furthered the need for increased education across care providers, coaches, and athletes. Orthopaedic surgeons, who commonly treat athletes for a variety of musculoskeletal injuries, must have a current knowledge base of what a concussion is, how a concussion is diagnosed, and how a concussion should be managed to properly address the full spectrum of sports-related injuries that they may encounter, even if this only means properly recognizing concussion symptoms and knowing when to refer an athlete with a concussion to an appropriate physician.

Epidemiology

The Centers for Disease Control and Prevention estimates that 1.6 to 3.8 million individuals in the United States sustain a sports-related mild traumatic brain injury each year.[4] A substantial portion of these sports-related mild traumatic brain injuries occur in children and adolescents, and the incidence of sports-related mild traumatic brain injuries has continued to rise with increased youth sports participation and improved concussion awareness and management. From 2001 to 2009, the number of hospital visits for sports- and recreation-related concussions that occurred in patients younger than 19 years increased by 62%, increasing from 153,375 to 248,418.[5] A recent systematic review reported that the concussion incidence in high school and college sports ranged from 0.1 to 21.5 per 1,000 athletic exposures, varying by sport, sex, and level of play[6-8] (**Table 1**).

Definitions

Concussion is a term that is used to describe clinical symptoms resulting from mild to moderate brain trauma that may not necessarily be related to a gross structural injury.[2] The Concussion in Sport Group, which included the authors of the 2012 Zurich Consensus statement, formally defined concussion as "a complex pathophysiological process affecting the brain, induced by biomechanical forces."[2] The Concussion in Sport Group further identified several key diagnostic elements that are common to concussions. A concussion may be caused by a direct blow to the head or by an indirect blow elsewhere on the body that transmits forces to the head and typically results in neuropathologic changes. These functional, rather than structural, neuropathologic changes are not detected via standard structural neuroimaging studies but may result in clinical and cognitive symptoms that typically resolve within a few days; however, in some patients, symptoms may take several weeks or more to resolve.[2] Echoing the definition of concussion that was developed by the Concussion in Sport Group, the authors of the 2013 American Academy of Neurology guideline on the evaluation and management of concussion in sports defined concussion as "a clinical syndrome of biomechanically induced alteration of brain function, typically affecting memory and orientation, which may involve loss of consciousness."[3]

Clinical Pathophysiology

Concussive trauma, which is sustained to the head or body, transmits impulsive forces to the brain.[9] These impulsive forces stretch and distort axonal networks and shear cell membranes, which results in indiscriminate ion efflux. This ion efflux leads to the widespread release of neurotransmitters, such as glutamate and other excitatory amino acids, which trigger widespread depolarization. In an attempt to restore a normal resting potential, sodium-potassium adenosine triphosphate pumps increase their activity, becoming hyperglycolytic, which drastically increases the brain's demand for glucose and oxygen. Although the energy demand increases, the cellular response to injury restricts cerebral blood flow, which results in a metabolic mismatch or an uncoupling between energy supply and demand.[10,11]

This metabolic mismatch between increased cerebral metabolic needs and reduced blood flow and glucose delivery makes the brain vulnerable in the acute period after a concussion and has been used to justify recommendations for physical and cognitive rest after an injury in patients who sustain a concussion. Under such a state of physiologic stress, neurons are more susceptible to secondary injury, which may result in substantial negative sequelae.[12] Animal models have demonstrated this concept of acute metabolic vulnerability. In a study of adult rats that sustained repeated concussive injuries, Prins et al[13] reported worse neurocognitive function and traumatic axonal injury in the rats that sustained concussive injuries that were separated by only 3 or 5 days compared with the rats that sustained concussive injuries that were separated by 7 days. Furthermore, second impact syndrome, which is a catastrophic complication (rapid brain swelling that may cause death) resulting from a closely timed repeat injury that occurs before healing, has furthered the need for circumspect management of concussion immediately postinjury.[14]

Media attention on professional athletes who sustain a concussion has focused on CTE, which is a neurodegenerative disease that is associated with head trauma. CTE is a postmortem histologic diagnosis that is characterized by the deposition of tau protein in neuronal tissue. Although previously believed to only affect boxers, CTE has been identified in former American football players, hockey players, wrestlers, and military veterans.[15] Despite the reported increase of CTE in high-profile athletes, the risk for CTE, apart from a history of repeated head trauma, remains unknown, and the claim that CTE risk may increase with the duration of years of professional American football played[16] has not been substantiated.[15] Complicating matters, comorbid neurodegenerative diseases may obscure a true diagnosis of CTE, and CTE has been diagnosed in autopsies of the brains of patients who had no history of CTE symptoms.[17] Given the lack of scientific evidence, studies are premature to conclude that playing contact sports will lead to CTE; however, further research on CTE is necessary, and orthopaedic surgeons must recognize the role that CTE and high-profile media reports have on the public's understanding of sports-related concussion.

Concussion management is complicated by not only a consideration of the long-term negative sequelae of repeated head injury but also the challenge of determining the point at which a full metabolic recovery has occurred. Although approximately 80% to 90% of concussions in humans tend to resolve symptomatically within 7 to 10 days,[2] uncertainty remains with regard to whether full symptom resolution indicates a full metabolic recovery. Currently, no biomarker or imaging study exists that indicates a complete metabolic recovery after a concussion, and several studies have reported continued deficits in balance, reaction time, and neurocognitive function in patients who sustained a concussion and in whom symptoms have resolved.[18,19] Moreover, some brain metabolites, such as N-acetylaspartate in the frontal white matter, that were studied with the use of magnetic resonance spectroscopy have been reported to require as many as 30 days postinjury before they return to normal levels.[20] The long-term negative sequelae of repeated head injury in combination with the subjective nature of a full metabolic recovery underlie the uncertainty associated with the management of postconcussion recovery and underscore the necessity of ensuring that a patient's brain has had the chance to reestablish neurometabolic equilibrium before being placed at risk for subsequent injury.

Evaluation and Management
Sideline Evaluation

Any athlete in whom a concussion is suspected should be removed from play and assessed by a licensed medical provider. If performing a sideline evaluation, clinicians must adhere to standard emergency management principles (airway, breathing, and circulation) and rule out an injury to the cervical spine. Sideline evaluation indications for the transfer of an athlete to an emergency department include, but are not limited to, a Glasgow Coma Scale score less than 15; deteriorating mental status; progressive, worsening, or new neurologic signs, such as repetitive emesis, extremity numbness, or seizure; and potential spinal injury.[2] After substantial injuries have been ruled out, clinicians should evaluate the athlete for a concussion. Both the mechanism of injury and concussion-related symptoms should be considered; however, neither should be used as the sole determinant of whether an athlete has sustained a concussion because concussions can occur in the absence of clear trauma, and symptoms may be delayed in onset or appear temporarily and then reappear hours to days later.[21]

Although athletes should be monitored for signs or symptoms of concussion, including headache, dizziness, disorientation, confusion, and memory loss, the acute evaluation of an athlete in whom a concussion is suspected depends on sideline assessment tools, which represent less comprehensive forms of neurocognitive tests that are used to assess a range of domains, including cognitive impairment and balance deficits. The Sport Concussion Assessment Tool–3rd Edition (SCAT3), which is the most well-known and widely used sideline assessment tool, consists of eight sections, including Glasgow Coma Scale score, Maddocks Score, symptom evaluation, cognitive assessment with the Standardized Assessment of Concussion, neck examination, balance examination with Modified Balance Error Scoring System (BESS) testing, coordination examination, and Standardized Assessment of Concussion Delayed Recall. A modified version of the SCAT3 exists for children aged 12 years or younger to account for age and the overall developmental stage of children within that age range.

The King–Devick test, which is a portable, 2-minute test that involves reading single digits that are displayed on cards, has been increasingly used as a sideline assessment tool. The King–Devick test assesses rapid eye movement and can be used in combination with the SCAT3 to detect subtle saccadic visual dysfunction that is associated with concussion.[22] Recent studies have reported that the King–Devick test, if used in combination with the Modified BESS test and the Standardized Assessment of Concussion, accurately identified 100% of concussions.[23,24]

Computerized neurocognitive testing, such as Immediate Post-Concussion Assessment and Cognitive Testing and Axon Sports/Cogstate Sport testing, also has been increasingly used as a sideline assessment tool. Computerized neurocognitive tests are frequently administered before the sporting season begins to establish an athlete's baseline values, which can then be referenced for comparison if an injury occurs. Van Kampen et al[25] reported that computerized neurocognitive testing improved the accuracy and sensitivity of concussion diagnosis in the immediate postinjury window if used in conjunction with self-reported symptoms, which further reinforces the potential utility of computerized neurocognitive testing as a sideline assessment tool.

Although sideline assessment tools can be used to assess a variety of domains, the sensitivity and reliability of these tools for the diagnosis of a concussion, especially without preinjury baselines for comparison, remain unknown.[26] Given the dangers of a secondary injury, the sideline evaluation of an athlete in whom a concussion is suspected should err on the side of caution, and return to play on the day of a concussive injury should never occur.[2] Ultimately, a licensed medical provider who is trained in the management of concussions should make the final determination with regard to an athlete's fitness to play.

Clinical Evaluation

Although clinical imaging modalities, such as CT and MRI, are useful to rule out more severe traumatic brain injury, they currently are insufficient to diagnose a concussion.[27] Although other imaging modalities, including functional MRI, diffusion tensor imaging, and positron emission tomography, have shown promise in detecting changes after mild traumatic brain injury, they are not yet routinely used in the clinical setting, primarily because of prohibitive cost and implementation barriers.[28] Therefore, the diagnosis of a concussion relies heavily on clinical judgment that is based on an athlete's injury history and physical examination. Clinicians must obtain details on the mechanism of injury, the onset and timing of symptoms, and the specific activities associated with the worsening of symptoms. Although objective baseline data on preinjury function typically are unavailable, clinicians should obtain an athlete's history of prior concussions and comorbid conditions, including attention-deficit/hyperactivity disorder, anxiety, depression, and migraines, all of which have been associated with a more complicated and prolonged recovery after a concussion.[29]

After an athlete's injury and medical history has been obtained, the clinician should perform a comprehensive physical examination, which is essential to properly diagnose and manage a concussion. After a thorough head, cervical spine, and neurologic examination has been performed, the physical examination should specifically target the vestibular and vision systems because they are most commonly affected by a concussion, and balance and vision deficits may be otherwise undetected.[30,31] Because substantial overlap exists in the underlying pathophysiology and effects of concussion on the vestibular and vision systems, the two systems often are assessed in tandem. The Vestibular/Ocular Motor Screening assessment, which was developed and validated by the University of Pittsburgh, assesses vestibular and ocular impairments via a suite of exercises, including smooth pursuit, horizontal and vertical saccades, near point of convergence, horizontal vestibular ocular reflex, and visual motion sensitivity.[32] The Vestibular/Ocular Motor Screening assessment demonstrated

internal consistency and sensitivity in the identification of patients with a concussion, and warrants further attention as a practical, clinically useful tool for the diagnosis of a concussion.

Static and dynamic balance testing can be used to clinically assess for balance or coordination deficits. The Modified BESS test, which is inexpensive, easily administered, and incorporated in the SCAT3, is commonly used to evaluate static balance; however, its potential limitations for clinical use recently have been scrutinized.[33,34] A dynamic tandem gait test, which asks a patient to walk forward and backward with his or her eyes open and closed, may offer clinicians a more reliable alternative to the Modified BESS test.[35]

Computerized neurocognitive testing, which also is used in the clinical setting, provides clinicians with a useful snapshot of a patient's neurocognitive function, which can be used as a supplementary tool for the diagnosis of a concussion and to monitor a patient's postconcussion recovery.[36] Athletes are increasingly required to take a preseason computerized neurocognitive test that will serve as a baseline for comparison if they sustain a head injury.[37] Even with baseline data for comparison, computerized neurocognitive testing is not sufficient to replace a patient's clinical history or physical examination because computerized neurocognitive test results may be greatly affected by confounding factors.

One of the primary difficulties in the clinical diagnosis and management of concussion stems from a lack of preinjury data. Although a variety of assessment tools, such as those previously discussed, are available to aid in the diagnosis of a concussion, clinicians should exercise caution in the

interpretation of test results because each patient has a different preinjury baseline for comparison. Therefore, clinicians can expect great individual variation in test results, and the comparison of test results with standardized normative values for different age groups may not be a reliable indicator of concussion. Given the difficulty of managing concussions without preinjury data, recent efforts have been made to incorporate multimodal assessment protocols in preseason baseline testing to help facilitate preinjury and postinjury comparisons for multiple areas of cognitive and physical function.[22,38]

The suite of assessment tools available to aid clinicians in the diagnosis of a concussion may help minimize clinician dependence on subjective symptom reports, which are subject to underreporting of symptoms by athletes who want to return to play or to overreporting of nonspecific symptoms as a result of factors other than concussion.[39] Although the severity and extent of an athlete's symptoms after a concussion may aid a clinician in managing and monitoring postconcussion recovery, symptom reports are most useful if other factors, such as an athlete's comorbid conditions, injury history, and physical examination as part of a comprehensive evaluation after a concussion, are considered.

Clinical Care Plan

Because a concussion is a heterogeneous injury, clinicians often develop an individualized clinical care plan to address a patient's specific symptoms and deficits, which are identified via a patient's clinical history and physical examination. Although clinical care plans may vary for each patient, certain clinical care plan elements are commonly

Table 2

2012 Zurich Consensus Statement Graduated Return-to-Play Protocol for Athletes With a Concussion

Rehabilitation Stage	Functional Exercise	Objective
1. No activity	Symptom-limited physical and cognitive rest	Recovery
2. Light aerobic exercise	Walking, swimming, or stationary cycling, keeping intensity <70% of maximum permitted heart rate; no resistance training	Increase heart rate
3. Sport-specific exercise	Skating drills in ice hockey, running drills in soccer; no head-impact activities	Add movement
4. Noncontact training drills	Progression to more complex training drills (eg, passing drills in football and ice hockey); may begin progressive resistance training	Exercise, coordination, and cognitive load
5. Full-contact practice	After medical clearance, participation in normal training activities	Restore confidence and assessment of functional skills by coaching staff
6. Return to play	Normal game play	

Adapted with permission from McCrory P, Meeuwisse WH, Aubry M, et al: Consensus statement on concussion in sport: The 4th International Conference on Concussion in Sport held in Zurich, November 2012. *Br J Sports Med* 2013;47(5):250-258.

and consistently used for all patients who sustain a concussion.

In the immediate acute postconcussion period, clinicians recommend physical and cognitive rest. In this vulnerable period after a concussion, rest allows a patient to avoid activities that may place his or her brain at risk for subsequent injury or that may exacerbate the metabolic mismatch previously discussed, both of which may prolong symptoms and delay recovery after a concussion. Although physical and cognitive rest have been the benchmark of concussion management and are still advised in the first few days postconcussion, recent studies have challenged the utility of prolonged rest, reporting that it may lead to secondary symptoms of fatigue, depression, and physiologic deconditioning.[40-42]

Recent guidelines on concussion management have advocated a graded return to activity after a patient is asymptomatic. The concussion management guidelines published by the Concussion in Sport Group in the 2012 Zurich Consensus statement advocate a graduated, stepwise return-to-play protocol (**Table 2**), in which athletes who sustain a concussion proceed through a graded, six-level program of exertion as their symptoms resolve.[2] Athletes for whom this stepwise return-to-play protocol is prescribed progress from aerobic exercise to sport-specific activities to full-contact practice. Given the danger of repeat head trauma that occurs during the window in which an athlete's brain is vulnerable after a concussion, return to full-contact practice and sport is the final step in this stepwise

return-to-play protocol. The concussion management guidelines published by the Concussion in Sport Group in the 2012 Zurich Consensus statement specify that an athlete should be symptom free for a 24-hour period before he or she advances from one level of the stepwise return-to-play protocol to the next; therefore, at least 1 week may be required for an athlete to progress through all six levels of the protocol and return to play.[2] If any postconcussion symptoms occur as an athlete progresses through the stepwise return-to-play protocol, he or she is advised to return to the previous asymptomatic level of the protocol, at which he or she should remain for an additional 24-hour period before attempting to progress to the next level of the protocol.[2] Because the return-to-play progression depends on an athlete's symptoms, which may be affected by factors other than concussion or masked by an athlete who wants to return to play, this stepwise return-to-play protocol should be led by an experienced healthcare professional who can properly gauge an athlete's performance and readiness to progress through each stage of the protocol and return to play. Recent studies have reported that athletes who sustain a concussion have an increased risk for musculoskeletal injuries after they return to full sport participation if they are not properly reconditioned or if subtle symptoms, balance deficits, or cognitive deficits that predispose them to subsequent injury remain.[43,44] This reinforces the need for sufficiently challenging tasks in return-to-play protocols that can aid in a patient's rehabilitation and assessment of recovery after a concussion.

Although the clinical care plan for athletes who sustain a concussion

Concussion in Sports: What Do Orthopaedic Surgeons Need to Know?

Chapter 45

primarily focuses on return to play, a return-to-learn plan also is critically important, especially for student athletes.[45] To avoid triggering or exacerbating postconcussion symptoms via an abrupt return to full cognitive activity, return-to-learn protocols, which mirror return-to-play protocols, have been designed to gradually integrate students athletes back to a full day of school and adult athletes back to a full day of work.[46,47] Similar to return-to-play protocols, the progression of an athlete through a return-to-learn protocol depends on the close monitoring of symptoms and the maintenance of symptoms below a threshold level as cognitive demands increase.

Ongoing Management

Although most concussions resolve within the first 2 weeks postinjury, a substantial subset of patients who sustain a concussion have symptoms that persist beyond the standard recovery period, and postconcussion syndrome may develop in some patients who sustain a concussion, with symptoms lasting for months after the concussion.[48,49] In addition, patients in whom symptoms resolve may have prolonged deficits in balance, reaction time, and neurocognitive function.[18,19] Given the lack of prognostic factors that can effectively identify postconcussion outcomes at the onset of care, clinicians are unable to grade the severity of a concussion or determine which patients will follow an atypical, delayed recovery after a concussion. Although no causal relationships have been identified, several factors, including a loss of consciousness during the injury, a history of concussion, younger age, female sex, a history of migraines, learning disorders, attention-deficit/hyperactivity

disorder, anxiety, and depression, are associated with a delayed recovery after a concussion.[50]

Patients who have symptoms and deficits beyond the standard postconcussion recovery period should be referred to a specialist who has extensive experience in the management of concussions. For patients with a delayed recovery after a concussion, a multimodal treatment plan that involves active rehabilitation may be necessary to target specific deficits. Several therapies, including aerobic, vestibular, vision, and cognitive behavioral therapy, have gained attention as promising approaches to help patients with a more complicated postconcussion recovery return to their preinjury baseline.[51,52] Experienced medical specialists can help identify the specific deficits of a patient who sustained a concussion and make appropriate and targeted treatment recommendations.

Because a concussion is not only a cognitive injury but also a physiologic injury that affects both the heart and the autonomic nervous system, emerging evidence has shown that aerobic exercise may aid in postconcussion recovery by improving autonomic balance and cerebral blood flow regulation.[53] Although exercise that is performed too soon or too intensively after a concussion has been associated with delayed recovery and is used to justify prolonged periods of rest, recent studies have reported that subsymptom exacerbation threshold exercise, or exercise that does not lead to substantial additional or worsening of postconcussion symptoms, can be performed to safely address prolonged concussion-related symptoms that are associated with physiologic dysfunction.[54,55] In addition, exercise has been reported to improve

memory by increasing brain-derived neurotrophic factor and is believed to specifically aid in the relief of several symptoms that are associated with concussion, such as anxiety and depression.[56,57]

Other treatment modalities should be considered in patients in whom physiologic disturbance is not the primary contributor to prolonged postconcussion deficits and symptoms. Cognitive behavioral therapy can help address psychologic changes after a concussion by identifying and altering maladaptive thinking or behavior that may exacerbate depression and anxiety symptoms.[58] Vestibular and vision therapies have gained recent attention as modes of active rehabilitation that may help facilitate recovery in patients with balance or visual deficits that are detected via a physical examination after a concussion.[59,60] Specialists who are trained in the management of concussions are increasingly using vestibular and ocular tests, such as the Vestibular/Ocular Motor Screening assessment, as part of the clinical evaluation of patients who sustain a concussion to detect and distinguish potential vestibular and vision problems. Vestibular therapy may be useful in patients with impairments on saccadic, gaze stability, or balance tests because it incorporates increasingly challenging tasks that are designed to re-train the vestibular and vision systems. Patients with vision abnormalities such as convergence insufficiency may require vision therapy beyond the simple vision exercises that are administered in vestibular therapy. In addition, given the amount of reading and close-visual work that is involved with school work, vision therapy is especially important in student-athletes who have prolonged postconcussion vision deficits.[61] Although each of these treatment modalities can be used in isolation to target specific postconcussion symptoms and deficits, they also can be used in combination for patients who require a multimodal approach to postconcussion recovery.

Summary

Although concussion management is not the primary responsibility of orthopaedic surgeons, the increased incidence of concussion and the multidisciplinary approach that is required to manage a concussion requires orthopaedic surgeons to have a baseline understanding of this injury. Although concussion research continues to rapidly evolve, orthopaedic surgeons must be aware of the clinical features, clinical tools, and consensus guidelines that currently guide the diagnosis and management of concussion, especially in athletes.

References

1. Guion P: NFL concussions: Federal judge approves up to $5 million per player in concussion settlement. *The Independent*. April 23, 2015. Available at: http://www.independent. co.uk/news/world/americas/ nfl-concussions-federal-judge-approves-up-to-5-million-per-player-in-concussion-settlement-10199372. html. Accessed April 20, 2016.

2. McCrory P, Meeuwisse WH, Aubry M, et al: Consensus statement on concussion in sport: The 4th International Conference on Concussion in Sport held in Zurich, November 2012. *Br J Sports Med* 2013;47(5):250-258.

3. Giza CC, Kutcher JS, Ashwal S, et al: Summary of evidence-based guideline update: Evaluation and management of concussion in sports. Report of the Guideline Development Subcommittee of the American Academy of Neurology. *Neurology* 2013;80(24):2250-2257.

4. Langlois JA, Rutland-Brown W, Wald MM: The epidemiology and impact of traumatic brain injury: A brief overview. *J Head Trauma Rehabil* 2006;21(5):375-378.

5. Gilchrist J, Thomas KE, Xu L, McGuire LC, Coronado VG: Nonfatal sports and recreation related traumatic brain injuries among children and adolescents treated in emergency departments in the United States, 2001–2009. *MMWR* 2011;60(39):1337-1342.

6. Clay MB, Glover KL, Lowe DT: Epidemiology of concussion in sport: A literature review. *J Chiropr Med* 2013;12(4):230-251.

7. Marar M, McIlvain NM, Fields SK, Comstock RD: Epidemiology of concussions among United States high school athletes in 20 sports. *Am J Sports Med* 2012;40(4):747-755.

8. Hootman JM, Dick R, Agel J: Epidemiology of collegiate injuries for 15 sports: Summary and recommendations for injury prevention initiatives. *J Athl Train* 2007;42(2):311-319.

9. Seifert T, Shipman V: The pathophysiology of sports concussion. *Curr Pain Headache Rep* 2015;19(8):36.

10. Giza CC, Hovda DA: The new neurometabolic cascade of concussion. *Neurosurgery* 2014;75(suppl 4):S24-S33.

11. Grady MF, Master CL, Gioia GA: Concussion pathophysiology: Rationale for physical and cognitive rest. *Pediatr Ann* 2012;41(9):377-382.

12. Maugans TA, Farley C, Altaye M, Leach J, Cecil KM: Pediatric sports-related concussion produces cerebral blood flow alterations. *Pediatrics* 2012;129(1):28-37.

13. Prins ML, Alexander D, Giza CC, Hovda DA: Repeated mild traumatic brain injury: Mechanisms of cerebral vulnerability. *J Neurotrauma* 2013;30(1):30-38.

14. McCrory P, Davis G, Makdissi M: Second impact syndrome or cerebral swelling after sporting head injury. *Curr Sports Med Rep* 2012;11(1):21-23.

15. Maroon JC, Winkelman R, Bost J, Amos A, Mathyssek C, Miele V: Chronic traumatic encephalopathy in contact sports: A systematic review of all reported pathological cases. *PLoS One* 2015;10(2):e0117338.

16. McKee AC, Stern RA, Nowinski CJ, et al: The spectrum of disease in chronic traumatic encephalopathy. *Brain* 2013;136(pt 1):43-64.

17. Ban VS, Madden CJ, Bailes JE, Hunt Batjer H, Lonser RR: The science and questions surrounding chronic traumatic encephalopathy. *Neurosurg Focus* 2016;40(4):E15.

18. Keightley ML, Saluja RS, Chen JK, et al: A functional magnetic resonance imaging study of working memory in youth after sports-related concussion: Is it still working? *J Neurotrauma* 2014;31(5):437-451.

19. Henry LC, Elbin RJ, Collins MW, Marchetti G, Kontos AP: Examining recovery trajectories after sport-related concussion with a multimodal clinical assessment approach. *Neurosurgery* 2016;78(2):232-241.

20. Vagnozzi R, Signoretti S, Tavazzi B, et al: Temporal window of metabolic brain vulnerability to concussion: A pilot 1H-magnetic resonance spectroscopic study in concussed athletes—part III. *Neurosurgery* 2008;62(6):1286-1296.

21. SCAT3. *Br J Spors Med* 2013;47(5):259.

22. Galetta KM, Morganroth J, Moehringer N, et al: Adding vision to concussion testing: A prospective study of sideline testing in youth and collegiate athletes. *J Neuroophthalmol* 2015;35(3):235-241.

23. Dhawan P, Starling A, Tapsell L, et al: King-Device Test identifies symptomatic concussion in real-time and asymptomatic concussion over time. *Neurology* 2014;82(10 suppl):S11.003.

24. Marinides Z, Galetta KM, Andrews CN, et al: Vision testing is additive to the sideline assessment of sports-related concussion. *Neurol Clin Pract* 2015;5(1):25-34.

25. Van Kampen DA, Lovell MR, Pardini JE, Collins MW, Fu FH: The "value added" of neurocognitive testing after sports-related concussion. *Am J Sports Med* 2006;34(10):1630-1635.

26. Nelson LD, LaRoche AA, Pfaller AY, et al: Prospective, head-to-head study of three computerized neurocognitive

assessment tools (CNTs): Reliability and validity for the assessment of sport-related concussion. *J Int Neuropsychol Soc* 2016;22(1):24-37.

27. Johnston KM, Ptito A, Chankowsky J, Chen JK: New frontiers in diagnostic imaging in concussive head injury. *Clin J Sport Med* 2001;11(3):166-175.

28. Kutcher JS, McCrory P, Davis G, Ptito A, Meeuwisse WH, Broglio SP: What evidence exists for new strategies or technologies in the diagnosis of sports concussion and assessment of recovery? *Br J Sports Med* 2013;47(5):299-303.

29. Miller JH, Gill C, Kuhn EN, et al: Predictors of delayed recovery following pediatric sports-related concussion: A case-control study. *J Neurosurg Pediatr* 2016;17(4):491-496.

30. Master CL, Grady MF: Office-based management of pediatric and adolescent concussion. *Pediatr Ann* 2012;41(9):1-6.

31. Matuszak JM, McVige J, McPherson J, Willer B, Leddy J: A practical concussion physical examination toolbox: Evidence-based physical examination for concussion. *Sports Health* 2016;1941738116641394.

32. Mucha A, Collins MW, Elbin RJ, et al: A brief vestibular/ocular motor screening (VOMS) assessment to evaluate concussions: Preliminary findings. *Am J Sports Med* 2014;42(10):2479-2486.

33. Caccese JB, Buckley TA, Kaminski TW: Sway area and velocity correlated with MobileMat Balance Error Scoring System (BESS) scores. *J Appl Biomech* 2016;32(4):329-334.

34. Hunt TN, Ferrara MS, Bornstein RA, Baumgartner TA: The reliability of the modified Balance Error Scoring System. *Clin J Sport Med* 2009;19(6):471-475.

35. Schneiders AG, Sullivan SJ, Handcock P, Gray A, McCrory PR: Sports concussion assessment: The effect of exercise on dynamic and static balance. *Scand J Med Sci Sports* 2012;22(1):85-90.

36. De Marco AP, Broshek DK: Computerized cognitive testing in the management of youth sports-related concussion. *J Child Neurol* 2016;31(1):68-75.

37. Kerr ZY, Snook EM, Lynall RC, et al: Concussion-related protocols and preparticipation assessments used for incoming student-athletes in National Collegiate Athletic Association member institutions. *J Athl Train* 2015;50(11):1174-1181.

38. Resch JE, Brown CN, Macciocchi SN, Cullum CM, Blueitt D, Ferrara MS: A preliminary formula to predict timing of symptom resolution for collegiate athletes diagnosed with sport concussion. *J Athl Train* 2015;50(12):1292-1298.

39. Master CL, Balcer L, Collins M: In the clinic: Concussion. *Ann Intern Med* 2014;160(3):ITC2-ITC1.

40. DiFazio M, Silverberg ND, Kirkwood MW, Bernier R, Iverson GL: Prolonged activity restriction after concussion: Are we worsening outcomes? *Clin Pediatr (Phila)* 2016;55(5):443-451.

41. Howell DR, Mannix RC, Quinn B, Taylor JA, Tan CO, Meehan WP III: Physical activity level and symptom duration are not associated after concussion. *Am J Sports Med* 2016;44(4):1040-1046.

42. Thomas DG, Apps JN, Hoffmann RG, McCrea M, Hammeke T: Benefits of strict rest after acute concussion: A randomized controlled trial. *Pediatrics* 2015;135(2):213-223.

43. Kemp S, Patricios J, Raftery M: Is the content and duration of the graduated return to play protocol after concussion demanding enough? A challenge for Berlin 2016. *Br J Sports Med* 2016;50(11):644-645.

44. Brooks MA, Peterson K, Biese K, Sanfilippo J, Heiderscheit BC, Bell DR: Concussion increases odds of sustaining a lower extremity musculoskeletal injury after return to play among collegiate athletes. *Am J Sports Med* 2016;44(3):742-747.

45. Master CL, Gioia GA, Leddy JJ, Grady MF: Importance of 'return-to-learn' in pediatric and adolescent concussion. *Pediatr Ann* 2012;41(9):1-6.

46. Halstead ME, McAvoy K, Devore CD, et al: Returning to learning following a concussion. *Pediatrics* 2013;132(5):948-957.

47. Gioia GA: Medical-school partnership in guiding return to school following mild traumatic brain injury in youth. *J Child Neurol* 2016;31(1):93-108.

48. McCrea M, Guskiewicz K, Randolph C, et al: Incidence, clinical course, and predictors of prolonged recovery time following sport-related concussion in high school and college athletes. *J Int Neuropsychol Soc* 2013;19(1):22-33.

49. Field M, Collins MW, Lovell MR, Maroon J: Does age play a role in recovery from sports-related concussion? A comparison of high school and collegiate athletes. *J Pediatr* 2003;142(5):546-553.

50. Zemek R, Barrowman N, Freedman SB, et al: Clinical risk score for persistent postconcussion symptoms among children with acute concussion in the ED. *JAMA* 2016;315(10):1014-1025.

51. Vidal PG, Goodman AM, Colin A, Leddy JJ, Grady MF: Rehabilitation strategies for prolonged recovery in pediatric and adolescent concussion. *Pediatr Ann* 2012;41(9):1-7.

52. Gagnon I, Grilli L, Friedman D, Iverson GL: A pilot study of active rehabilitation for adolescents who are slow to recover from sport-related concussion. *Scand J Med Sci Sports* 2016;26(3):299-306.

53. Leddy JJ, Kozlowski K, Fung M, Pendergast DR, Willer B: Regulatory and autoregulatory physiological dysfunction as a primary characteristic of post concussion syndrome: Implications for treatment. *NeuroRehabilitation* 2007;22(3):199-205.

54. Griesbach GS, Hovda DA, Molteni R, Wu A, Gomez-Pinilla F: Voluntary exercise following traumatic brain injury: Brain-derived neurotrophic factor upregulation and recovery of function. *Neuroscience* 2004;125(1):129-139.

55. Leddy JJ, Cox JL, Baker JG, et al: Exercise treatment for postconcussion syndrome: A pilot study of changes in functional magnetic resonance imaging activation, physiology, and symptoms. *J Head Trauma Rehabil* 2013;28(4):241-249.

56. Griffin ÉW, Mullally S, Foley C, Warmington SA, O'Mara SM, Kelly ÁM: Aerobic exercise improves hippocampal function and increases BDNF in the serum of young adult males. *Physiol Behav* 2011;104(5):934-941.

57. Dimeo F, Bauer M, Varahram I, Proest G, Halter U: Benefits from aerobic exercise in patients with major depression: A pilot study. *Br J Sports Med* 2001;35(2):114-117.

58. Al Sayegh A, Sandford D, Carson AJ: Psychological approaches to treatment of postconcussion syndrome: A systematic review. *J Neurol Neurosurg Psychiatry* 2010;81(10):1128-1134.

59. Pearce KL, Sufrinko A, Lau BC, Henry L, Collins MW, Kontos AP: Near point of convergence after a sport-related concussion: Measurement reliability and relationship to neurocognitive impairment and symptoms. *Am J Sports Med* 2015;43(12):3055-3061.

60. Alsalaheen BA, Mucha A, Morris LO, et al: Vestibular rehabilitation for dizziness and balance disorders after concussion. *J Neurol Phys Ther* 2010;34(2):87-93.

61. Master CL, Scheiman M, Gallaway M, et al: Vision diagnoses are common after concussion in adolescents. *Clin Pediatr (Phila)* 2016;55(3):260-267.

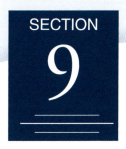

Orthopaedic Medicine

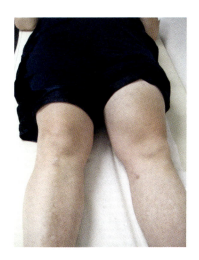

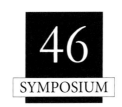

Key Concepts of Musculoskeletal Infection

Scott B. Rosenfeld, MD

Lawson A. Copley, MD, MBA

Megan Mignemi, MD

Thomas An, AB

Michael Benvenuti, BS

Jonathan Schoenecker, MD, PhD

Abstract

Over the past few decades, musculoskeletal infections have increased in both incidence and severity. The clinical manifestations of musculoskeletal infections range from isolated osteomyelitis to multisite infections with systemic complications. Although this increased incidence of musculoskeletal infections correlates with the increased incidence of methicillin-resistant Staphylococcus aureus *infections, other nonresistant infectious organisms have been associated with severe musculoskeletal infections; this finding supports the likelihood that an antibiotic resistance profile is not a major factor in bacterial virulence. Instead, a multitude of virulence factors allow infectious organisms to manipulate and evade the immune response of the host. Organisms such as* S aureus *and* Streptococcus pyogenes *are able to hijack the acute phase response of the host, which allows for protected proliferation and dissemination. The serum factors produced by the acute phase response, including interleukin-6, C-reactive protein, erythrocytes/fibrinogen, and platelets, can be used to assess musculoskeletal infection severity and monitor treatment. Bacterial genome sequencing has identified virulence factors in a wide variety of clinical manifestations of musculoskeletal infections and may help identify targets for clinical therapy. Currently, however, the management of musculoskeletal infections relies on accurate organism identification and a thorough recognition of the sites of infection and the tissues that are involved. MRI aids in the localization of musculoskeletal infection and identification of sites that require surgical débridement.*

Instr Course Lect 2017;66:569–584.

Over the past two decades, an evolution in the epidemiology and management of pediatric musculoskeletal infections has occurred. Evidence shows an increased incidence of musculoskeletal infections, which varies by region (**Figure 1**). In addition, several regional studies have reported an increased incidence of severe musculoskeletal infections in children.[1-6] This increased incidence of severe musculoskeletal infections in children is supported by reports of more severe associated complications, including deep vein thrombosis, septic pulmonary emboli, abscess, sepsis, and death. As the severity of musculoskeletal infections has increased, the workup and management of musculoskeletal infections have evolved. A better understanding of the human acute phase response (APR) has improved the ability of surgeons to assess and monitor musculoskeletal infections based on trends in laboratory tests, such as C-reactive protein (CRP) levels. To better understand the nature and location of musculoskeletal infections, MRI has become a key component in the workup of many patients in whom musculoskeletal infection is present.

Increasingly complex treatment options for the management of musculoskeletal infections, including more frequent surgical management, multiple surgeries, prolonged hospitalization,

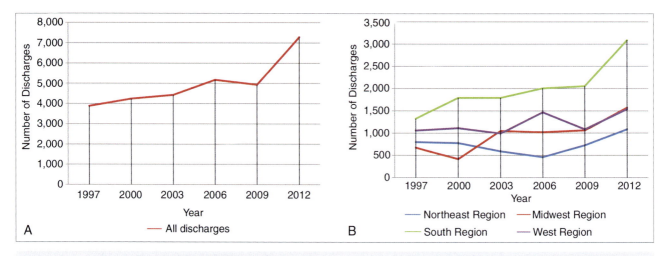

Figure 1 Line graphs from the Healthcare Cost and Utilization Project Kids' Inpatient Database show discharges of children (aged birth to 17 years) with a primary diagnosis of acute hematogenous osteomyelitis, septic arthritis, or pyomyositis from 1997 to 2012. **A,** All discharges. **B,** Regional variation in all discharges.

and critical care management, have been required; in addition, musculoskeletal infections have been associated with more adverse outcomes.[7-11] The increased incidence of musculoskeletal infections coincides with an increased incidence of methicillin-resistant *Staphylococcus aureus* (MRSA) infections.[1,3,5] Interestingly, although the incidence of severe musculoskeletal infections continues to increase, some studies have reported that most children who have osteomyelitis tend to respond quickly to antibiotic treatment and require minimal surgical intervention to manage musculoskeletal infections.[12,13] Clearly, more factors than just an antibiotic resistance profile are involved with regard to musculoskeletal infections. Patient-specific host characteristics, such as APR function, bacterial virulence factors, and regional variations

in bacterial epidemiology, likely contribute to the course of musculoskeletal infections.

Hijacking the APR

The APR, which is a systemic reaction to tissue injury, is mediated by the liver and characterized by the modulation of more than 1,000 genes (**Figure 2**). The APR results in the production of acute-phase reactants that prevent hemorrhage, combat infection, and stimulate tissue regeneration. Although the APR is essential for normal coagulation and immunity, dysregulation can lead to various complications, such as life-threatening hemorrhage, poor wound healing, and venous thromboembolism. These thromboembolic complications stem from the Virchow triad of venous stasis, endothelial injury, and hypercoagulability[14] (**Figure 2**).

Pathogenic bacteria possess an arsenal of virulence factors that allows them to invade, persist, and disseminate in the human body.[15] Virtually all bacteria exhibit selectivity for certain cells, tissues, or hosts. In the context of musculoskeletal infections, bacterial pathogens have developed a tropism for sites of tissue damage by hijacking specific acute phase reactants. The coagulation system is the universal phase of the APR that is hijacked by bacteria.

The Fibrin/DNA Web

In response to injury, the procoagulant arm of the coagulation system produces a fibrin/platelet web that seals off damaged musculoskeletal tissue both intravascularly and extravascularly.[16] After the injured compartment is sealed via coagulant processes, the fibrinolytic arm of the coagulation system breaks

Dr. Rosenfeld or an immediate family member serves as an unpaid consultant to OrthoPediatrics and serves as a board member, owner, officer, or committee member of the Pediatric Orthopaedic Society of North America. Dr. Copley or an immediate family member serves as an unpaid consultant to Epic and serves as a board member, owner, officer, or committee member of the Pediatric Orthopaedic Society of North America. Mr. An or an immediate family member has stock or stock options held in Merck and has received research or institutional support from Johnson & Johnson and Merck. Mr. Benvenuti or an immediate family member has stock or stock options held in Abbott, AbbVie, Bristol-Myers Squibb, GlaxoSmithKline, Johnson & Johnson, Pfizer, and Zimmer. Dr. Schoenecker or an immediate family member is a member of a speakers' bureau or has made paid presentations on behalf of OrthoPediatrics and has received research or institutional support from Ionis Pharmaceuticals. Neither Dr. Mignemi nor any immediate family member has received anything of value from or has stock or stock options held in a commercial company or institution related directly or indirectly to the subject of this chapter.

down fibrin/platelet clots and promotes efficient tissue regeneration. The protease plasmin is the principal mediator of this process, which occurs in a controlled manner to prevent unregulated loss of compartmentalization during tissue remodeling.[17,18]

In addition to isolating damaged tissue, the procoagulant arm of the coagulation system serves as the initial defense against bacterial invasion (**Figure 3, A**). Coagulation allows for antimicrobial activity by arresting bacteria within clots via a fibrin web (**Figure 3, B**) and recruiting macrophages (**Figure 3, C**) and neutrophils (**Figure 3, D**) to the site of infection.[19] In addition, neutrophils reinforce the fibrin web by emitting neutrophil extracellular traps (NETs; **Figure 3, D**), which are extracellular DNA fibers with associated proteins that function in a manner similar to that of fibrin, to immobilize and destroy pathogens.[20] Typically, this immediate innate immune response to pathogens is successful and staves off infection by most pathogens.

S aureus: Rearranging the NET

S aureus initially produces procoagulant factors to form an abscess of fibrin, in which it can proliferate without interference from the immune responses of a host (**Figure 4**). Coagulase, which is the most well-known *S aureus* virulence factor (**Figure 4, A**), associates with and activates prothrombin to thrombin[21] (**Figure 4, B**). The coagulase-thrombin complex catalyzes the cleavage of fibrinogen to fibrin[22] (**Figure 4, B**). von Willebrand factor-binding protein plays a similar role in *S aureus* virulence, associating with prothrombin to promote further fibrin formation[23] (**Figure 4, C**). The activation of

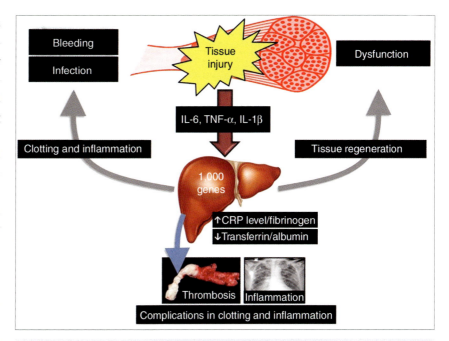

Figure 2   Illustration shows normal regulation of the acute phase response to tissue injury, which results in hemostasis and tissue regeneration; however, dysregulation of the acute phase response can lead to severe complications in clotting and inflammation. CRP = C-reactive protein, IL = interleukin, TNF = tumor necrosis factor.

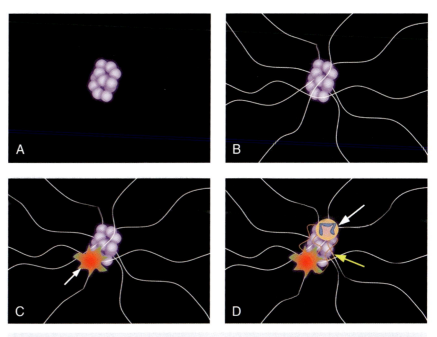

Figure 3   Computer-generated illustrations show how the fibrin/DNA web serves as a defense against bacterial infection. **A,** Bacteria in a human host. **B,** Bacteria is arrested in a fibrin web. **C,** A macrophage (arrow) is recruited to fight the infection. **D,** Neutrophils (white arrow) are recruited to fight the infection and emit neutrophil extracellular traps (yellow arrow).

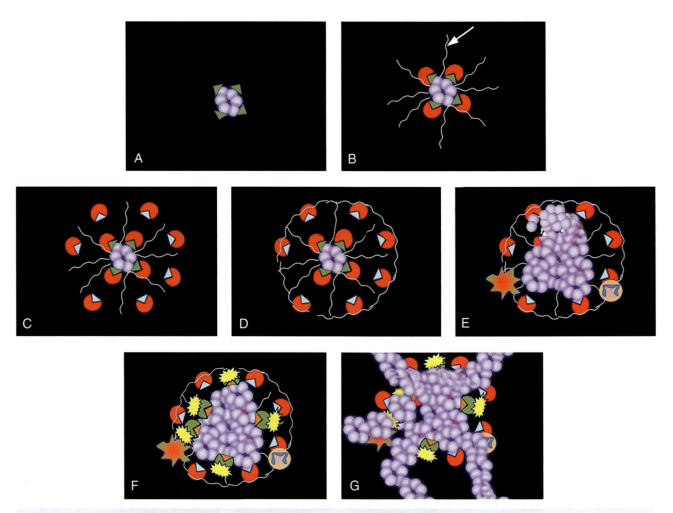

Figure 4 Computer-generated illustrations show the mechanism for *Staphylococcus aureus* proliferation. **A,** *S aureus* binds to virulence factor coagulase. **B** and **C,** Coagulase and von Willebrand factor-binding protein (vWBP) activation of prothrombin catalyzes the cleavage of fibrinogen to fibrin (arrow in panel **B**), which promotes clot and abscess formation. **D,** In the abscess, an inner pseudocapsule is formed by coagulase, and an outer meshwork is formed by vWBP. **E,** The pseudocapsule and outer meshwork create a barrier that prevents macrophage and neutrophil access. **F,** Nuclease and adenosine synthase are expressed to interfere with neutrophil extracellular traps. **G,** *S aureus* staphylokinase is expressed to promote fibrin degradation, abscess rupture, and dissemination. Blue triangles = von Willebrand factor-binding protein, green circles = plasmin, green triangles = coagulase, orange triangles = *S aureus* staphylokinase, red circles with cutout = prothrombin, yellow starbursts = plasmin cleaving fibrin.

prothrombin by both coagulase and von Willebrand factor-binding protein promotes clot and abscess formation[24] (**Figure 4, D**). Within an abscess, two concentric structures are formed: an inner pseudocapsule that is formed predominantly by coagulase and a thicker outer meshwork that depends on the von Willebrand factor-binding protein (**Figure 4, D**). Together, these redundant mechanisms generate a double-layer, fibrin-dependent protective barrier that prevents macrophage and neutrophil access and clearance[25] (**Figure 4, E**). *S aureus* further manipulates the immune system by expressing nuclease and adenosine synthase, which interferes with NETs[26] (**Figure 4, F**). This process allows *S aureus* to form its own compartment in the body by hijacking the normal coagulation response to the initial site of tissue injury. After the staphylococcal abscess reaches a quorum, which is a colony density that enables cell-to-cell communication and coordinated gene expression, *S aureus* expresses *S aureus* staphylokinase, which promotes fibrin degradation, abscess rupture, and dissemination[27] (**Figure 4, G**). Essentially, *S aureus* hijacks procoagulant factors to manipulate fibrin and form a protective abscess. After a quorum is reached,

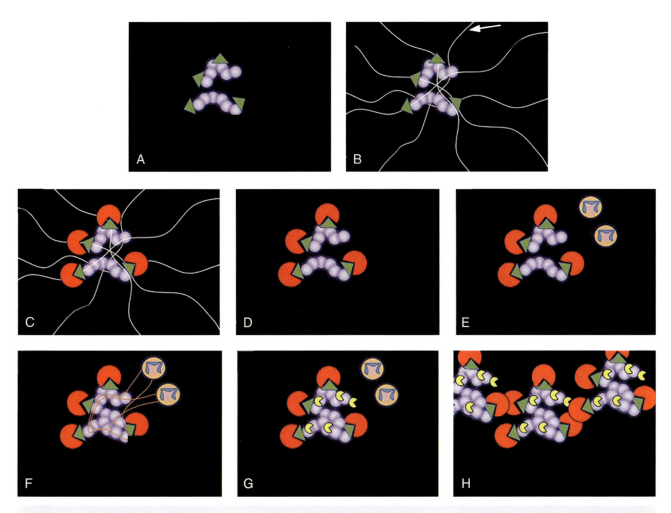

Figure 5   Computer-generated illustrations show the mechanism for *Streptococcus pyogenes* proliferation.
A, *S pyogenes* binds to virulence factor streptokinase. **B,** A fibrin web (arrow) is formed around *S pyogenes*. **C** and **D,** The streptokinase/plasmin complex activates plasmin, which leads to the rapid degradation of both fibrin and fibrinogen. The neutrophil extracellular traps that are produced by neutrophils (**E** and **F**) are evaded via DNAse expression (**G**). **H,** Dysregulation of the fibrinolytic system of the host leads to dissemination. Green triangles = streptokinase, red circles with cutout = plasmin, yellow circles with cutout = DNAse B.

S aureus activates the clot-busting activity of plasmin to break out of the abscess and disseminate.

Streptococcus pyogenes: Bypassing the NET

Streptococcus pyogenes uses a different approach for invasion and dissemination. *S pyogenes* bypasses the initial production of procoagulant factors to form an abscess and immediately expresses fibrinolytic proteins (**Figure 5**). The best studied of these fibrinolytic factors is streptokinase (**Figure 5, A**), which binds to and activates plasmin via conformational change (**Figure 5, B** and **C**). The resulting α-2 antiplasmin-resistant streptokinase/plasmin complex activates, circulating plasmin five times faster than tissue plasmin activator and 30 times faster than urokinase plasmin activator, which leads to the rapid degradation of both fibrin and fibrinogen[28] (**Figure 5, D**). The inability of a host to sequester *S pyogenes* infection is demonstrated by the invasiveness of necrotizing fasciitis infection, which disregards tissue planes, physiologic compartments, or extracellular matrix barriers.[29] To evade sequestration by the NETs that are produced by neutrophils (**Figure 5, E** and **F**), streptococci express DNAse to cleave neutrophils (**Figure 5, G**). Studies have reported a dose-dependent clearance of NETs in patients with *S pyogenes*.[30] In general, the virulence of *S pyogenes* depends heavily on dysregulation of the fibrinolytic system of the host, which allows

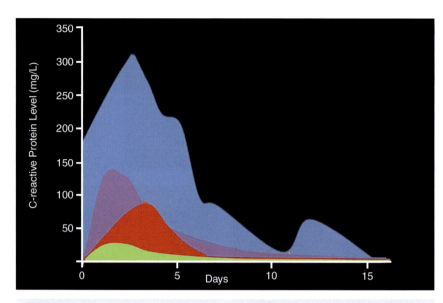

Figure 6   Graph shows a comparison of C-reactive protein levels in response to disseminated infection (blue), isolated osteomyelitis (red), total knee arthroplasty (purple), and periacetabular osteotomy (green).

for rapid invasion and dissemination (**Figure 5, H**).

Clinical Correlations for Musculoskeletal Infections

Correlation between pathogenic virulence mechanisms and clinical findings allows surgeons to accurately predict musculoskeletal infection severity and clinical outcomes. Musculoskeletal infections may be conceptualized as a continuous tissue injury that intensely activates the APR via the persistent production of interleukin-6. The tissue damage caused by musculoskeletal infections generates measurable increases of acute phase reactants in serum levels, and numerous studies have reported that inflammatory and coagulation markers (ie, CRP, erythrocytes/fibrinogen, and platelets) are sensitive indicators of musculoskeletal infection severity.[31] In addition, unpublished data from the authors of this chapter have demonstrated statistically significant differences in acute phase inflammatory

markers in patients who have disseminated musculoskeletal infections compared with patients who have compartmentalized musculoskeletal infections. Severe musculoskeletal infections lead to clinically relevant dysregulation of the coagulation system, which results in thromboembolism, sepsis, or disseminated intravascular coagulopathy. The area under the curve of the CRP level of a child who has isolated osteomyelitis is roughly equivalent to that of a patient who underwent total knee arthroplasty and greater than that of a patient who underwent periacetabular osteotomy (**Figure 6**). More impressively, a child with a disseminated musculoskeletal infection has CRP levels that are approximately equivalent to having undergone three total knee arthroplasties and six periacetabular osteotomies (**Figure 6**). An understanding of how pathogens dysregulate and exploit the coagulation system allows severe musculoskeletal infections to be diagnosed earlier when relevant indices (ie, fibrinogen,

D-dimer, international normalized ratio) are followed. Improved anticipation and diagnosis of systemic complications will lead to more timely and effective interventions and improved patient outcomes.

Severity of Illness Assessment and Bacterial Factors

Many recent studies have reported on the measurable severity of illness in children with musculoskeletal infections. Patients who have a MRSA infection experience more severe illness compared with those who have a methicillin-sensitive *S aureus* infection.[11,32-35] As such, a tendency exists to attribute the virulent behavior of a bacteria to the antibiotic resistance profile of the organism.[2,6,32,33] Current studies have described a variety of objective clinical parameters that can be used to differentiate musculoskeletal infection phenotypes;[11,32-35] unfortunately, many of these studies have potential flaws. Nearly all of these studies have been conducted in localized regions, and the microbiologic epidemiology of each of those regions likely differs substantially from that of other regions in which a musculoskeletal infection may occur. In addition, the studies used different parameters to assess the severity of illness. Therefore, it is a challenge to make meaningful conclusions in a comparison of these studies.

The heterogeneity observed in the results of these studies supports the notion that substantial differences may exist in the regional incidence and severity of musculoskeletal infections in children. National database search results further support this pattern of regional musculoskeletal infection variation, with a higher incidence of musculoskeletal infection discharges reported in regions that have temperate climates, such as the southern regions of the United States, and a lower incidence of musculoskeletal infection discharges reported in the northern regions of the United States.[36] This suggests that a spectrum of clinical disease, which may vary from community to community and from child to child, exists among children who have musculoskeletal infections. Such an epidemiologic phenomenon is likely the result of the combined behavior of the immune response of affected children and the virulence behavior of causative organisms.

Severity of Illness Assessment

In 2009, the concept of measurable comparative severity, which was used to illustrate increased virulence of MRSA osteomyelitis in children, was introduced.[11,32-35] Studies reported that differences in clinical factors could predict the likelihood of MRSA infection and potentially guide earlier antibiotic selection. However, independent analyses reported that these clinical predictive algorithms had relatively poor diagnostic performance in other regions.[34] Other studies reported that even patients who had methicillin-sensitive *S aureus* infections experienced more severe illness; however, severity of illness was not determined by the antibiotic resistance profile of the bacteria.

The cumulative results of these studies indicate the need for an objective manner in which surgeons can differentiate musculoskeletal infection phenotypes. An ideal scoring metric should be obtained at the earliest possible point of hospitalization, before substantial intervention occurs that may influence the response of a child

Table 1

Modified Severity of Illness Score for Children With Acute Hematogenous Osteomyelitis

Parameter	Point Value[a]
Initial CRP level (mg/dL)	
<10	0
10–15	1
>15	2
CRP level (mg/dL) 48 hours after presentation	
<5	0
5–10	1
>10	2
CRP level (mg/dL) 96 hours after presentation	
<5	0
5–10	1
>10	2
Band count (cells/μL)	
<1.5	0
≥1.5	1
Febrile days on antibiotics	
<2	0
≥2	1
ICU admission	
No	0
Yes	1
Disseminated musculoskeletal infection	
No	0
Yes	1

CRP = C-reactive protein, ICU = intensive care unit.
[a]Total scores range from 0 (mild) to 10 (severe).

to the intervention. This scoring metric must take into consideration the early evolution of musculoskeletal infection in an affected child, which may vary in severity via a rapid improvement or a decline in illness. Copley et al[35] proposed and validated such a scoring metric in a large retrospective cohort study of 56 children from the southwest United States who had acute hematogenous osteomyelitis. The scores correlated favorably with the causative organism, intensive care admission, surgeries, the length of hospitalization, readmission, and complications from the infection.[35] **Table 1** shows a modification of the scoring metric that was proposed by Copley et al,[35] which allows for a severity of illness score from 0 (mild) to 10 (severe). The modified severity of illness score has been used to guide clinical care and help reduce the length of hospitalization for children who have acute hematogenous osteomyelitis. The modified severity of illness score also has been helpful for musculoskeletal infection stratification in both gene expression studies and bacterial genome studies. Additional multicenter research is necessary to validate the modified severity of illness score.

Bacterial Genome Studies

In 2001, Kuroda et al[37] published entire genome sequences of two hospital-acquired strains of MRSA (N315 and Mu50) from Japan. The whole genome sequences illustrated the 2.8 million base pair circular chromosome of MRSA, which consists of a complex mixture of genes that seemingly are acquired via lateral gene transfer.[37] The authors identified 70 candidate virulence factors that reside in pathogenicity islands within the chromosome structure of MRSA.[37] Subsequently, Baba et al[38] published the entire genome sequence data of the community-acquired MW2 strain of MRSA (USA400) that was isolated from a 16-month-old girl from North Dakota who had fatal septic hip arthritis. The authors reported that this strain of MRSA carried a range of virulence genes that resided in genomic islands, but that these virulence genes were distinct from those of the N315 and Mu50 strains of MRSA.[38] In 2006, Diep et al[39] published the entire genome sequence data of the FPR3757 strain of USA300, which is the predominant clone of MRSA and a major source of community-acquired infection in the United States. The authors compared the entire genome sequence data of this isolate with that of 10 other staphylococcal strains, and reported that *S aureus* continues to evolve via the acquisition of mobile genetic elements, which enhances its long-term fitness and pathogenicity.[39]

Targeted Studies of Select Virulence Genes

Attempts to reveal the relative contribution of bacterial virulence genes to the pathogenesis of musculoskeletal infections has led to studies on a variety of specific genes via targeted polymerase chain reaction.[40-45] Currently, no consistent or definitive evidence exists that any one bacterial virulence gene plays a central role in the determination of virulence. Instead, the pathogenic behavior of *S aureus* is more likely predicated on a complex variety of bacterial virulence factors, which allows *S aureus* to survive and then thrive in a human host.[41,46] Iron metabolism is one mechanism via which *S aureus* survives and thrives in a human host. Less than 10 times[11] the amount of free iron sufficient for *S aureus* to survive is present in human blood.[47] As a result, *S aureus* must rapidly upregulate iron metabolism genes and liberate free iron from erythrocytes with the use of a variety of hemolysins, including gamma hemolysin.[48] Concurrently, *S aureus* avoids destruction by circulating neutrophils that are rapidly upregulated through gene expression via the innate immune response.[49] This neutrophil response may be deterred by necrotizing toxins, such as Panton-Valentine leukocidin.[36,43,44] Although studies have paid substantial attention to the association between Panton-Valentine leukocidin–positive MRSA and severe bone and joint infections, this mechanism is likely only one of many mechanisms in *S aureus'* arsenal via which *S aureus* survives and thrives in a human host.[42,48,49] In fact, *S aureus* has a highly redundant genome, particularly with regard to neutrophil defense, which results in automated cell death within 6 hours of bacterial phagocytosis by neutrophils.[50] After the

defenses of a host have been subverted, *S aureus* gains access to the deep tissues of bone, joint, or muscle, via microbial surface components recognizing adhesive matrix molecules, which bind to fibronectin, fibrinogen, elastin, collagen, and bone.[40,41,45] Local oxygenation rapidly becomes depleted in the deep tissues, particularly as the density of *S aureus* increases, and the overwhelming neutrophil response leads to abscess formation. This process leads to upregulation of bacterial genes to liberate local energy sources via proteolytic enzymes, lipolysis, gluconeogenesis, and the arginine deaminase pathway.[41,51,52]

Multigene Studies and Next-Generation Genome Sequencing

Multigene studies via either polymerase chain reaction or next-generation genome sequencing are used to assess genes that are more common in isolates that result in invasive musculoskeletal infections rather than in isolates that result in superficial musculoskeletal infections or nasal carriage in asymptomatic, healthy hosts.[53-55] These studies have delineated a variety of genes that appear to contribute independently, but possibly in a cumulative manner, to severe, invasive musculoskeletal infections. Subsequent studies reported substantial genomic heterogeneity of isolates in a single community, all of which resulted in acute hematogenous osteomyelitis in children who demonstrated a wide difference in clinical severity of illness.[56] The differences in clinical severity of illness were not the result of substantial insertions, deletions, or rearrangements but the result of single nucleotide polymorphisms, with a mean of 11 nonredundant, amino acid–changing single nucleotide polymorphisms per isolate.[56]

Table 2
Classification of Musculoskeletal Infections Based on Type of Tissue Infected

Diagnosis	Definition	Example(s)
Tissue injury of unknown origin	Diagnosis of exclusion Negative tissue and/or blood culture Joint effusion	Transient synovitis of the hip
Superficial abscess	Superficial to deep fascia of limb or located in the hand or foot	Septic prepatellar bursitis Superficial forearm abscess
Septic joint	Limited to joint space only; no extension to surrounding muscles or bone Synovial aspirate is grossly purulent with >50,000 cells, positive Gram stain, and/or positive bacterial culture	Septic knee
Osteomyelitis	Isolated to bone only; no extension to subperiosteal space or surrounding muscles or joints	Proximal femur osteomyelitis
Deep abscess/pyomyositis	Deep fascia of limb Isolated to muscle only; no extension to nearby bone or joints May include multiple muscle groups May be mild (edema only), moderate (phlegmon), or severe (abscess)	Obturator internus myositis Adductor and rectus femoris myositis
Complex musculoskeletal infection	Involves a combination of bone, muscles, and joints	Subperiosteal abscess Pericapsular myositis with ischial osteomyelitis Clavicular osteomyelitis with supra-clavicular abscess

Reproduced with permission from Mignemi M, Copley L, Schoenecker J: Evidence-based treatment for musculoskeletal infection, in Alshryda S, Huntley J, Banaszkiewicz PA, eds: *Paediatric Orthopaedics: An Evidence-Based Approach to Clinical Questions*. Heidelberg, Germany, Springer, 2017, pp 403-418.

The studies also reported that a higher percentage of single nucleotide polymorphisms were present in isolates that were obtained from children who had the highest clinical severity of illness.[56]

RNA Studies

An understanding of the genomic composition of causative organisms with regard to clinical severity of illness is valuable but leads to questions of which genes are actively expressed at which point in time during disease pathogenesis. Recent studies have reported differential gene expression in comparisons of in vivo and in vitro methods of gene expression analysis.[57,58] In vivo osteomyelitis studies of mice revealed genes that were more highly expressed in mice with acute and chronic osteomyelitis compared with mice with in vitro growth conditions.[58] Unsurprisingly, in vivo transcriptome-encoded proteins are involved in gluconeogenesis, proteolysis, iron acquisition, and evasion of the immune defenses of a host.[58]

Imaging of Musculoskeletal Infections

The thorough diagnosis and management of musculoskeletal infections are a challenge, partially because musculoskeletal infections represent a spectrum of clinical disease that is not always isolated to one tissue type or anatomic location. Although septic arthritis, osteomyelitis, and pyomyositis can occur in isolation, these musculoskeletal infections frequently occur in combination. A failure to recognize complex musculoskeletal infections that involve more than one tissue type and/or anatomic location can lead to delayed treatment, prolonged hospitalization, and an increased risk for complications. For these reasons, imaging has become a vital part of the diagnosis and management of musculoskeletal infections.

Workup

Traditionally, musculoskeletal infections were classified based on the type of tissue infected: superficial abscess, septic joint, osteomyelitis, deep abscess/pyomyositis, or complex musculoskeletal infections that involve multiple tissue types (**Table 2**; **Figure 7**).

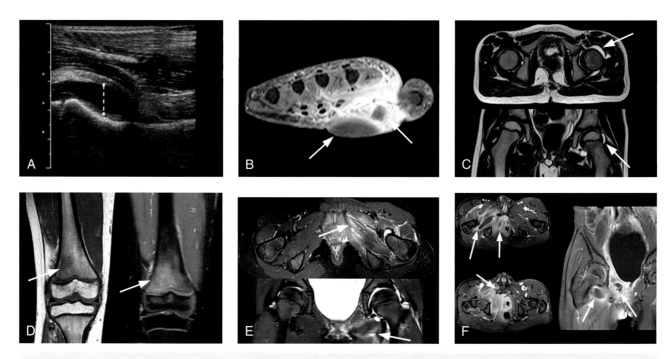

Figure 7 Images show classification of musculoskeletal infections based on the type of tissue infected. **A,** Ultrasonographic image of a hip shows an effusion (dashed yellow line), which represents a tissue injury of unknown origin. **B,** Axial T2-weighted MRI of a hand shows a superficial abscess (arrows). **C,** Axial (top) and coronal (bottom) T1-weighted MRIs of a pelvis show a septic hip (arrows). **D,** Coronal T1-weighted (left) and coronal T2-weighted (right) MRIs of a knee show osteomyelitis of the distal femur (arrows). **E,** Axial (top) and coronal (bottom) T2-weighted MRIs of a pelvis show deep abscess/pyomyositis of the obturator musculature (arrows). **F,** Axial (top left and bottom left) and coronal (right) T2-weighted MRIs of a pelvis show complex musculoskeletal infection (arrows).

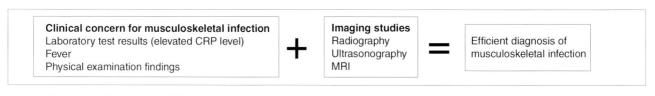

Figure 8 Equation shows the ideal workup for a patient with a suspected musculoskeletal infection, which includes a patient's history, physical examination findings, laboratory test results, and imaging studies. CRP = C-reactive protein.

This variability in presentation makes musculoskeletal infections a diagnostic challenge, which can lead to delayed treatment, prolonged hospitalization, and the overuse of hospital resources. The ideal clinical workup for patients in whom musculoskeletal infection is suspected includes a physical examination, laboratory tests, and appropriate imaging studies to make a quick and efficient diagnosis (**Figure 8**).

Specific Imaging Modalities
Radiography
Plain radiographs should be obtained in all patients in whom a concern for a musculoskeletal infection exists. Radiography, which is readily available and inexpensive, can be used to rule out trauma or other bone pathology, such as a tumor, that may have a similar clinical picture. Although plain radiographs typically appear normal in patients who

have acute musculoskeletal infections, joint space widening or joint effusions may be present (**Figure 9**). Soft-tissue swelling observed on radiographs may indicate an underlying musculoskeletal infection. Typically, bony destruction is unable to be observed on radiographs until an infection has been present for 7 to 14 days, which makes plain radiographs more useful for patients who have chronic musculoskeletal

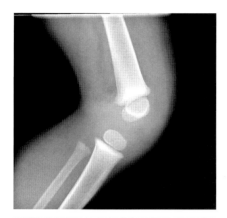

Figure 9 Lateral radiograph of a knee demonstrates joint effusion.

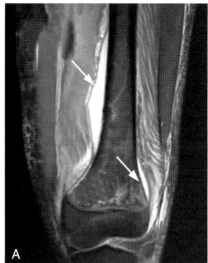
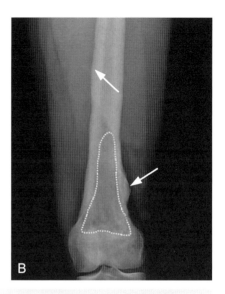

Figure 10 Images of a femur with osteomyelitis. **A,** Coronal T2-weighted MRI shows distal femur osteomyelitis and subperiosteal abscess (arrows). **B,** Follow-up AP radiograph demonstrates sequelae of infection, including sequestrum (dotted area) and involucrum (arrows).

infections. Radiographs also can be used to demonstrate sequelae of musculoskeletal infection, including involucrum/sequestrum, osteonecrosis, growth arrest, angular deformity, and joint destruction (**Figure 10**).

Ultrasonography

Similar to radiography, ultrasonography is a readily available, inexpensive imaging modality. Ultrasonography is most useful for the identification of fluid (joint effusions and superficial abscesses; **Figure 11**). Until recently, ultrasonography was the preferred imaging modality for the diagnosis of septic hip arthritis. However, ultrasonography has a limited ability to identify deep musculoskeletal infections, including those in bone and muscle, and, therefore, may miss contiguous periarticular musculoskeletal infections (ie, pericapsular hip pyomyositis with a septic hip joint). In the past decade, surgeons have widely accepted that many pediatric patients with a musculoskeletal infection have complex musculoskeletal infections that involve more than one tissue type or anatomic location (ie, septic hip arthritis with contiguous pyomyositis).[59,60] This in

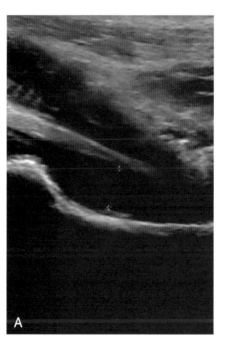
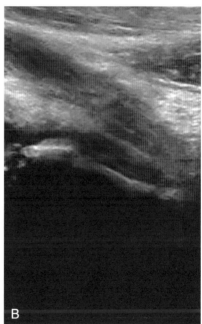

Figure 11 Ultrasonographic images of a patient's left hip (**A**), which shows an effusion, and right hip (**B**), which shows no effusion.

combination with the limitations of ultrasonography have made MRI the preferred imaging modality for pediatric patients in whom musculoskeletal infection is suspected.[61,62] However,

because of limitations in the availability and cost of MRI, many surgeons still rely heavily on ultrasonography for the workup of patients in whom musculoskeletal infection is suspected.

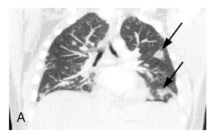 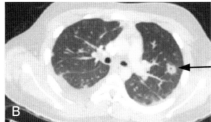

Figure 12 Coronal (**A**) and axial (**B**) chest CT scans demonstrate septic pulmonary emboli (arrows).

Computed Tomography

CT plays a limited role in the diagnosis of acute musculoskeletal infections. Although CT is able to detect large abscesses, its ability to evaluate early soft-tissue and bone infections is limited. CT requires considerable exposure to radiation and, therefore, should be avoided whenever possible in the pediatric population. However, a role for CT exists in the workup of patients who have chronic osteomyelitis or a disseminated musculoskeletal infection if concern for septic pulmonary emboli exists (**Figure 12**). CT also can be useful in the evaluation of sequelae of musculoskeletal infection, including involucrum/sequestrum, osteonecrosis, growth arrest, and joint destruction.[63]

Magnetic Resonance Imaging

With the increased recognition of more complex musculoskeletal infections that involve multiple tissue types and anatomic locations, MRI has become increasingly recognized as a key component in the workup of patients in whom musculoskeletal infection is suspected. MRI is able to detect fluid, from early inflammation to well-established musculoskeletal infections, and can be used to image many different tissue types, including bone, muscles, and joints (**Figure 13**). As a result, MRI is able to detect sites of musculoskeletal

infection, such as pericapsular pyomyositis adjacent to septic arthritis, that may be missed by other imaging modalities (**Figure 14**). Thus, for patients who have musculoskeletal infections that require surgical débridement, MRI is an essential tool for surgical or interventional radiology planning, which is used to identify all foci of a musculoskeletal infection that require débridement and/or drainage.

At many institutions, however, MRI is not readily available and is expensive, which limits its widespread use in the workup of patients in whom musculoskeletal infection is suspected. At the institution of the authors of this chapter, a fast spin-echo sequence protocol was initiated for pediatric patients in whom musculoskeletal infection is suspected to obtain nonsedated, noncontrast MRI in less than 30 minutes. The fast spin-echo sequence protocol includes a coronal T1-weighted short tau inversion recovery MRI and an axial T2-weighted MRI, both of which generally provide surgeons with enough detail to make an accurate diagnosis as well as identify any foci of musculoskeletal infection that are amenable to surgical or interventional radiology débridement and/or drainage (**Figure 15**). Gadolinium-enhanced MRI should not be routinely used in the evaluation of patients in whom musculoskeletal infection is

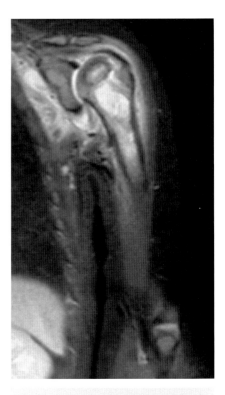

Figure 13 Coronal T2-weighted MRI of a left shoulder shows a complex musculoskeletal infection that affects multiple tissue types, including bone (osteomyelitis), joint (septic arthritis), and muscle (myositis).

suspected; however, MRI with contrast may increase the detection of small abscesses. In a study of 90 children with musculoskeletal infections in whom MRI was performed with and without contrast, Kan et al[64] reported that the abscesses of eight patients who required surgical intervention were identified only on MRIs with contrast. Musculoskeletal infection was not diagnosed in children with normal MRIs without contrast.

Whole Body Bone Scanning

Whole body bone scanning is a nuclear medicine imaging modality that uses a radioactive tracer to detect areas of inflammation (ie, musculoskeletal infection). Whole body bone scans can

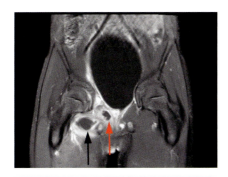

Figure 14 Contrast-enhanced, coronal, T2-weighted MRI of a pelvis shows pericapsular pyomyositis of a right hip that involves the obturator internus (red arrow) and obturator externus (black arrow) muscles.

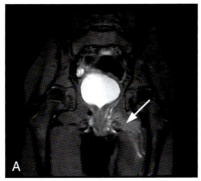

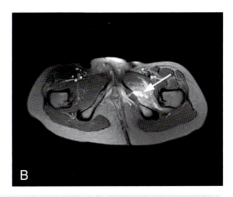

Figure 15 Images of a pelvis show a fast spin-echo sequence MRI protocol. **A,** Coronal, T1-weighted, short tau inversion recovery MRI shows a 1.22 cm × 1.04 cm abscess (arrow) in the obturator externus muscle. **B,** Axial T2-weighted MRI of the same abscess shown in panel **A.**

be a very useful tool for the workup of certain patients who have musculoskeletal infections. Specifically, whole body bone scans can be used to identify foci of a musculoskeletal infection in patients in whom the anatomic location of a musculoskeletal infection is not readily apparent (ie, patients who are too young to participate in the physical examination or patients who are critically ill). In addition, in patients in whom a disseminated musculoskeletal infection with multiple foci is suspected, a whole body bone scan can be used to identify possible sources of musculoskeletal infection; an MRI can then be obtained to evaluate those specific locations in detail.

Evidence for the Use of MRI

MRI is quickly becoming the preferred imaging modality for the diagnosis of musculoskeletal infections because of the variable presentation observed in patients with a suspected musculoskeletal infection. For example, most children who have septic arthritis demonstrate joint irritability with limited range of motion and refuse to bear weight; have a fever; have elevated

inflammatory markers such as CRP levels, erythrocyte sedimentation rate, and white blood cell count; and have joint effusion that is observed on ultrasonograms. Other pediatric musculoskeletal infections, especially those that occur around the hip joint, may mimic septic arthritis.

Although the Kocher criteria have long been used to differentiate septic hip arthritis and transient synovitis, recent studies have reported that the Kocher criteria are unable to distinguish septic arthritis from other types of musculoskeletal infections around the hip (osteomyelitis and pyomyositis).[65] For this reason, if concern exists for septic arthritis of the hip based on the clinical examination and elevated inflammatory markers, MRI should be performed as quickly as possible to evaluate the hip and the surrounding structures for contiguous musculoskeletal infection. In a study of 53 patients who were evaluated in the emergency department to rule out septic hip arthritis, Mignemi et al[66] reported that pelvic pyomyositis was twice as common as isolated septic hip arthritis based on MRI. Monsalve et al[67] reported that contiguous osteomyelitis was observed

on the MRIs of 70 of 103 patients who had septic arthritis.

Rosenfeld et al[59] found five variables to be predictive of adjacent musculoskeletal infection: age older than 3.6 years, CRP level greater than 13.8 mg/dL, duration of symptoms longer than 3 days, platelet count less than 314×10^3 cells/μL, and absolute neutrophil count greater than 8.6×10 cells/μL. The authors classified patients in whom three or more variables were present as high risk for septic arthritis with adjacent musculoskeletal infection (sensitivity, 90%; specificity, 67%; positive predictive value, 80%; negative predictive value, 83%). The authors recommended performing preoperative MRI in patients in whom at least three of these variables are present.[59] For patients in whom musculoskeletal infection is present adjacent to a joint in question, MRI can be used to direct the approach for joint aspiration. Usually, hip joint aspiration is performed via a medial approach, just posterior to the adductor longus tendon. However, in a substantial percentage of patients, pelvic pyomyositis affects the adductor musculature. Therefore, a theoretical risk for contamination of the hip joint exists if joint arthrocentesis is unknowingly performed via the standard medial approach.[66]

Postoperative MRI

After the initial management of a musculoskeletal infection, including antibiotic therapy, surgical radiology débridement and/or drainage, or interventional radiology débridement and/or drainage, patients should be carefully monitored for improved physical examination and inflammatory markers. Patients in whom appropriate clinical and laboratory improvements are not observed after the initiation of treatment should be carefully evaluated to determine if repeat MRI is necessary. Repeat MRI in the early postoperative setting is advised only if a surgeon believes previously unaddressed foci of musculoskeletal infection, either local or remote, are present. Otherwise, clinical and laboratory improvements should be used to guide the decision for repeat surgical management of known or previously addressed foci.[68-70]

In a study of 59 children with acute hematogenous osteomyelitis, Courtney et al[70] assessed 104 repeat MRIs with regard to the indications for repeat MRI and the effect on treatment. Twenty-eight of the repeat MRIs were obtained within 2 weeks of the index MRIs as a result of a worsening clinical course. Changes in treatment were prompted by eight of the repeat MRIs (29%) that were obtained within 2 weeks of the index MRIs compared with only three of the 76 repeat MRIs (3.9%) that were obtained more than 14 days after the index MRIs. Of the 11 children in whom repeat MRIs prompted a change in the ultimate treatment plan, CRP levels were increasing in seven children and were elevated or unchanged in four children. Thus, MRI is not recommended for the routine monitoring of musculoskeletal infection resolution because a prolonged inflammatory appearance observed on MRIs obtained after the surgical management of musculoskeletal infection may be difficult to interpret.

Summary

Musculoskeletal infections have evolved into complex multisystem musculoskeletal infections that have the potential to cause substantial morbidity and mortality. Multiple factors contribute to the spectrum of clinical presentation, including regional epidemiology, patient immune response, bacterial virulence factors, and antibiotic resistance profiles. A better understanding of the interplay between all these factors will allow for an increased ability to better assess and treat patients who have musculoskeletal infections. A better understanding of the regional variations of musculoskeletal infections is necessary to develop region-specific workup and treatment algorithms, which should include emerging treatment options that target the mechanisms that infecting organisms use to propagate and disseminate within a human host.

References

1. Gafur OA, Copley LA, Hollmig ST, Browne RH, Thornton LA, Crawford SE: The impact of the current epidemiology of pediatric musculoskeletal infection on evaluation and treatment guidelines. *J Pediatr Orthop* 2008;28(7):777-785.

2. Buckingham SC, McDougal LK, Cathey LD, et al: Emergence of community-associated methicillin-resistant Staphylococcus aureus at a Memphis, Tennessee Children's Hospital. *Pediatr Infect Dis J* 2004;23(7):619-624.

3. Hultén KG, Kaplan SL, Gonzalez BE, et al: Three-year surveillance of community onset health care-associated staphylococcus aureus infections in children. *Pediatr Infect Dis J* 2006;25(4):349-353.

4. Sarkissian EJ, Gans I, Gunderson MA, Myers SH, Spiegel DA, Flynn JM: Community-acquired methicillin-resistant staphylococcus aureus musculoskeletal infections: emerging trends over the past decade. *J Pediatr Orthop* 2016;36(3):323-327.

5. Martínez-Aguilar G, Avalos-Mishaan A, Hulten K, Hammerman W, Mason EO Jr, Kaplan SL: Community-acquired, methicillin-resistant and methicillin-susceptible Staphylococcus aureus musculoskeletal infections in children. *Pediatr Infect Dis J* 2004;23(8):701-706.

6. McCaskill ML, Mason EO Jr, Kaplan SL, Hammerman W, Lamberth LB, Hultén KG: Increase of the USA300 clone among community-acquired methicillin-susceptible Staphylococcus aureus causing invasive infections. *Pediatr Infect Dis J* 2007;26(12):1122-1127.

7. Gonzalez BE, Teruya J, Mahoney DH Jr, et al: Venous thrombosis associated with staphylococcal osteomyelitis in children. *Pediatrics* 2006;117(5):1673-1679.

8. Hollmig ST, Copley LA, Browne RH, Grande LM, Wilson PL: Deep venous thrombosis associated with osteomyelitis in children. *J Bone Joint Surg Am* 2007;89(7):1517-1523.

9. Gonzalez BE, Martinez-Aguilar G, Hulten KG, et al: Severe Staphylococcal sepsis in adolescents in the era of community-acquired methicillin-resistant Staphylococcus aureus. *Pediatrics* 2005;115(3):642-648.

10. Saavedra-Lozano J, Mejías A, Ahmad N, et al: Changing trends in acute osteomyelitis in children: Impact of methicillin-resistant Staphylococcus aureus infections. *J Pediatr Orthop* 2008;28(5):569-575.

11. Tuason DA, Gheen T, Sun D, Huang R, Copley L: Clinical and laboratory parameters associated with multiple surgeries in children with acute hematogenous osteomyelitis. *J Pediatr Orthop* 2014;34(5):565-570.

12. Peltola H, Unkila-Kallio L, Kallio MJ; The Finnish Study Group: Simplified treatment of acute staphylococcal osteomyelitis of childhood. *Pediatrics* 1997;99(6):846-850.

13. Peltola H, Pääkkönen M, Kallio P, Kallio MJ; Osteomyelitis-Septic Arthritis Study Group: Short- versus long-term antimicrobial treatment for acute hematogenous osteomyelitis of childhood: Prospective, randomized trial on 131 culture-positive cases. *Pediatr Infect Dis J* 2010;29(12):1123-1128.

14. Cray C, Zaias J, Altman NH: Acute phase response in animals: A review. *Comp Med* 2009;59(6):517-526.

15. Brunham RC, Plummer FA, Stephens RS: Bacterial antigenic variation, host immune response, and pathogen-host coevolution. *Infect Immun* 1993;61(6):2273-2276.

16. Mann KG, Brummel-Ziedins K, Orfeo T, Butenas S: Models of blood coagulation. *Blood Cells Mol Dis* 2006;36(2):108-117.

17. Yuasa M, Mignemi NA, Nyman JS, et al: Fibrinolysis is essential for fracture repair and prevention of heterotopic ossification. *J Clin Invest* 2015;125(8):3117-3131.

18. O'Keefe RJ: Fibrinolysis as a target to enhance fracture healing. *N Engl J Med* 2015;373(18):1776-1778.

19. Loike JD, el Khoury J, Cao L, et al: Fibrin regulates neutrophil migration in response to interleukin 8, leukotriene B4, tumor necrosis factor, and formyl-methionyleucyl-phenylalanine. *J Exp Med* 1995;181(5):1763-1772.

20. Krautgartner WD, Klappacher M, Hannig M, et al: Fibrin mimics neutrophil extracellular traps in SEM. *Ultrastruct Pathol* 2010;34(4):226-231.

21. Loeb L: The influence of certain bacteria on the coagulation of the blood. *J Med Res* 1903;10(3):407-419.

22. Rammelkamp CH, Hezebicks MM, Dingle JH: Specific coagulases of staphylococcus aureus. *J Exp Med* 1950;91(3):295-307.

23. Bjerketorp J, Nilsson M, Ljungh A, Flock JI, Jacobsson K, Frykberg L: A novel von Willebrand factor binding protein expressed by Staphylococcus aureus. *Microbiology* 2002; 148(pt 7):2037-2044.

24. Cheng AG, McAdow M, Kim HK, Bae T, Missiakas DM, Schneewind O: Contribution of coagulases towards Staphylococcus aureus disease and protective immunity. *PLoS Pathog* 2010;6(8):e1001036.

25. Guggenberger C, Wolz C, Morrissey JA, Heesemann J: Two distinct coagulase-dependent barriers protect Staphylococcus aureus from neutrophils in a three dimensional in vitro infection model. *PLoS Pathog* 2012;8(1):e1002434.

26. Berends ET, Horswill AR, Haste NM, Monestier M, Nizet V, von Köckritz-Blickwede M: Nuclease expression by Staphylococcus aureus facilitates escape from neutrophil extracellular traps. *J Innate Immun* 2010;2(6):576-586.

27. Mölkänen T, Tyynelä J, Helin J, Kalkkinen N, Kuusela P: Enhanced activation of bound plasminogen on Staphylococcus aureus by staphylokinase. *FEBS Lett* 2002;517(1-3):72-78.

28. Marcum JA, Kline DL: Species specificity of streptokinase. *Comp Biochem Physiol B* 1983;75(3):389-394.

29. Lin JN, Chang LL, Lai CH, Lin HH, Chen YH: Group A streptococcal necrotizing fasciitis in the emergency department. *J Emerg Med* 2013;45(5):781-788.

30. Buchanan JT, Simpson AJ, Aziz RK, et al: DNase expression allows the pathogen group A Streptococcus to escape killing in neutrophil extracellular traps. *Curr Biol* 2006;16(4):396-400.

31. Caird MS, Flynn JM, Leung YL, Millman JE, D'Italia JG, Dormans JP: Factors distinguishing septic arthritis from transient synovitis of the hip in children: A prospective study. *J Bone Joint Surg Am* 2006;88(6):1251-1257.

32. Highlander SK, Hultén KG, Qin X, et al: Subtle genetic changes enhance virulence of methicillin resistant and sensitive Staphylococcus aureus. *BMC Microbiol* 2007;7:99.

33. Ju KL, Zurakowski D, Kocher MS: Differentiating between methicillin-resistant and methicillin-sensitive Staphylococcus aureus osteomyelitis in children: An evidence-based clinical prediction algorithm. *J Bone Joint Surg Am* 2011;93(18):1693-1701.

34. Wade Shrader M, Nowlin M, Segal LS: Independent analysis of a clinical predictive algorithm to identify methicillin-resistant Staphylococcus aureus osteomyelitis in children. *J Pediatr Orthop* 2013;33(7):759-762.

35. Copley LA, Barton T, Garcia C, et al: A proposed scoring system for assessment of severity of illness in pediatric acute hematogenous osteomyelitis using objective clinical and laboratory findings. *Pediatr Infect Dis J* 2014;33(1):35-41.

36. Healthcare Cost and Utilization Project (HCUP): The Kids' Inpatient Database. Rockville, MD, Agency for Healthcare Research and Quality, February 2016. Available at: http://www.hcup-us.ahrq.gov/kidoverview.jsp. Accessed February 9, 2016.

37. Kuroda M, Ohta T, Uchiyama I, et al: Whole genome sequencing of meticillin-resistant Staphylococcus aureus. *Lancet* 2001;357(9264):1225-1240.

38. Baba T, Takeuchi F, Kuroda M, et al: Genome and virulence determinants of high virulence community-acquired MRSA. *Lancet* 2002;359(9320):1819-1827.

39. Diep BA, Gill SR, Chang RF, et al: Complete genome sequence of USA300, an epidemic clone of community-acquired meticillin-resistant Staphylococcus aureus. *Lancet* 2006;367(9512):731-739.

40. Massey RC, Kantzanou MN, Fowler T, et al: Fibronectin-binding protein A of Staphylococcus aureus has multiple, substituting, binding regions that mediate adherence to fibronectin and invasion of endothelial cells. *Cell Microbiol* 2001;3(12):839-851.

41. Peacock SJ, Moore CE, Justice A, et al: Virulent combinations of adhesin and toxin genes in natural populations of Staphylococcus aureus. *Infect Immun* 2002;70(9):4987-4996.

42. Vandenesch F, Lina G, Henry T: Staphylococcus aureus hemolysins, bi-component leukocidins, and cytolytic peptides: A redundant arsenal of membrane-damaging virulence factors? *Front Cell Infect Microbiol* 2012;2:12.

43. Dohin B, Gillet Y, Kohler R, et al: Pediatric bone and joint infections caused by Panton-Valentine leukocidin-positive Staphylococcus aureus. *Pediatr Infect Dis J* 2007;26(11):1042-1048.

44. Mitchell PD, Hunt DM, Lyall H, Nolan M, Tudor-Williams G: Panton-Valentine leukocidin-secreting Staphylococcus aureus causing severe musculoskeletal sepsis in children: A new threat. *J Bone Joint Surg Br* 2007;89(9):1239-1242.

45. Elasri MO, Thomas JR, Skinner RA, et al: Staphylococcus aureus collagen adhesin contributes to the pathogenesis of osteomyelitis. *Bone* 2002;30(1):275-280.

46. Gill SR, McIntyre LM, Nelson CL, et al: Potential associations between severity of infection and the presence of virulence-associated genes in clinical strains of Staphylococcus aureus. *PLoS One* 2011;6(4):e18673.

47. Malachowa N, DeLeo FR: Staphylococcus aureus survival in human blood. *Virulence* 2011;2(6):567-569.

48. DeLeo FR, Otto M, Kreiswirth BN, Chambers HF: Community-associated meticillin-resistant Staphylococcus aureus. *Lancet* 2010;375(9725):1557-1568.

49. Uhlemann AC, Kennedy AD, Martens C, Porcella SF, Deleo FR, Lowy FD: Toward an understanding of the evolution of Staphylococcus aureus strain USA300 during colonization in community households. *Genome Biol Evol* 2012;4(12):1275-1285.

50. Kobayashi SD, Braughton KR, Palazzolo-Ballance AM, et al: Rapid neutrophil destruction following phagocytosis of Staphylococcus aureus. *J Innate Immun* 2010;2(6):560-575.

51. Park B, Liu GY: Targeting the host-pathogen interface for treatment of Staphylococcus aureus infection. *Semin Immunopathol* 2012;34(2):299-315.

52. Suryadevara M, Clark AE, Wolk DM, Carman A, Rosenbaum PF, Shaw J: Molecular characterization of invasive staphylococcus aureus infection in central New York Children: Importance of two clonal groups and inconsistent presence of selected virulence determinants. *J Pediatric Infect Dis Soc* 2013;2(1):30-39.

53. Feil EJ, Cooper JE, Grundmann H, et al: How clonal is Staphylococcus aureus? *J Bacteriol* 2003;185(11):3307-3316.

54. Kennedy AD, Otto M, Braughton KR, et al: Epidemic community-associated methicillin-resistant Staphylococcus aureus: Recent clonal expansion and diversification. *Proc Natl Acad Sci U S A* 2008;105(4):1327-1332.

55. Shukla SK, Pantrangi M, Stahl B, et al: Comparative whole-genome mapping to determine Staphylococcus aureus genome size, virulence motifs, and clonality. *J Clin Microbiol* 2012;50(11):3526-3533.

56. Holden MT, Feil EJ, Lindsay JA, et al: Complete genomes of two clinical Staphylococcus aureus strains: Evidence for the rapid evolution of virulence and drug resistance. *Proc Natl Acad Sci U S A* 2004;101(26):9786-9791.

57. Gaviria-Agudelo C, Aroh C, Tareen N, Wakeland EK, Kim M, Copley LA: Genomic heterogeneity of methicillin resistant staphylococcus aureus associated with variation in severity of illness among children with acute hematogenous osteomyelitis. *PLoS One* 2015;10(6):e0130415.

58. Horst SA, Hoerr V, Beineke A, et al: A novel mouse model of Staphylococcus aureus chronic osteomyelitis that closely mimics the human infection: An integrated view of disease pathogenesis. *Am J Pathol* 2012;181(4):1206-1214.

59. Rosenfeld S, Bernstein DT, Daram S, Dawson J, Zhang W: Predicting the presence of adjacent infections in septic arthritis in children. *J Pediatr Orthop* 2016;36(1):70-74.

60. Montgomery CO, Siegel E, Blasier RD, Suva LJ: Concurrent septic arthritis and osteomyelitis in children. *J Pediatr Orthop* 2013;33(4):464-467.

61. Kim EY, Kwack KS, Cho JH, Lee DH, Yoon SH: Usefulness of dynamic contrast-enhanced MRI in differentiating between septic arthritis and transient synovitis in the hip joint. *AJR Am J Roentgenol* 2012;198(2):428-433.

62. Mazur JM, Ross G, Cummings J, Hahn GA Jr, McCluskey WP: Usefulness of magnetic resonance imaging for the diagnosis of acute musculoskeletal infections in children. *J Pediatr Orthop* 1995;15(2):144-147.

63. Gold RH, Hawkins RA, Katz RD: Bacterial osteomyelitis: Findings on plain radiography, CT, MR, and scintigraphy. *AJR Am J Roentgenol* 1991;157(2):365-370.

64. Kan JH, Young RS, Yu C, Hernanz-Schulman M: Clinical impact of gadolinium in the MRI diagnosis of musculoskeletal infection in children. *Pediatr Radiol* 2010;40(7):1197-1205.

65. Nguyen A, Kan JH, Bisset G, Rosenfeld S: Kocher criteria revisited in the era of MRI: How often does the Kocher criteria identify underlying osteomyelitis? *J Pediatr Orthop* 2015.

66. Mignemi ME, Menge TJ, Cole HA, et al: Epidemiology, diagnosis, and treatment of pericapsular pyomyositis of the hip in children. *J Pediatr Orthop* 2014;34(3):316-325.

67. Monsalve J, Kan JH, Schallert EK, Bisset GS, Zhang W, Rosenfeld SB: Septic arthritis in children: Frequency of coexisting unsuspected osteomyelitis and implications on imaging work-up and management. *AJR Am J Roentgenol* 2015;204(6):1289-1295.

68. Copley LA, Kinsler MA, Gheen T, Shar A, Sun D, Browne R: The impact of evidence-based clinical practice guidelines applied by a multidisciplinary team for the care of children with osteomyelitis. *J Bone Joint Surg Am* 2013;95(8):686-693.

69. Kan JH, Hilmes MA, Martus JE, Yu C, Hernanz-Schulman M: Value of MRI after recent diagnostic or surgical intervention in children with suspected osteomyelitis. *AJR Am J Roentgenol* 2008;191(5):1595-1600.

70. Courtney PM, Flynn JM, Jaramillo D, Horn BD, Calabro K, Spiegel DA: Clinical indications for repeat MRI in children with acute hematogenous osteomyelitis. *J Pediatr Orthop* 2010;30(8):883-887.

Soft-Tissue Tumors: A Pictorial- and Case-Based Guide to Diagnosis and Management

Valerae O. Lewis, MD
Adam S. Levin, MD
Ginger E. Holt, MD
Timothy A. Damron, MD
Scott D. Weiner, MD
Carol D. Morris, MD, MS

Abstract

General orthopaedic surgeons must learn how to appropriately evaluate patients with soft-tissue masses who present at their office. Although the incidence of benign soft-tissue sarcomas substantially outnumbers that of malignant soft-tissue sarcomas, the mismanagement of soft-tissue tumors markedly increases a patient's morbidity. The appropriate use of imaging modalities helps general orthopaedic surgeons accurately diagnose a soft-tissue mass, initiate appropriate management of a soft-tissue mass, and gain a better understanding of which patients with soft-tissue lesions should be referred to an orthopaedic oncologist.

Instr Course Lect 2017;66:585–617.

Presentation of Soft-Tissue Masses

The incidence of benign soft-tissue tumors greatly outnumbers the incidence of soft-tissue sarcomas (300 per 100,000 individuals and 3 per 100,000 individuals, respectively). Therefore, most patients with soft-tissue masses who present to orthopaedic surgeons have benign soft-tissue tumors.[1] Given this information, some studies have reported that as many as one-half of all soft-tissue sarcomas are identified after an unplanned excision.[2] Unplanned soft-tissue sarcoma excisions may lead to increased rates of local recurrence or amputation, and, ultimately, the need for advanced soft-tissue coverage of the affected area.[3] Therefore, although soft-tissue malignancies are rare, a comprehensive preoperative evaluation of patients with soft-tissue masses is essential to determine appropriate treatment.

The World Health Organization classifies soft-tissue masses based on the tissue that they most closely resemble on histologic images. More than 55 subtypes of soft-tissue sarcomas have been recognized by the World Health Organization. Clinically, soft-tissue masses tend to be painless, and although many patients may feel reassured by the

Dr. Lewis or an immediate family member has received research or institutional support from Stryker. Dr. Holt or an immediate family member serves as a board member, owner, officer, or committee member of the Musculoskeletal Tumor Society. Dr. Damron or an immediate family member has received research or institutional support from the Orthopaedic Research and Education Foundation and Stryker; and serves as a board member, owner, officer, or committee member of the American College of Surgeons and the Orthopaedic Research Society. Dr. Weiner or an immediate family member serves as a board member, owner, officer, or committee member of the American Academy of Orthopaedic Surgeons, the American Orthopaedic Association, the Musculoskeletal Tumor Society, and the Ohio Orthopaedic Society. Dr. Morris or an immediate family member serves as a board member, owner, officer, or committee member of the American Academy of Orthopaedic Surgeons and the Musculoskeletal Tumor Society. Neither Dr. Levin nor any immediate family member has received anything of value from or has stock or stock options held in a commercial company or institution related directly or indirectly to the subject of this chapter.

Table 1

Patterns of Mineralization Observed on Radiographs of Soft-Tissue Masses

Mineralization Pattern	Radiographic Example	Likely Diagnosis
Phleboliths		Hemangioma
Haphazard calcifications		Synovial sarcoma
Smooth, mature ossification that is more mature at the periphery		Myositis ossificans
Rounded areas of intra-articular calcification		Synovial chondromatosis

lack of discomfort from an enlarging soft-tissue mass, soft-tissue sarcomas, unlike osseous malignancies, rarely result in discomfort. Although a large, firm, fungating soft-tissue mass likely represents a malignancy, such a clinical scenario rarely occurs and does not present diagnostic difficulty. However, substantial overlap in the clinical and imaging features of most benign and malignant soft-tissue tumors exists. Recognition of the commonalities and differences between benign and malignant soft-tissue tumors is important to ensure the appropriate treatment of patients with soft-tissue masses.

A thorough patient history and physical examination will help surgeons identify clues to the diagnosis. In the examination of a patient with a soft-tissue mass, direct measurement of the diameter of the palpable mass and comparison of circumference measurements of the affected limb with those of the contralateral limb may help surgeons appreciate the size of a deep mass and objectively compare clinical findings over time. Approximately 85% of soft-tissue sarcomas are located deep to the investing fascia,[3] which is another factor that has been proposed as the reason for delay in the recognition and diagnosis of soft-tissue sarcomas. Surgeons should have a high index of suspicion for malignancy in patients with soft-tissue masses that are located deep to the fascia. Surgeons may be tempted to immediately focus on the mass itself; however, waiting until the end of the evaluation to examine the area of interest often helps ensure a thorough evaluation. Skin lesions, cutaneous nodules, satellite masses, and enlarged lymph nodes may aid in making the diagnosis. Diffuse swelling may suggest venous or lymphatic obstruction. Overlying skin changes or discoloration may represent a history of radiation therapy to the area of interest, which indicates additional diagnostic considerations.

Both benign and malignant soft-tissue tumors may grow over time. Rapid growth of a soft-tissue mass may indicate aggressiveness and may suggest a high-grade malignancy. However, some soft-tissue sarcomas, particularly synovial sarcoma and epithelioid sarcoma, may be so slow growing that they may be misinterpreted as benign soft-tissue masses. Many patients will recognize a soft-tissue mass after minor trauma and assume that the mass is a hematoma related to the trauma. If a soft-tissue mass does not resolve as would a hematoma, then imaging studies should be obtained. In addition, caution should be exercised in the management of spontaneous hematoma. Although a spontaneous hematoma can occur, a hematoma without an underlying cause should warrant suspicion and evaluation, especially if it does not resolve with equal spontaneity.

Diagnostic Modalities: Indications and Options

Several imaging modalities are available to guide the treatment of patients in whom a complete history and physical examination indicate an indeterminate or suspicious soft-tissue mass. Appropriate imaging studies often will help narrow the differential diagnosis and aid orthopaedic surgeons in determining which patients with soft-tissue masses to refer for oncologic evaluation and treatment.

Plain radiographs are an adequate initial imaging modality. Although most soft-tissue masses will not appear obvious on radiographs, plain radiography is advantageous. First, plain radiographs

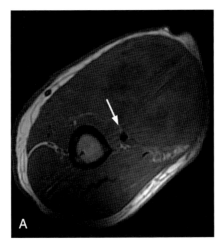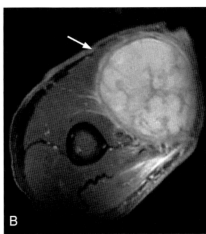

Figure 1   MRIs of an arm show the usefulness of MRI in defining soft-tissue masses. **A,** Axial T1-weighted MRI shows a mass (arrow) that is isointense to the adjacent muscle. The brachial artery and vein are clearly observed adjacent to the mass. **B,** Short tau inversion recovery MRI shows edema (arrow) around the pseudocapsule.

allow surgeons to determine the relationship of a soft-tissue mass to the underlying bone, demonstrating the extent of bony erosion and periosteal reaction. In some patients, plain radiographs may demonstrate that what was believed to be a soft-tissue mass actually is a mass arising from the bone. Second, plain radiographs are excellent at defining patterns of mineralization that may be present in soft-tissue masses (**Table 1**). In the absence of mineralization, the soft-tissue density of a mass can help distinguish lipomatous tumors from denser soft-tissue masses.

MRI is the most useful imaging modality for defining soft-tissue masses. Institutional preferences exist with regard to MRI sequences; however, T1-weighted, fat-suppressed T2-weighted, short tau inversion recovery, and gadolinium-enhanced MRIs are most often used by orthopaedic oncologists for diagnostic purposes and surgical planning. These MRI sequences help delineate the chemical composition, tissue composition, morphology, and

location of a soft-tissue tumor, all of which can help considerably narrow the differential diagnosis. T1-weighted MRIs are excellent at defining the anatomy of and the proximity of nerves, vessels, and other critical structures to a soft-tissue mass (**Figure 1, A**). Fat-suppressed T2-weighted MRIs are key to the evaluation of lipomatous masses. Soft-tissue masses that are composed entirely of fat uniformly suppress on fat-suppressed MRIs. Any areas of a soft-tissue mass that remain bright are not composed of fat and, therefore, warrant further investigation. Short tau inversion recovery MRIs are excellent for defining the extent of edema, which, in the classification of oncologic surgical margins, represents the reactive zone (**Figure 1, B**). Gadolinium enhancement is particularly helpful in defining solid versus cystic masses. The addition of contrast may be exceedingly beneficial in patients with small, homogeneous, periarticular masses, which are easily mistaken for cysts. Cystic masses will demonstrate peripheral enhancement of

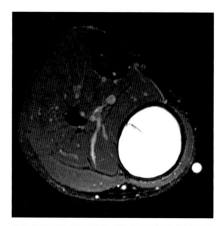

Figure 2 Axial T2-weighted, fat-saturated MRI of a right leg shows an intramuscular mass with internal septations and a thick peripheral rim, which is consistent with a hematoma. The patient had a remote history of trauma, and the mass had been present since the trauma occurred. He reported a history of bruising after the trauma that resolved.

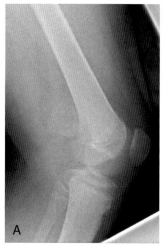
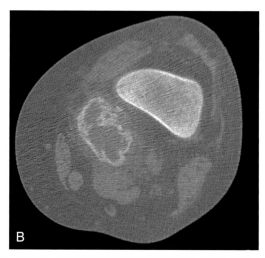

Figure 3 Images of the distal femur of a skeletally immature patient show myositis ossificans. **A,** Lateral radiograph demonstrates a peripheral zone of mineralization with a central fatty area or lucency. **B,** Axial CT scan demonstrates further definition of the peripheral mineralization and central lucency. No muscle fibers are observed. The patient had a history of an injury that was sustained while playing sports and difficulty walking and extending the knee, which was resolving.

only the capsule, whereas solid masses will demonstrate central enhancement throughout the mass. The addition of contrast also is helpful in distinguishing necrotic from viable tissue, which aids in biopsy planning and surgical planning after preoperative radiation therapy or chemotherapy for the management of known soft-tissue sarcomas. Any soft-tissue mass that is large (>5 cm), is located deep to the fascia, and demonstrates heterogeneous enhancement should be ruled a soft-tissue malignancy until proved otherwise.

CT is a reasonable alternative for patients with contraindications to MRI, such as those with pacemakers or electrical stimulators. The administration of intravenous contrast usually is required to provide a surgeon with adequate detail of a soft-tissue mass. CT is particularly advantageous in imaging the pelvis because motion artifact on MRIs of this anatomic area

may occasionally limit resolution. CT also is excellent for defining patterns of mineralization that may be present in soft-tissue masses and for determining the relationship of a soft-tissue mass to the underlying bone.

Compared with cross-sectional imaging, ultrasonography is a quick, easy, and inexpensive imaging modality. Ultrasonography is reliable for differentiating solid from cystic masses. Ultrasonography is ideal for young children, who often require anesthesia for MRI. However, ultrasonography likely is underutilized by orthopaedic surgeons because of a lack of expertise and familiarity in reading ultrasonograms.

Positron emission tomography is a nuclear medicine imaging modality that exploits the high metabolic activity of soft-tissue masses. The radiotracer most often used in positron emission tomography is fluorodeoxyglucose (fludeoxyglucose), which is an analog of glucose. Concentrations of the radiotracer will

indicate areas of high metabolic activity, which are observed as hot spots on positron emission tomography scans and quantified. Positron emission tomography should not be used as an initial imaging modality. Positron emission tomography is an advanced imaging modality that most often is used for staging purposes in patients in whom a malignancy has been diagnosed or to differentiate benign from malignant soft-tissue masses in patents who have diseases such as neurofibromatosis.

Nonneoplastic Soft-Tissue Masses That Mimic Soft-Tissue Sarcomas

Benign soft-tissue lesions are more common than soft-tissue sarcomas; however, nonneoplastic soft-tissue lesions are more common than benign soft-tissue masses.[4] Nonneoplastic soft-tissue lesions typically occur in a superficial location, and patients with nonneoplastic soft-tissue lesions typically have a

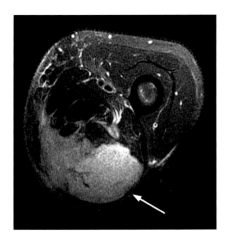

Figure 4   Axial T2-weighted, fat-suppressed MRI of a thigh shows a fluid collection with an irregular enhancing wall and an adjacent soft-tissue edema that enhanced with muscle fiber separation; these findings are consistent with a soft-tissue abscess (arrow). The patient had a fever, chills, and a rapidly enlarging thigh mass.

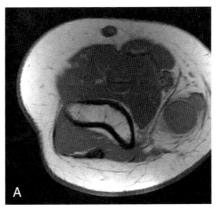

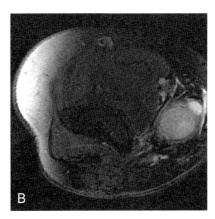

Figure 5   MRIs of a right epitrochlear lymph node show a mass in the subcutaneous tissues. A well-circumscribed rim is present around the lesion, which is observed to be isointense to muscle on an axial T1-weighted MRI (**A**) and hyperintense to muscle on an axial T2-weighted MRI (**B**). The patient was referred for evaluation of a soft-tissue sarcoma. On clinical examination, a large, mobile mass was palpated, and multiple scratches and open wounds on the distal extremity as a result of contact with a cat were observed.

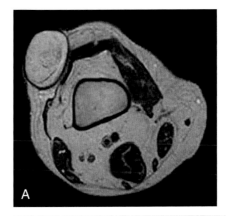

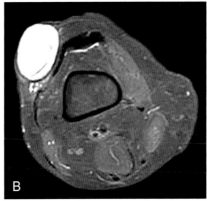

Figure 6   Axial MRIs of a left medial knee show a subcutaneous epidermal inclusion cyst. The lesion is located above the fascia, well-circumscribed, isointense to muscle on the T1-weighted MRI (**A**), and hyperintense to muscle on the T2-weighted MRI (**B**). The patient had a history of a pea-sized mass, which slowly enlarged over 25 years.

history of slow lesion growth or a history of trauma. Pain may be associated with a nonneoplastic soft-tissue lesion that results from trauma; however, pain in patients with nonneoplastic soft-tissue lesions typically demonstrates a pattern of resolution, whereas pain in patients with malignant soft-tissue lesions demonstrates progressive characteristics. Common benign, nonneoplastic soft-tissue lesions include hematomas (**Figure 2**), myositis ossificans (**Figure 3**), soft-tissue abscesses (**Figure 4**), lymph nodes (**Figure 5**), epidermal inclusion cysts (**Figure 6**), and bursa. The imaging characteristics of nonneoplastic soft-tissue masses that mimic soft-tissue sarcomas are defined in **Table 2**.[5]

Common Benign Soft-Tissue Masses

Benign soft-tissue tumors are important because they are far more common

than malignant soft-tissue tumors. Fewer than 1 in 100 soft-tissue masses that are examined by primary care physicians are deemed to be malignant.[6] At cancer centers, less than one-third of soft-tissue masses are deemed to be malignant. In a Swedish population-based study, only 18 in 1 million soft-tissue masses were deemed to be malignant.[7] Surgeons who recognize the features of common benign soft-tissue masses

should be able to determine which soft-tissue masses are not benign.

Commonly biopsied soft-tissue masses include lipomas, fibrous histiocytomas, nodular fasciitis, hemangiomas, fibromatoses, neurofibromas, and schwannomas. Soft-tissue masses that require a biopsy for diagnosis frequently appear indeterminate on imaging studies; however, several common benign soft-tissue masses should

Table 2

Imaging Characteristics of Nonneoplastic Soft-Tissue Masses That Mimic Soft-Tissue Sarcomas

Soft-Tissue Sarcoma Mimic	Imaging Characteristics
Hematoma	**Plain radiograph:** Soft-tissue density mass **Ultrasonogram:** Complex echogenic mass with septations **CT scan:** Complex mass without internal enhancement **MRI:** Complex mass with variable T1 and T2 signal and irregular rim enhancement; fluid-fluid levels may be present.
Myositis ossificans	**Plain radiograph:** Progressive pathognomonic ossification surrounding a clear central zone; typically located distant from adjacent bony structures. **CT scan:** Most sensitive means of detection; central fatty area with a zone phenomenon and peripheral ossification. **MRI:** Isointense on T1-weighted image and hyperintense on T2-weighted image; zone phenomenon appears as a hyperintense rim on gadolinium-enhanced, T1-weighted image. As the myositis ossificans miniature, the annular enhancement will become hypointense, representing mineralization; viable muscle fibers also will be observed in the lesion.
Soft-tissue abscess	**Plain radiograph:** Soft-tissue density mass **Ultrasonogram:** Complex echogenic mass with septations **CT scan:** Focalized fluid collection with a thick, irregular enhancing wall and adjacent soft-tissue edema that enhances with muscle fiber separation **MRI:** Same as CT scan and central nonenhancing matrix
Lymph node (epitrochlear, cat-scratch disease)	**Plain radiograph:** May reveal a shadow of a soft-tissue mass **Ultrasonogram:** Moderate echogenicity with sharp margins and central hyperemia but without necrosis or matting; soft-tissue edema and adjacent fluid collection may be observed. **CT scan:** Mass in subcutaneous tissues superficial to fascia; isointense with muscle. **MRI:** Mass in subcutaneous tissues; isointense on T1-weighted image and hyperintense on T2-weighted image.
Epidermal inclusion cyst	**Plain radiograph:** Normal **Ultrasonogram:** Well-circumscribed hypoechoic mass **CT scan:** Well-circumscribed lesion with a central density that is consistent with water **MRI:** Isointense on T1-weighted image and hyperintense on T2-weighted image; thin peripheral enhancement, with no central enhancement observed with the use of contrast.
Bursa	**Plain radiograph:** Typically normal **Ultrasonogram:** Fluid density with surrounding edema; no flow present. **CT scan:** Well-defined peripheral rim, with central homogeneous fluid collection observed with the use of peripheral contrast enhancement **MRI:** Fluid distention of the bursa, with intense enhancement (T2-weighted) of the wall and adjacent soft-tissue edema

be recognizable, or at least strongly suspected, before biopsy based on a patient's clinical examination and/or imaging studies. Nononcologic orthopaedic surgeons should be able to recognize these common benign soft-tissue lesions.

Lipoma

Lipomas are the most common soft-tissue masses. They are benign tumors of fatty origin. Lipomas comprise several histologic variants, including simple lipoma, angiolipoma, chondrolipoma, fibrolipoma, osteolipoma, hibernoma, and lipoblastoma. Atypical lipomatous tumors are a borderline low-grade malignant lesion that may mimic a lipoma. Most lipomas are small (<5 cm), doughy, superficial, and nontender. Most patients with lipomas have a painless soft-tissue mass, except for patients with an angiolipoma, which may result in some discomfort. Lipomas are fatty tumors that occur in adults. Lipoblastomas and hibernomas are fatty tumors that occur in children; however, they also may occur in adults.

Imaging studies of lipomas demonstrate nonenhancing homogeneous fat (**Figures 7** and **8**). In patients with subcutaneous lipomas, this nonenhancing homogeneous fat may be indistinct from the surrounding subcutaneous fatty signal. Intramuscular lipomas are well delineated from the surrounding muscle but demonstrate features that are identical to those of fat on all imaging studies. Although an atypical lipomatous tumor may be difficult to distinguish from a benign lipoma or lipoma variants via a physical examination and imaging studies, most higher grade lipomas will demonstrate considerable heterogeneity and enhancement on imaging studies (**Figures 9** and **10**). **Appendix, Figure 1** summarizes the evaluation and treatment of a patient in whom a lipoma is suspected.

Cysts

Cysts include synovial cysts and ganglia. Synovial cysts include Baker cysts, pediatric Baker cysts, parameniscal cysts, proximal tibiofibular cysts, and anterior and posterior paraglenoid cysts. Ganglia are common on the dorsal and volar aspects of the wrist.

Clinically, cysts typically fluctuate in size over time. Superficial cysts may transilluminate, confirming their fluid-filled nature. Ultrasonography helps distinguish purely cystic masses from solid masses; however, cysts that appear complex should raise suspicion. Cysts are characterized by a fluid signal on MRI. Cysts appear dark on T1-weighted MRIs, appear bright on T2-weighted and short tau inversion recovery MRIs, and demonstrate only peripheral enhancement (**Figures 11** and **12**). Synovial sarcomas and other soft-tissue sarcomas with cystic components may mimic soft-tissue cysts. **Appendix, Figure 2** summarizes the evaluation and treatment of a patient in whom a cystic lesion is suspected.

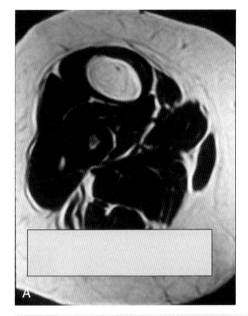
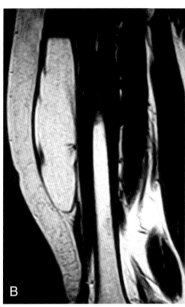

Figure 7   Axial (**A**) and sagittal (**B**) T1-weighted MRIs of a thigh show a homogeneous, fatty, bright signal, which is consistent with an intramuscular lipoma.

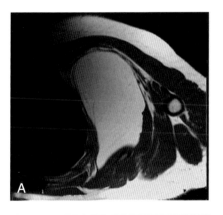
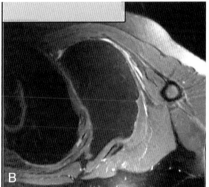
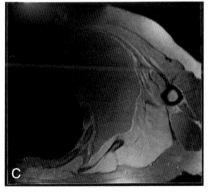
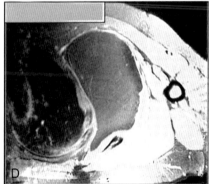

Figure 8   Axial MRIs of a large left axillary and chest wall lipoma show that benign lipomas do not demonstrate enhancement. A homogeneous, fatty signal is observed on T1-weighted (**A**); T2-weighted, fat-suppressed (**B**); and pre–gadolinium-enhanced (**C**) images, and enhancement is not observed on a post–gadolinium-enhanced MRI (**D**) after the administration of contrast.

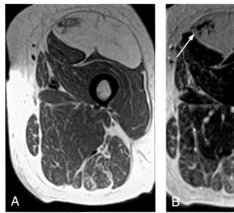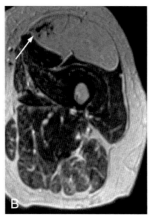

Figure 9 Axial T1-weighted MRIs of a thigh show that focal heterogeneity, although sometimes observed in patients with benign fatty tumors, should be a cause for concern. **A,** MRI shows an intramuscular, fatty tumor within the anterior aspect of the thigh. **B,** MRI shows a focal site of heterogeneity (arrow).

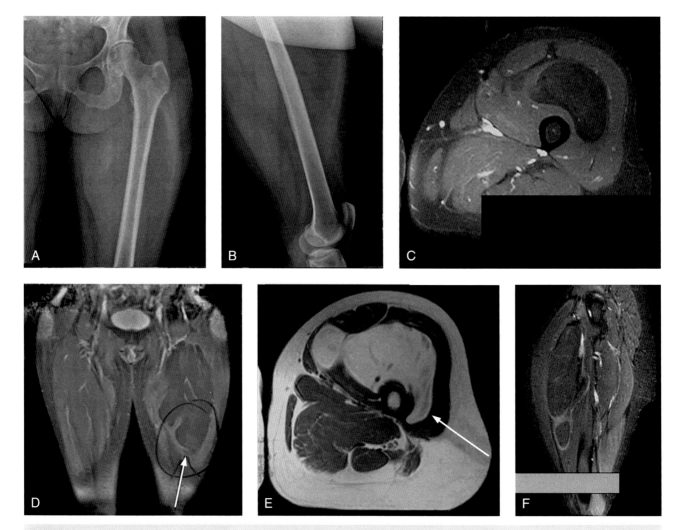

Figure 10 Images of the left thigh of a patient with a large lipoma show that focal heterogeneity may be observed in benign lipomas as a result of muscle stranding, which consists of benign strands of muscle that run through a tumor and create the appearance of heterogeneity on axial imaging. AP (**A**) and lateral (**B**) radiographs demonstrate a fatty soft-tissue shadow within the muscle of the thigh. Axial T1-weighted (**C**); coronal T1-weighted, fat-suppressed, postcontrast (**D**); axial T1-weighted, fat-suppressed, postcontrast (**E**); and sagittal T1-weighted, fat-suppressed, postcontrast (**F**) MRIs show predominantly homogeneous adipose tissue but with focal heterogeneity (arrow in panels **D** and **E**), which likely represents muscle strands that run through the tumor. The final histologic analysis revealed a benign intramuscular lipoma.

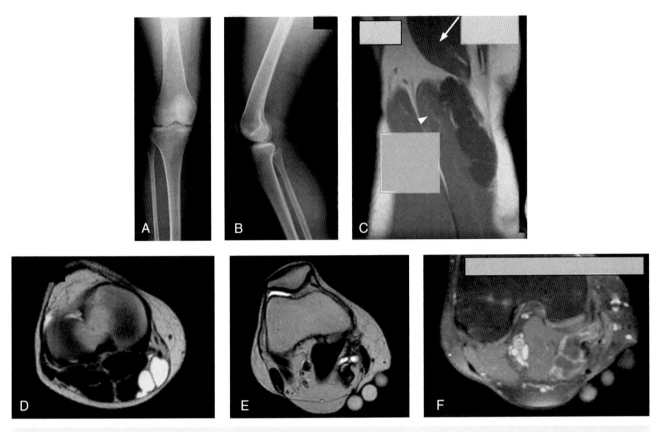

Figure 11   Images of the knee of an adult patient with a Baker cyst show peripheral enhancement after the administration of contrast, which is a typical feature of cysts. No central enhancement is present as a result of the lack of vascularity in this nonvascular tissue, which readily distinguishes cysts from solid tumors. AP (**A**) and lateral (**B**) radiographs demonstrate early degenerative changes. **C,** Coronal T1-weighted MRI shows a low-signal mass extending in the typical interval between the semimembranosus muscle/tendon (arrow) and the medial head of the gastrocnemius muscle (arrowhead). Axial T2-weighted MRIs (**D** and **E**) show the homogeneous, bright neck of the mass extending up toward the joint in the typical interval. **F,** Axial T1-weighted, fat-suppressed MRI taken after contrast was administered shows enhancement of the periphery of the mass, which confirms the cystic nature of the lesion.

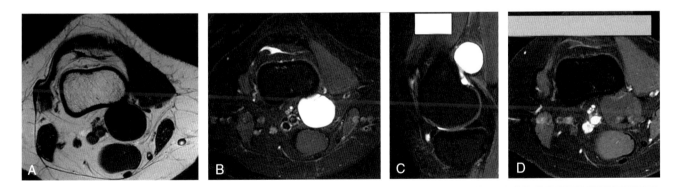

Figure 12   MRIs of a posterior distal femur show that some cysts lack characteristic features on imaging studies. Axial T1-weighted (**A**), axial T2-weighted (**B**), and sagittal T2-weighted (**C**) MRIs show a popliteal mass that is predominantly characterized by fluid signal, with slight heterogeneity observed on the T2-weighted MRIs. **D,** Axial T1-weighted, postcontrast MRI shows that the lesion appears complex. A biopsy is recommended for patients in whom a clinical examination and imaging studies are unclear.

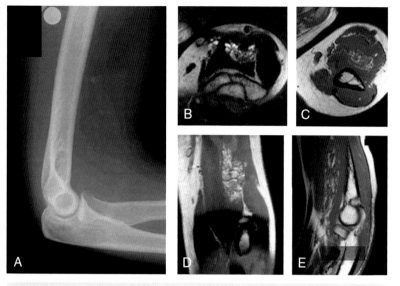
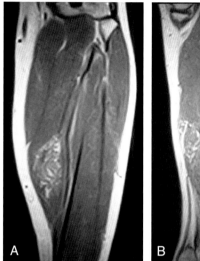
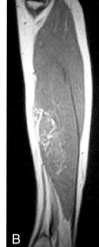

Figure 13   Images of the elbow of a 35-year-old woman who had aching pain in her upper arm that was associated with a soft-tissue mass. The pain and swelling fluctuated with activity, which are characteristic symptoms of an intramuscular hemangioma. **A**, Lateral radiograph demonstrates phleboliths, which obviate the need for a biopsy. Axial T1-weighted MRIs (**B** and **C**) show the intermixture of serpiginous vessels with fat. Coronal (**D**) and sagittal (**E**) T1-weighted MRIs show an infiltrative pattern within muscle.

Figure 14   Coronal (**A**) and sagittal (**B**) T1-weighted MRIs of a forearm show the intermixture of serpiginous vascular structures with fat and an infiltrative pattern, which are characteristic findings of an intramuscular hemangioma.

Hemangiomas and Vascular Malformations

Hemangiomas and vascular malformations are some of the most common pediatric soft-tissue tumors. Clinically, hemangiomas and vascular malformations frequently fluctuate in size, and symptoms of pain in patients with a hemangioma or vascular malformation vary depending on a patient's activity. Occasionally, the physical examination of a patient in whom a hemangioma or vascular malformation is suspected will reveal vascular markings, and superficial vascular tumors often will blanch with the application of pressure. Palpation of the soft-tissue mass will reveal a compressible mass rather than a firm mass.

Imaging studies of patients with an intramuscular hemangioma usually are diagnostic. Features that help confirm the diagnosis of a hemangioma include phleboliths that are observed on radiographs (**Figure 13, A**) and the intermixture of serpiginous vascular markings with fat and a pattern of infiltration rather than displacement within the surrounding structures that are observed on MRI (**Figure 13, B** through **E** and **Figure 14**). A history and physical examination that reveal characteristics of an intramuscular hemangioma obviate the need for a biopsy. However, a biopsy is recommended for patients in whom imaging studies indicate an indeterminate soft-tissue mass (**Figure 15**). Ultrasonography helps demonstrate flow, if present, and magnetic resonance angiography helps distinguish high-flow arterial vascular tumors from low-flow venous vascular tumors. Alveolar soft part sarcomas may mimic hemangiomas and vascular malformations. **Appendix, Figure 3** summarizes the evaluation and treatment of a patient in whom a vascular mass is suspected.

Hematomas

Hematomas typically are accompanied by visible bruising initially and should decrease in size over time. Hematomas are included in this chapter because they are among the more common benign soft-tissue masses that soft-tissue sarcomas mimic. Typically, patients with a hematoma have at least two, if not all three, of the following findings: (1) substantial trauma to the affected area, (2) external bruising initially, and (3) a history of anticoagulation at the time of injury. Most hematomas resolve over time. Hematomas generally do not enlarge or expand, and the diagnosis of an expanding hematoma should be viewed with considerable skepticism.

The features of a hematoma on imaging studies should evolve as the blood components within a hematoma evolve. Chronic hematomas are distinguished

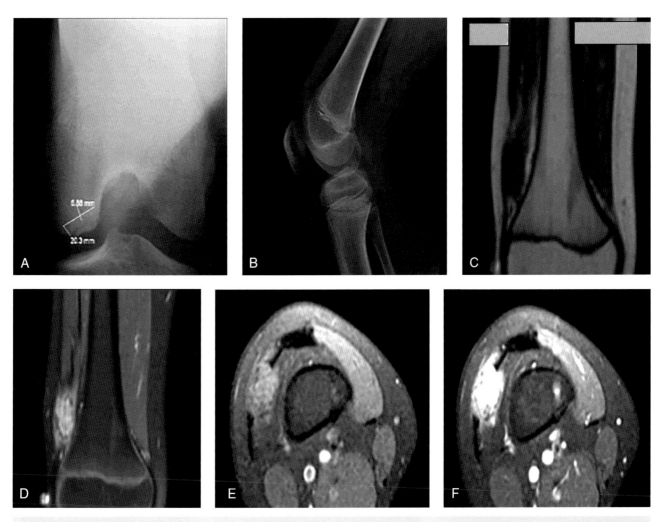

Figure 15   Images of the knee of a skeletally immature patient with a painful mass and progressive enlargement over the anterolateral distal thigh adjacent to the quadriceps tendon show that not all intramuscular hemangiomas are typical. AP (**A**) and lateral (**B**) radiographs do not demonstrate any phleboliths. Coronal T1-weighted (**C**); coronal proton density (**D**); axial T1-weighted, fat-saturated (**E**); and axial T1-weighted, fat-saturated, post-enhancement (**F**) MRIs show only an indeterminate, solid-enhancing, heterogeneous, deep mass involving the muscle and fascia of the lateral distal thigh.

by peripheral hemosiderin deposition, which creates a low-signal rim that is observed on imaging studies (**Figures 16** and **17**). Soft-tissue sarcomas may mimic hematomas (**Figure 18**).

Myositis Ossificans

Myositis ossificans, similar to hematoma, is characterized by a discrete injury and the subsequent development of mineralization in the soft tissues at the site of the injury. Persistent pain and a mass are typical in patients with

myositis ossificans. A history of injury should be obtained in patients in whom myositis ossificans is suspected based on imaging studies.

The imaging characteristics of myositis ossificans may be confusing because the mineralization that is characteristic of myositis ossificans is not apparent until a few weeks to months postinjury (**Figure 19, A** and **B**). Although mineralization may be observed on plain radiographs, CT is the best imaging modality to observe

the peripherally mature mineralization pattern that is characteristic of myositis ossificans (**Figure 19, E** and **F**). MRIs may be confusing, demonstrating extensive soft-tissue edema, which may engender concern for soft-tissue sarcoma (**Figure 19, C** and **D**). A biopsy is recommended for patients in whom imaging studies indicate an indeterminate soft-tissue mass (**Figure 20**).

Extraskeletal osteosarcoma, which typically has a more centrally mature, cumulus-cloud mineralization pattern;

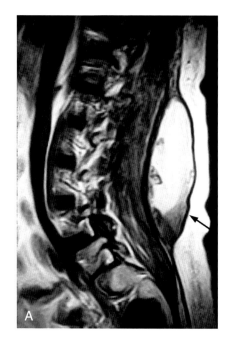

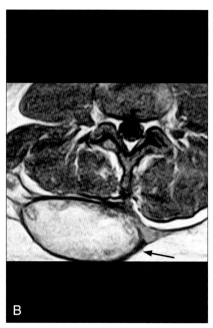

Figure 16 Sagittal (**A**) and axial (**B**) T1-weighted MRIs of the spine of a patient who sustained a blow to the flank from a baseball bat years prior, which left him with considerable bruising initially after the injury and an unchanging soft-tissue mass that has been present in the area since the injury. The images show a low-signal rim (arrows), which is characteristic of a chronic hematoma.

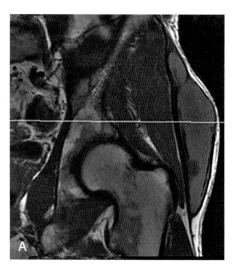

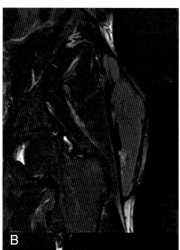

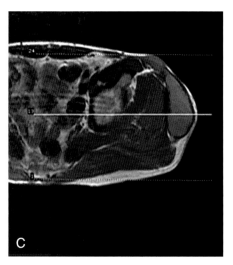

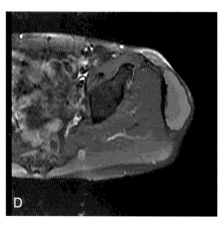

Figure 17 Coronal T1-weighted (**A**); coronal T1-weighted, postcontrast (**B**); axial T1-weighted (**C**); and axial T1-weighted, postcontrast (**D**) MRIs of a hip show a mass that is surrounded by a low-signal rim, which indicates chronic hemosiderin deposition and suggests a benign, expanding, chronic hematoma. To confirm the diagnosis, a biopsy was performed. The histologic analysis revealed evidence of only a chronic hematoma.

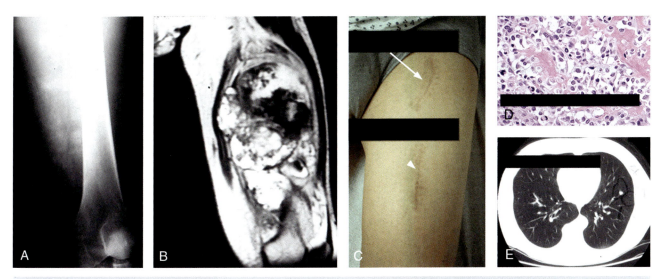

Figure 18   Images of a 56-year-old man who sustained an injury at work and experienced subsequent swelling of his thigh that persisted for 6 months, after which the patient underwent surgical treatment for an expanding hematoma. **A,** AP radiograph of the thigh demonstrates cloud-like mineralization in the soft tissues, which may be caused by myositis ossificans related to trauma. CT would have better distinguished between the classic peripheral rim of calcification that is characteristic of myositis ossificans and the centrally mature ossification that is characteristic of soft-tissue sarcomas, such as an extraskeletal osteosarcoma. **B,** Coronal T1-weighted MRI of the thigh shows a large, deep, heterogeneous mass that lacks the classic low-signal rim that is characteristic of a chronic hematoma. **C,** Clinical photograph of the thigh shows the scar from the surgical approach to the superficial femoral artery to manage uncontrollable bleeding (arrow) and the scar from the surgical incision to evacuate the expanding hematoma (arrowhead). **D,** Histologic image of the tissue that was obtained from the expanding hematoma shows a high-grade, extraskeletal osteosarcoma. **E,** Axial CT scan of the patient's chest taken after he underwent surgical treatment for the expanding hematoma demonstrates stage IV disease of the lungs.

synovial sarcoma, which has a patchy mineralization pattern; and extraskeletal mesenchymal chondrosarcoma are the most common soft-tissue sarcomas that may mimic myositis ossificans. However, any soft-tissue sarcoma may demonstrate mineralization on imaging studies. **Appendix, Figure 4** summarizes the evaluation and treatment of a patient in whom myositis ossificans is suspected.

Benign Peripheral Nerve Sheath Tumors

Benign peripheral nerve sheath tumors (BPNSTs) cannot be diagnosed based on a patient's clinical examination and imaging studies alone; however, a patient's clinical examination and imaging studies may demonstrate distinct characteristics that strongly suggest a BPNST, which can then be confirmed via biopsy. Clinically, BPNSTs may be painful or locally tender and may present as sporadic solitary tumors or occur in patients with neurofibromatosis or schwannomatosis. Schwannomas (neurilemmomas) and neurofibromas are the two most common types of BPNSTs.

The predilection of BPNSTs for the flexor surfaces of the extremities and increased discomfort or an electric shock–like pain that radiates distally on percussion may be clues to the diagnosis. The relationship of a BPNST to a nerve often prevents proximal-distal movement of the lesion but allows free medial-lateral movement of the lesion. In general, the diagnosis of a peripheral nerve sheath tumor is clearer in patients who have obvious manifestations of neurofibromatosis type 1; however, distinguishing BPNSTs from malignant peripheral nerve sheath tumors often is more challenging in patients with neurofibromatosis type 1.

Numerous features on imaging studies, including a fusiform-shaped lesion, with the longitudinal axis of the mass running along the limb; a target sign observed on axial MRIs, with a brighter signal around the periphery of the mass; a string sign, which results from the adjacent nerve running alongside or into and out of the mass; a fat-sail sign, with fat splayed apart at the proximal and distal poles of the mass; and a fascicular sign or a smudged, dirty appearance observed on axial MRIs, suggest the diagnosis of a BPNST (**Figures 21, 22, 23**, and **24**). Malignant peripheral nerve sheath tumors

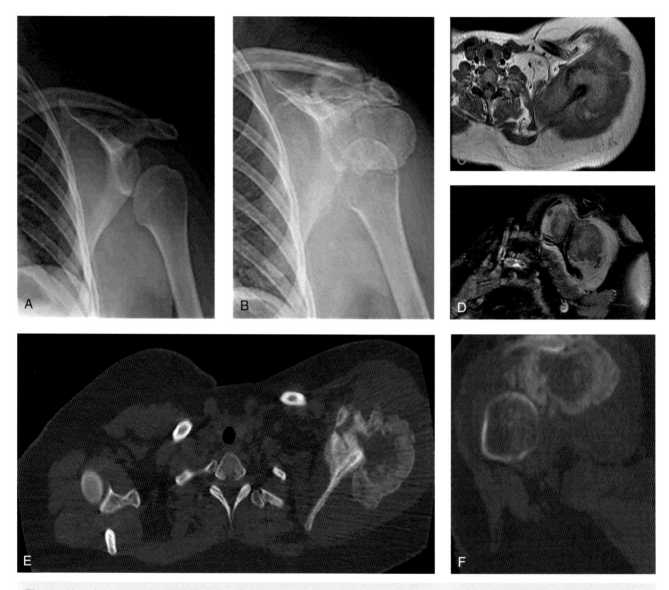

Figure 19   Images of the left shoulder of a young woman who sustained a minor injury while she was exercising. **A,** Initial AP radiograph does not demonstrate any mineralization in the soft tissue. **B,** AP radiograph taken 2 months after the initial radiograph was obtained demonstrates mineralization in the soft tissue. Axial T1-weighted (**C**) and axial T1-weighted, fat-suppressed, postcontrast (**D**) MRIs show a concerning appearance of the shoulder mass, which may be confusing because such an appearance is not specific to myositis ossificans and may indicate sarcoma. To distinguish between the peripherally mature rim of mineralization that is characteristic of myositis ossificans and the centrally mature ossification that is characteristic of soft-tissue sarcomas, such as an extraskeletal osteosarcoma, CT scans were obtained. Axial CT scans of the thorax (**E**) and the left shoulder (**F**) demonstrate the classic peripherally mature mineralization pattern that is characteristic of myositis ossificans.

and intraneural synovial sarcoma are the most common soft-tissue sarcomas that may mimic BPNSTs. **Appendix, Figure 5** summarizes the evaluation and treatment of a patient in whom a BPNST is suspected.

Tenosynovial Giant Cell Tumors

Tenosynovial giant cell tumors include localized and diffuse types of tumors, both of which demonstrate identical patterns under a microscope but have a predilection for different anatomic sites. The localized type of tumor is most commonly referred to as a giant cell tumor of the tendon sheath, and the diffuse type of tumor is commonly referred to as pigmented villonodular

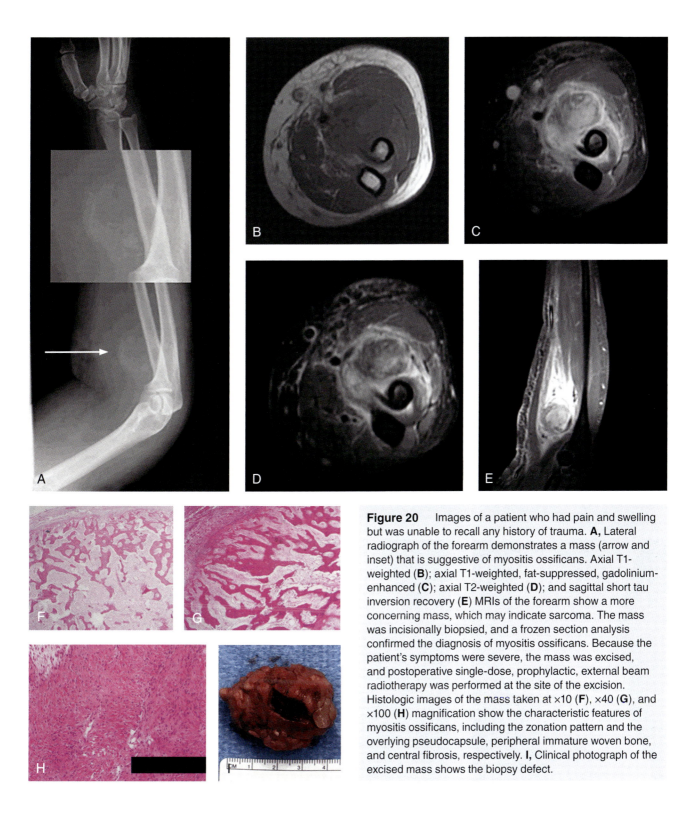

Figure 20   Images of a patient who had pain and swelling but was unable to recall any history of trauma. **A,** Lateral radiograph of the forearm demonstrates a mass (arrow and inset) that is suggestive of myositis ossificans. Axial T1-weighted (**B**); axial T1-weighted, fat-suppressed, gadolinium-enhanced (**C**); axial T2-weighted (**D**); and sagittal short tau inversion recovery (**E**) MRIs of the forearm show a more concerning mass, which may indicate sarcoma. The mass was incisionally biopsied, and a frozen section analysis confirmed the diagnosis of myositis ossificans. Because the patient's symptoms were severe, the mass was excised, and postoperative single-dose, prophylactic, external beam radiotherapy was performed at the site of the excision. Histologic images of the mass taken at ×10 (**F**), ×40 (**G**), and ×100 (**H**) magnification show the characteristic features of myositis ossificans, including the zonation pattern and the overlying pseudocapsule, peripheral immature woven bone, and central fibrosis, respectively. **I,** Clinical photograph of the excised mass shows the biopsy defect.

synovitis (PVNS). PVNS includes both nodular and diffuse forms.

Localized tenosynovial giant cell tumors (ie, giant cell tumors of the tendon sheath) are common neoplasms of the fingers and toes. Eighty percent of giant cell tumors of the tendon sheath occur on the flexor surfaces of the index, long, and ring fingers. Giant cell tumors of the tendon sheath are the most common soft-tissue masses that occur in the digits. Imaging studies of giant cell

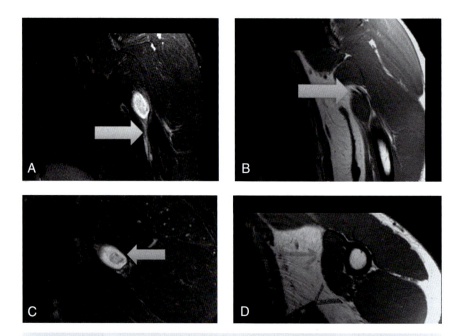

Figure 21 MRIs of an upper extremity show the classic features of benign peripheral nerve sheath tumors (BPNSTs). **A,** Axial T2-weighted image shows a string sign (arrow), which indicates a fusiform-shaped lesion with the nerve running immediately adjacent to it. **B,** Axial T1-weighted MRI image a split-fat sign or fat-sail sign (arrow), with fat splayed apart at the proximal and distal poles of the mass. **C,** Axial T2-weighted image shows a target sign (arrow), with a concentric circle of high signal around the mass, which can be observed on fluid-sensitive axial MRIs in particular. **D,** Axial T1-weighted image shows an appearance similar to that of both schwannomas and neurofibromas. This appearance, although strongly suggestive of a BPNST, is not diagnostic for a BPNST.

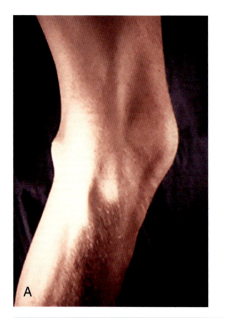
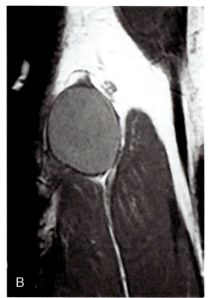
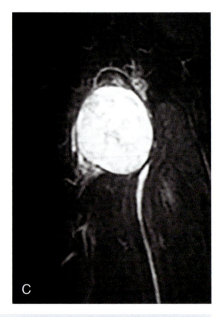

Figure 22 Images of a knee show that benign peripheral nerve sheath tumors (BPNSTs) typically occur on flexor surfaces. **A,** Clinical photograph of the posterior aspect of the knee shows a BPNST. Coronal T1-weighted (**B**) and T2-weighted (**C**) MRIs show a string sign, with the nerve exiting the caudal aspect of the BPNST.

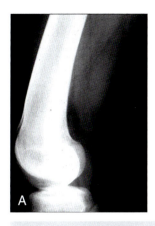
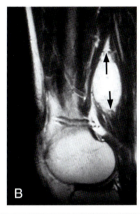
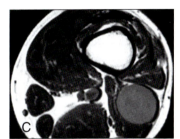
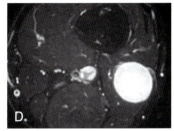

Figure 23   Images of a distal thigh show the typical features of benign peripheral nerve sheath tumors (BPNSTs). Lateral radiograph (**A**) and sagittal T1-weighted MRI (**B**) demonstrate a fusiform-shaped lesion, with split-fat signs observed proximally and distally (arrows) on the MRI. **C,** Axial T1-weighted MRI shows a lesion with a low signal appearance. **D,** Axial T2-weighted MRI shows a lesion with a bright signal appearance.

tumors of the tendon sheath are non-specific; however, bony erosions may be observed in 20% of patients with a giant cell tumor of the tendon sheath. A biopsy is necessary in patients in whom a giant cell tumor of the tendon sheath is suspected to confirm the diagnosis (**Figures 25** and **26**). Soft-tissue sarcomas may mimic giant cell tumors of the tendon sheath.

Diffuse tenosynovial giant cell tumors (ie, PVNS) includes both a solitary nodular form and a diffuse form. Eighty percent of diffuse tenosynovial giant cell tumors involve the knee. Patients with PVNS frequently have recurrent bloody effusions. The features of PVNS are recognizable on the imaging studies of many, but not all, patients; therefore, patients with PVNS, particularly the diffuse form, frequently are diagnosed via imaging studies. The hallmark finding of PVNS includes low signal areas within the synovium on all signal sequences, which suggests hemosiderin deposition as a result of chronic bleeding secondary to fragile, distended synovial fronds (**Figures 27, 28,** and **29**). Blooming artifact as a result of hemosiderin deposition in an intra-articular

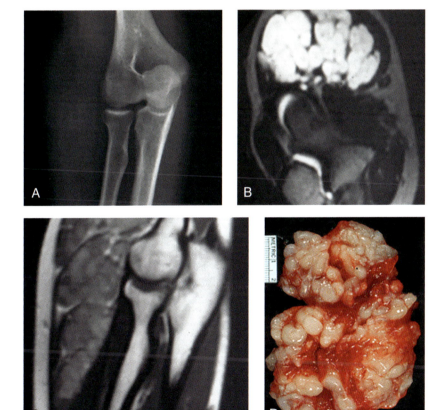

Figure 24   Images of a patient with a classic example of a plexiform neurofibroma, which is a unique benign peripheral nerve sheath tumor and is pathognomonic for peripheral neurofibromatosis type 1. **A,** AP radiograph of the elbow demonstrates a nonmineralized, soft-tissue mass over the radial proximal forearm. Axial T2-weighted (**B**) and sagittal T1-weighted (**C**) MRIs of the elbow show a soft-tissue mass with a bag-of-worms appearance. **D,** Clinical photograph of a gross specimen of the soft-tissue mass shows the bag-of-worms appearance.

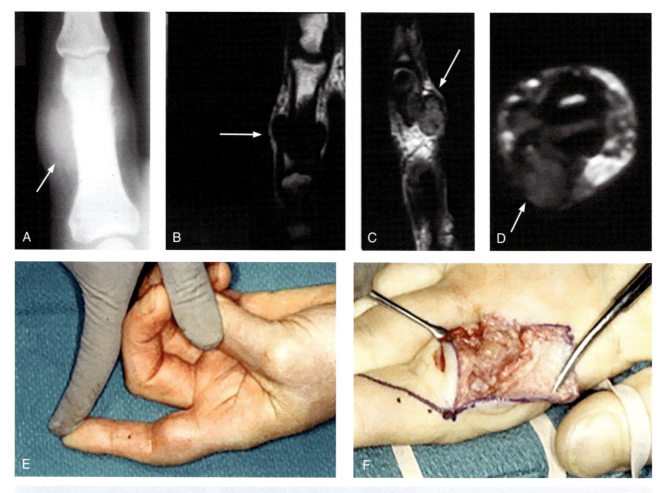

Figure 25 Images of the index finger of a 42-year-old man with a soft-tissue mass (arrows) overlying the proximal phalanx. **A,** AP radiograph demonstrates a nonmineralized mass, with apple-core, bony erosions around the distal aspect of the phalanx, which occur in 20% of patients with giant cell tumors of the tendon sheath. Coronal T1-weighted (**B**), sagittal proton density (**C**), and axial T1-weighted (**D**) MRIs are nonspecific, and a biopsy is necessary to confirm the diagnosis of a giant cell tumor of the tendon sheath. **E,** Clinical photograph shows the soft-tissue mass. **F,** Intraoperative photograph shows exploration of the soft-tissue mass, which has a rusty color that is characteristic of a giant cell tumor of the tendon sheath.

mass also suggests PVNS. Malignant degeneration of PVNS has been reported but is exceedingly rare. Typically, soft-tissue sarcomas do not mimic PVNS. **Appendix, Figure 6** summarizes the evaluation and treatment of a patient in whom PVNS is suspected.

Synovial Chondromatosis

Synovial chondromatosis, similar to PVNS, often is diagnosed via imaging studies. Typically, synovial chondromatosis involves large joints, and patients

with synovial chondromatosis have joint pain with loose-body symptoms. Plain radiographs and MRIs usually demonstrate calcified loose bodies (**Figure 30**) and will demonstrate loose bodies even if they are not calcified (**Figure 31**). Similar to PVNS, malignant degeneration of synovial chondromatosis is rare, and soft-tissue sarcomas typically do not mimic synovial chondromatosis; however, calcified areas that are located close to a joint should be ruled synovial sarcomas or extraskeletal mesenchymal

chondrosarcomas until proved otherwise. **Appendix, Figure 7** summarizes the evaluation and treatment of a patient in whom synovial chondromatosis is suspected.

Superficial Fibromatoses

Superficial fibromatoses are recognizable clinically; therefore, they are infrequently imaged or biopsied. Superficial fibromatoses are included in this chapter because, similar to lipomas, cysts, hemangiomas, and hematomas,

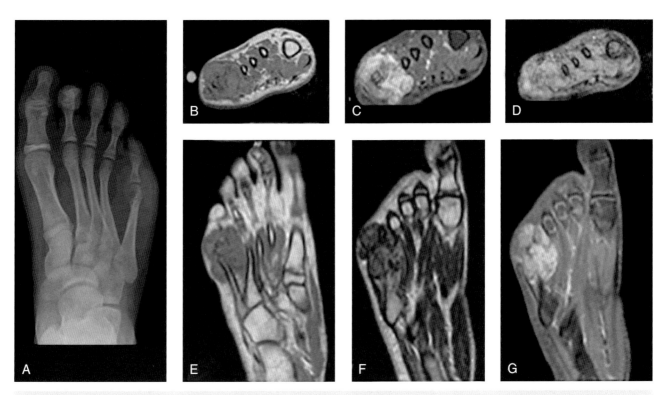

Figure 26   Images of a foot show a large soft-tissue mass encasing the distal aspect of the fifth metatarsal and overlapping the metatarsophalangeal joint. **A,** AP radiograph demonstrates a nonspecific soft-tissue mass and bony erosions. The position of the soft-tissue mass involving the joint and causing the bony erosions suggests that this is a diffuse giant cell tumor of the tendon sheath rather than a localized giant cell tumor of the tendon sheath. Coronal T1-weighted (**B**); coronal T2-weighted (**C**); coronal T1-weighted, fat-suppressed, postcontrast (**D**); axial T1-weighted (**E**); axial T2-weighted (**F**); and axial T1-weighted, fat-suppressed, postcontrast (**G**) MRIs show a nonspecific soft-tissue mass; therefore, a biopsy is recommended to confirm the diagnosis of a giant cell tumor of the tendon sheath.

soft-tissue sarcomas may mimic superficial fibromatoses. Superficial fibromatoses include those of the hand (palmar fibromatosis, Dupuytren disease of the palm; **Figure 32, A** and **B**), foot (plantar fibromatosis, Ledderhose disease; **Figure 32, C** and **D**), and penis (penile fibromatosis, Peyronie disease). Orthopaedic surgeons frequently treat patients with superficial fibromatoses of the hands and feet; nodules and cords have been well described in patients with these superficial fibromatoses. Soft-tissue sarcomas may mimic superficial fibromatoses by occurring in the same classic locations and having a similar appearance (**Figure 33**). **Appendix, Figure 8** summarizes the evaluation and treatment of a patient

in whom superficial fibromatosis is suspected.

Nodular Fasciitis

Nodular fasciitis frequently results in pain, often demonstrates more rapid enlargement compared with most noninfectious soft-tissue masses, and has a predilection for the subcutaneous or intrafascial tissues of the forearms and upper extremities. Nodular fasciitis may spontaneously regress after biopsy. Imaging studies of nodular fasciitis are nonspecific; however, MRIs may demonstrate a fascial tail sign that is suggestive of, but not specific to, nodular fasciitis. Therefore, a biopsy is necessary in patients in whom nodular fasciitis is suspected to confirm

the diagnosis (**Figures 34** and **35**). Although soft-tissue sarcomas may mimic nodular fasciitis, nodular fasciitis more frequently mimics soft-tissue sarcoma.

Algorithms for the Management of Soft-Tissue Masses

Algorithms for the management of soft-tissue masses rely on important features that help distinguish benign soft-tissue masses from malignant soft-tissue masses, including soft-tissue mass duration, change, size, and depth. Pain caused by a soft-tissue mass is notably absent from this list because it poorly distinguishes between benign soft-tissue masses and malignant soft-tissue masses. In fact,

The size and depth of a soft-tissue mass have been carefully evaluated epidemiologically with regard to benign versus malignant soft-tissue tumors. In general, soft-tissue tumors are classified into four categories based on a 2×2 grid, which accounts for size and depth. Tumors greater than 5 cm are classified as large, and depth is determined relative to the fascia (**Table 3**). Most soft-tissue tumors that are small and superficial are benign soft-tissue tumors, such as lipomas or cysts. The features of a soft-tissue mass in a superficial location usually are readily apparent on physical examination. Therefore, the doughy, palpable nature of a lipoma and the transilluminable nature of a cyst will be evident on physical examination. Conversely, one-third of soft-tissue sarcomas are small and superficial. Therefore, any small, superficial soft-tissue mass that does not feel doughy or does not transilluminate warrants suspicion, and imaging studies should be obtained. The remaining two-thirds of soft-tissue sarcomas fall into the other three quadrants of the 2×2 grid, being large and superficial, small and deep, or large and deep. Imaging studies should be obtained to better evaluate soft-tissue masses that may be soft-tissue sarcomas.

The aforementioned classification of soft-tissue tumors is the basis for the algorithm for the management of soft-tissue masses that was described by Simon and Finn[8] in 1993, which continues to be applicable (**Appendix, Figure 9**). Nandra et al[9] popularized a simpler algorithm for the management of soft-tissue masses based on soft-tissue mass size and growth, which simply states that "if your lump is bigger than a golf ball and growing, think sarcoma."

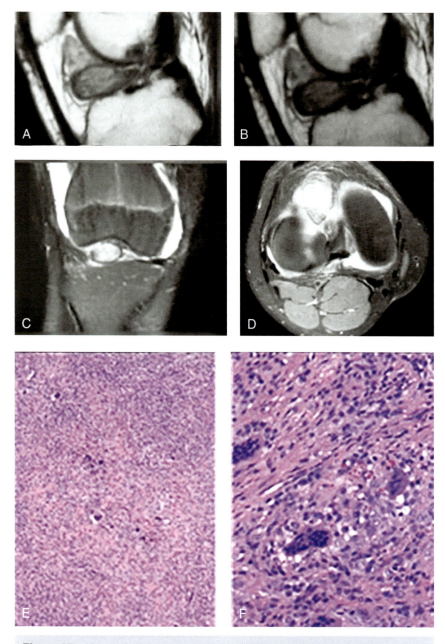

Figure 27 Images of a 23-year-old man with knee pain show nodular pigmented villonodular synovitis (PVNS). Sagittal T1-weighted (**A**), sagittal proton density (**B**), coronal T2-weighted (**C**), and axial T2-weighted (**D**) MRIs of the knee show a heterogeneous, intra-articular, soft-tissue mass with a consistently low-signal rim, which suggests hemosiderin deposition. Low-power (**E**) and high-power (**F**) histologic images of the soft-tissue mass are identical to those of a giant cell tumor of the tendon sheath. The patient underwent excision of the nodule.

most soft-tissue sarcomas are painless. Conversely, certain benign soft-tissue masses, such as hemangiomas, angiolipomas, and nodular fasciitis, are painful. Soft-tissue masses of a long duration that do not change are more likely to be benign; however, exceptions exist, such as synovial sarcoma.

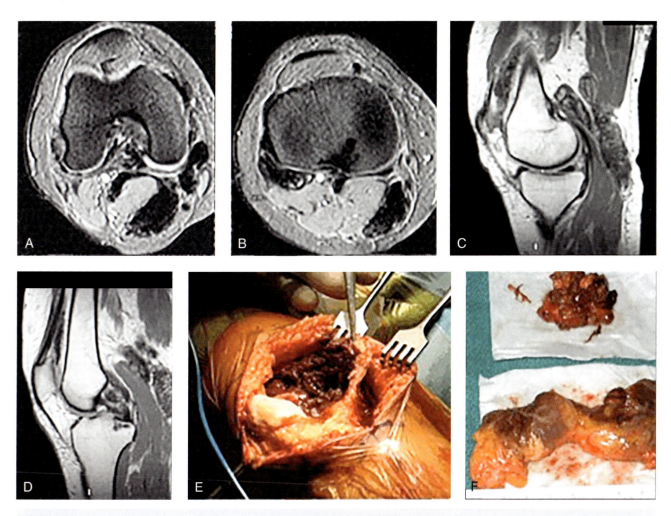

Figure 28   Images of a 44-year-old woman with chronic knee pain and swelling show diffuse pigmented villonodular synovitis (PVNS). Axial fat-suppressed (**A** and **B**) and sagittal T1-weighted (**C** and **D**) MRIs of the knee show a soft-tissue mass with a consistently low-signal rim. Most of the PVNS was located in the popliteal space and a Baker cyst; however, the anterior approach for open anterior and posterior synovectomy also revealed diffuse disease, which is shown in the intraoperative photograph of the knee (**E**). **F,** Clinical photograph shows the intra-articular appearance of the resected gross specimen, which has a rusty color that is characteristic of PVNS and a giant cell tumor of the tendon sheath.

Soft-Tissue Sarcomas

Approximately 10,000 soft-tissue sarcomas are diagnosed in the United States each year, and soft-tissue sarcomas contribute to an overall mortality rate of approximately 3,800 individuals each year. The most common sites of soft-tissue sarcomas are the extremities (60%), the trunk (19%), the retroperitoneum (15%), and the head and neck (9%). Metastasis of soft-tissue sarcomas is most likely to occur in the lungs; however,

soft-tissue sarcomas of the abdominal cavity are more likely to result in liver metastasis. Lymph node metastasis also can occur, and because certain subtypes of soft-tissue sarcomas (synovial sarcoma, epithelioid sarcoma, clear cell rhabdomyosarcoma, and undifferentiated pleomorphic sarcoma) have a predilection for lymph node metastases, the lymph node basin should always be examined. Local recurrence rates of 15% to 20% and 5-year mortality rates

of 50% to 60% have been reported in patients with soft-tissue sarcomas who undergo appropriate surgical resection with negative margins.[10]

Clinical Presentation and Staging

Typically, patients with soft-tissue sarcomas have painless, growing masses that, on physical examination, are found to be firmer than the surrounding muscle (**Figure 36**). In contrast to patients

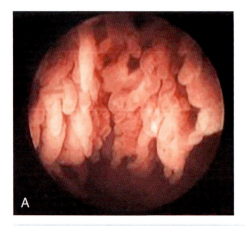 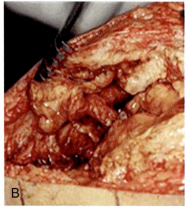 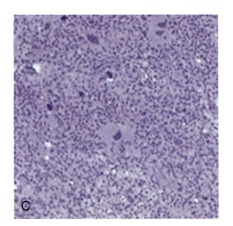

Figure 29   Images of a patient with diffuse pigmented villonodular synovitis (PVNS). **A,** Arthroscopic image of the knee shows distended, rusty-colored, engorged villi, which are characteristic of diffuse PVNS. **B,** Intraoperative photograph of the knee joint shows numerous distended fronds and lobules of a rusty-appearing synovium, which are classic findings of diffuse PVNS. **C,** Histologic image of the soft-tissue mass taken at ×100 magnification is identical to that of a giant cell tumor of the tendon sheath and shows scattered giant cells, large synoviocytes, smaller histiocytes, spindle cells, and macrophages.

with bone sarcomas, pain is not a reliable predictor of malignancy in patients with soft-tissue sarcomas. An MRI with contrast should be obtained to better define the internal characteristics of a concerning soft-tissue mass that is deep to the fascia (**Figure 37**). Typical MRI findings that are suggestive of a soft-tissue sarcoma include a soft-tissue mass that appears heterogeneous, is larger than 5 cm, is located deep to the investing fascia, appears dark on T1-weighted MRIs, and appears bright on T2-weighted MRIs. These same findings may be observed on MRIs of malignant tumors, which also can occur in the subcutaneous soft tissue; however, these lesions often are smaller in size. After the diagnosis of a soft-tissue sarcoma is confirmed via biopsy (discussed in the Management Principles section of this chapter), complete staging of the soft-tissue sarcoma should be performed via CT of the chest and evaluation of the regional lymph node basin (via either palpation or imaging studies) to evaluate for metastatic disease. Complete staging of a soft-tissue sarcoma is imperative for surgical planning.

Management Principles

The role of surgery in the diagnosis and management of soft-tissue sarcomas is twofold. Initially at presentation, a diagnostic biopsy of the suspected soft-tissue mass is necessary. In performing a biopsy, surgeons should remember that the center of a soft-tissue mass often is necrotic as a result of rapid centripetal growth. Therefore, biopsy tissue should be obtained from the periphery of the soft-tissue lesion, which can be accomplished via a variety of techniques, including fine-needle aspiration, core biopsy, and open biopsy. Fine-needle aspiration rarely is adequate for the biopsy of soft-tissue sarcomas; therefore, a core biopsy or an open biopsy is the best technique to identify the histologic patterns of soft-tissue sarcomas. A comparison of these biopsy techniques is beyond the scope of this chapter; however, any biopsy technique that yields an accurate diagnosis is appropriate. The amount of biopsy tissue

necessary to attain a diagnosis varies, and the surgeon should consult a pathologist to determine the amount of biopsy tissue required for any additional molecular studies that may be necessary. Percutaneous core biopsies yield a surprisingly adequate amount of diagnostic tissue.

The basic tenets of biopsy include making an incision that is in line with the future planned incision to allow for resection of the biopsy tract; attaining strict hemostasis to minimize contamination; placing a drain, if used, in line with the incision; and avoiding interfascial planes.[1] Complete removal of a soft-tissue sarcoma rarely is indicated at the time of a biopsy. Adherence to these principles results in the best patient outcomes. Improperly performed biopsies (via tumor seeding and improperly placed incisions) compromise patient outcomes; therefore, referral to a tertiary treatment center should be considered before a biopsy is performed in patients in whom a soft-tissue sarcoma is suspected. Biopsies are performed before soft-tissue sarcoma resection

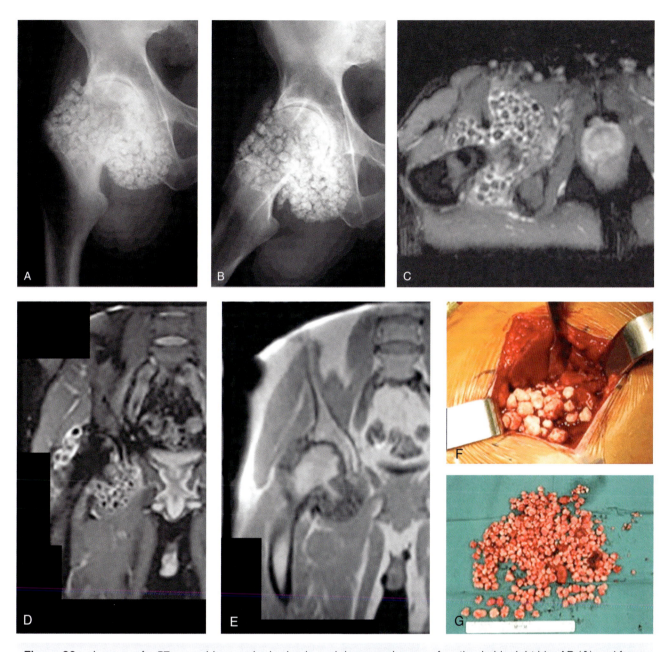

Figure 30   Images of a 57-year-old man who had pain and decreased range of motion in his right hip. AP (**A**) and frog-lateral (**B**) radiographs of the right hip demonstrate the classic radiographic appearance of synovial chondromatosis. Axial proton density (**C**), coronal proton density (**D**) and coronal T1-weighted (**E**) MRIs of the right hip show multiple loose bodies distending the hip joint. The patient underwent an arthrotomy with complete loose body removal and a synovectomy. Intraoperative photograph of the loose bodies (**F**) and photograph of the gross appearance of the loose bodies that were removed from the synovial chondromatosis (**G**).

in less than 50% of community-based practices.[11]

The management of soft-tissue sarcomas is multidisciplinary. Although surgical resection with negative margins is the mainstay of definitive treatment, multimodal treatment with the addition of radiation therapy and/or chemotherapy results in the best oncologic outcomes. Radiation therapy, which is indicated for patients with high-grade soft-tissue tumors, can be performed either preoperatively or postoperatively for improved local control; however, it should not be considered a substitute for re-resection if surgical margins are positive. The use of chemotherapy in the management of soft-tissue sarcomas

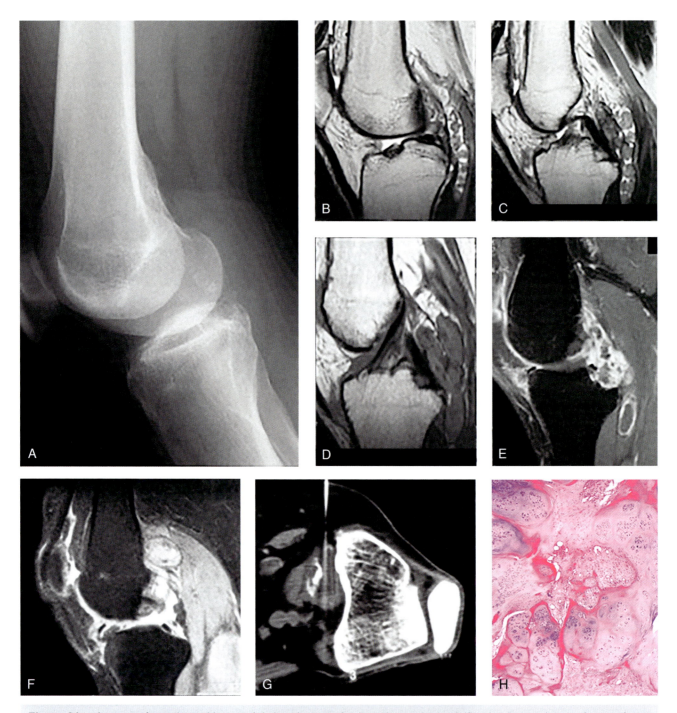

Figure 31   Images of a patient with synovial chondromatosis show that typical calcification is not always observed on radiographs. **A,** Lateral radiograph of the knee does not demonstrate mineralized loose bodies. Sagittal T1-weighted (**B, C,** and **D**) and sagittal T2-weighted (**E**) MRIs of the knee show numerous synovial chondromatous bodies in a popliteal cyst extending from the joint. Sagittal T2-weighted MRI (**F**), axial CT scan (**G**) taken at the time of image-guided needle biopsy, and low-power histologic image (**H**) of the lesion show that the benign lobules of cartilage are consistent with synovial chondromatosis. The patient underwent excision of the lesion, after which the patient's pain resolved.

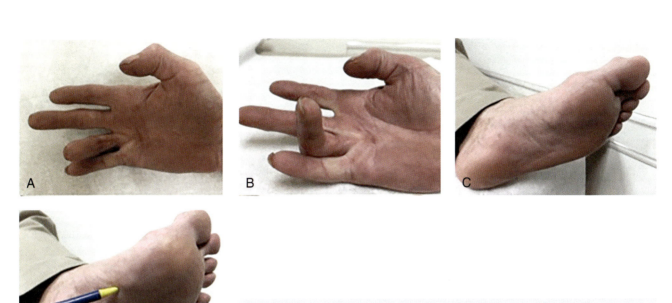

Figure 32   Clinical photographs show that superficial fibromatoses usually are easily recognizable. Dupuytren disease of the palm (palmar fibromatosis; **A** and **B**) and Ledderhose disease (plantar fibromatosis; **C** and **D**) are types of superficial fibromatoses.

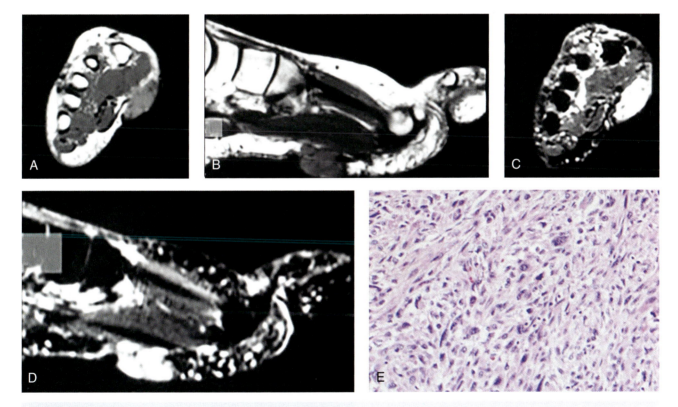

Figure 33   Images of a 54-year-old woman with a painless plantar mass located in the vicinity of the distal medial plantar fascia show that other lesions may mimic superficial fibromatoses by occurring in the same classic locations and having a similar appearance. Axial T1-weighted (**A**), sagittal T1-weighted (**B**), axial T2-weighted (**C**), and sagittal T2-weighted (**D**) MRIs of the foot show a heterogeneous lesion that is brighter on the T2-weighted MRIs and not in line with the plantar fascia, which gives it a nonspecific appearance that is inconsistent with plantar fibromatosis. Therefore, a biopsy was obtained to confirm the diagnosis. **E,** Histologic image of the mass taken at ×100 magnification shows a high-grade, soft-tissue sarcoma, which was diagnosed as a leiomyosarcoma via immunohistochemical analysis.

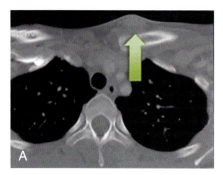
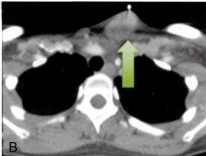
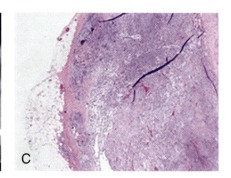

Figure 34   Images of a 20-year-old woman with a 3- to 4-week history of an enlarging and painful soft-tissue mass over the anterior aspect of her left clavicle. Axial CT scans (**A** and **B**) of the clavicle show a nonspecific soft-tissue mass (arrows). MRIs also would have revealed a nonspecific soft-tissue mass; therefore, a biopsy was performed. **C,** Low-power histologic image of the mass shows a teased-apart taffy candy appearance, sprinkles of inflammatory cells, and hemorrhage, which are characteristic features of nodular fasciitis.

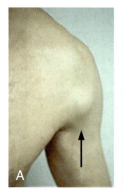
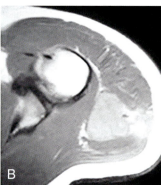
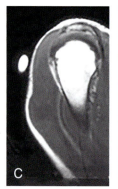
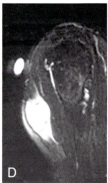
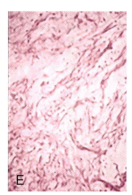

Figure 35   Images of a 30-year-old man with a 3-week history of a painful and enlarging soft-tissue mass over his left anterior shoulder. **A,** Clinical photograph of the shoulder shows the soft-tissue mass (arrow). Axial T1-weighted (**B**), sagittal T1-weighted (**C**), and sagittal T2-weighted (**D**) MRIs of the shoulder show a heterogeneous, enhancing, solid soft-tissue mass. Although the fascial tail sign that is shown in panel **D** has been described in patients with nodular fasciitis, it is not specific to nodular fasciitis; therefore, a biopsy was performed. **E,** Low-power histologic image of the mass shows the typical histologic appearance of nodular fasciitis.

remains controversial and may be considered in younger patients with high-grade, deep soft-tissue tumors or patients with metastatic disease.

Soft-tissue sarcomas grow in a centripetal fashion, compressing normal tissues that surround the tumor as it grows. This zone of compression is referred to as the reactive zone and, by definition, contains malignant cells. The goal of surgery is to resect the soft-tissue tumor, including the reactive zone, with a surrounding cuff of normal tissue (**Figure 38**). Anatomic constraints, such as major nerves, blood vessels, and bone, often limit and define the boundaries of the resection. The adequacy of the surgical margin is determined histologically; however, the definition of an adequate margin is controversial. At a minimum, the surgical margins should be microscopically negative (no ink at the cut surface). Limb salvage can be performed in more than 90% of patients.[1]

Despite adequate surgery and adjuvant therapies, the risk of

Table 3
2 × 2 Grid for the Triage of Soft-Tissue Masses

Size	Depth (Relative to the Fascia)	
	Superficial	**Deep**
≤5 cm	Typically benign lipomas or cysts	Warrants radiologic evaluation
>5 cm	Warrants radiologic evaluation	Highest concern for malignancy

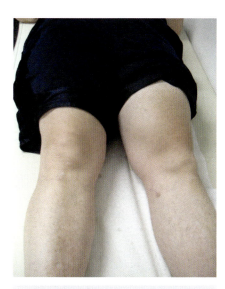

Figure 36 Clinical photograph of a lower extremity shows painless, growing masses that, on physical examination, were found to be more firm than the surrounding muscle.

local recurrence of soft-tissue sarcoma ranges from 5% to 10%, and the risk of distant metastases remains substantial in patients with high-grade soft-tissue tumors. Patients with high-grade soft-tissue tumors have the worst prognosis, whereas patients with superficial soft-tissue sarcomas tend to have a better prognosis. Therefore, frequent follow-up chest imaging and MRI of the affected area should be performed every 3 months for the first few years postoperatively and less frequently for many additional years postoperatively.

Summary

Orthopaedic surgeons often are required to evaluate soft-tissue masses. Most of these soft-tissue masses will be benign. However, the judicious use of available imaging modalities for the evaluation of soft-tissue masses and the use of the treatment algorithms that are presented in this chapter will aid physicians in avoiding pitfalls and result in the best possible outcomes for patients.

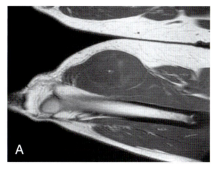

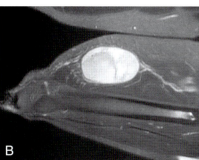

Figure 37 Coronal T1-weighted noncontrast (**A**) and coronal T1-weighted, fat-suppressed, postcontrast (**B**) MRIs of a thigh show that contrast is better for defining the internal characteristics of a mass in patients in whom a soft-tissue sarcoma is suspected.

References

1. Fletcher CDM, Bridge JA, Hogen-doorn PCW, Mertens F, eds: *WHO Classification of Tumours of Soft Tissue and Bone*. Lyon, France, International Agency for Research on Cancer, 2013.

2. Fiore M, Casali PG, Miceli R, et al: Prognostic effect of re-excision in adult soft tissue sarcoma of the extremity. *Ann Surg Oncol* 2006;13(1):110-117.

3. Italiano A, Le Cesne A, Mendiboure J, et al: Prognostic factors and impact of adjuvant treatments on local and metastatic relapse of soft-tissue sarcoma patients in the competing risks setting. *Cancer* 2014;120(21):3361-3369.

4. Bocklage TJ, Quinn RH, Schmit BP, Verschraegen CF: Benign mimics of bone and soft tissue tumors, in *Bone and Soft Tissue Tumors: A Multidisciplinary Review With Case Presentations*.

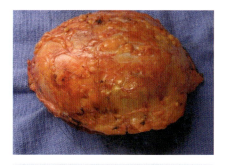

Figure 38 Clinical photograph shows a resected soft-tissue sarcoma, including the reactive zone with a surrounding cuff of normal tissue.

London, United Kingdom, JP Medical, 2014, pp 578-599.

5. Colman MW, Lozano-Calderon S, Raskin KA, Hornicek FJ, Gebhardt M: Non-neoplastic soft tissue masses that mimic sarcoma. *Orthop Clin North Am* 2014;45(2):245-255.

6. Rosenthal TC, Kraybill W: Soft tissue sarcomas: Integrating primary care recognition with tertiary care center treatment. *Am Fam Physician* 1999;60(2):567-572.

7. Gustafson P: Soft tissue sarcoma: Epidemiology and prognosis in 508 patients. *Acta Orthop Scand Suppl* 1994;259:1-31.

8. Simon MA, Finn HA: Diagnostic strategy for bone and soft-tissue tumors. *J Bone Joint Surg Am* 1993;75(4):622-631.

9. Nandra R, Forsberg J, Grimer R: If your lump is bigger than a golf ball and growing, think sarcoma. *Eur J Surg Oncol* 2015;41(10):1400-1405.

10. Gilbert NF, Cannon CP, Lin PP, Lewis VO: Soft-tissue sarcoma. *J Am Acad Orthop Surg* 2009;17(1):40-47.

11. Canter RJ, Smith CA, Martinez SR, Goodnight JE Jr, Bold RJ, Wisner DH: Extremity soft tissue tumor surgery by surgical specialty: A comparison of case volume among oncology and non-oncology-designated surgeons. *J Surg Oncol* 2013;108(3):142-147.

Appendix

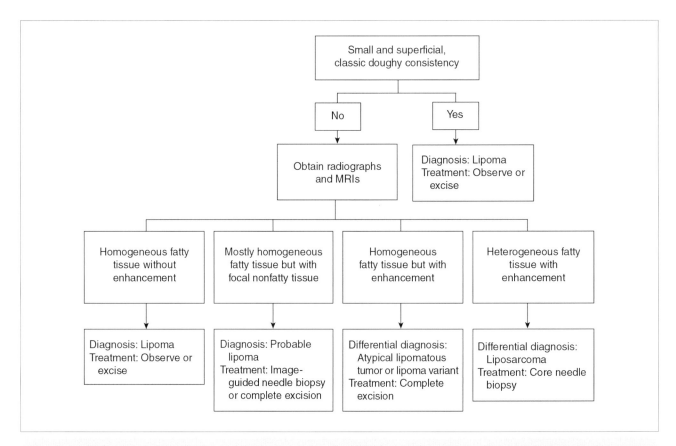

Figure 1   Suggested algorithm for the evaluation and treatment of a patient in whom a fatty tumor is suspected.

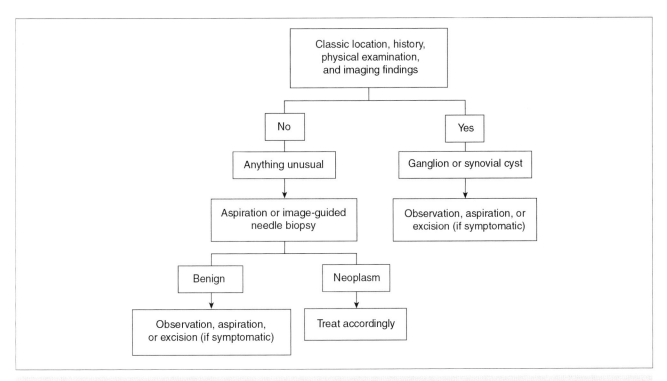

Figure 2   Suggested algorithm for the evaluation and treatment of a patient in whom a cystic lesion is suspected.

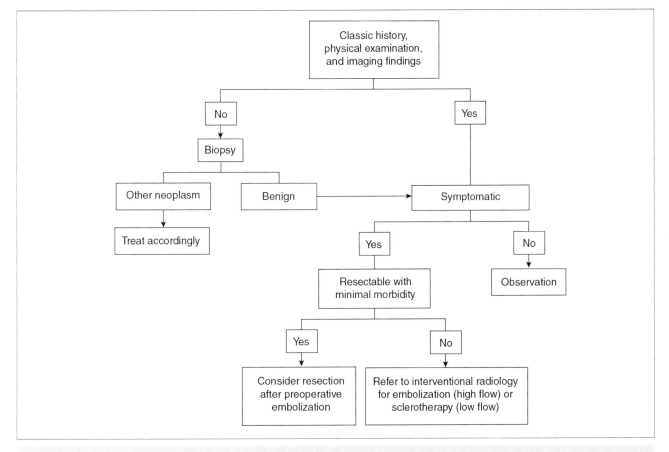

Figure 3   Suggested algorithm for the evaluation and treatment of a patient in whom a vascular mass is suspected.

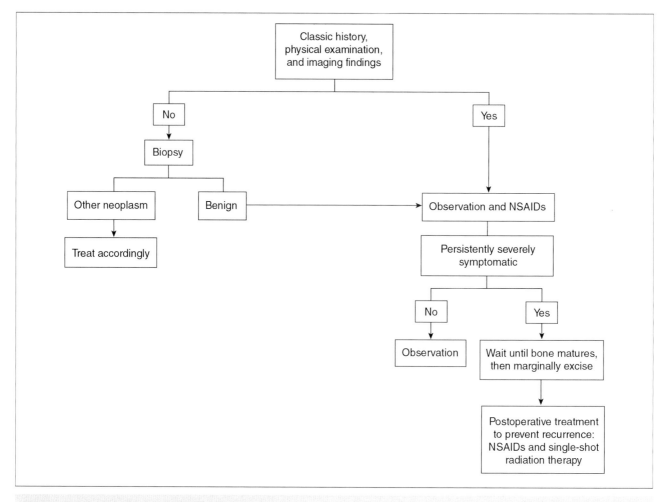

Figure 4 Suggested algorithm for the evaluation and treatment of a patient who has a lesion with patterns of mineralization, which suggests myositis ossificans.

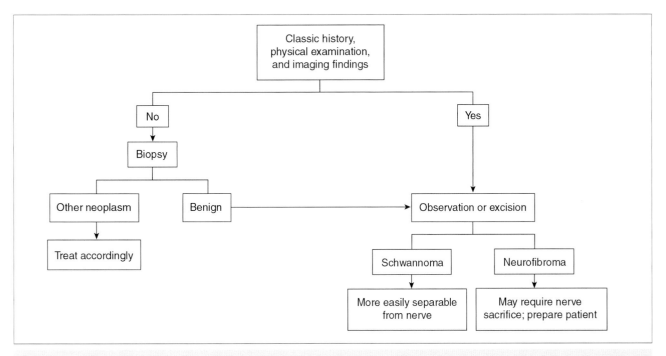

Figure 5   Suggested algorithm for the evaluation and treatment of a patient in whom a benign peripheral nerve sheath tumor is suspected

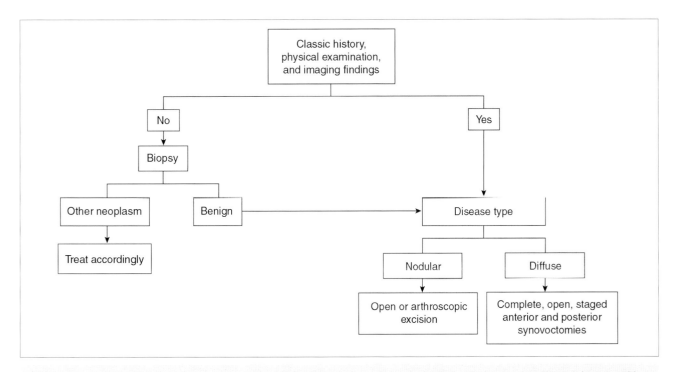

Figure 6   Suggested algorithm for the evaluation and treatment of a patient in whom pigmented villonodular synovitis is suspected.

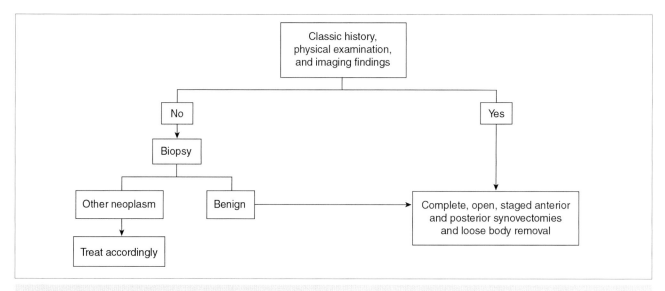

Figure 7   Suggested algorithm for the evaluation and treatment of a patient in whom synovial chondromatosis is suspected.

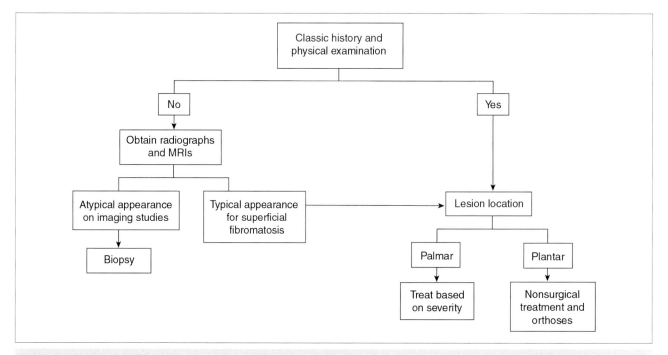

Figure 8   Suggested algorithm for the evaluation and treatment of a patient in whom superficial fibromatosis in the context of other potential orthopaedic oncology considerations is suspected.

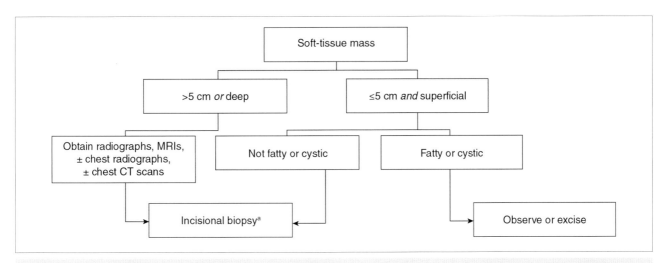

Figure 9   Algorithm for the management of soft-tissue masses, which was described by Simon and Finn[8] in 1993. [a]Biopsy is often done using a Tru-Cut needle (BD Worldwide).

What's Wrong With the Bone? An Overview of Metabolic and Neoplastic Bone Conditions

Richard L. McGough, MD
Michael P. Mott, MD
Kristy Weber, MD

Abstract

The evaluation of any orthopaedic condition often begins with obtaining plain radiographs. Fortuitously, plain radiographs provide surgeons with direct information on the biologic activity and, therefore, the aggressiveness of any bone lesion. More advanced imaging modalities may fail to elucidate the problem and may even obscure the diagnosis. The accurate interpretation of the aggressiveness of a bone lesion on plain radiographs is the first step in establishing a differential diagnosis for any bone lesion and, often, may result in a correct diagnosis without the need for additional imaging studies. A thorough understanding of the radiographic classification of bone lesions will allow surgeons to accurately diagnose and manage metabolic bone disease, benign bone lesions, and malignant bone lesions.

Instr Course Lect 2017;66:619–632.

The advent of plain radiography in the late 19th century revolutionized musculoskeletal diagnosis. Prior to the development of radiography, the main indicator of a fracture was crepitus, which was an inexact and painful means of diagnosis. Musculoskeletal imaging advanced dramatically in the 20th century, with planar tomography followed by nuclear medicine, CT, and MRI developed in the latter portion of the 20th century. Each of these imaging modalities provides surgeons with clues, which occasionally may be pathognomonic, that aid in establishing a musculoskeletal diagnosis. However, each of these imaging modalities has limitations, including lack of specificity, lack of sensitivity, exposure to radiation, and cost. Despite the recommendations of some radiologists and the demands of patients, newer imaging modalities are not always better with regard to establishing a musculoskeletal diagnosis. Plain radiography has many distinct advantages with regard to establishing a correct musculoskeletal diagnosis compared with other imaging modalities.

Plain radiography is ubiquitous and technically easy to perform. Plain radiography is accessible for patients, and radiographs can be obtained quickly at a relatively low cost. Plain radiography has specific advantages in patients with indwelling orthopaedic implants. Although metal-reducing technologies for CT or MRI can limit metallic artifact during imaging of an anatomic location that contains an implant, plain radiography of an anatomic location that contains an implant results in little to

Dr. McGough or an immediate family member serves as a paid consultant to Stryker; has received research or institutional support from Illuminoss; and serves as a board member, owner, officer, or committee member of the Musculoskeletal Tumor Society. Dr. Mott or an immediate family member serves as a board member, owner, officer, or committee member of the American Academy of Orthopaedic Surgeons and the Musculoskeletal Tumor Society. Dr. Weber or an immediate family member has received research or institutional support from Roche and serves as a board member, owner, officer, or committee member of the American Orthopaedic Association, the Musculoskeletal Tumor Society, the Orthopaedic Research Society, and the Ruth Jackson Orthopaedic Society.

Table 1
Miller Classification of Bone Lesions

Type	Description
A	Osteolytic lesion
A1	Geographic lesion
A1a	Well-defined lucency with sclerosis
A1b	Well-defined lucency without sclerosis
A1c	Poorly defined geographic lesion
A2	Moth-eaten lesion
A3	Permeative lesion
B	Sclerotic lesion
B1	Well-defined lucency containing mature bone
B2	Well-defined, calcified lesion
B3	Poorly defined lesion
C	Periosteal lesion
C1	Intrinsic lesion that originates from the periosteum or cortex
C1a	Well-defined periosteal lesion
C1b	Poorly defined periosteal lesion
C1c	Spiculated periosteal lesion
C2	Extrinsic lesion that originates from outside cortical region
C2a	Extrinsic lesion with sclerotic border
C2b	Extrinsic lesion with poorly defined border
D	Bony remodeling

Data from Miller TT: Bone tumors and tumorlike conditions: Analysis with conventional radiography. *Radiology* 2008;246(3):662-674.

Radiographic Classification of Bone Lesions

The memorization of complex alphanumeric bone lesion classification schemes does not necessarily promote knowledge or advance understanding. However, classification systems that organize bone lesions into recognizable groups may be useful. The simplest yet most complete classification of bone lesions was developed by Miller[1] (**Table 1**). This system classifies bone lesions into one of four categories: osteolytic lesions, sclerotic lesions, periosteal lesions, and bony remodeling. In classifying bone lesions into these four categories, the classification system organizes the spectrum of orthopaedic conditions into four biologic groups. Because the field of musculoskeletal oncology comprises more than 100 distinct biologic entities, the Miller classification of bone lesions enables surgeons to classify and organize biologic entities with the use of plain radiographs, which aid in diagnostic assessment.

no loss of image quality. Digital radiography, which, in the past two decades, has become the standard method via which plain radiographs are obtained, further enhances interpretative ability. The ability of a surgeon to window a radiograph to observe the bone around an implant allows for enhanced assessment of any adjacent bone lesions.

From a musculoskeletal oncology perspective, plain radiography has specific advantages with regard to the formation of a differential diagnosis compared with other imaging modalities. Plain radiography is a superior imaging modality for the assessment of cortical and cancellous bone. Plain radiographs allow surgeons to determine the biologic response of a bone to a lesion that is within or adjacent to it. Other imaging modalities may be inferior compared with plain radiography because of lack of specificity (eg, nuclear medicine) or sensitivity (eg, cortical bone is poorly observed on MRI, and MRIs may be distorted in patients with edematous processes). Radiographs, which clearly demonstrate the response of a bone to a lesion, allow surgeons to determine the aggressiveness of a bone lesion. In general, plain radiography should be the first imaging study ordered for children or adolescents in whom a bone lesion is suspected.

Osteolytic Lesions

Type A bone lesions are osteolytic lesions. Osteolytic lesions create radiolucencies of varying degrees of aggressiveness and are observed as dark holes in the bone on radiographs. A purely osteolytic lesion will have a homogeneous radiolucency. Unicameral bone cysts (before any healing) and multiple myeloma result in purely osteolytic lesions. Some osteolytic lesions have heterogeneous osteolysis, with some form of matrix (bone, calcification, or other) present within the lesion. An intraosseous hemangioma is an example of a lesion with heterogeneous osteolysis.

The rapidity of bony destruction and biologic aggressiveness increases from type A1 to type A3 bone lesions. Type A1 bone lesions are described as geographic lesions, which means that the lesion occupies a defined, recognizable space within the bone. Osteolytic lesions with a sclerotic border (type A1a bone lesions) are completely encapsulated by mature bone, which indicates an indolent, benign process. A long-standing synovial cyst in bone is an example of a type A1a lesion. Osteolytic lesions without a sclerotic border (type A1b bone lesions) may progress; however, even without a sclerotic border, most well-defined (narrow zone of transition) type A1b bone lesions remain benign. Poorly defined geographic osteolytic lesions (type A1c bone lesions) have a wide zone of transition, which indicates either malignancy or infection. Chronic osteomyelitis and metastatic bone disease are examples of type A1c bone lesions.

Type A2 bone lesions are described as moth-eaten lesions, which indicate biologic aggressiveness and a very wide zone of transition. Examples of type A2 bone lesions include osteosarcoma and some aggressive forms of osteomyelitis.

Type A3 bone lesions are described as permeative lesions. Type A3 bone lesions and aggressive type A2 bone lesions differ only in the rapidity via which bone is destroyed. Small blue-cell lesions, which rapidly destroy bone without producing any visible matrix (bone or cartilage), often cause permeation. Examples of type A3 bone lesions include Ewing sarcoma, lymphoma, and the most aggressive forms of osteomyelitis. Permeative bony changes often are accompanied by a large soft-tissue mass because the cellular process quickly proceeds through the bone and into the surrounding soft tissues.

Sclerotic Lesions

Type B bone lesions are sclerotic lesions. Sclerotic or osteoblastic lesions create a radiodensity on radiographs. This area of density is evidence of mineralization and may be comprised of bone (mature or immature), calcified cartilage, or amorphous calcification. Osteoblastic metastases, which are observed in patients with metastatic prostate or breast carcinoma, occur if metastatic cancer cells stimulate local osteoblasts to create immature bone.

The rapidity of bony destruction and biologic aggressiveness increases from type B1 to type B3 bone lesions. Type B1 and type B2 bone lesions differ only in content. Type B1 bone lesions contain mature bone (ossification), whereas type B2 bone lesions contain cartilage (calcification). Type B3 bone lesions are poorly defined, which indicates malignancy. Examples of a typical type B1 bone lesion include a bone island or enostosis. An enchondroma is an example of a calcified, benign, sclerotic type B2 bone lesion. Examples of a typical, poorly defined type B3 bone lesion include metastatic prostate or breast carcinoma.

Periosteal Lesions

Type C bone lesions are periosteal lesions. Periosteal lesions originate either from the bony cortex or periosteum (intrinsic lesions) or from the adjacent musculature (extrinsic lesions). As periosteal lesions progress, they grow into the bone and may extend into the medullary canal. Periosteal lesions are either intrinsic to the periosteum, such as a periosteal chondroma, or extrinsic to the periosteum, such as a mass that slowly erodes into (hemangioma) or frankly invades the cortex.

The same interpretive rules that apply to type A and type B bone lesions apply to type C bone lesions. Type C bone lesions with a well-defined or sclerotic border act in a biologically benign manner. Type C bone lesions with a wide zone of transition, moth-eaten edges, or permeation are more biologically aggressive.

Bony Remodeling

Type D bone lesions are the final category of bony change and include bony remodeling. Type D bone lesions include indolent processes and occur secondary to many factors. Age, osteoporosis, the presence of implants, metabolic processes, and various medical conditions may cause bony remodeling.

Metabolic Bone Disease

Metabolic bone disease is a term that encompasses a heterogeneous group of diseases that have one factor in common: all involve alterations of mineralization in some portion of the calcium/phosphate/vitamin D pathway or alterations in the function of osteoblasts/osteoclasts. All metabolic bone diseases have similar characteristics, including bony remodeling, endosteal scalloping, varus deformity of severely involved bone, and expanded bone circumference with relative osteopenia, that are observed on plain radiographs.[2-4]

Metabolic conditions can be distinguished from neoplastic conditions via several radiographic characteristics: polyostotic changes, whole-bone changes, and diffuse osteopenia. Although some neoplastic conditions may involve multiple bones, the involvement of every bone in a radiographic field is more likely to be the result of a systemic condition. Neoplastic conditions uncommonly involve all three segments of a long bone (the diaphysis, metaphysis, and epiphysis), whereas metabolic conditions frequently involve all three segments of a long bone. Unless a neoplastic condition is observed in an individual with senile osteoporosis or a metabolic condition, diffuse osteopenia generally is not severe. **Table 2** lists the most common metabolic conditions and their corresponding radiographic findings.[2-4]

Benign Bone Lesions

Benign bone lesions are extremely common in both children and adults. Many benign bone lesions can be definitively diagnosed using the principles discussed earlier. Benign bone lesions are broadly categorized based on the type of tissue that makes up the lesion (**Table 3**). Most benign bone lesions are more common in males, with the exception of fibrous dysplasia, aneurysmal bone cysts, and giant cell tumors, which are more common in females.

Bone-Forming Lesions
Osteoid Osteoma

An osteoid osteoma is a rare bone lesion. Patients with an osteoid osteoma have night pain that is relieved with NSAIDs. Radiographs will reveal a small lucent nidus (<1 cm) and a variable amount of surrounding reactive bone, which may obscure the underlying lesion. A thin-cut CT scan is the best imaging study to confirm a diagnosis of an osteoid osteoma. The lower extremity is the most common location of osteoid osteomas. In patients with an osteoid osteoma in other locations, a joint effusion or scoliosis may be observed. Radiofrequency ablation is the current standard of care that is used to eradicate the nidus and its associated pain. Less common treatment options

for patients with an osteoid osteoma include medical management or surgical excision.[5] The histologic analysis of an osteoid osteoma will reveal a cherry-red nidus with immature osteoid and woven bone admixed with a background of highly vascularized fibrous tissue.

Osteoblastoma

An osteoblastoma is a rare bone lesion that appears lytic and aggressive on radiographs, is larger (>1.5 cm) compared with an osteoid osteoma, and is commonly located in the posterior elements of the spine and sacrum. The histologic analysis of an osteoblastoma is similar to that of an osteoid osteoma; however, osteoblastomas have increased cellularity and vascularity.

Osteoma

Osteomas are 1- to 2-cm areas of dense normal bone. Typically, osteomas are asymptomatic, nonprogressive, and discovered incidentally. Osteomas that are large or growing must be distinguished

Table 2
Common Metabolic Conditions and Corresponding Radiographic Findings

Condition	Radiographic Findings
Osteomalacia	
Primary (parathyroid adenoma or hyperplasia)	Diffuse
	Phalangeal resorption
	Brown tumors
Secondary (nutritional or iatrogenic osteomalacia)	Diffuse osteopenia
Secondary (renal osteodystrophy)	Varus deformities (children)
	Widened physes (children)
	Endosteal/periosteal resorption
	Diffuse osteopenia
Rickets	
Nutritional	Dwarfism
	Varus deformities
	Costochondral enlargement
	Delayed dentition
	Physeal widening
	Metaphyseal cupping
	Looser lines
Vitamin D dependent	Similar to nutritional
Vitamin D resistant	Similar to nutritional
	No decrease in bone mass
Hypophosphatasia	Severe osteopenia
	Abrupt transition from normal diaphysis to undermineralized metaphysis
	Poorly healing stress fracture
Paget disease	Bony expansion/widening
	Cancellous disorganization
	Thickened trabeculae
	Secondary joint degeneration

Table 3

Types of Benign Bone Lesions

Type	Appearance	Cause for Concern If...	Common Treatment
Bone-forming lesions			
Osteoid osteoma	Small lucent lesion (nidus), abundance of mature reactive bone	Lesion enlarges, periosteal reaction becomes layered/aggressive	Percutaneous radiofrequency ablation
Osteoma	Dense, small sharp area of ossification	Enlarges, becomes painful	Observation
Fibrous lesions			
Nonossifying fibroma	Small, geographic, and nonprogressive, incidental finding	Painful periosteal reaction without known fracture/soft-tissue mass	Observation
Fibrous dysplasia	Single bone, incidental finding	Syndrome with multiple bone involvement, progressive femoral deformity, soft-tissue mass	Observation, syndrome management, fixation, or grafting of progressive proximal femoral deformity
Cartilage lesions			
Osteochondroma	Cartilage cap is small (<1.0 cm)	Cartilage cap enlarges, lesion grows after skeletal maturation	Observation Complete excision if mechanical symptoms
Enchondroma	Calcification without endosteal erosion	Substantial endosteal erosion or cortical thickening	Observation Curettage and grafting phalanx lesion with fracture
Chondroblastoma	Epiphyseal lesion, round, sclerotic border	Patient >25 years, large soft-tissue mass, poor zone of transition	Curettage and grafting
Bone cysts			
Simple/unicameral bone cyst	Sharp zone of transition, mild bone expansion, no pain	Weight-bearing bone with pain, progressive pain, periosteal reaction in absence of fracture	Observation or injection
ABC	Bone expansion with fluid-fluid levels without aggressive periosteal reaction	Only small portion of lesion appears to be ABC, soft-tissue mass, aggressive periosteal reaction	Biopsy confirmation, curettage, and grafting
Miscellaneous lesions			
Giant cell tumor	Epiphyseal lesion extending to subchondral surface	Poor zone of transition, large soft-tissue mass, aggressive periosteal reaction	Extended intralesional curettage and void filling ± fixation
Eosinophilic granuloma	Punched-out lesion with abundant periosteal reaction	Great imitator (always a concern), soft-tissue mass, adult age group	Biopsy ± observation, bracing, or steroid injection

ABC = aneurysmal bone cyst.

from an osteoblastic metastasis. Multiple osteomas have been associated with Gardner syndrome (familial polyposis). The histologic analysis of an osteoma will reveal dense normal bone that is distinctly separate from the surrounding cancellous spicules.

Fibrous Lesions
Nonossifying Fibroma
Nonossifying fibroma is a broad term that is synonymous with fibrous cortical defect, metaphyseal fibrous defect, and cortical desmoid. Nonossifying fibromas are found in as many as 30% of

skeletally immature individuals (**Figure 1**). The distal femur, the proximal tibia, the proximal fibula, and the distal tibia are the most common locations of nonossifying fibromas. Radiographs will reveal an eccentric, metaphyseal, osteolytic lesion with occasional mild

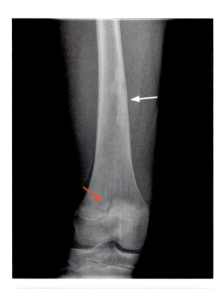

Figure 1   AP radiograph of the distal femur of a 14-year-old boy demonstrates a resolving nonossifying fibroma of the medial diaphysis of the femur (white arrow) and bipartite patella (red arrow). Note the eccentric location of the nonossifying fibroma with a scalloped sclerotic border.

expansion. Nonossifying fibromas will appear as a lucent area on CT scans and will have low T1 and intermediate T2 signal on MRIs. Nonossifying fibromas are most often managed with observation because they tend to involute and ossify with skeletal maturity. The histologic analysis of a nonossifying fibroma will reveal a swirling storiform pattern (whorled bundles), giant cells, and, during the involution process, occasional cholesterol clefts.

Fibrous Dysplasia

Fibrous dysplasia is a developmental hamartoma in which areas of the skeleton fail to mature and, instead, remain immature, poorly mineralized trabeculae. The genetic defect that is responsible for fibrous dysplasia is located in the G protein α subunit of the GNAS protein. Most likely present at birth, fibrous dysplasia may not be recognized for years, especially if patients have monostotic disease and are asymptomatic. In general, the skull, the maxilla, the proximal femur, and the tibia are the most common locations of fibrous dysplasia. Forms of fibrous dysplasia that involve multiple bones (polyostotic) tend to affect only one side of a patient's body (monomelic), and vertebral involvement is extremely rare. Polyostotic fibrous dysplasia is associated with McCune-Albright syndrome, which includes precocious puberty/endocrine abnormalities and café au lait spots (irregular, geographic coast of Maine pattern). Typically, radiographs will reveal a metaphyseal lesion that does not cross the growth plate, with cortical thinning, modest bone expansion, and a well-defined cortical rim. Often, fibrous dysplasia is described as having a ground or leaded glass appearance. Fibrous dysplasia will appear warm to hot on bone scans and have low T1 and moderately high T2 signal on MRIs.

Observation is acceptable for the treatment of asymptomatic patients with fibrous dysplasia. Disphosphonates have been used to treat patients with more severe fibrous dysplasia. Typically, aggressive curettage is reserved for patients with fibrous dysplasia who have progressive pain or deformity, especially in a weight-bearing limb. Internal fixation is frequently recommended for patients with symptomatic fibrous dysplasia of the femoral neck to prevent fracture and subsequent varus deformity. Notably, fibrous dysplasia heals with dysplastic bone; therefore, cortical allografts may be preferred for grafting procedures in patients with fibrous dysplasia because they tend to undergo resorption most slowly.[6] The histologic analysis of fibrous dysplasia will reveal a proliferation of fibroblasts, with spicules of woven bone that originate directly from the stroma without osteoblastic rimming.

Cartilage Lesions

Osteochondroma

Osteochondromas (exostoses) account for approximately 35% of all benign bone lesions. Osteochondromas may originate from aberrant cartilage on the bone surface. Osteochondromas grow with skeletal maturation and often are diagnosed in a patient's second decade of life. An osteochondroma is a firm, nonmobile mass about the distal femur, the proximal tibia, or the proximal humerus and may be associated with a snapping sensation, bursal swelling, or neurogenic symptoms. Multiple osteochondromas with skeletal dysplasia occur in patients with autosomal dominant multiple hereditary exostosis (MHE). Plain radiographs will reveal that osteochondromas share the cortex with the underlying bone, with intramedullary contents flowing into the lesion (**Figure 2**). Pedunculated osteochondromas point away from the joint. Although osteochondromas are sessile, tethering of the growth plate and bowing may occur. The cartilage cap of an osteochondroma is small (<1 cm) and variable in mineralization. Osteochondromas grow during childhood but should be quiescent after a patient reaches skeletal maturity. Malignant degeneration is incredibly rare in a solitary osteochondroma. In adults, a large cartilage cap or a growing osteochondroma warrants further evaluation. Patients with MHE have an increased risk for malignant transformation (1% to 10%). Patients with MHE have defects in the *EXT1*, *EXT2*, or *EXT3* tumor suppressor genes.[7] The management of a symptomatic benign osteochondroma involves complete removal of the lesion, including the perichondrium and cap.

Enchondroma

An enchondroma is a benign, intramedullary cartilage lesion. The hands, the feet, the proximal humerus, and the femur are the most common locations of enchondromas. Typically, enchondromas are solitary; however, they may be observed in patients with a skeletal dysplasia that involves enchondromas in multiple bones (Ollier disease). In the bones of the hand, a fracture may indicate an enchondroma. Radiographs will reveal variable cartilage calcification in a ring and arc pattern. Benign enchondromas in the long bones have minimal to no endosteal erosion, no cortical thickening, and no soft-tissue mass.[8,9] Enchondromas may cause increased uptake on a bone scan but not more than that observed at the iliac crests. Most enchondromas are asymptomatic and can be managed with observation. The histologic analysis of a benign enchondroma will reveal mature cartilage formation without substantial pleomorphism, nuclear atypia, mitotic figures, or invasion of bone.

Chondroblastoma

A chondroblastoma is a rare benign lesion. Typically, chondroblastomas are considered of cartilage origin because of chondroid matrix production; however, chondroblastoma tumor cells do not express type II collagen.[10] Eighty percent of chondroblastomas occur in patients younger than 25 years. The onset of a chondroblastoma is indolent and frequently attributed to local mechanical issues. Radiographs will reveal a true epiphyseal (apophyseal)

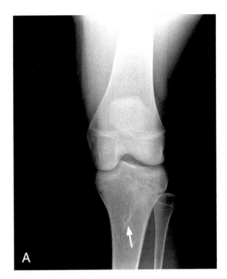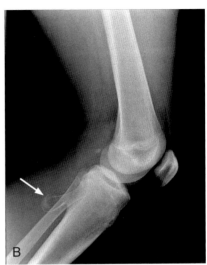

Figure 2   AP (**A**) and lateral (**B**) radiographs of the left knee of a 15-year-old boy demonstrate an osteochondroma of the proximal posterior tibia (arrow) and snapping neuromechanical pain.

lesion that occasionally crosses the physis. A chondroblastoma is a well-circumscribed lesion with a sclerotic rim. Extensive surrounding edema often is observed on the MRIs of patients with chondroblastomas. The management of a chondroblastoma consists of curettage and grafting, with adjuvants as indicated. Surgery may be technically challenging because of the adjacent joint and open growth plate.[11] The histologic analysis of a chondroblastoma will reveal round or polyhedral cells with elongated cleaved nuclei (coffee bean), a large number of multinucleated giant cells, areas of secondary aneurysmal bone cysts in one-third of patients, and lacey dystrophic calcification that results in a chicken-wire pattern.

Bone Cysts
Unicameral Bone Cyst
Unicameral (simple) bone cysts are commonly diagnosed in a patient's first two decades of life. Unicameral bone cysts are primarily located in the proximal humerus, with a lesser percentage of unicameral bone cysts located in the

proximal femur. Typically, unicameral bone cysts are asymptomatic unless a fracture occurs. Active (growing) unicameral bone cysts tend to be observed in patients younger than 10 years and located in close proximity to the epiphyseal plate. Radiographs will reveal a lucent lesion with mild bone expansion (not greater than the width of growth plate) and a sharp zone of transition. Minor, incomplete septations and fracture fragments that settle in the cavity (fallen leaf sign) may be observed. Initial treatment of a patient with a pathologic fracture through a humeral unicameral bone cyst involves management of the fracture and observation of the unicameral bone cyst because some unicameral bone cysts resolve with fracture healing. Stimulation of active unicameral bone cysts via aspiration and injection with the use of steroids or various types of filling material has been reported.[12] The histologic analysis of a unicameral bone cyst will reveal a simple cyst that consists of a thin rim of fibrous tissue with occasional multinucleated giant cells.

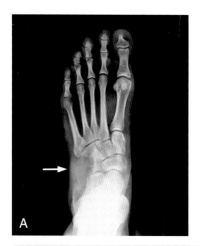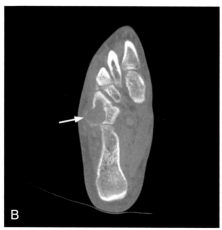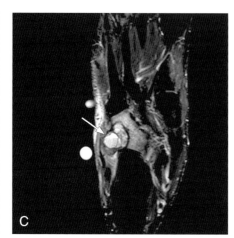

Figure 3 Images of the left foot of an 18-year-old woman with foot pain and an aneurysmal bone cyst of the cuboid. **A,** AP radiograph demonstrates an osteolytic lesion of the cuboid (arrow). **B,** Coronal CT scan demonstrates the eccentric, expansile nature of the lesion (arrow). **C,** Coronal, T2-weighted fat-saturated MRI shows the fluid-fluid levels within the lesion (arrow) and the surrounding bone edema.

Aneurysmal Bone Cyst

Aneurysmal bone cysts are more aggressive compared with unicameral bone cysts. Patients with an aneurysmal bone cyst have a unique genetic translocation of the *TRE17/USP6* oncogene.[13] Aneurysmal bone cysts may be primary (de novo) or secondary to underlying bone lesions. Pain is common in patients with an aneurysmal bone cyst. Aneurysmal bone cysts are more common in females compared with males. Eighty percent of aneurysmal bone cysts occur in a patient's first two decades of life (**Figure 3**). In general, the posterior elements of the spine, the femur, and the tibia are the most common locations of aneurysmal bone cysts. Radiographs will reveal an eccentric, expansive lesion that often is honeycombed and without mineralization. MRIs will reveal fluid-fluid levels. The differential diagnosis for an aneurysmal bone cyst includes telangiectatic osteosarcoma. The management of an aneurysmal bone cyst consists of extended intralesional curettage and grafting, with or without adjuvants and stabilization as indicated. The histologic

analysis of an aneurysmal bone cyst will reveal blood-filled, cystic, cavernous areas with surrounding fibrous tissue, absence of a true endothelial lining, and a large number of multinucleated giant cells.

Miscellaneous Lesions
Giant Cell Tumor

Giant cell tumors account for 5% of all primary bone lesions. Giant cell tumors are more common in females and older patients (90% older than 20 years). Patients with a giant cell tumor have insidious, progressive pain; swelling; and loss of motion. The distal femur, the proximal tibia, and the distal radius are the most common locations of giant cell tumors. Rarely, benign lung metastases will develop in patients with giant cell tumors (occurs in 2% of patients). Radiographs will reveal an eccentric lesion in the epiphysis (apophysis) with metaphyseal extension. The lesion extends to the subchondral surface and does not have a sclerotic rim. Giant cell tumors may cause increased uptake on a bone scan. Giant cell tumors

will demonstrate a lack of intralesional mineralization on CT scans and will appear as a low T1 and intermediate T2 signal on MRIs. The management of a giant cell tumor consists of extended intralesional curettage, with local adjuvants (phenol, liquid nitrogen, argon beam, peroxide) frequently applied to decrease the high rate of recurrence. Adequate visualization of the cavity and thorough lesion removal are critical. Large defects that result from curettage may be filled with bone graft or bone cement, with stabilization as indicated. Cementation does not decrease the rate of recurrence but aids in the detection of early recurrence. Patients with a giant cell tumor that causes joint destruction may require resection and joint arthroplasty (allograft or prosthesis). The use of denosumab has been approved for patients who have an unresectable giant cell tumor and has been reported to control symptoms.[14]

Eosinophilic Granuloma

An eosinophilic granuloma is a benign bone lesion that is observed in patients who have Langerhans cell histiocytosis. Eosinophilic granulomas can occur in any skeletal location but are most commonly located in the skull, the ribs, the vertebral column (thoracic more often than lumbar more often than cervical), the long bones, and the pelvis. Radiographs will reveal punched-out osteolytic lesions with a thick periosteal reaction. Vertebral body collapse (vertebra plana) is common in patients with an eosinophilic granuloma. Isolated eosinophilic granulomas can be managed with the use of intralesional steroid injections or biopsy alone. With the use of bracing alone, vertebra plana will spontaneously correct in 90% of patients with an eosinophilic granuloma. The histologic analysis of an eosinophilic granuloma will reveal that the pathognomonic cell is the Langerhans histiocyte (not the eosinophil) admixed among a variable number of histiocytes and a mixed inflammatory cell infiltrate.[15] Electron microscopy will reveal Birbeck granules (tennis racket–shaped inclusions) in histiocytes. The lesion also is CD1a positive.

Malignant Bone Lesions

Most bone lesions in children and adults are benign; therefore, surgeons may easily miss the less common malignant bone lesion. Primary malignant bone lesions account for approximately 3,000 of the more than 1.6 million new cases of cancer that occur each year.[16] This chapter discusses the clinical appearance, radiographic appearance, and management of the three most common malignant bone lesions.

Osteosarcoma

Osteosarcoma is the most common primary malignant bone lesion in children. Osteosarcoma is slightly more common in males. Osteosarcoma most frequently occurs in a patient's second decade of life. Pain in the extremities that is located close to a joint is the most common symptom of osteosarcoma; this may make the initial diagnosis of osteosarcoma difficult because the demographic in which osteosarcoma occurs actively participates in sports activities, which often lead to painful extremity injuries. Osteosarcoma is associated with mutations of the *P53* gene and the *RB1* gene, which is a tumor suppressor. Overall, osteosarcoma has a complex genetic profile and an overexpression of oncogenes, including *MDM2*, *HER2/neu*, c-*Myc*, and c-*Fos*. A second, late peak of osteosarcoma may occur in a patient's sixth decade of life. Osteosarcoma may be a secondary malignancy that is located in an area of prior radiation or associated with Paget disease.

In addition to pain, symptoms of osteosarcoma include swelling as a result of extraosseous extension of the lesion; decreased adjacent joint range of motion; and, depending on the location of the lesion, a limp.[17] In general, pain caused by a primary bone malignancy, such as an osteosarcoma, is progressive. Intermittent pain symptoms, which can be attributed to a recent injury, progress to constant pain (both at rest and at night) that often is unrelieved by anti-inflammatory medications. Assuming that pain is injury related, even as it worsens, is the most common mistake that both families and surgeons make in the initial evaluation of a young patient with pain. The initial management of a painful extremity or joint in an active patient, which includes the use of NSAIDs or activity modification, is symptomatic. However, imaging is required if the pain progresses. Plain radiographs should be obtained initially; more sophisticated imaging studies should be performed if a patient's symptoms do not improve.

Typically, plain radiographs of an osteosarcoma demonstrate a mixed appearance because of areas of bone formation and bone destruction (**Figure 4**). The metaphysis of the distal femur, proximal tibia, and proximal humerus are the most common skeletal locations of osteosarcoma. In skeletally immature patients, the epiphyseal plate may be a barrier against lesion growth. By the time of diagnosis, most osteosarcomas will have extended beyond a solely intraosseous location and form an adjacent soft-tissue mass. Typically, a Codman triangle of reactive bone is located adjacent to the lesion. A high-grade, intramedullary, osteoblastic osteosarcoma is the most common osteosarcoma subtype. Although less common, periosteal (surface lesion with a sunburst appearance and cartilaginous differentiation) and parosteal (surface lesion with a dense bone appearance and fibroblastic differentiation) osteosarcomas also exist. A telangiectatic osteosarcoma is a rare intramedullary osteosarcoma variant that has a purely osteolytic radiographic appearance. The histologic analysis of a telangiectatic osteosarcoma will reveal large, blood-filled spaces. The differential diagnosis for a telangiectatic osteosarcoma includes an aneurysmal bone cyst.

Often, a diagnosis of an osteosarcoma can be made with the use of plain radiographs alone; however, MRI can better delineate the extent of intramedullary marrow and soft-tissue involvement and assess the lesion in relation to the surrounding neurovascular structures. MRI also assists surgeons in both diagnosis and preoperative planning for

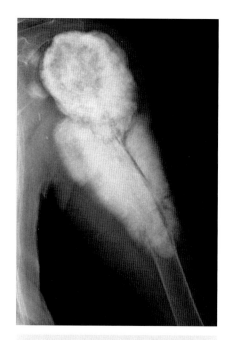

Figure 4 AP radiograph of a left proximal humerus demonstrates a bone-forming neoplasm. Note the dense ossification, which is consistent with the appearance of an osteosarcoma.

resection. CT scans can demonstrate mineralization of the lesion but do not provide surgeons with information in addition to that attained from MRI and only subject patients to additional radiation. Either a total-body technetium bone scan or a total-body positron emission tomography scan may be obtained as a staging study to assess for distant sites of metastases.

Patients with a clinical and radiographic evaluation that indicates osteosarcoma should undergo a biopsy to confirm a diagnosis of osteosarcoma. The biopsy can be performed as an image-guided needle biopsy or a surgical open incisional biopsy. If the lesion extends into the surrounding soft tissues, the leading edge rather than the intraosseous portion of the lesion should be biopsied. The histologic analysis of a classic osteosarcoma will reveal a frankly sarcomatous stroma-forming osteoid that permeates through and around existing bone trabeculae. The osteoblasts may be pleomorphic in appearance and form the neoplastic new bone.

Patients in whom osteosarcoma is diagnosed are treated with preoperative chemotherapy followed by surgical resection of the primary lesion, after which they are treated with additional postoperative chemotherapy.[18] Standard drugs for the management of osteosarcoma include methotrexate, doxorubicin, and cisplatin. More than 90% of patients with osteosarcoma are able to be treated with a limb-sparing procedure; however, amputation or rotationplasty are still performed, depending on the location of the lesion and the age of the patient.[19] The authors of this chapter are unable to discuss the multitude of options for reconstruction after resection of a lesion given the constraints of this chapter. Currently, most patients undergo reconstruction with either a modular, metal prosthesis if the lesion involves the adjacent joint or an intercalary allograft (with or without vascularized bone) if the tumor spares the adjacent joint.

The local recurrence rate of osteosarcoma in patients who undergo surgery is approximately 5%. The overall survival rate for patients with osteosarcoma has not substantially changed in the past 25 years and is approximately 70% at 5 years postoperatively for patients with osteosarcoma that is isolated to an extremity. Patients with osteosarcoma of the pelvis or metastatic osteosarcoma have a lower overall survival rate. The amount of necrosis observed in the primary lesion at the time of surgical resection (after neoadjuvant chemotherapy) is predictive of prognosis, with more than 90% necrosis being a good indicator. The most common site of osteosarcoma metastasis is the lungs, with osteosarcoma metastasis to the bone occurring less frequently. Aggressive management of lung metastasis with the use of a thoracotomy may increase long-term survival, especially in patients in whom the metastasis occurred more than 1 year after the completion of initial treatment.

Ewing Sarcoma

Ewing sarcoma is the second most common primary malignant bone lesion in children and is the most common diagnosis within the Ewing family of lesions. Approximately 80% of patients with Ewing sarcoma are younger than 20 years. Ewing sarcoma is slightly more common in males and is uncommon in African American and Chinese individuals. Similar to patients with osteosarcoma, the most common symptom in patients with Ewing sarcoma is pain, which also frequently occurs in this demographic as a result of more common etiologies, such as sports injuries. The genetics of Ewing sarcoma are less complex compared with the genetics of osteosarcoma, consisting primarily of a balanced chromosomal translocation (11;22), with *EWS/FLI1* being the most common fused gene. The specific cell from which Ewing sarcoma originates is unknown; however, some studies hypothesize Ewing sarcoma to be of neuroectodermal differentiation.

In addition to pain, symptoms of Ewing sarcoma include swelling as a result of extraosseous extension of the lesion; decreased adjacent joint range of motion; and, depending on the location of the lesion, a limp.[17] Many symptoms of Ewing sarcoma are similar to those of osteosarcoma; however, symptoms specific to Ewing sarcoma include fever and, occasionally, erythema. A diagnostic workup may reveal an elevated erythrocyte sedimentation rate, white blood count, or lactate dehydrogenase level. Fever or erythema as well as elevated laboratory values may lead to a misdiagnosis of osteomyelitis.

Additional imaging studies should be obtained because plain radiographs may appear deceptively normal. Lesions with a small, round, blue-cell histologic appearance may permeate through marrow as they grow, and obvious bone destruction may not be apparent until the lesion is more advanced. Findings of Ewing sarcoma on plain radiographs, if any, will consist of purely osteolytic bone destruction that is poorly marginated and permeative. In patients with a Ewing sarcoma that is more advanced, plain radiographs will reveal a periosteal reaction with a layered or onion-skin elevation (**Figure 5**). The diaphysis of long bones (femur, tibia, humerus) and the flat bones, such as the pelvis and scapula, are the most common skeletal locations of Ewing sarcoma. Patients with Ewing sarcoma often have a large soft-tissue mass that is not proportional with its innocuous appearance on plain radiographs; therefore, MRIs must be obtained to delineate the extent of marrow and surrounding tissue involvement. The differential diagnosis for Ewing sarcoma includes osteomyelitis, lymphoma, osteoid osteoma, Langerhans cell histiocytosis, and, occasionally, osteosarcoma.

Patients with a clinical and radiographic evaluation that indicates Ewing sarcoma should undergo a biopsy to confirm a diagnosis of Ewing sarcoma. The biopsy can be performed as an image-guided needle biopsy or a surgical open incisional biopsy. Given

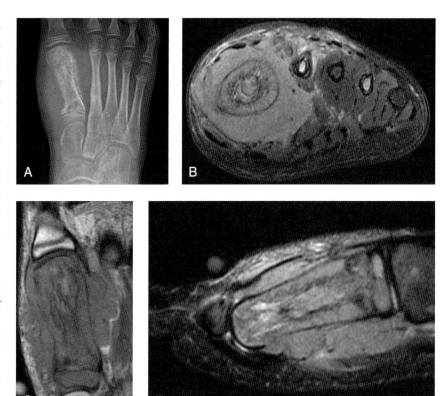

Figure 5   Images of the right first metatarsal of a patient show a Ewing sarcoma. **A,** AP radiograph demonstrates a permeative osteolytic lesion. Note the layered periosteal elevation of the entire diaphysis of the first metatarsal. Axial short tau inversion recovery (**B**), coronal T1-weighted (**C**), and sagittal short tau inversion recovery (**D**) MRIs show a circumferential mass around the first metatarsal. This mass is consistent with the appearance of a Ewing sarcoma, which is a small, round cell lesion.

that the symptoms of Ewing sarcoma and infection are similar, biopsied tissue should always be sent for both culture and pathologic review. The gross pathologic appearance of Ewing sarcoma may be of an almost liquid consistency, which mimics that of infection. The histologic analysis of a Ewing sarcoma will reveal a monotonous pattern of small, round, blue cells with round or oval nuclei. Prominent nucleoli and minimal cytoplasm will be present in each cell. The light microscopy findings of a Ewing sarcoma may be similar to those of lymphoma, osteomyelitis, alveolar rhabdomyosarcoma, neuroblastoma, or Langerhans cell histiocytosis.

The development of molecular testing for the 11;22 chromosomal translocation has allowed pathologists to accurately differentiate Ewing sarcoma from lesions that have a similar morphology.

Patients in whom Ewing sarcoma is diagnosed are treated with systemic chemotherapy followed by local control of the primary lesion, after which they are treated with additional chemotherapy.[20] Similar to children in the United States with osteosarcoma, most children in the United States who have Ewing sarcoma are treated under national protocols, which ensure standardized care and faster analysis of new drug regimens. The standard six-drug chemotherapy regimen for patients with Ewing sarcoma includes vincristine, doxorubicin, ifosfamide, etoposide, cytoxan, and actinomycin D. Local control of the primary lesion can be achieved via surgical resection or external beam radiation. Because of the side effects of high-dose radiation in younger children, which include growth disturbance, fibrosis, fracture, and secondary malignancy, most patients with a resectable and/or localized Ewing sarcoma undergo surgical resection. Often, patients with metastatic Ewing sarcoma or a primary site of Ewing sarcoma that would be difficult to resect with acceptable margins or would result in substantial morbidity undergo radiation. The reconstruction options for patients with Ewing sarcoma are similar to those for patients with osteosarcoma.

The overall survival rate for patients with Ewing sarcoma has not substantially changed in the past 25 years and is approximately 70% at 5 years postoperatively for patients with Ewing sarcoma that is isolated to an extremity. Patients with Ewing sarcoma of the pelvis or metastatic Ewing sarcoma have a lower overall survival rate. The amount of tumor necrosis observed in the primary lesion at the time of surgical resection (after neoadjuvant chemotherapy) is predictive of prognosis. The most common site of Ewing sarcoma metastasis is the lungs, with Ewing sarcoma metastasis to the bone or bone marrow indicating a worse prognosis.

Chondrosarcoma

Chondrosarcoma is the most common primary malignant bone lesion in adults. Chondrosarcoma is slightly more common in males. Typically, chondrosarcoma occurs in patients aged 40 to 75 years. Not enough information is known about the specific genetic abnormalities or targets for treatment in patients with chondrosarcoma; however, alterations in the *IHH/PTHrP* and *IDH1/IDH2* pathways have been identified in patients with chondrosarcoma. Many of the IDH mutations are functional and associated with epigenetic dysregulation of genes.[21] Mutations in the *EXT1* and *EXT2* genes have been observed in patients with MHE, which is a benign syndrome that predisposes patients to secondary chondrosarcoma.

Clinical symptoms common in patients with chondrosarcoma include pain and a slow-growing, firm mass. Depending on the location of a chondrosarcoma, patients may have bowel or bladder symptoms. Chondrosarcomas vary in grade; therefore, the rate of growth of a chondrosarcoma determines the timeframe of symptoms. Most chondrosarcomas are low grade and grow slowly, which may delay an accurate diagnosis. The pelvis, the proximal femur, the scapula, and the proximal humerus are the most common skeletal locations of chondrosarcoma. Chondrosarcoma can occur in the intramedullary aspect of a bone or on the surface of a bone. Chondrosarcoma may be primary or secondary to a preexisting enchondroma or osteochondroma (**Figure 6**). The benign preexisting lesion may be solitary or associated with multiple osteochondromas (eg, MHE) or enchondromas (eg, Ollier disease or Maffucci syndrome). Chondrosarcoma that originates from a solitary enchondroma or osteochondroma is extraordinarily rare and is indicated by a gradual increase in pain of a prolonged duration and/or slow, continued growth of an osteochondroma. Chondrosarcoma that is associated with multiple osteochondromas or enchondromas is more common, occurring in 1% to 10% of patients with MHE, 25% to 40% of patients with Ollier disease, and as many as 100% (including visceral malignancies) of patients with Maffucci syndrome.

Radiographs of a chondrosarcoma vary depending on the location and the grade of the lesion. A low-grade, intramedullary chondrosarcoma may appear similar to an enchondroma but will demonstrate extensive endosteal erosion/scalloping and/or cortical thickening. Typically, chondrosarcomas have mineralized (calcified) cartilage in the lesion with a ring-, arc-, or stipple-like appearance. By the time of diagnosis, a low-grade chondrosarcoma of the pelvis usually will have an extraosseous component. The soft-tissue mass may be quite large (>10 cm) and exert pressure along surrounding visceral or neurovascular structures. An intermediate or high-grade chondrosarcoma is less well defined compared with a low-grade chondrosarcoma, with obvious cortical destruction and a soft-tissue mass observed on imaging studies. Calcifications may be present in the soft-tissue mass. Secondary chondrosarcoma results from a preexisting enchondroma or osteochondroma, which often can be observed on radiographs. A dedifferentiated chondrosarcoma is a rare variant in which a high-grade sarcoma is located adjacent to a benign or low-grade malignant cartilage tumor. The zone of transition between the two types of tissue is sharply defined, with the high-grade sarcoma being a destructive osteolytic lesion. Advanced imaging modalities, such as CT or MRI, can help define marrow and soft-tissue involvement, especially in patients with chondrosarcoma of the pelvis.

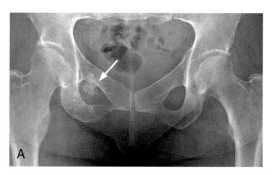 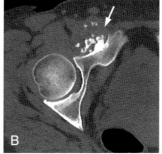 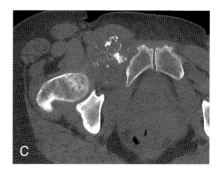

Figure 6   Images of the pelvis of a 61-year-old woman with multiple hereditary exostoses. **A,** AP radiograph demonstrates an enlarged painful mass (arrow) emanating from the right superior pubic ramus. **B** and **C,** Axial CT scans demonstrate a surface lesion with punctate calcification (arrow in panel **B**) within a surrounding soft-tissue mass, which is consistent with a chondrosarcoma secondary to an osteochondroma.

A needle biopsy is not required for patients in whom a low-grade chondrosarcoma is suspected. Diagnosis of chondrosarcoma is primarily radiographic, and the difference between an enchondroma and a low-grade chondrosarcoma may be difficult to observe based on the small amount of tissue obtained from a needle biopsy. Low-grade chondrosarcomas are grossly lobular, whereas high-grade chondrosarcomas have more myxoid areas. The histologic appearance of a chondrosarcoma will vary depending on the grade of the lesion. The histologic analysis of a low-grade chondrosarcoma will reveal a bland appearance; however, tumor cells will permeate and entrap the existing bony trabeculae. The histologic analysis of a high-grade chondrosarcoma will reveal a more hypercellular appearance, with binucleate cells and, occasionally, myxoid areas.

Because systemic chemotherapy, targeted treatments, and radiation therapy are not effective for the management of chondrosarcoma, most patients with chondrosarcoma undergo surgical resection alone.[22] Some controversy exists with regard to the extent of surgical resection required in patients with low-grade chondrosarcoma of an extremity, with some studies advocating careful intralesional curettage and other studies advocating wide resection. However, most surgeons acknowledge that patients with chondrosarcoma of the pelvis, regardless of the grade of the lesion, require wide resection.[23] Patients with intermediate or high-grade chondrosarcoma require wide resection.

The local recurrence rate of chondrosarcoma varies depending on the grade of the lesion, the margins of the original surgery, and the location of the lesion. The local recurrence rate of chondrosarcoma in patients with chondrosarcoma of the pelvis who undergo resection is approximately 15% to 20%. Repeated local recurrence of chondrosarcoma is associated with an increase in the grade and the aggressiveness of the lesion. The likelihood of chondrosarcoma metastasis and, subsequently, overall survival is correlated with the grade of the lesion. Chondrosarcoma progresses slowly; therefore, patients who undergo treatment for chondrosarcoma should be monitored for as long as 20 years postoperatively. The lungs are the most common site of chondrosarcoma metastasis, which is managed with the use of a thoracotomy. The overall 10-year survival rate for patients with chondrosarcoma is approximately 90% for patients with grade 1 chondrosarcoma, 60% to 70% for patients with grade 2 chondrosarcoma, and 30% to 50% for patients with grade 3 chondrosarcoma. Despite the use of chemotherapy, the 10-year survival rate for patients with dedifferentiated chondrosarcoma is less than 10%.

Summary

A thorough understanding of the clinical and radiographic appearance of bone lesions will allow surgeons to accurately diagnose and manage metabolic bone disease, benign bone lesions, and malignant bone lesions. Most bone lesions, especially those that occur in children, are benign and discovered incidentally. Most benign bone lesions are managed with observation because many resolve near or after a patient reaches skeletal maturity. Patients with aggressive benign bone lesions, such as giant cell tumor or chondroblastoma, require surgical treatment, which usually consists of intralesional curettage, to achieve local control of the lesion. Patients with malignant bone lesions require wide surgical resection. Malignant bone lesions that are common in children, such as osteosarcoma and

Ewing sarcoma, also are managed with systemic chemotherapy to increase a patient's likelihood of survival. Chondrosarcoma, which is primarily observed in adults, is managed with wide surgical resection alone.

References

1. Miller TT: Bone tumors and tumorlike conditions: Analysis with conventional radiography. *Radiology* 2008;246(3):662-674.

2. Marcus R: Diagnosis and treatment of hyperparathyroidism. *Rev Endocr Metab Disord* 2000;1(4):247-252.

3. Cohen-Solal M, Sebert JL: Renal osteodystrophy and hypercalcemia. *Curr Opin Rheumatol* 1993;5(3):357-362.

4. Zhang R, Alper B, Simon E, Florman S, Slakey D: Management of metabolic bone disease in kidney transplant recipients. *Am J Med Sci* 2008;335(2):120-125.

5. Rosenthal DI, Hornicek FJ, Torriani M, Gebhardt MC, Mankin HJ: Osteoid osteoma: Percutaneous treatment with radiofrequency energy. *Radiology* 2003;229(1):171-175.

6. Leet AI, Boyce AM, Ibrahim KA, Wientroub S, Kushner H, Collins MT: Bone-grafting in polyostotic fibrous dysplasia. *J Bone Joint Surg Am* 2016;98(3):211-219.

7. Pedrini E, Jennes I, Tremosini M, et al: Genotype-phenotype correlation study in 529 patients with multiple hereditary exostoses: Identification of "protective" and "risk" factors. *J Bone Joint Surg Am* 2011;93(24):2294-2302.

8. Hong ED, Carrino JA, Weber KL, Fayad LM: Prevalence of shoulder enchondromas on routine MR imaging. *Clin Imaging* 2011;35(5):378-384.

9. Wilson RJ, Zumsteg JW, Hartley KA, et al: Overutilization and cost of advanced imaging for long-bone cartilaginous lesions. *Ann Surg Oncol* 2015;22(11):3466-3473.

10. Söder S, Oliveira AM, Inwards CY, Müller S, Aigner T: Type II collagen, but not aggrecan expression, distinguishes clear cell chondrosarcoma and chondroblastoma. *Pathology* 2006;38(1):35-38.

11. De Mattos CB, Angsanuntsukh C, Arkader A, Dormans JP: Chondroblastoma and chondromyxoid fibroma. *J Am Acad Orthop Surg* 2013;21(4):225-233.

12. Pretell-Mazzini J, Murphy RF, Kushare I, Dormans JP: Unicameral bone cysts: General characteristics and management controversies. *J Am Acad Orthop Surg* 2014;22(5):295-303.

13. Oliveira AM, Hsi BL, Weremowicz S, et al: USP6 (Tre2) fusion oncogenes in aneurysmal bone cyst. *Cancer Res* 2004;64(6):1920-1923.

14. Thomas D, Henshaw R, Skubitz K, et al: Denosumab in patients with giant-cell tumour of bone: An open-label, phase 2 study. *Lancet Oncol* 2010;11(3):275-280.

15. DiCaprio MR, Roberts TT: Diagnosis and management of langerhans cell histiocytosis. *J Am Acad Orthop Surg* 2014;22(10):643-652.

16. Siegel RL, Miller KD, Jemal A: Cancer statistics, 2016. *CA Cancer J Clin* 2016;66(1):7-30.

17. Widhe B, Widhe T: Initial symptoms and clinical features in osteosarcoma and Ewing sarcoma. *J Bone Joint Surg Am* 2000;82(5):667-674.

18. Isakoff MS, Bielack SS, Meltzer P, Gorlick R: Osteosarcoma: Current treatment and a collaborative pathway to success. *J Clin Oncol* 2015;33(27):3029-3035.

19. Rougraff BT, Simon MA, Kneisl JS, Greenberg DB, Mankin HJ: Limb salvage compared with amputation for osteosarcoma of the distal end of the femur: A long-term oncological, functional, and quality-of-life study. *J Bone Joint Surg Am* 1994;76(5):649-656.

20. Gaspar N, Hawkins DS, Dirksen U, et al: Ewing sarcoma: Current management and future approaches through collaboration. *J Clin Oncol* 2015;33(27):3036-3046.

21. Samuel AM, Costa J, Lindskog DM: Genetic alterations in chondrosarcomas - keys to targeted therapies? *Cell Oncol (Dordr)* 2014;37(2):95-105.

22. Lee FY, Mankin HJ, Fondren G, et al: Chondrosarcoma of bone: An assessment of outcome. *J Bone Joint Surg Am* 1999;81(3):326-338.

23. Pring ME, Weber KL, Unni KK, Sim FH: Chondrosarcoma of the pelvis: A review of sixty-four cases. *J Bone Joint Surg Am* 2001;83(11):1630-1642.

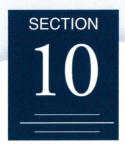

SECTION

10

The Practice of Orthopaedics

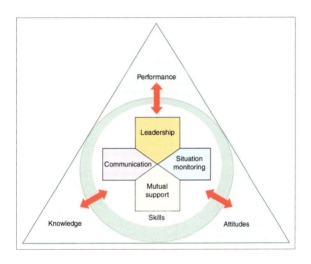

Implementation of TeamSTEPPS in Orthopaedic Surgery

Harpal S. Khanuja, MD
Zan A. Naseer, BS
Lynne C. Jones, PhD
James R. Ficke, MD, FACS
Dwight W. Burney III, MD

Abstract

An Institute of Medicine report published in 2000 brought attention to the devastating consequences of medical errors. The report estimated that 98,000 deaths occurred in US hospitals each year as a result of medical errors and spawned investigations into factors that are associated with medical errors as well as strategies to avoid them. Taking cues from high-reliability organizations, such as the airline industry, evidence-based tools were developed to minimize human risk factors and foster teamwork, communication, and other skills that are essential to patient safety and quality. Orthopaedic surgeons are in a unique position to advocate for patients and to lead healthcare teams through the cultural changes that are necessary to avoid harm and improve outcomes. The American Academy of Orthopaedic Surgeons has made a commitment to educate interdisciplinary healthcare teams and uses TeamSTEPPS to educate orthopaedic surgeons on the knowledge, skills, and attitudes that are necessary to develop teamwork and improve patient safety and the quality of care. Orthopaedic surgeons should understand the need for improved teamwork and the resources that are available to shape the cultural changes that are necessary to avoid harm and improve outcomes.

Instr Course Lect 2017;66:635–645.

The Institute of Medicine's (IOM's) report *To Err is Human* brought attention to the issue of medical errors.[1] The IOM's estimate of 98,000 deaths per year as a result of medical errors led to a patient safety movement that is focused on enhancing medical care in the United States. Subsequent studies reported that the number of deaths per year in the IOM's report was likely underestimated and may be closer to 400,000 preventable premature deaths per year.[2] These estimates do not include near-misses, many of which may go unreported. The IOM recommended a move in health care toward the principles practiced by high-reliability organizations, which are institutions that operate in highly complex and hazardous environments that have the potential to cause serious harm but only report a few errors over long periods of time.[3] Examples of high-reliability organizations include the airline industry, the nuclear industry, and the armed forces. Enhanced teamwork, communication, and leadership are essential for high-reliability organizations.[3] The IOM recommended that interdisciplinary team training programs be established to decrease the number of medical errors. Communication errors have been recognized as one of the most common causes of errors in orthopaedics, second only to equipment errors (24.7% and 29%, respectively).[4]

In response to the IOM's recommendation, the Agency for Healthcare Research and Quality and the Department of Defense developed an evidence-based program to enhance communication and team dynamics: Team Strategies and Tools to Enhance Performance and Patient Safety (TeamSTEPPS). In 2012, the American Academy of Orthopaedic Surgeons Board of Directors provided funding for TeamSTEPPS training to orthopaedic surgeons so they could set an example and serve as leaders for team performance and patient safety. The main goal of TeamSTEPPS is to develop the knowledge, skills, and attitudes of all of the individuals of a team so that the team can work more effectively and efficiently. TeamSTEPPS requires not only interdisciplinary team training but also administrative support and strong leadership. Orthopaedic surgeons can use TeamSTEPPS to lead and facilitate the cultural changes necessary to avoid harm and improve outcomes.

The TeamSTEPPS curriculum focuses on four skills: communication, leadership, situation monitoring, and mutual support (**Figure 1**). Establishing a team in a healthcare setting that includes individuals who have diverse backgrounds and roles is not intuitive. If team members are taught skills that are reinforced regularly, they will have the knowledge and attitude to enhance performance.

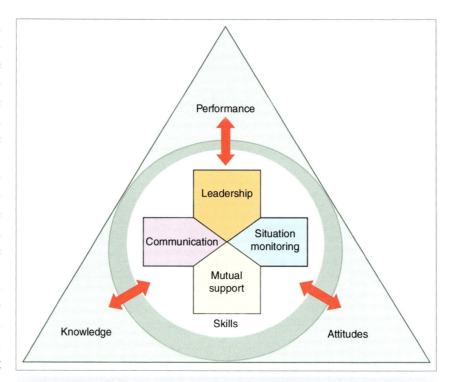

Figure 1 Diagram shows the TeamSTEPPS core patient-care team skills, which include communication, leadership, situation monitoring, and mutual support. With these skills, patient-care team members can develop the knowledge, attitudes, and performance attributes necessary to ensure patient safety. (Adapted with permission from TeamSTEPPS: Strategies and Tools to Enhance Performance and Patient Safety. Rockville, MD, the Agency for Healthcare Research and Quality, March 2016. http://www.ahrq.gov/professionals/education/curriculum-tools/teamstepps/index.html.)

TeamSTEPPS

The Team

A team is defined as two or more individuals who are working toward a common goal. In orthopaedics, there are multiple teams that include individuals who have different roles and areas of expertise, which is further complicated by multiple specialties, inconsistent team members, and, occasionally, personalities and egos that hinder positive team dynamics. In a healthcare setting, a team is defined as "two or more people who interact dynamically, interdependently, and adaptively toward a common and valued goal, have specific roles or functions, and have a time-limited membership."[5] The goal in a healthcare setting is to move health care from a "team of experts to an expert team."[6] Expert teams provide not only exceptional medical treatment but also have been trained in teamwork skills.[6] The optimal delivery of health care requires complete coordination between all providers. For example, in the operating room, the surgical, anesthesia, and nursing teams should be regarded not as independent entities but members who work interdependently with the common goal of a safe, effective, and efficient procedure. The entire medical and administrative teams as well as a patient's family are responsible for the care of a patient. A healthcare team is composed of all of the individuals who interact with a patient to provide care.[7]

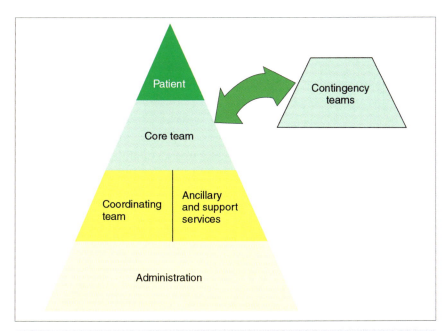

Figure 2 Diagram shows the TeamSTEPPS multisystem team, which is composed of a patient, a core team, contingency teams, a coordinating team, ancillary and support services, and administration. Each team functions independently but also collectively to ensure patient safety. (Adapted with permission from TeamSTEPPS: Strategies and Tools to Enhance Performance and Patient Safety. Rockville, MD, the Agency for Healthcare Research and Quality, March 2016. http://www.ahrq.gov/professionals/education/curriculum-tools/teamstepps/index.html.)

Team Structure and Function

A team is greater than the sum of its parts. Team synergy is influenced by leadership, cooperation, coordination, communication, and the situational awareness of each of the team members.[8,9] Team members must identify as a team and must have shared goals and mutual trust, both of which are established and maintained by team leadership. A team structure is determined by the number of team members as well as the role and expertise of each team member. Team dynamics may be different in small teams compared with large teams. For example, certain patients may require two or more attending surgeons. In this situation, it is important to determine which surgeon is taking the leadership role for the team. Larger teams can be affected by multiple distractions because different activities are coordinated simultaneously. In smaller teams, familiarity may be an advantage or disadvantage, depending on team dynamics. Each team member has a different skill set, knowledge, and experience. Each team member can perform interdependent tasks and function in a role that reflects their specific area of expertise yet still share the common goals of quality care and safety to ensure a successful patient outcome.[7,8]

Teamwork can be taught, encouraged, and rewarded; however, this rarely happens in a healthcare setting. The underlying philosophy of TeamSTEPPS is that patient care and safety necessitates that a team, including the patient and his or her support system, share a common goal for the care of the patient.

TeamSTEPPS can have a positive effect on the safety and outcome of the patient as well as team productivity.[10,11]

Multiteam System

Involvement of multiple teams is necessary to effectively care for patients. TeamSTEPPS consists of a multiteam system,[5] which involves several teams that work both independently and collaboratively to optimize the overall quality of care. The multiteam system is composed of a patient, a core team, contingency teams, a coordinating team, ancillary and support services, and administration[5] (**Figure 2**). The core team consists of all of the providers and staff who are directly responsible for the care of a patient. In the operating room, this may be the orthopaedic surgeons, scrub technician, circulating nurse, and anesthesiologist. The core team can be temporarily replaced with a contingency team, such as a rapid response team, in situations that require urgent treatment. The coordinating team consists of team members who are responsible for anticipating potential obstacles, providing resources, and creating an efficient workplace to support the core team. Ancillary and support services provide focused services that contribute to the "efficient, safe, comfortable, and clean healthcare environments, which affect the patient-care team, market perception, operational efficiency, and patient safety."[5] Administration fosters accountability and creates a patient safety culture for all teams that are responsible for the care of a patient.

Communication

The Joint Commission[12] identified breakdowns in communication as the third most common cause of failure in sentinel events. Communication, which must be bidirectional, is defined as "the process whereby information is clearly and accurately conveyed to another person using a method that is known and recognized by all involved. It includes the ability to ask questions, seek clarification, and acknowledge the message was received and understood."[5] The creation of an environment that allows questions to be asked and the comprehension of a message to be acknowledged is essential; it is the role of the team leader to establish this environment. Real or perceived hierarchies and poor team dynamics hinder effective communication. Effective communication is essential not only among providers but also between providers and the patient and his or her family, who must be given clear, concise, and comprehensible information so that informed decisions can be made.

Standards of Effective Communication

Effective communication between team members, including patients, is based on four fundamental principles: information must be complete, clear, brief, and timely. A balance must be maintained between providing an individual with enough yet not too much information.

Challenges to Communication

The recognition of challenges to communication, including language barriers, intense workloads, personality conflicts, lack of verified information, and communication style, is important.[5] Several strategies can be used to overcome these challenges to communication. Understanding the audience when relaying information is essential. The detail, quantity, and complexity of information

relayed should depend on each team member's level of involvement and understanding; being cognizant of this can lead to a more efficient and productive patient safety culture. The SBAR technique, the call-out technique, the check-back technique, and the IPASS handoff strategy are tools that are available to enhance communication.

SBAR Technique

The SBAR technique is a standardized framework used to efficiently communicate a patient's condition. For example, if information on a patient's newly developing symptoms needs to be relayed to a specific provider, a team member should first introduce the situation by providing a brief description of the event and its urgency. A concise and relevant medical background should be stated. The team member should then express his or her assessment and recommend a specific management plan. The SBAR acronym stands for situation (What is going on with the patient?); background (What is the clinical background or context?); assessment (What do I think the problem is?); and recommendation and request (What would I do to correct it?).[5]

The SBAR technique provides standardized principles for the communication of key information. These principles are flexible and can be individualized to a particular setting, the needs of each team, and each patient. The ultimate goal of the SBAR technique is to ensure that a reliable system for the exchange of information and ideas is available.

Call-Out Technique

A call-out technique is used to simultaneously relay urgent information to all team members, typically in an

emergency. The call-out technique is particularly effective in trauma settings, in which the timely distribution of important patient information, such as vital signs, breath sounds, and wound locations, is key. The call-out technique can be used in other settings, including the operating room. The call-out technique requires a team member to assume a leadership role and become responsible for the clear and firm communication of all information that is relevant to a situation. Any team member can perform the callout, which helps the team refocus to pertinent relevant information and anticipate future direction.

Check-Back Technique

The check-back technique is a closed-loop strategy in which a sender initiates a message; a recipient accepts the message and provides relevant feedback; and the sender confirms appropriate receipt of the message and acknowledges feedback. The check-back technique can prevent the misinterpretation of information between team members and can help clarify patient information, treatment plans, and goals. Although the check-back technique may seem redundant, it is an easy and simple verification tool (**Figure 3**).

IPASS Handoff Strategy

The handoff represents the period of time in the treatment of a patient in which care is transferred between team members. Both information and overall responsibility are transferred. Team members are responsible for fully informing their colleagues of potential plans and medical information with regard to a patient. The handoff transition point is vital. Lapses in efficient communication may result in substantial errors and harm.

The handoff period can provide staff, including physicians, nurses, and administrators, an opportunity to ask questions as well as confirm, clarify, and organize treatment plans. Several techniques to create structured handoffs are available. The IPASS acronym, which stands for introduction (introduce yourself and role/job [include patient]); patient (identify patient name, age, sex, location); assessment (present chief complaint, vital signs, symptoms, and diagnosis); situation (explain patient's current status/circumstances, including code status, level of [un]certainty, recurrent changes, and response to treatment); and safety (explain critical laboratory values/reports, socioeconomic factors, allergies, and alerts [falls, isolation, etc.]),[13] is one type of handoff strategy. Starmer et al[13] implemented the IPASS handoff strategy in nine pediatric residency programs. The authors reported that the use of the IPASS handoff strategy was associated with a statistically significant reduction in medical errors (24.5 errors versus 18.8 errors per 100 admissions).[13]

Keep the Patient Involved

Patients may be unintentionally excluded from important conversations about their care. Effective medical care is centered on the patient. Orthopaedic surgeons and the entire medical team should create an environment that is conducive to effective communication with patients. Often, patients are shy, intimidated, and nervous in a medical setting. Patients may not always ask questions or seek advice. Information on diagnosis and treatment plans may be communicated to patients haphazardly. Patients may not remember or comprehend the complexities of their condition or the goals of their treatment

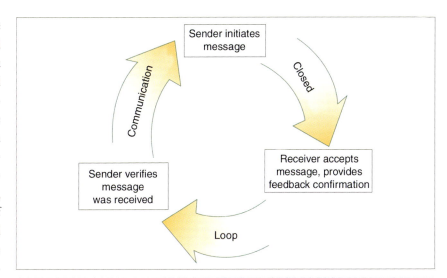

Figure 3   Diagram shows the TeamSTEPPS check-back technique, which is a closed-loop communication strategy that is used to verify and validate the exchange of information. (Adapted with permission from TeamSTEPPS: Strategies and Tools to Enhance Performance and Patient Safety. Rockville, MD, the Agency for Healthcare Research and Quality, March 2016. http://www.ahrq.gov/professionals/education/curriculum-tools/teamstepps/index.html.)

plan. Ineffective communication is often responsible for poor patient understanding and satisfaction. Ineffective communication can be overcome by articulating information to patients in simple, layperson terms. Medical jargon and assumptions on a patient's education level should be avoided. Asking patients if they have questions or are unclear on certain topics helps enhance the patient-provider relationship. Use of the check-back technique helps ensure that each patient is able to rearticulate his or her condition and treatment goals.

Leadership

Orthopaedic leaders are individuals who support the focus and success of their staff as well as take primary action and make key decisions with regard to a patient's treatment plan. Leadership is defined as the ability to motivate team members to work collectively to establish a common goal. In the operating room, orthopaedic surgeons maintain

the leadership role; however, effective leadership is only accomplished if orthopaedic surgeons create an environment that is conducive to feedback and encourages all team members to participate in the sharing of information.[14] Frequently, because of stress and/or complexities associated with a patient, the operating room environment may discourage effective communication. In these situations, orthopaedic surgeons must exhibit leadership qualities, including conflict resolution, the assignment of responsibilities, and the articulation of clear goals. A team leader must facilitate the flow of information; maintain team roles and responsibilities; ensure that expectations are met; motivate all team members, including himself/herself, to be involved in patient care; resolve conflicts; and provide constructive feedback.

It also is important to acknowledge designated and situational team leaders. Situational team leaders are those who are best equipped to lead a specific task. For example, although an orthopaedic surgeon may be the designated team leader for an orthopaedic case, an anesthesiologist is the situational team leader for the induction of anesthesia. TeamSTEPPS provides orthopaedic surgeons with several skills that are beneficial to leading a team and creating a synergistic and efficient team environment.

Defining the Plan

Achor and Ahn[15] reported that an orthopaedic surgeon needs to be a leader of the team in the operating room. The authors suggested that a strong leader maintains the confidence and trust of each team member; therefore, each team member feels comfortable bringing up observations and issues that could affect patient safety, which may be difficult in tense situations. Often, a surgeon will become frustrated if a particular surgical instrument is not available; an argument and/or outburst at this time may be extremely demoralizing and disadvantageous for the team dynamic.[15] As a leader of the operating room, the orthopaedic surgeon should acknowledge that no single team member is at fault in a particular situation. Orthopaedic surgeons should ensure that all team members are prepared preoperatively and account for all materials and instruments before surgery begins. This preoperative check sets expectations among team members and ensures that everyone is in agreement.[15]

Brief, Huddle, Debrief

A brief is a short meeting that is held for planning purposes. Briefs are meant to be concise (3 to 5 minutes) and include a discussion of action items and essential patient information. Information such as diagnosis, treatment plans, goals, and potential barriers also are discussed. A good brief before surgery includes identifying the individuals who will be in the room and their roles and responsibilities, understanding and agreeing on the goals of the surgery, and ensuring proper equipment is present. A discussion on the possible outcomes, the potential challenges, and the availability of additional resources that may be necessary (contingency strategies) is essential. A brief is not a timeout. A brief should be held before surgery to establish the appropriate environment and availability of expertise and resources.

A huddle is an ad hoc assessment and meeting that is held to re-establish goals and responsibilities as well as address specific issues that may have arisen during surgery.[5] In the operating room, a huddle may be held if there is a change in the procedure and the team needs to regroup and reallocate resources and responsibility. A huddle is appropriate if an intraoperative complication (surgical or medical) occurs.

A debrief is a meeting that is held after surgery, at which team members can ask for feedback and discuss strengths and weaknesses with the team leader. A debrief should begin with a discussion about what went well. A good debrief then identifies specific issues that should be addressed to improve patient safety in subsequent surgeries. These three team events (brief, huddle, and debrief) are not limited to use in the operating room and can be used throughout the day to reinforce the short-term and long-term goals that orthopaedic surgeons have for patients.[5]

Conflict Resolution and Modeling Teamwork

In any team, team members may not always be compatible, and conflicts may arise. These conflicts may be the result of differences in knowledge base, personalities, and work approach. Quick resolution of conflicts is essential to maintain the safe delivery of patient care. The team leader is responsible for facilitating mutual agreements and teaching team members strategies to resolve future conflicts. Furthermore, orthopaedic surgeons should become model team members by openly sharing information, providing constructive feedback, and facilitating the team dynamic.

Situation Monitoring/ Awareness

Situation monitoring is "the process of gaining and maintaining an understanding of what's going on around you."[5] Situation monitoring is an individual cognitive skill and a continual process. Similar to the way in which drivers continually scan the environment through their windshield, team members should scan the environment and share their perceptions to facilitate the formulation of a team's shared mental model.

Environmental signals must be perceived first and then comprehended. After comprehension is accomplished, likely scenarios can be forecasted.[16] Frequently, environmental signals are weak or ambiguous and, thus, are at risk for misinterpretation. If team members' perceptions of the environment are compared and frequently updated, the team's shared mental model (ie, collective comprehension) is strengthened (the wisdom of crowds), maintained, and updated and is more likely to accurately reflect the actual situation at any given time.

Surgery is a complex adaptive sociotechnical system and depends on the adaptability and ingenuity of humans to resolve emerging conditions that threaten patient safety. Even with safety processes and technology in place, only humans can understand emerging threats. In high-reliability organizations, situation monitoring is supported by the following characteristic ways of thinking: preoccupation with failure (accepting that human error is unavoidable); reluctance to simplify (not accepting the first likely explanation for an emerging situation); sensitivity to operations (understanding that actions have unpredictable reactions in complex systems); deference to expertise (ceding authority to the team member most qualified to manage the situation); and commitment to resilience (the organization's ability to function despite disruptive events or situations).

The evolution of crew resource management has led to the concept of "threat and error management" (**Figure 4**). Threats (factors with the potential to cause patient harm or an undesired patient state) are detected via situation monitoring (perception, comprehension, and forecasting, in the shared mental model), which leads to strategies for management. If human errors occur, resistance involves system defenses (alarms, checklists, standard operating procedures), but error resolution requires human intelligence and teamwork skills.[17] Constant monitoring, updating, and communicating of a situation allows self-organization in shifting situations.

Situation monitoring occurs at an individual team member level and at a team level. Another aspect of situation monitoring is cross monitoring, which involves assessing other team members' work and how that work

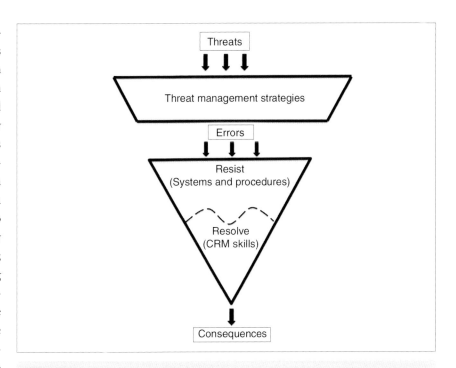

Figure 4   Diagram shows the concept of "threat and error management," which describes the relationship between threats, errors, and consequences. (Adapted with permission from the Australian Transport Safety Bureau: ATSB Transport Safety Report: Aviation Research & Analysis – AR-2006-156(2) Final. Perceived threats, errors and safety in aerial work and low capacity air transport operations. Canberra, Australian Capital Territory, Australia, Australian Transport Safety Bureau, 2009. https://www.atsb.gov.au/media/4182928/ar2006156.pdf.)

affects the team's progress. Cross monitoring is a natural part of the environmental scanning process. Barriers to cross monitoring include complacency, workload imbalance, and distractions. Task fixation or overload as well as underutilization or boredom can weaken the individual environmental scanning process. The communication style of a designated team leader (the orthopaedic surgeon) has a major effect on the team members' information exchange and, thus, the formulation of a team's shared mental model. In the operating room, orthopaedic surgeons communicate in an authoritative manner, which discourages team members from sharing their views and inhibits the formulation of the complex shared mental model that is necessary to ensure

optimal team efficiency.[18] For individual team members, the I'M SAFE acronym, which stands for illness; medication; stress; alcohol and drugs; fatigue; and eating and elimination, identifies potential causes of impaired function in a team member.

Team members also must realistically assess their own capacity and ability to perform. The STEP acronym, which stands for status of the patient (patient history, vital signs, medications, physical examination, plan of care, psychosocial issues); team members (fatigue, workload, task performance, skill, stress); environment (facility information, administrative information, human resources, triage acuity, equipment); and progress toward goal (status of team's patient[s], established goals of team, tasks/actions of team, plan still appropriate), helps identify potential causes of impaired function in the team as a whole.

Cross monitoring is a critical component of high functioning teams because it provides the team with a safety net that helps identify errors or oversights more quickly. Cross monitoring is not micromanagement but a way for team members to look out for one another. Situation monitoring is critical to achieve desired team outcomes, mutual trust, adaptability, shared mental models, and a team orientation. In addition, sense-making and self-organization are impossible to achieve without effective situation monitoring and information exchange.[19]

Mutual Support

Mutual support offers teams a tool kit to help them become high functioning, highly reliable, and resilient. Given that surgery is, perhaps, the ultimate team sport, these strategies and tools involve coaching and performance improvement as well as the collective sense-making and mindful organization that characterizes highly effective, resilient teams.[20] Mutual support among team members provides a high degree of psychologic safety.

Task Assistance

Task assistance, which involves providing task-related support and assistance, is an excellent example of mindful organization. Cross monitoring is an ongoing assessment of how team members are progressing toward task completion and goals. A strong team orientation exists if team members protect each other from work overload, expect each other to actively seek and offer assistance, and consider all offers and requests in the context of a patient's best interest (ie, patient safety).

Feedback

Feedback is information provided to team members to improve a team's performance. Feedback is a critique that involves a careful judgment in which an opinion is given on the positive and negative aspects of something and should be considered coaching because it is given with the intent of personal and team performance improvement. Wallace and Trinka[21] believe that "feedback is a gift" and that "ideas are the currency of our next success." Feedback must be considerate. The feedback sandwich (a positive comment followed by the need for specific performance improvement/behavior change followed by a positive comment) is respectful and considerate of the feelings of team members. Feedback also must be timely, given shortly after the behavior in question has occurred, and directed at a specific task or behavior.

Advocacy and Assertion

Advocacy and assertion are always undertaken in a patient's interest. In situations in which the viewpoints of team members do not coincide with those of the team leader, effective team members can assert a corrective action by making an opening (addressing the team leader by name), stating the concern, stating the problem (real or perceived), offering a solution (framed in terms of teamwork and patient safety), and reaching an agreement on the next steps.

The Two-Challenge Rule

The two-challenge rule empowers all team members to "stop the line" if they suspect or discover a safety breach. The two-challenge rule counters the tendency to use mitigated speech (the so-called "hint and hope")[22] by making information clear and unambiguous. A team member is responsible for assertively voicing concern at least two times to make sure that it is heard. The team member being challenged must acknowledge that the concern has been heard. If the safety issue is not addressed, the challenging member is responsible for moving the concern up the chain of command. Assertive statements should follow the CUS acronym, which stands for "I am concerned!"; "I am uncomfortable!"; "This is a safety issue!"; and "Stop the line!"

Interpersonal conflict in teams is inevitable; however, effective resolution techniques must be used to avoid the degradation of team function. Typical human reactions to interpersonal conflict (avoidance, deference, preservation of professional relationships) are inappropriate because the best interests of a patient are not the highest priority. The DESC acronym, which stands for describe the specific situation or behavior, provide concrete data; express how the situation makes you feel/what your concerns are; suggest other alternatives and seek agreement; and consequences should be stated in terms of impact on established team goals, strive for consensus, is similar to the SBAR technique and frames a concern in the context of patient safety.

The Authors' Experience With TeamSTEPPS

The authors of this chapter introduced TeamSTEPPS to several providers, including surgeons, anesthesiologists, and nurses in an orthopaedic surgery unit at an academic hospital. Each provider participated in 3 hours of didactic training on TeamSTEPPS, learning the fundamental concepts and strategies of TeamSTEPPS similar to those discussed in this chapter. Leadership and communication strategies were specifically reinforced during nursing staff meetings, orthopaedic surgeon meetings, and anesthesia grand rounds. In addition, reinforcement of the TeamSTEPPS' communication online module was accomplished via self-paced learning. Orthopaedic surgical teams were observed before and after the reinforcement activities. The authors of this chapter found that the implementation of TeamSTEPPS led to substantial improvements in both leadership and communication, which were topics that were heavily reinforced during training. The authors of this chapter believe that the implementation of a similar strategy across hospital systems can improve team dynamics and create a culture of patient safety.

Challenges to Implementation in Orthopaedics

The implementation of TeamSTEPPS in orthopaedic surgery requires overcoming specific barriers. The first challenge is scheduling a training meeting at which all members of the healthcare team can be present. This is a particular challenge in orthopaedics, which has three shifts of teams and rotating schedules. Furthermore, the continued education of the team members, which helps reinforce the knowledge gained at the initial training, can vary depending on the needs of the team members and may include updates and routine meetings, supplemental reading materials, or group activities.[10]

Another challenge may be the inconsistency of the team members. Experienced teams, which include team members who work together often, may have increased communication, effectiveness, and efficiency; however, many issues may influence the assignment of team members, such as nurses, anesthesiologists, and surgical assistants, to a specific patient.[23] This is further complicated by the addition of guests, such as students, visiting surgeons, or company representatives. In addition, the flow of information sharing between team members and ancillary support may be particularly complex. Given the tight schedules that are common in orthopaedic operating rooms, time and the streamlining of procedures are commodities that need to be balanced with safety and effectiveness. Two operating rooms in which procedures are performed simultaneously can be a particular obstacle to effective communication; therefore, strategies are necessary to enhance reporting between surgical teams.

The composition of a team has a large effect on its dynamic. There is a certain hierarchy within a team. Although an attending orthopaedic surgeon is often viewed as the leader of a team, the effectiveness of his or her leadership/coaching depends on his or her leadership skills. All team members influence the team dynamic because each team member brings a different temperament, knowledge base, and experience to the operating room. Factors that may affect the dynamic of a team include defensiveness, complacency, communication style, misinterpretation of cues, and preexisting or real-time conflicts, all of which may result in complications if the roles of team members are not specified before surgery. Other factors that may affect a team dynamic include fatigue, workload, illness, family situations, the weather (eg, snow), and a holiday schedule.

The Need for Orthopaedic Surgical Leadership

Surgical treatment is a complex undertaking that involves multiple teams of caregivers, multiple locations (clinic, emergency department, hospital, ambulatory surgical center, extended care facility, and the patient's home), and multiple transitions of care.[24] In each phase of care, the core team has a designated leader; however, situational leaders also play important roles in each phase of care. This "team of teams" concept[25] helps define an orthopaedic surgeon's leadership role in the surgical care process, an orthopaedic surgeon's obligation to the patient, and the importance of a shared consciousness in maintaining system resilience and helps make a patient's surgical treatment as safe as possible.

The TeamSTEPPS multiteam system model designates the patient and his or her family as critically important team members from the time of the decision to proceed with surgery through the preoperative, intraoperative, postoperative, and postdischarge phases of surgical treatment.[5] Because of the unique nature of the surgeon-patient relationship, the orthopaedic surgeon, regardless whether he or she is the designated team leader, also is a critically important team member in all phases of surgical care and must be adept at team membership. Leadership and communication are inextricably linked.[26] Orthopaedic surgeons must model positive communication and other teamwork behaviors. Without a strong commitment from the orthopaedic surgeon (who may not always be the designated team leader but is always a thought leader on a surgical team), teamwork initiatives will inevitably fail.[27] Several opportunities for improvement in surgical leadership exist.

Systems Approach

Traditional scope of practice boundaries and the value placed on first order problem solving inhibit the reporting culture that is critical to high-reliability organizations and system resilience.[28] Although local problem solving is critical, the failure to report local problems inhibits team and system learning and increases the likelihood that the same problems will recur. Nurses are more likely to report errors and near-misses compared with physicians.[29] Surgical care teams cannot be resilient if they cannot report, remember, learn, and predict.[19]

Transitions of Care

More than 80% of surgical harm to patients involves transitions of care and transfers of location.[30] Communication breakdowns are typically verbal, often involving ambiguity and status asymmetry in a one-on-one situation (resident to attending or attending to attending). Structured communication (SBAR technique, check-back technique) and handoff protocols (IPASS handoff strategy) help flatten hierarchy and decrease the risk of critical information loss, adverse events, and patient harm.[31,32]

Readmissions

Most unplanned readmissions for surgical patients involve complications that emerge after discharge.[33] Multiple patient factors predict a higher risk for readmission[34] and, if present, indicate the need for close follow up. Hazardous attitudes (macho, impulsive, antiauthority, resignation, invulnerable, and self-confident) are present

in approximately 40% of orthopaedic surgeons and are associated with higher readmission rates.[35] Orthopaedic surgeons should critically review their follow up protocols because many complications that lead to readmission can be managed without hospitalization if detected in a timely manner.

Communication

During the intraoperative phase of surgical care, orthopaedic surgeons communicate in an authoritative manner, which inhibits the free exchange of information among team members and impairs a team's ability to maintain an accurate shared mental model.[18] Disrespectful or disruptive communication, predominantly by attending surgeons, frequently occurs in the perioperative phase, which impairs teamwork and workflow and increases the likelihood of errors and adverse events.[36]

Surgical Safety Checklist

The World Health Organization Surgical Safety Checklist is a communication tool. Compared with surgeons in other specialties, orthopaedic surgeons are less compliant in ceasing activity and assessing the need for β-blockers and venous thromboembolism prophylaxis.[37] Full (as opposed to partial) use of the World Health Organization Surgical Safety Checklist is associated with a reduction in case-mix adjusted complications postoperatively.[38]

Summary

Orthopaedic surgeons have multiple opportunities to improve their teamwork and communication behaviors. Systems thinking, the use of structured and respectful communication, and improved situation monitoring during all phases of surgical care are

behavioral imperatives that should be considered unequivocal elements of professionalism and obligations of the surgeon-patient relationship. The implementation of the concepts and strategies of TeamSTEPPS in orthopaedic surgery can help promote a patient safety culture and help orthopaedic surgery team members efficiently and effectively care for their patients.

References

1. Kohn LT, Corrigan JM, Donaldson MS: *To Err Is Human: Building a Safer Health System*. Washington, DC, National Academies Press, 2000.

2. James JT: A new, evidence-based estimate of patient harms associated with hospital care. *J Patient Saf* 2013;9(3):122-128.

3. Baker DP, Day R, Salas E: Teamwork as an essential component of high-reliability organizations. *Health Serv Res* 2006;41(4 pt 2):1576-1598.

4. Wong DA, Herndon JH, Canale ST, et al: Medical errors in orthopaedics: Results of an AAOS member survey. *J Bone Joint Surg Am* 2009;91(3):547-557.

5. TeamSTEPPS: Strategies and Tools to Enhance Performance and Patient Safety. Rockville, MD, the Agency for Healthcare Research and Quality, March 2016. Available at: http://www.ahrq.gov/professionals/education/curriculum-tools/teamstepps/index.html.

6. Burke CS, Salas E, Wilson-Donnelly K, Priest H: How to turn a team of experts into an expert medical team: Guidance from the aviation and military communities. *Qual Saf Health Care* 2004;13(suppl 1):i96-i104.

7. Epps HR, Levin PE: The TeamSTEPPS approach to safety and quality. *J Pediatr Orthop* 2015; 35(5 suppl 1):S30-S33.

8. King HB, Battles J, Baker DP, et al: TeamSTEPPS: Team strategies and tools to enhance performance and patient safety, in Henriksen K, Battles JB, Keyes MA, Grady ML, eds: *Advances in Patient Safety: New Directions and*

Alternative Approaches. Rockville, MD, the Agency for Healthcare Research and Quality, 2008, vol. 3.

9. Hull L, Arora S, Kassab E, Kneebone R, Sevdalis N: Observational teamwork assessment for surgery: Content validation and tool refinement. *J Am Coll Surg* 2011;212(2):234-243.e1, 5.

10. Armour Forse R, Bramble JD, McQuillan R: Team training can improve operating room performance. *Surgery* 2011;150(4):771-778.

11. Capella J, Smith S, Philp A, et al: Teamwork training improves the clinical care of trauma patients. *J Surg Educ* 2010;67(6):439-443.

12. The Joint Commission: Sentinel Event Data: Root Causes by Event Type. 2004 – 2015. February 9, 2016. Available at: http://www.jointcommission.org/sentinel_event_statistics.

13. Starmer AJ, Spector ND, Srivastava R, et al: Changes in medical errors after implementation of a handoff program. *N Engl J Med* 2014;371(19):1803-1812 .

14. Weld LR, Stringer MT, Ebertowski JS, et al: TeamSTEPPS improves operating room efficiency and patient safety. *Am J Med Qual* 2015.

15. Achor TS, Ahn J: Becoming the "captain of the ship" in the OR. *J Orthop Trauma* 2014;28(suppl 9):S18-S19.

16. Endsley MR: Theoretical underpinnings of situation awareness: A critical review, in Endsley MR, Garland DJ, eds: *Situation Awareness Analysis and Measurement*. Boca Raton, FL, CRC Press, 2008, pp 3-32.

17. Gunther D: The airlines' perspective: Effectively applying crew resource management principles in today's aviation environment, in Kanki B, Helmreich R, Anca J, eds: *Crew Resource Management*. San Diego, CA, Academic Press, 2010, pp 427-434.

18. Bleakley A, Allard J, Hobbs A: 'Achieving ensemble': Communication in orthopaedic surgical teams and the development of situation awareness—an observational study using live videotaped examples. *Adv Health Sci Educ Theory Pract* 2013;18(1):33-56.

19. Ekstedt M, Cook RI: The Stockholm blizzard of 2012, in Wears RL, Hollnagel E, Braithwaite J, eds: *Resilient Health Care: Volume 2. The Resilience of Everyday Clinical Work*. Surrey, England, Ashgate Publishing, 2015, pp 59-74.

20. Sutcliffe KM, Weick KE: Mindful organising and resilient health care, in Wears RL, Hollnagel E, Braithwaite J, eds: *Resilient Health Care*. Surrey, England, Ashgate Publishing, 2013, pp 145-156.

21. Wallace L, Trinka J: *A Legacy of 21st Century Leadership: A Guide for Creating a Climate of Leadership Throughout Your Organization*. iUniverse. Lincoln, NE, 2007.

22. Gladwell M: *Outliers: The Story of Success*. New York, NY, Little, Brown and Company, 2008.

23. Tibbs SM, Moss J: Promoting teamwork and surgical optimization: Combining TeamSTEPPS with a specialty team protocol. *AORN J* 2014;100(5):477-488.

24. Kim FJ, da Silva RD, Gustafson D, Nogueira L, Harlin T, Paul DL: Current issues in patient safety in surgery: A review. *Patient Saf Surg* 2015;9:26.

25. McChrystal S, Collins T, Silverman D, Fussell C: *Team of Teams: New Rules of Engagement for a Complex World*. New York, NY, Penguin Random House, 2015.

26. Pugh CM, Cohen ER, Kwan C, Cannon-Bowers JA: A comparative assessment and gap analysis of commonly used team rating scales. *J Surg Res* 2014;190(2):445-450.

27. Morgan L, Hadi M, Pickering S, et al: The effect of teamwork training on team performance and clinical outcome in elective orthopaedic surgery: A controlled interrupted time series study. *BMJ Open* 2015;5(4):e006216.

28. Espin S, Lingard L, Baker GR, Regehr G: Persistence of unsafe practice in everyday work: An exploration of organizational and psychological factors constraining safety in the operating room. *Qual Saf Health Care* 2006;15(3):165-170.

29. Lyndon A, Sexton JB, Simpson KR, Rosenstein A, Lee KA, Wachter RM: Predictors of likelihood of speaking up about safety concerns in labour and delivery. *BMJ Qual Saf* 2012;21(9):791-799.

30. Greenberg CC, Regenbogen SE, Studdert DM, et al: Patterns of communication breakdowns resulting in injury to surgical patients. *J Am Coll Surg* 2007;204(4):533-540.

31. Frankel AS, Leonard MW, Denham CR: Fair and just culture, team behavior, and leadership engagement: The tools to achieve high reliability. *Health Serv Res* 2006;41(4 pt 2):1690-1709.

32. Starmer AJ, Sectish TC, Simon DW, et al: Rates of medical errors and preventable adverse events among hospitalized children following implementation of a resident handoff bundle. *JAMA* 2013;310(21):2262-2270.

33. Merkow RP, Ju MH, Chung JW, et al: Underlying reasons associated with hospital readmission following surgery in the United States. *JAMA* 2015;313(5):483-495.

34. Bernatz JT, Tueting JL, Anderson PA: Thirty-day readmission rates in orthopedics: A systematic review and meta-analysis. *PLoS One* 2015;10(4):e0123593.

35. Kadzielski J, McCormick F, Herndon JH, Rubash H, Ring D: Surgeons' attitudes are associated with reoperation and readmission rates. *Clin Orthop Relat Res* 2015;473(5):1544-1551.

36. Rosenstein AH, O'Daniel M: Impact and implications of disruptive behavior in the perioperative arena. *J Am Coll Surg* 2006;203(1):96-105.

37. Biffl WL, Gallagher AW, Pieracci FM, Berumen C: Suboptimal compliance with surgical safety checklists in Colorado: A prospective observational study reveals differences between surgical specialties. *Patient Saf Surg* 2015;9(1):5.

38. Mayer EK, Sevdalis N, Rout S, et al: Surgical Checklist Implementation Project: The impact of variable WHO checklist compliance on risk-adjusted clinical outcomes after national implementation. A longitudinal study. *Ann Surg* 2016;263(1):58-63.

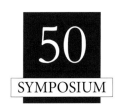

Patient-Reported Outcome Metrics in Total Joint Arthroplasty

Adam Rana, MD

Shaleen Vira, MD

Abstract

The Patient Protection and Affordable Care Act includes several provisions that focus on improving the delivery of health care in the United States. Reducing overall healthcare costs and improving the quality of care delivered are two overarching themes of the Patient Protection and Affordable Care Act. An evaluation of quality in total joint arthroplasty focuses on three main areas: complications, readmissions, and, more recently, patient-reported outcomes. Patient-reported outcomes allow surgeons and patients to objectively document pain relief and functional gain after total joint arthroplasty. Surgeons, groups, or hospitals that commit to the collection of patient-reported outcomes must consider which patient-reported outcomes to capture, the workflow and timing of postoperative patient-reported outcome collection, and how to minimize the burden of patient-reported outcome collection on both patients and surgeons.

Instr Course Lect 2017;66:647–652.

The American Association of Hip and Knee Surgeons and the American Association of Orthopaedic Surgeons have collaborated to develop physician performance measures that address the care of patients who undergo total hip replacement or knee replacement surgery. In addition, the American Association of Hip and Knee Surgeons and the American Association of Orthopaedic Surgeons have developed relationships with the Centers for Medicare & Medicaid Services and the Yale–New Haven Health Services Corporation/ Center for Outcomes Research and Evaluation to identify patient-reported outcome (PRO) measures that provide surgeons with appropriate assessments of outcomes in a manner that can be easily collected from patients. To successfully obtain appropriate assessments of outcomes, orthopaedic surgeons must build and maintain an electronic PRO database.

Identifying and Establishing an Electronic PRO Database or Joint Registry

Traditionally, the collection of PRO data occurred on paper, and PRO results were placed in a patient's chart. Without the appropriate office staff to electronically enter PRO data, data analysis was not possible. Therefore, the identification and acquisition of an electronic PRO database for the collection of PRO measures is imperative. Several different electronic health record software programs, such as Epic and Ortech Data Centre, are currently available. Although Epic is an electronic health record that covers all fields of medicine, Ortech Data Centre is an electronic health record that has a focus on orthopaedic surgery. Ortech Data Centre offers two modules: an

Neither of the following authors nor any immediate family member has received anything of value from or has stock or stock options held in a commercial company or institution related directly or indirectly to the subject of this chapter: Dr. Rana and Dr. Vira.

Table 1

Patient-Reported Outcome Measures Accepted by the American Joint Replacement Registry (AJRR)

Outcome Measure Type	Measure	Number of Items	Available as an AJRR Patient Portal Form	National Benchmarks Available via AJRR Dashboard
Health-related quality of life outcome measures	Veterans RAND 12-Item Health Survey	12	Yes	Yes
	Patient Reported Outcomes Measurement Information System Global Health 10-Item Short Form	10	Yes	Yes
	Medical Outcomes Study 12-Item Short Form	12	No, AJRR only accepts final scores	No
	Medical Outcomes Study 36-Item Short Form	36	Yes	No
	European Quality of Life-5 Dimensions Index and Visual Analog Scale	6	No, AJRR only accepts final scores	No
Joint-specific outcome measures	Hip Disability and Osteoarthritis Outcome Score, Joint Replacement	6	Yes	Yes
	Knee Injury and Osteoarthritis Outcome Score, Joint Replacement	7	Yes	Yes
	Hip Disability and Osteoarthritis Outcome Score	42	Yes	No
	Knee Injury and Osteoarthritis Outcome Score	42	Yes	No
	Oxford Hip Score	12	Yes	No
	Oxford Knee Score	12	Yes	No
	Knee Society Knee Scoring System	44	Yes	No
	Harris hip score	8	Yes	No
	Western Ontario and McMasters University Osteoarthritis Index	24	No, AJRR only accepts final scores	No

Adapted with permission from the American Joint Replacement Registry: AJRR's patient-reported outcome measures guide. Rosemont, IL, American Joint Replacement Registry, April 2016. Available at: http://www.ajrr.net/images/downloads/Data_elements/AJRR_PROMS_GUIDE_2016_FINAL.pdf. Accessed May 24, 2016.

operating room module, which is used for the collection of intraoperative data, and a clinical module, which allows for the collection of PRO data. Unfortunately, a substantial cost is associated with the acquisition of electronic health record software programs. The cost for Epic, which is typically purchased by large hospitals or healthcare systems, can range in the millions of dollars. In 2013, the Maine Medical Center (MMC) acquired Ortech Data Centre at an initial cost of $56,700 for six surgeons and pays an annual maintenance fee of $36,630.

Several joint registries, which are at different stages of PRO data collection, exist at the state, regional, and national levels. The American Joint Replacement Registry (AJRR) is the largest joint registry in the United States, including more than 650 participating hospitals. As of November 2015, hospitals participating in the AJRR may collect level 3 registry data (PRO data). **Table 1** demonstrates the PRO measures currently accepted by the AJRR. Function and Outcomes Research for Comparative Effectiveness in Total Joint Replacement (FORCE-TJR) is a federally funded research program that collects both surgical results and PRO data.[1] FORCE-TJR includes more than 130 orthopaedic surgeons who practice in a variety of settings (urban, rural, low-volume centers, and high-volume centers). The California Joint Replacement Registry (CJRR) and the Michigan Arthroplasty Registry Collaborative Quality Initiative are joint registries in California and Michigan, respectively, that collect PRO data (level 3 registry data), implant data (level 1 registry data), and adverse event data (level 2 registry data).

Determining Which PRO Measures to Collect

A substantial number of PROs are available for the evaluation of total hip replacement and total knee replacement outcomes. In August of 2015, the American Association of Hip and Knee Surgeons, the American Association of Orthopaedic Surgeons, the Centers for Medicare & Medicaid Services, the Yale–New Haven Health Services Corporation/Center for Outcomes Research and Evaluation, and several other stakeholders convened at the Patient Reported Outcomes Summit for Total Joint Arthroplasty.[2] The goal of the Patient Reported Outcomes Summit for Total Joint Arthroplasty was to agree on select health-related quality of life PRO measures and joint-specific PRO measures that could be used by the orthopaedic community. The summit workgroup selected validated PRO measures that had a minimal number of questions patients would need to answer and that were not associated with licensing fees. The summit workgroup recommended that either the Patient Reported Outcomes Measurement Information System Global Health 10-Item Short Form or the Veterans Rand 12-Item Health Survey be used to collect health-related quality of life information. The summit workgroup recommended that that the Hip Disability and Osteoarthritis Outcome Score (HOOS) Joint Replacement (six questions) or the Knee Injury and Osteoarthritis Outcome Score (KOOS) Joint Replacement (seven questions) be used to collect joint-specific information. All four of the PROs recommended by the summit workgroup are collected by the AJRR, which also collects three additional health-related quality of life PRO measures and seven additional joint-specific PRO measures, all of which are listed in **Table 1**.

FORCE-TJR collects PRO data from the Medical Outcomes Study 36-Item Short Form and the HOOS or the KOOS. The CJRR collects PRO data from the Medical Outcomes Study 12-Item Short Form, the HOOS or the KOOS, and the University of California–Los Angeles Activity Score.

Establishing a Workflow for PRO Data Collection

Establishing a workflow for PRO data collection is essential to successfully obtain appropriate assessments of outcomes. The determination of a preoperative PRO collection time point and set postoperative PRO collection time points is necessary. At the MMC, all hip arthroplasty and knee arthroplasty patients visit the office approximately 2 weeks before surgery so that their history can be obtained and a physical examination can be performed. After the patient's history has been obtained and the physical examination is complete, a physician assistant or nurse practitioner brings the patient to meet with a research analyst. The research analyst at the MMC devotes one full-time equivalent to maintaining the PRO database and joint arthroplasty registry. The patient is given a tablet, which includes his or her preentered demographic data, and completes the Patient Reported Outcomes Measurement Information System Global Health 10-Item Short Form, the HOOS Joint Replacement or the KOOS Joint Replacement, the University of California–Los Angeles Activity Score, and the visual analog scale pain score. The PRO measures take approximately 5 to 7 minutes for the patient to complete, and the research analyst is available to answer any questions the patient may have during the process. The patient also signs an electronic informed consent form, which allows the PRO data to be used for any future research-related work.

The patient's email address is captured for future electronic correspondence.

Postoperative PRO data are captured at 6 weeks, 1 year, 2 years, and 5 years postoperatively. Patients who have an email address in the MMC electronic database system are automatically emailed PRO measures 1 week before their scheduled office appointment. At the beginning of the week, the research analyst reviews each surgeon's and mid-level provider's daily clinic schedule to determine which patients have and have not completed their PRO measures. The research analyst flags all of the patients who have not completed their PRO measures, who are then sent a second email requesting that they complete their PRO measures. If the patients still do not complete their PRO measures, then the research analyst attempts to meet with them before their scheduled office appointment. In 2015, the preoperative and 1-year postoperative PRO measure capture rate at the MMC was 95% and 70%, respectively.

FORCE-TJR reports preoperative and postoperative PRO measure completion rates of 96% and 90%, respectively.[3] FORCE-TJR has joint registry staff who contact patients as necessary to ensure that complete PRO data have been submitted. **Figure 1** demonstrates the PRO survey collection workflow established by FORCE-TJR. The CJRR report that approximately 70% of patients who are scheduled to undergo total joint arthroplasty and approximately 30% of patients who have undergone total joint arthroplasty complete PRO measures.[4] The Michigan Arthroplasty Registry Collaborative Quality Initiative reported a preoperative and postoperative PRO measure collection rate of 20% and 10%, respectively, for total joint arthroplasty patients.[3] PRO

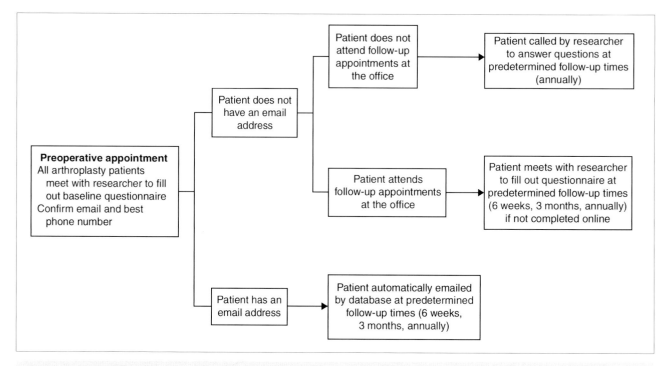

Figure 1 Algorithm shows the patient-reported outcome measure collection workflow established by Function and Outcomes Research for Comparative Effectiveness in Total Joint Replacement.

measures can be collected at postoperative visits or submitted by patients via a web portal.

Obstacles to PRO Data Collection

As highlighted previously, PRO collection rates vary considerably across joint registries. This disparity is a result of several obstacles that may be encountered during the PRO data capture process. The Michigan Arthroplasty Registry Collaborative Quality Initiative electronic health record reports multiple reasons for its low preoperative and postoperative PRO collection rates, including various settings for postoperative follow-up, different levels of surgeon involvement, and the limited use of e-mail and the Internet by patients.[5]

Conversely, FORCE-TJR attributes its excellent PRO completion rate to several factors. First, patient enrollment occurs in the surgeon's office and educates patients on the need for complete PRO data both before and after total joint arthroplasty. In addition, repeat mailings and phone calls are used after surgery to prompt patients to complete their postoperative PRO measures. The FORCE-TJR PRO measure collection workflow requires a dedicated clerical staff member to make reminder telephone calls each week; this level of office support is not always available across practices.

The CJRR developed innovative solutions to address several challenges that were encountered in the collection of complete PRO measures. The CJRR reported a 5% incidence of postoperative PRO measures being sent to incorrect email addresses and a 40% incidence of postoperative PRO measure emails being directed to spam filters.[6] The CJRR reformatted postoperative PRO measure emails so that they are sent from a patient's surgeon rather than the CJRR. The CJRR also created an outbound telephone calling program, which contacts patients who did not complete their postoperative PRO measures. Because of the diverse patient population in California (more than 18 languages are spoken), the CJRR made postoperative PRO measures available in languages other than English. Finally, to improve surgeon engagement, the CJRR holds surgeon webinars that are led by other surgeons to stress the importance of the joint registry. The CJRR also created a prescription pad for surgeons that contains information about the CJRR, the importance of PRO measures, the website of the CJRR, and a signature line.

Manners in Which PRO Data Can Be Used

Figure 2 demonstrates how the MMC graphically presents an individual

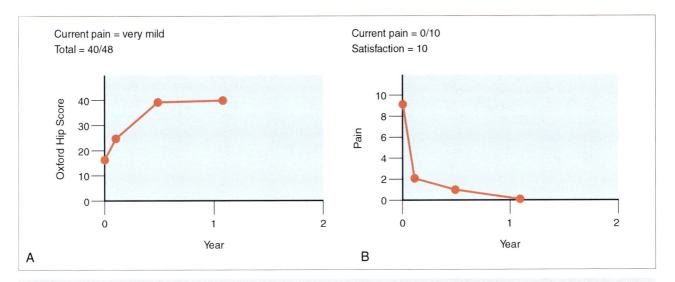

Figure 2   Graphs illustrate how the Maine Medical Center presents individual patient-reported outcome measure results. **A,** Oxford Hip Score. **B,** Visual analog pain scale score.

Table 2

Aggregate Patient-Reported Outcome Scores for Primary Total Hip Replacement and Primary Total Knee Replacement Patients by Surgeon

	Mean Preoperative Score			Mean 1-Year Postoperative Score			
	Oxford Hip Score	VAS pain score	UCLA	Oxford Hip Score	VAS pain score	UCLA	Satisfaction
Surgeon 1	23	5.9	4.5	44.6	0.7	6.5	9.5
Surgeon 2	22	6.3	4.1	42.7	1.0	6.1	9.3
Surgeon 3	18.2	6.4	3.8	42.6	0.8	5.8	9.2

UCLA = University of California–Los Angeles Activity Score, VAS = visual analog scale.

patient's PRO data at the follow-up office visit. Patients are able to see both their preoperative and postoperative functional, pain, and satisfaction scores. Providing patients this information in a visual manner has helped improve patient engagement at the follow-up office visit. As a result, the MMC has seen an increase in patient satisfaction; however, the MMC has yet to objectify this improvement in patient satisfaction. The MMC's PRO database also allows surgeons at the MMC to aggregate and analyze their PRO data overall, as a group, by variables of interest, or by surgeon. **Table 2** demonstrates

aggregate PRO scores for primary total hip replacement and primary total knee replacement patients by surgeon, and **Figure 3** demonstrates how the MMC graphically presents aggregate University of California–Los Angeles Activity Scores for primary total hip replacement and primary total knee replacement as a group.

The MMC has used data from their PRO database in different settings at the hospital, including monthly orthopaedic quality metric meetings that are attended by orthopaedic surgeons and representatives from the anesthesia, nursing, physical therapy, and case

management departments. In addition, the MMC uses data from their PRO database at quarterly group research meetings. Finally, data from the PRO database have been used to develop the MMC's annual Quality Outcomes Report, which highlights the MMC's surgical volume, complications, readmissions, length of hospital stay, discharge disposition, and PRO results from the previous year.[7] The MMC's Quality Outcomes Report is given to patients and primary care providers, and portions of the report are being used in discussions with insurances carriers.

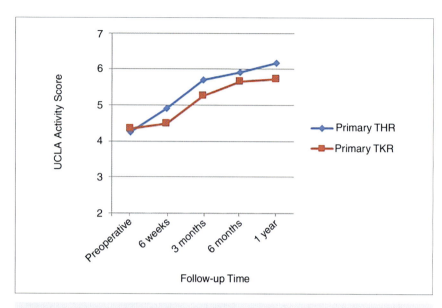

Figure 3 Graph illustrates how the Maine Medical Center presents aggregate University of California–Los Angeles (UCLA) Activity Scores for primary total hip replacement (THR) and primary total knee replacement (TKR) by follow-up time. (Adapted with permission from Maine Medical Partners – Orthopaedic & Sports Medicine Joint Replacement: 2015 Quality Outcomes Report. http://mainemedicalpartners.org/workfiles/MMP/MMP-Ortho-Book-QualityOutcomes2015.pdf.)

Summary

The creation of an electronic PRO database and participation in a joint registry to collect PRO data is a group undertaking and requires a physician champion. A considerable amount of work must be completed in advance to make the introduction of a PRO database a success. Establishing surgeon and hospital buy-in as well as a fluid workflow for PRO data collection are critical. A considerable investment for a PRO data collection program and for the training of office staff and possibly hiring additional staff, such as a research analyst, is necessary to establish an electronic PRO database. A determination of who will pay for an electronic PRO database (the hospital, the group, or both) is a discussion that must occur in advance of such an investment. A successful electronic PRO database can lead to improvements in quality via research, benchmarking, and improved patient engagement. A successful electronic PRO database also can answer the public mandate from the Centers for Medicare & Medicaid Services to improve the value of patient care amidst the current climate of healthcare reform.

References

1. Franklin PD, Allison JJ, Ayers DC: Beyond joint implant registries: A patient-centered research consortium for comparative effectiveness in total joint replacement. *JAMA* 2012;308(12):1217-1218.

2. American Association of Hip and Knee Surgeons: Patient reported outcomes summit for total joint arthroplasty report. August 31, 2015. Available at: http://www.aahks.org/wp-content/uploads/2015/09/pro-summit-report-2015.pdf. Accessed May 24, 2016.

3. Franklin PD, Lewallen D, Bozic K, Hallstrom B, Jiranek W, Ayers DC: Implementation of patient-reported outcome measures in U.S. Total joint replacement registries: Rationale, status, and plans. *J Bone Joint Surg Am* 2014;96(suppl 1):104-109.

4. California Joint Replacement Registry. Available at: http://caljrr.org. Accessed February 28, 2016.

5. Michigan Arthroplasty Registry Collaborative Quality Initiative. Available at: http://marcqi.org. Accessed February 28, 2016.

6. Chenok K, Teleki S, SooHoo NF, Huddleston J III, Bozic KJ: Collecting patient-reported outcomes: Lessons from the California Joint Replacement Registry. *EGEMS (Wash DC)* 2015;3(1):1196.

7. Maine Medical Partners – Orthopaedic & Sports Medicine Joint Replacement: 2015 Quality Outcomes Report. http://mainemedicalpartners.org/workfiles/MMP/MMP-Ortho-Book-QualityOutcomes2015.pdf. Accessed June 20, 2016.

Collaborative Orthopaedic Research Between and Within Institutions

Brian R. Wolf, MD, MS
Nikhil N. Verma, MD
Kurt P. Spindler, MD
Rick W. Wright, MD

Abstract

Collaborative research is common in many medical disciplines; however, the field of orthopaedics has been relatively slow to adopt this type of research approach. Collaborative research efforts can occur between multiple institutions and, in some instances, may benefit from subspecialty society sponsorship. Collaborative research efforts between several research spheres within a single institution also can be advantageous. Collaborative research has many benefits, including a larger number of patients in studies, more power in the research, and better generalizability. In addition, collaborative research efforts allow resources to be pooled within and between institutions. The challenges of collaborative research include data management, funding, and the publication of manuscripts that have many authors.

Instr Course Lect 2017;66:653–658.

Background

There is an increased trend toward collaboration in the field of orthopaedics with respect to both clinical and basic science research. Collaboration can occur between surgeons, between surgeons and scientists, between institutions, or between different entities within a single institution. The motivation for the move toward increased collaboration is likely related to the increased emphasis being placed on evidence-based medicine in all medical disciplines, including orthopaedics. Evidence-based medicine is possible only if high-level research is used to solve clinical problems; therefore, there has been a growing mandate for clinical researchers to conduct studies with the use of methods that will result in high-level evidence, which will, in turn, guide clinical practice. Several methodologic factors help generate high-level evidence in clinical research studies. The highest level of evidence in clinical research is assigned to prospective investigations that conduct either randomized clinical trials or cohort studies. As the emphasis on randomized clinical trials and cohort studies has increased, there has been a drive to develop large multisurgeon or multi-institution studies that include a greater number of patients. Research studies that include a greater number of patients allow for analysis of more variables and have more statistical power. Collaborative efforts for patient recruitment allow a greater number of patients to be recruited in a shorter period of time. Last, collaborative research that includes many clinicians may allow for better generalizability of study results.

The quality of orthopaedic research appears to have improved over time. A recent study reported that the number of level I and level II studies published in eight major orthopaedic journals between 2000 and 2010 increased approximately 50%.[1] The field of orthopaedics, however, may be lagging behind other medical disciplines. Brophy et al[2] reported that orthopaedic journals published fewer collaborative research studies compared with general medicine journals and other surgical subspecialty journals. The authors also reported that more institutions and more authors were typically involved in collaborative research studies published in general medicine journals and in other surgical subspecialty journals compared with collaborative research studies published in orthopaedic journals. The authors reported that collaborative multicenter research studies represented 24% to 40% of the articles published in the upper echelon medical journals that were analyzed (the *New England Journal of Medicine*, the *Lancet*, and the *Journal of the American Medical Association*) and 13% to 20% of the articles published in the surgical subspecialty journals that were analyzed (*Obstetrics & Gynecology*, *Ophthalmology*, and the *Journal of the Association for Research in Otolaryngology*). Conversely, collaborative multicenter research studies represented only 1.1% to 7.7% of the articles published in the orthopaedic journals that were analyzed (the *Journal of Bone and Joint Surgery*, *Spine*, and the *American Journal of Sports Medicine*).

The benefit of collaborative research is evident. Most major medical and scientific advances, including major scientific breakthroughs such as the Human Genome Project, have resulted from collaborative research efforts. Collaborative studies are cited in the literature more often than other types of research studies.[3] Although many challenges exist with regard to collaborative research, there has been an increase in the number of orthopaedic collaborative research groups, examples of which include the Lower Extremity Assessment Project, the Study to Prospectively Evaluate Reamed Intramedullary Nails in Patients with Tibial Fractures, the Anterior Total Hip Arthroplasty Collaborative, the Spine Patient Outcomes Research Trial, the Multicenter Orthopaedic Outcomes Network (MOON), the Multicenter ACL Revision Study (MARS), and the Major Extremity Trauma Research Consortium. In addition to collaborative research efforts across institutions, there is an increased trend toward collaboration between surgeons and scientists within research groups, which also allows for increased study size, power, and generalizability.

Surgeons should understand different types of collaborative research methods. Surgeons also should be aware of the challenges associated with various collaborative research settings and designs as well as the pearls for managing those challenges. The typical challenges of collaborative research efforts include organization of the research effort, data management, and group communication. In addition, collaborative research usually requires more funding for maintenance and personnel. Last, it may be challenging to reward researchers and investigators who participate in collaborative research efforts. Participation in collaborative research complicates an orthopaedic surgeon's clinical practice. Authorship on manuscripts that are produced from collaborative research efforts is the best reward for researchers and investigators who participate in collaborative research. Historically, most orthopaedic journals had limitations on the number of individuals who were allowed to be listed as authors on research publications. Fortunately, more journals are recognizing the importance of collaborative research studies that include many authors and are creating mechanisms to acknowledge numerous authors. For example, the *American Journal of Sports Medicine* allows a research group or a contributing authors paragraph to be included in a manuscript to recognize authors who are not listed in the main author byline. This contributing authors list is recognized by PubMed as well as other search engines and gives authorship credit to all of the individuals who participated in the research. The authors of this chapter hope that more mechanisms to recognize large groups of investigators who contribute to collaborative research efforts become available.

Dr. Wolf or an immediate family member serves as a paid consultant to or is an employee of CONMED Linvatec; has received research or institutional support from the Orthopaedic Research and Education Foundation; has received nonincome support (such as equipment or services), commercially derived honoraria, or other non-research–related funding (such as paid travel) from Arthrex; and serves as a board member, owner, officer, or committee member of the American Academy of Orthopaedic Surgeons, the American Orthopaedic Society for Sports Medicine, and the Mid-America Orthopaedic Association. Dr. Verma or an immediate family member has received royalties from Smith & Nephew; serves as a paid consultant to or is an employee of Minivasive, OrthoSpace, and Smith & Nephew; has stock or stock options held in CyMedica Orthopedics, Minivasive, and Omeros; has received research or institutional support from Arthrex, Smith & Nephew, Athletico Physical Therapy, CONMED Linvatec, MioMed, Mitek, Arthrosurface, and DJ Orthopaedics; and serves as a board member, owner, officer, or committee member of the Arthroscopy Association Learning Center Committee and the American Shoulder and Elbow Surgeons. Dr. Spindler or an immediate family member serves as a paid consultant to or is an employee of the Cytori Therapeutics Scientific Advisory Board and Mitek; has received research or institutional support from the National Institutes of Health (NIAMS & NICHD); and serves as a board member, owner, officer, or committee member of the American Academy of Orthopaedic Surgeons, the American Orthopaedic Society for Sports Medicine, the National Football League Charities Safety Panel, and the Orthopaedic Research Society. Dr. Wright or an immediate family member has received research or institutional support from the National Institutes of Health (NIAMS & NICHD); and serves as a board member, owner, officer, or committee member of the American Board of Orthopaedic Surgery, the American Orthopaedic Association, and the American Orthopaedic Society for Sports Medicine.

Collaborative research can occur in the field of orthopaedics via several methods, including the multicenter prospective cohort design model, the subspecialty society-based prospective cohort design model, and collaboration between surgeons and scientists within a large academic institution.

Collaborative Research Between Institutions: The Multicenter Prospective Cohort Model

The creation of a multicenter research group and initiative has many pearls. First and foremost, the participants who are involved in a multicenter research group are crucial. A multicenter research group must have a research leader who manages the mission, research goals, funding, and infrastructure of the group; this individual can be a clinician or a clinician scientist. The research leader must be able to manage all of the individuals in the multicenter research group and keep the group organized and focused on its mission. The research investigators at all of the research institutions must be team players and willing to put their personal agendas and egos aside to advance the mission of the multicenter research group.

Next, the research investigators must have a willingness to prioritize the group research effort and follow through on issues, such as enrollment, patient follow-up, completion of research data forms, and other tasks, or the group will suffer and may fail. Similar to team sports, a multicenter research group is only as successful as its weakest link; therefore, research investigators must meet established criteria to join a multicenter research group and meet established criteria and metrics to

continue their participation in a multicenter research group. If a research investigator is not fulfilling the established criteria and his or her expected duties, then he or she must be removed from the multicenter research group, which is a responsibility that often falls on the research leader. Removal of a research investigator is much easier if criteria are established early.

Last, each participating research institution must have research personnel who assist with the research study. The research personnel at each participating research institution assist with patient enrollment, Institutional Review Board (IRB) approval and modifications, and local research institution data monitoring, as well as communication with the central research institution.

A multicenter research effort requires a centralized research hub similar to the way in which an airline requires a main hub to coordinate flight operations. The research hub for a multicenter research group is the research institution at which most of the research personnel are located. A study coordinator who works with the research leader and is specifically trained in research methods, grant mechanisms, and statistics, as well as manuscript preparation and submission, is extremely useful. The study coordinator and the research hub help coordinate the research actions at all of the involved research institutions. Multicenter research groups should establish and use a manual of operations and procedures that outlines all of the details of the research study. The research hub establishes the primary IRB used for the research study and then assists the local research institutions with local IRB approval and modifications. Data management is the most important function of the research hub. There are

many mechanisms for the collection of data, including paper forms, forms that can be scanned via bar codes or other symbols, electronic forms, web-based forms that use proprietary technology, and university-and/or institution-based platforms. Data management is absolutely crucial to the success of a multicenter research study, and early due diligence is necessary to ensure that data are easily collected and stored in a usable and analyzable manner.

The MOON, which was established in 2002, is an example of a successful multicenter prospective collaborative research effort.[4] The study was established by Kurt P. Spindler, MD, and seven other orthopaedic sports medicine surgeons at seven institutions. In the past 13 years, the group has grown to include 18 surgeons at 7 institutions. The MOON research team exceeds 50 people and includes biostatistics and public health consultants as well as research assistants and coordinators. The MOON's research hub is located at Vanderbilt University in Nashville, TN; and the MOON's participating research institutions include the Cleveland Clinic Foundation in Cleveland, OH; The Ohio State University in Columbus, OH; the University of Iowa in Iowa City, IA; the University of Colorado in Boulder, CO; the Hospital for Special Surgery in New York, NY; and Washington University in St. Louis, MO. The focus of the MOON is a prospective cohort study of patients who underwent anterior cruciate ligament (ACL) reconstruction that aims to determine predictors of outcomes after ACL reconstruction surgery.

The MOON research effort demonstrates many of the benefits of collaborative research. By including numerous research institutions and research investigators, the MOON was able to enroll a substantial number of ACL patients in a relatively short amount of time. Approximately 3,000 patients who were undergoing ACL reconstruction were enrolled in the MOON between 2002 and 2010. The number of study participants allowed for a powerful and detailed analysis of multiple preoperative and intraoperative variables that were potentially related to patient outcomes. In addition, because of the numerous research investigators who were involved, there was, overall, good generalizability of the research results. Based on prospective cohort data, the MOON has reported on the 2-year and 5-year outcomes of the patients who were enrolled in the study and underwent ACL reconstruction and has published more than 45 level I and level II peer-reviewed studies on the outcomes of the patients who were enrolled in the study and underwent ACL reconstruction.

The MOON research effort also demonstrates many of the challenges of multicenter collaborative research. The inclusion of seven research institutions has required a tremendous amount of coordination. Each research institution has a research assistant who is dedicated to tasks related to the research study. Oversight of such a large research effort has been assisted by mandatory monthly research conference calls during which current research manuscripts, presentations, new research ideas, and other information are shared and discussed under the guidance of the research leader (Kurt P. Spindler, MD) and the main study coordinator. Group oversight also is assisted by biannual in-person MOON meetings that include a formal full-day agenda. Funding a collaborative research study

is another challenge. Clinical cohort studies are expensive because of the number of research personnel required for enrolling, contacting, and monitoring patients and data. A plethora of resources, including industry funding, internal institutional grants, small and large peer-reviewed grants, and national grants, are necessary to maintain a collaborative research study. In some research studies, there may be personal expenses on behalf of the research investigators to support the study at the various research institutions. The MOON obtained small-industry and competitive grant funding before it ultimately obtained grant funding from the National Institutes of Health. The definition of authorship criteria for manuscripts that are produced from a research study is another challenge of collaborative research. It is imperative that a multicenter research group establish authorship criteria that are known by all of the research study participants. Authorship on MOON research manuscripts mandates participation in patient enrollment and follow-up; completion of research data forms; participation in monthly research conference calls and biannual in-person meetings; and participation in manuscript writing, review, or editing.

Collaborative Research Between Surgeons: The Subspecialty Society-Based Prospective Cohort Model

Some research studies may benefit from the engagement and use of a subspecialty society for research initiatives. The subspecialty society-based prospective cohort model is very similar to the multicenter prospective cohort model. A subspecialty society is beneficial because it can offer participation in the

research group to its members, which may include private practice orthopaedists and academic center-based orthopaedists. Many orthopaedic subspecialty societies want to support the research projects of their members and, in some instances, can contribute monetary support until competitive grant funding is obtained. Access to the membership of a subspecialty society can help research groups that are investigating relatively rare clinical problems that individual practitioners do not see in a large number of patients. A subspecialty society can assist research groups in advertising for recruitment of research investigators, and many subspecialty societies can assist research groups in marketing for recruitment of study participants. A subspecialty society can help research groups obtain meeting space at society meetings, at which the research group can update the research participants and the subspecialty society on results of the research study.

Similar to a multicenter research group, a subspecialty society-based research group must have a research leader. Research investigators must meet established criteria to join and participate in a subspecialty society-based research group, and there must be strict data management; however, these requirements may be more difficult to achieve in subspecialty society-based research groups because many more research institutions and research investigators are likely to be involved.

Subspecialty society-based research groups have their own unique challenges. Most subspecialty society-based research groups require funding in addition to that provided by the subspecialty society; the maintenance of funding is a responsibility that often falls on the research leader. Subspecialty society-based research groups need to delineate who owns the research data and who is allowed to use the research data. The issue of authorship may be extremely challenging for subspecialty society-based research groups. Often, the appeal to participate in a subspecialty society-based research group is linked to the possibility of authorship credit. The recognition of dozens of research investigators on a peer-reviewed manuscript can be daunting, especially because many orthopaedic journals have limitations on the number of individuals who can be listed as authors on a publication. The research leader must establish authorship criteria at the beginning of the research study. Some journals and PubMed acknowledge large groups of authors or research groups by listing the name of the study group in the main author byline and then recognizing all of the contributing authors in a paragraph at the end of the manuscript.

The MARS is an example of a successful subspecialty society-based collaborative research effort.[5] The MARS was formed by members of the American Orthopaedic Society for Sports Medicine (AOSSM). ACL revision surgery is relatively uncommon given that the failure rate of primary ACL surgery is approximately 5%; therefore, most sports medicine and ACL surgeons perform relatively few ACL revisions, and the research literature on ACL revision surgery outcomes consist mainly of level IV data and small case series. The MARS research team includes 87 surgeons from the AOSSM. The MARS details, training, and updates are made available at the AOSSM's annual meeting and at subspecialty society meetings. The MARS is led by Rick W. Wright, MD, and the research hub is located at Washington University in St. Louis, MO. Approximately 1,000 patients who were undergoing ACL revision surgery were enrolled in the MARS, which was more patients than the total number of patients in all of the previous ACL revision surgery studies in the literature combined. The MARS obtained industry funding, small grant funding from the AOSSM, and small competitive funding before it ultimately obtained grant funding from the National Institutes of Health, which continues to be used to perform follow-up studies.

Collaborative Research Within an Institution

The benefits of collaborative research within a practice, a department, or an institution include the sharing of resources necessary for the research study; the sharing of data that are generated by the research study; and, ultimately, a higher quality and larger number of grants, presentations, and published manuscripts. Resources, such as funding and research personnel, often limit research productivity; however, many resources can be shared if collaborative research is performed within an institution. Shared resources for clinical research that is performed within an institution may include research personnel who assist with compliance and human subject approval, patient enrollment and follow-up, as well as data analysis. Shared resources for basic science research that is performed within an institution may include laboratory personnel and scientists. Durable laboratory equipment, computers, and other testing equipment are other resources that can be shared.

The quality of research also benefits from collaborative research within an institution. The participation of multiple research investigators in a research study allows for contributions to the research study from several perspectives. The participation of multiple research investigators in a research study can increase the number of clinical patients who are involved, which adds strength and generalizability to the outcomes of the research study. In addition, collaborative research within an institution allows for aspects of a research study to be divided among the research investigators, which enhances the efficiency of the research effort. Often, some research investigators may be skilled or more interested in specific parts of the research process, such as patient enrollment, manuscript writing and editing, or grant writing. In addition, collaborative research within an institution allows an entire team of research investigators to generate and receive credit for more research studies, presentations, publications, and grants.

The sports medicine program at Rush University Medical Center in Chicago, IL is an excellent example of a collaborative research effort within an institution that produces high-volume, high-quality research. Rush University Medical Center uses an organization chart to successfully coordinate basic science laboratory research as well as clinical outcomes research. The clinical research coordinator at Rush University Medical Center oversees the clinical outcomes research team and is a permanent, full-time research employee who handles IRB and compliance issues, coordinates patient cohort and randomized clinical trial studies, and manages clinical study budgets and funding. In parallel, the head basic scientist at Rush University Medical Center, who is a PhD, oversees the basic science research team. The head basic scientist oversees all laboratory projects as well as develops and optimizes all basic science protocols. The head basic scientist often has independent research interests and obtains some independent research funding. The laboratory manager, who works under the head basic scientist, is responsible for maintenance and operation of laboratory equipment, oversight of laboratory testing operations, as well as data preparation and analysis. Much of the day-to-day research is conducted by research assistants who are medical students, orthopaedic residents-in-training, or hired research assistant staff. The research assistants help manage assigned projects and assist with data analysis, manuscript preparation, presentations at national meetings, submissions to meetings and journals, as well as other tasks.

An organizational structure should be in place to oversee the process of collaborative research within an institution. The sports medicine program at Rush University Medical Center conducts research meetings at regular intervals to review and troubleshoot current research projects, brainstorm for new research projects, review data, and review the research mission and goals of the research team. Cooperation, leadership, and organization are inherent to the success of collaborative research within an institution.

Summary

Collaborative research is becoming more common in medicine and in orthopaedics. Collaborative research can occur via several methods, including the multicenter prospective cohort design model, the subspecialty society-based prospective cohort design model, and collaboration between clinicians and researchers within an institution. Multicenter prospective cohort research groups help generate high-level (level I or level II) research data that are powerful and generalizable and require a strong research leader as well as a team effort to be successful. Subspecialty society-based prospective cohort research groups help members of a subspecialty society contribute to research on relatively uncommon clinical problems. Collaboration within a department, an institution, or a practice can be very rewarding, can improve the quality and quantity of research performed, and allows for the sharing of key resources, such as facilities, research personnel, and funding. There are many challenges to collaborative research; however, appropriate planning, organization, and leadership can foster success.

References

1. Cunningham BP, Harmsen S, Kweon C, et al: Have levels of evidence improved the quality of orthopaedic research? *Clin Orthop Relat Res* 2013;471(11):3679-3686.

2. Brophy RH, Smith MV, Latterman C, et al: Multi-investigator collaboration in orthopaedic surgery research compared to other medical fields. *J Orthop Res* 2012;30(10):1523-1528.

3. Figg WD, Dunn L, Liewehr DJ, et al: Scientific collaboration results in higher citation rates of published articles. *Pharmacotherapy* 2006;26(6):759-767.

4. Spindler KP, Parker RD, Andrish JT, et al: Prognosis and predictors of ACL reconstructions using the MOON cohort: A model for comparative effectiveness studies. *J Orthop Res* 2013;31(1):2-9.

5. Wright RW, Huston LJ, Spindler KP, et al: Descriptive epidemiology of the Multicenter ACL Revision Study (MARS) cohort. *Am J Sports Med* 2010;38(10):1979-1986.

Surgeon–Patient Communication: The Key to Patient Satisfaction, Patient-Centered Care, and Shared Decision Making

Dwight W. Burney III, MD

Abstract

The surgeon–patient relationship is rapidly evolving from surgeon-centric to patient-centric. External forces, such as the Affordable Care Act and the unsustainable growth of healthcare costs in the United States, have disrupted the old model of medical care. Effective communication between surgeons and patients as well as patient satisfaction, treatment adherence, and shared decision making are essential components of the patient-centered care paradigm. Effective communication carries high stakes for surgeons, including increased surgeon satisfaction and a reduced risk of surgeon burnout and malpractice litigation. Communication skills are one of the six Accreditation Council for Graduate Medical Education core competencies, and an assessment of communication skills is now included in a surgeon's summative evaluations for employment, compensation, licensing, and maintenance of certification.

Instr Course Lect 2017;66:659–665.

The physician–patient relationship has always been at the center of medical care. The surgeon–patient relationship is particularly complex because it involves sense-making between a surgeon and a patient with regard to the reason for the referral,[1] the development of trust and mutual respect, a consideration of treatment options, shared decision making, and the navigation of a complicated multiphase care system if surgery is the selected treatment. The Affordable Care Act has prioritized patient empowerment. Some orthopaedic care is believed to be preference sensitive and driven by surgeon supply, which results in overutilization of surgical treatment in some patient populations and underutilization of surgical treatment in other patient populations. Consideration of a patient's goals, values, and preferences in the decision-making process allows for rational surgical care rather than rationed surgical care.[2]

Currently, patients are able to rate healthcare providers based on their experience of care as well as their satisfaction with the process and outcomes of care using the Consumer Assessment of Healthcare Providers and Systems survey. Clinician and Group Consumer Assessment of Healthcare Providers and Systems surveys and patient-reported outcome measures have become high-stakes evaluations of providers, especially surgeons, whose job security, salary, hospital privileges, and, even, medical license and board certification may be affected by a patient's rating of his or her care.

The change from physician-centric care to patient-centric care may be particularly stressful for surgeons. Surgeon burnout is a serious issue, and

Dr. Burney or an immediate family member serves as a board member, owner, officer, or committee member of the American Academy of Orthopaedic Surgeons.

Table 1

Elements of Patient-Centered Care

Exploring both the disease (differential diagnosis) and the illness experience (the patient's ideas, feelings, and expectations as well as the effect of the illness on function)

Understanding the entire patient (life history and social context, which includes family and others affected by the patient's illness, and the patient's physical environment)

Finding common ground with regard to management (problems and priorities, treatment goals, and patient and surgeon roles)

Incorporating prevention and health promotion (health enhancement, risk reduction, early detection, and ameliorating the effects of the disease)

Enhancing the physician–patient relationship (characteristics of the therapeutic relationship, sharing power, caring and healing relationship, self-awareness, transference, and countertransference)

Being realistic (time, resources, and team building)

Adapted with permission from Stewart M, Brown JB, Weston WW, McWhinney IR, McWilliam CR, Freeman TR: *Patient-Centered Medicine: Transforming the Clinical Method.* Thousand Oaks, CA, Sage Publications, 1995.

malpractice litigation remains a threat. Time and production pressures have increased as a result of the millions of newly insured patients who are seeking care. Language barriers (limited English proficiency) are a frequent source of frustration. Limited patient health literacy is a challenge for both surgeons and patients. A surgeon must effectively and efficiently evaluate a patient's health literacy and then translate information to a level that the patient can comprehend and use to make an informed decision.

A review of the medical literature revealed two major opportunities for improvement in surgeon–patient communication: a surgeon's willingness to discuss patient concerns and a surgeon's demonstration of empathy.[3] A study of Consumer Assessment of Healthcare Providers and Systems survey physician communication scores from a large multispecialty group revealed that orthopaedic surgery had the lowest scores of all the specialties that were surveyed.[4] A study of patient-reported

experience measures from mostly orthopaedic surgery patients revealed that patients who had a higher level of trust in and communication with their surgeon were much less likely to report a complication.[5] A study of hand surgery patients reported that surgeon empathy was the strongest driver of patient satisfaction, accounting for 65% of variance.[6]

A malpractice lawsuit is an indicator of patient dissatisfaction. Closed-claim studies of medical malpractice lawsuits consistently report communication failure as a major factor in a patient's decision to sue. Seventy-one percent of the malpractice claims reviewed by Beckman et al[7] involved dissatisfied patients who felt devalued, abandoned, poorly informed, or disrespected. Interestingly, in a study of surgeons' vocal tones, Ambady et al[8] correctly predicted the likelihood of whether a surgeon who had a dominant vocal tone (as opposed to a warm vocal tone) would be sued. In a study of orthopaedic-specific malpractice claims that primarily focused on

technical factors such as surgical error, Matsen et al[9] identified exploration of uncertainties with regard to surgical treatment as a missing component of surgeon–patient communication and informed consent.

Studies indicate a high prevalence of burnout among surgeons. Arora et al[10] reported that 50% to 60% of orthopaedic surgeons experience burnout. Regehr et al[11] reported that "interventions incorporating psychoeducation, interpersonal communication, and mindfulness meditation" were associated with decreased burnout rates among physicians. A survey of orthopaedic department chairs identified that stress management and self-management skills as well as practicing a set of work performance skills were effective preventive measures against surgeon burnout.[12] A key work performance skill is the surgeon–patient interview. In surgery and in orthopaedics, in particular, the surgeon–patient interview is viewed as a procedure (the most common procedure in any surgeon's career) that can be taught, learned, and improved.[13] Patient-centered care is not a new idea;[14] however, it has gained renewed emphasis as a result of the Affordable Care Act. The interrelated elements of patient-centered care are listed in **Table 1**.

The E4 Model of Surgeon–Patient Communication

Since 2001, the American Academy of Orthopaedic Surgeons, in partnership with the Institute for Healthcare Communication, has conducted more than 400 continuing medical education workshops on surgeon–patient communication that were attended by more than 7,000 orthopaedic residents, surgeons, and allied health providers.[15]

These workshops were based on the concepts of patient-centered care and shared decision making. The workshops were case-based as well as highly interactive and emphasized learning and practicing effective techniques to establish and strengthen the surgeon–patient relationship. The workshops used the E4 model of surgeon–patient communication (engage, empathize, educate, and enlist) to enhance the traditional differential-diagnosis–based surgeon-patient interview, which has been called the "find it and fix it" (biomedical) approach. The E4 model of surgeon–patient communication helps surgeons find not only the problem but also the patient-centered approach to fixing the problem. An awareness of differences in cultural health beliefs, which includes cultural humility, curiosity, sensitivity, and compassion, as well as an awareness of cultural biases, must be part of a surgeon's relationship with his or her patients regardless of ethnicity, race, and sex. A complete model of patient-centered care for orthopaedic surgeons incorporates all these elements.[14]

The E4 model of surgeon–patient communication incorporates the best clinical research evidence on physician behaviors to promote an effective surgeon–patient relationship. Effective first-impression techniques as well as empathic communication promote a sound surgeon–patient relationship and establish patient-centeredness. This sets the stage for effective education of the patient and his or her family and, finally, facilitates shared decision making to the extent determined by the patient.

E1: Engage

A surgeon must establish a human connection as efficiently as possible (**Table 2**). Humans arrive at a first

---

Table 2

Barriers to Surgeon–Patient Engagement

Time and production pressures

Interruptions

Number of patient complaints

Language barriers

Physical barriers (layout of the examination room, placement of furniture, and electronic health record)

Cultural barriers

Table 3

Getting in Character: The Greeting Ritual

Clear the mind of distractions to allow for full focus on the patient

Knock on the examination room door

Make eye contact; smile

On entry, greet the patient by name, introduce self and others (ie, residents) by name, and acknowledge others in the room

Make an appropriate social touch (handshake or neutral touch on upper arm/elbow)

Sit at or slightly below the patient's eye level (patients perceive that a physician has spent more time with them if seated)

Respect personal space; keep 3 to 4 ft between self and patient

---

impression of other humans within milliseconds of first meeting. Therefore, a surgeon must be in character and use an effective greeting ritual during each patient encounter. Studies have reported that patients have several desires in an encounter with a physician, including eye contact, a therapeutic touch, and respect (**Table 3**).

An open-ended question, such as "How can I help you today?", allows a patient to state the reason for his or her visit. Although it is somewhat daunting, a follow-up question, such as "Is there anything else today?", engages a patient's agenda and helps identify multiple complaints (the average orthopaedic patient has 3 to 12 complaints) proactively. Multiple problems will require negotiation and prioritization, which is done much more effectively up front. Familiarizing a patient with

the surgeon's agenda and how things work in the clinical setting decreases a patient's anxiety.

After a patient has stated the problem, an open-ended invitation ("Tell me more about that") followed by uninterrupted listening for 1 to 2 minutes allows the patient to discuss his or her experience of the illness and provides clues about the personal effects of the illness. If a patient stops short, facilitative comments, such as "OK," "go on," or "tell me more", can help draw out more information. Interrupting a patient's narrative prematurely (12 to 21 seconds) to get to the point (ie, the use of closed-ended questions to shape the differential diagnosis) is a common error.[16] Very few patients will return to their narrative after an interruption and, thus, valuable information will be lost. In addition, patients who are

Table 4
Barriers to Empathic Communication

Time and production pressures

Distractions

Language barriers

Unconscious biases

Physical barriers (electronic health record)

Blocking

Table 5
Empathic Stems

Stem	Example(s)
Reflective listening	"That must have been (frustrating/frightening/etc) for you."
	"So I hear you saying that…"
Self-disclosure	"I do not like to wait either."
Normalization	"Anyone/nobody would…"
Acknowledgment of nonverbal clues	"You seem (cheerful/sad/angry) today."

interrupted may believe that the surgeon does not value the importance of their story (the surgeon "does not listen"/"is too busy"/"does not care") and may feel disrespected.

Most patients will tell their stories within 2 minutes. A surgeon can then narrow the focus to closed-ended questions to complete the differential diagnosis. Successful engagement fosters a working relationship of trust between a surgeon and a patient, which is imperative for patient-centered care and shared decision making. In addition, effectively engaging a patient is a work performance skill that helps increase surgeon satisfaction and prevent surgeon burnout.

E2: Empathize

For the purposes of this chapter, empathy is defined as an understanding of another person's feelings and a communication of that understanding. Patients want to be seen, heard, accepted, and treated with respect. Empathic communication is a universal tool that can be used to achieve this connection with patients.[17] Every surgeon–patient encounter offers multiple opportunities for empathic communication; however, substantial barriers exist (**Table 4**).

Surgeons must understand that all humans communicate both verbally and nonverbally. Attentive listening and maintenance of eye contact with a patient are critically important to fully comprehend the content of the patient's statement. Nonverbal components of communication (eg, vocal tone, facial expressions, posture, and dress) represent more of the true content of communication than a patient's words. In a recent study of hand surgery patients, Menendez et al[6] reported that surgeon empathy was the most powerful driver of patient satisfaction. Surgeons, being human, also communicate nonverbally. If the verbal and nonverbal content of a surgeon's statements are not concordant, a patient may correctly or incorrectly perceive the surgeon's message as sarcastic or disrespectful.

A surgeon's acknowledgment of a patient's feelings also can be verbal or nonverbal. Verbal stems, such as those listed in **Table 5**, are useful; a surgeon should select one or more of these stems as go-to phrases. Nonverbal communication also can be empathic (eg, if a patient becomes tearful, a surgeon can stop the conversation and offer a box of tissues). Because empathic opportunities are commonly missed in surgeon–patient interviews, a strong emotion on behalf of a patient, if noted, must be acknowledged.[18] In addition, patients offer many clues about the effects of their illness (eg, mention of a person not present, such as "my wife" or "my boss"). The failure of a surgeon to acknowledge these clues may lead a patient to repeat them, which can lengthen the visit. Thus, the acknowledgment of clues is not only effective but also time efficient.[19]

Some surgeons may be hesitant to explore a patient's feelings and emotions because they fear losing control of time and are uncomfortable with discussing emotional issues. The model of clinical detachment that is still prevalent in surgery often leads to blocking behaviors that are used to fend off, discount, or ignore emotional content entirely and is counterproductive to and the antithesis of empathy[20] (**Table 6**). If surgeons use empathic communication and avoid blocking, patients will be more satisfied, more trusting of the surgeon, and more likely to adhere to a treatment plan. Empathic communication also is invaluable in dealing with angry patients. Surgeons who can listen without interruption, apologize if appropriate, avoid assigning blame, and acknowledge emotion with empathy (sometimes repeatedly) can usually defuse a patient's anger and de-escalate a confrontation.

E3: Educate

Education involves a surgeon sharing knowledge with a patient. In doing so, the surgeon helps the patient achieve a better knowledge and understanding of his or her illness, a greater capacity and better skills for self-management, and decreased anxiety. Patients want to know their diagnosis, the treatment plan (and why the recommended treatment plan is important), and what their role will be in management of the illness.[21]

Barriers to effective patient education are substantial (**Table 7**). Nearly one-half of Americans have trouble understanding health information (eg, reading prescription labels, appointment cards, and consent documents). Forty-three percent of patients in a hand surgery clinic study demonstrated limited health literacy.[22] Physicians compound the problem by using medical jargon that patients frequently do not understand and may misinterpret.[23] Only approximately one of eight Americans is fully health literate. Surgeons must efficiently assess a patient's health literacy, self-diagnosis, and prior knowledge before crafting a message that the patient will be able to comprehend.

The Agency for Healthcare Research and Quality recommended universal precautions for health literacy, which include providing written communication at an appropriate reading level (fifth grade) and using teach-back techniques to assess patient comprehension.[24] Several tools to assess health literacy, such as The Newest Vital Sign and the Test of Functional Health Literacy in Adults, can be administered by a clinical staff member. In particular, a response of "somewhat" or less with regard to the Test of Functional Health Literacy in Adults question that asks a patient his or her comfort with filling out forms has been correlated with limited health

literacy in both English- and Spanish-speaking patients. This question performed well across language, race/ethnicity, educational attainment, and age.[25]

Patients often use Internet resources for self-diagnosis but are reluctant to inform their surgeon that they have used such resources. Unfortunately, much of the printed patient-education material that surgeons use, including the content of patient-education websites, exceeds an average patient's reading level.[26] The Ask-Tell-Ask teach-back technique used in the E4 model of surgeon–patient communication determines what a patient already knows, which allows the surgeon to craft a message specifically for the patient, and assesses patient comprehension (**Table 8**). The teach-back technique is associated with increased patient satisfaction. Effective

education sets the stage for shared decision making.

E4: Enlist

Shared decision making, which is defined as using the best available evidence as well as a patient's values and preferences to reach a mutually agreed-on decision with regard to treatment, requires the surgeon to invite the patient to participate. Patients report a fear of being labeled as difficult if their physician's communication style is authoritarian; this impairs the shared decision-making process.[27] Because patients are much more likely to adhere to a treatment plan they helped make, the surgeon and the patient must agree on both the goals and the plan for treatment.

Barriers to shared decision making also exist (**Table 9**). A patient is much

---

Table 6
Blocking Behaviors

Offering advice and reassurance before the main problems have been identified

Explaining away distress as normal

Attending only to the physical aspects of the patient

Switching the topic

Jollying patients along (eg, "Cheer up!" and "Rome was not built in a day!")

Table 7
Barriers to Effective Patient Education

Time pressure

Emotional willingness of the surgeon and the patient

Health literacy (Does the patient understand?)

Human factors (Will the patient remember?)

Medical jargon

Table 8
"Ask-Tell-Ask" Teach-Back Technique

Ask what the patient already knows about the illness.

Tell the essential information; limit to three points, avoiding jargon (use the patient's own language level).

Ask the patient to repeat the message to assess comprehension. For example, "We have talked about a lot of information. To be sure I am doing a good job, could you repeat back to me what we talked about?" or "I know you will be talking to your (significant other) after you get home. Can you tell me what you will tell that person about our visit today?"

Table 9
Barriers to Shared Decision Making

Patient's preferences for participation (can range from "You are the doctor" to "My mind is made up")

Health literacy

Surgeon's (lack of) knowledge of patient preferences

Surgeon's willingness to share in decision making

Table 10
Shared Decision Making and Reality Testing

Acute versus chronic

Timeframe for treatment goals

Biologic variability/comorbidity

Financial concerns

Feasibility

Social supports

more likely to adhere to a treatment plan if the surgeon and the patient are able to discuss the patient's concerns, the patient is confident in his or her ability to follow through with the planned treatment, and the patient believes in the efficacy of the planned treatment. Critical flaws in shared decision making and the informed consent process are common in elective surgery.[28] In a study of patient satisfaction with treatment decision, Glass et al[29] reported that shared decision making strongly correlated with a patient's satisfaction with his or her treatment decision.

Shared decision making does not involve allowing a patient to select his or her treatment from a list of choices; instead, it creates a dialog between the surgeon and the patient. In a study on the practice of informed decision making in orthopaedic surgery, Braddock et al[30] reported that surgeons frequently discussed the nature of the treatment decision (92% of the time), alternatives (62% of the time), and risks and benefits (59% of the time) with patients; however, surgeons rarely discussed the patient's role in the treatment decision (14% of the time) with patients or assessed the patient's understanding of the treatment decision (12% of the time). Glass et al[29] reported that the strongest predictor of a patient's

satisfaction with his or her treatment decision was a positive response to question 5 from the 9-Item Shared Decision Making Questionnaire ("My doctor helped me understand all of the information").

Empathic communication is instrumental to shared decision making. Open-ended questions will help the surgeon understand a patient's situation. Exploration of a patient's concerns requires reflective listening, solicitation of the patient's concerns (general or specific, including costs and financial challenges), empathy, and, in some instances, asking the patient to explain why a certain choice may not be in his or her best interest (**Table 10**). Shared decision making is a collaboration between a surgeon and a patient. A written treatment plan and personalized handouts can help a patient. Financial issues should be routinely addressed because they may be a substantial reason for nonadherence.

Effective education and enlistment facilitate a true shared decision-making process, which results in increased patient satisfaction, improved adherence, and improved outcomes. Just as engagement fosters a greeting ritual for the patient encounter, a closing ritual also is important. Forecasting the end of the visit is part of the patient orientation

process. Follow-up on laboratory and imaging studies as well as how test results will be communicated with the patient should be part of the shared decision-making process. Finally, patients desire optimism from their physicians; therefore, an expression of hope with the farewell is appropriate.[31]

Summary

Effective techniques and tools exist to help surgeons refine and improve the surgeon–patient interview. The effective use of these tools and techniques requires work and practice on behalf of the surgeon but will result in worthwhile outcomes for both the surgeon and the patient.

Acknowledgment

The author gratefully acknowledges the leadership, dedication, and mentorship of John R. Tongue, MD, and Kathleen Bonvicini, MPH, EdD.

References

1. White SJ, Stubbe MH, Macdonald LM, Dowell AC, Dew KP, Gardner R: Framing the consultation: The role of the referral in surgeon-patient consultations. *Health Commun* 2014;29(1):74-80.

2. Youm J, Chenok KE, Belkora J, Chiu V, Bozic KJ: The emerging case for shared decision making in orthopaedics. *Instr Course Lect* 2013;62:587-594.

3. Levinson W, Hudak P, Tricco AC: A systematic review of surgeon-patient communication: Strengths and opportunities for improvement. *Patient Educ Couns* 2013;93(1):3-17.

4. Quigley DD, Elliott MN, Farley DO, Burkhart Q, Skootsky SA, Hays RD: Specialties differ in which aspects of doctor communication predict overall physician ratings. *J Gen Intern Med* 2014;29(3):447-454.

5. Black N, Varaganum M, Hutchings A: Relationship between patient reported experience (PREMs) and

patient reported outcomes (PROMs) in elective surgery. *BMJ Qual Saf* 2014;23(7):534-542.

6. Menendez ME, Chen NC, Mudgal CS, Jupiter JB, Ring D: Physician empathy as a driver of hand surgery patient satisfaction. *J Hand Surg Am* 2015;40(9):1860-5.e2.

7. Beckman HB, Markakis KM, Suchman AL, Frankel RM: The doctor-patient relationship and malpractice: Lessons from plaintiff depositions. *Arch Intern Med* 1994;154(12):1365-1370.

8. Ambady N, Laplante D, Nguyen T, Rosenthal R, Chaumeton N, Levinson W: Surgeons' tone of voice: A clue to malpractice history. *Surgery* 2002;132(1):5-9.

9. Matsen FA III, Stephens L, Jette JL, Warme WJ, Posner KL: Lessons regarding the safety of orthopaedic patient care: An analysis of four hundred and sixty-four closed malpractice claims. *J Bone Joint Surg Am* 2013;95(4):e201-e208.

10. Arora M, Diwan AD, Harris IA: Burnout in orthopaedic surgeons: A review. *ANZ J Surg* 2013;83(7-8):512-515.

11. Regehr C, Glancy D, Pitts A, LeBlanc VR: Interventions to reduce the consequences of stress in physicians: A review and meta-analysis. *J Nerv Ment Dis* 2014;202(5):353-359.

12. Saleh KJ, Quick JC, Sime WE, Novicoff WM, Einhorn TA: Recognizing and preventing burnout among orthopaedic leaders. *Clin Orthop Relat Res* 2009;467(2):558-565.

13. Lundine K, Buckley R, Hutchison C, Lockyer J: Communication skills training in orthopaedics. *J Bone Joint Surg Am* 2008;90(6):1393-1400.

14. Weston WW, Brown JB: Overview of the patient-centered clinical method, in Stewart M, Brown JB, Weston WW, McWhinney IR, McWilliam CR, Freeman TR, eds: *Patient-Centered Medicine: Transforming the Clinical Method.* Thousand Oaks, CA, Sage Publications, 1995, pp 21-30.

15. *Clinician-Patient Communication to Enhance Health Outcomes Workbook.* New Haven, CT, Institute for Healthcare Communication, 2014.

16. Beckman HB, Frankel RM: The effect of physician behavior on the collection of data. *Ann Intern Med* 1984;101(5):692-696.

17. Platt FW, Gordon GH: Building rapport: Empathy, the universal tool, in *Field Guide to the Difficult Patient Interview,* ed 2. Philadelphia, PA, Lippincott Williams & Wilkins, 2004, pp 21-29.

18. Easter DW, Beach W: Competent patient care is dependent upon attending to empathic opportunities presented during interview sessions. *Curr Surg* 2004;61(3):313-318.

19. Levinson W, Gorawara-Bhat R, Lamb J: A study of patient clues and physician responses in primary care and surgical settings. *JAMA* 2000;284(8):1021-1027.

20. Maguire P, Pitceathly C: Key communication skills and how to acquire them. *BMJ* 2002;325(7366):697-700.

21. National Patient Safety Foundation: Ask Me 3. July 7, 2014. Available at: https://npsf.site-ym.com/?page=askme3. Accessed January 19, 2016.

22. Menendez ME, Mudgal CS, Jupiter JB, Ring D: Health literacy in hand surgery patients: A cross-sectional survey. *J Hand Surg Am* 2015;40(4):798-804.e2.

23. Castro CM, Wilson C, Wang F, Schillinger D: Babel babble: Physicians' use of unclarified medical jargon with patients. *Am J Health Behav* 2007;31(suppl 1):S85-S95.

24. Cifuentes M, Brega AG, Barnard J, et al: Implementing the AHRQ Health Literacy Universal Precautions Toolkit: Practical Ideas for Primary Care Practices. AHRQ Publication No. 15-0023-1-EF. Rockville, MD, Agency for Healthcare Research and Quality, January 2015. Available at: http://www.ahrq.gov/sites/default/files/publications/files/healthlitguide_1.pdf. Accessed December 11, 2015.

25. Sarkar U, Schillinger D, López A, Sudore R: Validation of self-reported health literacy questions among diverse English and Spanish-speaking populations. *J Gen Intern Med* 2011;26(3):265-271.

26. Eltorai AE, Sharma P, Wang J, Daniels AH: Most American Academy of Orthopaedic Surgeons' online patient education material exceeds average patient reading level. *Clin Orthop Relat Res* 2015;473(4):1181-1186.

27. Frosch DL, May SG, Rendle KA, Tietbohl C, Elwyn G: Authoritarian physicians and patients' fear of being labeled 'difficult' among key obstacles to shared decision making. *Health Aff (Millwood)* 2012;31(5):1030-1038.

28. Ankuda CK, Block SD, Cooper Z, et al: Measuring critical deficits in shared decision making before elective surgery. *Patient Educ Couns* 2014;94(3):328-333.

29. Glass KE, Wills CE, Holloman C, et al: Shared decision making and other variables as correlates of satisfaction with health care decisions in a United States national survey. *Patient Educ Couns* 2012;88(1):100-105.

30. Braddock C III, Hudak PL, Feldman JJ, Bereknyei S, Frankel RM, Levinson W: "Surgery is certainly one good option": Quality and time-efficiency of informed decision-making in surgery. *J Bone Joint Surg Am* 2008;90(9):1830-1838.

31. Detsky AS: What patients really want from health care. *JAMA* 2011;306(22):2500-2501.

Surgeon–Patient Communication: Disclosing Unanticipated Medical Outcomes and Errors

Michael R. Marks, MD, MBA

Abstract

The disclosure of unanticipated medical outcomes and errors is essential as physicians strive to create a safer, higher quality healthcare delivery system. Physicians and other healthcare providers should use an organized approach to guide the disclosure of unanticipated medical outcomes and errors. An expression of sympathy or an apology on behalf of a physician depends on whether the medical outcome or error occurred after appropriate care (maloccurrence) or there was a deviation from the standard of care (malpractice).

Instr Course Lect 2017;66:667–671.

The Hippocratic Oath states "I will do no harm or injustice to them."[1] The American Medical Association Code of Medical Ethics states that physicians should: "deal honestly and openly with patients. Patients have a right to know... any mistaken beliefs concerning their conditions...in which a patient suffers significant medical complications that may have resulted from the physician's mistake or judgment...the physician is ethically required to inform the patient of all the facts necessary to ensure understanding of what has occurred. Only through full disclosure is a patient able to make informed decisions regarding future medical care...Concern regarding legal liability which might result following truthful disclosure should not affect the physician's honesty with a patient."[2]

In 2000, the Institute of Medicine analyzed hospital adverse events that led to death and reported adverse event rates as high as 13.6%. More than one-half of those adverse events resulted from preventable medical errors. If extrapolated to the more than 33.6 million admissions in US hospitals, the report suggested that more than 98,000 deaths per year are the result of medical errors.[3] Using new analytical tools, James[4] estimated that there were 210,000 to 400,000 deaths associated with preventable harm to patients and that serious harm appeared to be 10-fold to 20-fold more common than lethal harm. The author suggested that "fully engaging patients...during hospital care, systematically seeking the patients' voice in identifying harms, transparent accountability for harm, and intentional correction of root causes of harm will be necessary" to decrease medical harm. Physicians and healthcare institutions continue to struggle with the disclosure of unanticipated medical outcomes and errors to patients and their families; however, such disclosure is necessary to achieve a safer, patient-centric healthcare system.

Medical Training and Education

Physicians receive extensive technical training to become a doctor. This is especially true for orthopaedic surgeons and other proceduralists. A busy practicing hand surgeon may treat 1,000

Dr. Marks or an immediate family member serves as a paid consultant to or is an employee of Karen Zupko Associates and The Chartis Group and serves as a board member, owner, officer, or committee member of the American Academy of Orthopaedic Surgeons, the Connecticut Orthopaedic Society, the Institute for Healthcare Communication, and the CMIC Group.

patients per year. If that hand surgeon were to practice for 30 years, which may be a conservative estimate, he or she would perform 30,000 surgeries during his or her career. That same surgeon probably sees 120 patients per week. If that surgeon were to work 44 weeks per year for more than 30 years, he or she would have almost 160,000 patient encounters that require the use of nontechnical skills.

Most physicians' educational endeavors focused heavily on the technical rather than the nontechnical aspects of care. There are many potential reasons for this discrepancy. One of the more obvious reasons is that surgeons/proceduralists gravitate to hands-on rather than cognitive activities. The outcome after a procedure is very tangible. In addition, nontechnical skills have traditionally been viewed as soft science. In fact, thousands of studies have documented the scientific research that is the basis for embracing nontechnical skills.

Why mention nontechnical skills in a discussion on the disclosure of unanticipated medical outcomes and errors? The answer is simple: Nontechnical skills are imperative to properly disclose unanticipated medical outcomes and errors. These nontechnical skills include the E4 model of surgeon-patient communication (engage, empathize, educate, and enlist), which has been a focal point of the educational efforts of the American Academy of Orthopaedic Surgeons since 2001. Empathy is imperative in the disclosure of unanticipated medical outcomes and errors.

The Surgeon–Patient Relationship

No physician intentionally desires an unanticipated medical outcome;

however, every physician will have at least one unanticipated medical outcome, if not more, during his or her career. A physician's response to an unanticipated medical outcome will determine how a patient and his or her family respond, both emotionally and legally.

The way in which physicians are perceived and the surgeon–patient relationship have been altered as a result of several attitudinal and policy changes.[2-4] There has been a shift from a paternalistic surgeon–patient relationship to a patient-centric surgeon–patient relationship. This is in line with personalized medicine, in which treatment is tailored to a patient's condition rather than a one-size-fits-all approach.

Although many physicians would embrace a personalized approach to medicine, the current healthcare environment, which has been affected by the Patient Protection and Affordable Care Act,[5] the Health Information Technology for Economic and Clinical Health Act,[6] and other legislative acts, has made this more difficult. Traditionally, physicians have been at the top of the treatment pyramid. Currently, in many instances, physicians are grouped into a collective category called "providers" that includes all other individuals who treat patients. The government and insurance companies have created this expansion of individuals who can provide care for a patient. In some instances, physicians are viewed as part of a treatment team in which no single individual on that team is more important than any other individual. For many physicians, this impersonalized categorization of physicians has created internal confusion if an unanticipated medical outcome occurs. However, if an unanticipated medical outcome occurs, a patient's anger tends to focus on

those believed to be in charge or those who have the deepest pockets (ie, the hospital and the physicians). Physicians must remember that although insurance companies and the government have devalued the importance of the physician, patients and their families as well as the legal system still place primary responsibility for unanticipated medical outcomes on physicians.

Unanticipated Medical Outcomes and Errors

Medical education and postgraduate training rarely address the disclosure of unanticipated medical outcomes and errors. Surgeons may perceive that the disclosure of unanticipated medical outcomes and errors creates a conflict with clinical training that emphasizes perfection. The American Medical Association Code of Ethics, which was previously discussed, addresses the ethical aspect of this issue; however, the psychological aspect of a physician's self-preservation creates a conflict. To help resolve this conflict, 36 US states have apology laws that prohibit certain conversations related to the disclosure of unanticipated medical outcomes and errors from being admissible in a lawsuit.[7] Even with these laws in place, physicians are still uneasy with having disclosure discussions.

For hospitals (which also affects physicians), The Joint Commission requires institutions and practitioners to behave ethically as well as disclose mistakes and offer an apology to patients and, if appropriate, their family if the outcome of any treatment or procedure differs substantially from the anticipated outcome.[8] Unanticipated medical outcomes are the result of (1) uncorrected, unreasonable expectations; (2) biologic variability; (3) low-probability risks and side effects; (4) wrong judgments without negligence; and/or (5) individual, team, or system errors and equipment failures. With respect to medical negligence, only individual, team, or system errors and equipment failures are situations in which care is considered unreasonable and harm is preventable. The first four circumstances mentioned are instances in which care was reasonable and harm was not preventable and are cases of maloccurrence without medical negligence. A dichotomous approach to addressing unanticipated medical outcomes and errors is shown in **Figure 1**.

There are proper guidelines and approaches to appropriately resolve an unanticipated medical outcome with a patient and his or her family. Traditionally, healthcare providers and systems have approached unanticipated medical outcomes by trying to assign blame. This is a counterproductive approach. A better approach involves determining what contributed to the adverse outcome. Assigning blame and finding a scapegoat does not solve a patient's issues with the adverse outcome. In many instances, patients want to know if the adverse outcome can be avoided in the future.[9]

The concept of hindsight bias frequently results in an incorrect conclusion on the cause of an adverse outcome.[10] In some instances this has been called Monday–morning quarterbacking.[11] For example, if a coach knew a quarterback was going to throw an interception, then he or she would have called a running play. To avoid Monday–morning quarterbacking and to correct for hindsight bias, the substitution test should be used to answer the following question: What would a similarly trained physician do if he or she had the same information as the

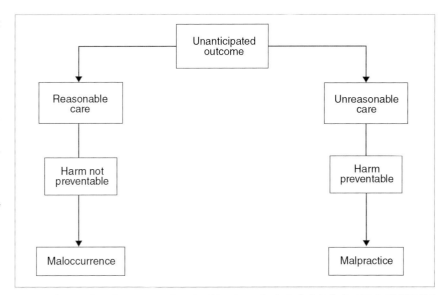

Figure 1   Algorithm shows a dichotomous approach to addressing unanticipated medical outcomes and errors.

treating physician?[12] Reviewing the adverse outcome from this perspective should help avoid "what if" scenarios.

If an examination of the facts demonstrates a medical or system error, then there may have been a deviation from the standard of care. From a medical and/or legal perspective, this may have been the result of a failure of a planned action to be completed as intended or the use of an incorrect plan to achieve a result. These errors are defined as acts of either commission or omission that would have been judged outside of the standard of care by skilled and knowledgeable peers at the time they occurred.[13]

All too frequently after an unanticipated medical outcome occurs, patients, in an effort to find an explanation, seek opinions and/or consultations from other physicians. It is imperative that outside physicians avoid Monday–morning quarterbacking. Outside physicians must have the maturity to appropriately discuss the situation with the patient and not make assumptions

about the intervention. More likely than not, a patient will ask what happened. Although difficult, the most appropriate response that an outside physician can provide involves redirecting the patient back to the treating physician and letting the patient know that he or she will contact the treating physician and convey the concerns the patient expressed with regard to his or her care and outcome.

Addressing Unanticipated Medical Outcomes and Errors

There is an acceptable, organized approach to addressing unanticipated medical outcomes and errors.[14] The acronyms AID (acknowledge, investigate, and disclose), ALEE (anticipate/adjust, listen, empathize, and explain), and TEAM (truth, transparency, and teamwork; empathy; apology and accountability; and manage until resolved) will help direct the process of addressing an unanticipated medical outcome. The specific process used will depend on whether the care was reasonable or unreasonable. In both circumstances, the process starts with AID. If the care was reasonable (maloccurrence), the physician should proceed with ALEE. If the care was unreasonable (malpractice), the physician should proceed with both ALEE and TEAM.

Immediately after the recognition of an adverse outcome, there are four tasks that must occur. (1) The physician and healthcare team must continue to care for the patient. The physician should not abandon the patient. The physician should make sure that all of the facts are charted and any pertinent materials are preserved for the investigation. (2) The physician's own emotions should be addressed. In many instances, the physician or healthcare team has been called the second victim.[15] (3) Discussions should include all team members so that everyone involved has clarity about what happened. (4) The physician should prepare for the discussion with the patient and his or her family.

A proper investigation of an adverse outcome within an institution should have the cooperation of both the physician and the institution. Being adversarial is not beneficial for anyone. The investigation should be performed in a timely manner, and the temptation to reach a conclusion on causation before the investigation is complete should be avoided.

The final step involves a formal disclosure of the adverse outcome. All appropriate members of the patient's family should be present. From the clinical side, the meeting should be led by a senior leader/facilitator who is skilled and comfortable with leading such a discussion. In addition, all individuals who had an accountable role in the adverse outcome should be present at the discussion. There should not be passive observers at the discussion because the patient and his or her family may ask why that person is present.

The approach for the formal disclosure depends on whether the care was reasonable or unreasonable. For situations in which the care was reasonable, the physician should proceed with ALEE. At the time a physician begins the formal disclosure, it is important to anticipate the emotions and questions that the patient and his or her family will ask. It is important for the physician to adjust his or her responses based on the questions asked. All formal disclosures should include some form of an apology. There are four elements to an apology: (1) admit wrong, (2) express remorse, (3) explain the changes that will be made to prevent future occurrences of the adverse outcome, and (4) provide restitution.[16]

If the care was reasonable, the process should begin with an expression of regret for the patient's experience. If the care was unreasonable, the process should begin with an apology for what the physician has done. There is a substantial difference between these two scenarios. In the former, a physician expresses sorrow for the patient's experience; in the latter, a physician apologizes for the harm he or she caused. Next, the physician must listen to the patient's story. The physician should invite the patient and his or her family to express their thoughts on the situation. In general, patients are angry after an adverse outcome because they feel that no one listened to them. It is important for the physician to empathize with the patient throughout the disclosure process so that the patient recognizes that he or she is being seen and heard and that his or her situation and concerns are understood by the physician. Finally, the formal disclosure should end with an explanation of the details. It is important for the physician to make sure that the patient and his or her family understand this explanation and the next steps that will be taken.

If the care was unreasonable, the physician should proceed with TEAM. It is important for the physician to tell the truth. The physician should answer all questions specifically by providing an explanation of what caused the mistake or contributed to the adverse outcome. The physician should present the truth as the facts were uncovered in the investigation. Transparency is important. The adage that it was not the event that worsened the problem but the cover-up of the facts has been shown to be true in politics and also applies to the disclosure of medical errors. A patient should not discover from an outside party that there was an error in his or her care. This situation can lead to great distrust and makes achieving an amicable resolution almost impossible because the patient will harbor too much anger to proceed appropriately with a resolution. To be successful in the disclosure of an adverse outcome, there must be a team approach; clinical staff, administrative staff, risk managers, and liability carriers must all be in agreement on the process that will be undertaken. Empathy for the medical, psychologic, and financial effects on the patient and his or her family must be demonstrated.

The apology must be sincere and heartfelt. Patients are interested in accountability for the adverse outcome, with a vested interest that other patients will not have to suffer or be injured in the future. The disclosure process is neither complete nor successful without managing to a resolution. This may include emotional support for all individuals involved; practical assistance, which may include financial restitution; and a plan for the future.

Summary

Appropriate disclosure of unanticipated medical outcomes is essential as the healthcare delivery system continues to evolve into a patient-centric model in which physicians strive to improve the quality and safety of the care provided. To appropriately disclose an unanticipated medical outcome, physicians must first decide whether an unanticipated outcome is a maloccurrence or malpractice. After this determination is made, the unanticipated medical outcome should be disclosed using the acronyms ALEE and/or TEAM.

References

1. National Library of Medicine: The Hippocratic oath, translated by Michael North, September 16, 2002. Available at: https://www.nlm.nih.gov/hmd/greek/greek_oath.html. Accessed December 8, 2015.

2. American Medical Association: AMA Code of Medical Ethics: Opinion 8.12–Patient information. Updated June 1994. Available at: http://www.ama-assn.org/ama/pub/physician-resources/medical-ethics/code-medical-ethics/opinion812.page. Accessed December 8, 2015.

3. Kohn LT, Corrigan JM, Donaldson MS; Committee on Quality of Health Care in America; Institute of Medicine: *To Err is Human: Building a Safer Health System.* Washington, DC, National Academy Press, 2000. Available at: https://iom.nationalacademies.org/Reports/1999/To-Err-is-Human-Building-A-Safer-Health-System.aspx. Accessed December 8, 2015.

4. James JT: A new, evidence-based estimate of patient harms associated with hospital care. *J Patient Saf* 2013;9(3):122-128.

5. Office of the Legislative Counsel: Compilation of Patient Protection and Affordable Care Act [as amended through May 1, 2010] including Patient Protection and Affordable Care Act Health-Related Portions of the Health Care and Education Reconciliation Act of 2010. May 2010. Available at: http://housedocs.house.gov/energycommerce/ppacacon.pdf. Accessed December 8, 2015.

6. U.S. Department of Health & Human Services: HITECH Act enforcement interim final rule. February 17, 2009. Available at: http://www.hhs.gov/ocr/privacy/hipaa/administrative/enforcementrule/hitechenforcementifr.html. Accessed December 8, 2015.

7. Sorry works! Making disclosure a reality for healthcare organizations: States with apology laws. Available at: http://www.sorryworks.net/apology-laws-cms-143. Accessed December 8, 2015.

8. Joint Commission Resources: Crafting an effective apology: What clinicians need to know. *Joint Comm Perspect Patient Saf* 2005;5(4):7-8.

9. Gallagher TH, Studdert D, Levinson W: Disclosing harmful medical errors to patients. *N Engl J Med* 2007;356(26):2713-2719.

10. Cherry K: What is a hindsight bias? About.com. Updated August 3, 2015. Available at: http://psychology.about.com/od/hindex/g/hindsight-bias.htm. Accessed December 8, 2015.

11. Merriam-Webster.com: Monday–morning quarterback. Available at: http://www.merriam-webster.com/dictionary/monday-morning%20quarterback. Accessed December 8, 2015.

12. Reason JT: *Managing the Risks of Organizational Accidents.* London, United Kingdom, Ashgate Publishing, 1997.

13. Wu AW, Cavanaugh TA, McPhee SJ, Lo B, Micco GP: To tell the truth: Ethical and practical issues in disclosing medical mistakes to patients. *J Gen Intern Med* 1997;12(12):770-775.

14. Institute for Healthcare Communications: Disclosing and Resolving Adverse Outcomes and Medical Errors. CME Instructional Course. New Haven, CT, Institute for Healthcare Communications, June 2011.

15. Wu AW: Medical error: The second victim. The doctor who makes the mistake needs help too. *BMJ* 2000;320(7237):726-727.

16. Lazare A: What an apology must do. Greater Good: The science of a meaningful life. September 1, 2004. Available at: http://greatergood.berkeley.edu/article/item/what_an_apology_must_do. Accessed December 8, 2015.

Getting Research Published and Achieving the Highest Impact Factor

Dia Eldean Giebaly, MBChB, MSc, MRCS

Fares S. Haddad, FRCS (Orth)

Abstract

High-quality surgical clinical trials are fundamental to the delivery of evidence-based orthopaedics; however, fewer than 1% of patients who undergo surgery worldwide are enrolled in surgical clinical trials. Advances in orthopaedic surgery depend on the creativity and innovation of researchers who investigate, develop, and execute local, national, and international surgical clinical trials, all of which will ultimately affect surgical practice and patient care. Surgeons should understand the challenges of surgical clinical trials, including identifying important research questions; getting support for ideas; establishing clinical research networks; collecting, collating, and analyzing data; as well as getting research published and achieving the highest impact factor. Surgeons also should understand how research material should be formatted and presented in a manuscript that is submitted for publication as well as the elements an editor seeks in a research manuscript.

Instr Course Lect 2017;66:673–679.

Traditionally, surgical innovations have been accepted based on endorsements by renowned experts or based on weak scientific evidence.[1,2] There has been a transition in research culture from eminence-based medicine to evidence-based medicine. A hierarchy of evidence has been created, with randomized controlled trials (RCTs), systematic reviews, and meta-analyses at the apex.[3] Although RCTs are well respected and often quoted in the field of orthopaedic surgery, there is a relative paucity of RCTs published in orthopaedic journals,[4] representing approximately 3% to 11% of studies published in the orthopaedic literature.[5-7]

The scarcity of RCTs in the orthopaedic literature may be greatly attributed to several perceived barriers that are associated with the design and execution of RCTs of surgical interventions. The process of developing a research idea into a formal hypothesis and a research grant submission followed by ethical/institutional review board approval and the creation of the infrastructure to conduct the research are difficult. In addition, there is the challenge of collecting, collating, and analyzing data, which can be very time consuming and, at times, complex and riddled with unexpected problems. After all of these challenges are overcome, great difficulties still exist in translating the research into a creditable, readable, and attractive manuscript that journals will accept for publication and that will be viewed favorably and subsequently cited.

Surgeons should understand how research material should be formatted and presented in a manuscript to more easily obtain publication in a journal with a high impact factor. There are

Dr. Haddad or an immediate family member has received royalties from Corin, MatOrtho, and Smith & Nephew; serves as a paid consultant to Smith & Nephew and Stryker; and has received research or institutional support from Smith & Nephew. Neither Mr. Giebaly nor any immediate family member has received anything of value from or has stock or stock options held in a commercial company or institution related directly or indirectly to the subject of this chapter.

many facets to getting research published and achieving the highest impact factor, including the basic quality of the research, the way the information is collated and transmitted, and the ability of a researcher to respond to queries and challenges. Surgeons should understand the current views on research methodologies and the best manner in which research material should be presented to ensure that it is acceptable for peer review. Surgeons also should be aware of the key issues with regard to the ethics of research and how to navigate increasingly complex regulations.

Identifying Important Research Questions

Research is, in essence, the search for the truth. Surgeons ask clinical questions to find truthful answers. In any research study, a clinician-scientist must first develop a research question. Although this may seem simple, clearly defining a primary research study question is difficult. The PICO (population, intervention, control, and outcomes) mnemonic may help clinician-scientists clearly define a primary research study question.[8,9] The identification of clinically relevant research questions within collaborative clinical research networks should be encouraged to promote a research culture in which RCTs are feasible and to ensure that the scarce funding resources for RCTs are used efficiently. The analysis of large datasets and registry data can help identify important research questions and hypotheses that can be tested in RCTs.[10,11]

Rangan et al[12] reviewed several studies on the role of research networks and societies in fostering collaboration among orthopaedic surgeons to identify and prioritize areas for future research. The studies suggested consulting active clinicians early in the research design process to unify the identification of research questions and, thus, prevent duplicated efforts. In addition, the studies suggested that the ability to access expertise from a wider pool of researchers and clinicians may benefit research trial design and decision making. Willett et al[13] used a Delphi approach to identify research questions that were believed to be most important to the orthopaedic trauma community based on a consensus between the faculty members of the AOUK, which is the United Kingdom section of the AO Foundation. The authors reported a clear interest in developing a collaborative research strategy and successfully identified 10 high-priority research questions thought to be important to the AOUK membership.[13]

Usually, research studies can be designed to answer only one question precisely and provide probable or possible answers to other secondary questions. A research study will have more support, be easier to publish, and engage the interest and attention of the reviewers if the research topic is novel and of interest to colleagues, collaborators, and the community at large. After a researcher has a clearly defined research question, the research protocol is usually easy to create.

Getting Support for Ideas

Clinical trials inevitably require funding, and a large number of funding opportunities are available for research. Broadly, funding opportunities can be classified as local funding, specialty society funding, charity funding, government funding, and industry funding.[14] Appropriate planning for the submission of a research funding application is vital to successfully secure funding, and, similar to manuscript submission to a scientific publication, the development of ideas is key. Factors such as investigator qualifications, success in pilot studies, and a research track record are important considerations in the peer review process of a research funding application.

Often, the closest and most accessible research funding resource is local institutions, such as universities or academic medical centers and departments, that have a small amount of seed dollars set aside for research or have start-up grants available for emerging clinician-scientists. Research foundations, specialty societies, and associations are another source of research funding; however, research funding from these resources may be limited by their size. Often, these organizations are specialty specific (eg, the Orthopaedic Research and Education Foundation and the Orthopaedic Trauma Association).

Research funding from charities that are dedicated to musculoskeletal research range from those that fund basic science and translational research to those that fund research that will have more immediate clinical benefits. Arthritis Research UK, which is the largest independent charity in the United Kingdom, awarded more than £20 million to research projects, ranging from laboratory science projects to clinical trials, in 2014.[15] Since 2004, Orthopaedic Research UK (formerly the Furlong Research Charitable Foundation), which is another charity in the United Kingdom that awards research funding, has supported more than 120 research projects and has awarded more than £1.1 million per year to postdoctoral fellows, clinical fellows, and students pursuing a medical degree or PhD who wished to conduct research projects.[16]

Larger amounts of research funding are available from government organizations that are interested in promoting clinical research. The American Academy of Orthopaedic Surgeons, the Canadian Institutes of Health Research, and the National Institutes of Health are three organizations that provide funding, occasionally in the millions of dollars, to well-designed clinical research trials. The American Academy of Orthopaedic Surgeons defined various research priorities for the Unified Orthopaedic Research Agenda, the mission of which is to "advance science and research in musculoskeletal care through a unified research strategy."[17] The National Institutes of Health award grant funding in broad areas, including research grants, research career development awards, research training and fellowships, program project/center grants, resource grants, and translational research programs. Current economic pressures, the aging population that has put a strain on healthcare organizations, and the increasing cost of clinical trials have made obtaining research funding increasingly difficult because government organizations worldwide are attempting to cut deficits. Orthopaedic surgeons may have particular difficulties in obtaining large-scale research funding because government organizations are less comfortable and less familiar with medical device and implant trials compared with pharmaceutical trials, which results in substantially less funding for surgical research.[18,19]

Perhaps the largest resource of research funding for orthopaedic clinical trials is industry. In the past decade, the number of clinical trials that were funded by industry substantially increased.[20,21] There is increasing evidence, however, that industry has become frustrated by the expense and administrative burdens that are associated with research conducted at academic medical centers and is shifting to clinical trials that are conducted at private organizations, such as contract research organizations.[22] In general, the academic–industry partnership is praised for promoting innovation and developing novel tools to fight disease and improve patient care;[21] however, several concerns were recently raised by a number of research articles and media reports. Disproportionately pro-industry research conclusions, biased research study designs, and the suppression of negative research results have contributed to the poor reputation associated with industry-funded research.[20] The disclosure of conflicts of interest, independent data gathering and statistical analysis, and the eradication of gag clauses that prevent the dissemination of research results are several strategies that help ensure mutually beneficial relationships between researchers and industry and prevent further disrepute.[20,21]

Establishing Clinical Research Networks

Orthopaedic research networks, such as orthopaedic associations, specialty associations, specialty societies, travelling fellowships, and clinical research networks, help researchers overcome the challenges of promoting RCTs in orthopaedic clinical practice. Although the structure of such collaborative clinical research networks vary from country to country, the underlying principles remain the same. An appropriate mix of individuals who have different skills, including clinicians, patients, trial methodologists, systematic reviewers, health economists, epidemiologists, and statisticians, is essential to effectively design and efficiently conduct RCTs. Individuals who have different skill sets are vital to the composition of a research team that has a proven track record in completing RCTs. Ownership of an RCT is key. A multicenter RCT is likely to be more successful and enjoyable if the members of the collaborative clinical research network think that they own the project. This ownership is fostered by the involvement and consultation of all members of the collaborative clinical research network at every stage of the research process, beginning with identification of the research question, and may involve the inclusion of orthopaedic consultants as well as trainees.

Since 2004, collaborative clinical research networks have been developed in the United Kingdom to support and coordinate high-quality clinical research and to facilitate RCTs and other studies within the United Kingdom National Health Service.[23] These collaborative clinical research networks, which have been established in each of the four nations of the United Kingdom and are funded by the United Kingdom Department of Health, were created as part of the government's "Best Research for Best Health" research and development strategy to provide a world-class infrastructure for clinical trials in all areas of disease and clinical need within the National Health Service and have streamlined the process of getting research centers "research ready."[12] In England, the National Institute for Health Research has six topic-specific clinical research networks (cancer, mental health, medicines for children, stroke, dementia, and neurodegenerative disease) and a primary care research network. In addition, there are 25 comprehensive local research networks that incorporate other specialties, including musculoskeletal disorders. The United Kingdom Clinical Research Network database currently has 950 musculoskeletal research studies in their portfolio.[12]

Support from comprehensive local research networks helps research associates who are employed by individual hospitals ensure that RCTs are run according to good clinical practice and appropriate research governance regulations. The more orthopaedic RCTs that use comprehensive local research networks, the more likely support will be available in the future and integrated into future job plans and appraisals.[13] Large United Kingdom-wide multicenter RCTs, such as the PROximal Fracture of the Humerus: Evaluation by Randomisation Trial, the United Kingdom Rotator Cuff Study, and the Distal Radius Acute Fracture Fixation Trial, have benefited considerably from research associate support from comprehensive local research networks.[23]

Training for investigators within the framework of collaborative clinical research networks is crucial. Trippel et al[24] highlighted the importance of orthopaedic specialty societies, such as the Pediatric Orthopaedic Society of North America, which established the Clinical Trials Network, in building research infrastructure through the development of guidelines and training for investigators. The authors of this chapter hope that greater involvement in clinical trials and collaboration with more experienced lead clinicians may help improve the infrastructure and research culture in orthopaedics. International fellowships, such as the American-British-Canadian Travelling Fellowship, have helped successfully promote

international collaboration.[23] Bhandari et al[25] urged orthopaedic surgeons who reside in countries that are proficient in conducting clinical trials to collaborate with international colleagues to promote a research culture, provide necessary training, and improve the external validity of clinical trials in specific settings.

Collecting, Collating, and Analyzing Data

Although statistics and clinical epidemiology are included in the core curriculum of medical schools and some residency programs, most clinicians have only limited knowledge in these areas. This limited proficiency in statistics and clinical epidemiology results not from a lack of training or interest but from a lack of frequent application and interpretation. Therefore, it is important for researchers to be familiar with the essential statistical and epidemiologic concepts as well as study design principles that are necessary to properly conduct and evaluate clinical research. Although it is impossible to comprehensively explain these essential statistical and epidemiologic concepts as well as study design principles within the scope of this chapter, many of the errors or flaws in clinical research result not from complex statistical or methodologic issues but from neglect of fundamental statistical or methodologic principles that are often forgotten.

Several organizational committees must exist to ensure the ethical and efficient execution of a clinical trial. Sprague et al[26] described the organization of a multicenter observational study that included a steering committee, a methods center, a data safety and monitoring board, a central adjudication committee, and a writing committee. A

description on the functions of each of these committees is beyond the scope of this chapter.

A steering committee is typically composed of the principal investigator as well as relevant clinical experts, biostatisticians, and research methodologists. A steering committee should be diverse enough to provide critical insight but small enough to prevent dysfunction and inefficiencies.[26]

In accordance with the ethical duties of all researchers, data safety and monitoring is necessary in every clinical research trial; however, a specific data safety and monitoring board may not be necessary in every clinical research trial to accomplish this goal.[27]

Good practices and transparency in the reporting of research methodologies is encouraged through the use of reporting guidelines. Reporting guidelines, such as the Consolidated Standards of Reporting Trials,[28-30] the Strengthening the Reporting of Observational Studies Epidemiology Statement,[31] the Preferred Reporting Items for Systematic Reviews and Meta-Analyses Statement,[32] and the Consolidated Health Economic Evaluation Reporting Standards Statement,[33] are well accepted in clinical trials, observational studies, meta-analyses, and health economic studies, respectively. These reporting guidelines have been shown to improve the quality of scientific reporting.[29] The development of international reporting guidelines is overseen by the Enhancing the Quality and Transparency of Health Research International Network,[34] which strives to ensure that scientific reporting is both transparent and accurate.[28]

A robust strategy for the dissemination of research findings is essential to maximize its effect, which will facilitate

Table 1

Four Basic Questions Every Manuscript Needs to Have Answered During the Peer Review Process

Is the manuscript scientifically sound?

Is the manuscript original?

Is the manuscript relevant?

Is the manuscript well presented?

the acceptance of research results and the translation of research into practice. An effective dissemination strategy should be incorporated into the earliest planning stages of a research study. Dissemination methods include the presentation of research findings at community, national, and international meetings of orthopaedic associations and specialty societies as well as the publication of research findings in journals that reach the target readership and are most likely to have the biggest effect on clinical practice. Systematic reviews and meta-analyses of RCTs help keep clinicians up to date on their specialty and are often used as a starting point for the development of clinical practice guidelines.[32] The Cochrane Collaboration is an international network that helps participants make well-informed decisions on health care by preparing, updating, and promoting the accessibility of systematic reviews.

Getting Research Published and Achieving the Highest Impact Factor

The publication of a scientific manuscript is one of the most rewarding achievements in a surgeon's career. The preparation of a manuscript is the culmination of the hard work that preceded it. The style of writing that is used in a manuscript is important.

Sentences should be short and clear, and the writing style should be scientific and pragmatic. The ability to get a manuscript published is largely related to the reviewers' and editors' perception of the quality of the manuscript, which is often made within reading the first few lines of the manuscript. The topic of a manuscript must be interesting, the research question must be clear, and the method used to answer the research question must be easy to follow and reproduce.

Authorship policies should be established relatively early in a research study so that all research participants are aware of how work will be credited. Authorship options include group authorship, representatives of a collaborative who are publishing on behalf of other research investigators (eg, Author A, Author B, and Author C on behalf of a group of research investigators), and individual authorship (eg, Author A, Author B, and Author C).

Although the peer review process is, to a degree, subjective and each reviewer approaches a manuscript in a different manner, there are four basic questions that every manuscript needs to have answered affirmatively before being accepted for publication (**Table 1**). To adequately evaluate any manuscript, a reviewer must understand the author's methodologic process. There is always disagreement among reviewers with regard to a manuscript; however, it is important that the reviewers use such disagreements to reach their final conclusions on a manuscript. Some manuscript topics may be rejected because they are too specialized; other manuscript topics may be accepted despite the presence of a so-called "fatal flaw."[35] It is uncommon for a manuscript to be accepted after the first review, and not

every manuscript needs to be the result of a RCT.[35] A manuscript may be well executed, but it may not be accepted in high-level journals if it does not have an effect on clinical practice.

A manuscript should be clear and concise, the key information should stand out, and the less important details should be hidden or omitted. Authors who are immersed in a manuscript fail to notice obvious mistakes. To spot errors in a manuscript that is ready for submission, many authors set the manuscript aside for a period of time, after which they review the manuscript again, inevitably finding errors because they are viewing their manuscript through the eyes of a reader. All of the authors of a collaborative manuscript should read the entire manuscript rather than just their own contribution to ensure that the manuscript does not have errors. The key to a successful manuscript is brevity without the omission of salient information. Words should be chosen carefully, with simple terms preferred instead of complicated language. An editing agency can help spot mistakes and errors and may be useful for authors whose first language is not English. Authors should carefully follow a journal's instructions to authors because deviations, no matter how minor, may lead to rejection of the manuscript.

Summary

Some of the barriers that orthopaedic researchers face are applicable to researchers in all medical specialties and other barriers are specific to researchers in certain surgical specialties. Surgeons are further challenged by the difficulty of blinding patients and surgeons to a particular treatment allocation, a strong surgeon-specific preference and expertise (lack of equipoise), institutional pressures on surgeons to increase clinical productivity, inadequate resources and structures to protect research time, and the unwillingness of patients to be randomized. Surgeons have obtained advanced degrees in clinical research and have developed prospective research programs at their institutions. Mentorship programs and role models at these institutions will help positively influence the career development of future orthopaedic clinician-scientists. The creation of collaborative clinical research networks that are allowed protected time free of clinical responsibilities is critical. Despite the many barriers that orthopaedic researchers face, more high-quality studies, including RCTs, are gaining momentum and being published in the orthopaedic literature. Several orthopaedic surgeons have led the way by developing collaborative clinical research networks to conduct multicenter RCTs.[12]

References

1. Wolf BR, Buckwalter JA: Randomized surgical trials and "sham" surgery: Relevance to modern orthopaedics and minimally invasive surgery. *Iowa Orthop J* 2006;26:107-111.

2. Cook JA: The challenges faced in the design, conduct and analysis of surgical randomised controlled trials. *Trials* 2009;10:9.

3. Oxford Centre for Evidence-Based Medicine: The Oxford Centre for Evidence-Based Medicine levels of evidence. Available at: www.cebm.net/ocebm-levels-of-evidence. Accessed March 23, 2016.

4. Campbell AJ, Bagley A, Van Heest A, James MA: Challenges of randomized controlled surgical trials. *Orthop Clin North Am* 2010;41(2):145-155.

5. Bhandari M, Richards RR, Sprague S, Schemitsch EH: The quality of reporting of randomized trials in the Journal of Bone and Joint Surgery from 1988 through 2000. *J Bone Joint Surg Am* 2002;84(3):388-396.

6. Poolman RW, Struijs PA, Krips R, et al: Reporting of outcomes in orthopaedic randomized trials: Does blinding of outcome assessors matter? *J Bone Joint Surg Am* 2007;89(3):550-558.

7. Obremskey WT, Pappas N, Attallah-Wasif E, Tornetta P III, Bhandari M: Level of evidence in orthopaedic journals. *J Bone Joint Surg Am* 2005;87(12):2632-2638.

8. AO Foundation: Case 3: How to use The Orthopedic Trauma Digest. Available at: https://www.aofoundation.org/Structure/research/clinical-research/case/using/Pages/3-orthopedic-trauma-digest.aspx. Accessed March 23, 2016.

9. Aslam S, Emmanuel P: Formulating a researchable question: A critical step for facilitating good clinical research. *Indian J Sex Transm Dis* 2010;31(1):47-50.

10. National Joint Registry: 12th Annual Report of the National Joint Registry for England, Wales, Northern Ireland and the Isle of Man. Hemel Hempstead, United Kingdom, National Joint Registry, 2015. Available at: www.njrcentre.org.uk/njrcentre/Portals/0/Documents/England/Reports/12th%20annual%20report/NJR%20Online%20Annual%20Report%202015.pdf. Accessed March 23, 2016.

11. Konan S, Haddad FS: Joint registries: A Ptolemaic model of data interpretation? *Bone Joint J* 2013;95(12):1585-1586.

12. Rangan A, Jefferson L, Baker P, Cook L: Clinical trial networks in orthopaedic surgery. *Bone Joint Res* 2014;3(5):169-174.

13. Willett KM, Gray B, Moran CG, Giannoudis PV, Pallister I: Orthopaedic trauma research priority-setting exercise and development of a research network. *Injury* 2010;41(7):763-767.

14. Rankin KS, Sprowson AP, McNamara I, et al: The orthopaedic research scene and strategies to improve it. *Bone Joint J* 2014;96(12):1578-1585.

15. Arthritis Research UK: Annual Report and Financial Statements: 31 March 2014. Available at: www.arthritisresearchuk.org/about-us/annual-report-and-accounts.aspx. Accessed March 23, 2016.

16. Orthopaedic Research UK: Research Impact Report: A decade of support. 2015. Available at: www.oruk.org/funding-research/research-projects. Accessed March 23, 2016.

17. Orthopaedic Research Society: Unified Orthopaedic Research Agenda. Available at: www.ors.org/unified-orthopaedic-research-agenda. Accessed March 23, 2016.

18. Mann M, Tendulkar A, Birger N, Howard C, Ratcliffe MB: National institutes of health funding for surgical research. *Ann Surg* 2008;247(2):217-221.

19. Rangel SJ, Efron B, Moss RL: Recent trends in National Institutes of Health funding of surgical research. *Ann Surg* 2002;236(3):277-287.

20. Okike K, Kocher MS, Mehlman CT, Bhandari M: Industry-sponsored research. *Injury* 2008;39(6):666-680.

21. Chopra SS: MSJAMA: Industry funding of clinical trials. Benefit or bias? *JAMA* 2003;290(1):113-114.

22. Bhattacharjee Y: U.S. research funding: Industry shrinks academic support. *Science* 2006;312(5774):671.

23. Rangan A, Brealey S, Carr A: Orthopaedic trial networks. *J Bone Joint Surg Am* 2012;94(suppl 1):97-100.

24. Trippel SB, Bosse MJ, Heck DA, Wright JG: Symposium: How to participate in orthopaedic randomized clinical trials. *J Bone Joint Surg Am* 2007;89(8):1856-1864.

25. Bhandari M, Sprague S, Schemitsch EH; International Hip Fracture Research Collaborative: Resolving controversies in hip fracture care: The need for large collaborative trials in hip fractures. *J Orthop Trauma* 2009;23(6):479-484.

26. Sprague S, Matta JM, Bhandari M, et al: Multicenter collaboration in observational research: Improving generalizability and efficiency. *J Bone Joint Surg Am* 2009;91(suppl 3):80-86.

27. Poolman RW, Hanson B, Marti RK, Bhandari M: Conducting a clinical study: A guide for good research practice. *Indian J Orthop* 2007;41(1):27-31.

28. Perry DC, Parsons N, Costa ML: 'Big data' reporting guidelines: How to answer big questions, yet avoid big problems. *Bone Joint J* 2014;96(12):1575-1577.

29. Plint AC, Moher D, Morrison A, et al: Does the CONSORT checklist improve the quality of reports of randomised controlled trials? A systematic review. *Med J Aust* 2006;185(5):263-267.

30. Moher D, Hopewell S, Schulz KF, et al: CONSORT 2010 explanation and elaboration: Updated guidelines for reporting parallel group randomized trials. *BMJ* 2010;340:c869.

31. von Elm E, Altman DG, Egger M, et al: Strengthening the Reporting of Observational Studies in Epidemiology (STROBE) statement: Guidelines for reporting observational studies. *BMJ* 2007;335(7624):806-808.

32. Moher D, Liberati A, Tetzlaff J, Altman DG; PRISMA Group: Preferred reporting items for systematic reviews and meta-analyses: The PRISMA statement. *J Clin Epidemiol* 2009;62(10):1006-1012.

33. Husereau D, Drummond M, Petrou S, et al: Consolidated Health Economic Evaluation Reporting Standards (CHEERS) statement. *BMJ* 2013;346:f1049.

34. Groves T: Enhancing the quality and transparency of health research. *BMJ* 2008;337:a718.

35. Villar RN: What an editor seeks. *Bone Joint J* 2013;95(5):577-577.

Index

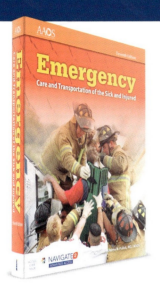
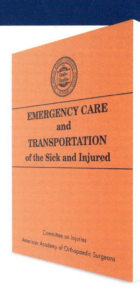
  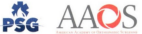
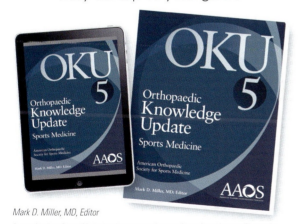
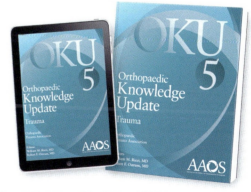

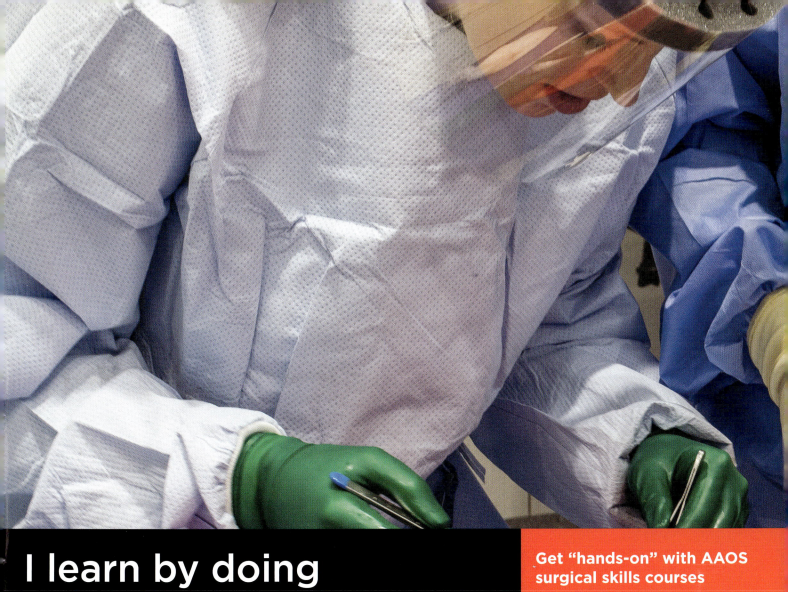

I learn by doing

AAOS surgical skills courses allow me to work side-by-side with the world's finest orthopaedic surgeons to learn new techniques and refine my skill level. I gain exceptional, unbiased instruction in a variety of orthopaedic procedures at the new, state-of-the-art OLC Education and Conference Center. That's why AAOS surgical skills courses are my top choice to ensure I provide the highest quality patient care.

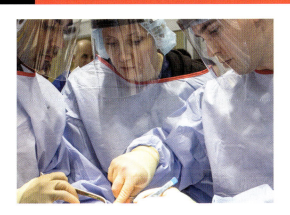

- Brand new, state-of-the art surgical skills facility

- 12 focused, hands-on skills courses 1:2 or 1:3 faculty-to-participant ratio

- Courses for residents through expert specialist level

Visit **aaos.org/courses** or call **1-800-626-6726** today

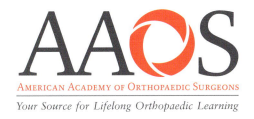

AAOS

AMERICAN ACADEMY OF ORTHOPAEDIC SURGEONS

Your Source for Lifelong Orthopaedic Learning